Orthotics & Prosthetics *in* REHABILITATION

THIRD EDITION

Orthotics & Prosthetics *in* REHABILITATION

Michelle M. Lusardi, PT, DPT, PhD
Professor Emerita
Department of Physical Therapy & Human Movement Science
College of Health Professions
Sacred Heart University
Fairfield, CT

Milagros "Millee" Jorge, PT, MA, EdD
Professor and Dean
Langston University
School of Physical Therapy
Langston, OK

Caroline Nielsen, BA, MA, Ph.D
Health Care, Education and Research Consultant
Bonita Springs, FL
Former Associate Professor and Director
Graduate Program in Allied Health
University of Connecticut
Storrs, CT

ELSEVIER
SAUNDERS

3251 Riverport Lane
St. Louis, Missouri 63043

ORTHOTICS & PROSTHETICS IN REHABILITATION, THIRD EDITION   978-1-4377-1936-9

978-1-4377-1936-9

Vice President: Linda Duncan
Content Manager: Kathy Falk
Senior Content Development Specialist: Christie M. Hart
Publishing Services Manager: Julie Eddy
Senior Project Manager: Andrea Campbell
Design Direction: Ashley Eberts

Printed in the United States of America

Last digit is the print number: 9   8   7   6   5   4   3

Dedication

To Lawrence Mario Lusardi
my husband and best friend
"To love someone deeply gives you strength. Being loved by
someone deeply gives you courage."—Lao Tzu
M.M.L.

To Mitchell B. Horowitz
In thanksgiving for our wonderful married life together
and in memory of my beloved brother William Jorge.
"The way to love anything is to realize that it may be lost."—G.K.
Chesterton
M.J.

To Svend Woge Nielsen
A true partner who nourishes my spirit and achievements with
his constant understanding and belief in me.
C.C.N.

Contributors

Elizabeth Ames, MD
Associate Professor, Residency Program Director, and
Coordinator of Orthopedic Curriculum
Dept. of Orthopaedics & Rehabilitation
UVM College of Medicine
Burlington, Vermont
Attending Surgeon
Dept. of Orthopaedics, Spine Institute
of New England
Fletcher Allen Health Care
Burlington, Vermont

Mark A. Anderson, PT, PhD, ATC
Professor
Department of Rehabilitation Sciences
University of Oklahoma Health Sciences Center
Oklahoma City, Oklahoma
Adjunct Professor
Health and Exercise Science
University of Oklahoma
Norman, Oklahoma

Noelle M. Austin, MS PT CHT
CJ Education & Cosulting LLC
Woodbridge, Connecticut
Certified Hand Therapist
ProPT
The Orthopaedic Group
Hamden, Connecticut

Ed Ayyappa, MS, CPO, FAAOP
Prosthetic Clinical Manager
Southern California Region
U.S. Department of Veteran Affairs
Health Care System
Long Beach, California

William J. Barringer, MS, CO
Department of Orthopedic Surgery
and Rehabilitation
University of Oklahoma
Oklahoma City, Oklahoma

Jennifer M. Bottomley, PT, MS, PhD
HEARTH–Homes for Elders at Risk Through Homes
Board of Directors, HEARTH
President, International Physical Therapists working with
Older People/WCPT
Adjunct Faculty
MGH Institute of Health Care Professions, Program
in Physical Therapy
Adjunct Faculty
Simmons College Program in Physical Therapy
Independent Educator and Geriatric Rehabilitation
Consultant
Boston, Massachusetts

Donna M. Bowers, PT, MPH, PCS
Clinical Associate Professor
Department of Physical Therapy
and Human Movement Science
Sacred Heart University
Fairfield, Connecticut

Kaia Busch, BS
Hanger Prosthetics and Orthotics
Seattle, Washington

Kevin Carroll, MS, CP, FAAOP
Vice President of Prosthetics
Hanger Prosthetics and Orthotics
Orlando, Florida

Joshua Carter, MD
Clinical Instructor
Orthopaedics and Rehabilitation Residency
Programs
South Burlington, Vermont

Mark D. Charlson, MD
Assistant Professor
Orthopaedics & Rehabilitation
University of Vermont College of Medicine
Burlington, Vermont

Kevin K. Chui, PT, DPT, PhD, GCS, OCS
Associate Professor
Department of Physical Therapy and
Human Movement Science
College of Health Professions
Sacred Heart University
Fairfield, Connecticut

Jeff Coppage, MD
Department of Orthopaedic Surgery and Rehabilitation
University of Vermont
Burlington, Vermont

Dana Craig, BS
Health System Specialist
Prosthetic Service Line, VISN 22
Dept. of Veterans Affairs
Long Beach, California

Barbara A. Crane, PhD
Assistant Professor
Physical Therapy Program
Department of Rehabilitation Sciences
University of Hartford
West Hartford, Connecticut

Carol P. Dionne, PT, DPT, PhD, OCS, Cert MDT
Association Professor
Department of Rehabilitation Sciences
University of Oklahoma Health Sciences Center
Oklahoma City, Oklahoma 73126-0901

Joan E. Edelstein, MA, PT, FISPO, CPed
Special Lecturer
Program in Physical Therapy
Columbia University
New York, New York

Juan C. Garbalosa, PT, PhD
Clinical Associate Professor of Physical Therapy
Quinnipac University
Hamden, Connecticut

Marylynn Jacobs, OTRL/C, CHT
Partner
Attain Therapy and Fitness
East Longmeadow, Massachusetts

Milagros Jorge, PT, MA, EdD
Director, Post-Professional DPT Program
Dean, School of Physical Therapy
Former
Langston University
Langston, Oklahoma

Carolyn B. Kelly, PT
Department of Rehabilitation
Hartford Hospital
Hartford, Connecticut

Anthony E. "Toby" Kinney, DPT, OCS, MBA
Clinical Assistant Professor/Associate ACCE
Physical Therapy & Rehabilitation Science
University of Montana
Missoula, Montana

David A. Knapp, BSME, MAEd
Practice Manager
Hanger Prosthetics and Orthotics
North Haven, Connecticut
Adjunct Faculty
College of Education
Department of Nursing and Health Professions
University of Hartford
Hartford, Connecticut
Clinical Instructor
Orthotics and Prosthetics
Newington Certificate Program
Newington, Connecticut

Géza F. Kogler, PhD, CO
Research Scientist
Clinical Biomechanics Laborator
School of Applied Physiology
Georgia Institute of Technology
Atlanta, Georgia

Donald S. Kowalsky, PT, EdD
Associate Professor and Chair
Department of Physical Therapy
School of Health Sciences
Quinnipiac University
Hamden, Connecticut

Michelle M. Lusardi, PT, DPT, PhD
Professor Emerita
Department of Physical Therapy & Human
Movement Science
College of Health Professions
Sacred Heart University
Fairfield, Connecticut

Edward Mahoney, PT, DPT, CWS
Assistant Professor
Physical Therapy, Program
School of Health Professions
Louisiana State University Health Sciences Center
Shreveport
Shreveport, Louisiana

John W. Michael, MEd, CPO, FISPO, FAAOP
President
CPO Servies, Inc.
Portage, Indiana

Olfat Mohammed, PhD, PT
Professor and Graduate Advisor
Department of Physical Therapy
California State University–Long Beach
Long Beach, California

Caroline Nielsen, BA, MA, Ph.D

Health Care, Education and Research Consultant
Bonita Springs, FL
Former Associate Professor and Director
Graduate Program in Allied Health
University of Connecticut
Storrs, Connecticut

Roberta Nole, MA, PT, CPed

President
Stride Orthotics, Inc.
Middlebary, Connecticut

Judith Pepe, MD

Senior Associate Director, Surgical Critical Care Surgery
Hartford Hospital
Hartford, Connecticut
Associate Professor of Surgery
University of Connecticut Medical Cehter
Farmington, Connecticut

Elicia Pollard, PT, PhD

Assistant Professor
School of Physical Therapy
Langston University
Langston, Oklahoma

Richard A. Psonak, MS, CPO, FAAOP

Director
Division of Prosthetics and Orthotics
Assistant Professor
Department of Orthopedics and Rehabilitation
School of Medicine
University of Mississippi
Medical Center
Jackson, Mississippi

John Rheinstein, CP, FAAOP

Hanger Prosthetics and Orthotics
New York, New York

Julie D. Ries, PT, PhD

Associate Professor
Department of Physical Therapy
Malek School of Health Professions
Marymount University
Arlington, Virginia

Melvin L. Stills, CO(E), HFISPO

New Virginia, Iowa

John Thompson, CO

Hanger Prosthetics and Orthotics
Oklahoma City, Oklahoma

Victor G. Vaughan, PT, DPT, MS, OCS

Clinical Manager
Sacred Heart Sports Medicine and Rehabilitation Centers
Fairfield, Connecticut
Clinical Instructor
Department of Physical Therapy and Human
Movement Science
College of Health Professions
Sacred Heart University
Fairfield, Connecticut

Scott Ward, PT, PhD

Professor and Chair
Department of Physical Therapy
University of Utah
Salt Lake City, Utah

Ellen Wetherbee, DPT, OCS

Associate Professor and Academic Coordinator
of Clinical Education
Physical Therapy Program
Department of Rehabilitation Sciences
University of Hartford
West Hartford, Connecticut

Margaret Wise, OTR, CHT, CCM, CVE

Director
Upper Extremity Specialists, Inc.
Dallas, Texas

Rita A. Wong, PT, EdD, FAPTA

Professor and Chair
Department of Physical Therapy
Malek School of Health Professions
Marymount University
Arlington, Virginia

Christopher K. Wong, PhD

Assistant Professor of Clinical Physical Therapy
Program in Physical Therapy
Columbia University
New York, New York

Heather N. Worden, MSOP, BSME, CP

Associate Professor
Loma Linda University
Entry Level Masters in Orthotics & Prosthetics
Loma Linda, California
Certified Prosthetist
VAMC
Long Beach, California
National Va Prosthetic Gait Lab
Long Beach, California

John R. Zenie, MBA, CPO

Guilford, Connecticut

Preface

The challenges facing health professionals who are dedicated to providing effective and efficient, evidence-based, rehabilitation care to individuals with conditions affecting their ability to engage in essential daily activities and participate in meaningful roles are many. These challenges include the ever more rapidly advancing technology that tests our ability to remain up to date about available prosthetic and orthotic options, expectations for productivity in practice reflected in the very real time constraints of daily patient care, and the need to be good stewards of the health care dollar while at the same time providing the best orthosis or prosthesis, and associated rehabilitation care so that the individual can meet his or her personal goals when using the device. Clearly, optimum care for these individuals and their family requires the combined expertise of health professionals from many different disciplines. The complexity of the health care delivery and reimbursement systems, at times, may make communication and collaboration problematic. We hope that this work addressed this complexity by providing information from the perspectives of many members of the rehabilitation team.

There have been incredible technical advances since publication of the second edition of this text, as evidenced by incorporation of stance-control knee units in knee ankle foot orthoses, the development of effective neuroprostheses as alternatives to traditional ankle foot orthoses, and the widespread adoption of microchip-enhanced knee unit in transfemoral prostheses. Military personnel surviving significant musculoskeletal and neuromuscular wounds or limb amputation in Operation Iraqi Freedom and Operation Enduring Freedom in Afghanistan have challenged expectations about what it is possible to accomplish while wearing a prosthesis, and prompted significant effort in research and development. The sacrifices of the service men and woman during war will have a positive long-term effect for all persons living with amputation or needing an orthosis for function and meaningful participation in activities of daily living. We are grateful for their military service, and appreciate the catalyst that their injuries and losses have been to research and development in the fields of prosthetics, orthotics, and rehabilitation.

The goal of this edition of *Orthotics and Prosthetics in Rehabilitation* is to present best available evidence for entry-level physical therapy and orthotic/prosthetic students exploring options, and to provide a positive model of clinical decision-making in the context of multidisciplinary and interdisciplinary care. We also intend the text to be a comprehensive and accessible reference for practicing clinicians; a resource for their person-centered examination, evaluation, intervention planning, and outcome assessment.

Our contributors are professionals from the fields of orthotics and prosthetics, physical and occupational therapy, and medicine and surgery. We present this text as an example of the value of collaborative and interdisciplinary patient care. Each contributor has carefully researched the developments in technology, examination, and intervention for the revised or new chapter presented in this third edition. We have incorporated concepts and language of the World Health Organization's International Classification of Functioning, Disability, and Health (ICF) to enhance communication across disciplines. We have updated the case examples, posing sequential relevant questions to provoke discussion of alternatives as a model of effective clinical decision-making. We have opted not to "answer" the questions posed, on the grounds that the general principles we present in the text must be adapted appropriately to meet individual needs, daring readers to work through the problem-solving process and debate the pros and cons of the various options with their peers. We seek to provide opportunity to "practice" the process of evidence-based clinical decision making, rather than present an absolute prescription or plan of care. We hope that this approach will provide a workable model, prompting reader to critically appraise evidence from a variety of sources, integrate this material with the clinical expertise of self and others, and include the individual and family's values and goals when making clinical decisions.

As in previous editions, we have chosen to use "person first" language in order to reflect the humanity and value of the individuals we care for. While phrased such as "person with stroke" or "person with amputation" may be cumbersome to say or read than "patient" or "amputee" we feel strongly that the use of person first language is well worth the extra time or effort required. We hope that this example assists students and clinicians using the text to embrace person centered care.

The text begins with a set of chapters that provide foundation and context for the care of persons who might benefit, in terms of function and of quality of life, from prescription of an orthosis or prosthesis. While chapters on exercise prescription for older adults, motor learning and motor control, and evidence-based practice may not initially seem to "fit" with the remaining chapters, they are written with the intent to apply these concepts to the rehabilitation of individuals using an orthosis or prosthesis, and we trust that those who read them will recognize their relevance. The chapters on assessment of the ability to walk, the methods of fabrication and fitting, and on footwear choices have obvious relevance.

The second part of the text takes us into the world of orthotic design and application, starting with orthoses for foot and lower limb, spine, and hand. We challenge our readers to think not only about selecting the most appropriate orthosis for persons with musculoskeletal or neuromuscular system problems, but to also design a rehabilitation intervention based on principles of motor learning that will facilitate the person's use of the orthoses and ability to participate in activities most meaningful to the individual. We then consider wheelchairs and seating as an orthosis-of-sorts, designed to enhance mobility for persons when functional walking is not a viable option.

The third part of the text focuses on the care of persons with amputation, beginning with consideration of why amputations are performed, care of those at risk of amputation (with prevention as a focus), how amputations are done, and post-operative/pre-prosthetic care. The following chapters provide overview of prosthetic options and alignment issues for those with partial foot, transtibial, transhumeral, and bilateral amputations. We then consider initial prosthetic rehabilitation, and have added chapters on advance skills for community function and of athletics following amputation. The chapter on children with limb deficiency prompts us to incorporate our understanding of motor, cognitive, and emotional development, as well as family dynamics, into prosthetic rehabilitation. We conclude with chapters on prosthetic options and rehabilitation for persons with upper extremity amputation; meant to provide exposure and "a place to start" rather than mastery of this less common, but perhaps more specialized aspect of prosthetic and rehabilitative care.

With this third edition of *Orthotics and Prosthetics in Rehabilitation*, we hope that our work will enhance collaboration, mutual respect, and communication, as well as broaden the knowledge base of health professionals involved in orthotic or prosthetic rehabilitation. It is our belief that collaborative and interdisciplinary care not only enriches clinical practice and teaching, but also insures the best possible outcomes for the individuals we provide rehabilitative care for.

Michelle M. Lusardi, PT, DPT, PhD
Milagros "Millee" Jorge, PT, MA, EdD
Caroline Nielsen, BA, MA, Ph.D

Contents

I

Building Baseline Knowledge

1

Orthotics and Prosthetics in Rehabilitation: Multidisciplinary Approach

CAROLINE C. NIELSEN AND MILAGROS JORGE

LEARNING OBJECTIVES

On completion of this chapter, the reader will be able to:
1. Describe the role of the orthotist, prosthetist, physical therapist, and other professionals in the rehabilitation of persons with movement dysfunction.
2. Describe the history and development of physical rehabilitation professions associated with the practice of orthotics and prosthetics in health care.
3. Identify the use of disablement frameworks in physical rehabilitation.
4. Discuss the role of the health professional in a multidisciplinary or interdisciplinary rehabilitation team.
5. Determine key attributes and attitudes that health professionals should possess to be successful members of interdisciplinary rehabilitation teams.

Allied health professionals work in health care settings to meet the physical rehabilitation needs of diverse patient populations. Today's health care environment strives to be patient-centered and advocates the use of best practice models that maximize patient outcomes while containing costs. The use of evidence-based treatment approaches, clinical practice guidelines, and standardized outcome measures provides a foundation for evaluating and determining efficacy in health care across disciplines. The World Health Organization International Classification of Functioning, Disability, and Health (ICF)[1] provides a disablement framework that enables health professionals to maximize patient/client participation and function while minimizing disability.

In this complex environment, current and evolving patterns of health care delivery focus on a team approach to the total care of the patient.

For a health care team to function effectively, each member must develop a positive attitude toward interdisciplinary collaboration. The collaborating health professional must understand the functional roles of each health care discipline within the team and must respect and value each discipline's input in the decision-making process of the health team.[2,3] Rehabilitation, particularly when related to orthotics and prosthetics, lends itself well to interdisciplinary teams because the total care of patients with complex disorders requires a wide range of knowledge and skills.[4] The physician, prosthetist, orthotist, physical therapist, occupational therapist, nurse, and social worker are important participants in the rehabilitation team. Understanding the roles and professional responsibilities of each of these disciplines maximizes the ability of the rehabilitation team members to function effectively to provide comprehensive care for the patient.

According to disability data from the American Community Survey 2003, 11.5% of civilian household populations aged 16 to 64 years reported having a disability.[5] Approximately 1.7 million people in the United States live with limb loss.[6] The U.S. military engagements in Iraq and Afghanistan have resulted in limb loss for more than 1000 soldiers.[7] The obesity epidemic in the United States has given rise to more people with diabetes who are at risk for dysvascular disease, such as peripheral arterial disease (PAD), which often results in musculoskeletal and neuromuscular impairments to the lower extremities. Ischemic disease can cause peripheral neuropathy, loss of sensation, poor skin care and wound formation, trophic ulceration, osteomyelitis, and gangrene, which can result in the need for amputation. Eight million Americans have PAD.[8]

Persons coping with illness, injury, disease, impairments, and disability often require special orthotic and prosthetic devices to help with mobility, stability, pain relief, and skin and joint protection. Appropriate prescription, fabrication, instruction, and application of the orthotic and prosthetic devices help persons to engage in activities of daily living as independently as possible. Prosthetists and orthotists are allied health professionals who custom-fabricate and fit prostheses and orthoses. Along with other health care professionals, including nurses, physical therapists, and occupational therapists, posthestists and orthotists are integral members of the rehabilitation teams responsible for returning patients to productive and meaningful lives. Definitions of disability continue to evolve. Current definitions consider social, behavioral, and environmental factors that affect the person's ability to function in society. These definitions have considerably broadened the original pathology model in which disability was a function of a particular disease or group of diseases.[9] The current, more inclusive model requires expertise from many sectors in rehabilitative care. This chapter discusses the developmental history of the art and science of orthotics, prosthetics, and physical therapy as professions dedicated to rehabilitating persons with injury and disability.

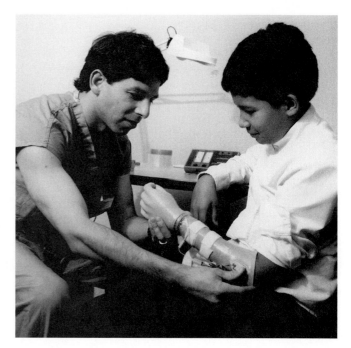

FIGURE 1-1 The prosthetist evaluates, designs, fabricates, and fits a prosthesis specific to a patient's functional needs. Here the prosthetist double-checks electrode placement sites for a myoelectrical upper extremity prosthesis in a child with amputation of the left forearm.

PROSTHETISTS AND ORTHOTISTS

Prosthetists provide care to patients with partial or total absence of limbs by designing, fabricating, and fitting prostheses or artificial limbs. The prosthetist creates the design to fit the individual's particular functional and cosmetic needs; selects the appropriate materials and components; makes all necessary casts, measurements, and modifications (including static and dynamic alignment); evaluates the fit and function of the prosthesis on the patient; and teaches the patient how to care for the prosthesis (Figure 1-1).

Orthotists provide care to patients with neuromuscular and musculoskeletal impairments that contribute to functional limitation and disability by designing, fabricating, and fitting orthoses, or custom-made braces. The orthotist is responsible for evaluating the patient's functional and cosmetic needs, designing the orthosis, and selecting appropriate components; fabricating, fitting, and aligning the orthosis; and educating the patient on appropriate use (Figure 1-2).

According to the U.S. Department of Labor, Bureau of Labor Statistics, in 2009, there were 5470 certified prosthetists and orthotists practicing in the United States.[10] An individual who enters the fields of prosthetics and orthotics today must complete advanced education (beyond an undergraduate degree) and residency programs before becoming eligible for certification. Registered assistants and technicians in orthotics or prosthetics assist the certified practitioner with patient care and fabrication of orthotic and prosthetic devices.

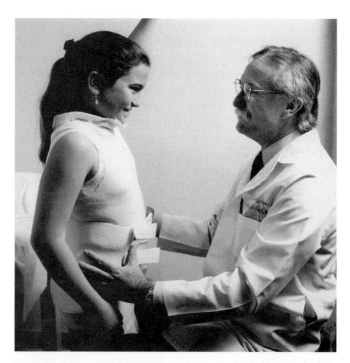

FIGURE 1-2 Once an orthosis has been fabricated, the orthotist evaluates its fit on the patient to determine whether it meets prescriptive goals and can be worn comfortably during functional activities or whether additional modifications are necessary. Here the orthotist is fitting a spinal orthosis and teaching his young patient about proper donning and wearing schedules.

HISTORY

The emergence of orthotics and prosthetics as health professions has followed a course similar to the profession of physical therapy. Development of all three professions is closely related to three significant events in world history: World War I, World War II, and the onset and spread of polio in the 1950s. Unfortunately, it has taken war and disease to provide the major impetus for research and development in these key areas of rehabilitation.

Although the profession of physical therapy has its roots in the early history of medicine, World War I was a major impetus to its development. During the war, female "physical educators" volunteered in physicians' offices and Army hospitals to instruct patients in corrective exercises. After the war ended, a group of these "reconstruction aides" joined together to form the American Women's Physical Therapy Association. In 1922, the association changed its name to the American Physical Therapy Association, opened membership to men, and aligned itself closely with the medical profession.[11]

Until World War II, the practice of prosthetics depended on the skills of individual craftsmen. The roots of prosthetics can be traced to early blacksmiths, armor makers, other skilled artisans, and even the individuals with amputations, who fashioned makeshift replacement limbs from materials at hand. During the Civil War, more than 30,000 amputations were performed on Union soldiers injured in battle; at least as many occurred among injured Confederate troops. At that time, most prostheses consisted of carved or milled wooden sockets and feet. Many were procured by mail order from companies in New York or other manufacturing centers at a cost of $75 to $100 each.[12] Before World War II, prosthetic practice required much hands-on work and craftsman's skill. D. A. McKeever, a prosthetist who practiced in the 1930s, described the process: "You went to [the person with an amputation's] house, took measurements and then carved a block of wood, covered it with rawhide and glue, and sanded it." During his training, McKeever spent three years in a shop carving wood: "You pulled out the inside, shaped the outside, and sanded it with a sandbelt."[13]

The development of the profession of orthotics mirrors the field of prosthetics. Early "bracemakers" were also artisans such as blacksmiths, armor makers, and patients who used many of the same materials as the prosthetist: metal, leather, and wood. By the eighteenth and nineteenth centuries, splints and braces were also mass produced and sold through catalogs. These bracemakers were also frequently known as "bonesetters" until surgery replaced manipulation and bracing in the practice of orthopedics. "Bracemaker" then became a profession with a particular role distinct from that of the physician.[14]

World War II and the period following were times of significant growth for the professions of physical therapy, prosthetics, and orthotics. During the war, many more physical therapists were needed to treat the wounded and rehabilitate those who were left with functional impairments and disabilities. The Army became the major resource for physical therapy training programs, and the number of physical therapists serving in the armed services increased more than sixfold.[15] The number of soldiers who required braces or artificial limbs during and after the war increased the demand for prosthetists and orthotists as well.

After World War II, a coordinated program for persons with amputations was developed. In 1945, a conference of surgeons, prosthetists, and scientists organized by the National Academy of Sciences revealed that little scientific effort had been devoted to the development of artificial limbs. A "crash" research program was initiated, funded by the Office of Scientific Research and Development and continued by the Veterans Administration. A direct result of this effort was the development of the patellar tendon-bearing prosthesis for individuals with transtibial (below-knee) amputation and the quadrilateral socket design for those with transfemoral (above-knee) amputation. This program also included educating prosthetists, physicians, and physical therapists in the skills of fitting and training of patients with these new prosthetic designs.[16]

The needs of soldiers injured in the military conflicts in Korea and Vietnam ensured continuing research, further refinements, and development of new materials. The development of myoelectrically controlled upper extremity prostheses and the advent of modular endoskeletal lower extremity prostheses occurred in the post–Vietnam conflict era. In 2008, the U.S. Department of Defense reported military operations in Iraq and Afghanistan (Operations Enduring Freedom and Iraq Freedom) have resulted in loss of limb for 1214 service men and women.[17] Veterans Health Administration Research Development is committed to exploring the use of new technology such as robotics, tissue engineering, and nanotechnology to design and build lighter, more functional prostheses that look, feel, and respond more like real arms and legs.[18]

The current term, *orthotics*, emerged in the late 1940s and was officially adopted by American orthotists and prosthetists when the American Orthotic and Prosthetic Association was formed to replace its professional predecessor, the Artificial Limb Manufacturers' Association. *Orthosis* is a more inclusive term than *brace* and reflects the development of devices and materials for dynamic control in addition to stabilization of the body. In 1948, the American Board for Certification in Orthotics and Prosthetics was formed to establish and promote high professional standards.

Although the polio epidemic of the 1950s played a role in the further development of the physical therapy profession, this epidemic had the greatest effect on the development of orthotics. By 1970, many new techniques and materials, some adapted from industrial techniques, were being used to assist patients in coping with the effects of polio and other neuromuscular disorders. The scope of practice in the field of orthotics is extensive, including working with children with muscular dystrophy, cerebral palsy, and spina bifida; patients of all ages recovering from severe burns or fractures; adolescents with scoliosis; athletes recovering from surgery or injury; and older adults with diabetes, cerebrovascular accident, severe arthritis, and other disabling conditions.

Like physical therapists, orthotists and prosthetists practice in a variety of settings. The most common setting is the private office, where the professional offers services to a patient on referral from the patient's physician. Many large institutions, such as hospitals, rehabilitation centers, and research institutes, have departments of orthotics and prosthetics with on-site staff to provide services to patients. The prosthetist or orthotist may also be a supplier or fabrication manager in a central production laboratory. In addition, some orthotists and prosthetists serve as full-time faculty in one of the 10 programs that are available for orthotic and prosthetic entry-level training or in one of the programs available at the master of science level.[19] Others serve as clinical educators in a variety of facilities for the year-long residency program required before the certification examination.

PROSTHETIC AND ORTHOTIC PROFESSIONAL ROLES AND RESPONSIBILITIES

With rapid advances in technology and health care, the roles of the prosthetist and orthotist have expanded from a technological focus to a more inclusive focus on being a member of the rehabilitation team. Patient examination, evaluation, education, and treatment are now significant responsibilities of practitioners. Most technical tasks are completed by technicians who work in the office or in the laboratory, or at an increasing number of central fabrication facilities. The advent and availability of modifiable prefabrication systems have reduced the amount of time that the practitioner spends crafting new prostheses and orthoses.

Current educational requirements reflect these changes in orthotic and prosthetic practice. Entry into professional training programs requires completion of a bachelor's degree from an accredited college or university, with a strong emphasis on prerequisite courses in the sciences. Professional education in orthotics or prosthetics requires an additional academic year for each discipline. Along with the necessary technical courses, students study research methodology, kinesiology and biomechanics, musculoskeletal and neuromuscular pathology, communication and education, and current health care issues. Orthotics and prosthetics programs are most often based within academic health centers or in colleges or universities with hospital affiliations. After completion of the academic program, a year-long residency begins, during which new clinicians gain expertise in the acute, rehabilitative, and long-term phases of pediatrics and adult care. On completion of the educational and experiential requirements, the student is eligible to sit for the certification examinations. In order to address the rehabilitation needs of individuals who will benefit from the art and science of the fields of prosthetics and orthotics, physical therapists, orthotists, prosthetists, and other members of the health care team must have discreet knowledge and skills in the management of persons with a variety of health conditions across the lifespan. Working as a rehabilitation team, physicians, nurses, prosthetists, orthotists, physical therapists, occupational therapists, social workers, patients, and family members seek to maximize function and alleviate disease, injury, impairments, and disability.

DISABLEMENT FRAMEWORKS

Historically, disability was described using a theoretical medical model of disease and pathology. Over time, various conceptual frameworks have been developed to organize information about the process and effects of disability.[20] Disablement frameworks in the past have been used to understand the relationship of disease and pathology to human function and disability.[20-23] The need to understand the impact that acute injury or illness and chronic health conditions have on the functioning of specific body systems, human performance in general, and on the typical activities of daily living from both the individual and a societal perspective has been central to the development of the disablement models. The biomedical model of pathology and dysfunction provided the conceptual framework for understanding human function, disability, and handicap as a consequence of pathological and disease processes.

The Nagi model was among the first to challenge the appropriateness of the traditional biomedical model of disability.[21] Nagi developed a model that looked at the individual in relationship to the pathology, functional limitations, and the role that the environment and society or the social environment played. The four major elements of Nagi's theoretical formulation included active pathology (interference with normal processes at the level of the cell), impairment (anatomical, physiological, mental, or emotional abnormalities or loss at the level of body systems), functional limitation (limitation in performance at the level of the individual), and disability. Nagi defined disability as "an expression of physical or mental limitation in a social context."[21] The Nagi model was the first theoretical construct on disability that considered the interaction between the individual and the environment from a sociological perspective rather than a purely biomedical perspective. Despite the innovation of the Nagi model in the 1960s, the biomedical model of disability persisted.

In 1980, the World Health Organization (WHO) developed the International Classification of Impairments, Disabilities, and Handicaps (ICIDH) to provide a standardized means of classifying the consequences of disease and injury for the collection of data and the development of social policy.[24] This document provided a framework for organizing information about the consequences of disease. However, it focused solely on the effects of pathological processes on the individual's activity level. Disability was viewed as a result of an impairment and considered a lack of ability to perform an activity in the normal manner. In 1993, the WHO began a revision of ICIDH disablement framework that gave rise to the concept that a person's handicap was less related to the health condition that created a disadvantage for completing the necessary life roles but rather to the level of participation that the person with the health condition was able to engage in within the environment. The concept of being handicapped was changed to be seen as a consequence of the level of participation for the person and the interaction within an environment.

The Institute of Medicine enlarged Nagi's original concept in 1991 to include the individual's social and physical environment (Figure 1-3). This revised model describes the environment as "including the natural environment, the built environment, the culture, the economic system, the political system, and psychological factors." In this model, disability is not viewed as a pathosis residing in a person but instead is a function of the interaction of the person with the environment.[25]

In 2001, ICIDH was revised to ICIDH-2 and renamed "International Classification of Functioning, Disability and Health" and is commonly referred to as ICF.[26] The ICF disablement framework includes individual function at the level of body/body part, whole person, and whole person within a social context. The model helps in the description of changes in body function and structure, what people with particular health conditions can do in standard environments (their level of capacity), as well as what they actually do in their usual environments (their level of performance).

One of the major innovations of the ICF model is the presence of an environmental factor classification that considers the role of environmental barriers and facilitators in the performance of tasks of daily living. Disability becomes an umbrella term for impairments, activity limitations, and participation restrictions. The ICF model emphasizes health and functioning rather than disability. The ICF model provides a radical departure from emphasizing a person's disability to focusing on the level of health and facilitating an individual's participation to whatever extent is possible within that level of health. In the ICF, disability and functioning are viewed as outcomes of interactions between health conditions (diseases, disorders, and injuries) and contextual factors (Figure 1-4).

The evolution of disablement frameworks from the biomedical models to the newer, contemporary models that include the biopsychosocial domains provides theoretical constructs that guide the rehabilitation professional in clinical practice. Input from all members of the rehabilitation team is essential in addressing the pathosis or disease process, impairments, functional limitations, and disabilities. Interrelationships among all four of these elements are the focus of the rehabilitation team. The physical therapist, orthotist, prosthetist, and other team members work together

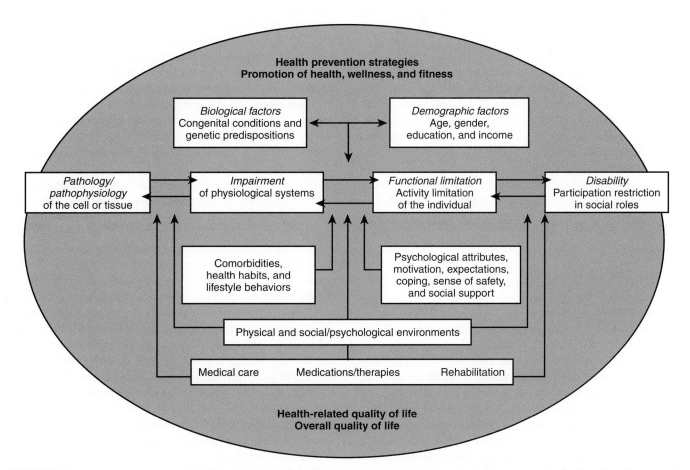

FIGURE 1-3 The revised Institute of Medicine/Nagi model of the disablement process considers the impact of pathological conditions and impairment as well as intraindividual and extraindividual factors that may influence functional limitation and disability affecting health-related and overall quality of life. (Modified from Guccione AA: Arthritis and the process of disablement. *Phys Ther* 1994;74[5]:410.)

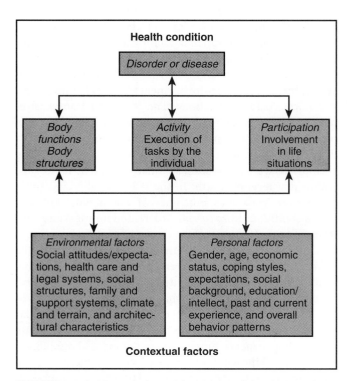

Health condition

Disorder or disease

Body functions Body structures

Activity Execution of tasks by the individual

Participation Involvement in life situations

Environmental factors Social attitudes/expectations, health care and legal systems, social structures, family and support systems, climate and terrain, and architectural characteristics

Personal factors Gender, age, economic status, coping styles, expectations, social background, education/intellect, past and current experience, and overall behavior patterns

Contextual factors

FIGURE 1-4 WHO uses a biopsychosocial model as the basis for its International Classification of Functioning, Disability and Health. (Modified from World Health Organization. *Towards a Common Language for Functioning, Disability and Health.* Geneva: World Health Organization, 2002. pp. 9-10.)

to create the most effective outcome for the patient by identifying and addressing pathological processes, functional limitations, impairments, and disability. The classification system developed by the WHO in the ICF document allows for data collection that can be useful in research leading to improved patient interventions, assessment of patient outcomes, and development of health and social policies. Implementation of this model of disability has been demonstrated to "improve considerably the quality of interdisciplinary work processes and contribute to a more systematic approach to rehabilitation tasks by the team members."[26]

CHARACTERISTICS OF REHABILITATION HEALTH CARE TEAMS

The complexity of the health care arena and the level of care required by individuals in rehabilitation care settings require the collaboration of many health care practitioners with varied professional skills who can form multidisciplinary, interdisciplinary, and transdisciplinary teams as needed. The multidisciplinary rehabilitation team is comprised of the different health professionals such as the physician, nurse, physical therapist, occupational therapist, prosthetist, orthotist, and social worker. Each professional operates with an area of specialization and expertise. The multidisciplinary team is hierarchically structured and typically led by the highest ranking member of the team.[27] Although the multidisciplinary team has varied representation of health providers, they may

or may not interact in a collaborative manner. The members of the multidisciplinary team work parallel to one another, and the medical record is the collecting source for the information gleaned and shared. Interdisciplinary teams also include the representatives of a variety of health disciplines, but there is interdependence among the professionals.[27] In the interdisciplinary team process, there is structure and organization that promotes program planning to support patient-centered care through effective communication and effective clinical management.[28] The interdisciplinary team members work to establish goals for the team that drive the rehabilitation process for the patient. Interdisciplinary teams traditionally follow a patient-centered approach to goal setting. Establishing the patient as the focus of the work for the team, the interdisciplinary team members collaborate to execute the goals and meet the desired outcomes. Most team processes in rehabilitation centers strive for an interdisciplinary team approach that promotes patient-centered care. Each discipline works within its scope of practice to optimize care through coordinated efforts.

Transdisciplinary teams are comprised of the same professional members identified in the multidisciplinary and transdisciplinary teams; however, the team members in the transdisciplinary model function differently in that they share clinical responsibilities and overlap in duties and responsibilities. In the transdisciplinary model of team building, the professional roles and responsibilities are so familiar to the team members that there is an interchange of tasks and functions.[27] Transdisciplinary teams engage in release of professional roles typical to the discipline in an effort to have the patient receive the interventions needed within a context that is supportive of the learning and the practice. The transdisciplinary model is operational in the management of infants and children who receive early intervention rehabilitation services and have an Individualized Family Service Plan (IFSP).

Two major issues emerging in health care that affect health care professionals include (1) the need for health care professionals with advanced education and training in specialty and subspecialty areas, and (2) the need for collaboration among health practitioners to ensure efficiency of patient management that results in best practice and improves patient outcomes. The information explosion in health care, particularly in rehabilitation, has led to increasing specialization and subspecialization in many fields. The interdisciplinary health care team concept has evolved, in part, because no single individual or discipline can have all the necessary expertise and specialty knowledge required for high-quality care, especially the care of patients with complex disorders. Interdisciplinary rehabilitation health care teams provide patient care management approaches that capitalize on clinical expertise by engaging members from diverse rehabilitation professions working together, collaborating, and communicating closely to optimize patient care.[28]

Collaboration is defined as a joint communication and decision-making process with the goal of meeting the health care needs of a particular patient or patient population.

Each participant on the rehabilitation team brings a particular expertise, and leadership is determined by the particular rehabilitation situation being addressed. The rehabilitation team has the opportunity to meet and engage in "asking the answerable questions" that are critical in clinical practice today when engaging in an evidence-based model of practice.[29] According to Sackett and colleagues,[29] evidence-based practice is the integration of the best research evidence, clinical expertise, and patient values. Evidence-based practice and clinical decision-making enhance the role of the rehabilitation team professionals as they share their clinical insights supported by historical and current evidence. Rehabilitation teams that are diverse in professional representation can bring a wide perspective of expertise on particular rehabilitation issues. With this perspective, clinical decision making becomes a more inclusive process.

The role of the health care professional on a rehabilitation team begins during professional education. Rehabilitation sciences health professionals must work at understanding, evaluating, and analyzing the many facets of health care that require specialized professionals who will work to meet the goals and objectives of the specialty and of health care delivery on the whole. The formation of a rehabilitation team provides a cohort of professionals who individually and collectively strive for effective and efficient management of patients. The team process allows for a deeper understanding of and appreciation for the contributions of the other rehabilitation disciplines in the assessment and treatment of the patient and management of patient problems.

In addition to discipline-specific skills and knowledge, health professionals must be aware of the interrelationships among health care workers. One of the major barriers to effective team functioning is a lack of understanding or misconception of the roles of different disciplines in the care of the whole patient.[30] A clear understanding of the totality of the health care delivery system and the role of each professional within the system increase the potential effectiveness of the health care team. A group of informed, dedicated health professionals working together to set appropriate goals and initiate patient care to meet these goals uses a model that exceeds the sum of its individual components.

Almost all rehabilitation health care today is provided in a team setting using a patient-centered approach. This integrated approach facilitates appreciation of the patient as a person with individual strengths and needs rather than as a dehumanized diagnosis or problem. The diverse perspectives and knowledge that are brought to the rehabilitation process by the members of the interdisciplinary team provide insight into all aspects of the patient's concerns. Conceptually, all members of the health care team contribute equally to patient care. The contribution of each is important and valuable; otherwise, quality of patient care and efficacy of intervention would be diminished. Although one member of the team may take an organization or management role, decision making occurs by consensus building and critical discussion. Professionals with different skills function together with mutual support, sharing the responsibility of patient care.

Effective team-based health care assumes that groups of health care providers representing multiple disciplines can work together to develop and implement a comprehensive, integrated treatment plan for each patient. This requires professionals, who have traditionally worked independently and autonomously, to function effectively in interdependent relationships with members of other disciplines.[31] However, this may not be an easy task to accomplish because of the considerable potential for dysfunction.

The Oxford English Dictionary defines *team* as "two or more persons working together."[32] Pearson and Jones define a *team* as "a small group of people who relate to each other to contribute to a common goal."[33] Much of our understanding of team function is drawn from organization and management research literature, the theories of which provide insight and information on how interdisciplinary teams operate and the factors that facilitate or inhibit their effectiveness. A number of factors are important influences on health professionals' perception of team membership that can be positive or negative to the team process.

Values and Behaviors

Some of the factors that tend to limit the effectiveness of a work group are large group size, poor decision-making practices, lack of fit between group members' skills and task demands, and poor leadership.[34-36] Other factors that influence team dynamics are classified as formal (tangible or visible) and informal (submerged). Formal factors include the policies and objectives of the group or its parent organization, the systems of communication available to the group, and the job descriptions of its members. Informal factors, which are often less obvious but equally influential on group process, include working relationships among team members; power networks within and external to the group; and the values, beliefs, and goals of individuals within the group (Box 1-1).[33] Team-building initiatives are often focused on

---

BOX 1-1 *Formal and Informal Factors That Influence Dynamics of the Multidisciplinary Work Group*

FORMAL (VISIBLE) INFLUENCES
Policies of the group or institution
Objectives of the group
Formal systems of communication
Job descriptions of group members

INFORMAL (SUBMERGED) INFLUENCES
Informal relationships among team members
Communication styles of team members
Power networks within the group
Individual values and beliefs
Goals/norms of individuals in the group

Modified from Pearson P, Jones K. The primary health care non-team? Dynamics of multidisciplinary provider groups. *BMJ* 1994;309(6966):1387-1388.

the formal, or visible, areas, but informal communication, values, and norms play key roles in the functioning of the health care team.

A variety of characteristics and considerations also enhance the effectiveness of the interdisciplinary health care team. In addition to having strong professional backgrounds and appropriate skills, team members must appreciate the diversity within the group, taking into account age and status differences and the dynamics of individual professional subgroups.[35] The size of the team is also important: the most capable and effective teams tend to have no more than 12 members. Team members who know each other and are aware of and value each other's skills and interests are often better able to set and achieve goals. Clearly defined goals and objectives about the group's purpose and primary task, combined with a shared understanding of each member's roles and skills, increase the likelihood of effective communication.

Values and behaviors that facilitate the collaborative team care model include the following:

- Trust among members that develops over time as members become more familiar with each other
- Knowledge or expertise necessary for the development of trust
- Shared responsibility for joint decision-making regarding patient outcomes
- Mutual respect for all members of the team
- Two-way communication that facilitates sharing of patient information and knowledge
- Cooperation and coordination to promote the use of skills of all team members
- Optimism that the team is indeed the most effective means of delivering quality care

In the early stages of development, it is essential that the team spend time developing goals, tasks, roles, leadership, decision-making processes, and communication methods. In other words, the team needs to know where it is going, what it wants to do, who is going to do it, and how it will get done.[37] One of the most important characteristics of an effective health care team is the ability to accommodate personal and professional differences among members and to use these differences as a source of strength. The well-functioning team often becomes a means of support, growth, and increased effectiveness and professional satisfaction for the physical therapist and other health professionals who wish to maximize their strengths as individuals while participating in professional responsibilities.[38]

Rehabilitation Teams

The interdisciplinary health care team has become essential in the rehabilitation of patients whose body function and level of participation in the tasks of daily living could be enhanced by assistive technology such as an orthosis or prosthesis. The complexity of the rehabilitation process and the multidimensional needs of patients frequently require the expertise of many different professional disciplines. The rehabilitation team is often shaped by the typical needs and characteristics of the patient population that it is designed

to serve. The individuals most often represented on the rehabilitation team include one or more physicians with specialties in rehabilitation medicine, orthopedics, vascular surgery or neurology, nurses, prosthetists and/or orthotists, physical therapists, occupational therapists, dietitians, social workers, vocational rehabilitation counselors, as well as patients and caregivers (Figure 1-5). Each member of the interdisciplinary team has an important role to play in the rehabilitation of the patient. Patient education is often one of the primary concerns of the team. Imparting information regarding the health condition, etiology, treatment, progression, management, and prognosis helps patients become active partners in the rehabilitation process rather than passive recipients of care. Patient education addresses prevention and treatment strategies; patients and their families are able to identify their needs and concerns and communicate them to the team members. Each member of the team has the responsibility for contributing to patient education, so that patients have the information needed for an effective partnership and positive outcome of rehabilitation efforts.

Research studies across a wide variety of medical conditions and health disciplines contain evidence that patients who feel prepared and informed are most likely to invest in and comply with recommended interventions and often have the most positive health outcome. Ideally, patient education about amputation and prosthetics begins in advance of, or at least immediately after, the amputation surgery.[39] A national survey of people with amputations (n = 109) revealed that information is often scarce at this crucial time.[40] Individuals with recent amputations are often caught in an information gap in the days between surgery and the initial process

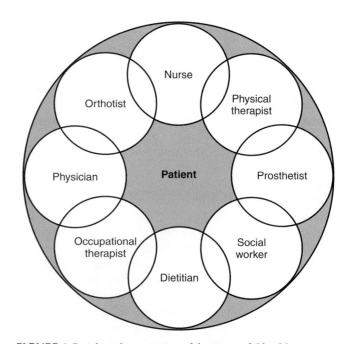

FIGURE 1-5 A key characteristic of the successful health care team is a clear understanding of the role, responsibilities, and unique skills and knowledge of each member of the rehabilitation team, combined with open and effective communication.

of prosthetic prescription and fitting. Only approximately 50% of patients with a new amputation received information about the timing and process of rehabilitation or about prosthetic options before or immediately after amputation.[40] Interestingly, the health professional most frequently cited as a provider of information at the time of amputation was the physical therapist (25%), followed by the physician (23%). The health professionals cited as most helpful after amputation were the prosthetist (65%) and the physical therapist (23%) (Table 1-1). Clearly, one of the most valued contributions of the physical therapist, in addition to the traditional role in facilitating a patient's mobility and independence, is as a provider of early information about the timing and process of the prosthetic fitting and training.

The respondents in this study desired to be active participants in treatment planning and rehabilitation decision-making in partnership with the health care team. The keys to the patient's successful participation in the rehabilitation team are efforts to provide more information and opportunity for open communication; both are likely to enhance patient satisfaction and compliance and the achievement of a positive clinical outcome.

Coordinated patient-centered care by an interdisciplinary rehabilitation team is just as essential for effective rehabilitation of children as it is for adults. For children with myelomeningocele or cerebral palsy, the broad knowledge base available through team interaction provides a stronger foundation for tailoring interventions to the ever-changing developmental needs of the child and family.[41,42] The optimal delivery of care for children is best provided in a comprehensive health care setting in which the various specialists can provide a truly collaborative approach. Orthopedic surgeons, neurologists, orthotists, prosthetists, physical therapists, occupational therapists, nurses, dietitians, social workers, psychologists, and special education professionals may all be involved in setting goals and formulating and carrying out plans for intervention and outcomes assessment.

The concept of a multidisciplinary pediatric clinic team was formulated as World War II came to an end.[43] This structure has evolved further over the years and is particularly effective for the more complex orthotic and prosthetic challenges. A "mini-team" consisting of the patient's physician, a physical therapist, and a prosthetist or orthotist can usually be assembled, even in a small town with few facilities. Regardless of its size, an effective team views the child and family from a holistic perspective, with the input from each specialty being of equal value. Under these circumstances, the setting of treatment priorities, such as whether prosthetic fitting or training in single-handed tasks is most appropriate at a child's current age or developmental level, is made on the basis of the particular needs of the individual.[44] Children with orthotic and prosthetic needs are followed in the community and within the school setting. As appropriate, a child may receive rehabilitation or habilitation services under the Individuals with Disabilities Education Act (IDEA).[45] The rehabilitation/educational team is a diverse group of health care professionals, educators, family, and caregivers, each with essential skills necessary to address the needs of the child that encourage maximum participation in tasks of daily living. Each member of the team works in a collaborative manner with the family and caregivers, and with the child's teachers and other health professionals to ensure that the goals of the Individualized Family Service Plan (IFSP) or the Individualized Education Plan (IEP) are addressed and met. Clear and frequent communication is essential for the team to function effectively and to achieve the desired outcomes for the child.

TABLE 1-1   *Health Professionals Cited as Sources of Information to Persons with Amputations (n = 109)*

Health Discipline	Provided Information at Time of Amputation	Most Helpful After Amputation
Physical therapist	24 (25%)	22 (23%)
Prosthetist	18 (19%)	63 (65%)
Surgeon/family physician	22 (23%)	28 (29%)
Others with amputation	21 (22%)	7 (7%)

Values are n (%).
Data from Nielsen CC. A survey of amputees: functional level and life satisfaction, information needs, and the prosthetist's role, *J Prosthet Orthot* 1991;3(3):125.

CASE EXAMPLE 1

Interdisciplinary Teams

P. G. is a 23-year-old man admitted to a level 3 trauma center two weeks ago after sustaining severe crush injuries to both lower extremities and a closed-head injury in an accident involving a motorcycle and a sport utility vehicle. Initially, unconscious with a Glasgow Coma Scale score of 8, P. G. was placed on life support in the emergency department. Radiographs revealed a severely comminuted fracture of the distal right femur and displaced fractures of the left tibia and fibula at midshaft. Examination revealed partial thickness "road burn" abrasions on the left anterior thorax and thigh; these were thoroughly cleaned and covered with semipermeable dressings. A computed tomography scan of his cranium and brain revealed a subdural hematoma over the left sylvian fissure and moderate contusion of the anterior pole and undersides of the frontal lobes. Arteriography indicated rupture of the right femoral artery 4 inches above the knee. Given the extent of the crush injuries, the trauma team determined P. G. was not a candidate for reconstructive surgery to salvage his right limb.

P. G. was taken to the operating room, where a standard length transfemoral amputation was performed on the right lower extremity. Simultaneously, orthopedic surgeons performed an open-reduction

Continued

internal fixation with an intramedullary rod in the tibia and used surgical plates and screws to repair the fibula. Neurosurgeons drained the subdural hematoma through a burr hole in his skull. P. G. was started on high-dose broad-spectrum antibiotics in the operating room. He was transferred to the surgical intensive care unit for postoperative care.

P. G. was weaned from the ventilator and is now functioning at a Rancho Los Amigos Scale level of 7. He is able to follow one- and two-step commands but becomes easily confused and angry in complex environments and when fatigued. His postoperative pain is currently being managed with Tylenol #3 as needed. His right lower extremity has been managed with soft dressings and elastic bandages; his residual limb is moderately bulbous, with resolving ecchymosis from the accident and surgery. Moderate serosanguineous drainage continues from the medial one third of the suture line. Although most of the skin abrasions show signs of regranulation, one area on his left thigh is red and hot, with yellowish drainage. When transferred (maximum assist of two) into a bedside recliner, P. G. tolerates 30 minutes in a 45- to 60-degree reclined position. He becomes lightheaded and has significant pain when sitting upright with his left lower extremity dependent. He has been referred to physical therapy for evaluation of rehabilitation potential and initiation of mobility activities.

Before his accident, P. G. was a graduate student in physics at a nearby university. He lived in a third floor walk-up apartment with his fiancé and his golden retriever. Besides his motorcycle, his interests and hobbies included long distance running and mountain climbing. His mother and father have traveled to be with him during the acute hospital stay.

Questions to Consider

- Who are the clinical specialists and health professionals needed to address the medical needs of the patient?
- What are the priorities, specific roles, and responsibilities for each potential member of the team? What team structure do you envision?
- How are the roles and responsibilities similar or different across the team?
- What external influences will affect team formation and functioning in a busy level 3 trauma center?
- What factors might facilitate team development?
- What factors might challenge the effectiveness of the team?
- As P. G. recovers from his injuries, how might the roles and responsibilities of the various team members change or evolve?
- When and how would you apply the ICF disablement model for P. G.?

CASE EXAMPLE 2

Interdisciplinary Teams

E. L. is a 73-year-old woman with a 10-year history of type 2 diabetes mellitus. She is insulin dependent. Two weeks before her most recent hospitalization, she and her husband (who is in the early stages of Alzheimer disease) moved from their home of 50 years to an assisted-living complex in a neighboring town. Although the furniture is set up and functional, they have not had the chance to fully unpack and make the apartment their own.

Over the past three years, E. L. has been monitored by her team of physicians for progressive polyneuropathy of diabetes and for moderate peripheral vascular disease. She had a transmetatarsal amputation of her right forefoot eight months ago because of nonhealing recurrent neuropathic ulcer. Despite wearing custom-molded shoes and accommodative orthoses, another ulcer of her first metatarsal head developed on the left foot two months ago. This new ulcer did not heal with conservative care and progressed to osteomyelitis two weeks ago. When vascular studies suggested inadequate circulation to heal the ulcer she received arterial revascularization intervention, but the ischemia persisted and E. L. underwent an elective transtibial amputation of her left lower extremity. Despite a short bout of postoperative delirium thought to be related to pain management with morphine, E. L. (5 days postoperatively) was adamant about returning to her new assisted-living apartment, using a wheelchair for mobility, and receiving home care until her residual limb is healed and ready for prosthetic fitting.

Currently she is able to ambulate two lengths of 15-foot-long parallel bars before needing to rest and has begun gait training with a "hop-to" gait pattern with a standard walker. She is able to transfer from sitting on a firm seating surface with armrests to standing with standby guarding and verbal cueing, and needs minimal assistance from low and soft seats without armrests. She believes that she and her husband will be able to manage at home because her bathroom has grab bars on the toilet, and a tub seat and handheld shower head are available from the "loaner closet" at her assisted-living facility.

At discharge, the suture line had one small area of continued moderate drainage, requiring frequent dressing changes. She is unable to move her residual limb into a position for effective visual self-inspection of the healing surgical wound without significant discomfort. Her husband, although attentive, becomes confused with the routine of wound care. E. L.'s postoperative limb volume and edema are being managed with a total contact cast, which she is able to don and doff independently. She had one late evening fall, when she awoke from a sound sleep having to go to the bathroom and was surprised when her left limb "wasn't really there" to stand on when she tried to get out of bed.

Since her amputation, E. L.'s insulin dosages have had to be adjusted frequently because of unpredictable changes in her serum glucose levels. She has lost 20 pounds (half of which can be attributed to her amputation) since admission.

Questions to Consider
- Who are the health care professionals likely to be involved in her care?
- Which team approach is most desirable for patient-centered care: multidisciplinary, interdisciplinary, or transdisciplinary? Why?
- What are the major challenges facing the team of care providers involved in the postoperative, preprosthetic care of E. L and her husband? How are these similar to or different from challenges and issues the trauma center team considered before her amputation?
- What strategies are currently in place or must be developed to ensure that E. L.'s care at home is comprehensive and coordinated?
- How will the roles and responsibilities of the team members evolve and change as she recovers from her surgery and is ready to begin prosthetic use?
- When and how would you apply the ICF disablement model for E. L.?

CASE EXAMPLE 3

Interdisciplinary Teams

M. S. is a 12-year-old girl with myelomeningocele (spina bifida) who uses a wheelchair for mobility. In the past year she has developed significant thoracolumbar scoliosis believed to be associated with a growth spurt. Concerned about the rate of increase in her S-shaped thoracolumbar curve, her parents sought the advice of an orthopedic surgeon who has been involved as a consultant in her care since birth. The surgeon recommends surgical stabilization of M. S.'s spine with Harrington rods and bony fusion to (1) prevent further progression of the curve and rib hump so that secondary impairment of the respiratory system will be minimized as she grows and (2) provide more efficient upright sitting posture for wheelchair propulsion in the years ahead.

M. S. currently attends classes in her neighborhood middle school where she receives related health services including physical therapy. Until two years ago, she ambulated for exercise by using a reciprocal gait orthosis during gym periods at school, but with recent spurts in growth the use of a manual wheelchair is more efficient for mobility (to keep up with her classmates). She is also followed up on a regular basis by a neurologist who monitors the operation of her ventriculoperitoneal shunt (commonly

used in the management of hydrocephalus associated with myelomeningocele).

In addition to their concerns about the risk of the surgical procedure, M. S.'s parents are quite concerned about how the anticipated four-month postoperative immobilization in a thoracolumbosacral orthosis will affect her capacity for self-care and independent wheelchair mobility. They are also concerned about how the surgery and postoperative period will potentially interrupt the effective bowel and bladder management routine for which M. S. has just begun to assume responsibility. As witnesses to their daughter's deconditioning and loss of stamina over the past six months, they are concerned that she might not be "physically ready" for the surgery and postoperative rehabilitation. They are also asking questions about whether this spinal surgery will ultimately improve the prognosis of a successful return to ambulation with her reciprocal gait orthosis.

Questions to Consider
- Who are the members of the rehabilitation team?
- What is the structure of the team that will best address the needs of the patient?
- What are the priorities, roles, and responsibilities of the health professionals involved in the care of this child and her family?
- How is the composition of M. S.'s rehabilitation team similar to or different from that of P. G.'s and E. L.'s teams?
- How will the health and education professionals support M. S. and her family through the postoperative recovery process?
- When and how would you apply the ICF disablement model to M. S.?

SUMMARY

Patient-centered care in in-patient rehabilitation and ambulatory community settings today relies on interdisciplinary rehabilitation teams that function to address the patient goals and maximize patient outcomes. The use of rehabilitation teams has evolved in part because no one person or discipline has the expertise in all the areas of specialty knowledge required for the established standards of care. This situation is particularly true for meeting the health care needs of persons in orthotic and prosthetic rehabilitation. The success of the rehabilitation team process requires health professionals to work together in a collaborative and cooperative manner. The rehabilitation team professional must demonstrate attitudes and attributes that foster collaboration, including[35]:

1. Openness and receptivity to the ideas of others
2. An understanding of, value of, and respect for the roles and expertise of other professionals on the team

3. Value interdependence and acceptance of a common commitment to comprehensive patient-centered care
4. Willingness to share ideas openly and take responsibility

This chapter introduces the topic of orthotics and prosthetics in rehabilitation and advocates for an multi and interdisciplinary approach to patient-centered care. There is a burgeoning demand for the use of orthotics and prosthetics, based on the traumatic injuries sustained by U.S. service men and women involved in military conflicts in the early years of this century and on the projected rise in the number of persons with chronic health conditions such as obesity, type 2 diabetes, and vascular disease. The WHO ICF is the current disablement framework endorsed by 191 countries.[46] Rehabilitation professionals including orthotists, prosthetists, physical, and occupational therapists will apply the ICF disablement model to maximize strategies for patient participation in the tasks of daily living through enhancement of environmental factors such as providing appropriate, cost-effective assistive technology including orthoses and prostheses. A rehabilitation model of patient-centered care that uses a transdisciplinary team approach to enhance communication, address goals and objectives, apply best practice, and improve patient outcomes is the current standard of care for persons in rehabilitation settings. Collaboration, mutual respect, and an understanding of the roles and responsibilities of colleagues engender productive teamwork and improved outcomes for the rehabilitation patient.

REFERENCES

1. World Health Organization. *International Classification of Functioning, Disability, and Health (ICF)*. http://www.who.int/classifications/icf/en/ Accessed 29.02.12.
2. Stubblefield C, Houston C, Haire-Joshu D. Interactive use of models of health-related behavior to promote interdisciplinary collaboration. *J Allied Health*. 1994;23(4):237–243.
3. Suddick KM, De Souza L. Therapists' experiences and perceptions of team work in neurological rehabilitation:reasoning behind the team approach, structure and composition of the team and teamworking processes. *Physiother Res Int*. 2006;11(2):72–83.
4. Nenedict SM, Scholten J. The Veterans' Health Administration's polytrauma system of care: rehabilitation for today's and tomorrow's veterans. *J Am Soc Aging*. 2010;34(2):106–108.
5. Stern S, Brault M. *Disability data from the American Community Survey: a brief examination of the effects of a question redesign in 2003*. U.S. Census Bureau, Housing and Household Economic Statistics Division; January 28, 2005. Available at: http://www.census.gov/acs/www/Downloads/library/2005/2005_Stern_01.pdf.
6. Limb Loss Information Centre. *Surge in war amputees drives improved prosthetic research*. http://limblossinformationcentre.com/2010/06/23/surge-in-war-amputees-drives-improved-prosthetic-research/ Accessed 29.02.12.
7. Stagnitti M. *The prevalence of obesity and other chronic conditions among diabetic adults in the U.S. community population, 2001*. AHRQ Statistical Brief #34. http://www.meps.ahrq.gov/mepsweb/data_files/publications/st34/stat34.pdf Accessed 29.02.12.
8. American Heart Association. *Peripheral arterial disease*. http://www.americanheart.org Accessed 29.02.12.
9. Ziegler-Graham K, MacKenzie EJ, Ephraim PL, et al. Estimating the prevalence of limb loss in the United States—2005 to 2050. *Arch Phys Med Rehabil*. 2008;89(3):422–429.
10. U.S. Department of Labor, Bureau of Labor Statistics. *Occupational Employment Statistics*. Available at: http://www.bls.gov/oes/current/oes292091.htm.
11. Myers RS. Historical perspective, assumptions, and ethical considerations for physical therapy practice. In: Myers RS, ed. *Saunders Manual of Physical Therapy Practice*. Philadelphia: Saunders; 1995:3–7.
12. Shurr DG, Michael JW. *Prosthetics and Orthotics*. 2nd ed. Norwalk, CT: Appleton & Lange; 2002: 1–5.
13. Retzlaff K. AOPA celebrates 75 years of service to O&P. *Orthotics and Prosthetics Almanac*. 1992;(Nov):45.
14. Hazenhyer IM. A history of the American Physiotherapy Association. Part IV: maturity, 1939-1946. *Phys Ther Rev*. 1946;26:174–184.
15. Wilson BA. History of amputation surgery and prosthetics. In: Bowker JH, Michael JW, eds. *Atlas of Limb Prosthetics: Surgical, Prosthetic and Rehabilitation Principles*. St. Louis: Mosby–Year Book; 1992:3–15.
16. Mishra R. Amputation rate for U.S. troops twice that of past wars. *Boston Globe*. December 9, 2004.
17. *Veterans Health Administration Research Advances: Facts About Prosthetics*. http://www.research.va.gov/resources/pubcs/docs/Prosthetics.pdf; January 2010 Accessed 29.02.12.
18. State of Virginia Research. *Improving Veterans' Lives*. Available at: http://www.research.va.gov/resources/pubs/docs/StateOfVAResearchApr2011.pdf; 2011 Accessed 29.02.11.
19. National Commission on Orthotic and Prosthetic Education. List of Schools. Available at: http://www.ncope.org/info_students/schools.asp.
20. Masala C, Donatella RP. From disablement to enablement: conceptual models of disability in the 20th century. *Disabil Rehabil*. 2008;30(7):1233–1244.
21. Nagi S. Some conceptual issues in disability and rehabilitation. In: Sussman M, ed. *Sociology and Rehabilitation*. Washington, DC: American Sociological Association; 1965:100–113.
22. Bornman J. The World Health Organisation's terminology and classification: application to serve disability. *Disabil Rehabil*. 2004;26(3):182–188.
23. Rimmer J. Use of the ICF in identifying factors that impact participation in physical activity/rehabilitation among people with disabilities. *Disabil Rehabil*. 2006;28(17):1087–1095.
24. *International Classification of Impairments, Disability, and Handicaps*. http://www.aihw.gov.au/publications/dis/dda-mnc/dda-mnc-c03.pdf; 1980 Accessed 29.02.12.
25. Nagi SZ. Disability concepts revisited: implications for prevention. In: Pope AM, Tarlov AR, eds. *Institute of Medicine Disability in America: Toward a National Agenda for Prevention*. Washington, DC: National Academy Press; 1991.
26. World Health Organization. *Towards a Common Language for Functioning, Disability and Health*. Geneva: World Health Organization; 2002.
27. Cooper BS, Fishman EF. *The Interdisciplinary Team in the Management of Chronic Conditions: Has Its Time Come? Partnerships for Better Solutions, In Retooling for an Aging America: Building the Health Care Workforce*. Washington, DC: The National Academies Press; 2008.
28. Hall P, Weaver L. Interdisciplinary education and teamwork: a long and winding road. *Med Educ*. 2001;35(9):867–875.

29. Sackett DL, Strauss SE, Richardson WS, et al. *Evidence-based Medicine.* 2nd ed. Toronto: Churchhill Livingston; 2000.

30. Strasser DC, Falconer JA, Martino-Saltzmann D. The rehabilitation team: staff perceptions of the hospital environment, the interdisciplinary team environment, and interprofessional relations. *Arch Phys Med Rehabil.* 1994;75(2):177–182.

31. Alexander JA, Lichtenstein R, Jinnet K, et al. The effects of treatment team diversity and size on assessment of team functioning. *Hospital Health Serv Admin.* 1996;41(1):37.

32. Oxford Dictionary Online. http://oxforddictionaries.com/definition/team?region=US$q=team.

33. Pearson P, Jones K. The primary health care non-team? Dynamics of multidisciplinary provider groups. *BMJ.* 1994;309(6966): 1387–1388.

34. Hackman JR. *Groups That Work (& Those That Don't): Creating Conditions for Effective Team Work.* San Francisco: Jossey-Bass; 1990.

35. Goodman PS, Devadas RA, Hughson TLG. Groups and productivity: analyzing the effectiveness of self-managing teams. In: Campbell JP, Campbell JR, eds. *Productivity in Organizations.* San Francisco: Jossey-Bass; 1988:295–327.

36. Van Norman G. *Interdisciplinary Team Issues. Ethics in Medicine.* Available at: http://depts.washington.edu/bioethx/topics/team.html; 2008 Accessed 29.02.12.

37. Fried B, Rundall T. Group and teams in health services organizations. In: Shortell SM, Kaluzny AD, eds. *Health Care Management, Organization, Design and Behavior.* 3rd ed. Albany, NY: Delmar; 1994.

38. Area Health Education Center, DC. *Models of Team Practice-Interdisciplinary Health Care Team Practice.* Available at: http://dcahec.gwumc.edu/education/session3/members.html Accessed 29.02.12.

39. Lopopolo RB. The relationship of role-related variable to job satisfaction and commitment to the organization in a restructured hospital environment. *Phys Ther.* 2002;82(10):984–999.

40. Nielsen CC. Factors affecting the use of prosthetic services. *J Prosthet Orthot.* 1989;1(4):242–249.

41. Nielsen CC. A survey of amputees: functional level and life satisfaction, information needs, and the prosthetist's role. *J Prosthet Orthot.* 1991;3(3):125–129.

42. Banta JV, Lin RS, Peterson M, et al. The team approach in the child with myelomeningocele. *J Prosthet Orthot.* 1990;2(4):365–375.

43. Wiart L, Darrah J. Changing philosophical perspectives on the management of children with physical disabilities: their effect on the use of powered mobility. *Disabil Rehabil.* 2002;24(9): 492–498.

44. Michael J. Pediatric prosthetics and orthotics. *Phys Occup Ther Pediatr.* 1990;10(2):123–146.

45. U.S.Department of Education. *Individuals with Disabilities Education Act.* http://idea.ed.gov/ Accessed 2.02.12.

46. World Health Organization. *International Classification of Functioning, Disability and Health.* Available at: http://www.who.int/classifications/icf/en/ Accessed 15.02.11.

2

Aging and Activity Tolerance:
Implications for Orthotic and Prosthetic Rehabilitation

KEVIN K. CHUI AND MICHELLE M. LUSARDI

LEARNING OBJECTIVES

On completion of this chapter, the reader will be able to do the following:

1. Describe the role of the cardiopulmonary and cardiovascular systems as "effectors" for goal-driven functional motor activity.
2. Define the key components of cardiopulmonary and cardiovascular systems as they relate to energy expenditure during functional activity.
3. Describe the functional consequences of age-related change in cardiopulmonary and cardiovascular structures, especially with respect to exercise and activity tolerance.
4. Apply principles of cardiopulmonary/cardiovascular conditioning to rehabilitation interventions for older or deconditioned individuals, or both, who will be using a prosthesis or an orthosis.
5. Weigh the benefits and limitations, with respect to energy cost and facilitation of daily function, in selecting an appropriate orthosis or prosthesis for an older or deconditioned individual.

Many individuals who rely on orthotic or prosthetic devices in order to walk or to accomplish functional tasks have impairments of the musculoskeletal or neuromuscular systems that limit the efficiency of their movement and increase the energy cost of their daily and leisure activities. The separate and interactive effects of aging, inactivity, and cardiac or pulmonary disease can also compromise the capacity for muscular "work," tolerance of activity, and ability to function.

Consider this example: a 79-year-old woman with insulin-controlled type 2 diabetes has been referred for physical therapy evaluation after transfemoral amputation following a failed femoral-popliteal bypass. She has been on bed rest for several weeks because of her multiple surgeries. The physical effort required by rehabilitation and prosthetic training may initially feel overwhelming to this woman. In her deconditioned state, preprosthetic ambulation with a walker is likely to increase her heart rate (HR) close to the upper limits of a safe target HR for aerobic training. What, then, is her prognosis for functional use of a prosthesis? What

are the most important issues to address in her plan of care? What intensity of intervention is most appropriate given her deconditioned state? In what setting and for how long will care be provided? These are questions without simple answers.

The physical therapist, orthotist, and prosthetist must recognize factors that can be successfully modified to enhance performance and activity tolerance when making decisions about prescription and intervention strategies. Aerobic fitness should be a key component of the rehabilitation program for those who will be using a prosthesis or orthosis for the first time. It is vitally important that rehabilitation professionals recognize and respond to the warning signs of significant cardiopulmonary or cardiovascular dysfunction during treatment and training sessions.

Although the anatomical and physiological changes in the aging cardiopulmonary system are important to our discussion, our focus is on the contribution of cellular and tissue-level changes to performance of the cardiopulmonary and cardiovascular systems and, subsequently, on the individual's ability to function. This view provides a conceptual framework for answering four essential questions:

- Is this individual capable of physical work?
- If so, what is the energy cost of doing this work?
- Is it possible for this individual to become more efficient or more able to do physical work?
- What impact does the use of an orthosis or prosthesis have on energy use and cost during functional activities for this person?

OXYGEN TRANSPORT SYSTEM

The foundation for the functional view of the cardiopulmonary system is the equation for the oxygen transport system (Figure 2-1). Aerobic capacity (VO_{2max}) is the body's ability to deliver and use oxygen (maximum rate of oxygen consumption) to support the energy needs of demanding physical activity. VO_{2max} is influenced by three factors: the efficiency of ventilation and oxygenation in the lungs, how much oxygen-rich blood can be delivered from the heart (cardiac output, or CO) to active peripheral tissues, and how well

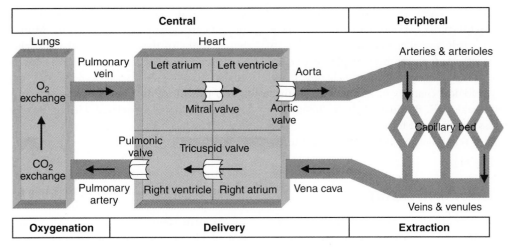

Work Capacity: $VO_2max = \underset{(HR \times SV)}{CO} \times \underset{(C_aO_2 - C_vO_2)}{AVO_2diff}$

FIGURE 2-1 Functional anatomy and physiology of the cardiorespiratory system. After blood is oxygenated in the lungs, the left side of the heart contracts to deliver blood, through the aorta and its branches, to active tissues in the periphery. Oxygen must be effectively extracted from blood by peripheral tissues to support their activity. Deoxygenated blood, high in carbon dioxide, returns through the vena cava to the right side of the heart, which pumps it to the lungs for reoxygenation. Aerobic capacity (VO_{2max}) is the product of how well oxygen is delivered to cardiac output (CO) and extracted by arterial-venous oxygen difference (AVO_{2diff}) active tissues. HR, Heart rate; SV, stroke volume.

oxygen is extracted from the blood to support muscle contraction and other peripheral tissues during activity (arterial-venous oxygen difference, or AVO_{2diff}).[1-3] Aerobic capacity can be represented by the following formula:

$$VO_{2max} = CO \times AVO_{2diff}$$

The energy cost of doing work is based on the amount of oxygen consumed for the activity, regardless of whether the activity is supported by aerobic (with oxygen) or anaerobic (without oxygen) metabolic mechanisms for producing energy. VO_{2max} provides an indication of the maximum amount of work that can be supported.[1-3]

CO is the product of two elements. The first is the HR, the number of times that the heart contracts, or beats, per minute. The second is stroke volume (SV), the amount of blood pumped from the left ventricle with each beat (measured in milliliters or liters). Cardiac output is expressed by the following formula (measured in milliliters or liters per minute):

$$CO = HR \times SV$$

As a product of HR and SV, CO is influenced by four factors: (1) the amount of blood returned from the periphery through the vena cava, (2) the ability of the heart to match its rate of contraction to physiological demand, (3) the efficiency or forcefulness of the heart's contraction, and (4) the ability of the aorta to deliver blood to peripheral vessels. The delivery of oxygen to the body tissues to be used to produce energy for work is, ultimately, a function of the central components of the cardiopulmonary system.[1-3]

The second determinant of aerobic capacity, the AVO_{2diff}, reflects the extraction of oxygen from the capillary by the surrounding tissues. The AVO_{2diff} is determined by subtracting the oxygen concentration on the venous (postextraction) side of the capillary bed (CvO_2) from that of the arteriole (preextraction) side of the capillary bed (CaO_2), according to the formula:

$$AVO_{2diff} = CaO_2 - CvO_2$$

The smaller vessels and capillaries of the cardiovascular system are involved in the process of extraction of oxygen from the blood by the active tissues. Extraction of oxygen from the blood to be used to produce energy for the work of the active tissues is a function of the peripheral components of the cardiopulmonary system.[1-3]

During exercise or a physically demanding activity, CO must increase to meet the need for additional oxygen in the more active peripheral tissues. This increased CO is the result of a more rapid HR and a greater SV: As the return of blood to the heart increases, the heart contracts more forcefully and a larger volume of blood is pumped into the aorta by the left ventricle. Chemical and hormonal changes that accompany exercise enhance peripheral shunting of blood to the active muscles, and oxygen depletion in muscle assists transfer of oxygen from the capillary blood to the tissue at work.[3,4]

The efficiency of central components, primarily of CO, accounts for as much as 75% of VO_{2max}. Peripheral oxygen extraction (AVO_{2diff}) contributes the remaining 25% to the process of making oxygen available to support tissue work.[5] In healthy adults, under most conditions, more oxygen is delivered to active tissues (muscle mass) than is necessary.[3,5] For those who are significantly deconditioned or who have cardiopulmonary or cardiovascular disease, the ability to deliver oxygen efficiently to the periphery as physical activity increases may be compromised. With normal aging, there are age-related physiological changes in the heart itself that limit maximum attainable HR. Because of these changes, it is important to assess whether and to what degree SV can be increased effectively if rehabilitation interventions are to be successful.

THE AGING HEART

The ability to plan an appropriate intervention to address cardiovascular endurance and conditioning in older adults who may need to use a prosthesis or orthosis is founded on an understanding of "typical" age-related changes in cardiovascular structure and physiology, as well as on the functional consequences of these changes.

Cardiovascular Structure

Age-related structural changes in the cardiovascular system occur in five areas: myocardium, cardiac valves, coronary arteries, conduction system, and coronary vasculature (i.e., arteries)[6–9] (Table 2-1). Despite these cellular and tissue level changes, a healthy older heart can typically meet energy demands of usual daily activity. Cardiovascular disease, quite prevalent in later life, and a habitually sedentary lifestyle can, however, significantly compromise activity tolerance.[10]

Myocardium

With advanced age, cells of the myocardium show microscopical signs of degeneration including increases in myocardial fat content (i.e., storage of triglyceride droplets within cardiomyocytes); however, the relationship between the quantity of fat and disease severity remains unclear.[11]

Unlike aging skeletal muscle cells, there is minimal atrophy of cardiac smooth muscle cells. More typically, there is hypertrophy of the left ventricular myocardium, increasing the diameter of the left atrium.[12–14] These changes have been attributed to cardiac tissue responses to an increased systolic blood pressure (SBP) and to reduced compliance of the left ventricle and are associated with an increase in weight and size of the heart.[13–17]

Valves

The four valves of the aged heart often become fibrous and thickened at their margins, as well as somewhat calcified.[18] Calcification of the aorta at the base of the cusps of the aortic valve (aortic stenosis) is clinically associated with the slowed exit of blood from the left ventricle into the aorta.[19] Such aortic stenosis contributes to a functional reduction in CO. A baroreflex-mediated increase in SBP attempts to compensate for this reduced CO.[20,21] Over time, the larger residual of blood in the left ventricle after each beat (increased end systolic volume, or ESV) begins to weaken the left ventricular muscle.[22] The left ventricular muscle must work harder to pump the blood out of the ventricle into a more resistant peripheral vascular system.[23,24]

Calcification of the annulus of the mitral valve can restrict blood flow from the left atrium into the left ventricle during diastole. As a result, end diastolic volume (EDV) of blood in the left ventricle is decreased because the left atrium does not completely empty. Over time, this residual blood in the left atrium elongates the muscle of the atrial walls and increases the diameter of the atrium of the heart.[23–25]

Coronary Arteries

Age-related changes of the coronary arteries are similar to those in any aged arterial vessel: an increase in thickness of vessel walls and tortuosity of its path.[26] These changes tend to occur earlier in the left coronary artery than in the right.[27]

TABLE 2-1   *Age-Related Changes in the Cardiovascular System*

Structure	Change	Functional Consequences
Heart	Deposition of lipids, lipofuscin, and amyloid within cardiac smooth muscle	Less excitability
	Increased connective tissue and fibrocity	Diminished cardiac output
	Hypertrophy of left ventricle	Diminished venous return
	Increased diameter of atria	Susceptibility to dysrhythmia
	Stiffening and calcification of valves	Reduction in maximal attainable heart rate
	Fewer pacemaker cells in sinoatrial and atrioventricular nodes	Less efficient dilation of cardiac arteries during activity
	Fewer conduction fibers in bundle of His and branches	Less efficient left ventricular filling in early diastole, leading to reduced stroke volume
	Less sensitivity to extrinsic (autonomic) innervation	Increased afterload, leading to weakening of heart muscle
	Slower rate of tension development during contraction	
Blood vessels	Altered ratio of smooth muscle to connective tissue and elastin in vessel walls	Less efficient delivery of oxygenated blood to muscle and organs
	Decreased baroreceptor responsiveness	Diminished cardiac output
	Susceptibility to plaque formation within vessel	Less efficient venous return
	Rigidity and calcification of large arteries, especially aorta	Susceptibility to venous thrombosis
	Dilation and increased tortuosity of veins	Susceptibility to orthostatic hypotension

When coupled with atherosclerosis, these changes may compromise the muscular contraction and pumping efficiency and effectiveness of the left ventricle during exercise or activity of high physiological demand.[2,3,28]

Conduction System

Age-related changes in the conduction system of the heart can have a substantial impact on cardiac function. The typical 75-year-old has less than 10% of the original number of pacemaker cells of the sinoatrial node.[29,30] Fibrous tissue builds within the internodal tracts as well as within the atrioventricular node, including the bundle of His and its main bundle branches.[29,30] As a consequence, the ability of the heart to coordinate the actions of all four of its chambers may be compromised.[29] Arrhythmias are pathological conditions that become more common in later life; they are managed pharmacologically or with implantation of a pacemaker/defibrillator.[31] Rehabilitation professionals must be aware of the impact of medications or pacemaker settings on an individual's ability to physiologically respond to exercise and to adapt to the intervention, whether it be a conditioning program or early mobility after a medical/surgical event, accordingly.[32]

Arterial Vascular Tree

Age-related changes in the arterial vascular tree, demonstrated most notably by the thoracic aorta and eventually the more distal vessels, can disrupt the smooth or streamline flow (i.e., laminar flow) of blood from the heart toward the periphery.[31,33] Altered alignment of endothelial cells of the intima creates rough or turbulence flow (i.e., nonlaminar flow), which increases the likelihood of deposition of collagen and lipid.[34] Fragmentation of elastic fibers in the intima and media of larger arterioles and arteries further compromises the functionally important "rebound" characteristic of arterial vessels.[35] Rebound normally assists directional blood flow through the system, preventing the backward reflection of fluid pressure waves of blood. This loss of elasticity increases vulnerability of the aorta, which, distended and stiffened, cannot effectively resist the tensile force of left ventricular ejection. Not surprisingly, the incidence of abdominal aortic aneurysms rises sharply among older adults, and stiffness (distensibility) of the ascending aorta is associated with severity of coronary artery disease.[36,37]

Cardiovascular Physiology

Although the physiological changes in the cardiovascular system are few, their impact on performance of the older adult can be substantial. The nondiseased aging heart continues to be an effective pump, maintaining its ability to develop enough myocardial contraction to support daily activity. The response of cardiac muscle to calcium (Ca^{++}) is preserved, and its force-generating capacity maintained.[38] Two aspects of myocardial contractility do, however, change with aging: the rate of tension development in the myocardium slows and the duration of contraction and relaxation is prolonged.[39,40]

Sensitivity Beta-Adrenergic

One of the most marked age-related changes in cardiovascular function is the reduced sensitivity of the heart to sympathetic stimulation, specifically to the stimulation of beta-adrenergic receptors.[40,41] Age-related reduction in beta-adrenergic sensitivity includes a decreased response to norepinephrine and epinephrine released from sympathetic nerve endings in the heart, as well as a decreased sensitivity to any of these catecholamines circulating in the blood.[41,42] Normally, norepinephrine and epinephrine are potent stimulators of ventricular contraction.

An important functional consequence of the change in receptor sensitivity is less efficient cardioacceleratory response, which leads to a lower HR at submaximal and maximal levels of exercise or activity.[43] The time for HR rise to the peak rate is prolonged, so more time is necessary to reach the appropriate HR level for physically demanding activities. A further consequence of this reduced beta-adrenergic sensitivity is less than optimal vasodilation of the coronary arteries with increasing activity.[41,44] In peripheral arterial vessels, beta-adrenergic receptors do not appear to play a primary role in mediating vasodilation in the working muscles.[45]

Baroreceptor Reflex

Age-related change in the cardiovascular baroreceptor reflex also contributes to prolongation of cardiovascular response time in the face of an increase in activity (physiological demand).[40] The baroreceptors in the proximal aorta appear to become less sensitive to changes in blood volume (pressure) within the vessel. Normally, any drop in proximal aortic pressure triggers the hypothalamus to begin a sequence of events that leads to increased sympathetic stimulation of the heart. Decreased baroreceptor responsiveness may increase an older individual's susceptibility to orthostatic (postural) and postprandial (after eating) hypotension, or compromise their tolerance of the physiological stress of a Valsalva maneuver associated with breath holding during strenuous activity.[46,47] Clinically, this is evidenced by lightheadedness when rising from lying or sitting, especially after a meal, or if one tends to hold one's breath during effortful activity.

The consequences of age-related physiological changes on the cardiovascular system can often be managed effectively by routinely using simple lower extremity warmup exercises before position changes. Several repetitions of ankle and knee exercises before standing up, especially after a prolonged time sitting (including for meals) or lying down (after a night's rest), help maximize blood return to the heart (preload), assisting cardiovascular function for the impending demand. In addition, taking a bit more time in initiating and progressing difficulty of activities may help the slowed cardiovascular response time reach an effective level of performance. Scheduling physical therapy or physical activity remote from mealtimes might also be beneficial for patients who are particularly vulnerable to postprandial hypotension.

Functional Consequences of Cardiovascular Aging

What are the functional consequences of cardiovascular aging for older adults participating in exercise or rehabilitation activities? This question can best be answered by focusing on what happens to the CO (Figure 2-2). The age-related structural and physiological changes in the cardiovascular system give rise to two loading conditions that influence CO: cardiac filling (preload) and vascular impedance (afterload).[3,20]

Preload

Cardiac filling/preload determines the volume of blood in the left ventricle at the end of diastole. The most effective ventricular filling occurs when pressure is low within the heart and relaxation of the muscular walls of the ventricle is maximal.[1,5] Mitral valve calcification, decreased compliance of the left ventricle, and the prolonged relaxation of myocardial contraction can contribute to a less effective filling of the left ventricle in early diastole.[48] Doppler studies of the flow of blood into the left ventricle in aging adults demonstrate decreased rates of early filling, an increased rate of late atrial filling, and an overall decrease in the peak filling rate.[5,22,48] When compared with healthy 45- to 50-year-old adults, the early diastolic filling of a healthy 65- to 80-year-old is 50% less.[5,22,49] This reduced volume of blood in the ventricle at the end of diastole does not effectively stretch the ventricular muscle of the heart, compromising the Frank-Starling mechanism and the myocontractility of the left ventricle.[50] The functional outcome of decreased early diastolic filling and the reduced EDV is a proportional decrease in SV, one of the determinants of CO and, subsequently, work capacity (VO_{2max}).[5,21,40]

Afterload

High vascular impedance and increased afterload disrupts flow of blood as it leaves the heart toward the peripheral vasculature. Increased afterload is, in part, a function of age-related stiffness of the proximal aorta, an increase in systemic vascular resistance (elevation of SBP, hypertension), or a combination of both factors.[40,51] Ventricular contraction that forces blood flow into a resistant peripheral vascular system produces pressure waves in the blood. These pressure waves reflect back toward the heart, unrestricted by the stiffened walls of the proximal aorta. The reflected pressure waves, aortic stiffness, and increased systemic vascular resistance collectively contribute to an increased afterload in the aging heart.[39,51] Increased afterload is thought to be a major factor in the age-associated

decrease in maximum SV, hypertrophy of the left ventricle, and prolongation of myocardial relaxation (e.g., slowed relaxation in the presence of a persisting load on the heart).[6,7,9]

An unfortunate long-term consequence of increased afterload is weakening of the heart muscle itself, particularly of the left ventricle. Restricted blood flow out of the heart results in a large residual volume (RV) of blood in the heart at the end of systole when ventricular contraction is complete. Large ESVs gradually increase the resting length of ventricular cardiac muscle, effectively weakening the force of contraction.[2,6,7,9,22,52]

Left Ventricular Ejection Fraction

Left ventricular ejection fraction (LVEF) is the proportion of blood pumped out of the heart with each contraction of the left ventricle, which is expressed by the following equation:

$$LVEF = (EDV - ESV) \div EDV$$

At rest the LVEF does not appear to be reduced in older adults. Under conditions of maximum exercise, however, the rise in LVEF is much less than in younger adults.[21,53,54] This reduced rise in the LVEF with maximal exercise clearly illustrates the impact that preload and afterload functional cardiovascular age-related changes have on performance.

A substantial reduction in EDV, an expansion of ESV, or a more modest change in both components may account for the decreased LVEF of the exercising older adult:

$$\downarrow EDV = \downarrow LVEF$$
$$\uparrow ESV = \downarrow LVEF$$

When going from resting to maximal exercise conditions, the amount of blood pumped with each beat for young healthy adults increases 20% to 30% from a resting LVEF of 55% to an exercise LVEF of 80%. For a healthy older adult, in contrast, LVEF typically increases less than 5% from rest to maximal exercise.[53,55] The LVEF may actually decrease in adults who are 60 years of age and older.[53,56] As LVEF and CO decrease with aging, so does the ability to work over prolonged periods (functional cardiopulmonary reserve capacity) because the volume of blood delivered to active tissue decreases (Figure 2-3). Functional reserve capacity is further compromised by the long-term effects of inactivity and by cardiopulmonary pathology.[21,28,57,58] The contribution of habitual exercise to achieving effective maximum exercise LVEF is not well understood but the decline may not be as substantial for highly fit older adults.[21]

PULMONARY FUNCTION IN LATER LIFE

Several important age-related structural changes of the lungs and of the musculoskeletal system have a significant impact on pulmonary function.[59] These include change in the tissues and structures making up the lungs and airways, alteration in lung volume, reduced efficiency of gas exchange, and a mechanically less efficient ventilatory pump related

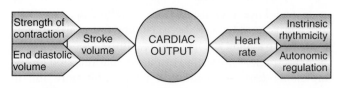

FIGURE 2-2 Factors affecting cardiac output are influenced by the aging process: If strength of contraction decreases and end diastolic volume increases, stroke volume is reduced. Coupled with alterations in heart rate response to increasing workload, activities that were submaximal in intensity at a younger age may become more physiologically demanding in later life.

Reserve capacity	Age-related loss	Age-related loss	Age-related loss
	Reserve capacity	Impact of inactivity	Impact of inactivity
		Reserve capacity	Impact of disease
			Reserve capacity
ADLs	ADLs	ADLs	ADLs
At rest	At rest	At rest	At rest
Healthy young adult	**Healthy older adult**	**Sedentary older adult**	**Older adult with disease**

FIGURE 2-3 Comparison of the effects of aging, inactivity, and cardiopulmonary disease on functional reserve capacity, expressed as cardiac output (CO in L/min). At rest, the heart delivers between 4 and 6 L/min of blood to peripheral tissues. This may double during many activities of daily living. In a healthy young person, the CO may increase to as much as 24 L/min to meet metabolic demands of sustained exercise. This reserve capacity decreases to approximately 18 L/min in healthy, fit adults after the age of 60 years. A sedentary lifestyle decreases functional reserve capacity further. Superimposed cardiopulmonary disease further limits the ability to do physical work, in some cases approaching or exceeding cardiopulmonary reserve capacity. (Modified from Irwin SC, Zadai CC. Cardiopulmonary rehabilitation of the geriatric patient. In Lewis CB [ed], *Aging: The Health Care Challenge*. Philadelphia: F.A. Davis, 1990. p. 190.)

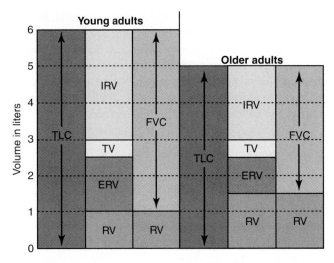

FIGURE 2-4 Changes in the distribution of air within the lungs (volume) have an impact on an older adult's efficiency of physical work. Loss of alveoli and increasing stiffness of the rib cage result in a 30% to 50% increase in residual volume (RV) and a 40% to 50% decrease in forced vital capacity (FVC). FVC includes three components: Inspiratory reserve volume (IRV) and expiratory reserve volume (ERV) tend to decrease with aging, whereas resting tidal volume (TV), the amount of air in a normal resting breath, tends to be stable over time. Total lung capacity (TLC) and inspiratory capacity (IRV + TV) also tend to decrease. Over time, the physiological consequences of these changes make the older adult more vulnerable to dyspnea (shortness of breath) during exercise and physically demanding activity.

to changes in alignment and posture[60] (Table 2-2). Although a healthy adult at midlife uses only 10% of the respiratory system capacity at rest, aging of the pulmonary system, especially when accompanied by chronic illness or acute disease, negatively affects the ability of the lungs to respond to increasing demands of physical activity[61] (Figure 2-4). Age-related changes in the pulmonary and musculoskeletal systems also contribute to an increase in the physiological work of breathing.

Changes within the Lung and Airway

The production of elastin, which is the major protein component of the structure of the lungs, decreases markedly in late life. The elastic fibers of the lung become fragmented, and, functionally, the passive elastic recoil or rebound important for expiration becomes much less efficient. The elastic fibers that maintain the structure of the walls of the alveoli also decrease in number. This loss of elastin means loss of alveoli and consequently less surface area for the exchange of oxygen, as well as an increase in RV associated with more "dead space" within the lung where air exchange cannot occur.[60,61]

TABLE 2-2 *Summary of Age-Related Changes in the Cardiopulmonary System and Functional Consequences*

Anatomical Changes	*Physiological Changes*	*Consequences*	*Change in Lung Function Tests*
Rearrangement and fragmentation of elastin fibers	Less elastic recoil for expiration	Greater airspace within alveoli, less surface area for O_2/CO_2 exchange thoracic cage	Increased functional residual capacity and residual volume tissue
Stiffened cartilage in compliant articulation of ribs and vertebrae	Greater compliance of lung		Shorter, less vital capacity, and forced expiratory volume in 1 second (FEV_1)
Increasing stiffness and compression of annulus fibrosis in intervertebral disks	Decreased vital capacity, forced More rigid thoracic cage	Increased work of breathing Less force during inspiration Less efficient cough	Decreased maximum inspiratory pressure, maximum expiratory pressure, and maximum voluntary
Reduction of strength and endurance of respiratory musculature	Decreased volume of maximum voluntary ventilation and maximum sustained ventilatory capacity Greater mismatch between ventilation and perfusion within lung	Diminished exercise tolerance Reduced resting PaO_2	ventilation

There may be as much as a 15% decrease in the total number of alveoli per unit of lung volume by the age of 70 years.[62]

With aging, there is also an increase in diameter of major bronchi and large bronchioles, as well as a decreased diameter of smaller bronchioles, often leading to a slight increase in resistance to air flow during respiration.[62] This contributes to greater physical work to breathe as age advances.

Starting at midlife and continuing into later life, there tends to be a growing mismatch between lung area ventilated with each breath and lung area perfused by pulmonary arterioles and capillaries, attributed to alteration in alveolar surface, vascular structures, and posture.[63] This mismatch compromises the efficiency of diffusion of oxygen across the alveoli into the capillary bed (i.e., decreasing arterial oxygen tension) within the lung becomes less efficient from midlife into later life.[60,63]

Changes in the Musculoskeletal System

The decreasing elastic recoil and alveolar surface area for oxygen exchange may be further compounded by increased stiffness (loss of flexibility), "barreling" of the thoracic rib cage that houses the lungs, and a decrease in height as intervertebral disks narrow and stiffen.[64] Much of the stiffness is attributed to changes in the articulation between rib and vertebrae, as well as decreased elasticity of intercostal muscle and soft tissue.[65] Although the stiffened rib cage may be as much a consequence of a sedentary lifestyle as of advancing age, lack of flexibility compromises inspiration and also decreases elastic recoil of expiration.[66] In addition, the forward head and slight kyphosis that tend to develop with aging alter rib and diaphragm position, decreasing mechanical efficiency of inspiration.[61,64,66] The net effect of a stiffer thoracic cage is an increase in the work of taking a breath since muscles of respiration must work harder during inspiration to counteract the stiffness.[61]

The striated muscles of respiration are composed of a combination of type I (slow twitch, fatigue resistant, for endurance) and type II (fast twitch, for power) fibers and are susceptible to the same age-related changes in strength and endurance that have been observed in muscles of the extremities.[67] Normally, type I muscle fibers are active during quiet breathing while recruitment of type II fibers is triggered by increasing physiological demand as activity increases. Age-related decrement in the strength and efficiency of the diaphragm, intercostals, abdominal muscles, and other accessory muscles of respiration affects the effectiveness and work of breathing.[61,68] Altered posture and higher RV within the lung also contribute to an increased work of breathing; when the diaphragm rests in less than optimal position and configuration for contraction, accessory muscles become active sooner, as physiological demand increases. Oxygen consumption in respiratory muscles, as in all striated muscle, decreases linearly with age, making older muscle more vulnerable to the effects of fatigue in situations of high physical demand, especially in the presence of lung disease or injury.[60]

Control of Ventilation

The rate of breathing (breaths per minute) is matched to physiological demand by input from peripheral mechanoreceptors in the chest wall, lungs, and thoracic joints, as well as centers in the brainstem of central nervous systems (CNS) and peripheral aortic and carotid bodies that are sensitive to concentration of CO_2, O_2, and hydrogen ions (pH) in the blood.[69] With aging, stiffness of the thorax tends to reduce efficiency of mechanoreceptors, and the CNS and peripheral nervous system (PNS) centers that monitor CO_2, O_2, and pH to detect hypoxia during activity slowly begin to decline.

Gradual loss of descending motor neurons within the CNS also occurs, with less efficient activation of neurons innervating muscles of respiration via the phrenic nerve to the diaphragm for inspiration and of spinal nerves to intercostals for expiration.[63] These three factors combine to compromise the individual's ability to quickly and accurately respond to increasing physiological demand and increase the likelihood of dyspnea during activity.

Functional Consequences of Pulmonary Aging

With less recoil for expiration and reduced flexibility for inspiration, the ability to work is compromised in two ways (see Figure 2-4). First, vital capacity (VC), the maximum amount of air that can be voluntarily moved in and out of the lungs with a breath, is decreased by 25% to 40%. Second, RV, the air remaining in the lungs after a forced expiration, is increased by 25% to 40%.[60] This combination of reduced movement of air with each breath and increased air remaining in the lung between breaths leads to higher lung-air carbon dioxide content and, eventually, lower oxygen saturation of the blood after air exchange. The increase in RV also affects the muscles of inspiration: the dome of the diaphragm flattens and the accessory respiratory muscles are elongated. As a result of these length changes, the respiratory muscles work in a mechanically disadvantageous range of the length-tension curve, and the energy cost of the muscular work of breathing rises.[61]

Functionally, the amount of air inhaled per minute (minute ventilation) is a product of the frequency of breathing times the tidal volume (volume of air moving into and out of the lungs with each usual breath). In healthy individuals, the increased ventilatory needs of low-intensity activities are usually met by an increased depth of breathing (i.e., increased tidal volume).[70] Frequency of breathing increases when increased depth alone cannot meet the demands of activity, typically when tidal volume reaches 50% to 60% of the VC.[70] For the older adult with reduced VC who is involved in physical activity, tidal volume can quickly exceed this level, so that frequency of breathing increases much earlier than would be demonstrated by a young adult at the same intensity of exercise.[71] Because the energy cost of breathing rises sharply with the greater respiratory muscle work associated with an increased respiratory rate, an important consequence of increased frequency of breathing is fatigue.[72] This early reliance on an increased frequency of breathing, combined with a large RV and its higher carbon dioxide concentration in lung air, results in a physiological cycle that further drives the need to breathe more frequently. Overworked respiratory muscles are forced to rely on anaerobic metabolism to supply their energy need, resulting in a buildup of lactic acid.

Because lactic acid lowers the pH of the tissues (acidosis), it is also a potent physiological stimulus for increased frequency of breathing.[72-74] The older person can be easily forced into a condition of rapid, shallow breathing (shortness of breath) to meet the ventilatory requirements of seemingly moderate-intensity exercise.

IMPLICATIONS FOR INTERVENTION

Rehabilitation professionals must consider two questions about the implications of age-related changes in the cardiovascular and cardiopulmonary systems on an older person's ability to do physical work. First, what precautions should be observed to avoid cardiopulmonary and cardiovascular complications? Second, what can be done to optimize cardiopulmonary and cardiovascular function for maximal physical performance?

Precautions

Because of the combined effects of the age-related changes in the cardiovascular and cardiopulmonary systems, the high incidence of cardiac and pulmonary pathologies in later life, and the deconditioning impact of bed rest and inactivity, older patients who require orthotic or prosthetic intervention may be vulnerable if exercise or activity is too physiologically demanding. Although most older adults can tolerate and respond positively to exercise, exercise is not appropriate in a number of circumstances (Table 2-3).

Estimating Workload: Heart Rate and Rate Pressure Product

One of the readily measurable consequences of the reduced response of the heart to sympathetic stimulation in later life is a reduction in the maximal attainable HR.[39,69,75] This reduction in

TABLE 2-3 *Signs and Symptoms of Exercise Intolerance*

Category	Cautionary Signs/Symptoms	Contraindications to Exercise
Heart rate	<40 bpm at rest >130 bpm at rest Little HR increase with activity Excessive HR increase with activity Frequent arrhythmia	Prolonged at maximum activity
ECG	Any recent ECG abnormalities	Prolonged arrhythmia or tachycardia Exercise-induced ECG abnormalities Third-degree heart block
Blood pressure	Resting SBP >165 mm Hg Resting DBP >110 mm Hg Lack of SBP response to activity Excessive BP response to activity	Resting SBP >200 mm Hg Resting DBP >110 mm Hg Drop in SBP >20 mm Hg in exercise Drop in DBP during exercise
Angina	Low threshold for angina	Resting or unstable angina New jaw, shoulder, or left arm pain
Respiratory rate	Dyspnea >35 breaths/min	Dyspnea >45 breaths/min
Blood gas values	O₂ saturation <90%	O₂ saturation <86%
Other symptoms	Mild to moderate claudication Onset of pallor Facial expression of distress Lightheadedness or mild dizziness Postactivity fatigue >1 hr Slow recovery from activity	Severe, persistent claudication Cyanosis, severe pallor, or cold sweat Facial expression of severe distress Moderate to severe dizziness, syncope Nausea, vomiting Increasing mental confusion Onset of ataxia, incoordination
Additional considerations	Fever >100°F Aortic stenosis Recent mental confusion Abnormal electrolytes (potassium) Known left main coronary artery disease Idiopathic hypertrophic subaortic stenosis Compensated heart failure	Any acute illness Digoxin toxicity Overt congestive heart failure Untreated second or third degree heart block Acute pericarditis <4 to 6 weeks after myocardial infarction <2 days after pulmonary embolism Acute thrombophlebitis Acute hypoglycemia

bpm, Beats per minute; DBP, diastolic blood pressure; ECG, electrocardiogram; HR, heart rate; SBP, systolic blood pressure.
Modified from Hillegass E (ed), *Essentials of Cardiopulmonary Physical Therapy*, 3rd ed. St. Louis: Elsevier Saunders, 2011, pp. 307, 564, 586.

maximal HR also signals that an older person's HR reserve, the difference between the rate for any given level of activity and the maximal attainable HR, is limited as well. For older patients involved in rehabilitation programs, the difference between resting and maximal HR is narrowed. One method of estimating maximal (max) attainable HR is the following[5]:

$$Max\ HR = 220 - age$$

For healthy individuals, the recommended target HR for aerobic conditioning exercise is between 60% and 80% of maximal attainable HR. For many older adults, especially those who are habitually inactive, resting HR may be close to the recommended range for exercise exertion.[76] Consider an 80-year-old individual with a resting HR of 72 beats per minute. His maximal attainable HR is approximately 140 beats per minute (220 − 80 years). A target HR for an aerobic training level of exertion of 60% of maximal HR would be 84 beats per minute. His resting HR is within 12 beats of the HR for aerobic training. Functionally, this means that an activity as routine as rising from a chair or walking a short distance on a level surface may represent physical work of a level of exertion equated with moderate- to high-intensity exercise. Because of the reduction in maximal attainable HR with age, older adults may be working close to their VO_{2max} range even in usual activities of daily living.[76,77]

Because HR essentially signals the work of the heart, with each beat representing ventricular contraction, increased HR relates closely to increased heart work and increased oxygen consumption by the myocardium.[75] Given that afterload on the heart increases with age, the overall work of the heart for each beat is likely greater as well.[21,38,39,40] A more representative way to estimate the work of the heart during activity for older adults is the rate pressure product (RPP),[78–80] using HR and SBP as follows:

$$RPP = HR \times SBP$$

The linear relationship between VO_{2max} and HR for younger adults actually levels off for older adults.[81] Because of this, HR alone cannot accurately reflect the physiological work that the older patient experiences; the RPP provides a clearer impression of relative work.[80] For older individuals with HR reserve limited by age, adjusting activity to keep the rise in HR within the lower end of the HR reserve is wise, especially for those with known coronary artery compromise.

Blood Pressure as a Warning Sign

An older person's blood pressure (BP) must also be considered. Hypertension, particularly increased SBP, is common in older adults. SBP also provides a relative indication of the level of afterload on the heart.[40,82,83] Resting BP can be used to indicate whether an older person can safely tolerate increased physiological work. Persons with resting BPs of more than 180/95 mm Hg may have difficulty with increased activity. A conservative estimate of the safe range of exercise suggests that exercise should be stopped if and when BP exceeds 220/110 mm Hg, although some consider 220 mm Hg too

conservative a limit for older adults.[75] SBP should rise with increasing activity or exercise.[84]

The older adult with limited HR reserve must increase SV to achieve the required CO.[21,39,53] SBP rises as SV increases and blood volume in the peripheral vasculature rises.[40] If SBP fails to rise or actually decreases during activity, this is a significant concern.[75] The drop or lack of change in SBP indicates that the heart is an ineffective pump, unable to contract and force a reasonable volume of blood out of the left ventricle. Continuing exercise or activity in the presence of a dropping SBP returns more blood to a heart that is incapable of pumping it back out to the body. Elevated diastolic blood pressure (DBP) suggests that the left ventricle is maintaining a higher pressure during the filling period.[39,40,69] Early diastolic filling during preload will be compromised,[40,49] and the heart will be unable to capitalize on the Frank-Starling mechanism to enhance the force of ventricular contraction.[21,53]

Respiratory Warning Signs

Dyspnea, or shortness of breath, is an important warning sign as well. Age-related changes in the pulmonary system increase the work of breathing, and breathing becomes less efficient as work increases.[72] Because an older person is prone to shortness of breath, recovering from shortness of breath during exercise may be difficult. Breathing more deeply requires a disproportionately greater amount of respiratory muscle work, which further increases the cost of ventilation.[73,74] The use of supplemental oxygen by nasal cannula for the postoperative or medically ill older adult who is beginning rehabilitation may be quite beneficial.

Oxygen supplementation may prevent or minimize shortness of breath, enabling an older person to tolerate increased activity better and to participate in rehabilitation more fully. During this oxygen-assisted time, any conditioning exercise to improve muscular performance (especially if combined with nutritional support) delivers blood to the working tissues and improves tissue oxygenation, ultimately aiding pulmonary function. Improved muscular conditioning and cardiovascular function may prevent or delay onset of lactic acidemia and the resultant increased desire to breathe that would trigger shortness of breath.[72,85]

Optimizing Cardiopulmonary Performance

For most older adults, conditioning or training is an effective way to improve function, although some may need a longer training period than younger adults to accomplish their desired level of physical performance.[86–90] Physical conditioning, in situations of acute and chronic illness, enables the older person to do more work and better accomplish desired tasks or activities.

Older adults, including those who are quite debilitated, experience improvement in physical performance as a result of conditioning exercises[88] (Figure 2-5). For some, significant gains are made as work capacity increases from an initial state below the threshold necessary for function, such that an older person appears to make greater gains than a younger individual in similar circumstances.[91,92] In many cases the cardiopulmonary system efficiency gained through conditioning means the difference between independence and

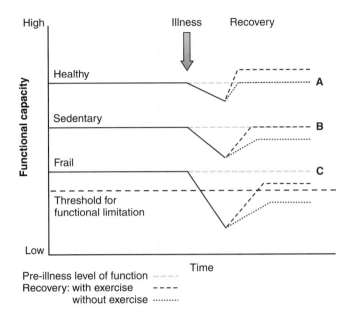

FIGURE 2-5 Comparison of the impact of illness or prolonged inactivity, or both, on functional status and of exercise on recovery of premorbid functional levels of healthy, sedentary, and frail older adults. Each individual's functional reserve is represented by the distance between the threshold for functional limitation and their functional capacity. **A,** Healthy older adults have the most functional reserve and may recover preillness functional capacity without conditioning exercise but often show improvement above baseline with exercise. **B,** Sedentary older adults may not resume preillness functional capacity without the benefit of conditioning exercise. **C,** Frail older adults have the least functional reserve, often fall below threshold for function when illness occurs, and tend to remain below this threshold without conditioning exercise. However, even frail older adults can regain functional status with conditioning exercise.

dependency, functional recovery and minimal improvement, life without extraordinary means and life support, and, for some older individuals, life and death.

The physiological mechanisms for achieving the conditioned responses of older adults may vary slightly from those of younger individuals. With increasing activity or exercise in the submaximal range, older adults demonstrate greater increases in SV and less rise in HR than do young adults.[21,40,49,53,75] This increase in SV is accomplished with an increased EDV, usually without change in the ESV.[21,40,49] Increasing the EDV enhances the force of ventricular contraction by the Frank-Starling mechanism, which, in turn, increases CO despite the age-related impairment of the cardioacceleratory responses, which limits the rise in HR.[21,39,40,49,53] An increased preload, which improves CO, is the usual outcome of training at any age because improved conditioning of the peripheral musculature prevents distal pooling of blood and increased resting tension of the muscles assists blood return.[75]

Preparation for Activity and Exercise

Simple lower extremity exercise as a warmup before any functional activity or training session enhances the preload of the heart. Any gentle, repetitive, active lower extremity motions (e.g., ankle "pumps" in dorsiflexion/plantar flexion, knee flexion/extension, or cycling movements of the legs) before transfer or ambulation activities, before upper trunk and upper extremity activities, or as part of the warmup portion of an aerobic or strength training exercise effectively improves the EDV. This increased EDV compensates in part for age-related preload problems, which might otherwise compromise work capacity.

Additionally, the muscular work of preliminary lower extremity exercise initiates the electrolyte and hormonal changes that promote the metabolic changes and vasodilation in peripheral tissues necessary to support aerobic metabolism for meeting energy demands of the task.[75,88] Peripheral oxygen exchange improves as much as 16% with regular exercise training.[21] The peripheral vasodilation associated with exercise helps to check the rise in afterload on the heart and also minimizes the development of lactic acidemia and the resulting drive to breathe more rapidly.[93]

As submaximal levels of exercise increase toward maximal exercise, SV continues to increase, maintaining CO.[21,49,53] When cardiopulmonary disease is present in addition to aging, however, this continued increase in SV is likely to be blunted.[39,75] Under these circumstances, the reduced sensitivity of the heart to sympathetic stimulation limits the force of contraction of the ventricle so that the ejection fraction decreases and the ESV rises slightly.[40]

Monitoring the Cardiorespiratory Response to Exercise

Consistent monitoring of the cardiopulmonary response is an essential component of rehabilitation interventions aimed at optimizing endurance or fitness of older frail or deconditioned individuals.[76,94] The positive effects of training only occur when the older person is appropriately challenged by the exercise or activity. According to the principle of overload, functional improvements occur only when the body is asked to do more than the customary workload for that individual.[5] For an individual who has been on prolonged bed rest and is quite deconditioned, simple lower extremity exercises while sitting upright may be as challenging as training for a marathon in a healthy young adult. The level of physiological exertion is relative to the individual's customary work. Providing the physiological overload necessary to produce improvements in performance, while avoiding a decline in performance because of exercise-induced fatigue or exhaustion, requires that the therapist monitor an individual's level of exertion.

Heart Rate and Blood Pressure

Maximum oxygen consumption (VO_{2max}) is the most accurate and sensitive measure of the individual workload, but the special equipment and technology necessary to determine VO_{2max} are not typically available in routine clinical practice.[75,76] Although the linear relationship between HR and VO_{2max} plateaus so that HR becomes an inaccurate reflection of the workload for older adults, HR does partially indicate the work of the heart.[75,81] For a rapid clinical impression of the physiological burden of an activity or exercise, HR is helpful as long as the clinician recognizes its limitations when using the measure with elders. Preexercise or activity BP provides some indication of likely afterload against which the heart will be working.[40,75,84] Continuing to monitor BP during the activity helps the clinician to recognize if the exercising cardiovascular system can meet the requirements of an increasing workload.[75] Calculation of the RPP (HR × BP) may be a more accurate estimate of cardiac workload for older adults.[79,80,84]

Perceived Exertion

Ratings of perceived exertion are also effective indicators of the level of physiological exertion experienced by patients who are exercising or involved in a strenuous physical activity[75,95,96] (Table 2-4).

These scales ask individuals to assess subjectively how much effort they are expending during an exercise session or activity, with higher ratings indicating greater effort. Similar scales have been developed to assess breathlessness, fatigue, and discomfort or pain during exercise (Table 2-5). In the clinical use of these ratings of perceived exertion, many older persons using ratings of perceived exertion tend to overestimate their true physiological stress, as indicated by their HR during exercise sessions.[75,95] Clinicians who appropriately recommend exercise for older adults relying on perceived exertion to limit the activity safely may find this phenomenon comforting.

Exercise Testing Protocols

Standard exercise testing protocols are appropriate for assessment of the status of conditioning of the cardiovascular system and exercise tolerance of older adults.[76,97] The "gold standard" treadmill test, a cycle ergometer, or a step test can be used in assessing cardiovascular performance of the older person, unless the specific clinical setting or associated musculoskeletal dysfunction (e.g., balance problems, arthritic joints, or lower extremity muscle weakness) precludes this type of testing.[76] Alternatives for individuals who can walk distances include the One-Mile Walk Test and the Six-Minute Walk Test.[98-100] A brief step test performed while sitting in a chair has been developed for individuals who cannot otherwise be safely tested on a treadmill, with an ergometer, or by distance walked.[75,101]

Careful monitoring of HR and BP before the sitting step test, at predetermined points during testing, at the completion of a brief bout of exercise, and a short while into recovery from the exercise bout provides a comprehensive picture of cardiovascular function of any given older patient. This information often proves important in clinical decision making and program planning. Similarly, careful monitoring of HR and BP before, during, and after a bout of exercise during rehabilitation allows the clinician to compare the pattern of responses with the expected pattern for conditioned adults.[102] Normal exercise-induced cardiovascular responses include a slow rate of rise of HR, a rise in SBP, and minimal (if any) rise in DBP during the exercise bout. For the conditioned older adult, HR and SBP should return toward preexercise values during the immediate postexercise recovery period, on the order of 50%

TABLE 2-4   *Borg Scales:Ratings of Perceived Exertion*

Linear Scale		Ratio Scale	
Value	Description	Value	Description
6	No exertion	0	No effort at all
7-8	Extremely light effort	1	Very little (very weak) effort
9-10	Very light effort	2	Light (weak) effort
11-12	Light effort	3	Moderate effort
13-14	Somewhat hard effort	4	Somewhat strong effort
15-16	Heavy or hard	5-6	Strong effort
17-18	Very hard effort	7-8	Very strong effort
19	Extremely hard effort	9	Extremely strong effort
20	Maximum exertion	10	Maximal exertion

Modified from Borg G, Ottoson D. *The Perception of Exertion in Physical Work*. London: Macmillan, 1986.

TABLE 2-5   *Ratio Scales of Perceived Breathlessness, Fatigue, or Discomfort During Exercise*

Value	Breathlessness/Dyspnea	Fatigue	Discomfort or Pain
0	No breathlessness at all	No fatigue at all	No pain or discomfort
1	Very light breathlessness	Very light fatigue	Very little (weak) pain
2	Light breathlessness	Light fatigue	Little (weak) discomfort
3	Moderate breathlessness	Moderate fatigue	Moderate discomfort
4	Somewhat hard to breathe	Somewhat hard	Somewhat strong discomfort
5-	Heavy breathing	Heavy work/fatigue	Strong discomfort or pain
7-8	Very heavy breathing	Very heavy fatigue	Very heavy discomfort
9	Very, very breathless	Very, very fatigued	Very, very hard discomfort
10	Maximum breathlessness	Maximally fatigued	Maximal discomfort or pain

Modified from Dean E. Mobilization and exercise. In Frownfelter D, Dean E (eds), *Principles and Practice of Cardiopulmonary Physical Therapy*, 3rd ed. St. Louis: Mosby, 1996, p. 282.

of the changes during exercise. The pattern of change in the RPP for the exercise bout and recovery period may be an even more descriptive measure of the cardiovascular response.

Expecting individuals who are significantly deconditioned, can barely tolerate sitting for 30 minutes, are short of breath after 10 repetitions of simple lower extremity exercises while sitting, or are fatigued after 5 minutes of a sitting step test to be fully able to participate in gait and balance training is unreasonable. How can older individuals who are working at 90% or more of their maximum target HR be truly concerned with much more than delivering oxygen to the working tissues? Deconditioned individuals who are working at a high intensity in simple, well-known tasks have seriously restricted energy reserves; they are likely to have difficulty with focus and attention, processing, and the therapist's directions and supporting muscle activity— all necessary components for motor learning in performing a new skill such as gait training with a prosthetic device. Under these circumstances emphasis must first be placed on improving cardiovascular conditioning, to improve energy reserves so that subsequent functional training with an orthosis or prosthesis has greater likelihood of a successful outcome.

Physical Performance Training

The same principles of training that are used with young adult athletes can be adapted and applied to frail or deconditioned older adults who are recovering from amputation in prosthetic rehabilitation or a neuromuscular or musculoskeletal event that necessitates use of an orthosis. The primary goals of conditioning for frail individuals are (1) to develop enough aerobic capacity to do work and (2) to ensure efficient muscle function to produce work.[75,76,103] These concepts can guide any single rehabilitation session, as well as the progression of the rehabilitation program over time. An understanding of exercise for improving fitness and of the few physiological age-related changes in cardiopulmonary function provide a foundation for exercise prescription, which then is individualized on the basis of current exercise tolerance of a specific older patient. This strategy can likely optimize the performance and recovery of older adults in rehabilitation.

An effective strategy to improve cardiopulmonary response to exercise and activity for older patients who are deconditioned by bed rest, acute illness, or sedentary lifestyle begins with a warmup of continuous alternating movements using large muscle groups, particularly of the lower extremities. The goal of such activity is facilitation of the preload and SV; any increase in SV realized through this training regimen helps an older patient maximize cardiovascular function despite age-associated limitations in HR, cardioacceleratory responses, and baroreceptor sensitivity.

For healthy young adults, the recommended regimen for aerobic conditioning and endurance training involves at least three sessions per week of 30 to 60 minutes' duration in activities that use large muscles (running, cycling, swimming, brisk walking) and keep HR in a target range between 60% and 80% of the individual's maximal attainable HR.[104] This may be unreasonable for an older adult who is recovering from an acute illness, habitually sedentary, or coping with age- or

pathology-related impairments of cardiac or pulmonary function. Evidence suggests that, for older adults who are deconditioned, slower but significant improvement in functional capacity can occur at exercise intensities as low as 40% of maximal HR.[87,105,106] Although high-frequency, high-intensity exercise can maximize increase in work capacity (VO_{2max}), high-intensity exercise performed less frequently and low-intensity exercise performed more frequently can also yield positive endurance training effects.[107] Evidence is also growing of improvement in oxygen extraction and muscle function when older adults are involved in regular endurance training.[106]

In addition to aerobic conditioning, the rehabilitation program might include exercises that focus on flexibility. One goal of stretching and flexibility exercise for older adults is to preserve or restore any limited joint mobility that would otherwise compromise essential functions.[108] As flexibility of the trunk and thorax improves, a more effective alignment of the diaphragm and improved elastic recoil of the chest wall will have a positive impact on VC and inspiratory reserve volume and minimize RV, reducing the work of breathing and improving ventilation. Availability of essential range of motion is especially important for energy-efficient gait with lower limb orthoses or prostheses. Contracture of the hip, knee, or ankle has an impact on the alignment of orthotic and prosthetic components and often leads to greater sway and smaller stride length during gait, significantly increasing the energy cost or workload of walking.

Muscle strengthening can begin as soon as the aerobic conditioning appears adequate to oxygenate the peripheral muscular tissue sufficiently. Assessment of the adequacy of peripheral oxygenation might include monitoring the coloring of the distal extremities before and during exercise and noting whether cramping or claudication occurs during exercise. One of the most sensitive indicators of appropriate intensity and duration of exercise is whether the activity can be increased without a marked rise in respiratory rate or onset of shortness of breath; a potent stimulus for frequency of breathing is the pH of the exercising tissues, with decreases as lactic acid builds up during anaerobic exercise.

Two factors should be considered when including strengthening exercises in a rehabilitation program.[94] First, is there adequate muscle strength for consistent and safe performance of the motor tasks needed for functional independence (including the use of assistive devices)? Second, is the muscle mass large enough to support a VO_{2max} that allows activities of daily living to represent a light to modest work intensity level? For many older people who have lost muscle mass (whether as a result of disuse and sedentary lifestyle or because of recent health problems that limit activity), development of more muscle mass increases lean body mass and improves the basal metabolic rate, improving overall health, fitness, and functional status.[109,110]

ENERGY COST OF WALKING

The human body is designed to be energy efficient during upright bipedal gait. Muscles of the trunk and extremities are activated by the CNS in a precise rhythmic cycle to move the body forward while maintaining dynamic stability, adapting stride length and walking speed to the constraints and demands of the task, the force of gravity, and the characteristics of the environment in which walking is occurring.[111,112] The advancing foot is lifted just enough to clear the surface in swing, and muscle activity at the stance-side hip and lower torso keeps the pelvis fairly level and the trunk erect, minimizing vertical displacement of the body's center of mass.[113] Normal arthrokinematic and osteokinematic relationships between body segments ensure a narrow base of support in quiet stance and relaxed walking, and reciprocal arm swing counterbalances the dynamic pendular motion of the lower extremities, ensuring that the center of mass progresses forward with minimal mediolateral sway.[113-116] Much of the energy cost of walking is related to the muscular work performed to keep the center of mass moving forward with a minimum of vertical and mediolateral displacement.[117]

Self-Selected Walking Speed

Because self-selected walking speed emerges from the interaction of the cardiovascular, pulmonary, musculoskeletal,

and neurological systems, it reflects the overall health and functional status of an individual.[118] Walking speed is recognized as a vital sign that not only captures current function, but also can be used to predict risk of functional decline, adverse health events and morbidity, length of stay and discharge location after hospitalization, and mortality.[119-128] Although self-selected walking speed tends to decrease with aging, multiple studies have demonstrated that even into the ninth and tenth decades of life, healthy older adults are able to walk at speeds at or greater than 1 m/sec (Table 2-6).[129-131] Values for typical walking speed are also becoming available for community living older adults with impaired mobility and physical frailty.[132,133] There is also evidence that the ability to increase walking speed is an indicator of functional reserve.[129,133,134]

Walking speed can be quickly and reliably measured using a stop watch and either a 20- or 6-m walkway (Figure 2-6). The indivudal is instructed to walk over the entire distance of the walkway but is timed only while walking the middle two thirds (10 or 4 m) of the distance so that steady-state speed is

TABLE 2-6   *Typical Self-Selected and Fast Walking Speeds for Community-Living Healthy and Mobility-Impaired Older Adults, Reported as Mean SD (m/sec)*

Researcher:		Chui et al[129]		Bohannon[131]		Steffen et al[130]		Lusardi et al[133]	
Population		Healthy		Healthy		Healthy		Mobility Impaired	
Gender	Age Group	SSWS	FWS	SSWS	FWS	SSWS	FWS	SSWS	FWS
Women	60-69	—	—	1.30 (0.21)	1.77 (0.25)	1.44 (0.25)	1.87 (0.30)	1.24 (0.12)	1.81 (0.17)
	70-79	1.34 (0.26)	1.69 (0.32)	1.27 (0.21)	1.79 (0.28)	1.33 (0.22)	1.71 (0.26)	1.25 (0.18)	1.80 (0.26)
	80-89	1.05 (0.12)	1.44 (0.17)	—	—	1.15 (0.21)	1.59 (0.28)	0.80 (0.16)*	1.20 (0.29)
	90-99	0.80 (0.17)	1.05 (0.22)	—	—	—	—	0.71 (0.23)†	1.05 (0.32)†
Men	60-69	—	—	1.36 (0.21)	1.93 (0.36)	1.59 (0.24)	2.05 (0.31)	—	—
	70-79	1.55 (0.58)	2.19 (0.78)	1.33 (0.20)	2.08 (0.36)	1.38 (0.23)	1.83 (0.44)	1.25 (0.23)	1.94 (0.26)
	80-89	1.30 (0.15)	1.75 (0.21)	—	—	1.21 (0.18)	1.65 (0.24)	0.88 (0.24)*	1.29 (0.38)*
	90-99	1.10 (0.38)	1.55 (0.66)	—	—	—	—	0.72 (0.14)†	1.27 (0.13)†

*29.4% of older adults in sample routinely used rolling walker, standard walker, or cane while walking.
†58.8% of older adults in sample routinely used rolling walker, standard walker, or cane while walking.
FWS, Fast walking speek; SSWS, self-selected walking speed.

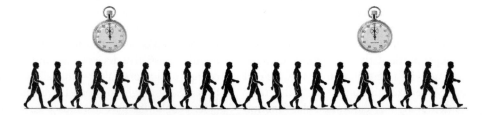

Acceleration Zone	Timed Walk	Deceleration Zone
1 meter	4 meters	1 meter
5 meters	10 meters	5 meters

FIGURE 2-6 Strategy for assessing self selected or fast walking speed timing either the central 10-m distance (10- m walk) or central 4-m distance (4-m walk) allowing for acceleration and deceleration at either end, so that steady state speed is better approximated.

more likely, and the impact of acceleration (at the start) and deceleration (at the end) are minimized. Reliability is strong at either distance for persons with amputation, stroke, and spinal cord injury, as well as physical frailty and other neurological pathologies.[135-138] Minimal detectable differences (MDD) have been consistently reported as between 0.08 m/sec to 0.1 m/sec for community-living persons, those with cognitive impairment, and those with hip fractures.[129,139,140] Minimal clinically important difference for walking speed following stroke is reported to be 0.16 m/sec.[141] Walking speed has been successfully used to evaluate the outcome of interventions for persons with cognitive impairments as well as those with hip fractures.[129,139,140]

Any musculoskeletal or neuromuscular pathology that interferes with the alignment of body segments, the carefully controlled sequential activation of muscles, or the effectiveness of muscle contraction increases the energy cost of walking. As vertical displacement and mediolateral sway increase and gait deviations occur, muscles must work harder to keep the center of mass moving forward despite extraneous displacing moments. As muscle work increases, the cardiopulmonary system responds to this physiological demand with increased HR, SV, and respiratory rate. Any orthosis or prosthesis that adds mass to or alters movement of the lower extremity potentially increases the work of walking. However, in individuals with amputation or neuromuscular dysfunction, walking with an appropriate prosthesis or orthosis may actually require less energy than walking without it.[117,142,143]

Measuring Energy Costs of Walking

Measurement of physiological energy expenditure by direct calorimetry is not realistic in all but the most sophisticated research laboratory settings. Instead, several indirect indicators have been found to be valid and reliable estimates of the energy cost and the efficiency of gait in research and clinical applications. These include calculation of oxygen consumption (VO_{2max}) and oxygen cost while walking, monitoring blood lactate levels, calculating the physiological cost index (PCI) of walking, and monitoring heart and respiratory rates during activity.

Oxygen Rate and Oxygen Cost

The most precise indirect measurements of energy and gait efficiency use special equipment (e.g., a portable spirometer or a Douglas bag) to monitor ventilatory volumes and to measure how much oxygen is taken in and carbon dioxide exhaled during physical activity. This type of testing is usually done while the subject or patient walks, runs on a treadmill or track, or cycles on a stationary bicycle. The rate of oxygen consumption (O_2 rate), measured as volume of oxygen consumed per unit of body weight in 1 minute (mL/kg/min), provides an index of intensity of physical work at any given time.[115,144] VO_{2max} is the highest rate of oxygen uptake possible and is determined by progressing the exercise test to the point of voluntary exhaustion, when the age-adjusted maximum attainable HR is approached or reached.[145,146]

If oxygen consumption during gait is low, an individual is likely to be able to walk long distances. If it is high, however, the distance of functional gait is likely to be limited. The oxygen cost of walking is determined by dividing the rate of oxygen consumption by the speed of walking. Oxygen cost is a precise indicator of efficiency of gait, the amount of energy expended to walk over a standard distance (mL/kg/m).[115] Most of what researchers currently understand about energy expenditure when using a prosthesis or orthosis is based on studies that have measured oxygen rate and oxygen cost of walking.

Serum Lactate

The energy efficiency of walking is also assessed by evaluation of serum carbon dioxide and lactate levels as indicators of anaerobic energy production. The energy (adenosine triphosphate [ATP]) required for muscle contraction during gait can be derived from a combination of aerobic oxidative and anaerobic glycolytic pathways.[147] The aerobic oxidative pathway, which depends on oxygen delivery to active muscle cells, is the most efficient source of energy, producing almost 19 times as much ATP as the anaerobic pathway. In healthy, fit individuals, this aerobic pathway is more than able to meet energy requirements of relaxed walking. If energy demands of an exercise or activity are met by aerobic oxidation, the activity can be sustained for long periods with relatively low levels of fatigue. As activity becomes strenuous (i.e., as walking speed or surface incline increases) and the need for energy begins to exceed the availability of oxygen for aerobic oxidation, additional energy is accessed through anaerobic metabolism.[148] This transition to anaerobic metabolism is reported to begin at work levels of 55% of VO_{2max} in healthy, untrained individuals but may begin at 80% of VO_{2max} in highly trained athletes.[149]

When the ability to deliver oxygen is compromised by the physical deconditioning of a sedentary lifestyle or by cardiac, pulmonary, or musculoskeletal pathology, anaerobic glycolysis becomes a primary source of energy at lower levels of work.[150] Whenever the anaerobic pathway is the major source of energy, blood levels of lactate and carbon dioxide rise, lowering blood pH and increasing the respiratory exchange ratio (CO_2 production/O2 consumption).[151] Under these conditions, the ability to sustain activity is limited, with an earlier onset of fatigue as workload increases. Serum lactate levels are most often used in studies of assisted ambulation using hybrid orthotic/functional electrical stimulation systems for those with spinal cord injury.

Heart Rate and Physiological Cost Index

High correlations between HR and oxygen consumption during gait have been reported for children and for healthy young adults at a variety of walking speeds.[152,153] Although this suggests that HR monitoring may be a reliable substitute for oxygen consumption, it should be used with caution in older adults because of the age-related changes in cardiopulmonary function discussed earlier in this chapter. This is especially true for older adults with heart disease who are being managed with medications that further blunt HR response.[154,155] The RPP or the PCI may be more appropriate indicators of the energy cost of walking in these circumstances. The PCI is calculated as follows[156]:

$$PCI = (HR\ walking - HR\ resting)/walking\ speed$$

Measured in beats per meter, the PCI reflects the effort of walking; low values suggest energy-efficient gait. The PCI was originally used to assess gait restrictions in adults with rheumatoid arthritis and similar inflammatory joint disease.[156] For children between 3 and 12 years of age, the mean PCI at self-selected or preferred walking speed has been reported to be between 0.38 and 0.40 beats per meter.[157] Typical PCI values for adolescents and young adults at usual walking speeds ranged from 0.3 to 0.4 beats per meter.[158] In a study of healthy adults older than age 65 years, the mean PCI value when walking on a flat 10-m track was 0.43 (SD = 0.13) beats per meter; when calculated while walking on a treadmill, mean PCI increased to 0.60 (SD = 0.26) beats per meter.[159]

The PCI has been used to assess the effect of different assistive devices on the effort of walking,[160] evaluate the short- and long-term impact on neuromuscular stimulation on the ability to walk and run in older adults and in children with hemiplegia, assess outcomes of orthopedic surgery in children with cerebral palsy, and evaluate the efficacy of reciprocal gait orthosis/functional electrical stimulation systems for individuals with spinal cord injury.[161–169] High correlation among the PCI, percent maximum HR, and oxygen rate (r = 0.91, P > .005) in able-bodied children and children with transtibial amputation supports its validity as an indicator of energy cost for children.[170] A similar study of energy cost of walking in young adults using a microprocessor-controlled transfemoral prosthesis suggests that PCI is comparable with oxygen uptake as an indicator of the energy cost of walking.[171] The PCI has also been used to compare energy cost of walking in different types of transfemoral prosthetic sockets and assess efficacy of a stance control knee orthosis.[172,173]

Studies of variability in PCI values on repeated measures have raised questions about its accuracy and sensitivity to change in energy cost of gait, as compared with monitoring of oxygen consumption and oxygen cost.[174–176] Although the relationship between PCI and the "gold standards" of oxygen consumption and oxygen cost may not be strong enough for researchers, it remains an important tool for clinicians who lack the resources necessary to directly monitor oxygen consumption and cost yet want to estimate the energy cost of walking and assess the impact of orthotic or prosthetic rehabilitation over time.

Energy Expenditure at Self-Selected Walking Speeds

The energy requirements of walking vary with age and walking speed.[176–182] Oxygen consumption is highest in childhood and decreases to approximately 12 mL/kg/min in healthy adults and elders.[177] When oxygen consumption during walking is expressed as a percent of VO_{2max}, a slightly different picture emerges. For a healthy, untrained young adult, oxygen consumption at a comfortable walking speed may be 32% of VO_{2max}, whereas for an older adult walking at a similar speed, oxygen consumption may be as much as 48% of VO_{2max}.[113,183] For functional gait, if walking is to cover long distances or is to be sustained over prolonged periods of time, oxygen consumption must be less than 50% of that individual's VO_{2max} so that aerobic oxidation will be used as the primary source of energy.[5] At comfortable walking speeds, older adults are working nearer the threshold for transition to anaerobic metabolism than are younger adults. If some form of gait dysfunction is superimposed, increasing the energy cost of gait, the work of walking will transition to anaerobic glycolysis unless a cardiovascular conditioning program is included in the rehabilitation program.[184]

For individuals without neuromuscular or musculoskeletal impairment, the relationship between the energy cost of walking and walking speed is nearly linear[185] (Figure 2-7). Gait is most efficient, as indicated by oxygen cost (O_2 rate/velocity), at an individual's self-selected or customary walking speed; energy requirements increase whenever walking speed is much slower or much faster.[185–188] The customary walking speed of most individuals with neuromuscular or musculoskeletal impairments is often much slower, a strategy that minimizes the rate of energy used during walking. As a result of slower speed, however, it takes longer to cover any given distance. Any impairment that reduces walking speed leads to increased oxygen cost, even if oxygen consumption remains close to normal.[189–194]

The weight and design of the prosthesis or orthosis are also determinants of energy cost of gait. The impact of added mass on the energy cost of gait depends on where the load is placed: Extra weight loaded on the trunk (e.g., a heavy backpack) changes oxygen rate during walking less than would a smaller load placed around the ankle.[195] This highlights the importance of minimizing weight of lower extremity orthoses and prostheses to keep the energy cost of walking within an individual's aerobic capacity.[196]

Work of Walking with an Orthosis

When discussing the energy cost of walking with an orthosis, it is important to remember that, for those with significant neuromuscular or musculoskeletal impairment, the energy cost of

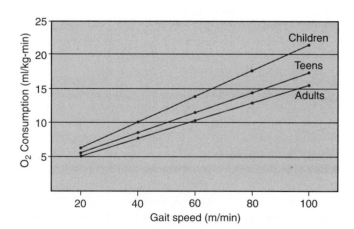

FIGURE 2-7 Relationship between walking speed and oxygen consumption (O_2 rate). The differences in O_2 rate between children and adults (20 to 80 years) are attributed, in part, to differences in body composition. (From gait-velocity regression formulas reported by R. L. Waters. Energy expenditure. In Perry J, Burnfield JM [eds], *Gait Analysis: Normal and Pathological Function*. Thorofare, NJ: Slack, 2010. pp. 483-518.)

walking without the orthosis is typically higher than walking with an appropriate orthosis.[197-199] One of the determinants of energy cost when walking with a cast or an orthosis is the degree of immobility that the orthosis imposes on the ankle, knee, and hip and the associated change in walking speed.[200] For individuals with restriction of knee motion because of a cast or orthosis, the energy cost of gait can be reduced by placing a shoe lift on the contralateral limb to improve swing limb clearance.[201]

For individuals with spinal cord injury, regardless of age, the potential for functional ambulation appears to be determined by four conditions: the ability to use a reciprocal gait pattern, the adequacy of trunk stability, at least fair hip flexor strength bilaterally, and fair quadriceps strength of at least one limb.[202,203] This corresponds to an ambulatory motor index (AMI) score of 18 of 30 possible points, or 60% of "good" lower extremity strength.[179] In this instance, gait may be possible with bilateral ankle-foot orthoses (AFOs) or an AFO and knee-ankle-foot orthosis combination. Those with spinal cord injury at mid to low thoracic levels with AMI scores of less than 60% often require bilateral knee-ankle-foot orthoses, with Lofstrand or axillary crutches in a swing-through gait pattern to ambulate. Waters[117] reports a near linear positive relationship between AMI scores and gait velocity, as well as a somewhat curvilinear inverse relationship between AMI score and oxygen rate (% above normal) and oxygen cost. For persons with spinal cord injury who have the potential for functional ambulation, continued cardiovascular conditioning after discharge from rehabilitation improves the efficiency of walking, as reflected in lower oxygen cost and improvement in walking speed.[203-205] The development of reciprocal gait orthoses and "parawalkers," at times augmented by functional electrical stimulation, has also made modified ambulation possible for those with injury at mid and upper thoracic levels.[206-214] The high energy cost of the intense upper extremity work using crutches to propel the body forward during swing and maintain upright position in stance, however, restricts functional ambulation as a primary means of mobility.

The movement dysfunction associated with stroke and other neuromuscular impairments tends to reduce walking speed, with the degree of slowing determined by the severity of neuromuscular impairment.[190,198,215] As abnormal movement patterns and impaired postural responses compromise the cyclic and dynamic flow of walking, the higher levels of muscle activity that are required to remain upright and to move forward increase the energy cost of gait.[216,217] Reduction of walking speed is a functional strategy to keep energy expenditure within physiological limits. Oxygen rate (consumption) of persons with stroke who walk at a reduced walking speed is close to that of older adults who walk at their customary walking speed; however, oxygen cost is significantly higher.[117,190,218] When compared with unimpaired individuals who walk at similar speeds, persons with hemiplegia wearing an AFO use 52% more energy; when they walk without an orthosis, their energy cost can increase to as much as 65% more than unimpaired gait.[219]

Work of Walking with a Prosthesis

The characteristics of gait and the energy cost of walking with a prosthesis are related to the etiology and the level of amputation.[220,221] The walking speed, stride length, and cadence of persons with lower extremity amputation who walk with a prosthesis are typically lower than those of individuals without impairment, regardless of the cause of amputation,[222] although individuals with traumatic etiology tend to walk faster than those with dysvascular etiology.[223,224] Additionally, biomechanical and energy efficiency of prosthetic gait decreases as amputation level increases. Therefore, preservation of the anatomical knee joint appears to be especially important.[222,225]

A classic study by Waters and colleagues[224] (Table 2-7) demonstrated that, for young adults with traumatic transtibial amputation, walking speed, oxygen rate, and oxygen cost were quite close to normal values reported by Perry.[113] For those with traumatic transfemoral or dysvascular amputation, diminishing walking speeds kept oxygen consumption close to that of normal adult gait; however, oxygen cost increased well beyond the normal value of 0.15 mg/kg/m.[200] Although walking speeds reported 20 years later by Torburn and colleagues[223] are much higher (most likely due to biomechanical advances in prosthetic components in the time between the studies), the difference in performance between traumatic and dysvascular groups was consistent. Other studies report oxygen costs of prosthetic gait at between 16% and 28% above normal

TABLE 2-7   *Walking Speed, Oxygen Consumption, and Oxygen Cost in Prosthetic Gait: Comparison of Etiology and Level of Unilateral Amputation*

Etiology and Level:	Traumatic		Dysvascular	
Parameter	Transtibial	Transfemoral	Transtibial	Transfemoral
Waters et al, 1976[224]				
Walking speed (m/min)	71	52	45	36
O₂ rate (mL/kg/min)	12.4	10.3	9.4	10.8
O₂ cost (mL/kg/m)	0.16	0.20	0.20	0.28
Torburn et al, 1995[223]				
Walking speed (m/min)	82.3	—	61.7	—
O₂ rate (mL/kg/min)	17.7	—	13.2	—
O₂ cost (mL/kg/m)	0.22	—	0.21	—

for individuals with transtibial amputation and between 60% and 110% above normal for individuals with transfemoral amputation.[226-230] Although the relationship between walking speed and oxygen rate (consumption) in prosthetic gait is linear, just as it is in unimpaired gait, the slope is significantly steeper.[231] The clinical implication of this relationship is that the rate of energy consumption and of cardiac work, at any walking speed, is higher for those with amputation and that the threshold for transition from aerobic to anaerobic metabolism is reached at lower walking speeds.[232]

Several explanations are possible for the differences in prosthetic gait performance after traumatic versus dysvascular amputation. Because those with dysvascular amputation are typically older than those with traumatic amputation, differences in performance may be the result of age-related changes and concurrent cardiovascular disease in the dysvascular group.[226,233,234] For many older patients with dysvascular amputation, the energy source for walking with a prosthesis may be anaerobic rather than the more efficient aerobic metabolic pathways.[223] A larger cardiac and respiratory functional reserve capacity in younger persons with traumatic transtibial amputation may permit them to meet the increased metabolic demands of prosthetic use because proximal muscle groups work for longer periods at higher intensities to compensate for the loss of those at the ankle.[223,231,235]

Importantly, for most individuals with unilateral transtibial and transfemoral amputation, regardless of age or etiology of amputation, the energy cost of walking with a prosthesis is less than that expended when walking without it using crutches or a walker.[224] For most persons with a new transtibial amputation, the ability to ambulate before amputation is the best predictor of tolerance of the increased energy cost of walking with a prosthesis after surgery.[233] For some older individuals with transfemoral amputation and concurrent cardiovascular or respiratory disease, and for those with bilateral amputation at transfemoral/transtibial or bilateral transfemoral levels, wheelchair mobility may be preferred.[236-239]

Since the 1990s, significant efforts have been made to reduce the energy cost of prosthetic gait by developing dynamic response (energy storing) prosthetic feet and cadence-responsive and microprocessor-controlled prosthetic knee units.[240-254] The flexible keels of most dynamic response prosthetic feet are designed to mimic those of normal ankle mobility, such that mechanical energy stored by compression during stance is released to enhance push-off in the terminal stance.[218] However, the impact of different prosthetic foot designs on the energy cost is not clear. For adults with transtibial amputation, the FlexFoot functioned more like an anatomical ankle than did four other dynamic response feet and the SACH foot, but little difference in stride, velocity, or energy cost was noted.[223,235,246] However, the materials and design of most dynamic response feet may enable transtibial prosthetic users to jump, run, and use a step-over step pattern in stair climbing; these activities are difficult or not possible with a traditional SACH foot.[224-251] Additionally, many individuals with transtibial amputation wear their prosthesis for longer periods during the day and report less fatigue in prolonged walking when using a prosthesis with a dynamic response foot.[233]

SUMMARY

An understanding of normal cardiopulmonary function and how it changes in aging, as a result of sedentary lifestyle or pathological conditions, provides a necessary foundation for rehabilitation professionals working with patients who require an orthosis or prosthesis to walk. This chapter reviews the anatomy and physiology of the cardiopulmonary system, with attention to age-related changes, energy expenditure, and principles of aerobic conditioning for older adults.

Optimal performance of the cardiopulmonary system is influenced by three interrelated factors. First, the patient must have sufficient flexibility and mobility of the trunk for efficient and uncompromised ventilation. Second, adequate mobility of the extremities and excursion of the joints must be present for efficient performance of functional tasks. Third, the individual must have enough muscle mass, strength, and endurance to support the performance of the activity and function of the heart. Immediate and ongoing interventions that functionally enhance preload by returning blood to the older heart and avoidance of conditions (e.g., isometric muscle contraction and Valsalva maneuvers) that unnecessarily increase afterload can result in marked improvement in physical performance of the older person. With these conditions, as well as compensation for the beta-adrenergic receptor-reduced sensitivity with a prolonged period of warmup exercises, an older person is capable of physical performance that is quite similar to that of younger counterparts and essential for the process of recovery of function for the optimal outcome of rehabilitation.

The energy cost and efficiency of gait are affected by aging, deconditioning of a sedentary lifestyle, and neuromuscular and musculoskeletal impairments that alter motor control or the biomechanics of walking. Although an orthosis that restricts joint motion increases the energy cost in unimpaired individuals, the same orthosis leads to more efficient gait in those with neuromuscular impairment. Determinants of efficiency of prosthetic gait include the level and etiology of the amputation. Reduction of walking speed when using an orthosis or prosthesis helps to maintain oxygen consumption at close to normal levels; however, this tends to compromise overall efficiency of gait, as indicated by oxygen cost. Attention to the principles of cardiovascular conditioning including monitoring the response to exercise so that patients are challenged appropriately optimizes the outcomes of rehabilitation programs.

REFERENCES

1. Des Jardins TR. *Cardiopulmonary Anatomy and Physiology: Essentials for Respiratory Care.* 5th ed. Clifton Park, NY: Delmar Publishers; 2008.
2. Phibbs B. *The Human Heart: A Basic Guide to Heart Disease.* 2nd ed. Philadelphia: Lippincott Williams & Wilkins; 2007.
3. Saltin B, Secher NH, Mitchel J, et al., eds. *Exercise and Circulation in Health and Disease.* Champaign, IL: Human Kinetics; 2000.
4. Ekblom B, Astrand P, Saltin B, et al. Effect of training on circulatory response to exercise. *J Appl Physiol.* 1968; 24(4):518–528.

5. Astrand P, Rodahl K, Dahl HA, et al. *Textbook of Work Physiology: Physiological Bases of Exercise.* 4th ed. Champaign, IL: Human Kinetics; 2003.

6. Bolton E, Rajkumar C. The ageing cardiovascular system. *Rev Clin Gerontol.* 2011;21(2):99–109.

7. Scalia GM, Khoo SK, O'Neill S. Age-related changes in heart function by serial echocardiography in women aged 40-80 years. *J Womens Health.* 2010;19(9):1741–1745.

8. Kojodjojo P, Kanagaratnam P, Markides V, et al. Age-Related changes in human left and right atrial conduction. *J Cardiovasc Electrophysiol.* 2006;17(2):120–127.

9. Aronow WS. Heart disease and aging. *Med Clin North Am.* 2006;90(5):849–862.

10. Alexander NB, Dengel DR, Olson RJ, et al. Oxygen uptake (VO2) kinetics and functional mobility performance in impaired older adults. *J Gerontol Biol Med Sci.* 2003;58(8):734–739.

11. Iozzo P. Myocardial, perivascular, and epicardial fat. *Diabetes Care.* 2011;34(suppl 2):S371–S379.

12. Lakatta EG, Sollott SJ. Perspectives on mammalian cardiovascular aging: humans to molecules. *Comp Biochem Physiol A Mol Integr Physiol.* 2002;132(4):699–722.

13. Elliott P, Spirito P. Prevention of hypertrophic cardiomyopathy-related deaths: theory and practice. *Heart.* 2008;94(10):1269–1275.

14. Rieck AE, Cramariuc D, Staal EM, et al. Impact of hypertension on left ventricular structure in patients with asymptomatic aortic valve stenosis (a SEAS substudy). *J Hypertens.* 2010;28(2):377–383.

15. Gosse P. Left ventricular hypertrophy as a predictor of cardiovascular risk. *J Hypertens.* 2005;23(S1):S27–S33.

16. Kubo T, Kitaoka H, Okawa M, et al. Hypertrophic cardiomyopathy in the elderly. *Geriatr Gerontol Int.* 2010;10(1):9–16.

17. Gradman AH, Alfayoumi F. From left ventricular hypertrophy to congestive heart failure: management of hypertensive heart disease. *Prog Cardiovasc Dis.* 2006;48(5):326–341.

18. Roberts WC, Shirani J. Comparison of cardiac findings at necropsy in octogenarians, nonagenarians, and centenarians. *Am J Cardiol.* 1998;82(5):627–631.

19. Selzer A. Changing aspects of the natural history of valvular aortic stenosis. *N Engl J Med.* 1987;317(2):91–98.

20. Seals DR, Monahan KD, Bell C, et al. The aging cardiovascular system: changes in autonomic function at rest and in response to exercise. *Int J Sport Nutr Exerc Metab.* 2001;11(suppl):S189–S195.

21. Rodeheffer RJ, Gerstenblith G, Becker LC, et al. Exercise cardiac output is maintained with advancing age in healthy human subjects: cardiac dilation and increased stroke volume compensate for a diminished heart rate. *Circulation.* 1984;69(2):203–213.

22. Ghali JK, Liao Y, Cooper RS. Left ventricular hypertrophy in the elderly. *Am J Geriatr Cardiol.* 1997;6(1):38–49.

23. Truong QA, Toepker M, Mahabadi AA, et al. Relation of left ventricular mass and concentric remodeling to extent of coronary artery disease by computed tomography in patients without left ventricular hypertrophy: ROMICAT study. *J Hypertens.* 2009;27(12):2472–2482.

24. Bluemke DA, Kronmal RA, Lima JA, et al. The relationship of left ventricular mass and geometry to incident cardiovascular events: The MESA (Multi-Ethnic Study of Atherosclerosis) study. *J Am Coll Cardiol.* 2008;52(25):2148–2155.

25. Okin PM, Gerdts E, Wachtell K, et al. Relationship of left atrial enlargement to persistence or development of ECG left ventricular hypertrophy in hypertensive patients: implications for the development of new atrial fibrillation. *J Hypertens.* 2010;28(7):1534–1540.

26. Campuzano R, Moya JL, Garcia-Lledo A, et al. Endothelial dysfunction, intima-media thickness and coronary reserve in relation to risk factors and Framingham score in patients without clinical atherosclerosis. *J Hypertens.* 2006;24(8):1581–1588.

27. Kitzman DW, Edwards WE. Age-related changes in the anatomy of the normal human heart. *J Gerontol Biol Med Sci.* 1990;45(1):33–39.

28. Binder EF, Schechtman KB, Ehsani AA, et al. Effects of exercise training on frailty in community dwelling older adults: results of a randomized controlled clinical trial. *J Am Geriatr Soc.* 2002;50(12):1921–1928.

29. Lakatta EG. Cardiovascular regulatory mechanism in advanced age. *Physiol Rev.* 1993;73(2):413–467.

30. Shiaishi I, Takamatsu T, Minamikawa T, et al. Quantitative histological analysis of the human sinoatrial node during growth and aging. *Circulation.* 1992;85(6):2176–2184.

31. Erol-Yilmaz A, Schrama TA, Tanka JS, et al. Individual optimization of pacing sensors improves exercise capacity without influencing quality of life. *Pacing Clin Electrophysiol.* 2005;28(1):17–25.

32. Squires RW. *Exercise Prescription for the High Risk Cardiac Patient.* Champaign, IL: Human Kinetics; 1998.

33. Tsakiris A, Doumas M, Nearchos N, et al. Aortic calcification is associated with age and sex but not left ventricular mass in essential hypertension. *J Clin Hypertens.* 2004;6(2):65–70.

34. Lindroos M, Kupari M, Valvanne J, et al. Factors associated with calcific aortic valve degeneration in the elderly. *Eur Heart J.* 1994;15(7):865–870.

35. Robert L. Aging of the vascular wall and atherosclerosis. *Exp Gerontol.* 1999;34(4):491–501.

36. Newman AB, Arnold AM, Burke GL, et al. Cardiovascular disease and mortality in older adults with small abdominal aortic aneurysms detected by ultrasonography: the cardiovascular health study. *Ann Intern Med.* 2001;134(3):182–190.

37. Yildiz A, Gur M, Yilmaz R, et al. The association of elasticity indexes of ascending aorta and the presence and the severity of coronary artery disease. *Coron Artery Dis.* 2008;19(5):311–317.

38. Wei JY, Epstein FH. Age and the cardiovascular system. *N Engl J Med.* 1992;327(24):1735–1739.

39. Kitzman DW. Aging and the heart. *Dev Cardiol.* 1994;1(1):1–15.

40. Lakatta EB, Mitchell JH, Pomerance A, et al. Human aging: changes in structure and function III. Characteristics of specific cardiovascular diseases in the elderly. *J Am Coll Cardiol.* 1987;10(2 suppl A):42–47.

41. Lakatta EG. Altered autonomic modulation of cardiovascular function with adult aging; perspectives from studies ranging from man to cells. In: Stone HL, Weglicki WB, eds. *Pathobiology of Cardiovascular Injury.* Boston: Martinus Nijhoff; 1985:441–460.

42. Turner MJ, Mier CM, Spina RJ, et al. Effects of aging and gender on cardiovascular responses to isoproterenol. *J Gerontol.* 1999;54A(9):B393–B400.

43. Lakatta EG. Cardiovascular regulatory mechanisms in advanced age. *Physiol Rev.* 1993;73(2):413–467.

44. Shimada K, Kitazumi T, Ogura H. Differences in age-dependent effects of blood pressure on baroreflex sensitivity between normal and hypertensive subjects. *Clin Sci.* 1986;70(5):763–766.

45. Guyton AC, Hall JE. *Textbook of Medical Physiology.* 12th ed. Philadelphia: Saunders Elsevier; 2011.

46. Mukai S, Lipsitz LA. Orthostatic hypotension. *Clin Geriatr Med.* 2002;18(2):253–268.

47. Vloet LCM, Pel-Little RE, Jansen PAF, et al. High prevalence of postprandial and orthostatic hypotension among geriatric patients admitted to Dutch hospitals. *J Gerontol A Biol Sci Med Sci.* 2005;60A(10):1271–1277.

48. Gardin JM, Arnold AM, Bild DE, et al. Left ventricular diastolic filling in the elderly: the cardiovascular health study. *Am J Cardiol.* 1998;82(3):345–352.

49. Kitzman DW, Higginbotham MB, Sullivan MJ. Aging and the cardiovascular response to exercise. *Cardiol Elderly.* 1993;1(6):543–550.

50. Green JS, Crouse SF. Endurance training, cardiovascular function, and the aged. *Sports Med.* 1993;16(5):331–341.

51. Cheitlin MD. Cardiovascular physiology—changes with age. *Am J Geriatr Cardiol.* 2003;12(1):9–13.

52. Steinberg DH. Diastolic dysfunction of the left ventricle. A review of the physiology, causes, diagnosis, treatment, and implications. *J Insur Med* 1997;29(2):12–125.

53. Port S, Cobb FR, Coleman E, et al. Effect of age on the response of the left ventricular ejection fraction to exercise. *N Engl J Med.* 1980;303(20):1133–1137.

54. Nichols WW, O'Rourke MF, Avolio AP. Effects of age on ventricular-vascular coupling. *Am J Cardiol.* 1985;55(9):1179–1184.

55. Devereux RB, Roman MJ, Paranicas M, et al. A population-based assessment of left ventricular systolic dysfunction in middle-aged and older adults: the Strong Heart Study. *Am Heart J.* 2001;141(3):439–446.

56. Lakatta EG. Changes in cardiovascular function with aging. *Eur Heart J.* 1990;11(suppl C):22–29.

57. Jurimae T, Jurimae J, Pihl E. Circulatory response to single circuit weight and walking training sessions of similar energy cost in middle-aged overweight females. *Clin Physiol.* 2000;20(2):143–149.

58. Vaitkevicius PV, Ebersold C, Muhammad S, et al. Effects of aerobic exercise training in community-based subjects aged 80 and older: a pilot study. *J Am Geriatr Soc.* 2002;50(12):2009–2013.

59. Amara CE, Koval JJ, Paterson DH, et al. Lung function in older humans: the contribution of body composition, physical activity, and smoking. *Ann Hum Biol.* 2001;28(5):522–537.

60. McRae H. Cardiovascular and pulmonary function. In: Spirduso WW, Francis KL, MacRae PG, eds. *Physical Dimensions of Aging.* 2nd ed. Champaign, IL: Human Kinetics; 2005:87–106.

61. LaPier T. Impaired aerobic capacity/endurance. In: Guccione AA, Avers D, Wong RA, eds. *Geriatric Physical Therapy.* 3rd ed. St. Louis: Mosby; 2012:229–247.

62. Rossi A, Ganassini A, Tantucci C, et al. Aging and the respiratory system. *Aging.* 1996;8(3):143–161.

63. Zaugg M, Lucchinetti E. Respiratory function in the elderly. *Anesthesiol Clin North America.* 2000;18(1):47–58.

64. Christiansen C. Impaird joint mobility. In: Guccione AA, Avers D, Wong RA, eds. *Geriatric Physical Therapy.* 3rd ed. St. Louis: Mosby; 2012:248–262.

65. Davidson WR, Fee EC. Influence of aging on pulmonary hemodynamics in a population free of coronary artery disease. *Am J Cardiol.* 1990;65(22):1454–1458.

66. Babb TG. Mechanical ventilatory constraints in aging, lung disease, and obesity: perspectives and brief review. *Med Sci Sports Exerc.* 1999;31(suppl 1):12–22.

67. Tolep K, Kelsen SG. Effects of aging in respiratory skeletal muscles. *Clin Chest Med.* 1993;14(3):363–378.

68. Brooks SV, Faulkner JA. Effects of aging on the structure and function of skeletal muscle. In: Roussos C, ed. *The Thorax.* New York: Academic Press; 1995:295–312.

69. Dias K. Physiology of the Cardiovascular and Pulmonary Systems. In: Hillegass E, ed. *Essentials of Cardiopulmonary Physical Therapy.* 3rd ed. St. Louis: Elsevier Saunders; 2011:27–46.

70. Zeleznik J. Normative aging of the respiratory system. *Clin Geriatr Med.* 2003;19(1):1–18.

71. Camhi SL, Enright PL. How to assess pulmonary function in older persons. *J Respir Dis.* 2000;21(6):395.

72. Stulberg M, Carrieri-Kohlman V. Conceptual approach to the treatment of dyspnea: focus on the role of exercise. *Cardiopulmonary Phys Ther.* 1992;3(1):9–12.

73. Spector N, Connolly MA, Carlson KK. Dyspnea: applying research to bedside practice. *AACN Adv Crit Care.* 2007;18(1):45–60.

74. Maher D, Hemming L. Palliative care for breathless patients in the community. *Br J Community Nurs.* 2005;10(9):414–418.

75. Pollock ML, Wilmore JH, eds. *Exercise in Health and Disease.* Philadelphia: Saunders; 1990.

76. VanBeveran PJ, Avers D. Exercise and physical activity for older adults. In: Guccione AA, Avers D, Wong RA, eds. *Geriatric Physical Therapy.* 3rd ed. St. Louis: Mosby; 2012:64–86.

77. Host HH, Sinacore DR, Turner MJ, et al. Oxygen uptakes at preferred gait velocities of frail elderly subjects. *Phys Ther.* 1996;76(4):S69.

78. Wanderley FAC, Oliveira J, Mota J, et al. Six-minute walk distance (6MWD) is associated with body fat, systolic blood pressure, and rate-pressure product in community dwelling elderly subjects. *Arch Gerontol Geriatr.* 2011;52(2):206–210.

79. Ellestad MH. *Stress Testing: Principles and Practice.* 5th ed. Oxford: Oxford University Press; 2003.

80. Housh TJ, Housh DJ, DeVries HA. *Applied Exercise and Sport Physiology.* 2nd ed. Scottsdale, AZ: Holcomb Hathaway; 2006.

81. Tonino RP, Driscoll PA. Reliability of maximal and submaximal parameters of treadmill testing for the measurement of physical training in older persons. *J Gerontol.* 1988;42(2):M101–M104.

82. Materson BJ. Isolated systolic blood pressure: new answers, more questions. *J Am Geriatr Soc.* 1991;39(12):1237–1238.

83. Applegate WB, Davis BR, Black HR. Prevalence of postural hypotension at baseline in the systolic hypertension in the elderly program (SHEP) cohort. *J Am Geriatr Soc.* 1991;39(11):1057–1064.

84. Naughton J. *Exercise Testing: Physiological, Biomechanical, and Clinical Principles.* Mount Kisco, NY: Futura; 1988.

85. Crawford K, McNamara SB, Vogel W, et al. Pulmonary medications. In: Hillegass E, ed. *Essentials of Cardiopulmonary Physical Therapy.* 3rd ed. St. Louis: Elsevier Saunders; 2011:515–533.

86. Matsuda PN, Shumway-Cook A, Ciol MA. The effects of a home-based exercise program on physical function in frail older adults. *J Geriatr Phys Ther.* 2010;33(2):78–84.

87. Tse MMY, Wan VTC, Ho SSK. Physical exercise: does it help in relieving pain and increasing mobility among older adults with chronic pain? *J Clin Nurs.* 2011;20(5/6):635–644.

88. Hagberg JM, Allen WK, Seals DR. A hemodynamic comparison of young and older endurance athletes during exercise. *J Appl Physiol.* 1985;58(6):2041–2046.

89. Ekstrum JA, Black LL, Paschal KA. Effects of a thoracic mobility and respiratory exercise program on pulmonary function and functional capacity in older adults. *Phys Occup Ther Geriatr.* 2009;27(4):310–327.

90. Steib S, Schoene D, Pfeifer K. Dose-response relationship of resistance training in older adults: a meta-analysis. *Med Sci Sports Exerc.* 2010;42(5):902–914.

91. Fleg JL, Morrell CH, Bos AG, et al. Accelerated longitudinal decline of aerobic capacity in healthy older adults. *Circulation.* 2005;112(5):674–682.

92. Yarasheski KE. Managing sarcopenia with progressive resistance exercise training. *J Nutr Health Aging.* 2002;6(5):349–356.

93. Casaburi R, Patessio A, Ioli F. Reductions in exercise lactic acidosis and ventilation as a result of exercise training in patients with obstructive lung disease. *Am Rev Respir Dis.* 1991;143(1):9–18.

94. Marcus RL, Westlen-Boyer K, LaStayo P. Impaired muscle performance. In: Guccione AA, Avers D, Wong RA, eds. *Geriatric Physical Therapy.* 3rd ed. St. Louis: Mosby; 2012:263–271.

95. Borg G. Perceived exertion as an indicator of somatic stress. *Scand J Rehabil Med.* 1970;2(3):92–97.

96. Borg G, Ottoson D. *The Perception of Exertion in Physical Work.* London: Macmillan; 1986.

97. Fletcher GF, Mills WC, Taylor WC. Update on exercise stress testing. *Am Fam Physician.* 2006;74(10):1749–1754.

98. Kline GM, Porcari JP, Hintermeister R, et al. Estimation of VO_{2max} from a one-mile track walk, gender, age, and body weight. *Med Sci Sports Exerc.* 1987;19(3):253–259.

99. Butland RJ, Pang J, Gross ER, et al. Two-, six-, and 12-minute walking tests in respiratory disease. *BMJ.* 1982;284(6329):1607–1608.

100. Guyatt GH, Sullivan MJ, Thompson PJ, et al. The 6-minute walk test: a new measure of exercise capacity in patients with chronic heart failure. *Can Med Assoc J.* 1985;132(8):9919–9923.

101. Smith EL, Gilligan C. Physical activity perception for the older adult. *Phys Sports Med.* 1993;11:91–101.

102. Prentice WE. *Armheim's Principles of Athletic Training: a Competency Based Approach.* 14th ed. New York: McGraw-Hill; 2011.

103. Durstine JL, Moore GE, Painter PL, et al. *ACSM's Exercise Management for Persons with Chronic Diseases and Disabilities.* 3rd ed. Champaign, IL: Human Kinetics; 2009.

104. Ehrman JK, deJong A, Sanderson B, et al., eds. *ACSM's Resource Manual for Guidelines for Exercise Testing and Prescription.* 6th ed. Philadelphia: Lippincott Williams & Wilkins; 2010.

105. Cress ME, Buchner DM, Prohaska T, et al. Best practices statement: physical activity programs and behavior counseling in older adult populations. *Med Sci Sports Exerc.* 2004;36(11):1997–2003.

106. Mandic S, Riess K, Haykowsky MJ. Exercise training for individuals with coronary artery disease or heart failure. *Physiother Can.* 2006;58(1):21–29.

107. Seals DR, Hagberg JM, Hurley BF, et al. Effects of endurance training on glucose tolerance and plasma lipid levels in older men and women. *JAMA.* 1984;252(5):645–649.

108. Lewis CB, Kellems S. Musculoskeletal changes with age: clinical implications. In: Lewis CB, ed. *Aging the Health Care Challenge.* 4th ed. Philadelphia: F.A. Davis; 2002:104–126.

109. Avers D, Brown M. Strength training for the older adult. *J Geriatr Phys Ther.* 2009;32(4):148–152, 158.

110. Hunter GR, McCarthy JP, Bamman MM. Effects of resistance training on older adults. *Sports Med.* 2004;34(5):329–348.

111. Palta AF. Neurobiomechanical bases for the control of human movement. In: Bronstein A, Brandt T, Woollacott M, eds. *Clinical Disorders of Balance, Posture, and Gait.* London: Arnold; 1996:19–40.

112. Bianchi L, Angelini D, Orani GP, et al. Kinematic coordination in human gait: relation to mechanical energy cost. *J Neurophysiol.* 1998;79(4):2155–2170.

113. Perry J, Burnfield JM. Basic functions. In: Perry J, Burnfield JM, eds. *Gait Analysis: Normal and Pathological Function.* 2nd ed. Thorofare, NJ: Slack; 2010:19–48.

114. Olney SJ, Eng J. Gait. In: Levangie PK, Norkin CC, eds. *Joint Structure and Function: A Comprehensive Analysis.* 5th ed. Philadelphia: F.A. Davis; 2011:524–567.

115. Winter DA, Quanbury AO, Reimer GD. Analysis of instantaneous energy of normal gait. *J Biomech.* 1976;9(4):252–257.

116. Rose J, Gamble JG. *Human Walking.* 3rd ed. Philadelphia: Lippincott Williams & Wilkins; 2005.

117. Waters RL. Energy expenditure. In: Perry J, Burnfield JM, eds. *Gait Analysis: Normal and Pathological Function.* 2nd ed. Thorofare, NJ: Slack; 2010:483–518.

118. Studenski S, Perera S, Kushang P, et al. Gait speed and survival in older adults, *JAMA.* 2011;305(1):50–58.

119. Fritz S, Lusardi M. White paper: walking speed: the sixth vital sign. *J Geriatr Phys Ther.* 2009;32(2):46–49.

120. Brach JS, VanSwearingen JM, Newman AB, et al. Identifying early decline of physical function in community-dwelling older women: performance-based and self-report measures. *Phys Ther.* 2002;82(4):320–328.

121. Cesari M, Kritchevsky SB, Newman AB, et al. Added value of physical performance measures in predicting adverse health-related events: results from the Health, Aging and Body Composition Study. *J Am Geriatr Soc.* 2009;57(2):251–259.

122. Cesari M, Kritchevsky SB, Penninx BW, et al. Prognostic value of usual gait speed in well-functioning older people—results from the health, aging and body composition study. *J Am Geriatr Soc.* 2005;53(10):1675–1680.

123. Brach JS, VanSwearingen JM, FitzGerald SJ, et al. The relationship among physical activity, obesity, and physical function in community-dwelling older women. *Prev Med.* 2004;39(1):74–80.

124. Brach JS, FitzGerald S, Newman AB, et al. Physical activity and functional status in community-dwelling older women: a 14-year prospective study. *AMA Arch Intern Med.* 2003;163(21):2565–2571.

125. Cawthon PM, Fox KM, Gandra SR, et al. Clustering of strength, physical function, muscle, and adiposity characteristics and risk of disability in older adults. *J Am Geriatr Soc.* 2011;59(5):781–787.

126. Purser JL, Weinberger M, Cohen HJ, et al. Walking speed predicts health status and hospital costs for frail elderly male veterans. *J Rehabil Res Dev.* 2005;42(4):535–545.

127. Rabadi MH, Blau A. Admission ambulation velocity predicts length of stay and discharge disposition following stroke in an acute hospital. *Neurorehabil Neural Repair.* 2005;19(1):20–26.

128. Studenski S, Perera S, Patel K, et al. Gait speed and survival in older adults. *JAMA.* 2011;305(1):50–58.

129. Chui KK, Lusardi MM. Spatial and temporal parameters of self-selected and fast walking speeds in healthy community-living adults aged 72-98 years. *J Geriatr Phys Ther.* 2010;33(4):173–183.

130. Steffen TM, Hacker TA, Mollinger L. Age- and gender-related test performance in community-dwelling elderly people: six-minute walk test, berg balance scale, timed up & go test, and gait speeds. *Phys Ther.* 2002;82(2):128–137.

131. Bohannon RW. Comfortable and maximum walking speed of adults aged 20-79 years. *Age Ageing.* 1997;26(1):15–19.

132. Wert DM, Brach J, Perera S, et al. Gait biomechanics, spatial and temporal characteristics, and the energy cost of walking in older adults with impaired mobility. *Phys Ther.* 2010;90(7):977–985.

133. Lusardi MM, Pellecchia GL, Schulman M. Functional performance in community living older adults. *J Geriatr Phys Ther.* 2003;26(3):14–22.

134. Ko S, Hausdorff JM, Ferrucci L. Age-associated differences in the gait pattern changes of older adults during fast-speed and fatigue conditions: results from the Baltimore Longitudinal Study of Ageing. *Age Ageing.* 2010;39(6):688–694.

135. Deathe AB, Miller WC. The L Test of Functional Mobility: measurement properties of a modified version of the timed "up & go" test designed for people with lower-limb amputations. *Phys Ther.* 2005;85(7):626–635.

136. Rossier P, Wade DT. Validity and reliability comparison of 4 mobility measures in patients presenting with neurologic impairment. *Arch Phys Med Rehabil.* 2001;82(1):9–13.

137. van Hedel HJ, Wirz M, Dietz V. Assessing walking ability in subjects with spinal cord injury: validity and reliability of 3 walking tests. *Arch Phys Med Rehabil.* 2005;86(2):190–196.

138. Studenski S, Perera S, Wallace D. Physical performance measures in the clinical setting. *J Am Geriatr Soc.* 2003;51(3):314–322.

139. Ries JD, Echternach JL, Nof L, et al. Test-retest reliability and minimal detectable change scores for the timed "up & go" test, the six-minute walk test, and gait speed in people with Alzheimer disease. *Phys Ther.* 2009;89(6):569–579.

140. Hollman JH, Beckman BA, Brandt RA, Merriwether EN, Williams RT, Nordrum JT. Minimum detectable change in gait velocity during acute rehabilitation following hip fracture. *J Geriatr Phys Ther.* 2008;31(2):53–56.

141. Tilson JK, Sullivan KJ, Cen SY, et al. Meaningful gait speed improvement during the first 60 days poststroke: minimal clinically important difference. *Phys Ther.* 2010;90(2):196–208.

142. Water RL, Mulroy SJ. Energy expenditure of walking in individuals with lower limb amputation. In: Smith DC, Michael JW, Bowker JH, eds. *Atlas of Amputations and Limb Deficiency: Surgical, Prosthetics and Rehabilitation Principles.* 3rd ed. Rosemont, IL: American Academy of Orthopedic Surgeons; 2004:395–408.

143. Perry J. Normal and pathological gait. In: Hsu JD, Michael JW, Fisk JR, eds. *AAOS Atlas of Orthoses and Assistive Devices.* 4th ed. Philadelphia: Mosby Elsevier; 2008:61–82.

144. Thompson WR, Gordon NF, Pescatello LS, eds. *ACSM's Guidelines for Exercise Testing and Prescription.* 8th ed.Philadelphia: Lippincott Williams & Wilkins; 2010.

145. Kalapotharakos VI. Aerobic exercise in older adults: effects on VO$_{2max}$ and functional performance. *Crit Rev Phys Rehabil Med.* 2007;19(3):213–225.

146. Sergi G, Coin A, Sarti S, et al. Resting VO2, maximal VO2 and metabolic equivalents in free-living healthy elderly women. *Clin Nutr.* 2010;29(1):84–88.

147. Leeuwenburgh C, Heinecke JW. Oxidative stress and antioxidants in exercise. *Curr Med Chem.* 2001;8(7):829–838.

148. Fleg JL, Morrell CH, Bos AG, et al. Accelerated longitudinal decline of aerobic capacity in healthy older adults. *Circulation.* 2005;112(5):674–682.

149. Saltin B, Blomquist G, Mitchell JH, et al. Response to submaximal and maximal exercise after bedrest and training. *Circulation.* 1968;38(suppl 7):1–78.

150. Davis JA. Anaerobic threshold: review of the concept and directions for future research. *Med Sci Sports Exerc.* 1985;17(1):6–8.

151. McArdle WD, Katch FI, Katch VL. *Exercise Physiology: Energy, Nutrition, and Human Performance.* 6th ed. Philadelphia: Lippincott Williams & Wilkins; 2006.

152. Rose J, Gamble JG, Medeiros J, et al. Energy cost of walking in normal children and in those with cerebral palsy: comparison of heart rate and oxygen uptake. *J Pediatr Orthop.* 1989;9(3):276–279.

153. Rose GK. Clinical gait assessment. *J Med Eng Technol.* 1983;7(6):273–279.

154. Eston R, Connolly D. The use of ratings of perceived exertion for exercise prescription in patients receiving beta-blocker therapy. *Sports Med.* 1996;21(3):176–190.

155. Faulhaber M, Flatz M, Burtscher M. Beta-blockers may provoke oxygen desaturation during submaximal exercise at moderate altitudes in elderly persons. *High Alt Med Biol.* 2003;4(4):475–478.

156. Steven MM, Capell HA, Sturrock RD, et al. The physiological cost of gait (PCG): a new technique for evaluating non-steroidal anti-inflammatory drugs in rheumatoid arthritis. *Br J Rheumatol.* 1983;22(3):141–145.

157. Butler P, Engelbrecht M, Major RE, et al. Physiological cost index of walking for normal children and its use as an indicator of physical handicap. *Dev Med Child Neurol.* 1984;26(5):607–612.

158. Nene AV. Physiological cost index of walking in able-bodied adolescents and adults. *Clin Rehabil.* 1993;7(4):319–326.

159. Peebles KC, Woodman-Aldridge AD, Skinner MA. The physiological cost index in elderly subjects during treadmill and floor walking. *N Z J Physiother.* 2003;3(1):11–16.

160. Hamzeh MA, Bowker P, Sayeqh A, et al. The energy cost of ambulation using 2 types of walking frames. *Clin Rehabil.* 1988;2:119–123.

161. Johnson CA, Burridge JH, Strike PW, et al. The effect of combined use of botulinum toxin type A and functional electrical stimulation in the treatment of spastic foot drop after stroke: a preliminary investigation. *Arch Phys Med Rehabil.* 2004;85(6):902–909.

162. Kottink AI, Oostendorp LJ, Buurke JH, et al. The orthotic effect of functional electrical stimulation on the improvement of walking in stroke patients with dropped foot: a systematic review. *Artif Organs.* 2004;28(6):577–586.

163. Burridge JH, Taylor PN, Hagan SA, et al. The effects of common peroneal nerve stimulation on the effort and speed of walking: a randomized controlled clinical trial with chronic hemiplegic patients. *Clin Rehabil.* 1997;11(3):201–210.

164. Burridge J, Taylor P, Hagan S, et al. Experience of clinical use of the Odstock dropped foot stimulator. *Artif Organs.* 1997;21(3):254–260.

165. Carmick J. Clinical use of neuromuscular electrical stimulation for children with cerebral palsy: lower extremity. *Phys Ther.* 1993;73(8):505–513.

166. Nene AV, Evans GA, Patrick JH. Simultaneous multiple operations for spastic diplegia: Outcome and functional assessment of walking in 18 patients. *J Bone Joint Surg Br.* 1993;75(3):488–494.

167. Yang L, Condie DN, Granat MP, et al. Effects of joint motion constraints on normal subjects and their implications on the further development of hybrid FES orthosis for paraplegic persons. *J Biomech.* 1996;29(2):217–226.

168. Nene AV, Jennings SJ. Physiological cost index of paraplegic locomotion using the ORLAU ParaWalker. *Paraplegia.* 1992;30(4):246–252.

169. Stallard J, Major RE. The influence of stiffness on paraplegic ambulation and its implications for functional electrical stimulation walking systems. *Prosthet Orthot Int.* 1995;19(2):108–114.

170. Engsberg JR, Herbert LM, Grimston SK, et al. Relation among indices of effort and oxygen uptake in below knee and able-bodied children. *Arch Phys Med Rehabil.* 1994;75(12):1335–1341.

171. Chin T, Sawamura S, Fujita H, et al. The efficacy of physiological cost index measurement of a subject walking with an intelligent prosthesis. *Prosthet Orthot Int.* 1999;23(10):45–49.

172. Hachisuka K, Umezu Y, Ohmine S, et al. Subjective evaluations and objective measurements of the ischial-ramal containment prosthesis. *J UOEH.* 1999;21(2):107–118.

173. Herbert JS, Liggins AB. Gait evaluations of an automatic stance control knee orthosis in a patient with post-poliomyelitis. *Arch Phys Med Rehabil.* 2005;86(8):1676–1680.

174. Hagberg K, Tranberg R, Zügner R, Danielsson A. Reproducibility of the Physiological Cost Index among individuals with a lower-limb amputation and healthy adults. *Physiother Res Int.* 2011;16(2):92–100.

175. Danielsson A, Willen C, Sunnerhagen KS. Measurement of energy cost by the physiological cost index in walking after stroke. *Arch Phys Med Rehabil.* 2007;88(10):1298–1303.

176. Genin JJ, Bastien GJ, Lopez N, et al. Does the physiological cost index reflect the cost of walking? *Arch Physiol Biochem.* 2004;112(suppl):73.

177. Morgan DW, Tseh W, Caputo JL, et al. Longitudinal stratification of gait economy in young boys and girls: the locomotion energy and growth study. *Eur J Appl Physiol.* 2004;91(1):30–34.

178. Waters RL, Hislop HJ, Thomas L, et al. Energy cost of walking in normal children and teenagers. *Dev Med Child Neurol.* 1983;25(2):184–188.

179. Waters RL, Lunsford BR, Perry J, et al. Energy-speed relationship of walking: standard tables. *J Orthop Res.* 1988;6(2):215–222.

180. Waters RL, Hislop HJ, Perry J, et al. Comparative cost of walking in young and old adults. *J Orthop Res.* 1983;1(1):73–76.

181. Aoyagi Y, Togo F, Matsuki S, et al. Walking velocity measured over 5 m as a basis of exercise prescription for the elderly: preliminary data from the Nakanojo Study. *Eur J Appl Physiol.* 2004;93(1–2):217–223.

182. Malatesta D, Simar D, Dauvilliers Y, et al. Aerobic determinants of the decline in preferred walking speed in healthy, active 65- and 80-year-olds. *Eur J Physiol [Pflugers Arch].* 2004;447(6):915–921.

183. Astrand A, Astrand I, Hallback I, et al. Reduction in maximal oxygen uptake with age. *J Appl Physiol.* 1973;35(5):649–654.

184. Binder EF, Schechtman KB, Ehsani AA, et al. Effects of exercise training on frailty in community-dwelling older adults: results of a randomized, controlled trial. *J Am Geriatr Soc.* 2002;50(12):1921–1928.

185. Corcoran PJ, Gelmanan B. Oxygen reuptake in normal and handicapped subjects in relation to the speed of walking beside a velocity controlled cart. *Arch Phys Med Rehabil.* 1970;51(2):78–87.

186. Holt KG, Hamill J, Andres RO. Predicting the minimal energy cost of human walking. *Med Sci Sports Exerc.* 1991;23(4):491–498.

187. Duff Raffaele M, Kerrigan DC, Corcoran PJ, et al. The proportional work of lifting the center of mass during walking. *Am J Phys Med.* 1996;75(5):375–379.

188. Hanada E, Kerrigan DC. Energy consumption during level walking with arm and knee immobilized. *Arch Phys Med Rehabil.* 2001;82(9):1251–1254.

189. Bruinings AL, van den Berg-Emons HJ, Buffart LM, et al. Energy cost and physical strain of daily activities in adolescents and young adults with myelomeningocele. *Dev Med Child Neurol.* 2007;49(9):672–677.

190. Detrembleur C, Dierick F, Stoquart G, et al. Energy cost, mechanical work, and efficiency of hemiparetic walking. *Gait Posture.* 2003;18(2):47–55.

191. Brophy LS. Gait in cerebral palsy. *Orthop Phys Ther Clin North Am.* 2001;10(1):55–76.

192. Patrick JH. The case for gait analysis as part of the management of incomplete spinal cord injury. *Spinal Cord.* 2003;41(9):479–482.

193. Jeans KA, Browne RH, Karol LA. Effect of amputation level on energy expenditure during overground walking by children with an amputation. *J Bone Joint Surg.* 2011;93(1):49–56.

194. Bell KL, Davies PS. Energy expenditure and physical activity of ambulatory children with cerebral palsy and of typically developing children. *Am J Clin Nutr.* 2010;92(2):313–319.

195. Inman VT, Ralston HJ, Todd F. *Human Walking.* Baltimore: Waverly; 1981.

196. Waters RL, Lunsford BR. Energy expenditure of normal and pathological gait: application to orthotic prescription. In: Bowker JH, Michael JW, eds. *Atlas of Orthotics.* St. Louis: Mosby; 1985:151–159.

197. Buckon CE, Thomas SS, Jakobson-Huston S, et al. Comparison of three ankle-foot orthosis configurations for children with spastic diplegia. *Dev Med Child Neurol.* 2004;46(9):590–598.

198. Franceschini M, Massucci M, Ferrari L, et al. Effects of an ankle-foot orthosis on spatiotemporal parameters and energy cost of hemiparetic gait. *Clin Rehabil.* 2003;17(4):368–372.

199. Kaufman KR, Irby SE, Mathewson JW, et al. Energy-efficient knee-ankle-foot orthosis: a case study. *J Prosthet Orthot.* 1996;8(3):79–85.

200. Waters RL, Campbell J, Thomas L, et al. Energy costs of walking in lower-extremity plaster casts. *J Bone Joint Surg Am.* 1982;64(6):896–899.

201. Abudulhadi HM, Kerrigan DC, LaRaia PJ. Contralateral shoe-lift: effect on oxygen cost of walking with an immobilized knee. *Arch Phys Med Rehabil.* 1996;77(7):760–762.

202. Morganti B, Scivoletto G, Ditunno P, et al. Walking index for spinal cord injury (WISCI): criterion validation. *Spinal Cord.* 2005;43(1):27–33.

203. Hussey RW, Stauffer ES. Spinal cord injury: requirements for ambulation. *Arch Phys Med Rehabil.* 1973;54(12):544–547.

204. Yakura JS, Waters RL, Adkins RH. Changes in ambulation parameters in spinal cord injury individuals following rehabilitation. *Paraplegia.* 1990;28(6):364–370.

205. Waters RL, Yakura JS, Adkins RH. Gait performance after spinal cord injury. *Clin Ortop.* 1993;228:87–96.

206. Johnston TE, Smith BT, Betz RR. Strengthening of partially denervated knee extensors using percutaneous electric stimulation in a young man with spinal cord injury. *Arch Phys Med Rehabil* 2005;86(5):1037–1042.

207. Johnston TE, Finson RL, Smith BT, et al. Technical perspective Functional electrical stimulation for augmented walking in adolescents with incomplete spinal cord injury. *J Spinal Cord Med.* 2003;26(4):390–400.

208. Brissot R, Gallien P, Le Bot M, et al. Clinical experience with functional electrical stimulation-assisted gait with parastep in spinal cord-injured patients. *Spine.* 2000;25(4):501–508.

209. Solomonow M, Baratta R, D'Ambrosia R. Standing and walking after spinal cord injury: experience with the reciprocating gait orthosis powered by electrical muscle stimulation. *Top Spinal Cord Inj Rehabil.* 2000;5(4):29–53.

210. Lam T, Eng JJ, Wolfe DL, et al. A systematic review of the efficacy of gait rehabilitation strategies for spinal cord injury. *Top Spinal Cord Inj Rehabil.* 2007;13(1):32–57.

211. Atrice MB. Lower extremity orthotic management for the spinal-cord-injured client. *Top Spinal Cord Inj Rehabil.* 2000;5(4):1–10.

212. Knutson J, Audu M, Triolo R. Interventions for mobility and manipulation after spinal cord injury: a review of orthotic and neuroprosthetic options. *Top Spinal Cord Inj Rehabil.* 2006;11(4):61–81.

213. Rasmussen AA, Smith KM, Damiano DL. Biomechanical evaluation of the combination of bilateral stance-control knee-ankle-foot orthoses and a reciprocating gait orthosis in an adult with a spinal cord injury. *J Prosthet Orthot.* 2007;19(2):42–47.

214. Yang L, Granat MH, Paul JP, et al. Further development of hybrid functional electrical stimulation orthoses. *Artif Organs.* 1997;21(3):183–187.

215. Ryerson SD. Hemiplegia. In: Umphred DA, ed. *Neurological Rehabilitation.* 5th ed. St. Louis: Mosby Elsevier; 2006:857–901.

216. da Cunha IT, Lim PA, Qureshy H, et al. Gait outcomes after acute stroke rehabilitation with supported treadmill ambulation training: a randomized controlled pilot study. *Arch Phys Med Rehabil.* 2002;83(9):1258–1265.

217. Chen G, Patten C, Kothari DH, et al. Gait deviations associated with post-stroke hemiparesis: improvement during treadmill walking using weight support, speed, support stiffness, and handrail hold. *Gait Posture.* 2005;22(1):57–62.

218. Courbon A, Calmels P, Roche F, et al. Relationship between maximal exercise capacity and walking capacity in adult hemiplegic stroke patients. *Am J Phys Med Rehabil.* 2006;85(5):436–442.

219. Mauritz KH, Hesse S. Neurological rehabilitation of gait and balance disorders. In: Bronstein AM, Brandt T, Woollacott MH, eds. *Clinical Disorders of Balance, Posture and Gait.* London: Arnold; 1996:236–250.

220. Ward KH, Meyers MC. Exercise performance of lower extremity amputees. *Sports Med.* 1995;20(4):207–214.

221. Lin-Chan S, Nielsen DH, Shurr DG, et al. Physiological responses to multiple speed treadmill walking for Syme vs. transtibial amputation—a case report. *Disabil Rehabil.* 2003;25(23):1333–1338.

222. Winter DA, Sienko SE. Biomechanics of below-knee amputee gait. *J Biomech.* 1988;21(5):361–367.

223. Torburn L, Powers CM, Guiterrez R, et al. Energy expenditure during ambulation in dysvascular and traumatic below-knee amputees: a comparison of five prosthetic feet. *J Rehabil Res Dev.* 1995;32(2):111–119.

224. Waters RL, Perry J, Antonelli D, et al. The energy cost of walking of amputees: influence of level of amputation. *J Bone Joint Surg.* 1976;58(1):42–46.

225. Esqienazi A. Geriatric amputee rehabilitation. *Clin Geriatr Med.* 1993;9(5):731–743.

226. Ganguli S, Datta SR, Chatterjee B. Performance evaluation of amputee-prosthesis system in below knee amputees. *Ergonomics.* 1973;16(6):797–810.

227. Gailey RS, Wenger MA, Raya M, et al. Energy expenditure of transtibial amputees during ambulation at self-selected pace. *Prosthet Orthot Int.* 1994;18(2):84–91.

228. Otis JC, Lane JM, Kroll MA. Energy cost during gait in osteosarcoma patients after resection and knee replacement and after above the knee amputation. *J Bone Joint Surg.* 1985;67A(4):606–611.

229. Fisher SV, Gullickson G. Energy cost of ambulation in health and disability: a literature review. *Arch Phys Med Rehabil.* 1978;59(3):124–133.

230. Jaeger SM, Vos LD, Rispens P, et al. The relationship between comfortable and most metabolically efficient walking speed in persons with unilateral above knee amputations. *Arch Phys Med Rehabil.* 1993;74(5):521–525.

231. Molen NH. Energy/speed relation of below knee amputees walking on a motor driven treadmill. *Int Z Angew Physiol.* 1973;31(3):173–185.

232. Czerniecki JM. Rehabilitation of limb deficiency. 1: Gait and motion analysis. *Arch Phys Med Rehabil* 1996;77(suppl 35): S29–S37, S81–S82.

233. May BJ. Lower extremity prosthetic management. In: *Amputation and Prosthetics: A Case Study Approach.* 2nd ed, Philadelphia: F.A. Davis; 2002.

234. Andrews KL. Rehabilitation in limb deficiency. 3: The geriatric amputee. *Arch Phys Med Rehabil* 1996;77(3):S14–S17.

235. Torburn L, Perry J, Ayyappa E, et al. Below knee amputee gait with dynamic elastic response feet: a pilot study. *J Rehabil Res Dev.* 1990;27(4):369–384.

236. Dubow LL, Witt PL, Kadaba MP, et al. Oxygen consumption of elderly persons with bilateral below knee amputation: ambulation vs. wheelchair propulsion. *Arch Phys Med Rehabil.* 1983;64(6):255–259.

237. Wu YJ, Chen SY, Lin MC, et al. Energy expenditure of wheeling and walking during prosthetic rehabilitation in a woman with bilateral transfemoral amputation. *Arch Phys Med Rehabil.* 2001;82(2):265–269.

238. Nissen SJ, Newman WP. Factors influencing reintegration to normal living after amputation. *Arch Phys Med Rehabil.* 1992;73(6):548–551.

239. Nitz JC. Rehabilitation outcomes after bilateral lower limb amputation for vascular disease. *Physiother Theory Pract.* 1993;9(3):165–170.

240. Hofstad C, Van der Linde H, Van Limbeek J, et al. *Prescription of Prosthetic Ankle Foot Mechanisms After Lower Limb Amputation.* Washington, DC: Cochrane Library; 2004. 003978.

241. Zmitrewicz RJ, Neptune RR, Walden JG, et al. The effect of foot and ankle prosthetic components on braking and propulsive impulses during transtibial amputee gait. *Arch Phys Med Rehabil.* 2006;87(10):1334–1339.

242. Gitter A, Czerniecki JM, DeGroot DM. Biomechanical analysis of the influence of prosthetic feet on below knee amputee walking. *Am J Phys Med Rehabil.* 1991;70(3):142–148.

243. Hsu MJ, Nielsen DH, Yack JH, et al. Physiological measurements of walking and running in people with transtibial amputations with 3 different prostheses. *J Orthop Sports Phys Ther.* 1999;29(9):526–533.

244. Pomeranz B, Adler U, Shenoy N, et al. Prosthetics and orthotics for the older adult with a physical disability. *Clin Geriatr Med.* 2006;22(2):377–394.

245. Barth DG, Shumacher L, Sienko-Thomas S. Gait analysis and energy cost of below-knee amputees wearing six different prosthetic feet. *J Prosthet Orthot.* 1992;4(2):63–75.

246. McFarlane PA, Nielsen DH, Shurr DG, et al. Gait comparisons for below-knee amputees using a FlexFoot versus a conventional prosthetic foot. *J Prosthet Orthot.* 1991;3(4):150–161.

247. Wirta RW, Mason R, Calvo K, et al. Effect on gait using various prosthetic ankle foot devices. *J Rehabil Res Dev.* 1991;28(2):13–24.

248. Czerniecki JM, Gitter A. The impact of energy storing prosthetic feet on below knee amputation gait. *Arch Phys Med Rehabil.* 1989;70(13):918.

249. Czerniecki JM, Gitter A, Murno C. Joint moment and muscle power output characteristics of below knee amputees

during running: the influence of energy storing prosthetic feet. *J Biomech.* 1991;24(1):63–75.

250. Casillas JM, Dulieu V, Cohen M, et al. Bioenergetic comparison of a new energy storing foot and SAHD foot in traumatic below-knee vascular amputations. *Arch Phys Med Rehabil.* 1995;76(1):39–44.

251. Torburn L, Schweiger GP, Perry J, et al. Below knee amputee gait in stair climbing: a comparison of stride characteristics using five different prosthetic feet. *Clin Ortop.* 1994;303:185–192.

252. Perry J, Burnfield JM, Newsam CJ, et al. Energy expenditures and gait characteristics of a bilateral amputee walking with C-leg prostheses compared with stubby and conventional articulating prostheses. *Arch Phys Med Rehabil.* 2004;85(10):1711–1717.

253. Hafner BJ, Smith DG. Differences in function and safety between Medicare Functional Classification Level-2 and -3 transfemoral amputees and influence of prosthetic knee joint control. *J Rehabil Res Dev.* 2009;46(3):417–433.

254. Berry D, Olson MD, Larntz K. Perceived stability, function, and satisfaction among transfemoral amputees using microprocessor and nonmicroprocessor controlled prosthetic knees: a multicenter survey. *J Prosthet Orthot.* 2009;21(1):32–42.

3

Motor Control, Motor Learning, and Neural Plasticity in Orthotic and Prosthetic Rehabilitation

Michelle M. Lusardi and Donna M. Bowers

LEARNING OBJECTIVES

On completion of this chapter, the reader will be able to:

1. Discuss the strengths, limitations, and implementation for practice of current models of motor control.
2. Compare and contrast the tenets of current motor learning theories.
3. Discuss the role physical therapy interventions based on knowledge of motor control and motor learning in augmenting neural plasticity after brain injury.
4. Apply principles of practice conditions in the design of therapeutic interventions for individuals using orthoses or prostheses.
5. Appropriately use augmented feedback in therapeutic situations with individuals using orthoses or prostheses.
6. Describe the role of mental practice and imagery on skill acquisition for individuals using orthoses or prostheses.

WHY THINK ABOUT MOTOR CONTROL, MOTOR LEARNING, OR NEUROPLASTCITY?

Physical therapists and colleagues in rehabilitation help individuals with movement dysfunction improve or adapt their ways of moving so that they are safe, efficient, and satisfied with their level of function in the activities they consider important for their quality of life.[1] Many different impairments, across any of the physiological structures and systems of the body, might lead to ineffective or abnormal patterns of movement and interfere with an individual's ability to carry out activities and participate effectively in their family and social roles.[2,3]

Several underlying principles influence current thinking about how people move.[4] The first is that *movement is goal directed*. Individuals move in order to accomplish a task or activity that they want to do, during self-care or other activities of daily living (ADLs), as part of their work role, or during leisure activities.[5] The second is that there are *many different ways to accomplish any task*: the central nervous system (CNS) organizes muscles and bodies using available physiological resources in the context of the environment to accomplish any given task; there is no single "best" way of moving.[6-8]

The third is that *each person develops preferential ways of moving*: although there are many possible movement strategies available, people tend to move in ways that are most efficient for their own, individual physical characteristics.[9] Preferential movement patterns, however, are not always optimal ways of moving. Repetitive motion injuries, for example, may be the result of preferential movement patterns that are not biomechanically effective, stressing tissues until inflammation or permanent deformation occurs.[10] Finally, emerging evidence suggests that appropriate interventions have the potential to *drive neural plasticity* and enhance recovery following insult to the CNS.

When there are impairments of musculoskeletal, neuromuscular, or cardiopulmonary systems, the resources that an individual can bring to movement may be altered, limited, or constrained.[11] Because movement is goal directed, an individual with impairments will find a way to accomplish movement goals that "work," often using a less effective or abnormal movement strategy. These altered strategies are recognized clinically as movement dysfunction.[12] The use of ineffective or abnormal movement patterns, over time, can lead to inflammation, tissue remodeling, or even deformity.[13] In an individual recovering from stroke who is walking, for example, an "abnormal" extensor synergy of the lower extremity may provide stance phase stability but will impair swing limb advancement, leading to a compensatory circumduction or vaulting step.[14] Abnormal tone may contribute to habitual plantar flexion and eventually an equinus deformity.[15] Someone with a painful knee or back will alter the way he or she uses those joints, as well as the limbs or trunk, when walking and moving between sitting and standing.[16-20] Over time, the individual may develop secondary musculoskeletal problems at distal or proximal joints or become physically deconditioned, compounding his or her movement dysfunction.[21,22] An individual with pain, shortness of breath, or a sense of fatigue (whether due to disease or deconditioning) may choose to be less active to "conserve" energy and, as a result, become even more deconditioned, develop soft tissue tightness that impairs flexibility, and lose muscle mass that limits functional strength.[23-27] Individuals who are concerned about pain, falling, or injury may also limit physical activity and have similar decrement in physiological capacity and resources.[28-30]

Physical and occupational therapists use various types of therapeutic exercise (e.g., strengthening, endurance programs, flexibility, balance activities), as well as functional training (often with assistive devices or ambulatory aids, orthoses, and prostheses), in order to minimize movement dysfunction and to remediate or accommodate the underlying impairments.[31] To be effective in these interventions, rehabilitation professionals must understand the principles of exercise and the effect that exercise has on the human body.[32-34] They must know both the purpose of an orthosis, prosthesis, or assistive device and how the design of the device will enhance or constrain movement and function.[35,36] If the goal of rehabilitation professionals is to help those with movement dysfunction learn more effective ways to accomplish what is important to them, they must also be aware of the process of learning, both on a cognitive and a motor level, and integrate this understanding into the interventions they plan and implement.[37]

This chapter provides an overview of recent thought on motor control, using a dynamic systems perspective. The chapter also reviews the tenets of motor learning and considers practice, augmented feedback, and mental imagery as tools to assist development of new or adapted movement skills. The chapter also consider how physical therapy intervention founded on knowledge of motor control and motor learning can augment neural plasticity and recovery after brain injury. The case studies at the end of the chapter are designed to help readers integrate growing understanding of the principles of motor control and of motor learning into the planning of interventions for movement dysfunction.

THEORIES OF MOTOR CONTROL

Human movement has traditionally been examined from two distinct fields of study: a neurophysiological control approach and a motor behavioral approach.[4,38-41] The traditional neurophysiological approach explained movement within a hierarchical system of control on the basis of the development of neural mechanisms within the central and peripheral nervous systems and the interaction of sensory and motor systems. The motor behavioral approach examined movement performance from the perspectives largely from the field of psychology. Only in the past few decades have the two fields of study interfaced to bring about newer theories regarding human movement that more fully explain human movement and performance.[4,41-43] Recently, there has been an increasing emphasis on the use of therapeutic intervention as a means of driving neural plasticity as a mechanism of recovery following brain injury.[44-46]

Dynamic Systems Perspectives

Rehabilitation professionals think about the human body as a complex biological system with many interacting elements and subsystems (Figure 3-1). These components have an infinite number of ways to work together in accomplishing a goal-directed motor act.[47-49] Because the human body is a dynamic, adaptive, and inherently complex set of subsystems, motor behaviors and ways of moving become more efficient with practice and experience: motor control systems can consistently generate simple and well-organized movement from a complex array of movement possibilities.[50,51] The dynamic systems perspective of motor control is founded on understanding of behaviors that physical systems of various types have in common: the ability to change over time, the ability to be adaptive yet have preference for habitual tendencies, and the context of interaction with the environment in which movement occurs.[43,52-54] In the human movement system, there is great "motor abundance"; each person has a wide variety of ways to accomplish an intended movement goal (i.e., solve a functional movement problem) in whatever environmental conditions or circumstances that function occurs.[55,56]

According to Bernstein's model of motor control, individuals have the capacity "to make a choice within a multitude of accessible trajectories... of a most appropriate trajectory."[57] Dynamic systems theory suggests that there are both opportunities and challenges presented by interaction of the environment and the individual's will to move.[57] Unlike systems that are purely physical, the human biological system is a smart, special-purpose machine able to instantaneously and efficiently work to meet the many parallel and serial functional demands.[58-60] In addition, biological systems such as the human body are self-organizing[59,61]; the mutually dependent and complex processes among the body's subsystems allow this wonderfully dynamic structure to enact efficient functional movement patterns. Even though it is an inherently multidimensional biological system, the human body prefers to be in a state of relative equilibrium.[62,63] This is likely to be the underlying reason that the gait cycle at self-selected (comfortable) walking speed tends to center around one cycle per second, and that most individuals transition from walk to run, as gait speed increases, at nearly the same velocity.[64] The human body, as a smart and dynamic biological system, is also intentional; there is a purposeful, goal-directed, and task-oriented nature in most motor behaviors.[65] The dynamic systems model defines an intention as a purposeful or desired act that influences (attracts) the human system to organize motor behavior toward the desired outcome, in the context of the environment in which the movement is occurring.[66] The organism and the environment are interdependent; each is defined with respect to the other.[58,65,66] Although the characteristics of the physical environment are the focus on many studies of goal-directed movement, the social-emotional environment can also influence the emergence of goal-directed movement.[67] The combination of resources available to the organism-environment interaction, in conjunction with the individual's intention, shapes (constrains) how task-oriented motor behavior is organized.

Motor control has been defined by Shumway-Cook and Woollacott as "the ability to regulate or direct the mechanisms essential to movement."[39] The interactive systems that provide resources that an individual uses to initiate and regulate goal-directed movement include the neurological,

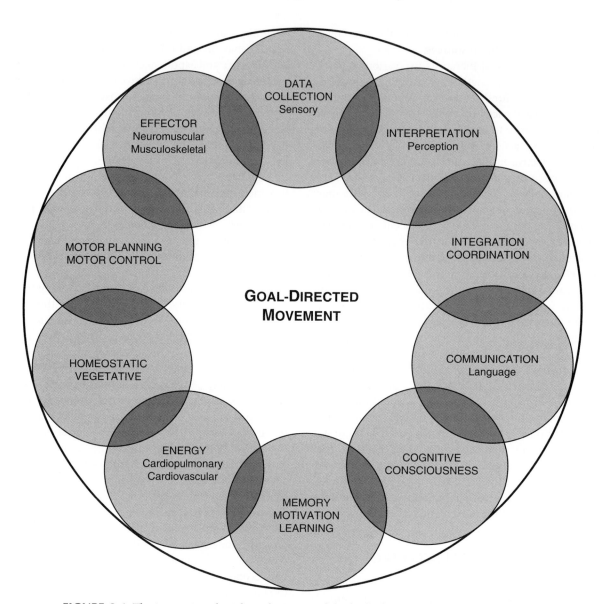

FIGURE 3-1 The interactive physiological systems of the body that contribute to an individual's ability to carry out during goal-directed (functional) movement. Sensory and perceptual systems contribute by monitoring the environment as well as the position and condition of the body during movement. Integrative, coordination, cognitive, memory, motivational, and planning systems work together to determine how a goal-directed task might be best implemented, corrected, or adapted for success. Homeostatic, vegetative, and energy systems anticipate physiological demand and insure that oxygen and glucose supplies are sufficient to meet task demands. The neuromuscular system fine tunes postural control, tone, and recruitment so that the musculoskeletal system can be used effectively to accomplish the movement goal. Continuous communication and interaction among physiological systems occurs before, during, and in response to movement so that both feed-forward and feedback can instantaneously influence task performance.

musculoskeletal, sensory/perceptual, cardiorespiratory, and cardiopulmonary, and the cognitive, learning, and memory systems. Human movement, or motor control, is a product of the interaction of the individual (with all of his or her subsystems), the characteristics of the environment, and the nature of the specific task or goal that the individual is involved in (Figure 3-2). Movement, then, is goal directed and purposeful; it makes use of the innate and learned resources available to the individual and is subject to the influences of the environment in which it is performed. By considering each of

these essential contributors to functional movement, rehabilitation professionals can assess potential sources of movement dysfunction, explore alternative movement strategies, and adapt or alter the task or environment to improve movement outcomes.[68,69]

Resources of the Individual

The first component to consider in this model of motor control is the individual, with his or her ability to think and reason, to sense and perceive, and to actively respond or initiate

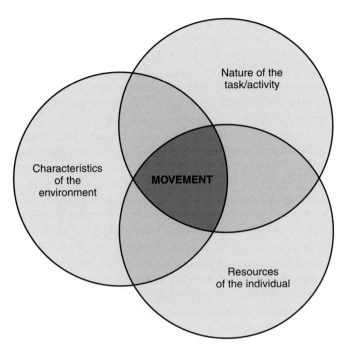

FIGURE 3-2 A contemporary model of motor control: movement emerges from the interaction of the individual, the environment, and the task being attempted. Therapists must consider how the characteristics, resources, and constraints of each influence the ability to move, and how each might be manipulated during intervention to enhance motor learning and effectiveness of movement.

movement (Figure 3-3). An individual's cognitive resources include the abilities to critically think and integrate concepts, organize and delay gratification, assign emotional meaning/significance to an activity or circumstance, problem solve, access and use memory, manage attention and focus (especially when engaged in concurrent tasks), and learn.[70-72] An individual's perceptual resources are the products of the ability to receive and process many different types of sensory information (i.e., data) and to integrate and interpret these data at both subcortical and cortical levels of information processing.[73-77] An individual's resources for action include the ability to motor plan and refine motion at cortical and subcortical levels; error control systems of the cerebellum; pyramidal and extrapyramidal motor systems; and the neuromuscular, musculoskeletal, and cardiopulmonary/cardiovascular contributors to "effector" systems.[78-93]

To illustrate how individual resources influence movement, consider two individuals who are walking to their cars after a major-league baseball game. Their pathway moves across a gravel-surfaced parking area with a slightly sloped and slightly unstable support surface. One person has the "stocking-glove" sensory and motor impairment typical of diabetic polyneuropathy. The other has consumed a few too many servings of beer in cheering his team to victory, making his thinking and motor behavior less efficient than normal. Both are likely to exhibit less efficient postural response and

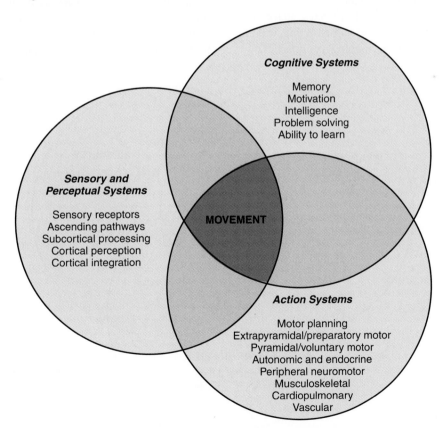

FIGURE 3-3 The individual resources that contribute to movement include those in the sensory/perceptual systems, the cognitive systems, and the action systems. For persons recovering from central nervous system insult, the therapist must understand whether dysfunction in any of these systems has occurred and consider how intervention might enhance neural plasticity and recovery of function in each of these areas.

unsteady gait patterns as they return to their vehicles, but for very different reasons. The quality of the sensory data that the individual with diabetic neuropathy can collect may not be sufficient for accurate perception of environmental conditions, and, complicated by distal weakness, her patterns of movement may not meet the challenges presented by the sloped and slightly movable ground surface. The individual who is tipsy has normal data collection ability; however, the temporary impairment in cognitive function (judgment and perception) and less efficient "error control" associated with alcohol consumption lead to motor behaviors that are not matched to environmental demands. Both baseball fans may stumble, walk with a wide base of support, or reach for the support of solid objects as they make their way toward their cars, but the underlying individual contributors to this motor outcome are quite different.

Nature of the Task

The task is the second essential component to the overall outcome or motor behavior performed. A functional task may require an individual to organize goal-directed movement to address one or more of the following motor control goals (Figure 3-4):

- Maintaining or adjusting antigravity posture (static, anticipatory, or reactionary postural control)[94-96]
- Transitioning from one stable position to another (quasimobility; e.g., moving from sitting to standing)[97-99]
- Moving a limb or the whole body through space (e.g., reaching, lifting, carrying, walking, stair climbing, walking on inclines, avoiding obstacles, hopping, running)[100-102]

- Using or manipulating tools appropriate to the task (e.g., assistive devices, objects needed for ADLs)[103,104]

Any task can be described along a number of different dimensions or continua: it can have *discrete* beginning and endpoints (e.g., transferring from bed to chair) or be *continuous* (e.g., walking or running over large distances). They can involve *stability* or require *mobility*, occur at *various speeds*, require different levels of *accuracy or precision*, and demand different levels of *attention or focus* (Box 3-1). Repetitive and overlearned tasks performed in predictable (closed or fixed) environments are often executed on a nearly automatic level, requiring little attention; this allows the individual to focus attentional resources on other prioriteis.[105] Tasks occurring in a changing (dynamic or open) environment must be flexible or adaptable to be successful and require a higher degree of attention during performance.[106,107] Finally, the complexity of the task and the attentional requirements for effective task performance must be considered.[108]

One way to understand the nature of a task (either broken into components or as a whole) is to examine or classify the task using Gentile's Taxonomy of Movement Tasks (Figure 3-5).[40] The first component considered in the taxonomy is the movement task's outcome goals: does the task primarily focus on stability of the body, transition between stable positions, or on transport (movement) of the body through space? As an example of a body stability task, consider the ability of an individual learning to use a transfemoral prosthesis to control hip and pelvic position while in single-limb stance on the prosthetic side, while slowly lifting the "intact" limb to place it on a stool or step placed in front of him or her.

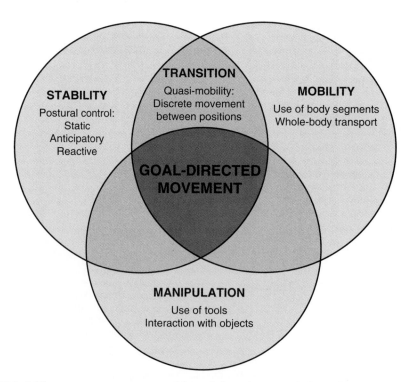

FIGURE 3-4 The components or nature of the task being attempted also influence the movement that emerges: The task can include or combine goals of stability, transitions, mobility, and manipulation of tools or objects.

BOX 3-1 *Descriptors of Movements Based on the Attributes/Nature of a Task*

- Discrete: The beginning or end point of movement, or both, as determined by the task itself (e.g., stepping onto a curb, donning a prosthesis, catching a ball).
- Serial: An ordered sequence of discrete movements, defined by the task itself (e.g., climbing a flight of stairs).
- Continuous: The beginning and end points of the task are determined and controlled by the individual (e.g., riding a bicycle, deciding when to start or stop).
- Stability: The primary task goal is to maintain position of body segments (often against gravity or in response to perturbation) or to keep the body's center of mass within the available base of support during functional activity (e.g., to provide a secure base in sitting or standing for subsequent skilled use of extremities).
- Transitional (quasimobility): The primary task goal is to move the body from a starting position of stability to a different ending position of stability (e.g., moving from sitting to standing, rolling from supine to prone, getting up from the floor).
- Mobility: The primary task goal is to move a body part, or the entire body, through physical space (e.g., rolling over in bed, walking or running, reaching for an object on a shelf or on the floor).
- Manipulation continuum: The degree to which a task requires the individual to use (manipulate) or interact with one or more external objects in order to complete the activity successfully (e.g., fastening buttons or handling clothes during dressing, donning/doffing a prosthesis or orthosis, opening doors during mobility, locking the brakes on a wheelchair).
- Automaticity: The degree to which the task is well understood and can be carried out automatically or requires attention because of high task demand (level of preciseness, consequence of error) or the changing nature of the task or environmental conditions (e.g., threading a sewing needle, walking down an icy sloping walkway, catching a thrown object).
- Variability in performance: The degree to which an individual is able to adapt the performance of a learned task in response to differences in environmental conditions or changes in task constraints; the flexibility to apply what has been learned to similar or novel situations.

A transitional (quasimobile) task for this person might be practicing moving between sitting and standing position from various seating surfaces or heights.[4] A body mobility task for the same individual might be to learn to use a cadence-responsive prosthetic knee unit by altering gait speed, changing direction, or navigating through a crowded public space.

The next consideration is whether the task involves use of, or interaction with, a tool or object (i.e., is object manipulation part of the task?). In working with persons with spinal cord injuries to develop postural control in sitting, for example, therapists often use catching and throwing activities with balloons and balls of various weights, thrown at different speeds and in varying directions, to provide opportunity to master this body stability skill.[109-111] Managing assistive devices (e.g., cane, crutches) during transfers or operating orthotic knee locks or prosthetic knee units during transfers are examples of object manipulation during transitional motor tasks. Learning to use an ambulatory assistive device (e.g., crutch walking in a four-point reciprocal pattern; managing crutches when ascending or descending stairs) is a prime example of a body mobility task that requires object manipulation.[112,113]

Characteristics of the Environment

The final component of the Shumway-Cook and Woollacott's model of motor control is the setting, environmental context, or conditions in which the goal-directed movement takes place (Figure 3-6). The physical therapist must examine (and, during intervention, purposefully manipulate) the environmental context in which functional movement occurs. Is the physical environment comfortable to be in while taking part in exercise and other rehabilitation interventions? Is it visually interesting and stimulating but not too distracting or challenging? Is the motor task occurring in an environment that is predictable (i.e., in a closed environment), or is there a degree of variability and possibility of change external to the individual (i.e., an open environment) that will require the individual to monitor and respond more carefully while performing the task?[114-116] Therapists must also consider the social-emotional context of the environment that is rooted in the interpersonal interaction: will the individual feel supported and encouraged as he takes risks and makes errors as part of the development of skill in salient activities? Or does the emotional environment contribute to anxiety about receiving negative criticism or a fear of failure?[117,118]

For the therapeutic application of environmental variables, therapists can consider both macroenvironmental influences (e.g., actual physical conditions that influence task demand, the therapeutic setting, or the involvement of family members), as well as microenvironmental influences (e.g., the level of visual and auditory "noise" present in the therapy room or variations in surfaces over which a client may be sitting or walking). Mastery of a motor task within a single, simple environment does not directly translate into safe performance of the same task under more complex and demanding environmental conditions. Navigating up and down a set of training steps in the physical therapy gym does not mean that the individual with stroke or paraplegic-level spinal cord injury will be functional and safe on a wet, leaf-covered, uneven brick staircase (with no railings) when entering or leaving his best friend's house or favorite neighborhood hangout.[119,120]

When working with persons with acquired brain injury functioning at the Rancho Los Amigos cognitive continuum

	BODY STABILITY		TRANSITION (Quasi-mobility)		BODY TRANSPORT	
	No object manipulation	Object Manipulation	No object manipulation	Object Manipulation	No object manipulation	Object Manipulation
CLOSED ENVIRONMENT — No variability	Stand in prosthesis unsupported in the parallel bars in a quiet PT gym	Stand in prosthesis unsupported while putting on jacket in a quiet PT gym	Practice the sit-to-stand transition from a single chair with armrests in a quiet PT gym	Practice the sit to stand transition from the same chair while managing axillary crutches	Walk the length of the parallel bars at comfortable speed, turn around, repeat	Walk forward with crutches using a 2-point gait pattern in an empty hallway
CLOSED ENVIRONMENT — Trial variability	Stand in prosthesis in parallel bars with diagonal weight shifts on command	Stand in prosthesis in parallel bars catching ball from different directions and speeds	Transfer to and from wheelchair, toilet, and shower seat, moving to left and right in random order	Transfer between seating surfaces of different heights while holding a full glass of water in a quiet PT gym	Practice stepping in different directions and distances in the parallel bars	Walk up to a closed door, opening it, and walking through while using a cane
OPEN ENVIRONMENT — No variability	Remain standing upright as people walk by at regular intervals from similar directions	Retrieve an object repeatedly from the same spot on the floor in a corner of a busy PT gym	Practice moving from standing to sitting using arms in a pre-positioned chair in the cafeteria of the rehabilitation hospital	Move from standing to sitting and vice versa from a rocking chair while managing crutches	Practice ascending and descending a set of training stairs in the corner of a busy PT gym	Approach and ascend a full flight of stairs in a quiet hallway, using bilateral canes
OPEN ENVIRONMENT — Trial variability	Remain upright while standing in line in a busy public area	Retrieve various randomly dropped objects throughout an active PT gym	Rise repeatedly from a seat in the movie theater so that other people (of various height and weight) can move past into the row	Scoot sideways while sitting, managing the blankets on a soft mattress so that grandchildren can climb into bed to hear a story	Ascend and descend stairs using the railing in a busy public space	Walk from car to supermarket door, pushing the grocery cart across the busy parking lot

FIGURE 3-5 Examples of therapeutic activities for an individual learning to use bilateral transtibial prosthesis, based on a modified version of Gentile's Taxonomy of Movement Tasks.

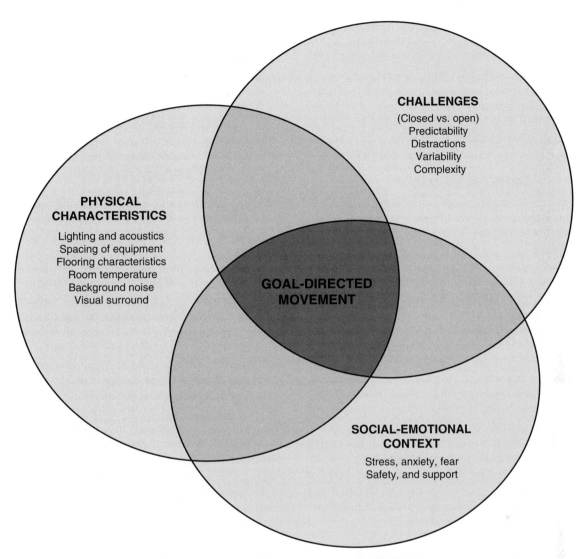

FIGURE 3-6 In considering the role of the environment on motor performance, the therapist must understand the challenges that it presents, the social-emotional context that might influence the individual's ability to move, and the physical characteristics of the movement space that affect the individual's safety and ability to move. Therapists often manipulate the social-emotional context by providing physical support and encouragement to create a situation where it is safe for the individual to attempt difficult movement and risk failure (error) as part of the motor learning process.

of 4 (confused and agitated), 5 (confused inappropriate), or 6 (confused appropriate), therapists must provide a structured and predictable environment for functional and rehabilitative activities, so that the demands of the environment do not exceed the individual's ability to monitor and respond to the challenges that the environment presents.[121-123] A complex environment can be overwhelming to the individual recovering from brain injury; the structured environment provides opportunity to complete key tasks with minimal frustration and behavioral complications. However, the complexity of the environment must be gradually increased as the individual prepares for discharge. Being able to cross the street safely at a crosswalk with real traffic is a more complex task than managing curbs and walking over a distance in the rehabilitation gym.

Gentile's taxonomy provides an organizational strategy for intervention planning by rehabilitation professions

working with individuals with musculoskeletal or neuromuscular impairments and limitations in performing functional activities. The primary goal of a man who has had a recent stroke may be to climb stairs so that he can return to his home, where the bedroom and bathroom are upstairs. In the early stages of rehabilitation, it may be necessary to first concentrate on static postural control and controlled weight shifting in sitting and standing on a firm support surface (body stability, no object manipulation, predictable environment). As the quality and control of these motor tasks become more consistent, intervention expands to include ambulation in the parallel bars (body mobility, no object manipulation, unvarying environment), then with an assistive device in a quiet hallway (body mobility, object manipulation, predictable environment), and finally in a busy rehabilitation gym in which the individual must anticipate and react to others in the environment (body mobility, object manipulation, changing environment). As postural control becomes more efficient on level surfaces, task demand is increased by increasing speed or attempting more challenging surfaces such as stairs, inclines, and stepping over obstacles; this may initially occur in a relatively predictable environment but must eventually occur in an "open" situation in which the individual must dynamically react to or navigate around other persons and objects.

Skill Acquisition Models

Movement has also been examined from the behavioral perspective, with a focus on quality of motor performance and acquisition of skilled behavior. Researchers with this perspective are interested in the influence of cognitive-information processing and cognitive psychology on motor behavior. They concentrate on the acquisition of skill, the learning processes associated with skills, and the refinement process of skills across applications. Early on, studies of skill acquisition focused on orientation to the task; as the field developed and expanded, focus shifted toward understanding the process of skill development. This led to formulation of the concepts of motor memory and schema. Adams' theory of feedback-based learning was a catalyst for later research, which gave rise to Schmidt's schema theory for motor learning.

Current motor control theory has become a blend of the various bodies of study presented in this section, integrating neurophysiological, dynamic systems/ecological, and behavioral models. This shared interest gave rise to the study of motor learning, which is concerned with the adaptation and application of movement strategies to altered or novel functional, behavioral, and environmental contexts.

THEORIES OF MOTOR LEARNING

Although models of motor control focus on how the biological system organizes and adapts movement as it occurs, models of motor learning consider how the individual comes to understand and consistently perform a particular behavioral task. The outcome of effective motor learning is mastery of skilled behaviors so that the individual can function appropriately in his or her physical and social environment. Most models of motor learning are founded on four distinct notions about learning:

1. Motor learning is a dynamic process that leads to acquisition of ability for skilled actions.
2. In order for motor learning to occur, there must be an opportunity to practice and build experience. Making errors is a necessary part of the learning process; as learning occurs motor memories are established.
3. Motor learning itself cannot be observed directly; it is inferred by observation of changes in motor behavior that become consistent over time.
4. Learning produces relatively permanent changes in the capability for skilled behavior, by building motor memory; as a result, what has been learned can be applied or adapted when altered task or environmental constraints occur.

In order to effectively master a novel motor task or recover from disease-disrupted motor function, the individual must[52,124]:

- Develop sensory and perceptual strategies for collecting information relevant to the task at hand and the environment in which is occurring
- Understand key features of the task, the performance environment, and any tools required to complete the task successfully
- Activate the components of the motor control system (anticipatory, guiding, corrective, and reactive) necessary for skillful performance of the task
- Apply (transfer) knowledge of the task, environment and tools in order to adapt skilled motor performance to situations that are different from the one in which learning took place

Rehabilitation professionals must be careful to distinguish between the concepts of motor learning and motor performance. *Motor performance* is the observable action or behavior that can be measured (rated) qualitatively or quantitatively by an observer.[41] As health care professionals who focus on function, therapists are quite skilled at examining motor performance, and determining whether an individual is moving normally or is coping with some form of movement dysfunction. Physical therapists use both subjective ratings (e.g., ratings of perceived exertion; using the terms "poor, fair, good, normal/excellent" to describe static postural control, dynamic balance ability, or endurance), and objective performance-based scales and measures (e.g., self-selected and fast walking speeds, Timed Up and Go times, Functional Reach distances, Dynamic Gait Index scores, 6-minute walk test distance, Gross Motor Functional Measure scores, among many others).[125-131]

In contrast, *motor learning* refers to the process that leads to changes in the quality, consistency, and efficiency of motor performance of a given individual. This process is not easily measured except by considering consistency or how other dimensions of performance of the task change over time. Comparisons of baseline performance to postintervention performance indicate changes in quality of performance. Although motor performance tends to transiently improve after a single practice session, we cannot be confident that learning has occurred until performance becomes consistent after multiple sessions over a period of time.[132,133] Improvement in motor performance to the level of consistency infers that effective motor learning has occurred. Motor learning has occurred when the task can be accomplished in various ways as situations demand.

Evolution of Models of Motor Learning

Initial models of motor learning were published in the early 1970s, the most prominent being Adams' closed-loop theory and Schmidt's schema theory.[134,135] Both models assume that, as a result of the motor learning process, the brain develops *generalized motor programs*: rules for timing and sequencing of muscle activity for key tasks.[132] The closed-loop theory proposes that sensory information generated from movements occurring during performance of functional tasks provides *feedback* necessary to build the memory and perceptual traces that guide and refine subsequent performance of the task.[134] In contrast, schema theory suggests that an open-loop process occurs, in which a general set of rules for a particular movement is developed (motor recall and sensory recognition schema) over time. Such schemas allow the individual to continuously compare actual outcomes of movement with anticipated (feedforward)/predicted outcomes via error detection and correction mechanism.[135,136] According to schema models, variability of practice must occur to establish and strengthen the movement schema over time.[137,138]

In the 1990s, Newell proposed an alternative ecological model of motor learning (resonant with Bernstein's dynamic systems model of motor control) that suggests individuals use a problem-solving approach to discover the optimal strategy to produce the task (performance) given both environmental and task influences.[139,140] By exploring the *perceptual motor workspace* during practice, individuals begin to recognize salient sensory/perceptual cues as they explore movement options that might lead to successful task completion. In viewing a demonstration, perceptual information helps the learner better understand the nature of the task and task-related movements that need to be mastered. Perception during (knowledge of performance) and perception after (knowledge of results) task-related movement provides intrinsic feedback that assists the problem solving process in the development of optimal strategies for the task at hand. Therapists can provide augmented information (explicit cues and extrinsic feedback) to facilitate an individual's search for optimal strategies. In this way, the perception (salient cues about the task and the environmental) and action (adaptive motor performance of the task.) are linked so that task-relevant connection is established.[145]

Refer to Shumway-Cook and Woollacott[132] and Schmidt and Lee[128] for a more detailed discussion of these theoretical models.

Temporal Considerations

Motor learning has also been explained through a temporal perspective in which learning occurs in stages over time. Various three- and two-stage models have been proposed to describe the process for acquisition of a skill and for adaptability or generalization/transfer of the skill (Table 3-1).

Three-stage models generally describe the earliest stage as the discovery stage, in which an understanding of the nature of a task is developed through trial and error, sometimes with guidance.[54,128,137-144] In this initial stage of motor learning, the need for attention is high, and there is significant trial and error-related variability in task performance early on, with an eventual understanding or selection of the best plan for the task for that individual. Once a plan has been settled on, the second stage of motor learning focuses on refinement of the performance; error during performance decreases while efficiency of performance increases, but attention is still required and distraction is often problematic, interfering with performance.[145] In the third and final stage of motor learning, the individual can generalize or adapt the learned skill to changing environmental demands;

much less attention to task is required, and the task can be performed effectively in various ways under multiple environmental demands.

Building on the work of Lereijken and colleagues, Shumway-Cook and Woollacott describe a system-oriented three-stage model, integrating principles of dynamic systems motor control, human development, and the ecological model of motor learning.[132,144] Early in motor learning, individuals constrain (freeze) the degrees of freedom among limb segments (joints) involved in the task as a means of reducing task difficulty; this freezing cocontraction around joints results in relatively accurate movement, although the movment typcially has a high energy cost.[146] As learning occurs, there is a tendency to "unfreeze" joints sequentially such that movement becomes more fluid and energy-efficient. With mastery, the individual employs freedom of movement to fluidly perform the task and can adapt to changing characteristics of the environment.[147]

Two-stage models of motor learning focus on (1) acquisition of the skill and (2) adaptation or application of the skilled motor behavior.[148] The initial phase consolidates the first two components of the three-stage models: Acquisition and refinement of performance occur within the same stage. Variability of performance occurs through internal demands within the individual's attempts to find and select a preferred action/strategy before refinement. In the second stage performance is variable due to external demands of the environment: The person must adapt the task accordingly; this is quite similar to the final component of each of the three-stage models.[149]

Implicit and Explicit Aspects of Motor Learning

To understand the process of motor learning, it is important to consider the principles underlying all learning processes: how new information is translated into memory to become useful. One can think about learning as the process of acquiring new information and new skills; memory then is the product or outcome of the learning process.[150] Learning is one of the major drivers of plasticity within the CNS, stimulating formation of new synapses as well as refinement of existing neural connections throughout the brain.[151,152] This plasticity is evident as information is moved from our short term (working) memory into initial long term memory stores which become better established, and more resistant to disruption, with practice and experience (Figure 3-7).[153]

Learning theorists describe two major categories of learning: implicit (nondeclarative) and explicit (declarative) learning (Figure 3-8).[154] Both categories lead to functional and physiological changes in synapses of involved areas of the spinal cord, brainstem, and forebrain.[155] One aspect of motor learning falls into the category of implicit procedural learning: it requires trial and error (discovery) in a relevant and functional context.[155] Consistently improved task performance over time and situation provide evidence of effective procedural learning. Neural structures thought to be necessary for implicit procedural learning include cortex

TABLE 3-1 Comparison of Concepts in the Major Models of Motor Learning

Models	Descriptive Stages/Movement Characteristics		
THREE-STAGE MODELS			
Fitts and Posner[142]	COGNITIVE Early skill acquisition through trial and error; performance highly variable to find most effective strategy for task	ASSOCIATIVE Refinement of skill; performance less variable and more efficient	AUTONOMOUS Low attention necessary for task; transfer or adapting skill to other environments; performance of skill during multiple task demands
Vereijken, Whiting, and Beek[54]	NOVICE Discovery of task constraints; restriction of degrees of freedom to simplify task	ADVANCED Release of some degrees of freedom to coordinate movement; adapt tasks to environmental demands	EXPERT All degrees of freedom released; exploitation of mechanical forces to complement environmental forces
Larin[144] (Refers to children)	DISCOVERY Verbal-cognitive stage; physical and verbal guidance necessary	INTERMEDIATE Motor stage; independent performance, greater consistency	AUTONOMOUS Skilled performance; economy of effort; task adaptable to environment
Shumway-Cook, Woollacott Systems Model[132]	STAGE 1 Co-contraction to constrain degrees of freedom to reduce the number of body segments or joints to be controlled during movement	STAGE 2 Gradual release of degrees of freedom of limb segments results in gradual increase in control and flexibility of the body during movement	STAGE 3 Mastery of the skilled movement with automaticity and variability during performance, allowing adaptation and transfer of skill in response to changing conditions/demands
TWO-STAGE MODELS			
Gentile[148]	EXPLICIT LEARNING Attainment of action-goal; conscious mapping of the movement's structure; rapid stabilization of performance	IMPLICIT LEARNING Dynamics of force generation; active and passive force components finely tuned unconsciously; gradual change in performance	
Manoel and Connolly[147]	ACQUISITION Formulation of the action plan; understanding task and how to accomplish it; stabilization of action	ADAPTATION Task and environment interaction; task is fluid with range of options to cope with new situations; breakdown of stable task and reorganization for new action plans	

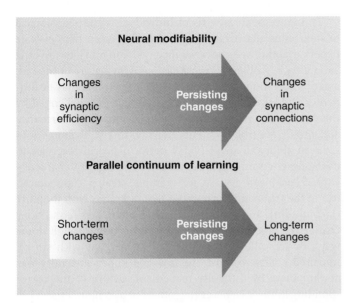

FIGURE 3-7 The gradual shift from short term (acquisition) to long term (retention) learning and memory is reflected in a move along the continuum of neural modifiability. Short-term changes, associated with an increased synaptic efficiency, persist and gradually give way to structural changes, the underpinnings of long-term learning. (From Shumway-Cook A, Woollacott MH [eds]. Motor Control: Translating Research into Clinical Practice, 4th ed. Philadelphia: Wolters Kluwer Lippincott Williams & Wilkins, 2012. p. 84.)

of the frontal and parietal lobes, nuclei of the basal ganglia, and cerebellar cortex and nuclie.[156-158] Recent work has also identified that the hippocampus in involved in perceptual components of procedural learning.[159] Explicit (declarative) learning is founded on attention and conscious thought and can be described or demonstrated by the learner.[160] Neural structures involved with explicit learning include prefrontal cortex, cingulate gyrus (limbic system), head of the caudate

nucleus, medial temporal lobes, and hippocampus.[161] The hippocampus plays a key role in motor learning because it contains a cognitive-spatial map of the typical areas in which humans function.[166] Early motor learning is strengthened, as evidenced by changes in output of the primary motor cortex, when explicit learning of sequences is associated with implicit learning.[162-164]

Once sequential aspects of the task are well understood, the need to pay close attention during motor performance diminishes, and the skill becomes less effortful as it transitions toward automaticity.[165] As automaticity increases, the ability to attend to simultaneous tasks also increases.[166,167] There is growing evidence that the transition from early motor learning of complex, sequentially organized tasks to automaticity requires more time and practice as a person ages.[168-171] Encouragement and feedback that focus on building perceptions of capability (self-efficacy) with respect to better performance than peers appears to enhance motor learning in both young and older adults.[172,173]

Key motor learning concepts that physical therapists working with individuals new to prosthetic or orthotic use include *practice* conditions and schedule; the role of *variability, contextual interference,* and *feedback* on skill acquisition; development of *automaticity* of performance; as well as *retention* and *transfer* of the newly learned motor skill (Box 3-2).[128,132] Each is discussed in the following section.

THE IMPORTANCE OF PRACTICE

Common to all models of motor learning is the concept of practice: Motor learning cannot occur unless the individual has an opportunity to gain experience through repeated attempts (both successful and unsuccessful) at accomplishing the desired movement task.[174] Much of the research literature in the area of motor learning is devoted to exploration

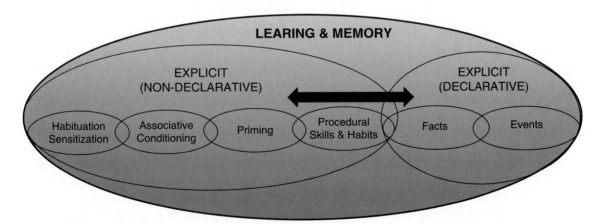

FIGURE 3-8 Learning is the process of acquiring information or skill while memory is the product of the learning process. Traditionally, the learning process has been described as having two separate domains: explicit or declarative learning, which is primarily involved in acquisition of knowledge about facts and events, and implicit or nondeclarative learning. Much of motor learning falls into the category of procedural implicit learning: the mastery of skills and habits. Recent research evidence using functional magnetic resonance imaging suggests that there are interactions between explicit and implicit processes *(arrow)* regardless of whether the focus is on fact or movement.

of practice and the optimal conditions or configurations in which it occurs. Conditions of practice can be classified or designed in several different ways. The type of practice used can influence the efficacy of motor learning that occurs, as well as its carryover or generalizability to similar tasks or environmental conditions.

Variability

In a complex and variable world, there are innumerable ways to respond to challenges that are encountered. Over the life span, typically developing individuals explore many movement options to accomplish salient task goals, developing a set of action plans that demonstrate both automaticity in performance and adaptability to variations in task or environmental constraints (i.e., the mastery of bipedal locomotion, over different surfaces, at various speeds, in closed versus open environments).[175,176] Discovery learning and the feedback/feedforward provided by error during repeated practice across conditions with differing constraints allows the individual to develop an understanding (perception) of the common elements of the task wherever and whenever it is performed.[174,177,178] This perception provides the flexibility to select from a range of task-specific options and adapt movement in response to variations encountered in daily life; variability in skilled movement is an adaptive resource responsive to variation in environmental demands.[179]

The movement patterns of individuals with neurological or neuromuscular dysfunction, however, often demonstrate hypervariability or hypovariability.[176,180] Too much or too little variability is problematic: Perception of the nature of the task and of interaction between task and environment may be limited or altered, and acquisition of skill may be challenged by the constraints associated with altered muscle performance and motor control.[181-183] Functionally, this contributes to a reduced ability to adapt (vary) performance in response to changing environmental conditions. The rigidity characteristic of Parkinson disease, for example, creates "super stability" of the trunk and extremities that interferes with mobility (locomotion) and postural control when task conditions change (i.e., the need to increase speed, walk through doorways, or to walk on inclines).[181,184] In persons with stroke, impaired ability to move the involved upper extremity was accompanied by difficulty recognizing action of the corresponding limb when observing others or a computer model.[185] In persons with right hemisphere stroke, impairments of attention and perception challenge the ability to develop the set of task-specific movement options necessary for adaptive function in response to variations in environment and context.[186,187] While implicit motor learning can be successful after a stroke, movement during acquisition stages is often slower and more variable in both blocked and random practice conditions.[188] Variability in movement is also altered in children with hypertonic and dyskinetic cerebral palsy, and in those with developmental coordination disorder.[179,182,189]

In rehabilitation, therapists set up opportunities for discovery motor learning for patients that are designed to enhance the likelihood of discovering, from among all possible movement options, the set of movements most likely to result in successful task performance.[175,176] This is accomplished by manipulating the environmental and task constraints in relevant and meaningful ways to actively engage the individual in iterations of the task, with the goal of promoting both perceptual understanding and a usable set of action options for completing the task.[175,190,191]

Practice Conditions: Blocked, Random, or Serial?

One way to describe practice is by whether it occurs in a blocked or random sequence. *Blocked practice* (also known as constant practice) is characterized by separate but subsequent repeated trials of the same task.[132,174] For blocked practice, the task is repeated under consistent environmental conditions. Modified blocked practice involves repeating the motor task three or more times in one condition before altering conditions or context in which practice of the same task is repeated. During blocked practice, the individual concentrates on performance of a single task; this focus reduces overall demand on working memory. As a result, quality of performance tends to improve substantially over successive bouts of blocked practice. In healthy adults, acquisition of skill appears to be effective (performance becomes more accurate over a single practice session) with blocked practice, however retention of the skill over time and transfer of the skill to differing conditions is not as strong.[192] Blocked practice appears to have a positive impact on retention of skill for children younger than 10 years; this is thought to be a function of emergence of information processing capability in late childhood and early adolescence.[193,194]

For the individual with transfemoral amputation working on stance control on the prosthetic limb, a blocked practice session might include stepping up onto a stool with the intact limb for 10 trials (repetitions), while standing in the parallel bars. The level of difficulty of the activity could be advanced by setting up an additional practice session, asking the individual to perform a similar task while supporting himself or herself with a straight cane to a practice curb or step outside the parallel bars. Theoretically, practice in the parallel bars would provide a model to use when performing a similar activity outside the parallel bars.

Random practice (also described as variable practice) is characterized as practicing a set of tasks in which order and perhaps difficulty of tasks varies across bouts of practice.[132,174] Because of the variation encountered during random practice, there is less improvement of performance in a given practice session (compared with blocked practice); however, there is greater retention of what has been learned over time. Theoretically, random practice creates *contextual interference* (the work of keeping many options available in working memory over time) that actually enhances learning and mastery over time despite poorer immediate performance.[174,192] While this may be counterintuitive, the efficacy of contextual interference on mastery of complex movement tasks is well supported.[195–199] One of the proposed mechanisms for enhanced retention in random practice is increased attentional demand that results in better use of perceptual understanding to prepare for movement.[197,199] The degree of similarity of tasks (distraction) undertaken during a practice session can also be a source of contextual interference; greater attention is required to discriminate between tasks with similar but distinct characteristics.[198] The improvement of retention occurs even when the context or characteristics of the task are somewhat altered; thus random variable practice may enhance transfer of learning.[174]

To practice the primary task of stance phase stability using a random practice order, the individual with a transfemoral prosthesis would be involved in an ongoing session of gait training. As this person walked the length of the parallel bars (or across the gym), he or she might be asked to step up onto a stool or over an obstacle at a different point in the walk and to change direction or speed on randomly delivered commands. The walk itself might be repeated 10 times (practice trials), with a step up onto or over the stool and changing speed and direction at a different point in each of the 10 trials of walking. These trials of stepping up or over and altering speed and direction do not occur sequentially but instead are interspersed throughout the entire ambulation event.

A third practice condition called *serial practice* can be thought of as a blending of the blocked and random practice order. Serial practice is a collection of different tasks performed sequentially, from a designated starting point to a defined ending point, always occurring in the same order, and repeated as a whole set of movement tasks.[132,174]

In a serial practice session for an individual learning to use a transfemoral prosthesis, the therapist may instruct him or her to repeat a specific sequence of movements such as the following:

1. Rise from a seated position and take three steps toward an obstacle in your pathway.
2. Step over the stool (obstacle) with your intact (right) foot, bringing your prosthetic limb around the object in a small arc.
3. Complete three more gait cycles and turn around to the right.
4. Walk back toward the obstacle, stepping over it with the prosthesis first on the return.
5. Continue walking back to the chair, turn, and sit down.
6. Rise to standing once again, and repeat the entire sequence until you have done it a total of × number of times.

The original task of stepping onto the stool with the right foot has been embedded into a series of different (but somewhat related) tasks performed in the same order over multiple trials.

Another way to classify practice is by the relative period of time spent in active practice versus rest time between practice sessions. In conditions of *massed practice*, there is more time spent over a practice trial than there is rest time between trials. Fatigue may be a factor in decreases in performance over repeated practice sessions if rest periods are insufficient. In conditions of *distributed practice*, the amount of practice time is less than or equal to the amount of rest time between trials.[132,174] Given evidence of better retention and transfer of skills with longer rest periods between practice trials (i.e., distributed practice), rest appears to be more than a period of physical recovery; it may also enhance consolidation of perceptual schemas and action rules associated with the skill that has been practiced into memory.[200] What is not yet understood is how much practice time and how much rest is optimal for tasks of different complexity or learners with various resources or impairments.

Part vs. Whole Task Training

Many functional tasks have sequential, recognizable subcomponents. The task of rising from a chair, for example, may require moving forward toward the edge of the seat, changing foot position, leaning forward to shift body weight from the ischial tuberosities toward the feet, lifting off the seat, accelerating quickly upward into standing, and then establishing postural control in the upright position.[201] The task of walking can be divided into stages including weight acceptance in early stance, stability during single limb stance, preparation for swing at the end of stance, and initiation through completion of limb advancement during swing phase.[202] When working with individuals who have neurological, neuromuscular, or musculoskeletal related movement dysfunction, therapists often use task analysis to determine what subcomponents of the task are problematic. The therapist might opt to practice the problematic components of the task to build skill before attempting the entire task (*part to whole training*) or to practice the entire task repeatedly (*whole task training*). In partial task training, the task is divided into separate parts, and each part is explained or modeled as distinct components of the task, while in whole task training the entire task is explained verbally or modeled (demonstrated) in entirety from beginning to end. The decision to structure training as part versus whole is influenced by level of difficulty of the task; the degree that the individual has already mastered some of the task components; the individual's ability to attend to the task, his or her level of motivation and frustration; and safety considerations as the task is attempted. Tasks that are serial in nature lend themselves in part to whole training; spending time practicing complex or difficult task components (ending the session by putting all of the components together to perform the whole task) often leads to better retention and transfer than the same amount of time spent practicing the entire task.[174,202,203] Tasks that are continuous, such as carrying a tray while walking through the cafeteria, are not as easily separated into components because of the degree of coordination and interplay necessary among task components. When coordination, timing, and interaction must be learned, whole task training appears to be more efficacious.[174,203,204]

Relationships: Practice, Retention, and Transfer

The effectiveness of the various practice conditions on motor learning has been the subject of many studies in psychology, movement science, and rehabilitation. As we consider the evidence that these studies present to us (to determine their clinical relevance and possible application), it is important to note the specific outcome of practice that is being investigated. Are the researchers focused on change in quality of performance during practice trials (i.e., skill acquisition within a session) or in carryover of understanding of the task from one practice session to another (i.e., postpractice performance or retention over time)? This distinction is particularly important for rehabilitation professionals to keep in mind.

How, then, do rehabilitation professionals determine whether the interventions they have implemented have resulted in effective motor learning and skill development? Rather than focusing on improvement in a single session, we look instead at the development of *automaticity* and the ability to adapt performance across sessions and circumstances. Although performance over repeated trials within a practice session is often observed, this is not a reliable indicator that motor learning has occurred. Consistency in motor behavior (as the product of the learning process) across sessions and over time suggests that there has been *retention* (consolidation), a relatively permanent change in motor behavior. The ability to *transfer* what has been learned and apply the set of movement options across situations appears to be related to the opportunity to practice under a variety of environment conditions and constraints.

Scientists who study motor learning hypothesize that individuals who develop flexible learning strategies through random practice and whole-task training are better able to transfer learned skills to novel situations. This is critical for the individuals we care for, who will ultimately need to perform skills beyond the rehabilitation practice environment (rehabilitation settings) as they return to the real world environment of their homes and community. Keeping this in mind, rehabilitation professionals need to carefully consider and choose the practice conditions that will lead to the best possible functional outcomes for individuals for whom they care.

INTRINSIC AND EXTRINSIC FEEDBACK

A second key concept in motor learning paradigms centers on the provision of feedback during practice trials (Box 3-3).[205] As movement occurs, it generates *intrinsic (inherent) feedback* that the CNS (especially the cerebellum as a system interested in coordination and error control) compares with the sensation that it "anticipates" (feedforward) will or should result from the movement. *Extrinsic (augmented) feedback* refers to information about the movement performance that is provided by an external source before, during, or after the movement. If rehabilitation professionals understand the "what, when, why, and how" of extrinsic feedback (and combine them with appropriately structured practice), they will be much more effective in facilitating motor learning as well as the individual's ability to problem solve or adapt a motor skill. Rehabilitation professionals must determine what type of information is most appropriate (knowledge of performance or knowledge of results) for the individual they are working with, as well as how and when the feedback would best be provided (feedback mode and schedule).

To initiate a therapy session, the therapist may ask an individual how he or she might approach a functional motor problem, and what they expect will happen when performing a task: for example, "We're going to practice moving from the bed to the chair. How can you prepare to do this? What is the first thing you need to do? Are you ready to do it?" This provides extrinsic augmented *feedforward* information aimed at engaging the person in the exploration of probable solutions for the initial steps of the transfer task. If the therapist asks the person to assess what he or she felt or experienced during the performance, they are providing *concurrent* extrinsic feedback. If the therapist asks or comments on performance after the task is completed, they are providing *terminal* extrinsic feedback. Therapists provide extrinsic feedback, sometimes without careful thought, in each intervention encounter when they say "Good job!" or "Did that work out the way you expected?" or "What might you do differently next time you try this?" In providing extrinsic information, the therapist calls the person's attention to, and enhances the use of, intrinsically generated feedback (or sometimes the substitution of an alternative source of information in the presence of sensory impairment).

Knowledge of Performance and Knowledge of Results

Extrinsic information can provide the individual who is learning a new motor strategy or skill with either knowledge of results (KR), information about the outcome of the movement

---

BOX 3-3 *Definitions for Feedback in Motor Learning*

BASIC DEFINITIONS

- Intrinsic (inherent): Sensations generated by movement of the body itself, monitored by sensory receptors (exteroception, proprioception, vestibular, visual, auditory), and transmitted to the brainstem and brain via sensory pathways.
- Extrinsic (augmented): Information provided about the movement task by sources external to the individual who is moving. Extrinsic feedback can be provided by another individual (e.g., the therapist or coach), or by an external device (e.g., biofeedback, other types of signals) that would not necessarily be present during usual performance of the task. It can be provided before, during, or after movement.

DIMENSIONS OF EXTRINSIC FEEDBACK

- Knowledge of performance (KP): Information about the quality of the movement, provided during or following performance.
- Knowledge of results (KR): Information about the outcome (success) of the movement or task, provided after it has been completed.

VARIATIONS OF EXTRINSIC FEEDBACK

- "Feedforward": Prompts or clues provided prior to movement to assist the learner's active engagement in problem solving or preparation for the motor task.
- Concurrent: KP information about the movement provided as it occurs.

- Terminal: KP or KR information provided after the movement task has been completed. This can be provided either as soon as the movement is finished (immediate) or after a period of time (delayed).
- Distinct: KP or KR information about one specific practice trial.
- Accumulated (summary): KP or KR information that reflects multiple attempts to perform the task or movement.

CHANNELS USED FOR EXTRINSIC FEEDBACK

- Verbal: Questions or statements made by the therapist or coach about the movement.
- Nonverbal: Gestures and facial expressions made by the therapist or coach; touch or guidance used to direct or redirect attention or movement; lights, whistles, or other sounds used to guide or influence the learning during or following the movement.

TIMING FOR EXTRINSIC FEEDBACK

- Consistent (100%): KR or KP distinct information provided after every practice trial.
- Reduced (50%, 33%, 25%): KR or KP distinct or summary information provided after every other, every third, or every fourth practice trial.
- For poor trials: Providing feedback for trials with large errors during practice.
- For good trials: Providing feedback for trials with relatively small or few errors during a practice trial.

(i.e., whether it was successful), or knowledge of performance (KP), information about the quality or execution of the movement (accuracy of the performance).[205] Much of the research on feedback in motor learning has focused on KR (outcome); however, in rehabilitation, we often use KP (quality; e.g., "Do you think that you were leaning far enough forward as you began to stand up?") to help individuals recognize and respond to movement errors.

Evidence in the literature suggests that, although KR does not necessarily lead to better performance during practice conditions, this type of augmented feedback information contributes to better task performance during retention tests.[133,205] The individual learning a new skill may benefit most by considering whether he or she has accomplished a movement goal (KR), especially in early and mid stages of motor learning, rather than how accurately or efficiently the goal was attained (KP). Early on, details about quality of performance may interfere with the individual's developing understanding of the nature of the task and ability to sort through possible strategies that might be used. In later stages of motor learning, when focus shifts to refinement or improved precision of performance, KP is probably a more appropriate and powerful form of feedback information, as long as the task is consistently accomplished.[206]

It appears that augmented and intrinsic KP feedback leads to better quality and consistency of performance during practice, but perhaps to less accurate performance in retention tests.[165,205] Although KP may not enhance retention as much as hoped, it has been found to be both effective and necessary in the acquisition of complex motor tasks, as compared with mastery of simple motor tasks.[206,207]

How and when Should Feedback be Used?

Another thread within the motor learning research literature explores the efficacy of different frequencies and timing in the provision of augmented information. Providing too much anticipatory prompting before initiation of the task or excessive feedback as the task proceeds and is completed can actually be detrimental to the learning process. Frequent KR-focused feedback, provided on almost each trial of the task, often contributes to dependence on external guidance and ultimately degrades performance on retention tests. Summarized KR-focused feedback given at infrequent intervals (after multiple trials) appears to improve performance during practice, as well as on retention testing.[208-210] Delaying the timing of KR appears to have a positive effect on performance during practice, as well as on retention tests. Providing feedback after trials that are relatively successful appears to enhance motor learning more than when trials are full of error.[211-213] Researchers have noted that KR, like random practice and whole training methods, better prepares individuals for adapting motor performance to changing environmental demands, resulting in better performance on retention tests. These findings are consistent across individuals with no neurological impairment; adults with stroke, head injury, and Parkinson's disease; children with cerebral palsy and developmental delay; and persons with mild cognitive impairment and early dementia.[214-219] There is gathering evidence that allowing individuals to pace or control feedback frequency also has a beneficial impact on the retention (effectiveness) of what has been learned.[220-222]

What Modality for Feedback is Appropriate?

Extrinsic feedback (augmented information) can be provided in a number of ways, using the visual system (e.g., demonstration and modeling, targets and other visual cues); the auditory system (e.g., informational verbal prompts or questions, use of tone of voice); and somatosensory-tactile systems (e.g., manual contacts, tapping/sweeping motions, compression of limb segments to cue stability response, traction/elongation of limb segments to cue mobility, appropriate resistance to guide movement).

Early in the motor learning process, therapists judiciously use all three modalities, keeping in mind that early stages of motor learning are periods of experimentation and trial/error as the individual becomes familiar with the nature of the task and problem solves strategies that lead to accomplishment of the task. Although it is tempting to explicitly direct and "tell" someone with movement dysfunction how to move more efficiently, prompting by using questions often can more effectively engage the individual in an active learning process. It appears that certain tasks are more responsive to particular modalities of feedback than others.[223,224] In persons with stroke, for example, visual feedback about weight distribution is useful for balance activities and auditory feedback about force production positively impacts on learning the sit to stand transition; efficacy of verbal and kinesthetic is not as well understood.[225,226]

Simple tasks appear to be learned more easily following demonstration or physical practice, with or without KP-focused feedback. The learning of more cognitively and motorically complex tasks, on the other hand, benefitted from a combination of demonstration and practice with KP feedback.[226] Many studies suggest that an *external focus* of attention (success or quality of the movement) has a more beneficial effect on motor learning than an internal (kinesthetic) focus of attention during practice.[227-230]

As individuals move into the later stages of motor learning, therapists must be aware of the need to wean the amount and frequency of augmented information as the individual moves toward becoming adept at the task. In the final stages of motor learning, augmented information becomes less and less essential or effective, as mastery of the motor task is achieved.

Using Normative Feedback

There is increasing evidence that providing information that is normative (social-comparative) has a positive impact on motor learning.[227] Providing feedback that suggests that the individual is doing as well or better than others in similar situations, when paired with KR information about outcomes of the individual's actual practice, appears to improve trial-to-trial performance as well as retention.[231,232] Making a statement at the start of a therapy session focused on a difficult motor task indicating persons facing similar challenges typically do well and are able to master the task with practice enhances the individual's expectations of their own ability (self-efficacy) and reduces anxiety associated with risk of failure; this enhances motor learning as well.[233]

Mental Practice and Imagery

Another resource available to assist the process of motor learning is the incorporation of mental practice and imagery into therapeutic interventions. Mental practice is defined as the imagined execution of a task-related movement without actual movement or muscle activation.[234] Mental practice of a motor task is thought to activate the same areas and networks of the CNS that actual movement does, especially if the task has been previously practiced.[234,235] Growing evidence in both the human performance and rehabilitation literature indicates that mental practice and the use of imagery enhance learning effects of physical practice and improves motor performance and retention.[236-238] Mental practice and motor imagery that focus on ease and quality of movement have been found to be particularly helpful in acquisition of motor skills in persons recovering from acute and chronic stroke.[239,240]

Imagery and mental practice appear to have a more powerful influence on improving performance during skill acquisition; their impact on retention of skills is not as well understood. This has implications for application to practice in therapeutic settings. Given high-volume patient case loads and the realities of multiple patients per therapist during sessions, mental imagery can be an effective tool for maintaining involvement of the client in the activity even when the therapist is attending to other patients.

Role of Sleep in Motor Learning

Newly acquired motor memory becomes more stable (more resistant to disruption or interference) during sleep.[241] The procedural memory consolidation process appears to reduce the need for neocortical (prefrontal lobe) input into the neuronal representation of the movement, making it easier to recall the movement and increasing efficacy of retention.[242] While early research suggested that consolidation during sleep actually improved learning (off-line learning) and enhanced motor performance, more recent work proposes that it instead provides protection against forgetting by counteracting both physical and neuronal fatigue associated with practice.[243,244] Whichever perspective will prove to be accurate, it appears that sleep is a key component in the motor learning process.

The positive effect of sleep on retention of newly learned skills appears to be true for motor skills that have been physically practiced as well as those reinforced by mental imagery, in both persons who are healthy and in persons with CNS pathology.[245,246] It is important that opportunity for uninterrupted overnight sleep for offline consolidation of motor memory is a key component of the rehabilitation process for persons with stroke.[247,248] Individuals with prefrontal lobe damage (e.g., after traumatic brain injury), who typically are quite challenged by novel motor tasks presented during rehabilitation, appear to benefit significantly from the opportunity for off-line learning and memory consolidation that occurs during a night of sound sleep.[248]

Importance of Patient/Client-Centered Goals

Rehabilitation goals focus on improving an individual's ability to participate in meaningful activities. One aspect of the motor learning process that is often taken for granted is the salience of the task to the learner; therapists may assume that the goals that they have developed for a given patient (e.g., to walk 150 feet safely and efficiently using an assistive device and a prosthesis or orthosis) are consistent with the goals of the individual with whom they are working, when in fact there may be a mismatch.[249,250] Emerging evidence suggests that focusing on the tasks that are most meaningful to the individual enhances motivation and attention, necessary components of the motor learning process as well as facilitators of neural plasticity and recovery after brain injury.[251,252] A sense of empowerment and increasing self-efficacy contributes to efficacy of learning when an individual works toward a goal that is particularly meaningful to that person.[253–255]

How does a rehabilitation professional assist an individual to identify salient personal goals and use these goals to inform design of appropriate opportunity for motor learning (Figure 3-9)? Framing goals at the level of activity and participation is the first step.[256] The next is to ensure that stated goals reflect consensus (as much as possible) of the patient and the health professional.[257] Such consensus is a key influence on the relationship between the patient and the health professional; being "on the same page" creates a level of trust that provides a solid foundation for risking failure in the rehabilitation learning environment.[257] Goals for motor learning are most effective if they reflect both expertise of the therapist and expectations of the individual beginning rehabilitation; at times, reaching consensus requires patient and family education as well as negotiation about priorities.[258–260] Effectively defined goals are (1) specifically related to the task to be accomplished or mastered; (2) measurable (i.e., use quantifiable metrics of distance, time, effort or difficulty, and frequency of performance), (3) ambitious yet achievable within the forecasted episode of care; (4) relevant, realistic, and congruent with the individual's potential and expectations; and (5) include a timeline for achievement.[261] Establishing clearly stated and measurable goals provides a framework for assessment of outcomes of interventions, as well as revision or progression of activities that will further improve functional capacity and ability to participate in meaningful activity. Such attention to early establishment of functional goals has been found to positively affect on outcome of rehabilitation for children with cerebral palsy and persons with spinal cord injury, stroke, and traumatic brain injury.[262–267]

Neural Plasticity in Motor Control and Motor Learning

Rehabilitation professionals are on the cusp of significant expansion in the understanding of the neurobiological/physiological basis of recovery after neurological and neuromuscular injury.[268,269] The developing science suggests that we can use our understanding of motor control and motor learning to *drive neural plasticity* in both acute and chronic stages of many neurological and neuromuscular diseases.[270–273] This science also challenges us to reevaluate whether our interventions are sufficient, in terms of therapeutic approach, intensity, and duration, to trigger the neuroplastic changes that will improve function and quality of life.[274–276]

The term *neural plasticity* refers to the dynamic ability of the brain to structurally and functionally reorganize neural circuits in response to activity and environmental demand: such plasticity occurs during development in children, during adulthood as one masters new motor skills and builds knowledge base, as well as after any type of brain injury or insult.[271,276] Plasticity is driven by (i.e., is dependent on) the process of learning, whether it be focused on new knowledge or skills, or relearning of skills disrupted by illness or injury. While the mechanisms underlying neuroplastic change are not fully understood, exposure to learning opportunities of sufficient intensity and duration contributes to remapping of motor, perceptual, and communication areas within the brain.[271–273,277] Early in rehabilitation, as the effects of inflammation and edema associated with CNS infarct or injury diminish, activity-based interventions may help revive and restore function in neural structures that were initially compromised; this is *neural recovery*.[278] Even if there is potential for neural recovery, at times the effort required to activate recovering neural circuits is intensely difficult and frustrating. Without encouragement and opportunity to practice, function may continue to be compromised due to *learned nonuse* of a body part.[279] As rehabilitation progresses, continued activity-based interventions may facilitate recruitment of intact neighboring neural structures to supplement function of damaged brain structures. Even though this is actually a mechanism of *neural compensation*, it may be perceived by the individual, family, and rehabilitation professionals as *functional recovery* at the level of WHO-ICF levels of body function and activity.[271] If brain injury has been so extensive that alternative ways of performing key functional tasks is necessary, retraining leads to *functional compensation*.[271]

Medical management of newly injured or compromised brains has traditionally focused on preventing or limiting secondary sequelae that result from insult, whether traumatic, ischemic, or infectious. Refer to Shumway-Cook & Woollacott, 2012, pp. 93-99 for a summary of the brain's cellular and functional responses to injury.[155] While evolving pharmacological or interventional strategies (e.g., transcranial stimulation) now target recovery of function, rehabilitation based on principles of motor learning is currently the most powerful facilitator or neural plasticity.[270,280,281] The behavioral, sensory/perceptual,

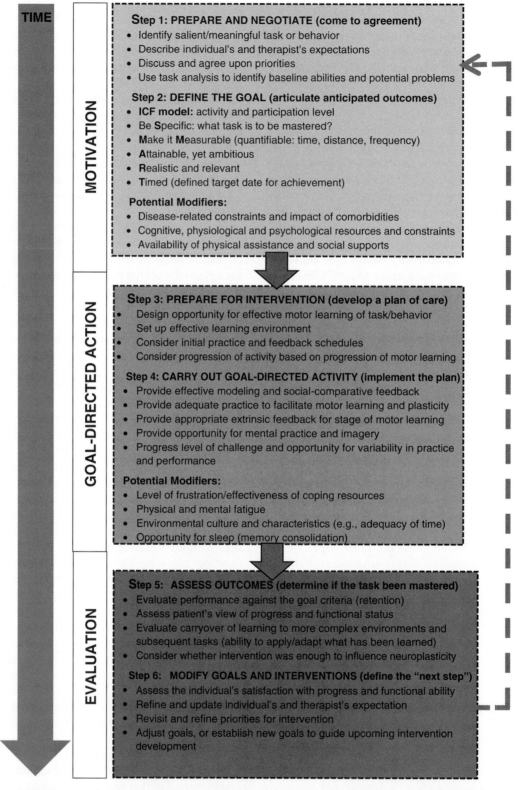

TIME

MOTIVATION

Step 1: PREPARE AND NEGOTIATE (come to agreement)
- Identify salient/meaningful task or behavior
- Describe individual's and therapist's expectations
- Discuss and agree upon priorities
- Use task analysis to identify baseline abilities and potential problems

Step 2: DEFINE THE GOAL (articulate anticipated outcomes)
- **ICF model:** activity and participation level
- Be **S**pecific: what task is to be mastered?
- **M**ake it **M**easurable (quantifiable: time, distance, frequency)
- **A**ttainable, yet ambitious
- **R**ealistic and relevant
- **T**imed (defined target date for achievement)

Potential Modifiers:
- Disease-related constraints and impact of comorbidities
- Cognitive, physiological and psychological resources and constraints
- Availability of physical assistance and social supports

GOAL-DIRECTED ACTION

Step 3: PREPARE FOR INTERVENTION (develop a plan of care)
- Design opportunity for effective motor learning of task/behavior
- Set up effective learning environment
- Consider initial practice and feedback schedules
- Consider progression of activity based on progression of motor learning

Step 4: CARRY OUT GOAL-DIRECTED ACTIVITY (implement the plan)
- Provide effective modeling and social-comparative feedback
- Provide adequate practice to facilitate motor learning and plasticity
- Provide appropriate extrinsic feedback for stage of motor learning
- Provide opportunity for mental practice and imagery
- Progress level of challenge and opportunity for variability in practice and performance

Potential Modifiers:
- Level of frustration/effectiveness of coping resources
- Physical and mental fatigue
- Environmental culture and characteristics (e.g., adequacy of time)
- Opportunity for sleep (memory consolidation)

EVALUATION

Step 5: ASSESS OUTCOMES (determine if the task been mastered)
- Evaluate performance against the goal criteria (retention)
- Assess patient's view of progress and functional status
- Evaluate carryover of learning to more complex environments and subsequent tasks (ability to apply/adapt what has been learned)
- Consider whether intervention was enough to influence neuroplasticity

Step 6: MODIFY GOALS AND INTERVENTIONS (define the "next step")
- Assess the individual's satisfaction with progress and functional ability
- Refine and update individual's and therapist's expectation
- Revisit and refine priorities for intervention
- Adjust goals, or establish new goals to guide upcoming intervention development

FIGURE 3-9 A patient-centered model for setting goals for effective motivation and facilitation of motor learning in rehabilitation. Initial efforts focus on building consensus between patient and therapist on establishment of appropriate meaningful goals, and articulation of such goals so that they can be later used to assess outcomes. Given understanding of motor learning, motor control, neuroplasticity, and recovery of function, the therapist then designs and implement task-specific, goal-directed rehabilitation interventions. Both the patient and therapist use agreed upon goals as markers of efficacy of intervention, and modify or progress therapeutic activities and practice based on achievement of the goals.

and cognitive aspects of functional and skilled movement appear to effectively trigger neuroplastic processes in damaged brains, in ways much like occurs in developing brains.[270]

Kleim and Jones[270] have developed a set of 10 principles that translates current best evidence about experience-dependent neural plasticity from animal and human basic science studies to inform development of motor learning-based interventions for clinical rehabilitation practice (Table 3-2). Discussion of each principle follows.

Use it or Lose it

Basic science research has clearly demonstrated that impaired performance and eventual loss of skill and ability is likely if neural circuits are not consistently activated by functional activity. This is the underlying assumption of the learned nonuse theory that forms the foundation for constraint-induced therapy targeting upper extremity use for adults and children with hemiplegia.[282,283] A similar principle has been described as an explanation for decline in muscle performance and endurance associated with sedentary lifestyle and bed rest.[284] Early in rehabilitation, individuals with

TABLE 3-2 *Kleim and Jones' Principles of Experience-Dependent Neural Plasticity*

Principle	Description
Use it or lose it	Failure to drive specific brain functions can lead to functional degradation
Use it and improve it	Training that drives a specific brain function can lead to enhancement of that function
Specificity	The nature of the training experience dictates the nature of the plasticity
Repetition matters	Induction of plasticity requires sufficient repetition
Intensity matters	Induction of plasticity requires sufficient training intensity
Time matters	Different forms of plasticity occur at different times during training
Salience matters	The training experience must be sufficiently salient to induce plasticity
Age matters	Training induced plasticity occurs more readily in younger brains
Transference	Plasticity in response to one training experience can enhance the acquisition of similar behaviors
Interference	Plasticity in response to one experience can interfere with acquisition of other behaviors

Adapted with permission from Kleim JA, Jones TA. Principles of experience-dependent neural plasticity: implications for rehabilitation after brain damage. J Speech Lang Hear Res 2008;51(1): S225-S239.

CNS dysfunction or disease may discover compensatory or alternative movement strategies that are less difficult or frustrating given their altered brain function, and the resulting paresis or altered muscle tone.[11] Moving differently also impacts muscle performance and flexibility, making development of secondary impairments more likely. Thus, over time, not only does neural circuitry necessary for normal movement degrade, but also the individual's physical resources for movement change. Both of these factors reinforce the altered or abnormal movement pattern and the loss of premorbid skill and activity.

Use it and Improve it

Animal models consistently show that, in both nonimpaired and impaired circumstances, consistent or extended training induces cortical plasticity as evidenced by reorganization of cortical motor and sensory mapping and synaptogenesis.[285] The expectation is that behavioral experience will optimize neural plasticity in humans as well.[273] Participating in extended training (i.e., practice, experience) of specific skills and functions enhances performance in areas of the brain associated with those functions; this is the outcome expectation for constraint-induced therapy and task-specific paradigms used in stroke, brain injury, and spinal cord injury rehabilitation programs.[282,286,287]

Specificity is Significant

In humans, the acquisition of particular motor skills (e.g., finger tapping) through physical practice leads to changes in neural activity only in particular areas of motor cortex and cerebellum (e.g., areas mapped to hand and fingers) as evidenced on functional magnetic imaging.[288] This demonstrates that the training experience that leads to acquisition of a specific behavioral skill determines the resulting type and extent of plasticity. Task-specific training has been evaluated extensively as an intervention for recovery of upper extremity function and of locomotion after stroke.[289,290] It is important to note, however, that neuroplastic changes associated with training of one skill does not necessarily contribute to improvement in other skills or changes in other areas of the brain. Nonskilled movement appears to have little, if any, impact on neural plasticity.

Repetition, Repetition, Repetition

One successful performance of a motor task does not mean that the task has been skillfully mastered. In motor learning, evidence of mastery is the transition to automaticity.[105,166] An individual moves toward automaticity only after many practice sessions. Sufficient repetition of new or relearned behaviors is necessary for neuroplastic changes to become well established. The underlying assumption is that the outcome of such repetition is the establishment of neural circuitry that makes the effectively learned behavior less likely to decay over time, when practice is infrequent.[270] The role of repetition for driving learning and neural plasticity is a critical one. Body weight–supported treadmill (TM) training is designed to provide opportunity for repeated practice of locomotion that would not be possible in overground walking early in rehabilitation after stroke and spinal cord injury.[291,292] TM training has the added benefit of inducing cardiopulmonary/cardiovascular fitness, adding to overall resources for movement available to the individual whose CNS dysfunction may carry an associated secondary risk of deconditioning.

Intensity is Important

In persons without brain injury, training intensity (dose, number of repetitions, number of practice sessions) influences both degree and stability of the neuroplastic change induced by practice.[270] Both constraint-induced therapy for upper extremity rehabilitation, and treadmill training for recovery of locomotion are high-intensity interventions. While the optimal "dosage" for rehabilitation intervention is not well defined and may differ across diagnoses, it is clear that outcomes of intervention are influenced by dose, with high-intensity programs having the largest effect.[293] Current rehabilitation practice models do not always provide the number of repetitions or dose intensity that might be necessary to induce neural plasticity and cortical reorganization.[294] Much of the research on intensity of intervention has involved persons who are medically stable, in the chronic period after their neurological event. These individuals appear to tolerate intense interventions with little adverse consequence. What is not well understood, however, is whether there may be sensitivity to overuse in newly injured brains that is detrimental after a threshold level of repetitions is exceeded.[270,295] In the absence of guidelines about level intensity for persons with recent CNS insult, careful monitoring for signs of activity intolerance of the brain and body (e.g., fatigue, irritability, distractibility, change in attention or alertness, as well as greater than anticipated decrement in performance, among others) may assist the therapist in keeping the intensity of intervention within safe ranges.

Time and Timing

There are many molecular, cellular, structural, and physiological contributors to the process of neuroplasticity; the relationships and timing of changes at each of these levels continues to be explored.[270] Consolidation of motor memory, for example, requires "off-line" time after practice for a newly learned skill to be effectively retained.[281] As in development, there may be windows of opportunity within the typical pattern of recovery when interventions targeting neuroplasticity are likely to be most effective.[295,296] Delaying intervention (or providing intervention at suboptimal levels of intensity) may allow abnormal compensatory movement patterns to become established; and rendering rehabilitation less effective.[270] Certainly, there is much more investigation needed regarding when neuroplasticity focused rehabilitation intervention would be best implemented during the course of recovery following CNS insult.

Salience is Substantial

Even a well-practiced activity will not successfully induce neural plasticity unless it is perceived as meaningful and important to the individual. Motivation, attention, and the ability to learn are influenced by the relevance of and perception of potential reward associated with a movement task.[297,298] Participation in rehabilitation interventions modelled on motor learning in the context of neural plasticity requires considerable investment and effort on the part of the patient. If the goal and level of effort needed to achieve it outweigh the perceived potential benefits or rewards of participation, is it any wonder that little will be accomplished in terms of skill development or facilitation of neural plasticity? It is essential that there be discussion and, optimally, consensus between the individual and the therapist about the likelihood of improved functional performance at a level that the individual perceives as valuable and important as a result of intervention. Salience (meaningfulness) appears to impact motor learning and recovery via the cholinergic system of the basal forebrain.[299]

Considering the Life Span

While the brain is clearly most "plastic" in early life during periods of rapid motor, perceptual, and cognitive development, the brains of older adults continue to be responsive to experience-driven catalysts of neural plasticity.[300–302] Rich physical, emotional, and cognitive experiences over the life span appear to protect the older individual against decrements in brain function typically thought to be the result of aging.[303,304] There are differences in the process of motor learning and neural plasticity, however, at both ends of the life span. Children may require longer periods of practice and a more gradual reduction in frequency of feedback for effective motor learning than adults to effect neuroplastic change and consolidation of newly learned skills.[305] Older adults also require longer periods of practice and increased number of repetitions, especially if attempting to replace competing compensatory movement strategies after CNS insult.[306] When compared with younger adults, efficacy of the motor learning process (and by extension, neural plasticity) appears to be somewhat less for older adults in both acquisition and retention of skilled sequential movements and retention.[307] This may be associated with age-related declines in visuospatial working memory and of attentional focus.[308] Nevertheless, older adults with stroke and other CNS diseases do respond to appropriately targeted complex motor skill training, demanding environmental contexts, and exercise interventions in both acquisition and reinforcement of skilled movement.[291,309–311]

Transference

Kleim and Jones[270] describe transference as the ability of plastic changes in one set of neural circuits to enhance concurrent or future neuroplastic changes in other neuronal circuits. Adding repetitive transcranial magnetic stimulation to physical practice of salient motor skills appears to enhance acquisition and retention of motor skills and promote more extensive return of function during acute and chronic stages while recovering from a stroke.[312,313] Animal studies suggest that living and functioning in complex enriched environments may also potentiate neuroplastic changes in the cortex after brain injury.[314] In humans, both enriched environments and physical exercise appear to have a potentiating neuroplastic effect on the damaged brain, brainstem, cerebellum, or spinal cord, contributing to angiogenesis mediated by the release of brain-derived neurotrophic factors during activity.[315,316] Repetitive physical activity and exercise during rehabilitation has the potential to enhance neural plasticity, as well as to improve muscle performance and cardiovascular/cardiopulmonary conditioning.

Interference

Just as some neuroplastic changes enable reorganization in the process of transference, they also may block, interfere with, or otherwise impede operation or reorganization of other circuits, with a negative impact on the ability to learn.[270] Kleim and Jones[270] define interference as the ability of plasticity in a particular neural circuit to impede the generation of novel circuits or enactment of established circuits. How does this translate into rehabilitation? The clearest example is the detrimental impact that self-discovered compensatory movement strategies (a neuroplastic change in which persons with stroke have learned to move functionally using alternate movement strategies) on learning more effective strategies of movement during therapy.[317,318] This interference has also been demonstrated in persons with acute or chronic pain who have learned to move in ways that avoid discomfort but are not kinematically effective and are associated with likelihood of additional dysfunction.[319,320]

Neuroplastic interference as described by Kleim and Jones is a different concept than the contextual interference that occurs during random practice discussed earlier in the chapter as a facilitator of motor learning. Contextual interference occurs as a result of the need to keep many options that might solve a motor problem available in working memory over time.[174,192] The increased attentional demand associated with contextual interference appears to augment, rather than interfere, with the learning (and hence the neuroplastic) process.[197-199] From a motor learning perspective, neuroplastic interference might occur if the type of practice or feedback provided during a rehabilitation session is not appropriate for a learner's specific needs or characteristics.[321,322] Another example of neuroplastic interference might be the impact of learning of an additional novel complex motor task soon after practice of a newly learned complex motor task; having little "off-line" time may interfere with motor memory consolidation of the newly learned task.[323,324]

Aerobic Exercise, Neuroplasticity, and Neuroprotection

Exercise may be a rehabilitation professional's most potent tool for facilitating neural plasticity. Fitness (aerobic) exercise causes a cascade of events, at both molecular and cellular levels, that support the health and development of neural circuits.[325] This is thought to be due to the interplay of central and peripheral mechanisms supporting energy metabolism and homeostatis.[326,327] During and for a short time following a bout of aerobic exercise, the level of circulating neurotrophic factors increases, and is more available for support of neuroplastic and neuroprotective changes in the brain.[325,328] Resistance (strengthening) exercise does not lead to the degree of increase in neurotrophic factors that aerobic exercise does.[329] While rehabilitation professionals typically endorse aerobic exercise as a means of building functional capacity and activity tolerance, we may not be as aware of the role that aerobic exercise may play in readiness of the brain to learn. These are two powerful reasons that aerobic activity should be included in plans of care for all persons with CNS dysfunction, as well as any individual who must develop new motor skills (e.g., learning to walk with a prosthesis).

Participation in treadmill training during rehabilitation after stroke or incomplete spinal cord injury enhances motor learning and neural plasticity in several ways: it is task-specific, provides repetitive practice at high dosage, builds cardiovascular/cardiopulmonary fitness and (as a result) readies the brain for functional modification of neural circuits.[291,325] Aerobic fitness is associated with greater neuroplasticity and better cognitive performance in persons with multiple sclerosis.[330,331] There is growing evidence that aerobic exercise can enhance motor performance and possibly slow progression of mobility impairment in persons with Parkinson's disease.[332-334] A bout of fitness exercise appears to transiently improve cognitive function in older adults, and participation in habitual cardiovascular fitness appears to have a neuroprotective effect on cognition and the ability to learn in later life.[335-337] The neuroplastic and neuroprotective effect of aerobic conditioning also appears to improve or stabilize cognitive function and learning in persons with mild cognitive impairment and dementia.[338-342]

Given current evidence about the ability of aerobic exercise to potentiate and protect brain health and function, rehabilitation programs that fail to incorporate a fitness or conditioning component may miss the opportunity to enhance motor learning and recovery of function. This applies to persons with neurological problems, as well as those who may be learning to use an orthosis or prosthesis as a result of neuromuscular and musculoskeletal impairment from trauma, overuse, or disease.

APPLICATION: CASE EXAMPLES

The following case examples are presented as opportunities for readers to apply the information presented in this chapter. Readers are urged to take time to develop an appropriate plan of care/therapeutic intervention within the framework of the ICF Model, using the interactive person-task-environment (systems) framework of motor control and principles of therapy/activity-driven neuroplasticity, in the context of the modified version of Gentile's Taxonomy of Movement Tasks presented in the chapter, and principles of goal-setting, practice and feedback for effective motor learning/acquisition of skills that have been discussed.

Questions to Consider

The authors suggest that readers consider the following strategies and questions to guide their planning.

Functional Considerations

- What tasks or activities are most appropriate or important to address in developing a physical therapy plan of care for the individual described in the case? (Prioritize three or four tasks to be targeted by physical therapy intervention.)
- How can the therapist incorporate the goals and priorities of the person into the development of goals and plan of care?

Motor Control Considerations

- What resources/buffers and impairments/constraints does this individual bring to the situation? In what ways are these helpful or constraining, given the person's neuromotor and musculoskeletal condition, cognitive and emotional status, and level of fitness?
- What is the nature of the tasks that have been selected (stability, mobility, or quasimobility with or without object manipulation)? What are the foundational skills necessary to perform the task? What skills or abilities may be difficult, given the impairments/constraints described in the case?
- Under what environmental conditions would this individual be best able to function at this time (closed/predictable versus open/variable)? In what type of environment does this individual need to be able to eventually function? How might you manipulate activities and environmental conditions to achieve function in the real environment?
- What is the emotional context of the environment? Can you manipulate the emotional context to facilitate better learning conditions? Does your patient require more "emotional press" to problem solve with you on the task? Does your patient require a stressful environmental context to be reduced in order to have an appropriate ready-to-learn context?
- How might you organize/prioritize a sequence of activities, using the modified Gentile's Taxonomy of Movement Tasks (Stability/Transitional/Mobility), to prepare or progress the individual toward safe independent function in the least restrictive environment?

Motor Learning Issues

Identify the purpose of the task trials that will be designed by the therapist:

- Is this a task that needs to be acquired (or reacquired postamputation or post-incidence) or is this a task that needs to be refined?
- In what stage of motor learning is the individual as related to the above defined task?
- Does the individual have an understanding or familiarity with the task, or is it completely novel?
- Is current task performance sufficient for the task to be functional?
- Is performance efficient or optimal?

- Is performance automated or variable? Can the individual use a variety of multiple motor strategies to accomplish or address this task?
- Can the person respond to changing environmental variables or task demands that warrant adaptability in performance?
- Can this task be broken into discrete parts? Would it be better to practice the task as a whole? Why or why not?
- Is performance of a particular part of the task problematic (mechanics of the task, fluidity between the components of the task)?
- Is performance of the task as a whole problematic (completion, speed, endurance)?

On the basis of your thoughts about the task trials, identify the best practice conditions for achieving the desired outcome:

- Is the primary goal of practice *retention* of motor behavior across practice sessions or *improving performance* within a practice session?
- Which practice condition or combination of practice conditions (blocked, random, or serial; massed or distributed; part- or whole-task training) would you use to assist retention of the skill? Why have you chosen these strategies?
- Which practice condition or combination of practice conditions (blocked, random, or serial; massed or distributed; part- or whole-task training) would assist improved performance? Why have you chosen these strategies?
- How might contextual interference influence the learning process?
- What type of augmented information should be included during practice of the tasks to achieve the desired outcome?
- What modes of information should be used for this individual (visual cues and demonstration, verbal prompting, physical prompt/facilitation)? Why has this augmented information strategy or combination of strategies been selected?
- What effect will the information have on the client's ability to recognize errors and self-correct motor behavior?
- What delivery scheme (KR or KP) should be used to provide augmented feedback?
- What is the anticipated effect of the selected delivery scheme (KR or KP) on retention versus performance of the motor skill being targeted?
- Can visual imagery or mental practice enhance the performance? What images would a rehabilitation professional want the client to visualize? What effect will imagery have on performance and on retention of the motor skill?
- What components can the client practice mentally? What effect will mental practice have on performance and on retention of the motor skill?
- How can the therapist incorporate understanding of neural plasticity into goal-directed activity and intervention?

What aspects of the task are most vulnerable to degradation associated with learned non-use?

- How do activities and tasks included in the plan of care solidify the desired neuroplastic changes to enhance recovery of function?

- Are the activities and tasks included in the plan of care sufficient in repetition and intensity to influence neural plasticity?
- What evidence is available to guide decisions about potential windows of opportunity to time intervention for optimal neuroplastic effect in patients with similar diagnoses?
- Are the activities and tasks included in the plan of care important (salient) and meaningful to the patient, so that both experience- and motor learning–related neural plasticity is likely to occur?
- How should the plan of care be influenced by the age of the patient, in terms of facilitation of motor learning and neural plasticity?
- What additional medical interventions, environmental conditions, or principles of exercise can potentiate motor learning and neural plasticity for recovery of function?
- Are there other factors or activities that may interfere with effective motor learning and neural plasticity for recovery of function? How might the plan of care be modified to reduce the influence of these interfering factors?

SUMMARY

This chapter explores the concepts that shape current understanding of human motor control, focusing on the dynamic and adaptive characteristics of the body as a biological system. Rehabilitation professionals use their understanding of (1) an individual's resources and characteristics, (2) environmental conditions, and (3) the nature and constraints of functional tasks to develop appropriate interventions aimed at improving or adapting individuals' abilities to move effectively, in ways that are safe and efficient, to accomplish what is important for them to do.

The chapter also considers the process of motor learning, the ways in which individuals come to understand and approach a novel task or adapt a familiar task in differing environmental conditions or following injury or illness that changes personal resources. Using their understanding of the stages of motor learning, the purpose of augmented information, types and timing of feedback/feedforward information, and types of practice conditions and other factors that enhance motor learning, physical therapists and other rehabilitation professionals can construct interventions that will effectively enhance retention of motor learning or refine performance for persons with movement dysfunction.

The chapter concludes with a discussion of the emerging field of neuroplasticity, which links recovery of motor control and motor learning, considering rehabilitation as a mechanism to trigger neural plasticity and recovery of function after insult or injury to the CNS. As understanding of neuroplasticity grows, rehabilitation professionals must reevaluate whether the interventions designed to enhance motor learning are sufficient to also drive neural plasticity and recovery of function for persons recovering from events and diseases that impact the structure and function of the brain.

Adult with Right Hemiparesis Who Is Learning to Use an Ankle-Foot Orthosis and Ambulatory Assistive Device

A. F. is a slightly obese 78-year-old African-American woman with a history of type 2 diabetes mellitus who had an ischemic stroke of the L middle cerebral artery 3 weeks ago. A computed tomography scan revealed a lacunar-shaped infarct from an embolic occlusion of a deep branch of the middle cerebral artery serving the internal capsule. A. F. was recently transferred to a skilled nursing facility for rehabilitation, particularly to address transfers and ambulation. She had just received a prefabricated solid ankle AFO before her arrival. She says that the brace is intended to help control her "bad knee" and "lazy foot" position so she can walk better. She has not had much opportunity to use the orthosis and is concerned that it may actually make it more difficult for her to walk. She indicates that she prefers to use a rolling walker, although her therapist in the hospital insisted she use a straight cane.

Chart review, interview, and physical therapy examination reveal the following:

- *Psychosocial*: A. F. lives alone in a two-story walk-up apartment. Her immediate family lives out of state. She retired 10 years ago from a position as a legal secretary and is heavily involved in the outreach ministry of her evangelical church.
- *Baseline vital signs*: heart rate: 82 beats per minute; blood pressure: 132/94 mmHg; respiratory rate: 16 breaths per minute.
- *Cognitive status*: alert and oriented times 3.
- *Communication*: some slurring of words; has trouble finding the words she wants to say, but comprehension appears intact.
- *Vision*: intact; typically wears trifocals.
- *Sensory system*: cranial nerves intact, normal responses to light touch, pin prick, proprioception all extremities.
- *Neuromotor status*:
  - *Tone*: moderate spasticity of right (R) upper extremity (UE) and lower extremity (LE); 1+ on the Modified Ashworth Scale.
  - *Range of motion (ROM)*: Passive ROM within normal limits for all extremities.
  - *Strength*: L extremities 4+/5 throughout.
  - *R UE*: shoulder elevation 2+/5; hand grip 2/5; elbow flexion 2/5; *R LE*: function strength grades include ankle pf 3/5; ankle dorsiflexion 1/5; knee extension 2+/5; knee flexion 3/5; hip flexion 3/5; hip extension 3/5; hip abduction 3/5; and hip adduction 3+/5.
  - *Postural control*: able to sit upright against gravity, asymmetrical weight distribution with more weight borne on left side. Anticipatory posture changes are adequate when reaching toward right, inadequate when reaching toward left. Stands with supervision; requires verbal and tactile cues to bear weight on R LE.

Continued

- *Functional activities*: rolls independently to both sides; supine to sit over edge of bed with supervision; transfers from bed to wheelchair with supervision; sit to stand transitions with supervision.
- *Ambulation*: uses straight cane with moderate assist, requiring both verbal cueing and physical prompt to improve loading response on right leg and to minimize genu recurvatum during forward advancement over right foot.

Design a physical therapy plan of care that will focus on development of motor skills necessary for safe and efficient locomotion using the AFO and straight cane.

CASE EXAMPLE 2

Child with Cerebral Palsy Who Has Just Received New (Bilateral) Articulating Ankle-Foot Orthoses

---

T. D. is a delightful 2½-year-old-boy with cerebral palsy with moderate severity spastic diplegia. He was born prematurely at 27 weeks' gestation and remained in the neonatal intensive care unit for 10 weeks. By the time he was 18 months old, there were increasing indications of developmental delay and abnormal motor control. He currently attends an early intervention program (EIP), receives individual home visits from a physical therapist, and attends a therapeutic play group run by an educator and occupational therapist weekly.

EIP examination findings include the following:

- *Social*: T. D. lives with both parents and an older brother in a two-story, single-family home. He interacts well with his family members and is on target for social development. He plays side by side with peers and occasionally interacts with them appropriately.
- *Cognition*: T. D. scores age appropriately for cognitive tasks including cause and effect, object permanence, means to end, early numeration, and sorting by categories. His play with objects includes variety and imagination.
- *Language*: T. D.'s comprehension, expression, and pragmatic use of language are on target for his age. He has an extensive vocabulary and uses language appropriately in various situations.
- *Fine motor/ADLs*: T. D.'s reach, grasp, and release skills are within the age-expected range. Bimanual skills and object manipulation are also on target. Feeding skills are appropriate; T. D. uses utensils and drinks from a cup as expected for his age. His dressing skills are slightly below age expectations largely due to balance concerns in standing for putting on pants.
- *Gross motor*: T. D.'s gross motor skills fall below age expectations. He has been walking independently with bilateral solid ankle-foot orthoses (AFOs) for 6 months. He can walk on multiple terrains including tile or wood floors, carpets, grass, asphalt, and woodchips. He has

some difficulty with stairs, requiring a railing or one hand held. Tripping and falling are issues with increasing speeds during ambulation and with attempts at running. T. D.'s mother is most concerned about his safety in ambulation at this point.

T. D. was having increasing difficulty with squatting and transitions into and out of standing from the floor. When discussing the problem, the rehabilitation team decided that articulating AFOs would increase the availability of ankle range of motion for these transition tasks. T. D. just received bilateral articulating AFOs with a plantar flexion stop set at 10 degrees. He is currently having trouble descending stairs in the new orthoses, refusing to go down stairs unless both hands are held. He also has increased frequency of tripping outside while ambulating on the grass and rock driveway at home.

Design a physical therapy plan of care to help him master locomotion and transitional activities with the less-constraining articulating AFOs in the environments of a typical 2½-year-old.

CASE EXAMPLE 3

Child with Congenital Upper Limb Deficiency Learning to Use a Myoelectric Prosthesis

---

T. L. is a 3-year-old girl who has had a congenital right upper extremity limb deficiency since birth. She has an intact humerus and musculature of the upper limb with a functional elbow joint. Her forearm is incomplete with a shortened ulna, missing radius, and no wrist or hand complex. T. L. has been wearing a prosthesis with a passive terminal device since she was 6 months old and uses her prosthesis well in mobility tasks and to stabilize objects against her body or a support surface during bimanual activities. T. L. began a preschool program 2 months ago and has adjusted well to socialization. She engages in play with her peers appropriately. She has good functional use of her left upper extremity (intact limb) and uses the residual limb to assist herself in tasks, particularly for stabilizing objects.

T. L. has been working with her prosthetist and therapists to learn to use a two-channel (voluntary closing/ voluntary opening) myoelectrically controlled terminal device for the past 2 weeks. When she wears the myoelectric prosthesis throughout the day, she primarily uses it as she did her previous passive prosthesis. She has not attempted to use the "hand" for play or ADLs unless prompted by her parents or therapists. During her therapy sessions, she is intrigued with her new ability to open and close her "hand" but is inconsistent in controlling force of grasp and has difficulty initiating release. In today's session, she practiced picking up 1-inch blocks and placing them in a bowl, achieving the desired result in two of five trials. She was unsuccessful (and became frustrated) at picking up pegs that were much narrower than the blocks. The rehabilitation team's goals for T. L. include functional use of the prosthesis for grasp and release of household objects for feeding and self-care and school objects for play and participation in preschool activities. The team would like to increase the use of bimanual manipulation of various-sized objects.

Design a rehabilitation plan of care to help T. L. master grasp and release of objects of various sizes and levels of durability in activities meaningful for a 3-year-old child.

CASE EXAMPLE 4

Adolescent with Transtibial Amputation Working on Returning to Competition in Track Events

W. P. is a 16-year-old junior in high school who has been a star track athlete since he was a freshman. He currently holds his high school records in the 100-meter and 200-meter events, which he achieved during his sophomore year. He also finished third in the state championships that same year.

Three months ago during the summer, W. P. was seriously injured when the garden tractor/lawnmower he was operating rolled over and down an embankment as he was making a fast turn while mowing the lawn. He sustained deep lacerations to his right foot and lower leg from the mower's blade, as well as third-degree burns from the muffler. His injured limb was pinned under the tractor in a pile of leaves and debris. In the emergency department, trauma surgeons thought he did not meet criteria for limb salvage and performed a long, open transtibial amputation. After an intensive course of antibiotics, W. P. returned to the operating room 1 week later for closure to the standard transtibial level, with equal anterior/posterior flaps. When his residual limb healed without difficulty, W. P. was fit with a patellar tendon–bearing prosthesis, with a sleeve and pin suspension, and a Seattle Systems, Inc., dynamic response foot. He quickly mastered ambulation without an assistive device and returned to school in the winter of his junior year.

W. P. is eager to return to track for his senior year. His prosthetist has fabricated a special prosthesis for him to wear in competition, an Otto Bock Healthcare Sprinter prosthetic foot designed for track and field athletes. He has begun training for his events and is pleased that he can run again. He has two goals: to decrease his performance time (hoping to meet the records he set last year) and to become much more efficient at leaving the starting block. He wants to master the new prosthesis this year so he can concentrate on conditioning for his senior year.

Develop a prosthetic training regimen focusing on improving his performance as he prepares to return to track competition.

REFERENCES

1. *Who are physical therapists? Guide to Physical Therapist Practice.* Alexandria, VA: American Physical Therapy Association. http://guidetoptpractice.apta.org.htt.
2. *Towards a Common Language for Functioning, Disability and Health: ICF The International Classification of Functioning, Disability and Health.* WHO/EIP/GPE/CAS/01. Geneva: World Health Organization; 2002.
3. Jette AM. Toward a common language of disablement. *J Gerontol A Biol Sci Med Sci.* 2009;64A(11):1165–1168.
4. Shumway-Cook A, Woollacott MH. Motor control: issues and theories. In: Shumway-Cook A, Woollacott MH, eds. *Motor Control: Translating Research into Clinical Practice.* 4th ed. Philadelphia: Wolters Kluwer Lippincott Williams & Wilkins; 2012:3–20.
5. Mastos M, Miller K, Eliasson AC, Imms C. Goal-directed training: linking theories of treatment to clinical practice for improved functional activities in daily life. *Clin Rehabil.* 2007;21(1):47–55.
6. Davids K, Glazier P. Deconstructing neurobiological coordination: the role of the biomechanics-motor control nexus. *Exerc Sport Sci Rev.* 2010;38(2):86–90.
7. Welsh TN, Elliott D. The effects of response priming on the planning and execution of goal-directed movements in the presence of a distracting stimulus. *Acta Psychol (Amst).* 2005;11(2):123–142.
8. Cornus S, Laurent M, Laborie S. Perception-movement coupling in the regulation of step lengths when approaching an obstacle. *Ecological Psychol.* 2009;21(4):334–367.
9. Chow JY, Davids K, Button C, Rein R. Dynamics of movement patterning in learning a discrete multi-articular action. *Motor Control.* 2008;12(3):219–240.
10. Sahrmann SA. *Diagnosis and Treatment of Movement Impairment Syndromes.* St. Louis: Mosby; 2002.
11. Shumway-Cook A, Woollacott MH. Constraints on motor control, an overview of neurological function. In: Shumway-Cook A, Woollacott MH, eds. *Motor Control: Translating Research into Clinical Practice.* 4th ed. Philadelphia: Wolters Kluwer Lippincott Williams & Wilkins; 2012:104–140.
12. Schenkman M, Deutsch JE, Gill-Body KM. An integrated framework for decision making in neurologic physical therapist practice. *Phys Ther.* 2006;86(12):1681–1702.
13. Mueller MJ, Maluf KS. Tissue adaptation to physical stress: a proposed "physical stress theory" to guide physical therapist practice. *Phys Ther.* 2002;82(4):383–403.
14. Pavlik AJ. The effect of long-term ankle-foot orthosis use on gait in the post-stroke population. *J Prosthet Orthot.* 2008;20(2):49–52.
15. Keenan MA. The management of spastic equinovarus deformity following stroke and head injury. *Foot Ankle Clin.* 2011;16(3):499–514.
16. Patsika G, Kellis E, Amiridis IG. Neuromuscular efficiency during sit to stand movement in women with knee osteoarthritis. *J Electromyogr Kinesiol.* 2011;21(5):689–694.
17. Christiansen CL, Stevens-Lapsley JE. Weight-bearing asymmetry in relation to measures of impairment and functional mobility for people with knee osteoarthritis. *Arch Phys Med Rehabil.* 2010;91(10):1524–1528.
18. Rutherford DJ, Hubley-Kozey CL, Stanish WD, Dunbar MJ. Neuromuscular alterations exist with knee osteoarthritis presence and severity despite walking velocity similarities. *Clin Biomech (Bristol, Avon).* 2011;26(4):377–383.

19. Shum GL, Crosbie J, Lee RYW. Effect of low back pain on the kinematics and joint coordination of the lumbar spine and hip during sit-to-stand and stand-to-sit. *Spine.* 2005;30(17):1998–2004.

20. Seay JF, Van Emmerik RE, Hamill J. Low back pain status affects pelvis-trunk coordination and variability during walking and running. *Clin Biomech (Bristol, Avon).* 2011;26(6):572–578.

21. Dunlop DD, Semanik P, Song J, et al. Risk factors for functional decline in older adults with arthritis. *Arthritis Rheum.* 2005;52(4):1274–1282.

22. Duque I, Parra JH, Duvallet A. Maximal aerobic power in patients with chronic low back pain: a comparison with healthy subjects. *Eur Spine J.* 2011;20(1):87–93.

23. Topinkova E. Aging, disability and frailty. *Ann Nutr Metab.* 2008;52(Suppl 1):6–11.

24. Michael K, Macko RF. Ambulatory activity intensity profiles, fitness, and fatigue in chronic stroke. *Top Stroke Rehabil.* 2007;14(2):5–12.

25. Dekker J, van Dijk GM, Veenhof C. Risk factors for functional decline in osteoarthritis of the hip or knee. *Curr Opin Rheumatol.* 2009;21(5):520–524.

26. Gill TM, Allore H, Guo Z. Restricted activity and functional decline among community-living older adults. *Arch Intern Med.* 2003;163(11):1317–1322.

27. Clark L, White P. The role of deconditioning and therapeutic exercise in chronic fatigue syndrome. *J Mental Health.* 2005;14(3):237–252.

28. Duque I, Parra JH, Duvallet A. Physical deconditioning in chronic low back pain. *J Rehabil Med.* 2009;41(4):262–266.

29. Gaxatte C, Nguyen T, Chourabi F, et al. Fear of falling as seen in the Multidisciplinary falls consultation. *Ann Phys Rehabil Med.* 2011;54(4):248–258.

30. Boyd R, Stevens JA. Falls and fear of falling: burden, beliefs and behaviors. *Age Ageing.* 2009;38(4):423–428.

31. American Physical Therapy Association. What are interventions? In: *Guide to Physical Therapist Practice.* Alexandria, VA: APTA. http://guidetoptpractice.apta.org/content/1/SEC6.

32. Thompson WR, Gordon NF, Pescatello LC, eds. *ACSM's Guidelines for Exercise Testing and Prescription.* Philadelphia: Wolters Kluwer Lippincott Williams & Wilkins; 2009.

33. Ratamess NA, Alvar PA, Evetoch TK, et al. Progression models in resistance training for healthy adults. *Med Sci Sports Exerc.* 2009;41(3):687–708.

34. Durstine J, Moore GE, Painter PL, Roberts SO, eds. *ACSM's Exercise Management for Persons with Chronic Diseases and Disabilities.* 3rd ed. Champaign, IL: Human Kinetics; 2009.

35. May BJ, Lockard MA. *Prosthetics & Orthotics in Clinical Practice: A Case Study Approach.* Philadelphia: FA Davis; 2011.

36. Edelstein J, Moroz A. *Lower-Limb Prosthetics and Orthotics: Clinical Concepts.* Thorofare, NJ: Slack; 2010.

37. Plack M, Driscoll M. *Teaching and Learning in Physical Therapy: From Classroom to Clinic.* Thorofare, NJ: Slack; 2011.

38. Schmidt R, Lee T. Evolution of a field of study. In: *Motor Control and Learning: A Behavioral Emphasis.* 5th ed. Champaign, IL: Human Kinetics; 2011.

39. Shumway-Cook A, Woollacott M. A conceptual framework for clinical practice. In: *Motor Control: Theory and Practical Applications.* 4th ed. Philadelphia: Lippincott Williams & Wilkins; 2012:141–158.

40. Gentile A. Skill acquisition: action, movement, and neuromotor processes. In: Carr J, Shepherd R, Gordon J, eds. *Movement Science: Foundation for Physical Therapy in Rehabilitation.* Rockville, MD: Aspen Systems; 1987:115.

41. Lehto NK, Marley TL, Exekiel HJ, et al. Application of motor learning principles: the physiotherapy client as a problem solver. IV future directions. *Physiother Can.* 2001;53(2):109–114.

42. Papavasiliou AS. Management of motor problems in cerebral palsy: a critical update for the clinician. *Eur J Paediatr Neurol.* 2009;13(5):387–396.

43. Turvey MT, Fonseca S. Nature of motor control: perspectives and issues. *Adv Exp Med Biol.* 2009;629:93–123.

44. Nudo RJ. Neural bases of recovery after brain injury. *J Commun Disord.* 2011;44(5):515–520.

45. Hallett M. Neuroplasticity and rehabilitation. *J Rehabil Res Devel.* 2005;42(4):xvii–xxi.

46. Callahan J, Parlman K, Beninato M, Townsend E. Perspective: impact of the III Step Conference on Clinical Practice. *J Neurol Phys Ther.* 2006;30(3):157–166.

47. Davids K, Bennett S, Newell K. *Movement System Variability.* Champaign IL: Human Kinetics; 2006.

48. Warren WH. The dynamics of perception and action. *Psychol Rev.* 2006;113(2):358–389.

49. Davids K, Glazier P. Deconstructing neurobiological coordination: the role of the biomechanics-motor control nexus. *Exerc Sport Sci Rev.* 2010;38(2):86–90.

50. Mastos M, Miller K, Eliasson AC, Imms C. Goal-directed training: linking theories of treatment to clinical practice for improved functional activities in daily life. *Clin Rehabil.* 2007;21(1):47–55.

51. Levac D, DeMatteo C. Bridging the gap between theory and practice: dynamic systems theory as a framework for understanding and promoting recovery of function in children and youth with acquired brain injuries. *Physiother Theory Pract.* 2009;25(8):544–554.

52. Stergiou N, Harbourne RT, Cavanaugh JT. Optimal movement variability: a new theoretical perspective for neurologic physical therapy. *J Neurol Phys Ther.* 2006;30(3):120–129.

53. Gibson J. *The Ecological Approach to Visual Perception.* Mahwah, NJ: Erlbaum; 1986.

54. Vereijken B, Whiting H, Beek W. A dynamical systems approach to skill acquisition. *Q J Exp Psychol A.* 1992;45(2):323–344.

55. Gera G, Freitas S, Latash M, Monahan K, Schoner G, Scholz J. Motor abundance contributes to resolving multiple kinematic task constraints. *Motor Control.* 2010;14(1):83–115.

56. Latash ML, Gorniak S, Zatsiorsky VM. Hierarchies of synergies in human movements. *Kinesiology.* 2008;40(1):29–38.

57. Bernstein N. Essay II: On motor control. In: Latash M, Turvey M, eds. *Dexterity and Its Development.* Mahway, NJ: Erlbaum; 1996:25–44.

58. Warren WH. The dynamics of perception and action. *Psychol Rev.* 2006;113(2):358–389.

59. Fajen BR, Diaz G, Cramer C. Reconsidering the role of movement in perceiving action-scaled affordances. *Hum Mov Sci.* 2011;30(3):504–533.

60. Coello Y. Spatial context and visual perception for action. *Psicologica.* 2011;26(1):39–59.

61. Mainzer K. The emergence of mind and brain: an evolutionary, computational, and philosophical approach. *Prog Brain Res.* 2008;168:115–132.

62. Feldman AG, Goussev V, Lagole A, Levin MF. Threshold position control and the principle of minimal interaction in motor actions. *Prog Brain Res.* 2007;165:267–281.

63. Martin V, Scholz JP, Schoner G. Redundancy, self motion, and motor control. *Neural Comput.* 2009;21(5):1371–1414.

64. De Smet K, Segers V, Lenoir M, De Clercq D. Spatiotemporal characteristics of spontaneous overground walk-to-run transition. *Gait Posture*. 2009;29(1):54–58.

65. Latash ML, Levin MF, Scholz JP, Schoner G. Motor control theories and their applications. *Medicina*. 2010;46(4):382–392.

66. Kaoru T, Toshikatsu O. Neurobiological basis of controlling posture and locomotion. *Adv Robotics*. 2008;22(15):1629–1663.

67. Smith ER, Collins EC. Contextualizing person perception: distributed social cognition. *Psycholog Rev*. 2009;116(2):343–364.

68. Jahiel RI, Scherer MJ. Initial steps towards a theory and praxis of person-environment interaction in disability. *Disabil Rehabil*. 2010;32(17):1467–1474.

69. Mastos M, Miller K, Eliasson AC, Imms C. Goal-directed training: linking theories of treatment to clinical practice for improved functional activities in daily life. *Clin Rehabil*. 2007;21(1):47–55.

70. Baker KS, Mattingley JB, Chambers CD, Cunnington R. Attention and the readiness for action. *Neuropsychologia*. 2011;49(12):3303–3313.

71. Lam WK, Masters RS, Maxwell JP. Cognitive demands of error processing associated with preparation and execution of a motor skill. *Conscious Cogn*. 2010;19(4):1058–1061.

72. Pellecchia GL, Shockley K, Turvey MT. Concurrent cognitive task modulates coordination dynamics. *Cognitive Sci*. 2005;29(4):531–557.

73. Rueschemeyer SA, Pfeiffer C, Bekkering H. Body schematics: on the role of the body schema in embodied lexical-semantic representations. *Neuropsychologia*. 2010;48(3):774–781.

74. Corradi-Dell'Acqua C, Tomasino B, Fink GR. What is the position of an arm relative to the body? Neural correlates of body schema and body structural description. *J Neurosci*. 2009;29(13):4162–4171.

75. Kitagawa N, Spence C. Audiotactile multisensory interactions in human information processing. *Jpn Psychologic Res*. 2006;48(3):158–173.

76. Bernier PM, Grafton ST. Human posterior parietal cortex flexibly determines reference frames for reaching based on sensory context. *Neuron*. 2010;68(4):776–788.

77. Beurze SM, Toni I, Pisella L, Medendorp WP. Reference frames for reach planning in human parietofrontal cortex. *J Neurophysiol*. 2010;104(3):1736–1745.

78. Makoshi Z, Kroliczak G, van Donkelaar P. Human supplementary motor area contribution to predictive motor planning. *J Motor Behavior*. 2011;43(4):303–309.

79. Iseki K, Hanakawa T, Shinozaki J, Nankaku M, Fukuyama H. Neural mechanisms involved in mental imagery and observation of gait. *Neuroimage*. 2008;41(3):1021–1031.

80. Liuzzi G, Hörniss V, Hoppe J, et al. Distinct temporospatial interhemispheric interactions in the human primary and premotor cortex during movement preparation. *Cereb Cortex*. 2010;20(6):1323–1331.

81. Buch ER, Mars RB, Boorman ED, Rushworth MF. A network centered on ventral premotor cortex exerts both facilitatory and inhibitory control over primary motor cortex during action reprogramming. *J Neurosci*. 2010;30(4):1395–1401.

82. Wolfensteller U. Juggling with the brain—thought and action in the human motor system. *Prog Brain Res*. 2009;174:289–301.

83. Turner RS, Desmurget M. Basal ganglia contributions to motor control: a vigorous tutor. *Curr Opin Neurobiol*. 2010;20(6):704–716.

84. Kreitzer AC, Malenka RC. Striatal plasticity and basal ganglia circuit function. *Neuron*. 2008;60(4):543–554.

85. Pollok B, Gross J, Kamp D, Schnitzler A. Evidence for anticipatory motor control within a cerebello-diencephalic-parietal network. *J Cogn Neurosci*. 2008;20(5):828–840.

86. Manto M, Bastian AJ. Cerebellum and the deciphering of motor coding. *Cerebellum*. 2007;6(1):3–6.

87. Molinari M, Restuccia D, Leggio MG. State estimation, response prediction, and cerebellar sensory processing for behavioral control. *Cerebellum*. 2009;8(3):399–402.

88. Salmi J, Pallesen KJ, Neuvonen T. Cognitive and motor loops of the human cerebro-cerebellar system. *J Cogn Neurosci*. 2010;22(11):2663–2676.

89. Lemon RN. Descending pathways in motor control. *Annu Rev Neurosci*. 2008;31:195–218.

90. Petersen NC, Butler JE, Taylor JL, Gandevia SC. Probing the corticospinal link between the motor cortex and motoneurones: some neglected aspects of human motor cortical function. *Acta Physiol (Oxf)*. 2010;198(4):403–416.

91. Falla D, Farina D. Neural and muscular factors associated with motor impairment in neck pain. *Curr Rheumatol Rep*. 2007;9(6):497–502.

92. Gates D, Dingwell J. The effects of neuromuscular fatigue on task performance during repetitive goal-directed movements. *Exp Brain Res*. 2008;187(4):573–585.

93. Borghuis J, Hof AL, Lemmink KAP. The importance of sensory-motor control in providing core stability: implications for measurement and training. *Sports Med*. 2008;38(11):893–916.

94. Chern J, Lo C, Wu C, Chen C, Yang S, Tang F. Dynamic postural control during trunk bending and reaching in healthy adults and stroke patients. *Am J Phys Med Rehabil*. 2010;89(3):186–197.

95. Girolami GL, Shiratori T, Aruin AS. Anticipatory postural adjustments in children with typical motor development. *Exp Brain Res*. 2010;205(2):153–165.

96. Bigongiari A, de Andrade e Souza F, Franciulli PM, Neto SE, Araujo RC, Mochizuki L. Anticipatory and compensatory postural adjustments in sitting in children with cerebral palsy. *Hum Mov Sci*. 2011;309(3):648–657.

97. Alexander NB, Grunawalt JC, Carlos S, Augustine J. Bed mobility task performance in older adults. *J Rehabil Res Dev*. 2000;37(5):633–895.

98. Guarrera-Bowlby PL, Gentile AM. Form and variability during sit-to-stand transitions: children versus adults. *J Mot Behav*. 2004;36(1):104–114.

99. Ganea R, Paraschiv-Ionescu A, Büla C, Rochat S, Aminian K. Multi-parametric evaluation of sit-to-stand and stand-to-sit transitions in elderly people. *Med Eng Phys*. 2011;33(9):1086–1093.

100. Michel J, Grobet C, Dietz V, van Hedel HJ. Obstacle stepping in children: task acquisition and performance. *Gait Posture*. 2010;31(3):341–346.

101. Hicheur H, Quang-Cuong P, Arechavaleta G, Laumond JP, Berthoz A. The formation of trajectories during goal-oriented locomotion in humans. I. A stereotyped behavior. *Eur J Neurosci*. 2007;26(8):2376–2390.

102. Zietz D, Hollands M. Gaze behavior of young and older adults during stair walking. *J Mot Behav*. 2009;41(4):357–366.

103. Nagengast AJ, Braun DA, Wolpert DM. Optimal control predicts human performance on objects with internal degrees of freedom. *PLoS Comput Biol*. 2009;5(6):1–15.

104. Botvinick MM, Buxbaum LJ, Bylsma LM, Jax SA. Toward an integrated account of object and action selection: a computational analysis and empirical findings from reaching-to-grasp and tool-use. *Neuropsychologia*. 2009;47(3):671–683.

105. Puttemans V, Wenderoth N, Swinnen SP. Changes in brain activation during the acquisition of a multifrequency bimanual coordination task: from the cognitive stage to advanced levels of automaticity. *J Neurosci.* 2005;25(17):4270–4278.

106. Hemond C, Brown RM, Robertson EM. A distraction can impair or enhance motor performance. *J Neurosci.* 2010; 30(2):650–654.

107. Wulf G, Shea C, Lewthwaite R. Motor skill learning and performance: a review of influential factors. *Med Educ.* 2010; 44(1):75–84.

108. Wulf G, Tollner T, Shea CH. Attentional focus effects as a function of task difficulty. *Res Q Exerc Sport.* 2007;78(3): 257–264.

109. Ashford D, Bennett SJ, Davids K. Observational modeling effects for movement dynamics and movement outcome measures across differing task constraints: a meta-analysis. *J Mot Behav.* 2006;38(3):185–205.

110. Fulk GD, Schmitz TJ, Behrman AL. Traumatic spinal cord injury. In: O'Sullivan SB, Schmitz TJ, eds. *Physical Rehabilitation.* 5th ed. Philadelphia: FA Davis; 2007:937–996.

111. Boswell-Ruys CL, Harvey LA, Barker JJ, Ben M, Middleton JW, Lord SR. Training unsupported sitting in people with chronic spinal cord injuries: a randomized controlled trial. *Spinal Cord.* 2010;48(2):138–143.

112. Krause D, Wunnemann M, Erlmann A. Biodynamic feedback training to assure learning partial load bearing on forearm crutches. *Arch Phys Med Rehabil.* 2007;88(7):901–906.

113. Pasquini SM, Peterson ML, Rattansi SM, et al. The impact of assistive device prescription on gait following total knee replacement. *J Geriatr Phys Ther.* 2010;33(2):64–70.

114. Richardson JK, Thies SB, DeMott TK, Ashton-Miller JA. Gait analysis in a challenging environment differentiates between fallers and nonfallers among older patients with peripheral neuropathy. *Arch Phys Med Rehabil.* 2005;86(8):1539–1544.

115. Shumway-Cook A, Patla AE, Stewart A, Ferrucci L, Ciol MA, Guralnik JM. Environmental demands associated with community mobility in older adults with and without mobility disabilities. *Phys Ther.* 2002;82(7):670–681.

116. Tieman B, Palisano RJ, Gracely EJ, Rosenbaum PL. Variability in mobility of children with cerebral palsy. *Pediatr Phys Ther.* 2007;19(3):180–187.

117. Psychosocial aspects of adaptation and adjustment during various phases of neurological disability. In: Umphred DA, ed. *Neurological Rehabilitation.* 5th ed. St. Louis: Mosby; 2007:119–148.

118. Dickinson HO, Colver A. Quantifying the physical, social and attitudinal environment of children with cerebral palsy. *Disabil Rehabil.* 2011;33(1):36–50.

119. Kimberley TJ, Samargia S, Moore LG, Shakya JK, Lang CE. Comparison of amounts and types of practice during rehabilitation for traumatic brain injury and stroke. *J Rehabil Res Dev.* 2010;47(9):851–861.

120. Musselman KE, Fouad K, Misiaszek JE, Yang JF. Training of walking skills overground and on the treadmill: case series on individuals with incomplete spinal cord injury. *Phys Ther.* 2009;89(6):601–616.

121. Kelly F, Nikopoulos CK, Brooks N, Harrington H. Facilitating independence in personal activities of daily living after a severe traumatic brain injury. *Int J Ther Rehabil.* 2010;17(9):474–482.

122. Winkler PA. Traumatic brain injury. In: Umphred DA, ed. *Neurological Rehabilitation.* 5th ed. St. Louis: Mosby; 2007:532–566.

123. Fulk GD. Traumatic brain injury. In: O'Sullivan SB, Schmitz TJ, eds. *Physical Rehabilitation.* 5th ed. Philadelphia: FA Davis; 2007:895–935.

124. Wolpert DM, Flanagan JR. Motor learning. *Curr Biol.* 2010; 20(11):467–472.

125. Borg G. Psychophysical scaling with applications in physical work and the perception of exertion. *Scand J Work Environ Health.* 1990;16(suppl 1):55–58.

126. Fritz S, Lusardi MM. Walking speed: the sixth vital sign. *J Geriatr Phys Ther.* 2009;32(2):2–5.

127. Podsiadlo D, Richardson S. The timed up and go: a test of functional mobility for frail elderly persons. *J Am Geriatr Soc.* 1991;39(2):142–148.

128. Schmidt RA, Lee TD. The learning process. In: Schmidt RA, Lee TD, eds. *Motor Control and Learning: A Behavioral Emphasis.* Champaign, IL: Human Kinetics; 2011:429–460.

129. Shumway-Cook A, Baldwin M, Pollissar NL, Gruber W. Predicting probability for falls in community-dwelling older adults. *Phys Ther.* 1997;77(8):812–819.

130. Guyatt GH, Sullivan MJ, Thompson PJ, et al. The 6-minute walk: a new measure of exercise capacity in patients with chronic heart failure. *Can Med Assoc J.* 1985;132(8):919–923.

131. Russell DJ, Rosenbaum PL, Avery LM, et al. *Gross Motor Functional Measure User's Manual.* London: MacKeith Press; 2002.

132. Shumway-Cook A, Woollacott MJ, eds. *Motor learning and recovery of function. In Motor Control: Translating Research into Clinical Practice.* 4th ed. Philadelphia: Wolters Kluwer Lippincott Williams & Wilkins; 2012:21–44.

133. Schmidt RA, Lee TD. Retention and transfer. In: Schmidt RA, Lee TD, eds. *Motor Control and Learning: A Behavioral Emphasis.* Champaign, IL: Human Kinetics; 2011:461–490.

134. Adams JA. Closed loop theory of motor learning. *J Mot Behav.* 1971;3(2):111–150.

135. Schmidt RA. A schema theory of discrete motor skill learning. *Psychol Rev.* 1975;82(4):225–260.

136. Schmidt RA, Lee TD, eds. *Motor Control and Learning: A Behavioral Emphasis.* 5th ed. Champaign, IL: Human Kinetics; 2011:327–346.

137. Shea CH, Wulf G. Schema theory: a critical appraisal and reevaluation. *J Mot Behav.* 2005;37(2):85–101.

138. Sherwood DE, Lee TD. Schema theory: critical review and implications for the role of cognition in a new theory of motor learning. *Res Q Exerc Sport.* 2003;74(4):376–382.

139. Hamilton ML, Pankey R, Kinnunen D. *Constraints of Motor Skill Acquisition: Implications for Teaching and Learning.* Available at: http://www.eric.ed.gov/contentdelivery/servlet/ERICServlet?accno=ED471196; 2002.

140. Newell KM. Motor skill acquisition. *Annu Rev Psychol.* 1991;42(1):213–237.

141. Chow JY, Davids K, Button C, Rein R, Hristovski R, Koh M. Dynamics of multi-articular coordination in neurobiological systems. *Nonlinear Dynamics Psychol Life Sci.* 2009;13(1):27–55.

142. Fitts PM, Posner MI. *Human Performance.* Belmont, CA: Brooks/Cole; 1967.

143. Vereijken B, van Emmerik REA, Whiting HTA, Newell KM. Freezing degress of freedom in skill acquisition. *J Mot Behav.* 1992;24(1):133–142.

144. Larin H. Motor learning: a practical framework for paediatric physiotherapy. *Physiother Theory Pract.* 1998;14(1):33–47.

145. Luft AR, Buitrago MM. Stages of motor skill learning. *Mol Neurobiol.* 2005;32(3):205–216.

146. Konczak J, vander Velden H, Jaeger L. Learning to play the violin: motor control by freezing, not freeing degrees of freedom. *J Mot Behav.* 2009;41(3):243–252.

147. Manoel E, Connolly K. Variability and the development of skilled action. *Int J Psychophysiol.* 1995;19(2):129–147.

148. Gentile A. Implicit and explicit processes during acquisition of functional skills. *Scand J Occup Ther.* 1998;5(1):7–16.

149. Caillou N, Nourrit D, Deschamps T, Lauriot B, Delignieres D. Overcoming spontaneous patterns of coordination during the acquisition of a complex balancing task. *Can J Exp Psychol.* 2002;56(4):283–293.

150. Coch D, Fischer KW, Dawson G, eds. *Human Behavior, Learning, and the Developing Brain: Typical Development.* New York: Guilford Publications; 2010.

151. Taubert M, Draganski B, Anwander A, et al. Dynamic properties of human brain structure: learning-related changes in cortical areas and associated fiber connections. *J Neurosci.* 2010;30(35):11670–11677.

152. May A. Experience-dependent structural plasticity in the adult human brain. *Trends Cogn Sci.* 2011;15(10):475–482.

153. van Merriënboer JJ, Sweller J. Cognitive load theory in health professional education: design principles and strategies. *Med Educ.* 2010;44(1):85–93.

154. Bastalbe S, Gramet P, Jacobs K, Sopczyk D. *Health Professional as Educator: Principles of Teaching and Learning.* Burlington, MA: Jones & Bartlett; 2010.

155. Shumway-Cook A, Woollacott MH. Physiological basis of motor control and recovery of function. In: Shumway-Cook A, Woollacott MH, eds. *Motor Control: Translating Research into Clinical Practice.* 4th ed. Philadelphia: Wolters Kluwer Lippincott Williams & Wilkins; 2012:83–103.

156. Park J, Kim Y, Jang SH, Chang WH, Park C, Kim ST. Dynamic changes in the cortico-subcortical network during early motor learning. *Neuro Rehabil.* 2010;26(2):95–103.

157. Seger CA. The basal ganglia in human learning. *Neuroscientist.* 2006;12(4):285–290.

158. Saywell N, Taylor D. The role of the cerebellum in procedural learning—are there implications for physiotherapists' clinical practice? *Physiother Theory Pract.* 2008;24(5):321–328.

159. Rose M, Haider H, Salari N, Büchel C. Functional dissociation of hippocampal mechanism during implicit learning based on the domain of associations. *J Neurosci.* 2011;31(39):13739–13745.

160. Sweatt JD. *Mechanisms of Memory.* 2nd ed. Burlington, MA: Academic Press; 2010.

161. Kandel ER. Cellular mechanism of learning and the biological basis of individuality. In: Kandel ER, Schwart JH, Jessell TM, eds. *Principles of Neural Science.* 4th ed. New York: McGraw-Hill Medical; 2000:1247–1279.

162. Degonda N, Mondadori CR, Bosshardt S, et al. Implicit associative learning engages the hippocampus and interacts with explicit associative learning. *Neuron.* 2005;46(3):505–520.

163. Sun R, Zhang X, Slusarz P, Mathews R. The interaction of implicit learning, explicit hypothesis testing learning and implicit-to-explicit knowledge extraction. *Neural Netw.* 2007; 20(1):34–47.

164. Vidoni ED, Boyd LA. Achieving enlightenment: what do we know about the implicit learning system and its interaction with explicit knowledge? *J Neurol Phys Ther.* 2007;31(3):145–154.

165. Milton JG, Small SS, Solodkin A. On the way to automatic; dynamic aspects in the development of expertise. *J Clin Neurophysiol.* 2004;21(3):134–143.

166. Poldrack RA, Saab FW, Foerde K, et al. Neural correlates of motor skill automaticity. *J Neurosci.* 2005;25(22):5356–5364.

167. Wu T, Hallett M. The influence of normal human aging on automatic movements. *J Physiol.* 2005;526(2):605–615.

168. Verwey W, Abrahamse E, Ruitenberg M, Jiménez L, Kleine E. Motor skill learning in the middle-aged: limited development of motor chunks and explicit sequence knowledge. *Psychol Res.* 2011;75(5):406–422.

169. Fraser SA, Li KZ, Penhune VB. A comparison of motor skill learning and retention in younger and older adults. *Exp Brain Res.* 2009;195(3):419–427.

170. Nemeth D, Janacsek K. The dynamics of implicit skill consolidation in young and elderly adults. *J Gerontol B Psychol Sci Soc Sci.* 2011;66(1):15–22.

171. Shea CH, Park JH, Braden HW. Age-related effects in sequential motor learning. *Phys Ther.* 2006;86(4):478–488.

172. Wulf G, Chiviacowsky S, Lewthwaite R. Altering mindset can enhance motor learning in older adults. *Psychol Aging.* 2011; Advance online publication. doi:10.1037/a0025718.

173. Badami R, Vaez M, Wulf G, Namazizadeh M. Feedback after good trials enhances intrinsic motivation. *Res Q Exerc Sport.* 2011;82(2):360–364.

174. Schmidt RA, Lee TD. Conditions of practice. In: Schmidt RA, Lee TD, eds. *Motor Control and Motor Learning.* 5th ed. Champaign, IL: Human Kinetics; 2011:347–392.

175. Stergiou N, Harbourne RT, Cavanaugh JT. Optimal movement variability: a new theoretical perspective for neurologic physical therapy. *J Neurol Phys Ther.* 2006;30(3):120–129.

176. Fetters L. Perspective on variability in the development of human action. *Phys Ther.* 2010;90(12):1860–1867.

177. Turvey MT. Action and perception at the level of synergies. *Hum Mov Sci.* 2007;26(4):657–697.

178. Sparrow WA, Shinkfield AJ, Day RH, Hollitt S, Jolley D. Visual perception of movement kinematics and the acquisition of "action prototypes". *Motor Control.* 2002;6(2):146–165.

179. Hadders-Algra M. Variation and variability: key words in human motor development. *Phys Ther.* 2010;90(12):1823–1837.

180. Fetters L, Ellis T. A perception-action framework for physical therapy for persons with neurological dysfunction: use of therapeutic affordance and unit less ratio. *J Neurol Phys Ther.* 2006;30(3):142–147.

181. Dimitrova D, Horak FB, Nutt JG. Postural muscle responses to multidirectional translations in patients with Parkinson's disease. *J Neurophysiol.* 2004;91(1):489–501.

182. Sanger TD. Arm trajectories in dyskinetic cerebral palsy have increased random variability. *J Child Neurol.* 2006;21(7):551–557.

183. Sanger TD, Kaiser J, Placek B. Reaching movement in childhood dystonia contain signal-dependent noise. *J Child Neurol.* 2005;6:489–496.

184. Cowie D, Limousin P, Peters A, Day BL. Insights into the neural control of locomotion from walking through doorways in Parkinson's disease. *Neuropsychologia.* 2010;48(9):2750–2757.

185. Serino A, De Filippo L, Casavecchia C, Coccia M, Shiffrar M, Ladavas E. Lesions to the motor system affect action perception. *J Cogn Neurosci.* 2010;22(3):413–426.

186. Rengachary J, He BJ, Shulman GL, Corbetta M. A behavioral analysis of spatial neglect and its recovery after stroke. *Front Hum Neurosci.* 2011;5:29. www.frontiersin.org/human%20 neuroscience/10.3389/fnhum.2011.00029.

187. Kerkhoff G, Rossett Y, Pérennou D. Postural disorders and spatial neglect in stroke patients: a strong association. *Restor Neurol Neurosci.* 2006;24(4/6):319–334.

188. Pohl PS, McDowd JM, Filion D, Richards LG, Stiers W. Implicit learning of a motor skill after mild and moderate stroke. *Clin Rehabil.* 2006;20(3):246–253.

189. Barela JA, Focks GM, Hilgeholt T, Barela AM, Carvalho RP, Savelsbergh GJ. Perception-action and adaptation in postural control of children and adolescents with cerebral palsy. *Res Dev Disabil.* 2011;32(6):2075–2083.

190. Mulder T, Hochstenbach J. Adaptability and flexibility of the human motor system: implications for neurological rehabilitation. *Neural Plast.* 2001;8(1–2):131–140.

191. Fell DW. Progressing therapeutic intervention in patients with neuromuscular disorders: a framework to assist clinical decision making. *J Neurol Phys Ther.* 2004;28(1):35–46.

192. Kruisselbrink LD, Van Gyn GH. Task characteristics and the contextual interference effect. *Percept Mot Skills.* 2011;113(1):19–37.

193. Jarus T, Gutman T. Effects of cognitive processes and task complexity on acquisition, retention, and transfer of motor skills. *Can J Occup Ther.* 2001;68(5):280–289.

194. Pollock BJ, Lee TD. Dissociated contextual interference effects in children and adults. *Percept Mot Skills.* 1997;84(3):851–858.

195. Boutin A, Blandin Y. On the cognitive processes underlying contextual interference: Contributions of practice schedule, task similarity and amount of practice. *Hum Mov Sci.* 2010;29(6):910–920.

196. Porter JM, Magill RA. Systematically increasing contextual interference is beneficial for learning sport skills. *J Sports Sci.* 2010;28(12):1277–1285.

197. Cross ES, Schmitt PJ, Grafton ST. Neural substrates of contextual interference during motor learning support a model of active preparation. *J Cogn Neurosci.* 2007;19(11):1854–1871.

198. Kruiselbrink LD, Van Gyn GH. Task characteristics and the contextual interference effect. *Percept Mot Skills.* 2011;112(4):19–37.

199. Magnuson CE, Wright DL. Random practice can facilitate the learning of tasks that have different relative time structures. *Res Quart Ex Sport.* 2004;75(2):197–202.

200. Bock O, Thomas M, Grigorova V. The effect of rest breaks on human sensorimotor adaptation. *Exp Brain Res.* 2005; 163(2):258–260.

201. Lord SR, Murray SM, Chapman K, Munro B, Tiedemann A. Sit-to-stand performance depends on sensation, speed, balance, and psychological status in addition to strength in older people. *J Gerontol A Biol Sci Med Sci.* 2002;57(8):M539–M543.

202. Ayyappa E, Mohammed O. Clinical assessment of pathological gait. In: Lusardi MM, Nielsen CC, eds. *Orthotics and Prosthetics in Rehabilitation.* 2nd ed. St. Louis: Saunders// Elsevier; 2007:35–68.

203. Park JH, Wilde H, Shea CH. Part-whole practice of movement sequences. *J Motor Behav.* 2004;36(1):51–61.

204. Fontana FE, Furtado O, Mazzardo O, Gallagher JD. Whole and part practice: a meta-analysis. *Percept Mot Skills.* 2009;109(2): 517–530.

205. Schmidt R, Lee T. *Augmented feedback.* In *Motor Control and Learning: A Behavioral Emphasis.* 5th ed. Champaign, IL: Human Kinetics; 2011.

206. Viitasalo JT, Era P, Konttinen N, Mononen H, Mononen K, Norvapalo K. Effects of 12-week shooting training and mode of feedback on shooting scores among novice shooters. *Scand J Med Sci Sports.* 2001;11(6):362–368.

207. Thorpe DE, Valvano J. The effects of knowledge of performance and cognitive strategies on motor skill learning in children with cerebral palsy. *Pediatr Phys Ther.* 2002;14(1):2–15.

208. Butki BD, Hoffman SJ. Effects of reducing frequency of intrinsic knowledge of results on the learning of a motor skill. *Percept Mot Skills.* 2003;97(2):569–580.

209. Bruechert L, Lai Q, Shea CH. Reduced Knowledge of Results Frequency Enhances Error Detection. *Res Q Exerc Sport.* 2003;74(4):467–472.

210. Anderson DI, Sekiyam H, Magill RA, Ryan G. Support for an Explanation of the Guidance Effect in Motor Skill Learning. *J Mot Behav.* 2005;37(3):231–238.

211. Chiviacowsky S, Wulf G, Wally R. Knowledge of Results after Good Trials Enhances Learning in Older Adults. *Res Q Exerc Sport.* 2009;80(3):663–668.

212. Chiviacowsky S, Wulf G. Feedback after Good Trials Enhances Learning. *Res Q Exerc Sport.* 2007;78(2):40–47.

213. Anderson DI, Magill A, Sekia H. Motor learning as a function of KR schedule and characteristics of task-intrinsic feedback. *J Mot Behav.* 2001;33(1):59–66.

214. Subramanian SK, Massie CL, Malcolm MP, Levin MF. Does provision of extrinsic feedback result in improved motor learning in the upper limb post stroke? A systematic review of the evidence. *Neurorehabil Neural Repair.* 2010;24(2):113–124.

215. Onla-or S, Winstein CJ. Determining the optimal challenge point for motor skill learning in adults with moderately severe Parkinson's disease. *Neurorehabil Neural Repair.* 2008;22(4):385–395.

216. Hemayattalab R, Rostami LR. Effects of frequency of feedback on the learning of motor skill in individuals with cerebral palsy. *Res Dev Disabil.* 2010;31(1):212–217.

217. Rice MS, Hernandez HG. Frequency of knowledge of results and motor learning in persons with developmental delay. *Occup Ther Int.* 2006;13(1):35–48.

218. Rice MS, Fertig PA, Maitra KK, Miller BK. Reduced feedback: motor learning strategy in persons with Alzheimer's disease. *Phys Occup Ther Geriatr.* 2008;27(2):122–138.

219. van Halteren-van Tilborg IA, Scherder EJ, Hulstijn W. Motor-skill learning in Alzheimer's disease: a review with an eye to the clinical practice. *Neuropsychol Rev.* 2007;17(3):203–212.

220. Wulf G. Self-controlled practice enhances motor learning: implications for physiotherapy. *Physiother.* 2007;93(2):96–101.

221. Hansen S, Pfeiffer J, Patterson JT. Self-control of feedback during motor learning: accounting for the absolute amount of feedback using a yoked group with self-control over feedback. *J Mot Behav.* 2011;43(2):113–119.

222. Chiviacowsky S, Wulf G, de Medeiros FL. Research self-controlled feedback in 10-year-old children: higher feedback frequencies enhance learning. *Q Exerc Sport.* 2008;79(1):122–127.

223. Ronsse R, Puttemans V, Coxon JP, et al. Motor learning with augmented feedback: modality-dependent behavioral and neural consequences. *Cereb Cortex.* 2011;21(6):1283–1294.

224. Liu T, Jensen JL. Effectiveness of auditory and visual sensory feedback for children when learning a continuous motor task. *Percept Mot Skills.* 2009;109(3):804–816.

225. van Vliet PM, Wulf G. Extrinsic feedback for motor learning after stroke: what is the evidence? *Disabil Rehabil.* 2006;28(13–14): 831–840.

226. Piron L, Turolla A, Agostini M, et al. Motor learning principles for rehabilitation: a pilot randomized controlled study in post stroke patients. *Neurorehabil Neural Repair.* 2010;24(6):501–508.

227. Wulf G, Shea C, Lewthwaite R. Motor skill learning and performance: a review of influential factors. *Med Educ.* 2010;44(1):75–84.

228. Emanuel M, Jarus T, Bart O. Effect of focus of attention and age on motor acquisition, retention, and transfer: a randomized trial. *Phys Ther.* 2008;88(2):251–260.

229. Wulf G, Chiviacowsky S, Schiller E, Avila LT. Frequent external-focus feedback enhances motor learning. *Front Psychol.* 2010;1:190. http://frontiersin.org/Movement_Science_and Sport_Pschology/10.3389/fpsyg.2010.00190/full.

230. Chiviacowsky S, Wulf G, Wally R. An external focus of attention enhances balance learning in older adults. *Gait Posture.* 2010;32(4):572–575.

231. Wulf G, Chiviacowsky S, Lewthwaite R. Normative feedback effects on learning a timing task. *Res Q Exerc Sport.* 2010;81(4):425–431.

232. Lewthwaite R, Wulf G. Social-comparative feedback affects motor skill learning. *Q J Exp Psychol.* 2010;63(4):738–749.

233. Wulf G, Chiviacowsky S, Lewthwaite R. Altering mindset can enhance motor learning in older adults. *Psychol Aging.* 2011. Advance online publication. doi:10.1037/a0025718.

234. Mulder T. Motor imagery and action observation: cognitive tools for rehabilitation. *J Neural Transm.* 2007;114(10):1265–1278.

235. Lacourse MG, Turner JA, Randolph-Orr E, Schandler SL, Cohen MJ. Cerebral and cerebellar sensorimotor plasticity following motor imagery-based mental practice of a sequential movement. *J Rehabil Res Dev.* 2004;41(4):505–523.

236. Gentili R, Papaxanthis C, Pozzo T. Improvement and generalization of arm motor performance through motor imagery practice. *Neuroscience.* 2006;137(3):761–772.

237. Spittle M, Kremere P. Mental practice and the retention of motor learning; a pilot study. *Percept Mot Skills.* 2010;110(3):888–896.

238. Tunney N, Billings K, Blakely BG, Burch D, Hill M, Jackson K. Mental practice and motor learning of a functional motor task in older adults: a pilot study. *Phys Occ Ther Geriatr.* 2006;24(3):63–80.

239. Page SJ, Szaflarski JP, Eliassen JC, Pan H, Cramer SC. Cortical plasticity following motor skill learning during mental practice in stroke. *Neurorehabil Neural Repair.* 2009;23(4):382–388.

240. McEwen SE, Huijbregts MP, Ryan JD, Polatajko HJ. Cognitive strategy use to enhance motor skill acquisition post-stroke: A critical review. *Brain Inj.* 2009;23(4):263–277.

241. Diekelmann S, Born J. One memory, two ways to consolidate? *Nat Neurosci.* 2007;10(9):1085–1086.

242. Fischer S, Nitschke MF, Melchert UH, Erdmann C, Born J. Motor memory consolidation in sleep shapes more effective neuronal representations. *J Neurosci.* 2005;25(49):11248–11255.

243. Rickard TC, Cai DJ, Rieth CA, Jones J, Ard MC. Sleep does not enhance motor sequence learning. *J Exper Psychol Learning Memory Cognition.* 2008;34(4):834–842.

244. Sheth BR, Janvelyan D, Khan M. Practice makes imperfect: restorative effects of sleep on motor learning. *PLoS One.* 2008;3(9):e3190.

245. Debarnot U, Creveaux T, Collet C, et al. Sleep-related improvements in motor learning following mental practice. *Brain Cogn.* 2009;69(2):398–405.

246. Siengsukon CF, Boyd LA. Perspective. Does sleep promote motor learning? Implications for physical rehabilitation. *Phys Ther.* 2009;89(4):370–383.

247. Siengsukon CF, Boyd LA. Sleep enhances implicit motor skill learning in individuals post stroke. *Top Stroke Rehabil.* 2008;15(1):1–12.

248. Siengsukon CF, Boyd LA. Sleep to learn after stroke: Implicit and explicit off-line motor learning. *Neurosci Lett.* 2009;451(1):1–5.

249. Gzil F, Lefeve C, Cammelli M, Pachoud B, Ravaud JF, Leplege A. Why is rehabilitation not yet fully person-centered and should it be more person-centered? *Disabil Rehabil.* 2007;29(20/21):1616–1624.

250. Bloom LF, Lapierre NM, Wilson KG, Curran D, Deforge DA, Blackmer J. Concordance in goal setting between patients with multiple sclerosis and their rehabilitation team. *Am J Phys Med Rehabil.* 2006;85(10):807–813.

251. Cramer SC, Sur M, Dobkin BH, et al. Harnessing neuroplasticity for clinical applications. *Brain J Neurol.* 2011;134(6):1591–1609.

252. Kee YH, Liu. Effects of dispositional mindfulness on the self-controlled learning of a novel motor task. *Learning Individual Diff.* 2011;21(4):468–471.

253. Taylor RR. Extending client-centered practice: the use of participatory methods to empower clients. *Occup Ther Mental Health.* 2003;19(2):57–75.

254. Gauggel S, Fischer S. The effect of goal setting on motor performance and motor learning in brain-damaged patients. *Neuropsychol Rehabil.* 2001;11(1):33–44.

255. Eschenfelder VG. Shaping the goal setting process in OT: the role of meaningful occupation. *Phys Occup Ther Geriatr.* 2005;23(4):67–81.

256. Harty M, Griesel M, van der Merwe A. The ICF as a common language for rehabilitation goal-setting: comparing client and professional priorities. *Health Qual Life Outcomes.* 2011;9:87. http://www.hqlo.com/content/9/1/87.

257. Playford ED, Siegert R, Levack W, Freeman J. Areas of consensus and controversy about goal setting in rehabilitation: a conference report. *Clin Rehabil.* 2009;23(4):334–344.

258. Leach E, Cornwell P, Fleming J, Haines T. Patient centered goal-setting in a subacute rehabilitation setting. *Disabil Rehabil.* 2010;32(2):159–172.

259. Scobbie L, Dixon D, Wyke S. Goal setting and action planning in the rehabilitation setting: development of a theoretically informed practice framework. *Clin Rehabil.* 2011;25(5):468–482.

260. Scobbie L, Wyke S, Dixon D. Identifying and applying psychological theory to setting and achieving rehabilitation goals. *Clin Rehabil.* 2009;23(4):321–333.

261. Bovend'Eerdt TJ, Botell RE, Wade DT. Writing SMART rehabilitation goals and achieving goal attainment scaling: a practical guide. *Clin Rehabil.* 2009;23(4):352–361.

262. Löwing K, Bexelius A, Carlberg EB. Goal-directed functional therapy: a longitudinal study on gross motor function in children with cerebral palsy. *Disabil Rehabil.* 2010;32(11):908–916.

263. Löwing K, Bexelius A, Carlberg EB. Activity focused and goal directed therapy for children with cerebral palsy—do goals make a difference? *Disabil Rehabil.* 2009;31(22):1808–1816.

264. Spooren AI, Janssen-Potten YJ, Kerckhofs E, Bongers HM, Seelen HA. ToCUEST: a task-oriented client-centered training module to improve upper extremity skilled performance in cervical spinal cord-injured persons. *Spinal Cord.* 2011;49(10):1042–1048.

265. Laver K, Halbert J, Stewart M, Crotty M. Patient readiness and ability to set recovery goals during the first 6 months after stroke. *J Allied Health.* 2010;39(4):e149–e154.

266. Gustafsson L, McLaughlin K. An exploration of clients' goals during inpatient and outpatient stroke rehabilitation. *Int J Ther Rehabil.* 2009;16(6):324–330.

267. Levack WM, Siegert RJ, Dean SG, McPherson KM. Goal planning for adults with acquired brain injury: how clinicians talk about involving family. *Brain Inj.* 2009;23(3):192–202.

268. Hallett M. Guest editorial: neuroplasticity and rehabilitation. *J Rehabil Res Dev.* 2005;42(4):xvii–xxi.

269. Callahan J, Parlman K, Bennato M, Townsend E. Perspective: impact of the IIIStep Conference on clinical practice. *J Neurol Phys Ther.* 2006;30(3):157–166.

270. Kleim JA, Jones TA. Principles of experience-dependent neural plasticity: implications for rehabilitation after brain damage. *J Speech Lang Hear Res.* 2008;51(1):S225–S239.

271. Kleim JA. Neural plasticity and neurorehabilitation: teaching the new brain old tricks. *J Commun Disord.* 2011;44(5):521–528.

272. Landers M. Treatment-induced neuroplasticity following focal injury to the motor cortex. *Int J Rehabil Res.* 2004;27(1):1–5.

273. Wittenberg GF. Experience, cortical remapping, and recovery in brain disease. *Neurobiol Dis.* 2010;37(2):252–258.

274. Purton J, Golledge J. Establishing an effective quantity of physiotherapy after stroke: a discussion. *Int J Ther Rehabil.* 2007;14(7):318–323.

275. Teasell R, Bitensky J, Foley N, Bayona NA. Training and stimulation in post stroke recovery brain reorganization. *Top Stroke Rehabil.* 2005;12(3):37–45.

276. Damiano DL. Rehabilitative Therapies in Cerebral Palsy: The Good, the Not As Good, and the Possible. *J Child Neurol.* 2009;24(9):1200–1204.

277. Kolb B, Muhammad A, Gibb R. Searching for factors underlying cerebral plasticity in the normal and injured brain. *J Commun Disord.* 2011;44(5):503–514.

278. Cramer SC. Repairing the human brain after stroke; I. Mechanisms of spontaneous recovery. *Ann Neurol.* 2008; 63(3):272–287.

279. Oujamaa L, Relave I, Froger J, Mottet D, Pelissier JY. Rehabilitation of arm function after stroke. Literature review. *Ann Phys Rehabil Med.* 2009;52(3):269–293.

280. Carey JR, Bhatt E, Nagpal A. Neuroplasticity promoted by task complexity. *Exerc Sport Sci Rev.* 2005;33(1):24–31.

281. Kantak SS, Sullivan KJ, Fisher BE, Knowlton BJ, Winstein CJ. Neural substrates of motor memory consolidation depend on practice structure. *Nat Neurosci.* 2010;13(8):923–925.

282. Sunderland AT, Tuke A. Neuroplasticity, learning and recovery after stroke: a critical evaluation of constraint-induced therapy. *Neuropsychol Rehabil.* 2005;15(2):81–96.

283. Huang H, Fetters L, Hale J, McBride A. Bound for success: a systematic review of constraint-induced movement therapy in children with cerebral palsy supports improved arm and hand use. *Phys Ther.* 2009;89(11):1126–1141.

284. Hanson ED, Srivatsan SR, Agrawal S, et al. Effects of strength training on physical function: influence of power, strength, and body composition. *J Strength Cond Res.* 2009;23(9):2627–2637.

285. Kleim JA, Hogg TM, VandenBerg PM, Cooper NR, Bruneau R, Remple M. Cortical synaptogenesis and motor map reorganization occur during late but not early, phase of motor skill learning. *J Neurosci.* 2004;24(3):628–633.

286. DeFina P, Fellus J, Polito MZ, et al. The new neuroscience frontier: promoting neuroplasticity and brain repair in traumatic brain injury. *Clin Neuropsychol.* 2009;23(8):1391–1399.

287. Behrman AL, Bowden MG, Nair PM. Neuroplasticity after spinal cord injury and training: an emerging paradigm shift in rehabilitation and walking recovery. *Phys Ther.* 2006;86(10):1406–1425.

288. Nyberg L, Eriksson J, Larsson A, Marklund P. Learning by doing versus learning by thinking: an fMRI study of motor and mental training. *Neuropsychologia.* 2006;44(5):711–717.

289. Hubbard IJ, Parsons MW, Neilson C, Carey LM. Task-specific training: evidence for and translation to clinical practice. *Occup Ther Int.* 2009;16(3–4):175–189.

290. Sullivan KJ, Brown DA, Klassen T, et al. Effects of task-specific locomotor and strength training in adults who were ambulatory after stroke: results of the STEPS randomized clinical trial. *Phys Ther.* 2007;87(12):1580–1607.

291. Forrester LW, Wheaton LA, Luft AR. Exercise-mediated locomotor recovery and lower-limb neuroplasticity after stroke. *J Rehabil Res Dev.* 2008;45(2):205–220.

292. van Hedel HJ, Dietz V. Rehabilitation of locomotion after spinal cord injury. *Restor Neurol Neurosci.* 2010;28(1):123–134.

293. Byl NN, Pitsch EA, Abrams GM. Functional outcomes can vary by dose: learning-based sensorimotor training for patients stable post stroke. *Neurorehabil Neural Repair.* 2008;22(5):494–504.

294. Kimberley TJ, Samargia S, Moore LG, Shakya JK, Lang CE. Comparison of amounts and types of practice during rehabilitation for traumatic brain injury and stroke. *J Rehabil Res Dev.* 2010;47(9):851–861.

295. Kerr AL, Cheng SY, Jones TA. Experience-dependent neural plasticity in the adult damaged brain. *J Commun Disord.* 2011;44(5):538–548.

296. Cramer SC, Sur M, Dobkin BH, et al. Harnessing neuroplasticity for clinical applications. *Brain.* 2011;134(6):1591–1609.

297. Umphred DA, Hall M, West TM. The limbic system: influence over motor control and learning. In: Umphred DA, ed. *Neurological Rehabilitation.* 5th ed. St. Louis: Mosby Elsevier; 2007:71–118.

298. Min-Fang K, Grosch J, Fregni F, Paulus W, Nitsche MA. Focusing effect of acetylcholine on neuroplasticity in the human motor cortex. *J Neurosci.* 2007;27(52):14442–14447.

299. Anderson V, Spencer-Smith M, Wood A. Do children really recover better? Neurobehavioural plasticity after early brain insult. *Brain J Neurol.* 2011;134(8):2197–2221.

300. Landi D, Rossini PM. Cerebral restorative plasticity from normal ageing to brain diseases: a "never ending story". *Restor Neurol Neurosci.* 2010;28(3):349–366.

301. Heuninckx S, Wenderoth N, Swinnen SP. Systems neuroplasticity in the aging brain: recruiting additional neural resources for successful motor performance in elderly persons. *J Neurosci.* 2008;27(53):91–99.

302. Goh JO, Park DC. Neuroplasticity and cognitive aging: the scaffolding theory of aging and cognition. *Restor Neurol Neurosci.* 2009;27(5):391–403.

303. Kramer AF, Erickson KI. Capitalizing on cortical plasticity: influence of physical activity on cognition and brain function. *Trends Cogn Sci.* 2007;11(8):342–348.

304. Sullivan KJ, Kantak SS, Burtner PA. Motor learning in children: feedback effects on skill acquisition. *Phys Ther.* 2008;88(6):720–732.

305. Brosseau J, Potvin MJ, Rouleau I. Aging affects motor skill learning when the task requires inhibitory control. *Dev Neuropsychol.* 2007;32(1):597–613.

306. Boyd LA, Vidoni ED, Siengsukon CF. Multidimensional motor sequence learning is impaired in older but not younger or middle-aged adults. *Phys Ther.* 2008;88(3):351–362.

307. Bo J, Borza V, Seidler RD. Age-related declines in visuo-spatial working memory correlate with deficits in explicit motor sequence learning. *J Neurophysiol.* 2009;102(5):2744–2754.

308. Harvey RL. Improving post stroke recovery: neuroplasticity and task-oriented training. *Curr Treat Options Cardiovasc Med.* 2009;11(3):251–259.

309. Muir AL, Jones LM, Signal NE. Is neuroplasticity promoted by task complexity? *N Z J Physiother.* 2009;37(3):136–144.

310. Dimyan MA, Cohen LG. Neuroplasticity in the context of motor rehabilitation after stroke. *Nat Rev Neurol.* 2011;7(2):76–85.

311. Khedr EM, Abdel-Fadeil MR, Farghali A, Qaid M. Role of 1 and 3 Hz repetitive transcranial magnetic stimulation on motor function recovery after acute ischemic stroke. *Eur J Neurol.* 2009;16(12):1323–1330.

312. Khedr EM, Etraby AE, Hemeda M, Nasef AM, Razek AA. Long-term effect of repetitive transcranial magnetic stimulation on motor function recovery after acute ischemic stroke. *Acta Neurol Scand.* 2010;121(1):30–37.

313. Will B, Galani R, Kelche C, Rosenzweig MR. Recovery from brain injury in animals: relative efficacy of environmental enrichment, physical exercise, or formal training. *Prog Neurobiol.* 2004;72(3):167–182.

314. Knaepen K, Goekint M, Heyman EM, Meeusen R. Neuroplasticity—exercise-induced response of peripheral brain-derived neurotrophic factor: a systematic review of experimental studies in human subjects. *Sports Med.* 2010;40(9):765–801.

315. Bekinschtein P, Oomen CA, Saksida LM, Bussey TJ. Effects of environmental enrichment and voluntary exercise on neurogenesis, learning and memory, and pattern separation: BDNF as a critical variable? *Semin Cell Dev Biol.* 2011;22(5):536–542.

316. Bekinschtein P, Oomen CA, Saksida LM, Bussey TJ. Effects of environmental enrichment and voluntary exercise on neurogenesis, learning and memory, and pattern separation: BDNF as a critical variable? *Semin Cell Dev Biol.* 2011;22(5):536–542.

317. Celnik PA, Cohen GL. Modulation of motor function and cortical plasticity in health and disease. *Neurol Neurosci.* 2004;22(3–5):261–268.

318. Fregni F, Pascual-Leone A. Hand motor recovery after stroke: tuning the orchestra to improve hand motor function. *Cogn Behav Neurol.* 2006;19(1):21–33.

319. van Vliet PM, Heneghan NR. Motor control and the management of musculoskeletal dysfunction. *Man Ther.* 2006;11(3):208–213.

320. Langevin HM, Sherman KJ. Pathophysiological model for chronic low back pain integrating connective tissue and nervous system mechanisms. *Med Hypotheses.* 2007;68(1):74–80.

321. Boyd LA, Winstein CJ. Explicit information interferes with implicit motor learning of both continuous and discrete movement tasks after stroke. *J Neurol Phys Ther.* 2006;30(2):46–57.

322. Boyd LA, Winstein CJ. Impact of explicit information on implicit motor-sequence learning following middle cerebral artery stroke. *Phys Ther.* 2003;83(11):976–989.

323. Aberg KC, Herzog MH. Does perceptual learning suffer from retrograde interference? *PLoS One.* 2010;5(12):e14161.

324. Krakauer JW, Shadmehr R. Consolidation of motor memory. *Trends Neurosci.* 2006;29(1):58–64.

325. Knaepen K, Goekint M, Heyman EM, Meeusen R. Neuroplasticity—exercise-induced response of peripheral brain-derived neurotrophic factor: a systematic review of experimental studies in human subjects. *Sports Med.* 2010;40(9):765–801.

326. Michelini LC, Stern JE. Exercise-induced neuronal plasticity in central autonomic networks: role in cardiovascular control. *Exp Physiol.* 2009;94(9):947–960.

327. Mueller PJ. Exercise training and sympathetic nervous system activity: evidence for physical activity dependent neural plasticity. *Clin Exp Pharmacol Physiol.* 2007;34(4):377–384.

328. Vaynman S, Gomez-Pinilla F. License to run: exercise impacts functional plasticity in the intact and injured central nervous system by using neurotrophins. *Neurorehabil Neural Repair.* 2005;19(4):283–295.

329. Rojas Vega S. Effect of resistance exercise on serum levels of growth factors in humans. *Horm Metab Res.* 2010;42(13):982–986.

330. Prakash RS, Snook EM, Erickson KI, et al. Cardiorespiratory fitness: a predictor of cortical plasticity in multiple sclerosis. *Neuroimage.* 2007;34(3):1238–1244.

331. White LJ, Castellano V. Exercise and brain health—implications for multiple sclerosis: part 1— neuronal growth factors. *Sports Med.* 2008;38(2):91–100.

332. Ahlskog JE. Does vigorous exercise have a neuroprotective effect in Parkinson disease? *Neurol.* 2011;77(3):288–294.

333. Petzinger GM, Fisher BE, Van Leeuwen JE, et al. Enhancing neuroplasticity in the basal ganglia: the role of exercise in Parkinson's disease. *Mov Disord.* 2010;25(Suppl 1):S141–S145.

334. Hirsch MA, Farley BG. Exercise and neuroplasticity in persons living with Parkinson's disease. *Eur J Phys Rehabil Med.* 2009;45(2):215–229.

335. Kamijo K, Hayasi Y, Sakai T, Yahiro T, Tanaka K, Nishihira Y. Acute effects of aerobic exercise on cognitive function in older adults. *J Gerontol B Psychol Sci Soc Sci.* 2009;64B(3):356–363.

336. Muscari A, Giannoni C, Pierpaoli L, et al. Chronic endurance exercise training prevents aging-related cognitive decline in healthy older adults: a randomized controlled trial. *Int J Geriatr Psychiatry.* 2010;25(10):1055–1064.

337. Lindwall M, Rennemark M, Berggren T. Movement in mind: the relationship of exercise with cognitive status for older adults in the Swedish National Study on Aging and Care (SNAC). *Aging Mental Health.* 2008;12(2):212–220.

338. Geda YE, Roberts RO, Knopman DS, et al. Physical exercise, aging, and mild cognitive impairment: a population-based study. *Arch Neurol.* 2010;67(1):80–86.

339. Baker LD, Frank LL, Foster-Schubert K, et al. Effects of aerobic exercise on mild cognitive impairment: a controlled trial. *Arch Neurol.* 2010;67(1):71–79.

340. Foster PP, Rosenblatt KP, Kuljiš RO. Exercise-induced cognitive plasticity, implications for mild cognitive impairment and Alzheimer's disease. *Front Neurol.* 2011;2:e28. www.frontiersin.org/dementia/10.3389/fneur.2011.00028; Accessed 16.11.11.

341. Ahlskog JE, Geda YE, Graff-Radford NR, Petersen RC. Physical exercise as a preventive or disease-modifying treatment of dementia and brain aging. *Mayo Clin Proc.* 2011;86(9):876–884.

342. Liu-Ambrose T, Eng JJ, Boyd LA. Promotion of the mind through exercise (PROMoTE): a proof-of-concept randomized controlled trial of aerobic exercise training in older adults with vascular cognitive impairment. *BMC Neurol.* 2010;10(special section):1–9.

4

An Evidence-Based Approach to Orthotic and Prosthetic Rehabilitation

KEVIN CHUI, RITA A. WONG, AND MICHELLE M. LUSARDI

LEARNING OBJECTIVES

On completion of this chapter, the reader will be able to do the following:

1. Describe the basic principles of evidence-based practice and apply these principles to orthotic and prosthetic rehabilitation.
2. Ask well-formulated, clearly defined, and clinically important questions applicable to orthotic and prosthetic rehabilitation.
3. Efficiently locate meaningful research specific to orthotic and prosthetic rehabilitation.
4. Critically appraise the evidence for validity and clinical importance.
5. Use the orthotic and prosthetic research evidence to make evidence-based clinical judgments that affect your practice.
6. Describe strategies to encourage practitioners to engage in greater use of evidence to inform their clinical decision making and thus practice.

WHAT IS EVIDENCE-BASED PRACTICE?

Providing effective health and rehabilitative care requires that practitioners be well informed about advances in assessment, medical management, technology, theory, and rehabilitation interventions. Relying on past experience or on the opinion of experts is not enough. An effective health care provider must also regularly update his or her knowledge base by accessing the ever-growing information generated by clinical researchers and their basic science colleagues.[1] Providers in all health care disciplines face a number of challenges, however, in efficiently and accurately locating, appraising, and applying scientific evidence in the midst of their increasingly hectic clinical practice schedules.[2-4] Health care providers who routinely use such skills and strategies demonstrate an evidence-based approach to patient care. This chapter provides guidance to the practitioner in overcoming these challenges to engaging in evidence-based practice (EBP).

David Sackett, MD, the father of evidence-based medicine, described this approach as the "integration of best research evidence with clinical expertise and patient values."[4] EBP is a broader concept that applies Sackett's physician-oriented concepts to a wide range of health professions.[4] Both models identify three major elements of evidence that are interactive and valuable, as well as a set of skills necessary to integrate each resource into an effective and informed clinical decision (Figure 4-1). The three major elements are the following:

1. Best available information from up-to-date, clinically relevant research
2. The skilled and experienced practitioner who can accurately perform diagnostic procedures and interventions, integrate findings to efficiently determine correct diagnosis, and engage in reflective clinical practice
3. The integration of the patient's and family's issues, concerns, and hopes into the care plan

All three elements are equally important for an effective clinical decision making process; optimal health care outcomes are grounded on integration of perspectives and priorities that each source of information brings to bear.

To make an informed clinical decision, the evidence-based rehabilitation professional must possess the skills to do the following:

1. Effectively search for and access relevant scientific evidence in the professional literature.[5]
2. Assess the strength and value of the scientific evidence that will support the decision to be made.[6]
3. Apply results of an accurate clinical examination, as well as the evidence from the literature, in the process of diagnosis, evaluation, prognosis, and development of an appropriate plan of care.[7]
4. Assess and incorporate the patient's or client's values, knowledge, preferences, and motivation into the intervention and anticipated outcomes.[8]

THE PROCESS OF EVIDENCE-BASED PRACTICE

EBP is essentially an orientation to clinical decision making that incorporates the best available sources of evidence into the process of assessment, intervention planning, and evaluation of outcomes. The skill set necessary for effective EBP develops over time, with practice and experience.

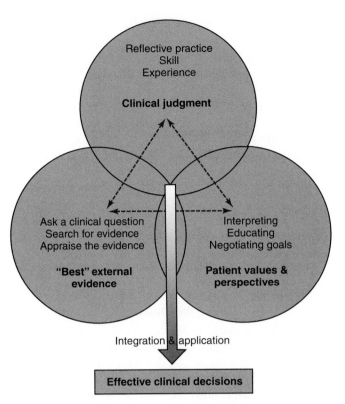

FIGURE 4-1 Model of three essential and interactive components necessary for effective evidence-based health care approach to guide clinical decision making, as well as the dimensions of each.

An EBP approach to the scientific literature is a systematic process with four primary steps[1,4,9]:

1. Posing a well-formulated, clinically important question
2. Locating meaningful research that is well targeted to the question (i.e., developing effective and efficient search strategies)
3. Critically appraising the available evidence for validity and clinical importance
4. Using the findings to make an evidence-based clinical judgment about examination or intervention options on the basis of the clinical relevance of the information applied to the needs of the individual patient

STEP 1: FORMULATING AN ANSWERABLE CLINICAL QUESTION

The questions posed by researchers and the questions posed by clinicians, while similar in many respects, are asked and answered at quite different levels. Research questions combine information from groups (samples) of individuals to develop evidence about relationships among characteristics, effectiveness of examination strategies, or effectiveness of intervention strategies for the group as a whole.[10] In contrast, clinical questions seek to apply this knowledge to a single person with individual characteristics.[4,5,9] For example, clinicians ask, "Which examination strategy will provide the information most important for the clinical decision-making process for this particular individual?" and "Which intervention is likely to have the optimal outcome for this particular individual?"

The first essential step in the EBP process is developing a well-formulated, clinically important question. Sackett identifies two categories of clinical questions: broad background questions and specifically focused foreground questions.[4] *Background questions* expand our knowledge or understanding of a disorder, impairment, or functional limitation; they are often concerned with etiology, diagnosis, prognosis, or typical clinical course. Patients and their family members often ask health care practitioners background questions. Answers to background questions expand the general knowledge base used in clinical decision making. Students and novice clinicians ask many background questions as they develop expertise in their field. Even expert clinicians routinely need to seek answers to basic background questions when they encounter an unfamiliar pathology or novel category of intervention. Answers to background questions do not, however, provide the specific evidence necessary to make individualized patient care decisions. Examples of broad background questions that might be asked by clinicians providing prosthetic and orthotic rehabilitation care include the following:

- What is the typical postsurgical rehabilitation program following a dysvascular transtibial amputation?
- What is peripheral arterial disease and why can it lead to limb amputation?
- What neurological functions are affected with a C7 spinal cord injury?
- What are the typical motor milestones of the first two years of life, and when is the achievement of these milestones considered delayed?

Foreground questions, in contrast, seek specific information to help guide management for an individual patient.[4,5,9] The most effective way to frame an answerable foreground clinical question follows the "PICO" model (Figure 4-2). It identifies the patient population of interest (P), noting specific characteristics (e.g., age, gender, diagnosis, acuity, severity) that will link the evidence to the patient care situation prompting the question. It then identifies the predictive factor, examination, or intervention (I) that is being considered. If appropriate, it

P	Patient	Patient diagnostic category or key characteristic
I	Intervention	Treatment group, or diagnostic tool, or prognostic marker
C	Comparison	Applicable if comparison is wanted between or among interventions, diagnostic tools, or prognostic markers
O	Outcome	What is the outcome of interest: presence or absence of disease? impairment? functional limitation? of disability?

FIGURE 4-2 The PICO system for formulating clinical questions includes consideration of the patient (P) who is receiving care; the intervention (I) being considered; and, if available, the "gold standard" it is being compared with (C) and the anticipated outcomes (O) (positive and negative) of the intervention being considered.

identifies what comparisons (C) are being made to inform choice of examination or intervention. Finally, it clearly defines the outcomes (O) that might be expected for the given patient on the basis of the best available evidence. Using the PICO model, foreground questions that rehabilitation professionals might ask as they care for a specific individual in need of a prosthesis or orthosis include the following:

- How much does advanced age (I) affect the ability to become a functional ambulator (O) in an individual who has a dysvascular transtibial amputation (P)?
- Does supported treadmill gait training (I) improve ambulation endurance with a prosthesis (O) in older patients with dysvascular transtibial amputation (P)?
- Does the addition of functional neuromuscular stimulation (I) to a typical early rehabilitation intervention (C) enhance active muscle control (O) in individuals with incomplete spinal cord injury (P)?
- What factors predict (I) ambulation ability (O) in a young child with spastic diplegic cerebral palsy (P)?

Patient Characteristics (P)

A well-focused clinical question narrows the scope of possible patient characteristics to ones most applicable to a specific clinical problem or situation.[4,9] It defines the key characteristics that will best differentially guide the search for evidence. Characteristics or categories that help focus a clinical question related to orthotic or prosthetic management are summarized in Table 4-1.

Intervention (I)

The term *intervention* is used broadly in the evidence-based literature. In the EBP paradigm the intervention (I) and comparison intervention (C), described according to the PICO system, refer to the central issue for which the clinician is seeking an answer. This issue can typically revolve around an intervention, a diagnosis, or a prognosis.

1. Intervention: a procedure or technique (e.g., a physical modality, surgical procedure, medication) (I) that is compared with alternative procedures or techniques (C).[11,12]
2. Diagnostic test: a test or measure (e.g., a bone mineral density test for identification of osteoporosis; the Berg Balance Scale for identification of fall risk) (I) that correctly differentiates patients with and without a specific condition (C).[13,14]
3. Prognostic marker: a specific set of characteristics or factors (I) that effectively predicts an outcome (O) for a given patient problem (P).[15]

Defining the Outcome (O)

A good clinical question focuses on the outcome that is most relevant to the patient care situation at hand. The Nagi model of disablement or the World Health Organization International Classification of Function (ICF) model provide frameworks for clinicians to define the outcome they are most interested in: pathology or disease at the cellular level, impairment of a physiological system, functional limitation at the level of the individual, or disability or handicap that interferes with the normal social role[16,17] (see Figure 1-3).

CASE EXAMPLE 1

An Elderly Woman with Recent Transtibial Amputation

F. H. is an 89-year-old woman who had an elective transtibial amputation 4 days prior, due to peripheral arterial disease (PAD) unrelated to diabetes. Her postoperative pain is being managed with a narcotic, and she has been mildly disoriented and distractible during rehabilitation visits. At present she requires moderate assistance in rising to standing and minimal assistance and directive cues to ambulate in a "hop to" pattern with a rolling walker. Her medical history includes mild congestive heart failure managed effectively with diuretics, hypertension managed effectively with beta-blockers, and a compression fracture (2 years ago) of the midthoracic spine secondary to osteoporosis. She recently had lens implants for cataracts. Before her hospitalization, she lived somewhat independently in an assisted living complex, walking long functional distances within the sprawling facility using a straight cane and eating her noon and evening meals in the communal dining room. She served as vice-chair of the Resident Council, and was the organizer of an active bridge club and book discussion group. Her nearest living relative is a granddaughter who is finishing medical residency at the hospital.

The amputation/prosthetic clinic team has been charged with developing a plan for prosthetic rehabilitation, including determining her potential for prosthetic use, the optimal setting for rehabilitation intervention,

the likely duration of rehabilitative care, and preliminary prosthetic prescription.

Questions to Consider

Possible clinical questions that the team would ask in order to guide her plan of care include the following:

- Which strategies (pharmacological and nonpharmacological) for postamputation pain management (I, C) will minimize risk of delirium and assist motor and cognitive learning (O) in elderly individuals with multiple comorbidities (P)?
- Which functional and cognitive characteristics (I) provide the best indication of potential for prosthetic use (O) in elderly individuals with multiple comorbidities?
- What intrinsic and extrinsic factors (I) influence the duration of preprosthetic and prosthetic care (O) for older adults with recent transtibial amputation (P)?
- Which prosthetic foot option (nonarticulating, articulating, or dynamic response) (C, I) and suspension system (silicone suspension sleeve with pin, supracondylar cuff, waist belt, and forked-strap extension aid) (C, I) would maximize potential for safe community ambulation (O) in older patients with transtibial amputation, impaired postural control, and limited cardiovascular endurance (P)?

TABLE 4-1 *Patient Characteristics that may be Used to Help Focus Literature Searches for Prosthetic and Orthotic Rehabilitation*

Domain	Characteristics	Search Terms
Underlying condition	Etiology	Acquired (traumatic injury, infectious process, autoimmune disease, ischemia, vascular disease, neoplasm, cancer)
		Congenital condition
		Developmental delay
		Hereditary disease
	Systems affected	Musculoskeletal
		Neuromuscular
		Cardiovascular
		Pulmonary, respiratory
		Integumentary
		Endocrine
		Systemic physiological
	Nature of condition	Chronic
		Progressive
		Degenerative
		Developmental
		Requiring remediation
		Requiring accommodation
	Comorbid conditions	Peripheral vascular disease
		Diabetes mellitus
		Systemic infections
		Cancer care, chemotherapy, radiation
		Heart disease
		Pulmonary disease
		Obesity
		Depression, anxiety
		Cognitive dysfunction
		Smoking
	Confounding factors	Alcohol use
		Other substance abuse
		Nutritional status
Family and lifespan development	Age category	Infant
		Toddler
		School-age child
		Adolescent
		Young adult
		Midlife adult
		Older adult
	Family system	Roles
		Responsibilities
		Caregiver
Fitness/conditioning	Level of activity	Frail
		Sedentary
		Active
		Elite athlete
Mobility	Use of assistive device	None
		Ambulatory aid (cane, crutch, walker)
		Wheelchair
		Adaptive equipment
		Requiring human assistance
Environmental issues	Environment	School
		Home
		Work
		Leisure
		Accessible/inaccessible
	Living arrangements	Community dwelling (alone, independent, with caregivers or family)
		Assisted living setting
		Skilled nursing

A Young Adult with Incomplete Spinal Cord Injury

S. K. is a 19-year-old with incomplete C7 level spinal cord injury who has just been admitted to the rehabilitation facility, 2 weeks after injury. S. K. was a backseat passenger injured in a driving-under-the-influence motor vehicle accident following a Thanksgiving homecoming football game victory at his high school. He was unconscious at the scene and for several hours afterward. He was given methylprednisolone in the emergency department 2 hours after injury. Radiographs revealed an anterior wedge fracture of C6 vertebra. After intubation, he was admitted to the neurological intensive care unit; 2 days later he had surgical fusion of C4 through C8, with immobilization in a cervical halo. During the postoperative period, pneumonia developed, has since resolved. Sensation is intact in all sacral and lumbar 3 to 5 dermatomes, and he has 2/5 strength in dorsiflexion and plantar flexion bilaterally, with hyperactive deep tendon reflex at the knee. He can tolerate sitting in a bedside recliner or high-back reclining wheelchair for approximately 45 minutes. He is anxious to know whether he will be able to walk again, and although frightened by what has occurred, appears to be motivated to begin his rehabilitation.

Before his injury, S. K. lived at home while attending a nearby state university as a biology major. His intention was to eventually apply to medical school to become an orthopedic surgeon. His parents and younger sister are involved in his care; a family member is with him for most of the day. He has a cousin, now in law school, who was born with spina bifida and uses a wheelchair for primary mobility.

Questions to Consider

Possible clinical questions that the team might ask to guide his plan of care might include the following:

- What are the most powerful indicators (I) of potential for return to functional ambulation (O) in patients with incomplete cervical spinal cord injury (P)?
- Which physical therapy interventions (I, C) will best improve functional lower extremity strength (O) in patients with incomplete cervical spinal cord injury who are immobilized in a cervical halo (P)?
- What strategies (pharmacological and nonpharmacological) (I, C) are effective in managing abnormal tone without compromising potential for strengthening (O) in patients with incomplete cervical spinal cord injury (P)?
- Will functional neuromuscular stimulation (I) reduce orthotic need and improve quality of gait (O) in patients with incomplete cervical spinal cord injury (P)?

A Toddler with Spastic Diplegic Cerebral Palsy

E. C. is an 18-month-old with spastic diplegic cerebral palsy being cared for by an interdisciplinary early intervention team. E. C. was born prematurely at 34 weeks of gestation after her mom's high-risk first pregnancy. Her course in the neonatal intensive care unit was relatively uneventful: She did not require ventilatory assistance but did have periodic episodes of apnea and bradycardia until she reached a weight of 4 lb. She was discharged to home at 3 weeks of age and appeared to be developing fairly typically until about 8 or 9 months of age. Her parents noted increasing "stiffness" of her lower extremities when in supported standing, a tendency toward "bunny hop" rather than reciprocal creeping, and overreliance on upper extremities to pull to stand (as compared with her cousins and babies in her playgroup). Her pediatrician referred the family to a pediatric neurologist, who found mild to moderate hyperreflexia and decorticate pattern hypertonicity in her lower extremities. She has been followed in the early intervention program for 7 months; the team is charged with determining whether this is an appropriate time for orthotic intervention, because she is ready to begin gait training.

Questions to Consider

Questions that might be asked to guide her plan of care include the following:

- What are the minimal levels of muscle performance and range of motion at the hip and knee (I) necessary for effective ambulation with an articulating ankle-foot orthosis (AFO) (O) in children with spastic diplegic cerebral palsy (P)?
- Which type of therapeutic activity or approach (e.g., neurodevelopmental [NDT], sensory integration, proprioceptive neuromuscular facilitation [PNF]) (I) is most effective in assisting dynamic postural control of the lower trunk and lower extremities during transitional and locomotor tasks (O) in children with spastic diplegic cerebral palsy (P)?
- What accommodations or adaptations of the home environment (I) will best assist safety, as well as developmental progression (O), in children with spastic diplegic cerebral palsy (P)?

STEP 2: LOCATING AND ACCESSING THE BEST EVIDENCE

Once the clinical question has been clearly identified and articulated, the next step is to search the rehabilitation research literature for relevant information. The second step is to access full text articles, access their quality, and read those might that inform decision making .[18-21] Among the many ways to find citations and (hopefully) the full text of the article are the following:

- Regularly visit key journal websites to review what has been recently published or published ahead of print that might be relevant to the question. The Journal of Prosthetics and Orthotics (http://www.oandp.org/jpo), for example, allows full access to any journal article published in the years previous to the current year. This strategy can be somewhat "hit or miss" in terms of effectiveness.
- Use the index in the back of up-to-date textbooks as a reliable secondary source of information; this can be especially useful to answer background questions.
- Use an Internet search engine such as Google.scholar (http://scholar.google.com; free access), which provides both unjuried and juried resources and requires the ability to carefully assess the quality of the source and of the information that has been located.
- Use electronic databases of peer-reviewed journals such as PubMed/Medline/OVID (http://www.ncbi.nlm.nih.gov/pubmed; free access), or the Physiotherapy Evidence Database (PEDro; http://www.pedro.org.au/; free access) using appropriate key words. Professional organizations such as the American Physical Therapy Association provide links to search engines (http://www.apta.org/OpenDoor), abstracted article reviews (http://www.hookedonevidence.org) or synthesized evidence (http://www.apta.org/PTNow) for organization members. Many medical libraries maintain subscriptions to multiple medical databases through services such as EBSCO (http://www.ebscohost.com/biomedical-libraries; subscription access) or ProQuest (http://www.proquest.com/en-US/catalogs/databases/detail/pq_health_med_comp.shtml), among others.

- Subscribe to online Table of Content (eTOC) alerts from research journals relevant to their practice areas. For example, the Physical Therapy Journal (http://ptjournal.apta.org/site/subscriptions/etoc.xhtml), the Journal of Geriatric Physical Therapy (www.jgpt.org), the Journal of Neurologic Physical (www.jnpt.org), Clinical Biomechanics (http://www.clinbiomech.com/user/alerts), and the Archives of Physical Medicine and Rehabilitation (http://www.archives-pmr.org/user/alerts/savetocalert), among many others will send table of contents for current issues to email, cell phone, iPads, e-readers, and other devices.

Each strategy has pros and cons in terms of efficiency and availability. Health professionals who use an evidence-based approach to patient care develop, over time, an information seeking strategy that works within their time constraints and accessible resources.[22-24]

Sources of Evidence

Clinicians can access information from the research literature in a variety of formats and from a variety of sources. One of the most accessible formats is a journal article.[25,26] Table 4-2 provides a list of the journals particularly relevant to orthotic and prosthetic rehabilitation. These journals often contain original clinical research, reviews of the literature, and case reports focused on issues most relevant to the particular professional group.

The medical literature is divided into primary and secondary sources of information. Primary sources are the reports of original scientific work, commonly published as journal articles. Secondary sources are summary reviews of the primary literature on given topics. Secondary sources include textbooks, review articles, systematic reviews such as meta-analyses, critical reviews of individual articles, clinical practice guidelines, and website summaries. Research studies are the foundation of meaningful evidence. Academic textbooks, biomedical journals, and Internet websites aimed at health professionals and biomedical researchers are common sources of research evidence.

TABLE 4-2 *Journals Relevant to Orthotic and Prosthetic Rehabilitation*

Journal Title	Abbreviation
American Journal of Occupational Therapy	Am J Occup Ther
American Journal of Physical Medicine & Rehabilitation	Am J Phys Med Rehabil
American Journal of Podiatric Medicine	Am J Podiatr Med
American Journal of Surgery	Am J Surg
American Rehabilitation	Am Rehabil
Annals of Physical Medicine	Ann Phys Med
Archives of Neurology	Arch Neurol
Archives of Physical Medicine and Rehabilitation	Arch Phys Med Rehabil
Archives of Surgery	Arch Surg
Assistive Technology	Assist Tech
Athletic Training	Athletic Training
Australian Journal of Physical Therapy	Aust J Physiother

(Continued)

TABLE 4-2   *Journals Relevant to Orthotic and Prosthetic Rehabilitation—cont'd*

Journal Title	Abbreviation
Biomechanics	Biomechanics
British Journal of Sports Medicine	Br J Sports Med
Bulletin of Prosthetic Research	Bull Prosthet Res
Canadian Journal of Occupational Therapy	Can J Occup Ther
Clinical Biomechanics	Clin Biomech
Clinics in Orthopedics and Related Research	Clin Orthop Rel Res
Clinics in Podiatric Medicine and Surgery	Clin Podiatr Med Surg
Clinics in Prosthetics and Orthotics	Clin Prosthet Orthot
Developmental Medicine & Child Neurology	Dev Med Child Neurol
Diabetes Care	Diabetes Care
Diabetic Foot	Diabe Foot
Diabetic Medicine	Diabe Med
Disability and Rehabilitation	Disabil Rehabil
Foot and Ankle Clinics	Foot Ankle Clin
Foot and Ankle International	Foot Ankle Int
Gait and Posture	Gait Posture
Interdisciplinary Science Reviews	Interdisc Sci Rev
International Journal of Rehabilitation Research	Int J Rehabil Res
Journal of Allied Health	J Allied Health
Journal of Applied Biomechanics	J Appl Biomech
Journal of Biomechanical Engineering	J Biomech Eng
Journal of Biomechanics	J Biomech
Journal of Bone and Joint Surgery	J Bone Joint Surg
Journal of Geriatric Physical Therapy	J Geriatr Phys Ther
Journal of Head Trauma and Rehabilitation	J Head Trauma Rehabil
Journal of Medical Engineering and Technology	J Med Eng Tech
Journal of Musculoskeletal Medicine	J Musculoskel Med
Journal of Neurologic Physical Therapy	J Neuro Phys Ther
Journal of Orthopaedic and Sports Physical Therapy	J Orthop Sports Phys Ther
Journal of Pediatric Orthopedics	J Pediatr Orthop
Journal of Prosthetics and Orthotics	J Prosthet Orthot
Journal of Rehabilitation	J Rehabil
Journal of Rehabilitation Medicine	J Rehabil Med
Journal of Rehabilitation Research and Development	J Rehabil Res Dev
Journal of Spinal Disorders	J Spinal Disord
Journal of the American Geriatrics Society	J Am Geriatr Soc
Journal of the American Medical Association	JAMA
Journal of the American Podiatry Association	J Am Podiatry Assoc
Journal of Trauma	J Trauma
Medical and Biological Engineering	Med Biol Eng Comp
Orthopedic Clinics of North America	Orthop Clin North Am
Paraplegia	Paraplegia
Physiotherapy Canada	Physiother Can
Physical and Occupational Therapy in Geriatrics	Phys Occup Ther Geriatr
Physical and Occupational Therapy in Pediatrics	Phys Occup Ther Pediatr
Physical Medicine & Rehabilitation Clinics of North America	Phys Med Rehabil Clin N Am
Physical Medicine & Rehabilitation: State of the Art Reviews	Phys Med Rehabil State Art Rev
Physical Therapy	Phys Ther
Physiotherapy	Physiotherapy
Physiotherapy Research International	Physiother Res Int
Prosthetics and Orthotics International	Prosthet Orthot Int
Rehabilitation Nursing	Rehabil Nurs
Rehabilitation Psychology	Rehabil Psychol
Scandinavian Journal of Rehabilitation Medicine	Scand J Rehabil Med
Spinal Cord	Spinal Cord
Spine	Spine
Topics in Stroke Rehabilitation	Top Stroke Rehabil

Textbooks

Academic textbooks can be a good starting point for locating background information, particularly for content areas that change slowly (e.g., gross anatomy or biomechanics). Evidence-based textbooks are well referenced, go through a review process, and are typically updated every 3 to 5 years. They summarize clinical studies and opinions of experts, and analyze/synthesize the impact of the research and expert opinion on the topic. Some textbooks are now available online, which provides the advantage of frequent updating of specific sections as new research evidence emerges and allows the reader to immediately hyperlink to primary research article sources. The website FreeBooks4Doctors! (www.freebooks4doctors.com) provides hyperlinks to many key medical textbooks free of charge online. Many other online textbooks are available for purchase. Box 4-1 lists key indicators of quality in academic textbooks.

Primary Sources: Journal Articles

Journal articles may serve as either primary or secondary literature sources. They can be useful for both background and foreground clinical questions. Primary research articles are those in which the author presents the findings of a specific original study.[27,28] It is best to use this category of evidence when dealing with rapidly evolving areas of health care (which many clinical practice questions fall into). Identifying two or three high-quality primary research articles that, in general, provide similar supporting evidence offers strong evidence on which to base a clinical decision. Searching, critiquing, and synthesizing primary research sources is a time-intensive task.

Secondary Sources: Integrative and Systematic Review Articles

Use of high-quality secondary source journal articles to guide evidence-based determinations can be a time-efficient strategy for clinicians.[29,30] Quality indicators for secondary source articles include a comprehensive search of the literature (using an explicit search strategy) to identify existing studies, an unbiased analysis of these studies, and objective conclusions and recommendations on the basis of the analysis and synthesis.[31] Secondary sources are available in a variety of formats: integrative narrative review, systematic review, meta-analysis, and clinical practice guideline (CPG). Each of these summative resources can be an effective and time-efficient method to obtain a critical assessment of a specific body of knowledge. However, there are benefits and drawbacks associated with each type of summative resource.

In an *integrative review article* the author reviews and summarizes, and sometimes analyzes or synthesizes, the work of a number of primary authors.[32] These narrative reviews are often broad in scope, may or may not describe how articles were chosen for inclusion in the review, and present a qualitative analysis of previous research findings. The quality (validity) of the narrative review varies with the expertise of the reviewer and requires careful assessment by the reader.

Systematic reviews are particularly powerful secondary sources of evidence that typically analyze and synthesize controlled clinical trials.[29,31,33] Well-done systematic reviews are valuable sources of evidence and should always be sought when initiating a search. Box 4-2 lists key indicators of a quality systematic review. Systematic reviews are typically focused on a fairly narrow clinical question, are based on a comprehensive search of relevant literature, and use well-defined inclusion and exclusion criteria to select high-quality studies (typically randomized controlled trials) for inclusion in the review. Each study included in the review is carefully appraised for quality and relevance to the specific clinical topic. The author attempts to identify commonalities among study methods and outcomes, as well as account for differences in approaches and findings. A good systematic review is labor intensive to prepare; thus only about 1.5% of all journal articles referenced in Medline are true systematic reviews.[34] Although the numbers are low, increasing numbers of systematic reviews are being published, including ones on topics relevant to orthotics and prosthetics. For example, a PubMed search from 2006 to July 2011 of the literature using the terms "limb amputation AND rehabilitation" combining the limits (a) review and (b) English yielded 49 applicable reviews (Appendix 4-1).

A *meta-analysis* is a type of systematic review that quantitatively aggregates outcome data from multiple studies to analyze treatment effects (typically using the "odds ratio" statistic) as if the data represented one large sample (thus with greater statistics power) rather than multiple small samples of individuals.[29,31,35] The limitation to performing a meta-analysis is that, in order to combine studies, the category of patients, the interventions, and the outcome measures across the studies must all be similar. Meta-analyses can provide more powerful statements of the strength of the evidence either supporting or refuting a given treatment effect than the separate assessment of each study. Because of the difficulty in identifying studies with enough similarity to combine data, only a small subset of systematic

---

BOX 4-1	***Quality Indicators for Textbooks and Internet Sources of Evidence***

- Credentials of the authors
- Quality of references
- Recent/regular updating
- Endorsement by respected groups
- Peer reviewed
- Disclosure of funding source

BOX 4-2	***Quality Indicators for Systematic Review Articles***

- Exhaustive search for evidence
- Clearly identified quality criteria for inclusion
- Multiple authors with independent judgments
- Impartial, unbiased summary
- Clearly stated conclusions: ready for clinical application
- If meta-analysis: statistical manipulation across studies

reviews have been carried to the level of a meta-analysis. One meta-analysis was identified in PubMed using the terms "limb amputation AND rehabilitation" combined the limits a) meta-analysis, b) English, and c) published in last 5 years.[36]

Secondary Sources: Clinical Practice Guidelines

Another secondary resource for clinicians may be CPGs that have been developed for application to clinical practice on the basis of the best available current evidence.[37] Most existing CPGs have been developed for screening, diagnosis, and intervention in medical practice. CPGs are intended to direct clinical decision making about appropriate health care for specific diseases among specific populations of patients. The best available evidence upon which CPGs are typically based combines expert consensus and review of clinical research literature.[38] Most are interpreted as prescriptive, using algorithms to assist decision making for appropriate examination and intervention strategies for patients with given characteristics. Examples of CPGs that may be relevant to orthotic and prosthetic rehabilitation are listed in Appendix 4-2. The National Guidelines Clearinghouse is the most comprehensive database in the United States for CPGs (www.guidelines.gov).

Electronic Resources and Search Strategies

A number of electronic databases can assist clinicians in quickly locating primary and secondary sources of evidence to guide clinical decision making (Table 4-3). When seeking articles, it is often helpful to use several different databases. The American Physical Therapy Association provides access to many electronic resources described below as a service to APTA members via its Open Door portal on the website www.APTA.org.

Using an electronic database effectively is a two-step process. First, the searcher must locate applicable citations that provide the title of the article, author, and other key identifying information (e.g., journal, issue, year, pages). Most often, these citations also provide an abstract of the article. Sometimes the searcher can gather enough information about the applicability of the article for his or her needs purely on the basis of the information found in the title and abstract. Most often, however, the searcher must access the full-text article in order to adequately assess the findings of the study. Citations and abstracts are readily available free of charge from numerous databases. However, access to the full text of articles often requires a paid subscription to search databases.

Locating Citations

The National Library of Medicine, through the database PubMed, produces and maintains Medline, the largest publicly available database of English language biomedical references in the world. PubMed references more than 4600 journals including many key non–English language biomedical journals. These journals, in the aggregate, include more than 15 million individual journal article citations. This database is also a rich source of citations for quality systematic reviews.

TABLE 4-3   *Electronic Databases Used to Search for Relevant Evidence*

Acronym	Database Information	Access
—	Academic Search Premier	By library access
Best Evidence	ACP Journal Club and Evidence Based Medicine (critical and systematic reviews)	http://hiru.mcmaster.ca/acpjc/acpod.htm
CCTR	Cochrane Controlled Trials Register	By subscription or library access
CDSR	Cochrane Database of Systematic Reviews	By subscription or library access
CHID	Combined Health Information Data Base (titles, abstracts, resources, program descriptions not indexed elsewhere)	www.chid.nih.gov
CINAHL	Cumulative Index of Nursing and Allied Health Literature (citations and abstracts)	By subscription or library access (www.cinahl.com)
DARE	Cochrane Database of Abstracts of Reviews of Effectiveness	By subscription or library access
EBM Online	Evidence-based Medicine for Primary Care and Internal Medicine (critical reviews and systematic reviews)	By subscription (www.ebm.bmjjournals.com)
Embase	Embase/Elsevier Science (Citations and abstracts)	By subscription (www.embase.com)
—	Hooked on Evidence/American Physical Therapy Association (citations, abstracts, annotations)	By membership in American Physical Therapy Association (www.apta.org)
Medline	National Library of Medicine (abstracts)	By library access
OVID	A collection of health and medical subject databases (abstracts and full text)	By subscription or library access (www.gateway.ovid.com)
PEDro	The Physiotherapy Evidence Database (systematic reviews)	www.pedro.fhs.usyd.edu.au/index.html
PubMed	National Library of Medicine (abstracts)	www.ncbi.nlm.nih.gov/entrez (no charge)

Journals indexed in PubMed must meet rigorous standards for their level of peer review and the quality of the articles published in the journal; this gives the searcher some confidence in the information that is located through PubMed. PubMed can be accessed through the National Library of Medicine's website (www.nlm.nih.gov). OVID is another Medline resource; it is typically accessed via library subscription and often links full text articles.

The Cumulative Index of Nursing and Allied Health Literature (CINAHL) includes journal citations from a larger pool of nursing and allied health fields than is found in Medline. Many of these journals have a much smaller circulation than the typical Medline cited journals, and the quality of these smaller circulation journals may not meet PubMed requirements. Thus the reader must be aware that closer scrutiny of validity and methodological quality may be necessary. However, the greater inclusion of rehabilitation-focused journals in the CINAHL database makes this an important database for rehabilitation professionals. This database is only available to paid subscribers (library or individual subscriptions).

Hooked on Evidence is a database of the American Physical Therapy Association (APTA) and is available free of charge to members of the association (www.hookedonevidence.com). Presently Hooked on Evidence consists of primary intervention studies only. Articles in Hooked on Evidence have been reviewed and abstracted by physical therapy academicians and researchers, graduate students, and clinicians. These abstracts may be sought by selecting a practice pattern group, condition, and clinical scenario.

PEDro is a database of the Centre for Evidence-based Physiotherapy at the University of Sydney, Australia, and is available to the public free of charge (www.pedro.org.au). PEDro lists clinical practice guidelines, systematic reviews, and clinical trials. An advanced search allows the searcher to select the type of therapy, problem, body part, and subdiscipline. Both the Hooked on Evidence and PEDro databases focus exclusively on high-quality studies related to physical therapy. Their benefit is ease of identifying citations applicable to physical therapy and rehabilitation. To search either database successfully, the research question should be fairly broad, using synonyms that represent words in the title. Both databases contain only a fraction of the citations found in PubMed; all of the citations, however, are directly applicable to rehabilitation. A search of PEDro using "orthoses" identified one practice guideline, 23 systematic reviews, and 26 clinical trials, all relevant to physical therapy (Appendix 4-3). A similar search in Hooked on Evidence found 77 reviews of clinical trials, 29 of which were published since 2006 (Appendix 4-4).

The Cochrane Database of Systematic Reviews (www.cochrane.org/cochrane-reviews) is widely accepted as the gold standard for systematic reviews. Groups of experts perform comprehensive and quantitative analysis and synthesis of the existing research on well-focused topics and distill the findings into scientifically supported recommendations. Cochrane reviews use a standardized format and carefully follow rules to decrease bias in the choice of articles to review and in the interpretation of the evidence. Although few address physical therapy exclusively, rehabilitation procedures and approaches are a component of many of these reviews. The findings are reported in structured abstracts that summarize the key aspects of the full review including the authors' conclusions about the strength of the evidence and their recommendations. These structured abstracts are available free online. Access to full-text review articles requires a paid subscription, however.

Finding valuable secondary references on the web is increasingly possible. However, searchers must carefully scrutinize these materials as there is wide variability in accuracy and objectivity of the published information.[39] This evidence represents such varied sources as reports of original research, research reviews from trusted experts, student summaries that are non–peer reviewed, marketing advertisements (sometimes presented visually to appear to be a peer-reviewed research report), and lobbying groups' perspectives and persuasive arguments. There are many patient-focused sites and fewer practitioner-focused ones. The quality indicators identified in Table 4-2 are applicable to Internet websites as well as textbooks.

Executing Search Strategies

Often, the first search for citations results in one of two extremes: hundreds or thousands of citations, with only a few related to the clinical question being asked, or almost no citations focused on the topic of interest.[18,40,41] Searchers should look carefully at the citations that result from a search. In the search that is too broad, the searcher must examine closely what he or she is really looking for, comparing titles and key words that have resulted from the search. Often, the search is repeated, by rewording or setting limiters to narrow results and omit the previously identified unrelated citations. A searcher who uses the search term *prosthesis* may find that the results the search include articles about such diverse topics as joint prostheses, dental prostheses, and skin prostheses, as well as limb prostheses. Search terms should be as applicable to the specific clinical question being posed as possible; using more precise search terms such as *limb prosthesis, leg prosthesis, arm prosthesis,* or *artificial limb may* be more effective.

Searchers should recognize that the search engine is simply matching the search words that the searcher has entered with subject headings linked to the article by the database administrator or librarian using predefined medical subject heading names or words included in the title or abstract. Searchers may need to adjust search terms to find applicable references. For example, a PubMed (www.ncbi.nlm.nih.gov/pubmed/) search of the English language literature published in the past 5 years (between July 2006 and July 2011) using the search terms *below-knee amputation* combined with the search term *prosthetic rehabilitation* yielded five citations. The same search using the term *transtibial amputation* rather than *below-knee amputation* yielded 45 citations, with no overlap between the two sets of citations. A third search using the term *trans-tibial amputation* in place of *transtibial amputation* yielded 12 citations, none of which overlapped with the first search and one that overlapped with the second search.

A search can be unforgiving to misspellings or, as described earlier, slight differences in search terms. If the searcher finds one citation that is on target for the topic of interest, repeating the search using terms from that article's title or abstract, as well as subject headings (key words), may yield additional appropriate citations. Using a variety of synonyms or Medical Subject Headings (www.ncbi.nlm.nih.gov/mesh) when repeating the search can help the searcher be more confident that the correct concepts are being targeted. Searchers should note the search terms that result in successful searches so that future searches can be most efficient. Searchers using PubMed can set up a permanent search by establishing a "cubby." This service is free and fully available via Internet connection to PubMed. Online directions help users set up cubbies that save search terms. Searchers can periodically check their cubbies and ask for literature updates on the topic.

In addition to the search topic, a good clinical question will often focus on one of three broad categories of clinical questions: treatment/intervention/therapy, diagnosis, or prognosis.[42] Searchers can use these terms to narrow their search as needed. Searchers must recognize that each database uses its own set of key words and may (or may not) include the title words, abstract words, or common sense clinical terms in their electronic search process. Familiarity with key headings used by the database can minimize frustration during the search process; combining words from the title or abstract (e.g., by using Boolean operators such as "AND," "OR," or "NOT"), as well as using synonyms for the clinical terms or concepts of interest, can also assist the search process. In many databases, searchers can choose to limit the search to systematic reviews addressing their topic of interest.

Searching for Interventions

Words that are likely to limit the search to studies that focus on interventions include the following[43]:

- Therapeutic use
- Clinical trials
- Therapy
- Comparative studies
- Randomized controlled trial (to limit search to articles of highest quality, only if there are many relevant articles)
- Rehabilitation

Examples of search terms for therapeutic interventions commonly used in prosthetics and orthotics include the following:

- Prosthetic rehabilitation
- Orthotic use
- Physical therapy techniques
- Prosthetic fitting
- Prosthetic training
- Gait training
- Therapeutic exercise
- Edema management
- Balance training
- Skin care
- Strength training

Diagnosis as the Intervention

If the primary clinical question relates to making an accurate and efficacious diagnosis about some aspect of the patient's condition, or on screening patients to determine the need for more specific assessment, the health practitioner may search the "diagnosis" literature for relevant studies. General search terms that help limit the search to general studies focusing on diagnosis include the following[42]:

- Diagnosis (actual disease or disorder)
- Diagnostic use (tool used in diagnosis)
- Diagnosis, differential
- Sensitivity
- Specificity
- Accuracy
- Predictive value
- Construct validity

Natural History or Prognosis

Studies of the prognosis of medical pathologies and impairments are becoming increasingly available. Such studies attempt to predict who is most likely to benefit from specific treatment interventions or determine whether specific characteristics of patients or their environment predict outcomes. Search terms that are likely to limit the citations to those focused on the general category of prognosis include the following[43]:

- Experimental cohort studies
- Prognosis
- Prognostic factors
- Disease progression
- Recurrence
- Morbidity
- Mortality
- Incidence
- Prevalence
- Clinical course
- Outcomes

Systematic Review

Currently PubMed does not identify systematic review as a specific "publication type." The searcher must use the limits "meta-analysis" or "review" under the Type of Article option. When "systematic review" is used as a search term, several types of reviews are retrieved, not limited to actual systematic reviews. Articles commonly identified as review-academic, CPGs, review-tutorial, meta-analysis, guideline, and consensus development conference are all categorized in PubMed under the term systematic review. Search terms that are likely to limit the citations to ones focused on true systematic reviews include the following:

- Systematic review (as a title word [tw])
- Systematic (as a key word)
- Meta-analysis

- Development
- Validation
- Cochrane database of systematic reviews (as a journal name [jn])

Locating Full-Text Articles

Once appropriate citations have been found via a search of the literature, the next step is to locate the full text of articles that appear to be most closely related to the clinical question of concern. Individual journals are published and owned by publishing companies that support themselves by paid journal subscriptions. Each journal has its own mechanism for providing access to the articles it contains. If the journal is published by a specific professional organization, members of that organization typically have access to a delivered hard copy of the journal or access via the organization's website (by entering an assigned user name and password).

Libraries purchase hard copy and online access to specific journals, either bundled together as part of an intermediary company service (e.g., EBSCO or Proquest), as stand-alone subscriptions, or as a publisher aggregated offering of several or all of its journals at a specified price. Libraries make the online copies of these journals available to their library patrons, either free of charge or for a specified library fee. Some journals provide full text free to the public via the Internet, either for all issues or for articles published after a certain period of time (e.g., 1 to 2 years after publication). Most journals provide full text of individual articles for a fee; this fee may be as much as $20 to $25 per article. One benefit of searching the literature on PubMed is that this database provides a link to any online access to a specific citation, both those with free access sources and those with a fee attached. The website www.freemedicaljournals.com lists the various biomedical journals that provide full text free, provides the hyperlink to the journal website, and identifies any limitations to free access (often time since publication). Health care practitioners should search out the availability of full-text biomedical journal articles (either hard copy or online) from the libraries to which they have regular access. Access will vary widely on the basis of the work setting and the mission of the library at the health facility or in the community.

STEP 3: CRITICALLY APPRAISING THE EVIDENCE

Once the clinician has located and screened the article to ensure that it is reasonably focused on the clinical research question of interest and applicable to the patients in his or her clinical practice, the clinician must critically appraise the methodological and analytical quality of the research process used in the study.[44] This is a skill that clinicians can develop with consistent practice, over time, and is well worth the effort involved.[22,23] Participation in study groups or journal clubs often helps development of this useful EBP skill.[45,46]

Overall Methodological Quality

The best quality research evidence comes from studies with a carefully articulated research question, an appropriate design and methodology, and a sample representative of the population of interest. No clinical research study or article is perfect, and the critical appraiser of the research literature must develop skills to *weigh the evidence* that an article provides to determine whether the information is accurate, relevant, and clinically important for his or her patients.[44,47] Just because something is published and in print does not ensure that it provides valuable or accurate information. Whether the clinical study focuses on treatment/intervention, prognosis, or diagnosis, the overall purpose of critical appraisal is to determine the extent to which threats to internal and external validity of the study bias, and potentially invalidate, the findings of the study.[48] The clinician is interested in determining whether, and to what degree, the findings of the study truly represent the answer to the research question asked in the study. Box 4-3 lists a series of questions about the overall quality and applicability of primary research studies. Some questions are applicable across all categories of primary research; others are specific to certain categories. Box 4-4 identifies quality assessment questions applicable to the secondary source category of systematic review.

The Sample: Adequacy and Appropriateness

Sample size must be considered when making judgments about the methodological quality of a study. In studies with small sample sizes, a few nonrepresentative subjects can skew data substantially and lead to statistical findings that are nonrepresentative of the parent group.[49] Additionally, the natural variability between subjects may end up masking real differences when sample size is low. There is no absolute minimum number of subjects identified quantitatively as the minimum needed for a legitimate study. However, research textbooks often recommend 8 to 15 subjects per group as a minimum number to ensure that the statistical analysis has at least a reasonable opportunity of demonstrating real differences or real relationships if they are present.[10,50] The larger the sample size, the more likely that the sample will represent the population from which it has been drawn.

Researchers, as well as readers of research articles, can use a power analysis to evaluate adequacy of the sample size. A power analysis provides an objective estimate of the minimum sample size necessary to demonstrate real differences or relationships, between and among groups.[51-53] Inclusion of a power analysis as a standard part of the research design is a fairly new concept. Thus although the presence of a power analysis is helpful in assessing the adequacy of the sample size, lack of a specifically identified power analysis—particularly in older studies—does not necessarily indicate a weak study.

A power level (β) of 0.8 (80%) is generally considered acceptable in assuring that, if real group differences (or relationships) are present, the study design is sensitive enough to pick them up. A power analysis considers five factors in the

BOX 4-3   *Questions to Consider in the Critical Appraisal of a Research or Review Article*

FOR ALL STUDIES

- What criteria were in place in the database used to find the study? (e.g., journal referenced in PubMed have met stringent quality criteria)
- How up to date (recent) is the study?
- Is the purpose of the study clearly stated? How closely does the purpose of the study address the clinical question of concern?
- How comprehensive is the review of the literature? How up to date and relevant are the references cited in the article? Does the review of the literature support the need for the study that is being reported?
- Are the outcome measurement tools used in the study described sufficiently? Are they appropriate to the clinical question of concern?
- Is evidence of the reliability and validity of each outcome measurement tool presented? Is the evidence adequate for the clinical question of concern?

FOR STUDIES OF INTERVENTIONS/ TREATMENTS/THERAPY

- Have subjects been randomly assigned to groups?
- Is there a control group (or placebo or standard care group) used to compare with the experimental group?

- Are the researchers collecting outcome data blind to subject group assignment?
- As feasible, subjects should be blinded to their group assignment?
- How similar are the experiment and control groups? Optimally, the only difference should be the intervention.
- Do confounding variables make the groups different before intervention?

FOR STUDIES CONCERNED WITH PROGNOSIS

- Are the researchers collecting outcome data blind to each subject's score on prognostic factors?
- Is the period of follow-up sufficiently long to ensure that the outcome of interest is captured?
- Is there evidence from repeated analysis with a second group of subjects, with similar results, to provide confirmation of the prognostic factors being investigated?

FOR STUDIES CONCERNED WITH DIAGNOSIS

- Has the new diagnostic test been compared with an accepted gold standard?
- Is the researcher performing the new diagnostic test blind to each subject's score on the gold standard?
- Is there evidence from repeated analysis with a second group of subjects, with similar results, to provide confirmation of the accuracy of the new diagnostic test?

BOX 4-4   *Questions Used to Assess Quality of a Systematic Review*

FORMULATION OF OBJECTIVES

- Is the topic (purpose of the review) well defined?
- The intervention
- The patients
- The outcomes of interest

LITERATURE SEARCH FOR STUDIES

- Was the search for papers thorough?
- Use of search terms that fully capture key concepts
- Identification of databases or citation sources used
- Search methods exhaustive, international in scope
- Search methods described in enough detail to replicate
- International in scope
- Search terms that fully capture search concepts

STUDY SELECTION

- Were study inclusion criteria clearly described and fairly applied?
- Explicit inclusion and exclusion criteria
- Criteria should be applicable to the topic
- Selection criteria are applied in a manner that limits bias
- Account for studies that are rejected

ASSESSING QUALITY OF DESIGN AND METHODS

- Was study quality assessed by blinded or independent reviewers?
- Was missing information sought from the original study investigators?

- Do the included studies seem to indicate similar effects?
- Were the overall findings assessed for their robustness?
- Was the play of chance adequately assessed?

DATA GATHERING

- Was information from each article extracted using a standardized format?
- Does the information gathered from each article include the following?
- Type of study (e.g., randomized, controlled trial)
- Characteristics of the intervention for experimental and control groups
- Key demographics of all subjects
- Primary outcome of importance
- An accounting for missing data

POOLING METHOD

- Are selected studies similar enough to be pooled for analysis?
- In design
- In interventions
- In operational definition of outcome variable

DISCUSSION, CONCLUSIONS, RECOMMENDATIONS

- Are recommendations based firmly on the quality of the evidence presented?
- Are conclusions and recommendations justified on the basis of the analysis performed?

determination of power. Knowing any four of these five factors allows the reader to calculate the final factor.[52] The five factors include the following:

1. The significance level (α coefficient) set for the statistical analysis of the outcome variable
2. Anticipated variance (e.g., standard deviation) within each group of subjects related to the outcome variable
3. Sample and group size
4. The anticipated effect size for the intervention or relationship; how large a difference or a correlation does there need to be to ensure than the outcome under review is important or clinically meaningful?
5. The desired level of power (β coefficient), an estimate of the likelihood that a real difference between groups will be demonstrated if it exists (avoiding a type II error)

Power analysis performed in preparation for a study (i.e., before subject recruitment, data collection, or analysis) identifies the ideal number of subjects that should be in each group.[29] When a power analysis is performed after the data analysis has been completed, it is used to determine the likelihood that small sample size affected the statistical analysis when insignificant findings occurred.[54]

When a power analysis is performed before implementation of a study, most employ a significance level of $\alpha = 0.05$ or lower and the power level of $b = 0.8$ or higher. The score for effect size and anticipated group variance will be study specific. Typically, researchers provide references from prior research or their own pilot data to justify their choices of effect size and variance. This use of power analysis provides evidence of a rigorous research design and helps the clinician trust the findings of the study.

The next important appraisal of the sample concerns its representativeness: to what extent are the subjects in the sample similar to (and therefore representative of) the "population" of interest and to the individual for whom the clinician is caring? The goal of all research studies is to make decisions about a general population of people on the basis of the findings of a representative sample from that population. How well a sample represents the larger group to which results will be generalized is a function of subject recruitment, selection, and retention.[55,56] In appraising an article to use as evidence for clinical decision making, the health professional must consider how subjects were selected and assigned to groups (hopefully randomly), what criteria were used to determine whether a possible subject was included or excluded from the study, and the reasons that subjects who started the study may have dropped out before data collection was completed. Study results will be biased if the sample used for the study is not representative of the underlying population. Small variations, randomly occurring across all subject groups, may be acceptable. Larger variations, particularly ones that systematically affect one subject group more than others, may introduce unacceptable amounts of bias.

As a critical appraiser of the research, the evidence-based practitioner must be on the alert for sampling bias.[57,58] In the ideal world, any subject in the patient population of interest should be equally likely to be chosen to be a subject in the study. Realistically, this is rarely the case. No one researcher has access to each older adult who has had a transtibial amputation, each child with cerebral palsy, or each young adult with an incomplete spinal cord lesion. The researcher should provide enough evidence in his or her discussion of the study's methodology that the reader can be reasonably comfortable that the methods implemented for choosing subjects provided access to subjects reasonably representative of the breadth of subjects with the target characteristics under investigation.

The article typically provides descriptive evidence from previous studies of the common characteristics of patients with the pathology of interest. The researcher then compares these known characteristics with the descriptive characteristics of subjects in their particular study. Any differences should be identified and discussed in the article. The critical appraiser must use professional judgment to determine the extent to which potential biasing factors influence the methodological rigor of the study. If inequalities were detected, it is possible to add steps to the statistical analysis to account for the inequality. This should be reported in the study.

Attrition (subject dropout rate) also influences the researcher's ability to generalize the findings of the study to the larger population of individuals with the diagnosis or impairment. A useful rule of thumb for readers who are critically appraising an article is that, if more than a 20% dropout rate has occurred, then findings of the study are likely suspect. In a strong research article, the researchers explain why and when subjects were lost. Evidence-based practitioners want to know whether subjects chose to leave the study because intervention made them worse or because the intervention was too difficult or painful to overcome its potential benefits. Another situation that may lead to attrition is based on a research design so burdensome or difficult that subjects were unable to meet participation requirements (so that only the most persistent individuals in the sample completed the study). Researchers attempt to account for dropouts either by performing an "intention-to-treat" analysis or presenting descriptive statistics that compare key characteristics of subjects who completed the study with those who did not complete the study.[59] If the researcher can confirm that both groups of subjects are not significantly different, particularly in terms of any characteristic that might bias outcomes, then a study may still be identified as having adequate methodological quality.

In an intention-to-treat analysis, all subjects who started a study but did not finish it are assigned the most negative outcome likely to occur with the measurement tool for the purposes of statistical analysis.[60] If a statistically significant finding still occurs in the presence of an intention-to-treat analysis, then even assuming that all dropouts had a bad outcome, the study still demonstrated significant effects.

Outcome Measures

In assessing methodological quality of a study's outcome measurement tools, three questions must be addressed:

- Are the outcome tools described well enough for the evidence-based practitioner to make an informed and realistic judgment about their appropriateness for assessing the variables of interest for this study?

- Are the outcome tools reasonably valid and reliable?
- Are the outcome tools reasonably responsive and sensitive to change?

A high-quality study describes the outcome measures in enough detail for the reader to understand exactly what was measured and to determine whether the tools are appropriate to answer the research questions addressed in the study.

The article should also provide sufficient detail to confirm reliability and validity of each outcome measurement tool. Reliability represents the consistency with which scores are reproduced given repetition of the test with the same tester or across numerous testers.[61,62] Validity represents the accuracy with which the measurement tool taps into the construct or characteristics that the test is purported to measure.[61,63–65] Table 4-4 lists the various aspects of reliability and validity.

TABLE 4-4   *Validity and Reliability*

DETERMINATION OF A TEST OR MEASURES RELIABILITY

Type of Reliability	*Question Being Addressed*
Intra-rater	Will the same examiner make consistent ratings of the same individual?
Test-retest	Is the measure stable/accurate over time?
Interrater	Will different examiners make consistent ratings of the same individual?
Internal consistency	How well do each of the items contribute or reflect what the test intends to measure (how well do the items hang together)?
Parallel forms	Are different versions of the test or measure equivalent?

RELIABILITY COEFFICIENTS

Parametric Analyses			*Nonparametric Analyses*	
Strategis for Continuous Measures	*Types of Reliability Evaluated*	*Strategies for Nominal Measures*	*Strategies for Ordinal Measures*	*Types of Reliability Evaluated*
Pearson product moment (Pearson's r) (association) (.0 to 1.0)	Intra-rater Test-retest Interrater Parallel forms	Percent agreement (includes chance agreement)	Percent agreement (includes chance agreement)	Intrarater Test-retest Interrater Parallel forms
Coefficient of Variation (SD/mean) (< 10% suggests reliability)	Intrarater Interrater	Kappa coefficient (agreement beyond chance)	Weighted percent agreement (magnitude of disparity) (includes chance agreement)	Intrarater Test-retest Interrater Parallel forms
Intraclass correlation coefficient (ICC) (association and agreement)	Intrarater Test-retest Interrater Parallel forms		Weighted kappa (agreement beyond chance)	Intrarater Test-retest Interrater Parallel forms
Cronbach's alpha	Internal consistency			

DETERMINATION OF A TEST OR MEASURE'S VALIDITY

Type of Validity	*Question Being Addressed*	*Continuous Measures*
Content	How well are items on the test sample from the domain being evaluated?	Content expert review of items
Concurrent or Criterion	How well does the measure reflect a particular event, characteristic, or outcome?	Correlation (with gold standard measure of characteristic or construct)
Predictive	How well does the measure predict a future event or outcome?	Correlation (with outcome variable, measured after a period of time)
Construct	Does the test measure a single underlying theoretical concept or construct? How many underlying constructs are included in the measure?	Correlation (with variables theoretically related to the construct of interest) Confirmatory factor analysis
Discriminant or Divergent	How well does the test or measure differentiate between/among groups?	T-test or analysis of variance

If a test is reliable, it should perform consistently under similar testing situations regardless of who performs the test. Studies of reliability usually report either correlation coefficients or intraclass correlation coefficients as the statistical measure of the accuracy with which scores are reproduced.[66] There is no absolute standard of minimally acceptable reliability.[67] A score of 1 indicates a complete reliability (and is rarely achieved); a score of 0 represents a complete lack of reliability. A general benchmark is that a score of r = 0.9 or better is strong evidence of reliability of that measure. Coefficients between 0.75 and 0.89 suggest that the measure has moderate risk of error but may be acceptable. Correlations of less than r = 0.75 are not typically perceived as having acceptable reliability.

The researchers who are reporting their study should provide an adequate description of the methodology of the study for the critical appraiser to determine which aspects of reliability are most important in this study (and therefore to determine whether the authors provided evidence of the appropriate reliability). Intertester reliability should be reported when more than one tester measures the same outcome, and intratester reliability should be reported when the same tester measures outcomes on more than one occasion. Test-retest reliability provides evidence that the test performs consistently when repeated under similar conditions.

In addition, readers are interested in whether the validity of the measure has been assessed. To be considered valid, there must be sufficient evidence to demonstrate that the test or tool measures what it is purported to measure.[63-65] The researchers who have written the article must provide this evidence about the measure so that the critical appraiser can be comfortable that concerns about validity have been adequately addressed. Just because a tool is reliable (consistent in its measurement properties) does not mean that it is also valid (measures what it intends to measure). A tool cannot be valid, however, if it is not reliable in its measurement.[61] Ideally, the tests or measures used in the study demonstrate great consistency with high reproducibility (i.e., reliability) and accurately assess the targeted characteristic (validity).

Evidence of validity is especially important when the test or tool measures an abstract concept (e.g., quality of life or functional independence) rather than a physiological phenomenon (e.g., heart rate, range of motion). A valid test or measure contains enough items or questions related to the concept or characteristic being evaluated that the clinician can be confident that the results of testing will represent the subject's status in relationship to the construct being assessed. A test or measure found to be reliable in one patient population is not automatically reliable in other populations.[61]

STEP 4: APPLICABILITY TO PATIENTS AND CLINICAL PRACTICE

The final component of an EBP approach to rehabilitative care is just as essential to provision of quality care as the ability to access and use available evidence and clinical expertise. Without consideration of the unique goals, expectations, values, and concerns that an individual in our care brings to the health care encounter, even the "perfect" plan of action will not be as efficacious as it might otherwise be. An individual's perspective and values are influenced by a number of factors including developmental issues and their position in the lifespan, their family system and culture, their work roles and responsibilities, their coping styles and strategies, their willingness or ability to access whatever resources might be available in their social support network, and their socioeconomic and educational resources.[68,69] To be as effective as possible in providing care, evidence-based practitioners must consider what the pathology, impairment, functional limitation, or disability means to the individual with respect to self-concept and sociocultural roles.[70]

Clinical Relevance

Assessing clinical importance of a study has both objective and subjective considerations. The clinician must look beyond the statistical significance of the findings.[71] Often this assessment is based on professional judgment about the impact of the extent of change. Does a statistically significant change in a functional test score or pain level translate into a change that the patient will perceive as important in daily life? Does long-term follow-up occur? That is, does the author examine the effectiveness of a given intervention 3 months, 6 months, or 1 year following the intervention? If the article only provides evidence of short-term benefits of the intervention, are these short-term benefits worth the time and effort in the long run? Would other interventions have had a better long-term outcome?

Making the decision to implement new approaches to care supported by the research literature requires the evidence-based practitioner to answer several questions related to his or her specific clinical environment[72]:

- How similar are the subjects used in the study to those in his or her clinical practice?
- How do the patient's values and expectations interact with or relate to effort, risks, and likely outcomes of the intervention being considered?

For studies of interventions/therapy/treatment consider the following:

- How likely is it that the patient will be willing and able to comply with intervention activities suggested in the study?

For studies of diagnosis consider the following:

- Is the diagnostic test adequately available, affordable, accurate, and precise for use in the clinician's setting?
- Is it likely that the patient will be willing and able to comply with the testing procedures?

For studies of prognosis consider the following:

- Will knowing the predictor factors make a clinically important difference in the way the clinician will care for his or her patients?

INTEGRATING CLINICAL EXPERTISE AND SKILL

Although research literature is a valuable and important resource for evidence-based decision making, using evidence from the literature is not sufficient for effective EBP. Practitioners must also have strong examination, evaluation, and diagnostic skills and should be able to incorporate these skills into reflective past experience and current research findings.[73]

What is clinical expertise? In rehabilitation, it is the combination and integration of (1) a multidimensional knowledge base that is grounded in basic science, medical science, psychological/sociocultural sciences, and movement sciences; (2) effective clinical reasoning skills and an orientation toward function; (3) well-developed and efficient psychomotor skills for examination and intervention; and (4) the desire or commitment to help the individuals clinicians provide care for[74-76] (Figure 4-3).

The first chapter of this text explores the educational preparation, roles, and responsibilities of individual health professionals involved in orthotic and prosthetic rehabilitation. Each has a particular body of knowledge to bring to the care of individuals needing a prosthesis or orthosis, as well as shared understanding (albeit at various depths) of anatomy, kinesiology, biomechanics, gait analysis, mobility training, motor control and motor learning, and principles of exercise. The authors have established that effective interdisciplinary teaming, in which each profession's perspective interacts so that the team becomes "more than the sum of its parts," is an essential component in the provision of successful orthotic or prosthetic rehabilitative care.

The background knowledge important in orthotic and prosthetic rehabilitation that enables clinicians to ask sound clinical questions and apply evidence to patient care includes a strong foundation in the following areas:

- Anatomy and physiology of the musculoskeletal, neuromuscular, cardiovascular, and cardiopulmonary systems
- Kinesiology and biomechanics of the human body

- Properties of orthotic and prosthetic materials
- Principles of motor control and motor learning
- Lifespan development
- Exercise prescription and assessment of exercise tolerance
- Determinants of normal gait and methods of gait assessment

How does the clinician gain knowledge necessary for expert practice? Entry-level professional education is the baseline, while on-the-job experience via trial and error practice and discussion/debate/collaboration with colleagues moves clinicians from students toward novices.[74,76] They become more competent in their roles and responsibilities as their experience grows; they support and enhance their developing mastery and expertise with continuing education, participation in journal clubs and perusal of the clinical research literature, and postgraduate education. Another important component of increasing competence and developing expertise is the ability to actively listen to the hopes and concerns of those they work with and incorporate these into decision making and plans of care.

Clinical expertise, then, allows health care providers to quickly and efficiently identify an individual's rehabilitation diagnosis and, based on their constellation of impairments and functional limitations, select the strategies for remediation or accommodation that will assist the individual's return to a preferred lifestyle.

Staying Current with the Literature

One proactive way that a clinician can keep informed about new studies focused on his or her area of practice is to sign up for an online service that automatically sends weekly or monthly electronic updates of new articles from journals that

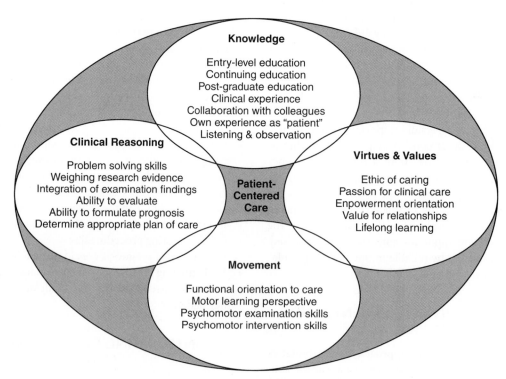

FIGURE 4-3 Expert patient-centered physical therapy practice requires integration and interaction of a provider's underlying knowledge, values, examination and intervention skills, and clinical reasoning.

the clinician feels are important to read or content areas that he or she wants to stay informed about. Professional organizations often offer this service as a membership benefit. Many journals allow readers to sign up for a service that electronically sends the table of contents via email whenever a new issue of the journal is released. Another valuable service (without charge) for evidence-based practitioners is available from an information management company, Amedeo (www.amedeo. com). When an evidence-based practitioner subscribes to Amedeo, he or she chooses from a list of topics for notification of newly published articles linked to those selected topics. Amedeo topics include rehabilitation, pain management, vascular surgery, and stroke, among many others. Amedeo routinely searches a large variety of high-quality journals for new publications on the topics selected by subscribers and sends weekly updates via email. This is a valuable resource for busy clinicians who may not have ready access to a medical library.

Two strategies, if routinely used, help health professionals to update and expand their expertise. The first is to select two or three journals (see Table 4-2) that are particularly appropriate for the clinician's area of professional interest and practice and arrange (via the journal's website) to receive an electronic copy of the table of contents of each issue. When the update arrives, it will be well worth the clinician's time and effort to scroll through the listing of articles and authors to determine which would be worth tracking down to read. The second strategy is to use whatever electronic literature update service is available through professional organizations, PubMed cubby, or Amedeo to arrange to be notified regularly of research reports published in the clinician's area of interest. The final step is to actually (and consistently) make time to read the resources that have been identified and discuss and debate them with colleaguesin order to effectively integrate the new information into clinical practice.

SUMMARY

This chapter explores the concepts underlying evidence-based health care practice and illustrates strategies to develop clear clinical questions, relevant to an individual patient who is receiving care. The chapter also identifies various sources of evidence available to clinicians and illustrates how electronic databases can assist the search process. The authors suggest strategies that clinicians can use to develop critical appraisal skills and to update and expand their clinical expertise. Although much of the chapter focuses on evidence available in the research literature, it is the integration of the best available scientific evidence; clinical expertise and judgment; and the concerns, values, and expectations of the individual who the clinicians care for that determines the effectiveness of clinical decision making.

APPENDIX 4-1

Reviews Published from 2006 to July 2011, Identified by Searching PubMed Electronic Research Database Using Search Terms "Limb Amputation AND Rehabilitation" and with the limits: a) review and b) English

Title	Authors	Journal
Moderators' summary: perceived performance differences; limb salvage versus amputation in the lower extremity (session II)	Andersen RC, Swiontkowski MF	J Am Acad Orthop Surg 2011;19 Suppl 1:S20-2
The clinical aspects of mirror therapy in rehabilitation: a systematic review of the literature	Rothgangel AS, Braun SM, Beurskens AJ, Seitz RJ, Wade DT	Int J Rehabil Res 2011;34(1):1-13
Neural interfaces for control of upper limb prostheses: the state of the art and future possibilities	Schultz AE, Kuiken TA	PM R 2011;3(1):55-67
Traumatic and trauma-related amputations: Part II: Upper extremity and future directions	Tintle SM, Baechler MF, Nanos GP, Forsberg JA, Potter BK	J Bone Joint Surg Am 2010;92(18):2934-45
Phantom limb pain: theories and therapies	Weeks SR, Anderson-Barnes VC, Tsao JW	Neurologist 2010;16(5):277-86
Evolving techniques in foot and ankle amputation	Ng VY, Berlet GC	J Am Acad Orthop Surg 2010;18(4):223-35
The role of physical therapy and occupational therapy in the rehabilitation of pediatric and adolescent patients with osteosarcoma	Punzalan M, Hyden G	Cancer Treat Res 2009;152:367-84
Bone sarcomas: Overview of management, with a focus on surgical treatment considerations	Lietman SA, Joyce MJ	Cleve Clin J Med 2010;77 Suppl 1:S8-12
Recent advances in lower extremity amputations and prosthetics for the combat injured patient	Fergason J, Keeling JJ, Bluman EM	Foot Ankle Clin 2010;15(1):151-74
Biomechanical parameters of gait among transtibial amputees: a review	Soares AS, Yamaguti EY, Mochizuki L, Amadio AC, Serrao JC	Sao Paulo Med J 2009;127(5):302-9
Phantom limb related phenomena and their rehabilitation after lower limb amputation	Casale R, Alaa L, Mallick M, Ring H	Eur J Phys Rehabil Med 2009;45(4):559-66
Mental practice for relearning locomotor skills	Malouin F, Richards CL	Phys Ther 2010;90(2):240-51
Advances in lower-limb prosthetic technology	Laferrier JZ, Gailey R	Phys Med Rehabil Clin N Am 2010;21(1):87-110
Systematic review of the effectiveness of mirror therapy in upper extremity function	Ezendam D, Bongers RM, Jannink MJ	Disabil Rehabil 2009;31(26):2135-49
Peripheral arterial disease in women	Aronow WS	Maturitas 2009 Dec 20;64(4):204-11
Prosthetic rehabilitation issues in the diabetic and dysvascular amputee	Uustal H	Phys Med Rehabil Clin N Am 2009;20(4):689-703
Clinical features and electrodiagnosis of diabetic peripheral neuropathy in the dysvascular patient	Wooten K	Phys Med Rehabil Clin N Am 2009;20(4):657-76

Title	Authors	Citation
One-stage osteoplastic reconstruction of the thumb	Cheema TA, Miller S	Tech Hand Up Extrem Surg 2009;13(3):130-3
What's new in orthopaedic rehabilitation	Hosalkar H, Pandya NK, Hsu J, Keenan MA	J Bone Joint Surg Am 2009;91(9):2296-310
Predicting walking ability following lower limb amputation: a systematic review of the literature	Sansam K, Neumann V, O'Connor R, Bhakta B	J Rehabil Med 2009;41(8):593-603
Treatment strategies for peripheral artery disease	McCann AB, Jaff MR	Expert Opin Pharmacother 2009;10(10):1571-86
Selection of outcome measures in lower extremity amputation rehabilitation: ICF activities	Deathe AB, Wolfe DL, Devlin M, Hebert JS, Miller WC, Pallaveshi L	Disabil Rehabil 2009;31(18):1455-73
Outcome measures in amputation rehabilitation: ICF body functions	Hebert JS, Wolfe DL, Miller WC, Deathe AB, Devlin M, Pallaveshi L	Disabil Rehabil 2009;31(19):1541-54
Assessment of health-related quality of life after bone cancer in young people: easier said than done	Eiser C	Eur J Cancer 2009;45(10):1744-7
Prosthetic feet: state-of-the-art review and the importance of mimicking human ankle-foot biomechanics	Versluys R, Beyl P, Van Damme M, Desomer A, Van Ham R, Lefeber D	Disabil Rehabil Assist Technol 2009;4(2):65-75
Sexuality and amputation: a systematic literature review	Geertzen JH, Van Es CG, Dijkstra PU	Disabil Rehabil 2009;31(7):522-7
Carbon fibre prostheses and running in amputees: a review	Nolan L	Foot Ankle Surg 2008;14(3):125-9
A systematic review of outcomes and complications of reconstruction and amputation for type IIIB and IIIC fractures of the tibia	Saddawi-Konefka D, Kim HM, Chung KC	Plast Reconstr Surg 2008;122(6):1796-805
On the use of longitudinal intrafascicular peripheral interfaces for the control of cybernetic hand prostheses in amputees	Micera S, Navarro X, Carpaneto J, Citi L, Tonet O, Rossini PM, Carrozza MC, Hoffmann KP, Vivó M, Yoshida K, Dario P	IEEE Trans Neural Syst Rehabil Eng 2008; 6(5):453-72
Patient rehabilitation following lower limb amputation	Kelly M, Dowling M	Nurs Stand 2008;22(49):35-40
Internal pedal amputations	Koller A	Clin Podiatr Med Surg 2008;25(4):641-53, ix
Ipsilateral total hip arthroplasty in a dysvascular below-knee amputee for advanced hip osteoarthritis: a case report and review of the literature	Mak J, Solomon M, Faux S	Prosthet Orthot Int 2008;32(2):155-9
Review of secondary physical conditions associated with lower-limb amputation and long-term prosthesis use	Gailey R, Allen K, Castles J, Kucharik J, Roeder M	J Rehabil Res Dev 2008;45(1):15-29
Controversies in lower extremity amputation	Pinzur MS, Gottschalk F, Pinto MA, Smith DG	Instr Course Lect 2008;57:663-72
MOC-PS(SM) CME article: lower extremity reconstruction	Reddy V, Stevenson TR	Plast Reconstr Surg 2008;121(4 Suppl):1-7
Prevention and management of complications of the Ilizarov treatment method	Sella EJ	Foot Ankle Spec 2008;1(2):105-7
Pain management in the traumatic amputee	Ketz AK	Crit Care Nurs Clin North Am 2008;20(1):51-7, vi
Return to work after lower limb amputation	Burger H, Marincek C	Disabil Rehabil 2007;29(17):1323-9

(Continued)

Reviews Published from 2006 to July 2011, Identified by Searching PubMed Electronic Research Database Using Search Terms "Limb Amputation AND Rehabilitation" and with the limits: a) review and b) English—cont'd

Title	Authors	Journal
Partial hand amputation and work	Burger H, Maver T, Marincek C	Disabil Rehabil 2007;29(17):1317-21
Prosthetic rehabilitation of persons with lower limb amputations due to tumour	Kauzlaric N, Kauzlaric KS, Kolundzic R	Eur J Cancer Care 2007;16(3):238-43
Posttraumatic finger reconstruction with microsurgical transplantation of toes	Wallace CG, Wei FC	Hand Clin 2007;23(1):117-28
Skin problems in lower limb amputees: an overview by case reports	Meulenbelt HE, Geertzen JH, Dijkstra PU, Jonkman MF	J Eur Acad Dermatol Venereol 2007;21(2):147-55
Complex limb salvage or early amputation for severe lower-limb injury: a meta-analysis of observational studies	Busse JW, Jacobs CL, Swiontkowski MF, Bosse MJ, Bhandari M	J Orthop Trauma 2007;21(1):70-6
Peripheral arterial disease	Aronow WS	Geriatrics 2007;62(1):19-25
Best practice in the assessment and management of diabetic foot ulcers	Delmas L	Rehabil Nurs 2006;31(6):228-34
Intermittent claudication	Cassar K	BMJ 2006;333(7576):1002-5
Physical capacity and walking ability after lower limb amputation: a systematic review	van Velzen JM, van Bennekom CA, Polomski W, Slootman JR, van der Woude LH, Houdijk H	Clin Rehabil 2006;20(11):999-1016
Lower extremity reconstruction	Heller L, Kronowitz SJ	J Surg Oncol 2006;94(6):479-89
Prosthetic rehabilitation for older dysvascular people following a unilateral transfemoral amputation	Cumming JC, Barr S, Howe TE	Cochrane Database Syst Rev 2006;(4):CD005260

APPENDIX 4-2

Examples of Clinical Practice Guidelines Available from the National Guideline Clearinghouse (www.guideline.gov)

Title	NGC#	Sponsoring Professional Organization(s)
SEARCH TERMS: ORTHOSIS OR ORTHOTIC AND REHABILITATION		
Best evidence statement (BESt). Lower extremity orthoses for children with hemiplegic cerebral palsy.	NGC:007670	Cincinnati Children's Hospital Medical Center - Hospital/Medical Center
Diagnosis and management of Duchenne muscular dystrophy, part 2: implementation of multidisciplinary care.	NGC:007681	DMD Care Considerations Working Group - Independent Expert Panel
Heel pain - plantar fasciitis: clinical practice guidelines linked to the International Classification of Functioning, Disability, and Health from the Orthopaedic Section of the American Physical Therapy Association.	NGC:007274	The Orthopaedic Section of the American Physical Therapy Association, Inc. - Medical Specialty Society
Clinical practice guidelines for gait training.	NGC:005309	Ottawa Panel - Independent Expert Panel
Best evidence statement (BESt). Intensive partial body weight supported treadmill training.	NGC:008168	Cincinnati Children's Hospital Medical Center - Hospital/Medical Center
Evidence-based care guideline for therapy management of congenital muscular torticollis in children age 0 to 36 months.	NGC:007301	Cincinnati Children's Hospital Medical Center - Hospital/Medical Center
Improving outcomes for people with sarcoma.	NGC:004878	National Collaborating Centre for Cancer - National Government Agency [Non-U.S.]
Diagnosis and treatment of forefoot disorders. Section 2. Central metatarsalgia.	NGC:007478	American College of Foot and Ankle Surgeons - Medical Specialty Society
Guideline for the evidence-informed primary care management of low back pain.	NGC:007704	Institute of Health Economics - Nonprofit Research Organization; Toward Optimized Practice - State/Local Government Agency [Non-U.S.]
VA/DoD clinical practice guideline for the management of stroke rehabilitation.	NGC:008250	American Heart Association - Professional Association; American Stroke Association - Disease Specific Society; Department of Defense - Federal Government Agency [U.S.]; Department of Veterans Affairs - Federal Government Agency [U.S.]; Veterans Health Administration - Federal Government Agency [U.S.]
European Federation of Neurological Societies/Peripheral Nerve Society guideline on management of chronic inflammatory demyelinating polyradiculoneuropathy: report of a joint task force of the European Federation of Neurological Societies and the Peripheral Nerve Society – first revision.	NGC:007904	European Federation of Neurological Societies - Medical Specialty Society; Peripheral Nerve Society - Disease Specific Society
Osteoporosis and fracture prevention in the long-term care setting.	NGC:007637	American Medical Directors Association - Professional Association
VA/DoD clinical practice guideline for rehabilitation of lower limb amputation.	NGC:006060	Department of Defense - Federal Government Agency [U.S.]; Department of Veterans Affairs - Federal Government Agency [U.S.]; Veterans Health Administration - Federal Government Agency [U.S.]
Ankle & foot (acute & chronic).	NGC:008511	Work Loss Data Institute - For Profit Organization.

(Continued)

Examples of Clinical Practice Guidelines Available from the National Guideline Clearinghouse (www.guideline.gov)—cont'd

Title	NGC#	Sponsoring Professional Organization(s)
Rehabilitation. In: Clinical guidelines for stroke management 2010.	NGC:008108	National Stroke Foundation (Australia) - Nonprofit Organization
Occupational therapy practice guidelines for adults with traumatic brain injury.	NGC:007509	American Occupational Therapy Association, Inc. - Professional Association
Diagnosis and treatment of forefoot disorders. Section 4. Tailor's bunion.	NGC:007480	American College of Foot and Ankle Surgeons - Medical Specialty Society
Evidence-based care guideline for serial casting of the lower extremity.	NGC:007161	Cincinnati Children's Hospital Medical Center - Hospital/Medical Center
Management of patients with stroke: rehabilitation, prevention and management of complications, and discharge planning. A national clinical guideline.	NGC:007955	Scottish Intercollegiate Guidelines Network - National Government Agency [Non-U.S.]
Evidence-based care guideline for pediatric constraint induced movement therapy (CIMT).	NGC:007162	Cincinnati Children's Hospital Medical Center - Hospital/Medical Center
EFNS guideline on diagnosis and management of limb girdle muscular dystrophies.	NGC:006935	European Federation of Neurological Societies - Medical Specialty Society
Occupational therapy practice guidelines for adults with neurodegenerative diseases.	NGC:007508	American Occupational Therapy Association, Inc. - Professional Association
Diabetic foot disorders: a clinical practice guideline.	NGC:005270	American College of Foot and Ankle Surgeons - Medical Specialty Society
Pressure ulcer prevention and treatment. Health care protocol.	NGC:007847	Institute for Clinical Systems Improvement - Nonprofit Organization
Management of diabetes. A national clinical guideline.	NGC:007892	Scottish Intercollegiate Guidelines Network - National Government Agency [Non-U.S.]
Metastatic spinal cord compression. Diagnosis and management of adults at risk of and with metastatic spinal cord compression.	NGC:007194	National Collaborating Centre for Cancer - National Government Agency [Non-U.S.]
Clinical practice guideline for the management of rheumatoid arthritis in Spain.	NGC:006691	Advanced Research Techniques in the Health Services - For Profit Research Organization; Spanish Society of Rheumatology - Medical Specialty Society
Traumatic brain injury: diagnosis, acute management and rehabilitation.	NGC:005397	New Zealand Guidelines Group - Nonprofit Organization
SEARCH TERMS: PROSTHESIS OR AMPUTATION AND REHABILITATION		
VA/DoD clinical practice guideline for rehabilitation of lower limb amputation.	NGC:006060	Department of Defense - Federal Government Agency [U.S.]; Department of Veterans Affairs - Federal Government Agency [U.S.]; Veterans Health Administration - Federal Government Agency [U.S.]
ACR Appropriateness Criteria® imaging after total knee arthroplasty.	NGC:005538	American College of Radiology - Medical Specialty Society
The diagnosis of periprosthetic joint infections of the hip and knee.	NGC:007976	American Academy of Orthopaedic Surgeons (AAOS) - Medical Specialty Society
Chronic wounds of the lower extremity.	NGC:005966	American Society of Plastic Surgeons - Medical Specialty Society
Long-term follow-up guidelines for survivors of childhood, adolescent, and young adult cancers. Sections 107-132: surgery.	NGC:007572	Children's Oncology Group - Medical Specialty Society
Ankle & foot (acute & chronic).	NGC:008511	Work Loss Data Institute - For Profit Organization

Guideline	NGC Number	Developer
Shoulder (acute & chronic).	NGC:008320	Work Loss Data Institute - For Profit Organization
Surgical site infection: prevention and treatment of surgical site infection.	NGC:006827	National Collaborating Centre for Women's and Children's Health - National Government Agency [Non-U.S.]
American Academy of Orthopaedic Surgeons clinical guideline on prevention of symptomatic pulmonary embolism in patients undergoing total hip or knee arthroplasty.	NGC:005665	American Academy of Orthopaedic Surgeons (AAOS) - Medical Specialty Society
Improving outcomes for people with sarcoma.	NGC:004878	National Collaborating Centre for Cancer - National Government Agency [Non-U.S.]
Clinical practice guideline for the management of rheumatoid arthritis in Spain.	NGC:006691	Advanced Research Techniques in the Health Services - For Profit Research Organization; Spanish Society of Rheumatology - Medical Specialty Society
Diabetic foot disorders: a clinical practice guideline.	NGC:005270	American College of Foot and Ankle Surgeons - Medical Specialty Society
ACR Appropriateness Criteria claudication — suspected vascular etiology.	NGC:007810	American College of Radiology - Medical Specialty Society
(1) Reducing foot complications for people with diabetes. (2) Reducing foot complications for people with diabetes 2007 supplement.	NGC:006572	Registered Nurses' Association of Ontario - Professional Association
Forearm, wrist, & hand (acute & chronic), not including carpal tunnel syndrome.	NGC:008311	Work Loss Data Institute - For Profit Organization
Warfarin therapy - management during invasive procedures and surgery.	NGC:008152	Medical Services Commission, British Columbia - National Government Agency [Non-U.S.]
ACR Appropriateness Criteria® acute shoulder pain.	NGC:007928	American College of Radiology - Medical Specialty Society
Prevention of venous thrombosis.	NGC:006599	Finnish Medical Society Duodecim - Professional Association
VA/DoD clinical practice guideline for the management of stroke rehabilitation.	NGC:008250	American Heart Association - Professional Association; American Stroke Association - Disease Specific Society; Department of Defense - Federal Government Agency [U.S.]; Department of Veterans Affairs - Federal Government Agency [U.S.]; Veterans Health Administration - Federal Government Agency [U.S.]
Palliative treatment of cancer.	NGC:005820	Finnish Medical Society Duodecim - Professional Association. View all guidelines by the developer(s) Compare Selected
EFNS guidelines on neurostimulation therapy for neuropathic pain.	NGC:005909	European Federation of Neurological Societies - Medical Specialty Society
NKF-KDOQI clinical practice guidelines for vascular access: update 2006.	NGC:005331	National Kidney Foundation - Disease Specific Society
Guideline for management of wounds in patients with lower-extremity arterial disease.	NGC:006521	Wound, Ostomy, and Continence Nurses Society - Professional Association
Assessment and management of stage I to IV pressure ulcers.	NGC:005793	Registered Nurses' Association of Ontario - Professional Association

APPENDIX 4-3

*Results of Search Using PEDro Database**

Type of Study	Title	Authors	Source
Clinical Practice Guideline	Non-drug treatment (excluding surgery) in rheumatoid arthritis: Clinical practice guidelines	Forestier R, Andre-Vert J, Guillez P, Coudeyre E, Lefevre-Colau MM, Combe B, Mayoux-Benhamou MA	Joint Bone Spine 2009;76(6):691-698
Systematic Review	Foot orthoses for patellofemoral pain in adults	Hossain M, Alexander P, Burls A, Jobanputra P	Cochrane Database Syst Rev 2011;Issue 1
Systematic Review	The efficacy of foot orthoses in the treatment of individuals with patellofemoral pain syndrome: a systematic review	Barton CJ, Munteanu SE, Menz HB, Crossley KM	Sports Med 2010;40(5):377-395
Systematic Review	Non-surgical interventions for paediatric pes planus	Rome K, Ashford RL, Evans A	Cochrane Database Syst Rev 2010;Issue 7
Systematic Review	Does the use of orthoses improve self-reported pain and function measures in patients with plantar fasciitis? A meta-analysis	Lee SY, McKeon P, Hertel J	Phys Ther Sport 2009;10(1):12-18
Systematic Review	Rehabilitation interventions for foot drop in neuromuscular disease	Sackley C, Disler PB, Turner-Stokes L, Wade DT, Brittle N, Hoppitt T	Cochrane Database Syst Rev 2009;Issue 3
Systematic Review	Diagnosis and management of deformational plagiocephaly	Robinson S, Proctor M	J Neurosurg Pediatr 2009;3(4):284-295
Systematic Review	The real risks of steroid injection for plantar fasciitis, with a review of conservative therapies	Tatli YZ, Kapasi S	Curr Rev Musculoskel Med 2009;19;2(1):3-9
Systematic Review	Evaluation of the scope and quality of systematic reviews on nonpharmacological conservative treatment for patellofemoral pain syndrome	Barton CJ, Webster KE, Menz HB	J Orthopaed Sports Phys Ther 2008;38(9):529-541
Systematic Review	Review of selected physical therapy interventions for school age children with disabilities	Effgen SK, McEwen IR	Phys Ther Rev 2008;13(5):297-312
Systematic Review	Efficacy of ankle-foot orthoses on gait of children with cerebral palsy: systematic review of literature	Figueiredo EM, Ferreira GB, Moreira RCM, Kirkwood RN, Fetters L	Pediatr Phys Ther 2008;20(3):207-223
Systematic Review	Custom-made foot orthoses for the treatment of foot pain	Hawke F, Burns J, Radford JA, du Toit V	Cochrane Database Syst Rev 2008;Issue 3
Systematic Review	Effectiveness of foot orthoses for treatment and prevention of lower limb injuries: a review	Hume P, Hopkins W, Rome K, Maulder P, Coyle G, Nigg B	Sports Med 2008;38(9):759-779
Systematic Review	Exercise therapy and orthotic devices in rheumatoid arthritis: evidence-based review	Oldfield V, Felson DT	Curr Opin Rheumatol 2008;20(3):353-359

Type	Title	Authors	Source
Systematic Review	Treatment for Charcot-Marie-Tooth disease	Young P, de Jonghe P, Stogbauer F, Butterfass-Bahloul T	Cochrane Database Syst Rev 2008;Issue 1
Systematic Review	Head shape measurement standards and cranial orthoses in the treatment of infants with deformational plagiocephaly	McGarry A, Dixon MT, Greig RJ, Hamilton DR, Sexton S, Smart H	Dev Med Child Neurol 2008;50(8):568-576
Systematic Review	Interventions for the prevention and treatment of pes cavus	Burns J, Landorf KB, Ryan MM, Crosbie J, Ouvrier RA	Cochrane Database Syst Rev 2007;Issue 4
Systematic Review	An evaluation of research evidence for selected physical therapy interventions for plantar fasciitis	de vera Barredo R, Menna D, Farris JW	J Phys Ther Sci 2007;19(1):41-56
Systematic Review	A systematic review of the efficacy of gait rehabilitation strategies for spinal cord injury	Lam T, Eng JJ, Wolfe DL, Hsieh JTC, Whittaker M	Topics Spinal Cord Inj Rehabil 2007;13(1):32-57
Systematic Review	Evaluating interventions to improve gait in cerebral palsy: a meta-analysis of spatiotemporal measures	Paul SM, Siegel KL, Malley J, Jaeger RJ	Dev Med Child Neurol 2007;49(7):542-549
Systematic Review	Effectiveness of upper and lower limb casting and orthoses in children with cerebral palsy: an overview of review articles	Autti-Ramo I, Suoranta J, Anttila H, Malmivaara A, Makela M	Am J Phys Med Rehabil 2006;85(1):89-103
Systematic Review	A critical review of foot orthoses in the rheumatoid arthritic foot	Clark H, Rome K, Plant M, O'Hare K, Gray J	Rheumatology 2006;45(2):139-145
Systematic Review	A review of the literature pertaining to KAFOs and HKAFOs for ambulation	Fatone S	J Prosthet Orthot 2006;18(3 S):137-168
Systematic Review	Conservative therapy for plantar fasciitis: a narrative review of randomized controlled trials	Stuber K, Kristmanson K	J Can Chiropract Assoc 2006;50(2):118-133
Clinical Trial	Effective orthotic therapy for the painful cavus foot	Burns J, Crosbie J, Ouvrier R	Australas J Podiatr Med 2006;40(3):61-66
Clinical Trial	Effective orthotic therapy for the painful cavus foot: a randomized controlled trial	Burns J, Crosbie J, Ouvrier R, Hunt A	J Am Podiatr Med Assoc 2006;96(3):205-211
Clinical Trial	Effectiveness of foot orthoses to treat plantar fasciitis: a randomized trial	Landorf KB, Keenan A, Herbert RD	Arch Intern Med 2006 26;166(12):1305-1310
Clinical Trial	Effectiveness of prefabricated and customized foot orthoses made from low-cost foam for non-complicated plantar fasciitis: a randomized controlled trial	Baldassin V, Gomes CR, Beraldo PS	Arch Phys Med Rehabil 2009;90(4):701-706
Clinical Trial	Foot orthoses and physiotherapy in the treatment of patellofemoral pain syndrome: randomised clinical trial	Collins N, Crossley K, Beller E, Darnell R, McPoil T, Vicenzino B	Br Sports Med 2009;43(3):169-176
Clinical Trial	Neutral functional realignment orthosis prevents hand pain in patients with subacute stroke: a randomized trial	Burge E, Kupper D, Finckh A, Ryerson S, Schnider A, Leemann B	Arch Phys Med Rehabil 2008;89(10):1857-1862

(Continued)

Results of Search Using PEDro Database*—cont'd

Type of Study	Title	Authors	Source
Clinical Trial	Foot orthoses and physiotherapy in the treatment of patellofemoral pain syndrome: randomised clinical trial	Collins N, Crossley K, Beller E, Darnell R, McPoil T, Vicenzino B	BMJ 2008;337(7677):a1735
Clinical Trial	Influence of foot orthoses on plantar pressures, foot pain and walking ability of rheumatoid arthritis patients — a randomised controlled study	Novak P, Burger H, Tomsic M, Marincek C, Vidmar G	Disabil Rehabil 2009;31(8):638-645
Clinical Trial	A randomized controlled trial of two types of in-shoe orthoses in children with flexible excess pronation of the feet	Whitford D, Esterman A	Foot Ankle Int 2007;28(6):715-723
Clinical Trial	Foot orthoses for the treatment of plantar fasciitis	Roos E, Engstrom M, Soderberg B	Foot Ankle Int 2006;27(8):606-611
Clinical Trial	Static progressive stretch brace as a treatment of pain and functional limitations associated with plantar fasciitis: a pilot study	Sharma NK, Loudon JK	Foot Ankle Spec 2010;3(3):117-124
Clinical Trial	Use of low-frequency electrical stimulation for the treatment of plantar fasciitis	Stratton M, McPoil TG, Cornwall MW, Patrick K	J Am Podiatr Med Assoc 2009;99(6):481-488
Clinical Trial	The effect of rigid versus flexible spinal orthosis on the clinical efficacy and acceptance of the patients with adolescent idiopathic scoliosis	Wong MS, Cheng JC, Lam TP, Ng BK, Sin SW, Lee-Shum SL, Chow DH, Tam SY	Spine 2008;33(12):1360-1365
Clinical Trial	Comparison of 3 preventive methods to reduce the recurrence of ankle inversion sprains in male soccer players	Mohammadi F	Am J Sports Med 2007;35(6):922-926
Clinical Trial	Effect of treadmill training and supramalleolar orthosis use on motor skill development in infants with down syndrome: a randomized clinical trial	Looper J, Ulrich DA	Phys Ther 2010;90(3):382-390
Clinical Trial	The immediate effect of orthotic management on grip strength of patients with lateral epicondylosis	Jafarian FS, Demneh ES, Tyson SF	J Orthopaed Sports Phys Ther 2009;39(6):484-489
Clinical Trial	Nonsurgical management of posterior tibial tendon dysfunction with orthoses and resistive exercise: a randomized controlled trial	Kulig K, Reischl SF, Pomrantz AB, Burnfield JM, Mais-Requejo S, Thordarson DB, Smith RW	Phys Ther 2009;89(1):26-37
Clinical Trial	The effect of dynamic ankle foot orthoses on function in children with cerebral palsy	Bjornson KF, Schmale GA, Adamczyk-Foster A, McLaughlin J	J Pediatr Orthopaed 2006;26(6):773-776
Clinical Trial	Immediate effects of an individually designed functional ankle-foot orthosis on stance and gait in hemiparetic patients	Pohl M, Mehrholz J	Clin Rehabil 2006;20(4):324-330
Clinical Trial	Plantar fasciopathy treated with dynamic splinting: a randomized controlled trial	Sheridan L, Lopez A, Perez A, John MM, Willis FB, Shanmugam R	J Am Podiatr Med Assoc 2010;100(3):161-165

Clinical Trial	Foot orthoses in the prevention of injury in initial military training	Franklyn-Miller A, Wilson C, Bilzon J, McCrory P	Am J Sports Med 2011;39(1):30-37
Clinical Trial	Effect of foot orthoses contour on pain perception in individuals with patellofemoral pain	McPoil TG, Vicenzino B, Cornwall MW	J Am Podiatr Med Assoc 2011;101(1):7-16
Clinical Trial	Does orthotic use affect upper extremity support during upright play in infants with down syndrome?	Looper J, Ulrich D	Phys Occup Ther Pediatr 2011;23(1):70-77
Clinical Trial	Kinematic features of rear-foot motion using anterior and posterior ankle-foot orthoses in stroke patients with hemiplegic gait	Chen C, Hong W, Wang C, Wu KP, Kang C, Tang SF	Arch Phys Med Rehabil 2010;91(12):1862-1868
Clinical Trial	Changes in gait economy between full-contact custom-made foot orthoses and prefabricated inserts in patients with musculoskeletal pain: a randomized clinical trial	Trotter LC, Pierrynowski MR	J Am Podiatr Med Assoc 2008;98(6):429-435
Clinical Trial	The short-term effectiveness of full contact custom-made foot orthoses and prefabricated shoe inserts on lower-extremity musculoskeletal pain: a randomized clinical trial	Trotter LC, Pierrynowski MR	J Am Podiatr Med Assoc 2008;98(5):357-363

*Key word: orthoses (limited to articles/abstracts published January 2006 – July 2011).

APPENDIX 4-4

Results of Search Using Hooked on Evidence, APTA*

Title	Author	Sources
Effects of carbon fibre spring orthoses on gait in ambulatory children with motor disorders and plantarflexor weakness	Bartonek A, Eriksson M, Gutierrez-Farewik EM	Dev Med Child Neurol 2007; 49(8): 615-620
The effect of dynamic ankle foot orthoses on function in children with cerebral palsy	Bjornson KF, Schmale GA, Adamczyk-Foster A, McLaughlin J	J Pediatr Orthop 2006; 26(6): 773-776
Effects of ankle-foot orthoses on ankle and foot kinematics in patient with ankle osteoarthritis	Huang YC, Harbst K, Kotajarvi B, Hansen D, Koff MF, Kitaoka HB, Kaufman KR	Arch Phys Med Rehabil 2006; 87(5): 710-716
Changes in gait economy between full-contact custom-made foot orthoses and prefabricated inserts in patients with musculoskeletal pain: a randomized clinical trial	Trotter LC, Pierrynowski MR	J Am Podiatr Med Assoc 2008; 98(6): 429-435
Effectiveness of prefabricated and customized foot orthoses made from low-cost foam for noncomplicated plantar fasciitis: a randomized controlled trial	Baldassin V, Gomes CR, Beraldo PS	Arch Phys Med Rehabil 2009; 90(4): 701-706
Foot orthoses and physiotherapy in the treatment of patellofemoral pain syndrome: randomised clinical trial	Collins N, Crossley K, Beller E, Darnell R, McPoil T, Vicenzino B	BMJ 2008; 337(7677): 1034-1036
Nonsurgical management of posterior tibial tendon dysfunction with orthoses and resistive exercise: a randomized controlled trial	Kulig K, Reischl SF, Pomrantz AB, Burnfield JM, Mais-Requejo S, Thordarson DB, Smith RW	Phys Ther 2009; 89(1): 26-37
Reach performance and postural adjustments during standing in children with severe spastic diplegia using dynamic ankle-foot orthoses	Naslund A, Sundelin G, Hirschfeld H	J Rehabil Med 2007; 39(9): 715-723
Use of strutter orthoses for an adolescent with myelodysplasia	Magee JA, Kenney DM	Pediatr Phys Ther 2008; 20(1): 81-88
Impact of ankle-foot orthoses on static foot alignment in children with cerebral palsy	Westberry DE, Davids JR, Shaver JC, Tanner SL, Blackhurst DW, Davis RB	J Bone Joint Surg Am 2007; 89(4): 806-813
Foot orthoses for the treatment of plantar fasciitis	Roos E, Engstrom M, Soderberg B	Foot Ankle Int 2006; 27(8): 606-611
Does orthotic use affect upper extremity support during upright play in infants with down syndrome?	Looper J, Ulrich D	Pediatr Phys Ther 2011; 23(1): 70-77
Use of foot orthoses and calf stretching for individuals with medial tibial stress syndrome	Loudon JK, Dolphino MR	Foot Ankle Spec 2010; 3(1): 15-20
Do ankle orthoses improve ankle proprioceptive thresholds or unipedal balance in older persons with peripheral neuropathy?	Son J, Ashton-Miller JA, Richardson JK	Am J Phys Med Rehabil 2010; 89(5): 369-375
Use of low-frequency electrical stimulation for the treatment of plantar fasciitis	Stratton M, McPoil TG, Cornwall MW, Patrick K	J Am Podiatric Med Assoc 2009; 99(6): 481-488

Title	Authors	Citation
Effective orthotic therapy for the painful cavus foot: a randomized controlled trial	Burns J, Crosbie J, Ouvrier R, Hunt A	J Am Podiatr Med Assoc 2006; 96(3): 205-211
Ankle bracing, plantar-flexion angle, and ankle muscle latencies during inversion stress in healthy participants	Kernozek T, Durall CJ, Friske A, Mussallem M	J Athl Train 2008; 43(1): 37-43
Comparison of 3 preventive methods to reduce the recurrence of ankle inversion sprains in male soccer players	Mohammadi F	Am J Sports Med 2007; 35(6): 922-926
Use of a postoperative lumbar corset after lumbar spinal arthrodesis for degenerative conditions of the spine. a prospective randomized trial	Yee AJ, Yoo JU, Marsolais EB, Carlson G, Poe-Kochert C, Bohlman HH, Emery SE	J Bone Joint Surg Am 2008; 90(10): 2062-2068
Short- and long-term influences of a custom foot orthotic intervention on lower extremity dynamics	MacLean CL, Davis IS, Hamill J	Clin J Sport Med 2008; 18(4): 338-343
The influence of foot orthoses on the function of a child with developmental delay	George DA, Elchert L	Pediatr Phys Ther 2007; 19(4): 332-336
Changes in joint kinematics in children with cerebral palsy while walking with and without a floor reaction ankle-foot orthosis	Lucareli PR, Lima Mde O, Lucarelli JG, Lima FP	Clinics 2007; 62(1): 63-68
Changes in muscle activity in children with hemiplegic cerebral palsy while walking with and without ankle-foot orthoses	Romkes J, Hell AK, Brunner R	Gait Posture 2006; 24(4): 467-474
The effect of fixed ankle foot orthoses in children with cerebral palsy	Butler PB, Farmer SE, Stewart C, Jones PW, Forward M	Disabil Rehabil Assist Technol 2007; 2(1): 51-58
A comparison of the thoracolumbosacral orthoses and providence orthosis in the treatment of adolescent idiopathic scoliosis: results using the new SRS inclusion and assessment criteria for bracing studies	Janicki JA, Poe-Kochert C, Armstrong DG, Thompson GH	J Pediatr Orthop 2007; 27(4): 369-374
The effect of custom-made braces for the ankle and hindfoot on ankle and foot kinematics and ground reaction forces	Kitaoka HB, Crevoisier XM, Harbst K, Hansen D, Kotajarvi B, Kaufman K	Arch Phys Med Rehabil 2006; 87(1): 130-135
Effects of ankle-foot orthoses on ankle and foot kinematics in patients with subtalar osteoarthritis	Huang YC, Harbst K, Kotajarvi B, Hansen D, Koff MF, Kitaoka HB, Kaufman KR	Arch Phys Med Rehabil 2006; 87(8): 1131-1136
Effectiveness of foot orthoses to treat plantar fasciitis: a randomized trial	Landorf KB, Keenan AM, Herbert RD	Arch Intern Med 2006; 166(12): 1305-1310
Effects of wearing foot orthosis with medial arch support on the fifth metatarsal loading and ankle inversion angle in selected basketball tasks	Yu B, Preston JJ, Queen RM, Byram IR, Hardaker WM, Gross MT, Davis JM, Taft TN, Garrett WE	J Orthop Sports Phys Ther 2007; 37(4): 186-191

*Key word: orthoses (listed articles/abstracts published January 2006 – July 2011).

REFERENCES

1. Wong RA, Barr JO, Farina N, et al. Evidence-based practice: a resource for physical therapists. *Issues Aging.* 2000;23(3):19–26.
2. McCluskey A, Home S, Thompson L. Becoming an evidence-based practitioner. In: Law M, MacDermid J, eds. *Evidence-Based Rehabilitation: A Guide to Practice.* 2nd ed. Thorofare, NJ: Slack; 2008:35–62.
3. MacDermid J, Law M. Evaluating the evidence. In: Law M, MacDermid J, eds. *Evidence-Based Rehabilitation: A Guide to Practice.* 2nd ed. Thorofare, NJ: Slack; 2008:121–142.
4. Straus SE, Richardson WS, Glasziou P, et al. *Evidence-based Medicine: How to Practice and Teach EBM.* 3rd ed. Edinburgh: Elsevier/Churchill Livingstone; 2005.
5. Donald A, Greenhalgh T. *A Hands-on Guide to Evidence-based Health Care: Practice and Implementation.* Oxford, UK: Blackwell Science; 2000.
6. Batavia M. *Clinical Research for Health Professionals: A User Friendly Guide.* Boston: Butterworth-Heinemann; 2001.
7. Who are physical therapists, and what do they do? In: American Physical Therapy Association, ed. *Guide to Physical Therapist Practice.* Revised 2nd ed. Alexandria, VA: APTA; 2003:31–42.
8. Kassirer JP. Incorporating patient's preferences into medical decisions. *N Engl J Med.* 1994;330(26):1895–1896.
9. Guyatt G, Haynes B, Jaeschke R, et al. The foundations: the philosophy of evidence-based medicine. In: Guyatt G, Rennie D, Meade M, et al., eds. *Users' Guide to the Medical Literature: A Manual for Evidence-Based Clinical Practice.* 2nd ed. Chicago: AMA Press; 2008:9–16.
10. Portney LG, Watkins MP. *Foundations of Clinical Research: Applications to Practice.* 3rd ed. Upper Saddle River, NJ: Prentice-Hall; 2009.
11. Greenhalgh T. Papers that report trials of drug treatments and other simple interventions. In: Greenhalgh T, ed. *How to Read a Paper: The Basics of Evidence Based Medicine.* 4th ed. London: BMJ Books; 2010:78–89.
12. Guyatt G, Cook D, Devereaux PJ, et al. Therapy (randomized trials). In: Guyatt G, Rennie D, Meade M, Cook D, eds. *Users' Guide to the Medical Literature: A Manual for Evidence-Based Clinical Practice.* 2nd ed. Chicago: AMA Press; 2008:67–86.
13. Greenhalgh T. Papers that report diagnostic or screening tests. In: Greenhalgh T, ed. *How to Read a Paper: The Basics of Evidence Based Medicine.* 4th ed. London: BMJ Books; 2010:98–112.
14. Fritz JM, Wainner RS. Examining diagnostic tests, an evidence-based perspective. *Phys Ther.* 2001;81(9):1546–1564.
15. Randolf A, Bucher H, Richardson WS, et al. Prognosis. In: Guyatt G, Rennie D, Meade M, et al., eds. *Users' Guide to the Medical Literature: A Manual for Evidence-Based Clinical Practice.* 2nd ed. Chicago: AMA Press; 2008:509–522.
16. On what concepts is the guide based? In: American Physical Therapy Association, ed. *Guide to Physical Therapist Practice.* Revised 2nd ed. Alexandria, VA: APTA; 2003:19–25.
17. World Health Organization. *Toward a Common Language for Functioning, Disability, and Health.* Geneva: World Health Organization; 2002.
18. Helewa A, Walker JM. Where to look for evidence. In: Helewa A, Walker JM, eds. *Critical Evaluation of Research in Physical Rehabilitation, Toward Evidence-Based Practice.* Philadelphia: Saunders; 2000:33–48.
19. Walker-Dilks C. Searching the physiotherapy evidence-based literature. *Physiother Theory Pract.* 2001;17(3):137–142.
20. Maher CG, Serrington C, Elkins M, et al. Challenges for evidence-based physical therapy: accessing and interpreting high-quality evidence on therapy. *Phys Ther.* 2004;84(8):644–654.
21. Greenhalgh T. Searching the literature. In: Greenhalgh T, ed. *How to Read a Paper: The Basics of Evidence Based Medicine.* 4th ed. London: BMJ Books; 2010:15–30.
22. Herbert RD, Sherrington C, Maher C, et al. Evidence-based practice—imperfect but necessary. *Physiother Theory Pract.* 2001;17(3):201–211.
23. Jette DU, Bacon K, Batty C, et al. Evidence-based practice: beliefs, attitudes, knowledge, and behaviors of physical therapists. *Phys Ther.* 2003;93(9):786–805.
24. Turner P. Evidence-based practice and physiotherapy in the 1990s. *Physiother Theory Pract.* 2001;17(2):107–121.
25. Maher C, Moseley A, Sherrington C, et al. Core journals of evidence-based physiotherapy practice. *Physiother Theory Pract.* 2001;17(3):143–151.
26. Bohannon RW. Core journals of physiotherapy. *Physiotherapy.* 1999;85(6):317–321.
27. Jada A. *Randomized Controlled Clinical Trials; A User's Guide.* London: BMJ Publishing Group; 1998.
28. Helewa A, Walker JM. The nuts and bolts of research: terms, concepts, and designs. In: Helewa A, Walker JM, eds. *Critical Evaluation of Research in Physical Rehabilitation: Towards Evidence-based Practice.* Philadelphia: Saunders; 2000:1–32.
29. Greenhalgh T. Papers that summarize other papers (systematic reviews and meta-analysis). In: Greenhalgh T, ed. *How to Read a Paper: The Basics of Evidence Based Medicine.* 4th ed. London: BMJ Books; 2010:113–131.
30. Cook DJ, Mulrow CD, Haynes RB. Systematic reviews: synthesis of best evidence for clinical decisions. *Ann Intern Med.* 1997;126(5):376–380.
31. Montori VM, Swiontkowski MF, Cook DJ. Methodologic issues in systematic reviews and meta-analyses. *Clin Orthop Relat Res.* 2003;413:43–54.
32. Bradley L, Law M. Systematically reviewing the evidence. In: Law M, MacDermid J, eds. *Evidence-based Rehabilitation: A Guide to Practice.* 2nd ed. Thorofare, NJ: Slack; 2008:143–160.
33. Lau J, Ionnidis JPA, Schmid CH. Quantitative synthesis in systematic reviews. *Ann Intern Med.* 1997;127(9):820–826.
34. Montori VM, Wilczynski NL, Morgan D, et al. Optimal search strategies for retrieving systematic reviews from Medline: analytical survey. *BMJ.* 2005;330(7482):68–71.
35. Lewis S, Clarke M. Forest plots: trying to see the wood and the trees. *BMJ.* 2001;322:1479–1480.
36. Busse JW, Jacobs CL, Swiontkowski MF, et al. Complex limb salvage or early amputation for severe lower-limb injury: a meta-analysis of observational studies. *J Orthop Trauma.* 2007; 21(1):70–76.
37. MacDermid J. Practice guidelines, algorithms, and clinical pathways. In: Law M, MacDermid J, eds. *Evidence-based Rehabilitation: A Guide to Practice.* 2nd ed. Thorofare, NJ: Slack; 2008:227–262.
38. Philadelphia panel evidence-based clinical practice guidelines on selected rehabilitation interventions: overview and methodology. *Phys Ther.* 2001;81(10):1629–1640.
39. *A User's Guide to Finding and Evaluating Health Information on the Web.* Medical Library Association. http://www.mlanet.org/resources/userguide.html.
40. Shojania KG, Bero LA. Taking advantage of the explosion of systematic reviews: an efficient search strategy. *Eff Clin Pract.* 2001;4(4):157–162.

41. O'Rourke A, Booth A. Another fine MeSH: clinical medicine meets information science. *J Info Sci*. 1999;25(4):275–281.

42. Snowball R. Using the clinical question to teach search strategy: fostering transferable conceptual skills in user education by active learning. *Health Libr Rev*. 1997;14(3):167–172.

43. McKibbon KA, Richardson WS, Walker-Dilks C. EBM notebook: finding answers to well built questions. *Evid Based Med*. 1999;4(6):164–167.

44. Greenhalgh T. Assessing methodological quality. In: Greenhalgh T, ed. *How to Read a Paper: The Basics of Evidence-based Medicine*. 4th ed. London: BMJ Books; 2010:47–60.

45. Fink R, Thompson CJ, Bonnes D. Overcoming barriers and promoting the use of research in practice. *J Nurs Adm*. 2005; 35(3):121–129.

46. Turner P, Mjolne I. Journal provision and the prevalence of journal clubs: a survey of physiotherapy departments in England and Australia. *Physiother Res Int*. 2001;6(3):157–169.

47. Urschel JD. How to analyze an article. *World J Surg*. 2005; 29(5):557–560.

48. Crombie IK. *The Pocket Guide to Critical Appraisal*. London: BMJ Publishing Group; 1998.

49. Kinnear PR, Gray CD. *IBM SPSS Statistics 18 Made Simple*. New York: Psychology Press; 2011.

50. Carter R, Lubinsky J, Dumholdt E. *Rehabilitation Research: Principles and Applications*. 4th ed. Philadelphia: Saunders; 2011.

51. Archibald CP, Lee HP. Sample size estimation for clinicians. *Ann Acad Med Singapore*. 1995;24(2):328–332.

52. Livingston EH, Cassidy L. Statistical power and estimation of required subjects for a study based on the t-test; a surgeons primer. *J Surg Res*. 2005;126(2):149–159.

53. Chow SC, Shao J, Wang H. *Sample Size Calculation in Clinical Research*. 2nd ed. Boca Raton, FL: Taylor & Francis; 2008.

54. Faul F, Erdfelder E, Lang A-G, Buchner A. G*Power 3: A flexible statistical power analysis program for the social, behavioral, and biomedical sciences. *Behav Res Methods*. 2007;39(2): 175–191.

55. Daunt DJ. Ethnicity and recruitment rates in clinical research studies. *Appl Nurs Res*. 2003;16(3):189–195.

56. Larson E. Exclusion of certain groups from clinical research. *Image J Nurs Sch*. 1994;26(3):185–190.

57. Sitthi-amorn C, Poshyachinda V. Bias. *Lancet* 1993;342 (8866):286–288.

58. Morabia A. Case-control studies in clinical research: mechanism and prevention of selection bias. *Prev Med*. 1997;25(5 Pt 1): 674–677.

59. Kruse RL, Alper BS, Reust C, et al. Intention-to-treat analysis: Who is in? Who is out? *J Fam Pract*. 2002;51:969–971.

60. Montori VM, Guyatt GH. Intention to treat principle. *Can Med Assoc J*. 2001;165(10):1339–1341.

61. Salkind NJ. Just the truth: An introduction to understanding reliability and validity. In: *Statistics for People Who (Think They) Hate Statistics*. 4th ed. Los Angeles, CA: Sage Publications; 2011:101–124.

62. Shultz KS, Whitney DJ. Classical true score theory and reliability, module 5. In: *Measurement Theory in Action*. Thousand Oaks, CA: Sage Publications; 2005:69–85.

63. Shultz KS, Whitney DJ. Content validation, module 6. In: *Measurement Theory in Action*. Thousand Oaks, CA: Sage Publications; 2005:87–100.

64. Shultz KS, Whitney DJ. Criterion-related validation, module 7. In: *Measurement Theory in Action*. Thousand Oaks, CA: Sage Publications; 2005:101–118.

65. Shultz KS, Whitney DJ. Construct validation, module 8. In: *Measurement Theory in Action*. Thousand Oaks, CA: Sage Publications; 2005:119–134.

66. Eliasziw M. Statistical methodology for the concurrent assessment of interrater and intrarater reliability: using goniometric measurements as an example. *Phys Ther*. 1994;74(8):777–788.

67. Stratford PW. Getting more from the literature; estimating standard error of measurement from reliability studies. *Physiother Can*. 2004;56(1):27–30.

68. Fell DW, Burnham JF. Access is key: teaching students and physical therapists to access evidence, expert opinion, and patient values for evidence based practice. *J Phys Ther Educ*. 2004;18(3):12–23.

69. Lockwood S. "Evidence of me" in evidence based medicine. *BMJ*. 2004;329(7473):1033–1035.

70. Spector RE. *Cultural Diversity in Health and Illness*. 7th ed. Upper Saddle River, NJ: Prentice-Hall; 2008.

71. Foster N, Barlas P, Chesterton L, et al. Critically appraised topics: one method of facilitating evidence-based practice in physiotherapy. *Physiotherapy*. 2001;87(4):179–190.

72. Greenhalgh T. Getting evidence into practice. In: Greenhalgh T, ed. *How to Read a Paper: The Basics of Evidence-based Medicine*. 4th ed. London: BMJ Books; 2010:199–220.

73. Jensen GM, Dwyer J, Shepard K, et al. Expert practice in physical therapy. *Phys Ther*. 2000;80(1):28–43.

74. Hack LM. Fostering evidence-based practice in physical therapy: clinical decision making frameworks. In: Wong R, ed. *Evidence-Based Healthcare Practice, Proceedings of a Consensus Conference "EBP: Where Are We Today? Where Are We Going? How Do We Get There?"*. Arlington, VA: Marymount University; 2001:22–30.

75. Resnik L, Jensen GM. Using clinical outcomes to explore theory of expert practice in physical therapy. *Phys Ther*. 2003;83(12):1090–1106.

76. Jensen GM, Gwyer J, Hack L, et al. *Expertise in Physical Therapy Practice*. 2nd ed. St. Louis, MO: Saunders Elsevier; 2007.

5

Clinical Assessment of Gait

OLFAT MOHAMED, DANA CRAIG, HEATHER WORDEN, AND EDMOND AYYAPPA

LEARNING OBJECTIVES

On completion of this chapter, the reader will be able to:

1. Describe the major functional tasks of the gait cycle and their corresponding subphases.
2. Identify the muscle activity, ground reaction forces, and joint angles during each of the subphases of the gait cycle.
3. Define the time and distance parameters used to describe and assess normal gait.
4. Describe common pathological gait patterns, including contributing factors, compensatory deviations, and when these are likely to occur in the gait cycle.
5. Compare and contrast the type and quality of information gathered with various quantitative, qualitative, instrumented, and function-based gait assessment tools.
6. Differentiate between pathological and compensatory gait characteristics typically observed in patients with lower motor neuron disease, hemiplegia, spastic diplegic cerebral palsy, and spina bifida.
7. Discuss how prosthetic components and alignment influence the efficacy and quality of gait for individuals with amputation at the transtibial and transfemoral levels.

WHY DO WE ANALYZE GAIT?

The first attempts to analyze gait, recorded in the *Rig Veda* more than 3500 years ago, most likely was an attempt to enhance mobility through early orthotic or prosthetic intervention. This classic prose chronicles the story of Vispala, a fierce female warrior whose leg, lost in battle, was replaced by an iron prosthesis that enabled her return to the front to fight again.[1]

Gait assessment describes the patterns of movement that control the progression of the body in walking. Bipedal gait requires a combination of automatic and volitional postural components. This can result in either asymmetric reciprocal movements of the lower limbs (seen in walking or running) or symmetric, simultaneous two-legged hopping. Kangaroos are bipeds that are successful two-legged hoppers.[2] Homo sapiens have reached the zenith of movement efficiency in bipedal walking and running by using reciprocal patterns of motion.

Walking requires numerous physiological systems to work congruently. Normal walking requires stability to provide body weight support against gravity during stance, mobility of body segments, and motor control to sequence multiple segments while transferring body weight from one limb to the other. The primary goal in gait is energy efficiency in forward progression by using a stable kinetic chain of joints and limb segments working congruently to transport its passenger unit, consisting of the head, arms, and trunk (HAT) in a continuously changing environment and task demands.

Understanding the process of walking is essential to critically evaluate examination findings and suggest effective intervention plans to help patients improve their walking ability. Clinical gait assessment identifies primary or pathological gait problems and helps differentiate them from compensatory strategies. It is necessary for selection of appropriate orthotic or prosthetic components, alignment parameters, and identification of other variants that might enhance an individual's ability to walk. Clinical gait assessment also contributes to the development of a comprehensive treatment plan, with the ultimate goal of optimal energy efficiency and appropriate pathomechanical control, balancing cosmesis and overall function.

KINEMATIC DESCRIPTORS OF HUMAN WALKING

Step length, stride length, cadence, and velocity are important quantitative, interrelated kinematic measures of gait. Step length and stride length are not synonymous. *Step length* is the distance from the floor-contact point of one (ipsilateral, originating) foot in early stance to the floor-contact point of the opposite (contralateral) foot: in normal individuals the distance from right heel contact to left heel contact. *Stride length* is the distance from floor contact on one side to the next floor contact on that same side: the distance from right heel contact to the next right heel contact. A reduction in functional joint motion or the presence of pain or muscle weakness can result in decreased stride or step length, or both. Pathological gait commonly produces asymmetries in step length between the two lower limbs.

Cadence is the number of steps taken in a given unit of time, most often expressed in steps per minute. *Velocity* is the distance traveled in a given unit of time (the rate of forward progression) and is usually expressed in centimeters per second or meters per minute. Velocity is the best single index of walking ability. Decreased joint motion, pain and/ or muscle weakness can reduce cadence or velocity or both. Velocity can also be qualitatively categorized as free, slow, or fast. Free walking (self-selected) speed is an individual's normal self-selected (comfortable) walking velocity. Fast walking speed describes the maximum velocity possible for a given individual while being safe. Slow walking speed describes a velocity below the normal self-selected walking speed. For healthy individuals, a fast walk velocity may be as much as 44% faster than free or self-selected walking speed.[3] In people with musculoskeletal and neuromuscular impairments that affect gait, often much less difference is found between free and fast gait velocity.

Double limb support is the period of time when both feet are in contact with the ground. It occurs twice during the gait cycle, at the beginning and the end of each stance phase. As velocity increases, double limb support time decreases. When running, the individual has rapid forward movement with little or no period of double limb support. Individuals with slow walking speeds spend more of the gait cycle in double support.

Step width, or width of the walking base, typically measures between 5 and 10 cm from the heel center of one foot to the heel center of the other foot.[4] A wide walking base may increase stability but also reduces energy efficiency of gait.

Ground reaction force (GRF) vector is the mean load-bearing line, which takes into account the forces acting in all three planes. It has magnitude as well as directional qualities. The spatial relation between this line and a given joint center influences the direction of its rotation. The rotational potential of the forces that act on a joint is called a *torque* or *moment*.

GAIT CYCLE

A variety of conceptual approaches describe the walking process. Saunders and colleagues[5] and Inman and colleagues[5] define the functional task of walking as translation of the center of gravity through space in a manner that requires the least energy expenditure. They identify six determinants, or variables, that affect energy expenditure in sustained walking: pelvic rotation, pelvic tilt, knee flexion in stance phase, foot interaction with the knee, ankle interaction with the knee, and lateral pelvic displacement. Individually and collectively, these determinants have an impact on energy expenditure and the mechanics of walking. Although they help us understand the process of walking, the determinants do not themselves offer a practical clinical solution to address the problems of gait assessment.

A comprehensive system to describe normal and abnormal gait has been developed by the Pathokinesiology and Physical Therapy Departments at Rancho Los Amigos Medical Center over the past several decades.[4,7,8] The Rancho Los Amigos system serves as the descriptive medium for this chapter (Figure 5-1). Because velocity affects many parameters of walking, the description of normal gait assumes a comfortable self-selected velocity. At free walking velocity, the individual naturally recruits strategies and assumes the speed that provides maximum energy efficiency for their physiological system.

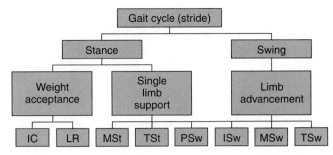

FIGURE 5-1 A complete gait cycle divided into three functional tasks of weight acceptance, single limb support, and limb advancement. The gait cycle can also be described in phasic terms of initial contact (IC), loading response (LR), midstance (MSt), terminal stance (TSt), preswing (PSw), initial swing (ISw), midswing (MSw), and terminal swing (TSw). The PSw phase is a transitional phase between single limb support and limb advancement.

The gait cycle is the period between any two identical events in the walking cycle. Initial contact is traditionally selected as the starting and completing event of a single cycle of gait. Each cycle is divided into two periods: stance phase and swing phase. *Stance* is the time when the foot is in contact with the ground; it constitutes approximately 60% of the gait cycle. *Swing* denotes the time when the foot is in the air; it constitutes the remaining 40% of the gait cycle. There are five subphases within the stance period: initial contact (IC), loading response (LR), midstance (MSt), terminal stance (TSt), and preswing (PSw). Swing phase is divided into three subphases: initial swing (ISw), midswing (MSw), and terminal swing (TSw). Because PSw prepares the limb for swing advancement, many consider PSw to be a preparatory component of swing phase.

Three functional tasks are achieved during these eight gait phases: weight acceptance in early stance, single limb support in mid-to terminal stance, and limb advancement during swing.

Functional Task 1: Weight Acceptance

IC and LR are the subphases of stance where weight acceptance is accomplished. Effective transfer of body weight onto the limb as soon as it makes contact with the ground requires initial limb stability, shock absorption, and the preservation of forward momentum.

Initial Contact

IC is the instant that the foot of the leading lower limb touches the ground. Most motor function during IC is preparation for LR. At IC, the ankle is in neutral position, the knee is close to full extension, and the hip is flexed 30 degrees. The sagittal plane GRF vector lies posterior to the ankle joint, creating a plantar flexion moment (Figure 5-2). Eccentric contraction of the pretibial muscles (tibialis anterior and long toe extensors) holds the ankle and subtalar joint in neutral position. At the knee, the GRF vector is anterior to the joint axis, which creates a passive extensor torque. Muscle contraction activity of the three vasti of the quadriceps and hamstring muscle groups continues from the previous TSw to preserve the neutral position of the knee joint. A flexion moment is present around the hip joint because the

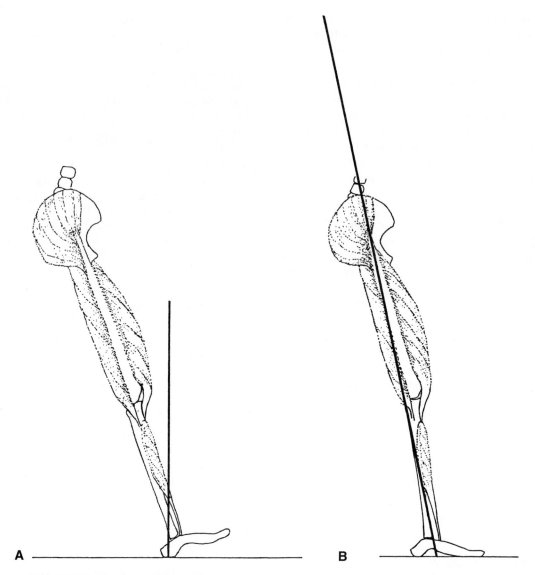

FIGURE 5-2 The two subphases of gait involved with the functional task of weight acceptance are initial contact (IC) and loading response (LR). **A,** At IC, the ground reaction force (GRF) line is posterior to the ankle and anterior to the knee and hip with activation of pretibial, quadriceps, hamstring, and gluteal muscles. Note that the length of the GRF line represents its magnitude. **B,** The LR phase results in an increased magnitude of the vertical force, which ultimately exceeds body weight. Activity of the same muscle groups elicited at IC increases steadily with the vertical force.

GRF vector falls anterior to the joint axis. Gluteus maximus and hamstring muscles are activated to restrain the resultant flexion torque.

Loading Response

LR occupies approximately 10% of the gait cycle and constitutes the period of initial double limb support (see Figure 5-2B). Two functional tasks occur during LR: controlled descent of the foot toward the ground and shock absorption as weight is transferred onto the stance limb.

The momentum generated by the fall of body weight onto the stance limb is preserved by the *heel rocker* (first rocker) of stance phase. Normal IC at the calcaneal tuberosity creates a fulcrum about which the foot and tibia move. The bony segment between this fulcrum and the center of the ankle rolls toward the ground as body weight is loaded onto the stance foot, preserving the momentum necessary for forward progression. Eccentric action of the pretibial muscles regulates the rate of ankle plantar flexion, and the quadriceps vasti contract to limit knee flexion. The action of these two muscle groups provides controlled forward advancement of the lower extremity unit (foot, tibia, and femur). During the peak of LR, the magnitude of the vertical GRF exceeds body weight. To absorb the impact force of body weight and preserve forward momentum, the knee flexes 15 to 18 degrees and the ankle plantar flexes to 10 degrees. The hip maintains its position of 30 degrees of flexion. Contraction of the gluteus maximus, hamstrings, and adductor magnus prevents further flexion of the hip joint.

Functional Task 2: Single Limb Support

Two phases are associated with single limb support: MSt and TSt. During this period, the contralateral foot is in swing phase, and body weight is entirely supported on the stance limb. Forward progression of body weight over the stationary foot while maintaining stability must be accomplished during these two subphases of stance.

Midstance

MSt begins when the contralateral foot leaves the ground and continues as body weight travels along the length of the stance foot until it is aligned over the forefoot at approximately 20% of the gait cycle (Figure 5-3). This pivotal action of the *ankle rocker* (second rocker) advances the tibia over the stationary foot. Forward movement of the tibia over the foot is controlled by the eccentric contraction of the soleus assisted by the gastrocnemius.

During this phase, the ankle moves from its LR position of 10 degrees of plantar flexion to approximately 5 degrees of dorsiflexion. The knee extends from 15 degrees of flexion to a neutral position. The hip joint moves toward extension, from 30 to 10 degrees of flexion. With continued forward progression, the body weight vector moves anterior to the ankle, creating a dorsiflexion moment. Eccentric action of the plantar flexors is crucial in providing limb stability as contralateral toe-off occurs, transferring body weight onto the stance foot. By the end of MSt, the body weight vector moves anterior to the knee (creating passive extensor stability at the knee) and posterior to the hip (reducing the demand on the hip extensors). The gluteus maximus, active in early MSt, ceases its activity and now stability relies on passive structures as the hip nears vertical alignment over the femur. Vertical GRF is reduced in magnitude at MSt

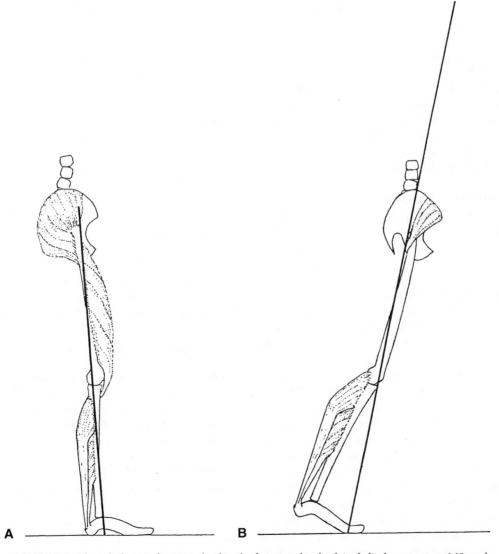

A ———————   **B** ———————

FIGURE 5-3 The subphases of gait involved in the functional task of single limb support are MSt and TSt. **A,** In early MSt, the vertical force begins to decrease and the triceps surae, quadriceps, and gluteus medius and maximus are active. **B,** During TSt, there is a second peak in vertical force, exceeding body weight, with high activity of the triceps surae, which maintain the third rocker. The tensor fascia lata restrains the increasing posterior hip vector. MSt, Midstance; TSt, terminal stance.

because of the upward momentum of the contralateral swing limb. In the coronal plane, activity of hip abductors during MSt is essential to provide lateral hip stability and almost a level pelvis.

Terminal Stance

TSt, the second half of single limb support, begins with heel rise of the stance limb and ends when the contralateral foot makes contact with the ground. As the body vector approaches the metatarsophalangeal joint, the heel rises and the phalanx dorsiflexes (extends). The metatarsal heads serve as an axis of rotation for body weight advancement (see Figure 5-3B). This is referred to as the *forefoot* or *toe rocker* (third rocker). The forefoot rocker serves as an axis around which progression of the body vector advances beyond the area of foot support, creating the highest demand on calf muscles (gastrocnemius and soleus). During TSt, the ankle continues to dorsiflex to 10 degrees. The knee is fully extended, and the hip moves into slight hyperextension. Forward fall of the body moves the vector further anterior to the ankle, creating a large dorsiflexion moment. Stability of the tibia on the ankle is provided by the eccentric action of the gastrocsoleus muscles.

The trailing posture of the limb and the presence of the vector anterior to the knee and posterior to the hip provide passive stability at hip and knee joints. The tensor fascia lata serves to restrain the posterior vector at the hip. At the end of TSt, the vertical GRF reaches a second peak greater than body weight, similar to that which occurred at the end of LR.

Functional Task 3: Limb Advancement

Four phases contribute to limb advancement: PSw, ISw, MSw, and TSw. During these phases the stance limb leaves the ground, advances forward, and prepares for the next IC.

Preswing

PSw, the second period of double limb support in gait, comprises the last 10% of the stance phase. It begins when the contralateral foot makes contact with the ground and ends with ipsilateral toe-off. During this period, the stance limb is unloaded and body weight is transferred onto the contralateral limb (Figure 5-4). The ankle moves rapidly from its TSt dorsiflexion into 20 degrees of plantar flexion. During this subphase, plantar flexor muscle activity decreases as the limb is unloaded. Toward the end of PSw, the vertical force is diminished such that plantar flexors rapidly decrease their activity to complete quiescence. There is no active muscle contraction for "push off" in normal reciprocal free walk bipedal gait.[6] The knee also flexes rapidly to achieve 35 to 40 degrees of flexion by the end of PSw. The GRF vector is at the metatarsophalangeal joints and posterior to the knee, creating passive knee flexion with toe clearance. Knee flexion during this phase prepares the limb for toe clearance in the swing phase. PSw hip flexion is initiated by the rectus femoris and the adductor longus, which also decelerates the passive abduction created by contralateral body weight transfer. The sagittal vector extends through the hip as the hip returns to a neutral position.

Initial Swing

Approximately one third of the swing period is spent in ISw. It begins the moment the foot leaves the ground and continues until maximal knee flexion (60 degrees) occurs, when the swinging extremity is directly under the body (see Figure 5-4B). Concentric contraction of pretibial muscles initiates foot dorsiflexion from its initial 20 degrees to 5 degrees of plantar flexion. This is necessary for toe and foot clearance as swing phase begins. Knee flexion, resulting from action of the short head of the biceps femoris, also assists in toe clearance. The knee continues to flex until it reaches a position of 60 degrees of flexion. Contraction of the iliacus advances the hip to 20 degrees of flexion. Contraction of the gracilis and sartorius muscles during this phase assists hip and knee flexion.

Midswing

During MSw, limb advancement and foot clearance continue. MSw begins at maximum knee flexion and ends when the tibia is vertical. Knee extension, coupled with ankle dorsiflexion, contributes to foot clearance while advancing the tibia (see Figure 5-4C). Continued concentric activity of pretibial muscles ensures foot clearance and moves the foot toward the neutral position. Momentum creates an extension moment, advancing the lower leg toward extension from 60 degrees to 30 degrees of flexion, with the quadriceps quiescent. Mild contraction of hip flexors continues to preserve the hip flexion position.

Terminal Swing

In the final phase, TSw, the knee extends fully in preparation for heel contact (see Figure 5-4D). Eccentric contraction of the hamstrings and gluteus maximus decelerates the thigh and restrains further hip flexion. Activity of the pretibial muscles maintains the ankle at neutral to prepare for heel contact. In the second half of TSw, the rectus femoris is quiescent but the rest of the quadriceps vasti become active to facilitate full knee extension. Hip flexion remains at 30 degrees.

DESCRIBING PATHOLOGICAL GAIT

Clinicians often use qualitative descriptive terms to characterize gait deviations and compensations. Some of these terms help identify specific primary problems; others describe compensatory strategies used by patients to solve gait difficulties created by various primary impairments.

Common Gait Deviations Observed During Stance

Trendelenburg gait occurs in the stance phase, when the trunk leans to the same side as the hip pathology (ipsilateral lean). This is a compensatory strategy used when the gluteus medius muscle and its synergists (gluteus minimus and tensor fascia lata) cannot adequately stabilize the pelvis during stance.[9] Normally the drop of the contralateral pelvis is limited to 5 degrees by the eccentric control of the strong hip abductor muscles. To support the pelvis, the hip abductor muscles must generate a force that is 1.5 times the body weight.[10] Weak or

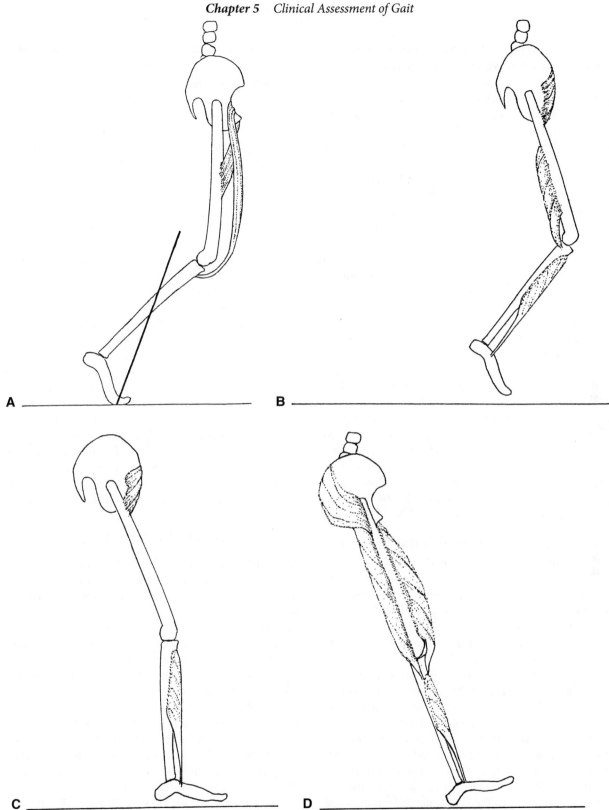

FIGURE 5-4 The subphases of gait involved in the functional task of swing limb advancement include preswing (PSw), initial swing (ISw), midswing (MSw), and terminal swing (TSw). **A,** During PSw, contralateral loading results in limited muscle activity in the limb transitioning from stance to swing. The rectus femoris and adductor longus initiate hip flexion. Knee flexion is passive, resulting from the planted forefoot and mobile proximal segments. **B,** During ISw, the pretibial muscles, short head of the biceps femoris, and iliacus are active in initiating limb advancement and providing swing clearance. **C,** A vertical tibia signals the end of the period of MSw. Here contraction of the iliacus preserves hip flexion while pretibial muscle activity maintains foot clearance. **D,** At TSw, the gluteus maximus, hamstrings, quadriceps, and pretibial muscles are active to prepare for limb placement and the ensuing loading response.

absent gluteus medius muscle leads to a postural substitution of an ipsilateral trunk lean over the weight-bearing hip joint. This reduces the external adductor moment created by a GRF line that falls medial to the joint center. Without this postural compensation, clearance becomes a problem for the swinging contralateral limb. Rarely, Trendelenburg gait is caused by overactive hip adductors (adductors longus, magnus, brevis, and gracilis).

Vaulting is exaggerated heel elevation of the stance foot, occasionally occurring with simultaneous stance limb hip and knee extension, with the goal of raising the pelvis to clear the contralateral swing limb. It occurs when the functional length of the swing limb is relatively longer than that of the stance limb. It also occurs when swing limb advancement is impaired or delayed by inadequate motor control of hip or knee flexion, or both, or in the presence of a plantar flexion contracture of the swing leg. It may compensate for pelvic obliquity or leg length discrepancy.

Antalgic gait is a strategy used to avoid pain during walking. It is frequently observed in LR when the patient reduces single limb support time on the affected limb. If the pain occurs during a particular interval in stance, that time interval is avoided. Antalgic gait caused by pain that originates around the hip might translate into a lateral lean to permit the patient to get the center of gravity over the support point, the head of the femur. If the pain occurs during the extreme end range of a particular joint motion, that motion is diminished. For example, if full extension produces pain, the knee would be maintained in slight flexion throughout the gait cycle.

Common Gait Deviations Observed During Swing

Circumducted gait is a swing phase deviation in which hip abduction is combined with a wide arc of pelvic rotation, most often occurring as a compensatory pattern when there is a relatively longer swing limb compared with the stance limb. This action is most likely to happen when there is limited motion or impaired motor control affecting ankle dorsiflexion, knee flexion, or hip flexion. A plantar flexion contracture at the foot or a stiff knee or hip joint can necessitate a circumduction pattern during swing in an effort to achieve toe and foot clearance. This combination of abduction and pelvic rotation is a compensatory strategy to advance the limb.

Circumduction can be observed as a lateral arc of the foot in the transverse plane that begins at the end of PSw and ends at IC on the same limb. The arc reaches the apex of its lateral movement at MSw. The typical pattern is a mixture of a wide base of support with the foot abnormally outset and may include an ipsilateral pelvic drop. It is possible for a contracture of the contralateral adductors to create this deviation by pulling the pelvis toward the contralateral femur and demanding a compensatory ipsilateral abducted position relative to the pelvis. A severe leg length discrepancy can result in an exaggerated pelvic tilt from the contralateral stance leg, which obligates the swing limb to an increased abduction position. Circumduction and abduction create a significant energy cost penalty, increasing lateral displacement of the center of gravity.

Gait Deviations Associated with Abnormal Muscle Tone

A variety of abnormal gait patterns are associated with abnormal muscle tone (spasticity, rigidity, hypotonicity, or abnormal motor control) or muscle weakness. *Scissors gait* describes a pattern of poor control in limb advancement or tracking of the swing leg often characterized by the crossing, or scissoring (hip adduction, flexion and medial rotation), of the lower limbs. It is most often observed in patients with spastic or paretic pathological conditions such as hemiplegia, spastic diplegia, and cerebral palsy. *Steppage gait* occurs when there is weakness or paralysis of the dorsiflexor musculature, such as in persons with peroneal palsy or peripheral neuropathy, demands exaggerated hip and knee flexion of the proximal joints to accomplish swing clearance. It is most easily observed in late MSw.

In *crouch gait* exaggerated knee and hip flexion occurs throughout the gait cycle. Crouch gait is often seen in combination with a toe-walking stance in children and adults with spastic diplegic cerebral palsy. It has been attributed to a combination of overactivity of the hamstrings and weakness of calf muscles. Although orthosis use can successfully control abnormal motion in the sagittal plane (e.g., in steppage gait), orthoses are less effective in controlling the abnormal transverse, rotational, or coronal limb placement problems observed in scissoring or crouched gait pattern.

In *ataxic gait* there is a failure of coordination or irregularity of muscular action of the limb segments commonly caused by cerebellar dysfunction. Ataxia often becomes accentuated when the eyes are closed or vision is impaired or distracted.

QUALITATIVE GAIT ASSESSMENT

Qualitative methods for identification and recording of gait deviations have played a role in patient care for decades. In 1925, Robinson[11] described pathological gait patterns and attempted to correlate them with specific disease processes. In 1937, Boorstein[12] identified 14 disease processes that could be diagnosed with gait assessment. He described seven major gait deficit groups, attributing the term *steppage gait* to the French physician Charcot and the identification of *waddling gait* in hip dysplasia to Hippocrates. In the late 1950s, Blair Hangar, the founder of Northwestern University's School of Prosthetics and Orthotics, and Hildegard Myers, a physical therapist at Rehabilitation Institute of Chicago, collaborated to develop the first comprehensive system of clinical gait analysis for persons with transfemoral amputation.[13] They identified 16 gait deviations and suggested numerous clinical and prosthetic causes for each. Their work, developed into an educational film and handbook in 1960, has been a model for subsequent instructional videos and assessment systems in prosthetics.[14] Brunnstrom's[15] comprehensive gait analysis form for hemiplegic gait, published in 1970, is a checklist of 28 deviations seen at the ankle, knee, and hip that are common after stroke.

Early work in observational gait analysis received a significant impetus from Perry[16] as an outgrowth of basic research data published in 1967. In the late 1960s, Perry and a group of physical therapists from the Rancho Los Amigos Medical Center Physical

Therapy Department developed an organized format for systematically applied observational gait analysis. Their work initially focused on the development of an in-house training program for students and personnel who were new to the rehabilitation hospital. The first Normal and Pathological Gait Syllabus was published by the Professional Staff Association of Rancho Los Amigos Hospital in 1977.[7] Subsequent revisions have included additional gait data and gait interpretation.[17] This syllabus uses parameters of normal gait as a comparative standard for abnormal or pathological gait. It focuses on identifying gait deviations that affect the three functional tasks of walking: weight acceptance, single limb support, and swing limb advancement. A form listing the most commonly occurring gait deviations in each subphase of gait is used to record any observed gait deviations that interfere with these functional tasks (Figure 5-5). Problems in each of the six major body segments are noted with a check in one of the boxes, beginning with the toes, then the ankle, knee, hip, pelvis, and trunk. This format allows the clinician to consider systematically the following questions:

- Are the toes up, inadequately extended, or clawed?
- Is there forefoot-only contact (toe walking), foot-flat contact, foot slap, excess plantar flexion, or dorsiflexion? Is heel-off, foot drag, or contralateral vaulting present?
- Is knee flexion adequate, absent, limited, or excessive? Is extension inadequate? Does the knee wobble, hyperextend, or produce an extension thrust (recurvatum)? Is varus or valgus present, or is excessive contralateral flexion seen?
- Is hip flexion adequate, absent, limited, or excessive? Is adequate extension seen? Is retraction of the thigh during TSw from a previously attained degree of flexion seen? Can internal or external rotation, abduction, or adduction be observed?
- Does the pelvis hike? Does it tilt anteriorly or posteriorly? Is forward or backward rotation seen? Does it drop to the ipsilateral or contralateral side?
- Does the trunk lean or rotate backward or forward? Does it lean laterally to the right or left?

Qualitative gait assessment is an important component of preorthotic assessment because it assists the clinician in identifying the functional task and the subphase of gait that are problematic and can be addressed with orthotic intervention. Similarly, deviations observed during gait analysis can identify the need for adjustment of prosthetic alignment.

INSTRUMENTED GAIT ANALYSIS

Instrumented gait analysis records the process of walking with measurable parameters collected through the use of equipment. Such basic techniques would have enabled measurement of walking velocity (distance traversed per unit of time) and cadence (steps per unit of time). Marks,[18] a New York City prosthetist, offered a more precise qualitative description of pathological gait in 1905, when he described the gait process in eight organized phases and discussed the implications of prosthetic component design on walking function. Marks praised "kinetoscopic" photography as a potential diagnostic tool for optimizing pathological gait.

Today we record gait parameters with instruments as common as a stopwatch or as complex as the simultaneous integration of three-dimensional kinematics, kinetics, and electromyographic (EMG) methods. The primary emphasis of clinical assessment has been on accessible techniques and inexpensive technologies. A simple, inexpensive footprint mat has been used for decades to record barefoot plantar pressures. Clinics use individual or multiple mats to record step and stride length as well as walking base width. Early on, video technology with slow-motion capabilities made more precise qualitative description of the gait cycle possible. The continued development of inexpensive video gait assessment software has made clinical quantitative applications more practical as well. Most quantitative and qualitative video systems, however, measure joint angles in two dimensions, which does not offer a complete analysis of the three-dimensional walking activity.

Technology in Gait Assessment

The high-tech side of quantitative gait analysis has traversed a surprisingly long road. The birth of instrumented kinematic, EMG, and temporal performance analysis began in the 1870s with E. J. Marey, who first performed movement analysis of pathological gait with photography.[19] He also developed the first myograph for measuring muscle activity and the first foot-switch collection system for measuring gait events related to the temporal parameters. The foot-switch system was an experimental shoe that measured the length and rapidity of the step and the pressure of the foot on the ground. Eadweard Muybridge,[20] working at Stanford University in the 1880s, used synchronized multiple camera photography with a scaled backdrop to record on film and assess the motion of subjects walking. Scherb made other major advances in instrumented gait analysis in 1920 by performing manual muscle palpation on individuals while using a treadmill. Additionally, in 1925 Adrian advocated the use of EMG to study the dynamic action of muscles.[21]

Modern gait technology began in 1945, when Inman and colleagues initiated the systematic collection of gait data for individuals without impairment and with amputation in the outdoor gait laboratory at the University of California at Berkeley.[5] Since then, researchers and clinicians have increasingly used the wide array of gait technologies to measure the parameters of human performance in normal and pathological gait. A full-service gait laboratory gathers information on six performance parameters in walking: temporal, metabolic, kinematic, kinetic, EMG, and pressure.[22]

Measuring Temporal and Distance Parameters

Temporal (time, distance) parameters enable the clinician to summarize the overall quality of a patient's gait. Temporal data collection systems might be one of the most effective components available for assessment in the clinical setting. In the gait laboratory, microswitch-embedded pads taped to the bottom of a patient's shoes or feet can record the amount of time that the patient spends on various anatomical landmarks over a measured distance. Portable pressure-sensitive gait mats, connected to a laptop computer with gait analysis software for time and distance parameters are also commercially available to use in clinical settings (Figure 5-6).[23,24] For example, the GAITRite system, which consists of an electronic walkway connected to

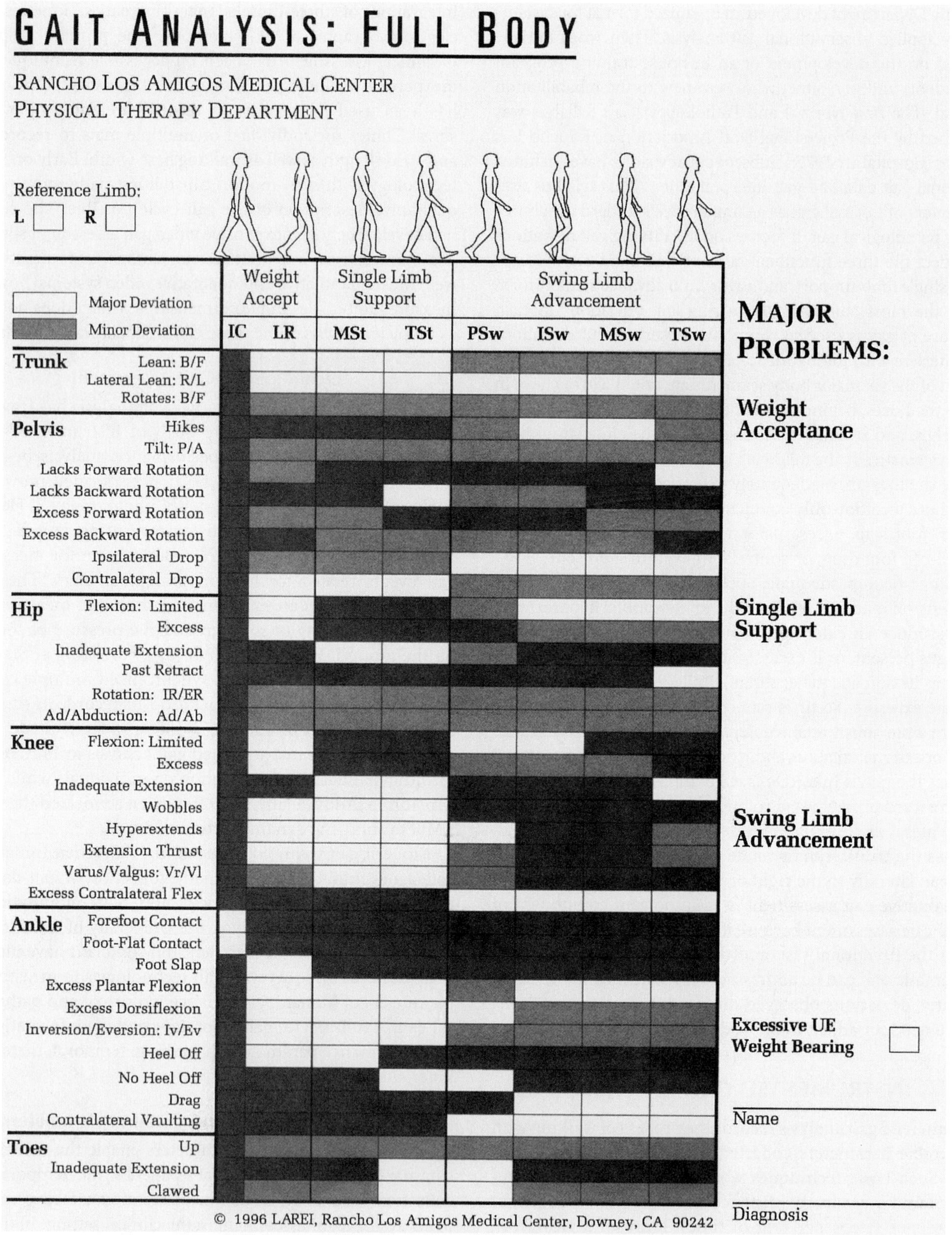

GAIT ANALYSIS: FULL BODY

RANCHO LOS AMIGOS MEDICAL CENTER
PHYSICAL THERAPY DEPARTMENT

Reference Limb:
L ☐   R ☐

☐ Major Deviation
▨ Minor Deviation

	Weight Accept		Single Limb Support		Swing Limb Advancement			
	IC	LR	MSt	TSt	PSw	ISw	MSw	TSw
Trunk Lean: B/F								
Lateral Lean: R/L								
Rotates: B/F								
Pelvis Hikes								
Tilt: P/A								
Lacks Forward Rotation								
Lacks Backward Rotation								
Excess Forward Rotation								
Excess Backward Rotation								
Ipsilateral Drop								
Contralateral Drop								
Hip Flexion: Limited								
Excess								
Inadequate Extension								
Past Retract								
Rotation: IR/ER								
Ad/Abduction: Ad/Ab								
Knee Flexion: Limited								
Excess								
Inadequate Extension								
Wobbles								
Hyperextends								
Extension Thrust								
Varus/Valgus: Vr/Vl								
Excess Contralateral Flex								
Ankle Forefoot Contact								
Foot-Flat Contact								
Foot Slap								
Excess Plantar Flexion								
Excess Dorsiflexion								
Inversion/Eversion: Iv/Ev								
Heel Off								
No Heel Off								
Drag								
Contralateral Vaulting								
Toes Up								
Inadequate Extension								
Clawed								

MAJOR PROBLEMS:

Weight Acceptance

Single Limb Support

Swing Limb Advancement

Excessive UE Weight Bearing ☐

Name _____

Diagnosis

© 1996 LAREI, Rancho Los Amigos Medical Center, Downey, CA 90242

FIGURE 5-5 The Rancho gait analysis system facilitates recording any observable activity that interferes with the three functional tasks of walking: weight acceptance, single limb support, and swing limb advancement. (Reprinted with permission from Los Amigos Research and Education Institute, Rancho Los Amigos Medical Center. Observational Gait Analysis Handbook. Downey, CA: Los Amigos Research and Education Institute, Rancho Los Amigos Medical Center, 1989. pp. 55.)

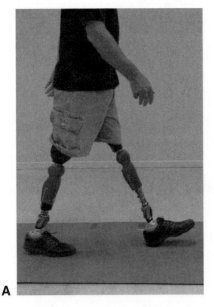

Parameters	
Distance (cm)	281.9
Ambulation time (sec)	2.50
Velocity (cm/sec)	112.7
Mean normalized velocity	1.44

Functional ambulation profile: 99	
Cadence (steps/min)	120.0
Step time differential (sec)	0.01
Step length differential (cm)	0.36
Cycle time differential (sec)	0.01

Walk # / footfall #	L/R	Mean (%CV)	All ages
Step time (sec)	L	0.494 (2)	
	R	0.504 (3)	0.53 0.59
Cycle time (sec)	L	0.994 (3)	
	R	1.007 (1)	1.06 1.18
Swing time (sec)	L	0.356 (2) /35.8	
/ %GC	R	0.382 (2) /37.9	36 44
Stance (sec)	L	0.638 (3) /64.2	
/ %GC	R	0.625 (0) /62.1	56 64
Single support (sec)	L	0.382 (2) /38.4	
/ %GC	R	0.356 (2) /35.4	38 42
Double support (sec)	L	0.269 (3) /27.1	
/ %GC	R	0.269 (3) /26.7	16 24
Step length (cm)	L	56.587 (5)	
	R	56.229 (3)	58 85
Stride length (cm)	L	113.665 (2)	
	R	112.429 (1)	116 170
Base of support (cm)	L	9.56 (36)	
	R	11.41 (17)	
Toe in / out (deg)	L	7 (33)	
	R	11 (13)	

FIGURE 5-6 A, The GAITRite system is an example of a portable pressure-sensitive walkway used to assess temporal and distance parameters of gait. **B,** The walkway is connected to a laptop computer, and the operator is able to quickly generate values for velocity, stride and step lengths, cadence, time and percent of cycle spent in stance, single and double limb support, and swing.

a computer, records the temporal and spatial characteristics of patients while walking as well as while performing other functional or occupational tasks. The GAITRite mat is flexible and can be rolled and transported in a hard case, which enables data collection at different clinics or sites. Wening and colleagues used the GAITRite system to validate the effect of using an ankle-foot orthosis (AFO) on the walking pattern of patients with stroke.[25] In this study, they compared stride length, velocity, cadence, percentage of the gait cycle spent in single and double limb support, as well as general stance progression patterns. Gait deviations related to excessive inversion, eversion, or prolonged heel-only time can be recognized and considered when modifying the alignment or components of prostheses or orthoses. A temporal data collection system is particularly cost effective and clinically meaningful. Temporal data are usually a product of another measuring system such as EMG or motion analysis. Temporal data systems are commercially available covering a wide range of cost, technical sophistication, and time required to analyze the summarized data. Some of the temporal parameters, however, can be recorded, to a lesser degree of accuracy using a stopwatch and video camera.[26]

Assessing the Energy Cost of Walking

Metabolic data reflect the physiological "energy cost" of walking. The traditional measures of energy cost are oxygen consumption, total carbon dioxide generated, and heart rate. Other relevant factors include volume of air breathed and respiratory rate. All these parameters are viewed in relation to velocity and distance walked over the collection period.

Historically, metabolic data were collected while the patient walked on a treadmill, wearing umbilical devices. In recent years, because of the known influence of treadmill collection in altering normal gait velocity, energy cost data are more likely to be obtained on an open track of a measured distance with the patient ambulating in a free walk or natural cadence (Figure 5-7). With the cardiopulmonary device market continually growing and advancing, there is a wide array of versatile testing equipment to choose from. This equipment allows the patient to negotiate their normal environments with little or no interruption due to the testing and collection setups. Some of the newest products on the market couple the traditional oxygen and carbon dioxide (Vo_2 and Vco_2) measurement with the capability of collecting telemetry data, indirect calorimetry, and integrated electrocardiogram among other add-ons to standard systems. The primary limitation of energy cost as an assessment tool is that, although it can inform the investigator about body metabolism relative to the patient's gait, it cannot explain why or how an advantage or disadvantage was obtained. Waters[27] demonstrated that an individual with Syme's level amputation uses less oxygen to traverse a given distance than someone with a transtibial amputation but could not explain why. For that explanation, other gait parameters must be examined. Energy cost measures cannot easily identify widely variant prosthetic foot designs worn by the same patient, whereas kinematic, kinetic, and EMG data typically can.[28] The Oxycon Champion respirometry system has been used in many studies; one involved measuring the step-by-step metabolic consumptions of amputees. This

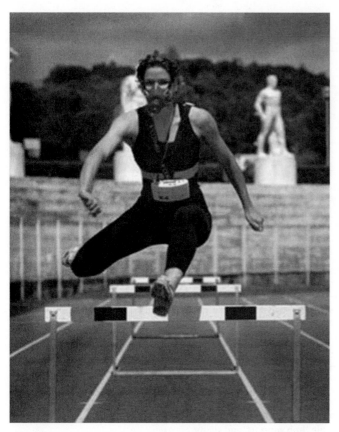

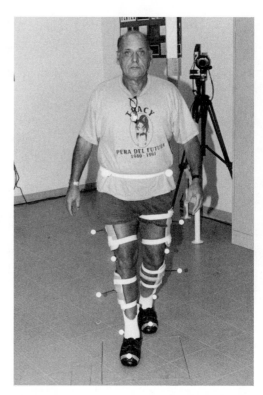

FIGURE 5-8 This individual is wearing reflective spheres. An infrared camera system can track limb segment motion as the patient walks across the field of view.

FIGURE 5-7 The Cosmed K4b2 method is an example of a portable pulmonary gas exchange system, which records and analyzes data on a breath-by-breath basis. Heart rate and other metabolic variables are monitored through integrated telemetry. (Courtesy of COSMED-Pulmonary Function Equipment, Rome, Italy.)

system allowed for unrestricted locomotion which made the data collection easier and more relevant to everyday situations of the participant.[29] The CPX by Medgraphics, a breath-by-breath analysis system for cardiopulmonary exercise testing, was used to record similar data relating to the biomechanics of lower-limb amputee gait and metabolic data.[30]

Perhaps the best kept secret in the energy cost arsenal is the *physiological cost index* (PCI). It is easily calculated as follows:

$$PCI = (walking\ pulse - resting\ pulse)/gait\ speed$$

The PCI is one of the most sensitive indicators of energy cost of gait. Winchester and colleagues[31] compared two different orthotic designs by measuring a wide variety of metabolic parameters as well as the PCI. Their results demonstrated statistically significant difference in PCI between the two devices when all other measured parameters failed to produce such differences. Pulse and respiratory rate taken at rest and after timed intervals during normal comfortable gait can also help assess exertion levels.

Kinematic and Kinetic Systems

Most *kinematic* systems provide joint and body segment motion in graphic form. This information includes sagittal, coronal, and transverse motions that occur at the ankle,

knee, hip, and pelvis. The patient is instrumented with reflective spheres that are placed on well-recognized anatomical landmarks (Figure 5-8). Typically, an infrared light source is positioned around each of several cameras. This light is directed to the reflective spheres, which in turn are reflected into the cameras. Each field of video data is digitized, an operator manually identifies the markers, and the coordinates of the geometric center of each marker are calculated with computer software. Resultant data are displayed as animated stick figures that represent the actual motions produced by the patient. The operator can freeze any frame and enlarge the image at any joint to examine gait patterns in greater depth. The operator can extract raw numbers that represent joint placement and motion in space or produce a printout showing joint motion in all planes plotted against the percentage of the gait cycle (Figure 5-9). Angular velocities, accelerations, and joint and segment linear displacements can be calculated. Data from other systems (force platforms and EMG) collected during the same time sequence as the motion data are often integrated with the kinematics. Advanced systems like these can be a very expensive component of the gait lab, but the data collected provides some of the most in-depth and valid data. In the gait lab or a clinical lab, the motion system setup serves as the technological core. A variety of Vicon motion systems have been used to evaluate the joint motion in patients with spastic diplegic cerebral palsy and various other patient populations.[32] Similarly the EvaRT motion analysis system has been used to collect data comparing mechanical and microprocessor knees in patients with gait and balance deficits.[33]

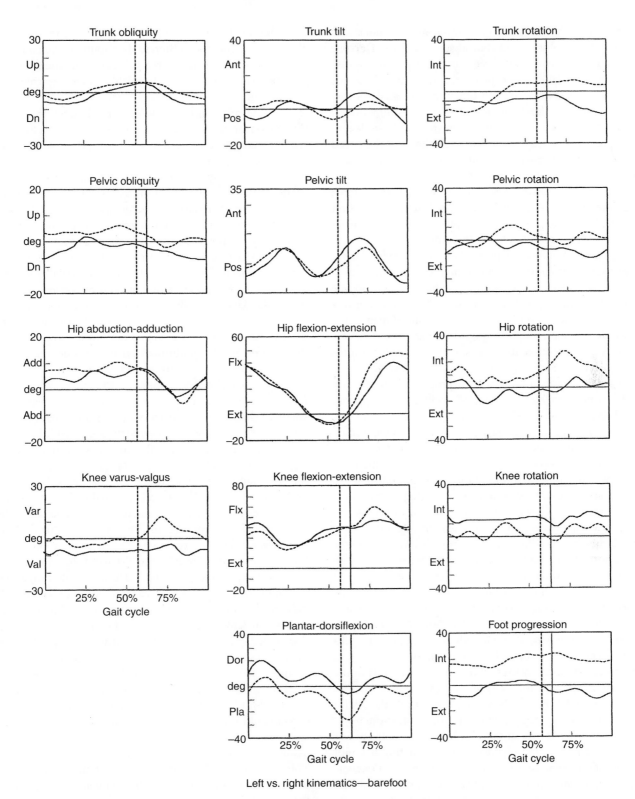

Left vs. right kinematics—barefoot

FIGURE 5-9 The output generated by a computer-based motion analysis system includes graphs of the mean range of motion at each body segment or joint (trunk, pelvis, hip, knee, and ankle) in coronal (left column), sagittal (middle column), and transverse (right column) planes as the individual being evaluated progresses through multiple gait cycles. This is the output of an 8-year-old child with spastic diplegic cerebral palsy. (Courtesy of the Center for Motion Analysis, Connecticut Children's Medical Center, Hartford, Conn.)

The Dartfish system is another motion analysis tool that is used in gait laboratories and clinical settings.[34] The Dartfish system allows for two- and three-dimensional joint motion analysis. It is portable, less expensive, and requires less time to set up when compared with other motion analysis systems. Dartfish has been used to record and immediately evaluate the effects of various prosthetic feet on knee flexion during normal walking. These tools can allow for improved technique and transmission of information to patients and optimally a decrease in recovery time.[35]

When an individual takes a step, he is exerting force against the surface he is walking on. This *kinetic* information is obtained from one or more force platforms, which collect data on the three components of the ground reaction force: vertical, fore-aft (anterior-posterior), and medial-lateral (Figure 5-10). The contribution of kinetic data can be significant. Fore-aft shear is quite useful in establishing appropriate transtibial prosthetic alignment in the sagittal plane. For this purpose the clinician would anticipate a balanced magnitude and timing of the braking and propulsive patterns. Data collection from two consecutive steps, one gait cycle, requires dual force plates. Some kinetic software packages also offer specialized programs for specific purposes such as stability analysis, which provides information about center of gravity shift relative to time.

While the typical force platform system provides data about forces and moments occurring at the ground, or center of pressure progression, it can be combined with kinematic data to provide additional information. By combining these two data sets, the moments and power acting at the joints can be calculated. This information is useful in measuring the dynamic joint control of an individual throughout stance, particularly when used in conjunction with EMG. Similarly, information about joint moments, sometimes referred to as *torque*, is also often reported as an outcome measure in research studies. While this information can be potentially important in the evaluation of pathological gait, it is also necessary to have a basic understanding of how these values are derived. As mentioned, as an individual ambulates, the individual exerts force on the walking surface; differing degrees of this force are similarly exerted on each of the joints in the lower extremity. With the exertion of these forces comes an associated moment that is also acting at the joint, along with a power value. In its most basic form, a moment is the result of a force multiplied by a distance or lever arm.[6] Joint power is then calculated by multiplying the moment acting at a joint by the joint's angular velocity. Additionally, the moment acting on a particular segment is most frequently calculated with reference to the center of mass of that segment. This means that the lever arm is the distance from where the forces are acting at the joint to the center of mass of the segment. In order to calculate these values, the lower extremity must be broken down into segments, often the ankle, shank or calf, and thigh. By doing this, a link-segment model is being applied and the parameters of interest can be calculated.[36]

To further illustrate, the interrelated nature of these measures, the calculation path for forces, moments, and power is also presented (Figure 5-11). It is important to note within the diagram where the different data sources originate. There are very few directly measured values that are then combined with biomechanical models to calculate these variables.

The calculation process begins with the determination of the ground reaction forces, which are obtained through the direct measurement of an individual stepping on a force platform. Once that information is available, it is combined with kinematic data, derived from a two- or three-dimensional motion capture system for each lower extremity body segment, so that the joint reaction forces can be calculated. As the forces at each of the joints are determined, then the associated moments acting on each segment can also be calculated. Ultimately, the power can be calculated as well (Figure 5-12).

In many cases, instrumented kinetic and kinematic systems have included an inverse dynamics model that is applied to determine the forces acting at each of the lower extremity joints. Like virtually all biomechanics models, certain assumptions must be made in order for the calculation to be carried out in a practical manner. With assumptions come the opportunity for additional error introduction throughout the process. This is why it is important to understand the limitations associated with them. A fundamental point is that frequently these calculations all rely upon data that are calculated using general body proportions and anthropometric models for whole bodied individuals. Because of this, certain assumptions are made about the mechanical properties of the segments and joints being evaluated. For example, many of the commonly used models assume that the subject has no limb deficiencies and essentially normal musculature. While this may be acceptable for evaluations of individuals without pathology, these assumptions can become a source of error when evaluating an individual with an amputation or other limb dysfunction. There is also the issue that the knee and ankle joints are frequently modeled as simple hinge joints. By doing this it makes the calculations more practical to perform but does not completely represent the anatomical reality. Particularly in the case of the knee, the joint center does not stay in a fixed position during stance, but many of the models for calculating joint moments assume that it does (Figure 5-13). As a result, there can be variation in the distance used to calculate the moment at the knee. Considering the physical location, even a small variation in the estimated joint center could result in a significant change in the value calculated. Because many of the calculations rely upon the model assumptions, the inherent errors can be easily compounded. This is not to say that these variables should be ignored but that their value should be tempered with an understanding of the process for obtaining them.

Electromyography

Muscle action beneath skin and subcutaneous tissue cannot be directly measured, but through the use of EMG, the activity can be approximated and studied in relation to the action, size of muscle, and signals obtained. EMG records the muscle activity by the electrical signal detected from the contraction and chemical stimulation of the respective musculature.[6]

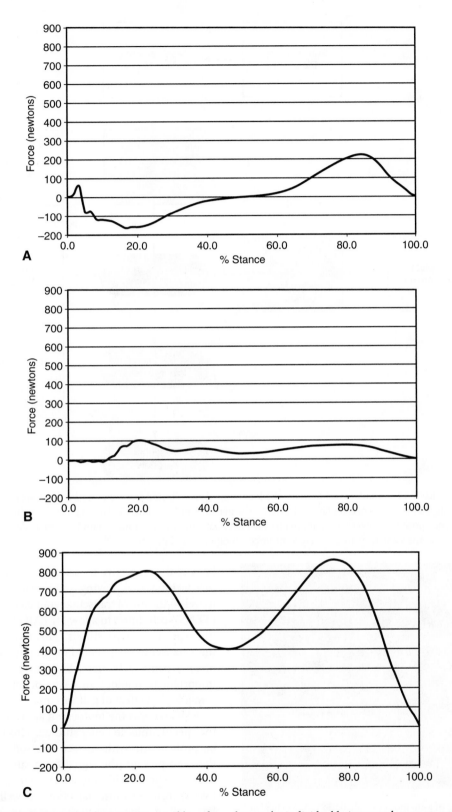

FIGURE 5-10 Example of output generated by a forceplate as the individual being tested progresses through stance phase. **A,** The anteroposterior component of the ground reaction force (GRF). **B,** The medial lateral component of the GRF. **C,** The vertical component of the GRF. (Output courtesy of the Motion Analysis Laboratory, Department of Physical Therapy and Human Movement Science, Sacred Heart University, Fairfield, Conn.)

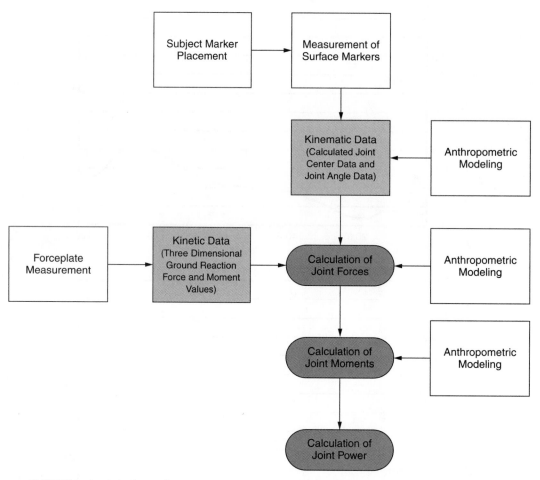

FIGURE 5-11 Calculation flowchart: the kinematic data collected from the motion analysis system is entered into series of calculations based on the person's anthropometric data to produce the instantaneous position of every joint and segment. These data are then combined with force plate data collected at the same time to calculate joint forces, moments, and powers.

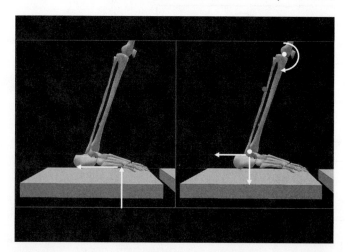

FIGURE 5-12 Example of joint moment calculation. **A,** Vertical and anteroposterior ground reaction forces recorded from a force plate. **B,** Joint moments are calculated by combining ground reaction forces and kinematic data, taking into account the segment's center of mass.

EMG instrumentation can vary, such as is seen with surface EMG or fine-wire EMG. With surface EMG the electrode pad is adhered to the skin above the muscle being studied, while fine-wire EMG uses wire electrodes directly inserted into the belly of the respective muscle. Intrasocket EMG is a relatively new technique employing traditional surface EMG techniques as well as the use of transcutaneous electrical nerve stimulation (TENS) techniques to allow for EMG to be worn by amputees underneath their prosthesis. This technique allows for EMG information to be gathered on amputees during walking and other dynamic activities.[37] EMG data may be the single most important technology in terms of understanding the direct physiological effect of gait variants.

EMG records the motor unit activation of muscle fibers in the specific muscle being studied. This is very useful but can be problematic with surface electrode applications, in that they can pick up the signal from surrounding musculature during testing. EMG characterization allows for timing, relative intensity of muscular effort, as well as resultant muscle force, all of which are necessary to understand normal and pathological gait. EMG data are normalized against maximum contraction data for each respective muscle. Without normalization, the data collected may be invalid and can lead to erroneous interpretation. Maximum contraction is dependent on joint angle as well as the duration of the contraction, both of which are influential to the overall information extracted from analysis.

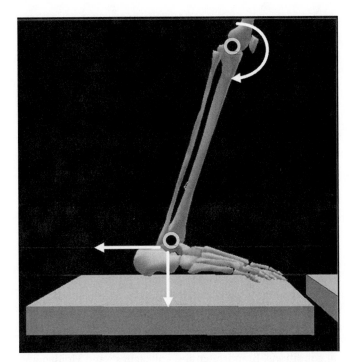

FIGURE 5-13 Soft tissues and joint geometry differences between the anthropometric model and the actual individual being, introduce a potential error in calculating joint moments. In this example, the outer circle indicates the potential range of location of the actual joint center, compared to where the model ultimately defines it (inner circle).

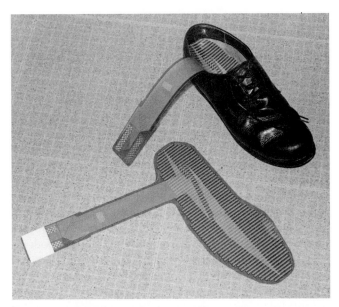

FIGURE 5-14 An in-shoe pressure-sensing array can help identify areas of high pressure concentration. This information assists in the design of an orthosis to modify pressure dynamics during the stance phase of gait.

Patterns of muscle activity in patients with abnormal gait are compared with well-established norms. Knowledge of the timing and intensity of the muscle activity throughout the gait cycle may guide gait training, orthotic or prosthetic prescription, and dynamic orthotic or prosthetic alignment aimed at reduction of excessive, ill-timed, or prolonged muscle activity. EMG is exceedingly adaptable with the most basic function of superficial muscle activity data to intramuscular fine wire sensor technology, which is all cohesive to the implementation of many other complex clinical or gait lab technologies.[26] EMG data are also helpful in guiding decisions about surgical intervention (dorsal rhizotomy, tendon lengthening, or osteotomy) in children with cerebral palsy.

Pressure-Sensing Technology

Pressure-sensing technologies offer the clinician tremendous insights into the treatment of patients at risk for amputation because of vascular disease and diabetic neuropathy. They can also assist vascular surgeons and orthopedic foot specialists in limb salvage through more appropriate custom-designed prophylactic orthoses. In some systems, a thin plastic array can slip nearly unnoticed between the plantar surface of the foot and an orthosis or insole of the shoe (Figure 5-14). This array, connected to a computer by a lead wire, can measure dynamic pressure patterns and record critical events throughout the walking cycle. A prosthetic version can provide various measurements at 60 individual sites within a socket and

record those measurements during multiple events of the gait cycle. Pressure is expressed in terms of a force over the area at which the force is acting.

$$Pressure = Force/Area$$

Cavanaugh and colleagues state that "Pressure measurement offers a way to help the clinician break out of the cycle of trial and error that is so often necessary to find the correct solution to a patient's problem."[38] Currently surface pressure measurement systems exist in various forms ranging from in-shoe, barefoot, seating and positioning, joint, and prosthetic and orthotic floor-based models. Over the years, Perry and colleagues have collected data on the most common types of pressure testing systems that consist of a "force plate" that uses ink and paper to record the areas of peak pressures during ambulation. This type of system is inexpensive and provides reliable, easily interpreted data. Instrumented insoles, however, are positioned inside the patient's shoes and worn during ambulation and activity performance. The insoles record pressures and various forces on the plantar surface of the foot through an integrated array of sensors.[6] The diversity of treatment applications has promoted these systems to one of the most valuable in the laboratory setting.[26] An example of the application of pressure sensing technology is the development of the dynamic gait stability index, which is based on plantar pressure and utilized the F-Scan insole sensors from Tekscan Inc. The compiled data was used to evaluate dynamic gait stability through six different parameters and were then indexed across different walking conditions, terrains, and speed.[39-41] This area is one of the more recent and clinically promising technologies for the assessment team.

CHOOSING THE APPROPRIATE ASSESSMENT TOOL

Over the past several decades, technologies have advanced and aided in providing a significantly improved understanding of pathological gait. They have also assisted clinicians in providing strong evidence for the efficacy of various treatment approaches and ultimately helped enhance patient care. Advocates of a more universal application of the high-end technologies in the clinical setting have made a compelling case for implementation in gait laboratories and clinical settings alike across the field of rehabilitative care. Determining the extent and necessity for various high-end devices, such as full featured motion analysis systems, in the clinical setting can be a very extensive process requiring the evaluation of the advantages and disadvantages to both the patient and the clinic, particularly in the current climate of cost containment. Perhaps the strongest argument for gait technology in our present era lies in its use for outcome measurement to justify legitimate therapeutic treatment approaches as well as orthotic and prosthetic applications.

Recognizing the need, benefits, and drawbacks of technology in the clinical setting is very important. Appropriate instrumented evaluations will need to be made by the rehabilitation team to help optimize patient outcomes.

FUNCTION-BASED ASSESSMENT

Task-oriented tests or functional measures are performance based tools directly related to specific activities and linked to "real-world" domains of function. For example walking in the community requires meeting the demand of varied distance, terrain, illumination, obstacles, stair-climbing, and multitasking. These tests usually measure performance of the individual against established norms for a specific population. Results of functional measures serve as a baseline to establish goals and benchmarks and evaluate progress after intervention.

Holden and colleagues[42] suggest that gait performance goals for patients with neurological impairments are best measured against values from impaired rather than healthy subjects. Treatment goals are adjusted for the individual patient's diagnosis, etiologic factor, ambulation aid, and functional category. In separate studies, Brandstater and colleagues[43] and Holden and colleagues[42] found that patients with the greatest number of gait deviations did not have the lowest temporal values. A great deal of energy is often expended by physical therapists, prosthetists, and orthotists in an attempt to help patients achieve optimal gait patterns. Holden and colleagues[42] suggest that hard-won qualitative gait improvements may cause secondary losses in time-distance parameters, such as slower velocity and reduced step length. The fundamental issue is whether temporal gait efficiency or cosmesis should be the preferred goal. Certainly, in cases in which patients are nominal walkers and in which therapy, surgery, and orthotics or prosthetics have optimized, gait efficiency is far more important than reducing in compensatory gait deficits.

In the past, symmetry and reciprocal movement patterns have been significant treatment goals. Wall and Ashburn[44] maintain that "an ideal objective in the functional rehabilitation of hemiplegia is the reduction of the asymmetrical nature of movement patterns." Measuring pathological gait against normal gait values is a useful means of providing an overall clinical picture. In setting treatment goals, however, measuring a patient's performance against their own best possible outcome is more reasonable. How can a given patient's best possible outcome be anticipated? This requires collection of accurate data to establish pre-treatment and post-treatment profiles for a wide variety of involvement levels within each pathological condition. Olney and Richards[45] suggest that large groups of instrumented studies be undertaken to identify clusters of biomechanical features associated with functional performance during walking

Time-distance parameters have enormous potential for setting outcome goals. Variations in time-distance values are often specific to pathological condition. Asymmetries in hemiplegia, for example, are obviously greater than in most other types of pathological conditions. Variables that are reported to affect temporal measurements in normal healthy subjects include age, gender, height, orthotic use, or type of assistive device. In separate studies of patients with pathological conditions, Brandstater and colleagues[43] and Holden and colleagues[42] found no significant difference in temporal performance based on gender or age.

Corcoran and colleagues[46] measured temporal parameters of subjects with hemiplegia under two gait conditions: with and without their AFO. Patients with hemiplegia had significantly faster gait velocity when wearing their orthoses than when walking without them.[46] Another similar study of healthy unimpaired subjects wearing AFOs found reduced step length. Apparently subjects without central nervous system involvement altered their movement strategy to decrease movements at the knee in an effort to minimize shearing forces in the AFO.[47] Reduced step length can minimize force exerted by the brace along the posterior aspect of the calf band.[48]

Functional Measures

A wide variety of functional measures are available to provide information about ambulatory function of individuals with neuromuscular, musculoskeletal, cardiopulmonary, or metabolic diseases and conditions. Most of these measures do not require specialized equipment or instrumentation. Some of the principal functional measures currently in use are (1) Functional Ambulation Classification System (FAC); (2) Functional Independence Measure locomotion and mobility subscales (FIM); (3) Gait Abnormality Rating Scale (GARS); (4) Timed Up and Go Test (TUG); and (5) Dynamic Gait Index (DGI). These measures provide information about how gait impairments affect function in the person's environment, rather than about specific gait problems or deviations. Most of these measures require some degree of practice or training so that testers may develop accuracy in using the tool and can apply all of its psychometric implications.

Walking Speed

Walking speed (WS) (or gait velocity) is the fundamental walking measure which defines the person's basic walking ability.[6] It is the time required for a person to traverse a specific distance. The term velocity indicates not only the speed of travel but also the specific direction of travel. Since walking is usually measured in the forward direction, the distinction between speed and velocity is not significant. On level ground people without pathology consistently walk at a preferred/comfortable or "self-selected" walking speed. This speed is the most efficient for that person; faster or slower speed will cost more energy.[49,50] In the gait laboratory, this preferred speed is referred to as "free walking velocity" to be distinguished from "fast walking velocity."

Walking speed as a functional measure is highly reliable and sensitive regardless of the method of measurement. In a group of frail elderly individuals, Van Iersel demonstrated that 5% change in walking speed had a sensitivity of 92% to detect clinically relevant change.[51] Walking speed also correlates with functional ability and physiological changes.[52] Several studies demonstrated that walking speed is a predictor of important aspects of health status and future events including hospitalization, discharge location, and mortality.[53-57]

Numerous factors contribute to walking speed including joint mobility, muscle strength, sensory function, neural control, cognitive status, and energy level, so it can reflect overall health. Fritz and Lusardi suggested considering walking speed as the "sixth vital sign" in older adults. The NIH Toolbox for the Assessment of Neurological and Behavioral Function includes walking speed as a measure of motor function.[58]

In gait laboratory, researchers have used a variety of state-of-the-art equipment including portable computerized walkways, motion analysis systems, and foot switches to measure walking speed. Clinicians, however, can reliably measure walking speed in almost any clinical setting using a stopwatch and a walkway. Most published reports measured walking speed for the middle 6 m of a 10-m walkway to avoid the acceleration and deceleration phases and capture the steady walking speed. Suggested walkway distance varied greatly between studies, however; a walkway as short as 6 m (recording zone is the central 4 m) is still a reliable measure (NIH). Fritz and Lusardi suggest a 10-m test with added 5 m for acceleration and 5 m for deceleration.[59]

In people without pathology, several factors affect walking, including age, gender, lower extremity length, strength, and spontaneous variability between individuals.[59] To follow the International Standards of Measurement, Gait Speed should be expressed in m/sec. Collectively the range for normal walking speed for adults is between 1.2 and 1.4 m/sec. Others reported walking speeds in m/min to be compatible with other energy and cadence measurement. Waters and colleagues reported a similar average of 82 m/min for adults.[60]

Functional Ambulation Classification

Holden and colleagues[42] suggest that grouping subjects by motor ability or functional category is more important than grouping by other indicators of gait. They have developed the Massachusetts General Hospital (MGH) FAC.[61] Six functional categories are defined in their system. A score of 0 indicates nonfunctional ambulation. Patients who require significant and constant assistance of another person for support and balance receive a score of 1. A score of 2 indicates that light touch or intermittent physical assistance is required, and 3 means

that the patient needs verbal cueing or occasional safety assistance. To be scored as a 4, the patient must be independent in ambulation on level surfaces, and a score of 5 means the patient is independent in ambulation on level and nonlevel surfaces, including stairs and inclines. Although the FAC is a general ambulation test, its scores showed a positive linear relationship with such variables as gait velocity and step length.

The FAC has been used most extensively in the assessment of functional locomotion and as a rehabilitation outcome measure for individuals recovering from stroke.[62-64] In a Rausch analysis of discriminant validity of measures used to assess outcome of stroke rehabilitation intervention, however, FIM motor scores and walking speed were better discriminators of outcome than FAC scores.[65] The FAC has also been helpful in assessing concurrent reliability of new mobility measures in stroke rehabilitation and portable instrumented pressure-sensitive monitors.[66,67]

Functional Independence Measure

Initially developed to assess burden of care for staff caring for patients in acute care settings, the FIM is a multidimensional scale that assesses locomotion as one dimension of overall functional status.[68] In the last decade, it has come into wide use as a tool to assess outcomes of rehabilitation interventions for patients with musculoskeletal conditions such as hip fracture and total joint replacement and for those with neuromuscular conditions such as spinal cord injury, myelopathy from spinal stenosis, and stroke.[69-75] The WeeFIM is a version of the FIM intended for use with children with cerebral palsy and other developmental disabilities, acquired brain injury, and other neuromuscular and musculoskeletal impairments.[76-79] The reliability and validity of the FIM have also been assessed in home care and assisted living settings for frail and disabled older adults.[80,81] There is both a performance-based and interview-based version of the FIM.[82,83]

The FIM has two domains of function: motor and cognitive.[82] The motor subscale has four dimensions: *self-care* (eating, grooming, bathing, dressing upper body, dressing lower body, and toileting), *sphincter control* (bladder and bowel management), *ability to transfer* (bed-chair-wheelchair, toilet, tub or shower), and *locomotion* (ambulation or wheelchair use, stair management). The cognitive subscale includes *communication* (comprehension and expression) and *social cognition* (social interaction, problem solving, and memory). The range of possible scores for each component of the subscales is 1 (total assistance required) to 7 (completely independent without any assistive device). Each component has specifically defined criteria. The scoring criteria for the ambulation component of the locomotion subscale are summarized in Table 5-1. The evidence of the measure's validity is strongest when a composite FIM score or motor/cognitive subscale scores are used, although component scores are sometimes used in documentation and record keeping.[81]

Gait Abnormality Rating Scale

Wolfson and colleagues[84] developed the original GARS in an effort to quantify abnormal gait performance of frail institutionalized older adults and identify those most at risk of falling. The

TABLE 5-1   *Scoring Criteria for the Locomotion Component of the Functional Independence Measure*

Score	Score Criteria
7	Able to walk at least 150 feet (50 m) *completely independently*, without any type of assistive device or wheelchair, safely and within a reasonable (functional) period of time
6	Able to walk at least 150 feet (50 m) *independently, but requires an assistive device* (orthosis, prosthesis, wheelchair, special shoes, cane, crutches, walker), or takes more than reasonable time, or has safety concerns
5	Requires *standby supervision*, cueing, or coaxing to walk or propel wheelchair at least 150 feet (50 m)
4	Requires *minimum contact assistance* (patient contributes 75% effort) to walk or propel wheelchair at least 150 feet (50 m)
3	Requires *moderate assistance* (patient contributes 50% to 74% effort) to walk or propel wheelchair a minimum of 150 feet (50 m)
2	Requires *maximal assistance* of one person (patient contributes 25% to 49% effort) to walk or propel wheelchair 50 feet (17 m)
1	Requires *total assistance* (patient contributes less than 25% effort) or requires assistance of more than one helper, or is unable to walk or propel wheelchair at least 50 feet (17 m)

scale has since been modified (GARS-M) by VanSwearingen and colleagues[85] for use in community settings.

In the GARS-M, a videotape of a patient walking on a level surface is scored on seven dimensions: variability, guardedness, staggering, foot contact, hip range of motion, shoulder extension, and synchrony of arm movement and heel strike. The measure uses a four-point criterion-based rating scale (0 to 3). Total GARS-M scores range from 0 to 21, with high scores indicating less efficient or safe performance. Gait variability is one of the unique measures of the GARS-M, which has been linked to increased fall risk in older adults. Huang and colleagues[86] documented the validity of the GARS-M by comparing its scores with those recorded on a computerized walkway. Evidence of interrater and intrarater reliability, and concurrent validity (compared with temporal and distance parameters of gait) and discriminate validity (between fallers and nonfallers) have been reported.[85,87]

Timed Up and Go

The TUG test is commonly used with frail older adults with limited mobility. Patients are asked to rise from a seated position in a standard height chair, walk 3 m on a level surface, turn, walk back to the chair, and return to a seated position, moving as quickly as they are safely able. Although the original get up and go test used a somewhat subjective 0 to 5 rating to score each component of the task, performance is now based on total time to complete the task.[88,89] In both versions, individuals being evaluated are instructed to move as quickly as they are safely able to move. Importantly, the TUG is a measure of overall functional mobility, assessing the ability to transfer, walk, and change direction.

Several studies documented reference ranges for the TUG in community-dwelling older adults.[90-93] Bohannon consolidated data from 21 studies for meta-analysis on the TUG reference values in people older than 60 years of age.[94] The mean TUG time for individuals at least 60 years of age was 9.4 (8.9 to 9.9) seconds. When the data were divided into three age subgroups, the mean for those 60 to 69 years was 8.1 seconds, for 70 to 79 years was 9.2 seconds, and for 80 to 99 years was 11.3 second. Several other studies documented the higher mean of the TUG values as age increased and for women compared to men.[92,93] Intrarater and interrater reliability of the TUG is excellent, Intraclass Correlation Coefficients range between 0.97 and 0.99.[90] Although the TUG does not specifically assess walking speed, it assesses the more functional components of mobility and transfer from sit to stand.[95]

The TUG times increased when healthy older adults were tested using an assistive device.[96,97] Reference range for the TUG times in patients who use assistive devices is not available. Higher TUG times are associated with functional impairment in individuals with arthritis, amputation, hip fracture, and Parkinson's disease.[98-104]

Dynamic Gait Index

The dynamic gait index (DGI) is a useful test in patients with vestibular and balance problems.[105] It includes eight items, walking on level surfaces, changing speeds, head turns in horizontal and vertical directions, walking and turning 180 degrees to stop, stepping over and around obstacles, and stair ascent and descent. Each item is scored on a scale of 0 to 3, with 3 indicating normal performance and 0 representing severe impairment. The best possible score on the DGI is a 24. Several studies demonstrated its high intrarater and interrater reliability in older adults and in different patient populations.[106-108] A score of less than 19 indicates a risk for falling.[107]

A short form of the DGI includes only four items: walking on level surfaces, changing speeds, and head turns in horizontal and vertical directions.[109] Anything less than the maximum score of 12 on the short form identified individuals with balance deficit and those who scored less than 10 were at risk for falls.[95]

CHOOSING AN ASSESSMENT STRATEGY

Recognizing similarities and differences in purpose and design of the various gait assessment methods is important. Gait-based methods, such as the Rancho Los Amigos observational gait assessment, seek to identify and differentiate pathological versus compensatory mechanisms and therefore guide the specific surgical, therapeutic, orthotic, or prosthetic interventions for a particular patient. Functional indexes, such as the MGH FAC, the FIM, or the TUG, may be a means of evaluating treatment efficacy, disease-related decline, or improvement over time. The cost of gait assessment through comprehensive instrumented procedures often precludes its general use in the clinical arena. Observational analysis through gait-based assessment will remain a viable and important contribution to clinical care for many years to come.

CLINICAL EXAMPLES OF GAIT DEFICIENCIES: IMPACT OF FUNCTIONAL TASKS DURING GAIT

The following case examples illustrate gait deficiencies associated with pathological conditions that commonly alter gait performance: pretibial flaccid paralysis, hemiplegia, cerebral palsy, and spina bifida. As might be expected, each example demonstrates common gait characteristics specific to the particular pathological condition while presenting variants from that profile. The discussion is based on information gathered by foot-switch stride and kinematic and observational gait analysis.

CASE EXAMPLE 1

A Patient with Flaccid Paralysis of Pretibial Muscles

J. J. is a 37-year-old man with inherited sensorimotor neuropathy (Charcot-Marie-Tooth disease) who has been referred to the gait assessment clinic for evaluation of his orthotic intervention. Examination of muscle function and strength reveals relatively symmetrical distal impairment. Manual muscle test scores include "trace" activity of dorsiflexion muscles bilaterally, "poor" plantar flexion on the left, and "fair+" plantar flexion on the right. Knee and hip strength is "normal."

Questions to Consider
- Given J. J.'s pattern of weakness, what types of primary difficulties or deviations might you predict during the functional task of (1) weight acceptance (IC and LR), (2) single limb support (MSt and TSt), and (3) swing limb advancement (PSw, ISw, MSw, and TSw)?

- Given J. J.'s pattern of weakness, what compensatory strategies (pathological gait deviations) might he use to accomplish these functional tasks of gait?
- What quantitative measures, indicators of energy cost, qualitative measures, or function-based assessments would you use to determine whether a change in orthoses would be warranted? Why would you select those measures?

Examination and Evaluation

During a foot-switch stride analysis, J. J. walks without his usual orthoses. In the trailing left limb, the posterior compartment fails to support the forefoot lever arm so that the tibia progresses forward with limited heel-off in late stance (Figure 5-15). This creates excessive knee flexion and limits the step length of the contralateral limb. The net effect of this

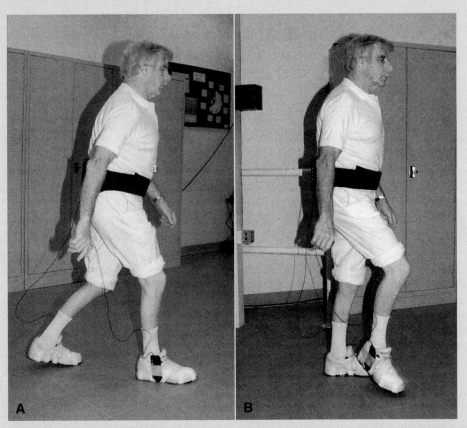

FIGURE 5-15 A patient with Charcot-Marie-Tooth disease demonstrates shortened right stride length because of inadequate support at the foot and ankle in late stance of the left limb (**A**), and the use of a compensatory steppage gait to ensure swing clearance in the presence of dorsiflexion weakness (**B**).

Continued

inadequate forefoot rocker is a reduction in velocity. Lack of support of the trailing forefoot allows depression of the center of gravity. At the same time, dorsiflexion weakness on the right creates early, abrupt plantar flexion (foot slap) with premature contact of the first metatarsal. The variance between plantar flexor strength of the left and right limbs is demonstrated by difference in single-limb support times. The stronger right calf participates in 39.8% (0.416 sec) of the gait cycle, whereas the weaker left calf commits itself to only 31.4% (0.328 sec). This subtle timing discrepancy in gait was not readily identifiable in observational analysis.

In right MSw, while the left foot is in a supporting posture, the classical steppage gait characteristics of a flail forefoot are observed: Compensatory swing clearance is accomplished through excessive hip and knee flexion (see Figure 5-12B).

When J. J. wears his orthoses (a dorsiflexion assist thermoplastic AFO on the right and a dorsiflexion stop–plantar flexion resist thermoplastic AFO on the left), results of foot-switch temporal analysis are quite different. Velocity,

cadence, and stride length increase slightly. The asymmetry between right and left single limb support times decreases because the AFO provides external support of the trailing left limb. The energy-inefficient steppage gait and unsightly foot slap are diminished as well.

Questions to Consider

- What specific problems do the examination and evaluation identify in each of the functional tasks of gait: weight acceptance (IC and LR), single limb support (MSt and TSt), and swing limb advancement (PSw, ISw, MSw, and TSw)?
- In what ways do J. J.'s orthoses address the functional problems observed when he walks without his orthoses in each of the functional tasks of the gait cycle: weight acceptance (IC and LR), single limb support (MSt and TSt), and swing limb advancement (PSw, ISw, MSw, and TSw)? In what ways do his orthoses potentially limit each of the functional tasks of gait? Do the benefits outweigh the limitations?

Clinical Characteristics of Gait in Hemiplegia

For most patients who are recovering from stroke—cerebrovascular accident (CVA)—improvement in the quality of gait is related to the natural history of the pathological process and the impact of gait retraining in rehabilitation. In the week immediately after CVA, only 24% to 38% of patients are able to ambulate independently.[110] After weeks of rehabilitation, more than 50% are able to walk without assistance, especially if using an appropriate AFO and assistive device.[111] At the 6-month mark, more than 80% of patients with CVA are functionally independent in ambulation.[112]

The many variations of limb control observed during the gait of patients who are recovering from a CVA can be explained by one or more of the following factors: primitive locomotor patterns, impaired postural responses, abnormal postural tone with various degrees of spasticity and rigidity, inappropriately timed muscle contractions, and diminished muscle strength. One of the primary determinants of gait dysfunction in post-CVA hemiplegia is whether the patient has some degree of selective control of specific muscles rather than activation of abnormal synergy patterns (mass flexion or extension). Patients with hemiplegia often have difficulty grading the magnitude of a particular muscle contraction with respect to other muscle contractions. Because of hyperactivity of muscle spindle/stretch reflex in the presence of spasticity, the ability to move toward dorsiflexion with forward progression of the tibia during stance may be counteracted by contraction of plantar flexors into a position of equinus. Spasticity, although difficult to measure, can be described for clinical purposes with the Ashworth Spasticity Scale.[113] The baseline level 0 indicates no measurable tone. A designation of level 1, mild tone, is given when a muscle "catches" with an abrupt passive movement into flexion or extension. A level

2 designation indicates marked abnormal tone but flexible range of motion and level 3 is characterized by pronounced tone and difficult passive movement. Level 4 denotes a limb that is held rigidly in either flexion or extension.

The orthotic goal for patients with hypertonicity of the lower extremity after a CVA is to control ankle motion and preposition for tibial advancement. Two orthotic strategies are commonly used: (1) provision of an AFO with a locked ankle component set in slight dorsiflexion or (2) use of an articulated AFO that allows slight ankle motion around the neutral position. When ankle joint motion is limited or blocked by an orthosis, stability in stance improves; however, forward progression of the tibia is compromised, and step length is reduced. Modifications to the shoe, such as application of a rocker bottom sole or elevation of the heel, can compensate by mimicking the second rocker of gait.

Over the course of rehabilitation, the patient with hemiplegia often experiences changes in tone, joint flexibility, pain or discomfort, fear or confidence, motor strength or weakness, and quality of proprioception. Six stages of motor recovery in hemiplegia have been identified by Brunnstrom.[15] In the first stage, no voluntary movement of limbs is present. In the second, movement reappears but is limited by pronounced muscle weakness or spasticity, or both. The patient is usually not yet ready for functional ambulation. In the third stage, spasticity coexists with limb synergy motion. Typically a mass extensor pattern is seen in the lower limb. As the patient continues to improve in the fourth stage, spasticity may be reduced as the patient begins to move out of stereotypical synergy patterns. In stage 5, selective control outside mass synergy patterns becomes more consistent and more functional. With recovery complete, in stage 6 the patient may achieve coordinated controlled movement. Because of the dynamic nature of the recovery process, the ability to adjust or alter orthotic alignment or characteristics is very desirable. It is not unusual that an orthosis prescribed early in rehabilitation becomes inappropriate or creates further gait dysfunction at a later stage. Once rehabilitation is complete and the patient has achieved stability in walking patterns, definitive biomechanical needs are identified and the adjustability of the orthosis is less important.

The extension synergy pattern places the lower extremity in excessive extension at the hip and knee and the foot in equinovarus. This reduces the amount of knee flexion and dorsiflexion during swing, necessitating a compensatory strategy, such as circumduction, to provide swing phase clearance.[114] Rigidity of the ankle leaves the patient with inadequate dorsiflexion mobility as well as vastly reduced plantar flexion excursion during PSw and early swing. Stance time is considerably reduced on the hemiplegic/paretic side, and the quadriceps, gastrocnemius, gluteus maximus, and semitendinous muscles are inappropriately active throughout stance.[115] Activity of lower limb muscle groups on the hemiplegic/paretic side is increased compared with normal patterns of muscle activation. Excessive hip flexion at MSt on the hemiplegic/paretic side shifts the GRF line anteriorly, producing a knee extension moment that interferes with forward progression. The hemiplegic/paretic side also displays less hip adduction in single limb support, which compromises lateral shift toward the affected side.[116] Brandstater and colleagues[42] describe reduced velocity, cadence, stride length, and single limb support time on the affected side, with consequent increased single limb support and reduced step length on the sound side. Hirschberg and Nathanson[115] demonstrated that an appropriate AFO improves the quality of gait by increasing step length and stance time as well as reducing swing time of the affected side. Velocity of gait improves when the AFO is placed in slight dorsiflexion. When spasticity is not problematic, an AFO that permits some plantar flexion normalizes IC to LR timing and prevents an unstable knee flexion moment in early stance. Because knee extensor strength often equals or exceeds hip extensor strength after CVA, most patients with hemiplegia can be effectively managed with an AFO rather than a knee-ankle-foot orthosis.[116] Muscle strengthening is less important in achieving improved walking characteristics in hemiplegia than is the retraining of normal movement patterns in gait.[117]

CASE EXAMPLE 2

A Patient with Hemiplegia

M. G. is a 67-year-old man referred to the gait laboratory for evaluation 13 months after a CVA damaged the sensorimotor cortex of the left hemisphere. Currently he is a community ambulator (MGH functional ambulation classification level 6) who walks with the aid of an AFO and quad cane (FIM locomotion score 6). In the clinical examination, his spasticity becomes apparent when his ankle moves toward a neutral position (Ashworth spasticity scale level 3). The orthosis he received early in rehabilitation, and continues to use, is a traditional double upright, which locks his ankle in slight plantar flexion. Although this ankle angle delays tibial advancement and forward progression in stance, the patient has come to rely on its contribution to stability at proximal joints.

Questions to Consider
- Given M. G.'s pattern of spasticity and weakness, what types of primary difficulties or deviations might you predict, when he is not wearing his orthosis, during the functional task of weight acceptance (IC and LR)? Of single limb support (MSt and TSt)? Of swing limb advancement (PSw, ISw, MSw, and TSw)?
- Given M. G.'s pattern of spasticity and weakness, what compensatory strategies (pathological gait deviations) might he use to accomplish these functional tasks of gait?

- What additional quantitative measures, indicators of energy cost, qualitative measures, or function-based assessments would you use to determine if a change in orthosis would be warranted? Why would you select those measures?

Examination and Evaluation
M. G.'s gait with the AFO is evaluated by foot-switch testing. Extensor synergy patterns contribute to function by providing a degree of stability in stance but also reduce efficiency of gait by limiting normal stance progression beginning with the first rocker period (Figure 5-16). Duration heel-only time of the first rocker (IC to the foot-flat position at the end of LR) is approximately one sixth of a second on the hemiplegic side, which is significantly less than normal heel-only time. Heel-only time on the intact side is roughly three times greater than that on the hemiplegic side. Forward progression during MSt is halted at the second rocker when spasticity prevents the necessary dorsiflexion of the ankle (see Figure 5-13). As M.G. moves into TSt, when metatarsophalangeal break (concurrent with heel-off) should allow progression onto the forefoot, the third rocker is also relatively blocked. This lack of mobility of the metatarsophalangeal joints, and inadequate third rocker, result in a loss of knee flexion, necessary for an effective PSw, for which the patient is unable to compensate. Of the 60 degrees of knee

Continued

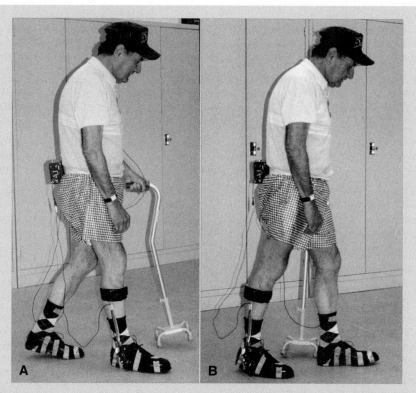

FIGURE 5-16 A patient with hemiplegia after cerebral vascular accident, the first rocker from initial contact to foot flat (**A**) is abrupt as a result of extensor patterns and limb rigidity. Extensor pattern at the ankle (**B**) translates into a failure to yield into dorsiflexion toward the end of the second rocker. Third rocker heel elevation will also be reduced, and lack of mobility reduces the step length of the contralateral limb.

flexion necessary for the swing phase clearance, 35 degrees should be achieved passively during PSw. For patients with hemiplegia, the loss of this positional flexion is an additional challenge to clearance, beyond that produced by the equinus position of the ankle. Any attempts to compensate by "hip hiking" are likely to be inefficient and unsuccessful. These rocker limitations reduce step length of the sound side, leading to premature double limb support. The corresponding MSw knee flexion on the hemiplegic side is also reduced. MG demonstrates a much reduced stance time on the affected side (62% gait cycle) versus the sound side (71% gait cycle) and a reduced single limb support time on the affected side (28% gait cycle) versus the sound side (38% gait cycle).

Questions to Consider

- What specific problems has the examination and evaluation identified in each of the functional tasks of gait: weight acceptance (IC and LR), single limb support (MSt and TSt), and swing limb advancement (PSw, ISw, MSw, and TSw)? How do these problems relate to his abnormal tone and motor control?
- In what ways does M. G.'s orthosis address or constrain each of the functional tasks of the gait cycle: weight acceptance (IC and LR), single limb support (MSt and TSt), and swing limb advancement (PSw, ISw, MSw, and TSw)?

Clinical Characteristics of Gait in Spastic Diplegic Cerebral Palsy

Children with spastic diplegic cerebral palsy often have significant spasticity and marked weakness of the antigravity muscles in both lower extremities. This combination is a precursor of joint contracture. The clinical term often used to describe the typical gait of a patient with diplegia is *crouched gait*. In crouched gait, marked internal rotation of the femur and tibia occurs throughout the gait cycle, the knees remain in flexion throughout stance, and the ankles remain in plantar flexion during stance (toe walking) and swing. Gage[118] clearly documented the high energy cost of flexed knee gait. The pathological

combination of an equinus ankle, positive Trendelenburg hip, and stiff knee gait often produces various combinations of compensatory hiking of the pelvis, external rotation of the foot, and circumduction of the swing limb. This pattern has been attributed to tightness and overactivity of the distal hamstrings, alone or in combination with the hip flexors.[119]

Some patients with diplegia ambulate with a *jump gait* pattern, using somewhat less hip and knee flexion than do patients with crouch gait but with excessive ankle dorsiflexion rather than plantar flexion.[120] Jump gait is often a postoperative manifestation of bilateral Achilles tendon lengthening without concurrent release of hip and knee contractures. Common compensatory strategies in jump gait include vaulting and circumduction. In crouch and jump gait, the GRF line falls progressively behind the knee joint center during single limb support of the stance phase. This creates an excessive demand on the quadriceps for stance phase stability. One surgical strategy used to correct jump gait combines hip flexion releases, hip flexion release lengthening of the distal hamstrings, and correction of external rotation. Postoperatively, the patient is fitted for floor reaction AFOs.[121] Ideally, the Achilles tendon is lengthened to neutral dorsiflexion position and the patient protected in AFOs for 1 year postoperatively.

The *scissoring* pattern, which is also a common gait deviation in children with diplegia, is aggravated by spastic hip flexors and adductors because the smaller base of support reduces the efficiency of their line of pull. Orthotic solutions provide limited assistance in limb tracking and rotational control. Those that attempt to control rotation must cross the hip joint, adding significant weight and bulk and increasing difficulty in donning and doffing.

A Patient with Spastic Diplegic Cerebral Palsy

K. E. is a 10-year-old boy with spastic diplegic cerebral palsy who has been referred to the gait laboratory for evaluation to assist his orthopedist in deciding whether corrective surgery is indicated. The boy currently ambulates independently, without assistive devices, wearing bilateral solid ankle AFOs (WeeFIM locomotion score of 6).

Questions to Consider
- Given K. E.'s pattern of spasticity and weakness, what types of primary difficulties or deviations might you predict when he is not wearing his orthoses during the functional task of weight acceptance (IC and LR)? Of single limb support (MSt and TSt)? Of swing limb advancement (PSw, ISw, MSw, and TSw)?
- Given K. E.'s pattern of spasticity and weakness, what compensatory strategies (pathological gait deviations) might he use to accomplish these functional tasks of gait?
- What additional quantitative measures, indicators of energy cost, qualitative measures, or function-based assessments might help determine whether surgical orthopedic intervention is warranted? Why would you select those measures?

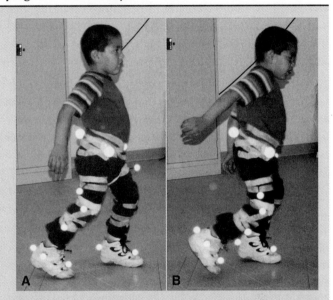

FIGURE 5-17 A child with spastic diplegia, classic crouch gait (**A**) is characterized by increased hip and knee flexion in combination with toe walking. Postural substitutions in crouch gait (**B**) may include increased lumbar lordosis, trunk extension, and posterior arm placement.

Examination and Evaluation
K. E. is fitted with reflective markers for three-dimensional motion analysis of this gait. A typical crouch gait pattern is observed during observational gait analysis while his gait is being recorded for more detailed kinematic and kinetic analysis by computer software. Foot-switch analysis confirms diminished heel contact with no heel-only time on the left and no heel contact at all on the right.

Clinical examination of K. E.'s lower extremity function reveals a combination of overactive hamstrings and weak gastrocnemius and soleus (Figure 5-17). The flexion of hips and knees increases the need for proximal stabilization, resulting in compensatory hyperextension of the trunk and posterior arm placement (see Figure 5-14B). Because the ankles are held in equinus, the final rocker propels tibial advancement despite limitation in ankle mobility. K. E. spends most of the stance phase in TSt and PSw; consequently, double limb support time is vastly increased.

K. E. has not had previous surgical release of his gastrocnemius muscles. Even with surgery, impairment of motor control may continue to be problematic, so that dorsiflexion may not work in concert with the knee flexion to provide a heel-toe gait pattern. Gastrocnemius release without concurrent release of the hip and knee contractures usually leads to short step lengths with a compensatory increase in cadence. Spastic hip flexors, also serving as adductors, create a mild scissors effect during each swing limb advancement. Ambulation with bilateral AFOs, which the patient prefers, increases step length and reduces knee flexion compared with ambulation with no orthosis.

Continued

Clinical Characteristics of Gait in Children with Spina Bifida

Spina bifida (myelomeningocele) occurs when vertebral arches fail to unite very early in gestation. Clinically, this leads to partial or complete paralysis at or below the level involved. The most common impairment is a flaccid paralysis, with loss of proprioception and exteroception (pain, temperature sensation, light touch, and pressure sensation). Many children with spina bifida have significant ambulatory deficiencies; more than 50% require an orthosis of some kind to ambulate.[122] Assessment for orthotic support begins as soon as the child attempts to gain an erect posture.

Severity of gait dysfunction depends on the level of involvement of the spinal cord. When the L-5 and S-1 nerve roots are affected, the gluteus maximus, hip abductors, and triceps surae are lost; the hamstrings are present but weak; and sensory loss is limited to the plantar surface of the feet. The plantar flexor deficit requires setting limits to dorsiflexion range of motion through orthotic joint control. This limitation of dorsiflexion allows the patient to establish hip stability through hip extension accomplished with exaggerated trunk lordosis. Without it, the patient would fall forward unopposed. Lateral stability is achieved through crutches and a wide walking base.

When the L-3 and L-4 root nerves are affected, hamstring function, hip extension, knee flexion, plantar flexion, and dorsiflexion are completely lost. The resulting foot drop cannot be adequately compensated for in swing by hip and knee flexion. Hip flexion, adduction, and knee extension are intact but may be weak. At the L-3 level, weak knee flexion from the gracilis may also be present. These children benefit early from standing frames; later, they often are able to ambulate with orthotic assistance . Adequate stabilization of the foot and ankle is achieved through orthotic application of a locked ankle in neutral or slight dorsiflexion. Trunk lordosis is a compensatory strategy used to stabilize the hip during stance. The muscular imbalance at the hip increases the likelihood of flexion contracture, which in turn amplifies the need for even more compensatory lordosis. Extreme hip flexion contracture may ultimately preclude ambulation. If contractures at the hip, knee, and ankle are minimal and the child gains trunk control, he or she will be able to stand erect but will rely on trunk alignment for static balance and forearm crutches for further stability.

A child with lesions that involve L-1 and L-2 levels has little lower limb function other than weak hip flexors. Such children often begin upright function with a parapodium or swivel walker and can later progress to reciprocal gait orthoses. The swing-through gait with bilateral hip-knee-ankle-foot orthosis has been shown to be less efficient than a reciprocal gait orthosis for thoracic level spinal bifida.[123]

CASE EXAMPLE 4

A Child with Spina Bifida

N. P. is an active 9-year-old boy with myelomeningocele at L-5 who returns to the gait laboratory as part of an ongoing research study to document changes in gait characteristics over time. He currently ambulates wearing bilateral AFOs set in a neutral ankle position, using Loftstrand crutches in a four-point reciprocal gait pattern.

Questions to Consider
- Given N. P.'s pattern of weakness and sensory loss, what types of primary difficulties or deviations might you predict when he is not wearing his orthoses, during the functional task of weight acceptance (IC and LR)? Of single limb support (MSt and TSt)? Of swing limb advancement (PSw, ISw, MSw, and TSw)?

- Given N. P.'s pattern of weakness and sensory loss, what compensatory strategies (pathological gait deviations) might he use to accomplish these functional tasks of gait?
- What additional quantitative measures, indicators of energy cost, qualitative measures, or function-based assessments might help determine if surgical orthopedic intervention is warranted? Why would you select those measures?

Examination and Evaluation

Comparative foot-switch testing reveals that, without crutches, stride length and velocity are reduced. External rotation of both limbs is present throughout the gait cycle

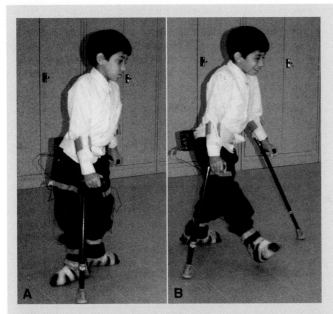

FIGURE 5-18 In this child with myelomeningocele, weakness at the hip results in external rotation of the limbs in both stance and swing phase **(A)**, which contributes to altered forward progression from the heel to the medial forefoot, with minimal weight bearing on the lateral foot **(B)**.

(Figure 5-18). With or without crutches, he has no measurable fifth metatarsal or toe contact on either limb in his typical stance phase weight-bearing patterns. Passive external rotation is present at the hip as well as abducted limb placement as he advances over the forefoot. His abducted limb placement and wide-based gait provide increased stability at a cost of excessive loading on the posteromedial aspect of the feet (see Figure 5-15B). Like many children with spina bifida, he spends excessive time in heel contact, largely to the exclusion of lateral forefoot weight bearing. This loading and shear pattern often leads to callusing and eventual neuropathic breakdown in adult life. His fastest gait velocity (55 m/min) is approximately 60% of normal free-gait velocity. During swing phase, external rotation of the limb is marked. The flail foot is held in slight dorsiflexion during TSw through the support of the AFO.

Questions to Consider
- What specific problems does the examination and evaluation identify in each of the functional tasks of gait: weight acceptance (IC and LR), single limb support (MSt and TSt), and swing limb advancement (PSw, ISw, MSw, and TSw)? How do these problems relate to N. P.'s flaccid paralysis and sensory impairment?
- In what ways do N. P.'s orthoses address or constrain each of the functional tasks of the gait cycle: weight acceptance (IC and LR), single limb support (MSt and TSt), and swing limb advancement (PSw, ISw, MSw, and TSw)? What is the interaction of his flaccidity and sensory with his orthoses on the efficacy and energy cost of his walking?

GAIT PATTERNS IN INDIVIDUALS WITH AMPUTATION

Qualitative observational gait analysis is a broadly accepted approach to achieving a clinically optimal gait in individuals with amputation. Instrumented gait analysis provides a more repeatable accurate assessment of prosthetic function. In its broadest scope, the data derived increasingly serve as foundation guidelines for both prosthetic design and clinical application. The daily practice of assessment and management of prosthetic gait, however, depends on the subjective skills of the prosthetist and the targeted treatment protocol of the therapist.

The University of California at Berkeley prosthetic project, which began in the mid 1950s, represented the most concentrated period of prosthetic advancement. The comprehensive basic gait studies and their application to the biomechanics of amputee gait for transtibial and transfemoral amputations established fundamental design criteria.[124] Contributions of subsequent investigators continue to be largely based on the Berkeley criteria.

Extensive calculations and interpretations were required to relate normal and prosthetic gait data to the problems of prosthetic design. Data reduction was a slow process before relatively recent technological advancements because all motion measurements had to be performed by hand. There were no automated film analyzers to identify the motion patterns and no computers to perform rapid data processing. Therefore, the number of subjects studied was limited. The project also had the additional depth of considering all three planes of motion, in contrast to prior studies that analyzed only the sagittal plane of gait progression.[6,125] Subsequent investigators, with the aid of more advanced instrumentation, have replicated and expanded the Eberhart-Inman work but have not found it in error.

Transtibial Prosthetic Gait

In 1957 the Berkeley project was specifically commissioned to reconsider transtibial prosthetic gait and biomechanics; with that goal, an advisory conference was held.[126] Basic transtibial prosthesis at that time was attached to the limb with a thigh lacer that included articulated knee joints and a foot with an articulated ankle. Detailed review of the normal and transtibial amputee-gait data resulted in a totally new approach that led to two developments: the patellar tendon-bearing (PTB) prosthesis and the solid-ankle, cushion heel foot.[127-129] The improved transtibial socket was a PTB design that closely followed the contours of the proximal tibia.[130] The PTB prosthesis replaced the thigh lacer with supracondylar fixation, again with the advantage of anatomical contour and total contact.

Prosthetic Feet During Stance

Compressible heel prosthetic feet have a solid plastic keel embedded in the proximal portion of a stiff foam foot that allows a slight degree of forefoot flexibility while the cushion heel lessens the impact of initial floor contact and through vertical compression simulates articulated ankle plantar flexion. Material compressibility replaced the mechanical joint of the single-axis foot. Foot contour, alignment, and elasticity facilitated progression onto the forefoot. This design followed careful analysis of the essential degrees of mobility. The compressible heel foot has become the standard terminal device for most individuals with amputation, though hybrids incorporating both low- and high-performance feet with multidirectional articulated ankles hold a significant place in clinical use as well.

Transtibial Alignment

The positional relation between the socket and prosthetic foot is critical to achieve optimal progression in stance, yet also highly subjective. The goal is to encourage tibial progression in stance and place the knee in a stable (minimally flexed) weight-bearing posture without causing hyperextension in late stance and to have the lower limb follow a normal path of motion in swing.

Static or "bench" alignment uses the subcutaneous crest of tibia (tibial blade) to establish alignment of the residual limb within the prosthesis. In the sagittal plane, this landmark, at its origin at the tibial tubercle, is typically angled approximately 5 degrees forward of the perpendicular to the tibial plateau that serves as the supporting surface for the knee joint. Hence, if the socket is aligned by the tibial blade, the socket is set so that the tibia is tilted slightly forward to avoid a backward thrust during stance. This angular posture of the prosthetic socket, in conjunction with a deliberate anterior displacement (translation) of the socket relative to the foot, generally succeeds in encouraging tibial progression.

Even with this alignment, the individual with dysvascular transtibial amputation who typically exhibits some degree of weakness will shift the weight line anterior to the knee by simply leaning forward during LR in a postural movement akin to a quad avoidance gait. This results in reduced knee flexion throughout stance phase and delayed flexion in swing (Figure 5-19). A hesitation of stance progression (the MSt dead spot) is a common phenomenon. A delay in the rollover pattern, common to the dysvascular transtibial amputee, is reflected in the shear pattern (see Figure 5-19B).

Final positioning of the socket-foot relation is determined by observational analysis of the subject's gait and feedback from the individual with an amputation. This process, referred to as dynamic alignment, examines smoothness of the rollover pattern and medial-lateral verticality of the foot, avoiding both extremes of inversion or eversion during progression. The absence of abnormal motions in swing such as a whip, compensatory motions to avoid scuffing the foot in swing (e.g., degree of pelvic elevation or vaulting), and an erect trunk posture are additional observational criteria used for assessment. Comfort and ease of walking

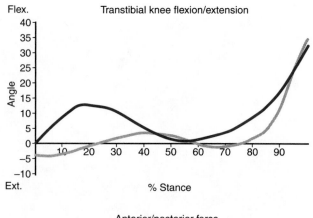

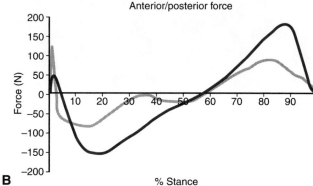

FIGURE 5-19 A, Patients with dysvascular transtibial amputation typically shift the weight line anterior to the knee early in stance, which results in reduced knee flexion throughout stance phase and delayed flexion in swing. **B,** Patients with dysvascular transtibial amputation typically shift the weight line anterior to the knee early in stance, which results in typical midstance (MSt) hesitation in the progression of rollover, reflected in the shear pattern. (Courtesy of VA Long Beach Gait Laboratory.)

are criteria of the individual with amputation. A one-subject study of repeated realignment by an experienced prosthetist over a 2-year period documented inconsistencies in the alignment accepted as being good, a decision confirmed each time by three other prosthetists.[131,132] A range of alignment variation satisfactory to both the prosthetist and amputee was defined.

In optimizing the alignment in the coronal plane, there is an attempt to mimic the slight varus moment seen at the knee during MSt of normal human locomotion. This moment is usually achieved by a slight medial inset of the prosthetic foot relative to the socket, taking advantage of the good weight-bearing areas in the proximal-medial and lateral-distal regions of the residual limb. Pressure in these areas is well tolerated. Inadequate inset of the foot, or worse, outset of the foot will generally result in excessive pressure on the very superficial cut end of the tibia (medial-distal) and the perineal nerve and bony prominence of the head of the fibula (lateral-proximal). Although observational analysis is appropriate for general clinical care, the alignment of individuals with amputation with complex fitting problems is best resolved through objective confirmation with forceplate and motion data.

Studies of Transtibial Prosthetic Gait

Most instrumented studies of individuals with transtibial amputation have focused on foot design, with the general exclusion of alignment. Prosthetic foot designers attempt to passively reproduce, by material quality, the normal dynamic functional balance between mobility and stability provided by the anatomical foot. The greatest difference is between the relatively rigid compressible heel–type feet and the mobile hinge of the single-axis foot.[133] Motion analysis has shown that the articulated ankle improves weight acceptance stability by providing significant plantar flexion, allowing an earlier foot flat posture[134] however, the arc of knee flexion and the timing and intensity of the quadriceps do not differ from that of the compressible heel–type foot.[135] Stance phase limb progression is enhanced by an articulating ankle in two ways. In footswitch analysis, the mobile ankle had a longer period of single limb stance time, whereas total stance time was shorter compared with solid-ankle designs.[135] In addition, there was more prolonged hamstring action with the compressible heel foot; this implies that a forward lean was used to improve progression over the less yielding foot. These functional advantages of a mobile prosthetic foot would be significant in a marginal walker, but the heaviness of a single-axis foot creates an energy-cost penalty that also must be considered.

Beginning in the 1980s, the use of elastic materials and designs has been increasingly applied to prosthetic feet. The initial objective was to facilitate running because the presence of normal knee control gives the transtibial individuals with amputation considerable functional potential.[136] Foot designs all emphasize controlled dorsiflexion mobility for greater push-off. It has been assumed that these dynamic, elastic prosthetic feet would be advantageous for the average walker by reducing the greater-than-normal energy cost currently experienced by individuals with amputation.[137] The most mobile designs, in terms of dorsiflexion range, are those with a long-bladed shaft such as the Flexfoot and Springlite. These bladed shaft designs have not lessened the muscular demands of weight acceptance. Their simulated "ankle plantar flexion" during limb loading is no better than the solid-ankle, cushion-heel foot. Both result in a plantar flexion that is markedly less than the normal controlled, yet rapid, ankle plantar flexion of 12 degrees used to reduce the propulsive effect of the heel rocker by allowing early forefoot contact. Both prosthetic feet cause a significant delay in attaining the stability of foot flat.[138]

The intact limb uses a modest arc (15 to 20 degrees) of knee flexion to absorb the shock of floor contact.[4] Prosthetic feet rely on a cushion heel. The time needed for adequate cushion compression delays the drop of the forefoot to the floor. This perpetuates an unsteady, heel-only source of support that requires increased active muscular control of the knee and hip to ensure weight-bearing stability. This subtle source of instability is obscured by two findings. Displacement of the customary heel marker gives a false reading of plantar flexion.[139] Heel cushion compression delays the rate of initial tibial advancement, resulting in reduced weight acceptance knee flexion for the transtibial amputee compared with normal. This difference is reflected in calculations of subnormal moments and powers.[140,141] These findings have been interpreted as a sign of reduced muscle demand, and a corresponding conservation of energy has been attributed to the dynamic elastic-response feet. Direct EMG recordings, however, show significantly higher than normal muscle demand for five different feet tested.[142]

CASE EXAMPLE 5

A Patient with a Unilateral Transtibial Amputation

W. T. is a 59-year-old transtibial amputee secondary to peripheral vascular disease. He underwent the amputation in September 2009 and subsequently experienced a fall, causing secondary injuries to the residual limb. Previously, he underwent bilateral total knee arthroplasty, most recently on the right side in 2007. W. T. started physical therapy for gait training in March 2010 and completed it in July 2010. He has been referred for a gait evaluation due to complaints of right knee pain as he has continues to become ambulatory with the prosthesis.

Questions to Consider

- Considering the gait deviations associated with transtibial amputees, how could this impact his affected side in conjunction with the total knee arthroplasty?
- What type of options could be considered to minimize the impact on his intact joints? With this, consider the role of patient education and possible compliance issues.
- What type of qualitative and quantitative information would you use to support your decision(s)?

Examination and Evaluation

On the day of evaluation, W. T. presented using a single point cane and after discussion with the staff complained of intermittent pain at the distal end of his residual limb. A further chart review revealed that since the time that he completed physical therapy multiple prosthetic feet have been trialed, along with additional modifications to the prosthetic socket to help increase comfort. There were also documented issues of patient noncompliance, particularly in terms of the prosthesis wear schedule. The patient had periodically developed areas of redness on his residual limb

Continued

and was advised to pay particular attention this area and to document it when it occurred.

An initial assessment with video-based data collection was determined to be an appropriate first step. During the evaluation, the patient was asked to walk multiple times over level ground at his self-selected walking speed while being videotaped. The principal findings were as follows: (1) Periodic knee hyperextension during midstance on the involved side, (2) the involved side knee is often not fully extended at initial contact, and (3) for the times that the knee is flexed going into stance there is a rapid extension during midstance.

Taking into consideration the patient's history and current complaints about exacerbated knee pain with ambula-

tion, it was determined that a trial of a custom knee brace modified to fit in conjunction with his prosthesis would be the next alternative. He was subsequently casted over the prosthesis to help ensure that the device would contour appropriately and not interfere with its function. By doing this, the brace would provide additional support when combined with the single point cane.

Questions to Consider

- Given the situation with this patient, would further, instrumented, kinetic, and kinematic testing be warranted?
- If so, how would you conduct the testing session and in which specific variables would you look for changes?

Transfemoral Prosthetic Gait

Initial research of transfemoral amputation by the Berkeley group focused upon unilateral amputation because the problems of this group appeared more critical at that time.[124]

Motion analysis showed a fully extended knee starting in TSw and continuing through stance. The inadequate ankle plantar flexion that followed heel strike and threatened knee stability was attributed to dependence on an ankle bumper in place of the lost pretibial muscle control. Active ipsilateral thigh control and postural adaptation by the sound limb and trunk were identified as the variable mechanisms used by the individual with transfemoral amputation to ensure knee extension stability. Rotation of the fully extended limb rolling over the ankle before heel rise causes a maximum rise of the hip (and thus center of gravity), which was interpreted as vaulting. Compensatory actions by the sound limb were identified.

In swing, the inability of the prosthetic foot to generate a propelling force to initiate limb advancement was interpreted as a need to restrict the weight of the prosthesis so that the work of hip flexors would not be excessive. The individual with transfemoral amputation also demonstrated rapid hip extension in TSw to use tibial inertia as a means of completing knee extension in preparation for stance. These findings of excessive knee extension in stance and excessive hip action in swing formed the basis for others to design more sophisticated knee joints to replace the then-dominant single-axis constant friction joint.

The biomechanical response to the problem of residual limb discomfort was twofold. Torque absorbers were designed, but the solution was the combination of improved socket design in addition to more normal joint mechanics. The loss of knee control creates compensatory kinematic and kinetic changes that result in asymmetries reflected in a variety of gait parameters. As the individual wearing transfemoral prosthesis with a compressible heel-type foot levers over the heel rocker during LR, the knee may be at

an increased risk of destabilization. When challenged by the potential for knee instability, the prosthetic wearer will attempt to preposition the hip before LR with a change in body mechanics to shift the GRF to a more anterior position. These typical compensatory patterns can be measured directly through EMG, kinematics, or kinetics or inferred by measuring heel-only load-bearing time through a temporal analysis.

Temporal Values

There are a several temporal values for which individuals with transfemoral amputation differ compared with those without amputation. A retrospective footswitch gait study conducted at the National VA Prosthetics Gait Lab, Long Beach, California, measured the self-selected velocity in 10 individuals with traumatic transfemoral amputation and compared it with the self-selected velocity of individuals without amputation. The individuals with amputation demonstrated a mean stride length of 1.16 meters compared with an average of 1.59 meters for individuals without amputation.[143] Overall timing of the transfemoral prosthetic gait cycle was slower for the individuals with amputation, requiring a mean of 1.25 seconds from IC to subsequent IC compared with 1.08 seconds for individuals without amputation. The mean velocity of the individuals with amputation was 55.8 m/min versus 88.3 m/min for individuals without amputation. James and Oberg[144] found that a longer, slower gait cycle on the prosthetic side combined with a reduced step length on the sound side resulted in a velocity that was only 38% of non-amputee velocity. As profound as these differences are, they are probably still subtle enough to remain unremarkable in a typical clinical environment. Murray[145] measured transfemoral gait with a younger group of individuals with amputation and found similar but slightly more subtle differences between individuals with amputation and those without amputation.

Initial Contact and Loading Response

The initiation of heel contact at the beginning of stance phase in transfemoral gait has been reported to be characteristically delayed on the prosthetic side, which typically demonstrates a longer swing phase.[145] Contemporary hydraulic knee units, particularly those that provide a programmable chip that can establish optimal swing phase timing characteristics, have the potential to overcome this limitation. However, probably because of cost, they do not represent a typical prosthetic. Early gait studies of single-axis prosthetic feet showed that as the prosthetic limb made contact with the ground and began to load, an exaggerated knee extension was seen in the prosthetic limb that continued throughout early stance.[145] This phenomena depends somewhat on knee design. There is little evidence that polycentric knees, such as four- and six-bar linkage knee units, and others that have been designed to be stable with a few degrees of built-in flexion compliance during stance, provide normal kinematics of the knee in stance. Most individuals with transfemoral amputation who use the polycentric designs walk with a nearly extended knee.

The total vertical forces occurring on the prosthetic side are less during the initial double limb support period than on the contralateral side during the terminal double limb support period. It has been theorized that this loading restraint requires costly compensations of the sound limb.[146] Knee instability, which produces these costly compensations, generally results from inappropriate positioning of the knee joint relative to the socket and prosthetic foot. The individual with transfemoral amputation relies on hip extensor strength and the reduced lever arm of the transected femur to stabilize the prosthetic knee by restraining the limb during LR. Profound hip extensor weakness can be catastrophic and preclude functional ambulation. Anterior translation of the prosthetic socket relative to the knee and foot has the effect of shifting the GRF anterior to the knee joint axis, thereby increasing stability. Socket flexion affects knee stability as well. Because efficient use of the gluteus maximus as a hip extensor requires the muscle group to be on stretch, the prosthetist deliberately places the socket in a position of flexion. Five degrees of socket flexion are generally considered clinically optimal in a patient with no contracture at the hip. In cases of hip contracture, the amount of flexion is limited by the length of the femoral remnant.[124]

Stability of the knee joint is unquestionably the most important factor in considering a knee unit. Uncontrolled knee flexion renders an otherwise perfect prosthesis useless. Thiele and colleagues[147] investigated possible neurophysiological reasons for weakness in individuals with transfemoral amputation by recording EMG activity of the quadriceps during gait. His team did not find abnormal recordings and concluded that muscle weakness is caused by biomechanical, rather than neurophysiological, factors. This supports the long-held clinical view that apart from the patient's general muscle tone, residual limb length is a crucial factor because of its effect as a lever arm against the

socket wall and as a result of intact or ablated insertions of the hamstring tendons and their obvious detrimental effect on extensor strength. A slight degree of socket flexion is also a factor affecting stability because socket flexion slightly elongates hip extensors, rendering them more effective. The relative positions of the prosthetic foot, knee, and socket to this line significantly affect stability of the knee when the patient walks. When the ground reaction line passes posterior to the knee center, the knee will collapse unless resisted by another force, usually the hip extensors forcing the femur against the socket wall.

Another potential destabilizing factor is limitation of free plantar flexion at heel contact, which may produce a knee flexion moment in early stance. This is why an articulated prosthetic foot (as opposed to a prosthetic foot, which attains a plantar grade position by means of heel compression) provides increased stability for those with transfemoral amputation. A general clinical guideline on a patient who demonstrates minimal knee stability is that the prosthetic foot should reach foot-flat position (mimicking plantar flexion during LR) as quickly as possible, short of demonstrating a foot slap characteristic. As soon as the foot plantarflexes fully during stance phase, the ground reaction line moves anteriorly from the point of foot-floor contact at the heel to approximately midfoot, enhancing stability at the knee. Because of this, a single or multiaxis foot with a soft plantar flexion bumper is preferred for those with a short transfemoral residual limb, who have limited muscular control for knee stability. At times, the single-axis function can be combined with that of dynamic response, such as with the College Park foot.

Midstance

As the individual using a transfemoral prosthesis moves into MSt, sound side hip elevation and trunk lean toward the affected side provide balance, limit the force on the lateral aspect of the residual limb, and reduce the demands of the residual limb abductors. The transition from braking to propulsive shear on the ipsilateral limb is characteristically delayed and unsteady (Figure 5-20).

When both limbs are intact, the momentum of the contralateral swing limb results in a reduced vertical force at MSt of the stance limb. This is not so, however, for those with dysvascular transfemoral amputation, in which the reduced upward velocity and momentum of the contralateral swing limb does not have the vigor necessary to decrease vertical force of the prosthetic limb during MSt (see Figure 5-20B). Even in those with traumatic amputation, maximum knee flexion of the sound side during swing phase reaches only 51 degrees, approximately 10 degrees less than normal gait.[148]

Stance phase knee flexion of the affected side is significantly reduced throughout stance (see Figure 5-20 C). During PSw, delayed and reduced knee flexion and consequent reduced heel rise on the ipsilateral limb are characteristic of the transfemoral amputee. Except in the case of those fitted with microprocessor stance control knees, it can be

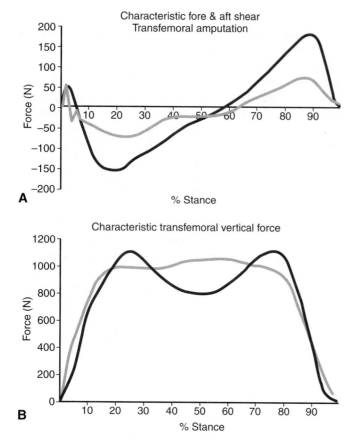

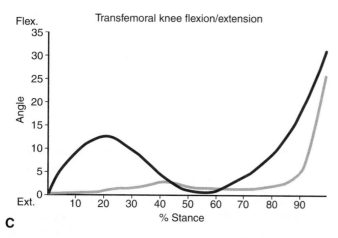

FIGURE 5-20 A, The transition from braking to propulsive shear on the ipsilateral limb during transfemoral prosthetic gait is characteristically delayed and unsteady. **B,** Although there is a reduction in vertical force at midstance (Mst) of the sound limb as the prosthetic limb advances in swing, the prosthetic transfemoral limb demonstrates reduced upward velocity because the momentum of the contralateral swing limb lacks the vigor to lessen the vertical force of the affected stance limb during MSt. **C,** Knee flexion of transfemoral prosthetic limb is reduced throughout stance. During preswing (PSw), delayed and reduced knee flexion and consequent reduced heel rise on the ipsilateral limb is characteristic. (Courtesy of VA Long Beach Gait Laboratory.)

anticipated that many individuals with transfemoral amputation will progress through MSt with a nearly extended knee. Microprocessor-controlled hydraulic knees, particularly the Otto Bock version, have shown a trend toward improvements in stance knee flexion as well as increased velocity in stair descent.[149,150] This is an important development because it may provide increased energy efficiency in gait and avoid compensatory mechanisms such as prepositioning of the femur before LR and MSt.

Terminal Stance

TSt on the prosthetic limb is noted for its premature cessation. The prosthetic side generally shows a decrease in single-limb support time, whereas the sound side shows a concurrent increase in single-limb support time.[148] There is a persistence of knee extension on the prosthetic limb during contralateral sound side deceleration.[151] Delayed and reduced knee flexion, and consequent reduced heel rise on the ipsilateral limb, are characteristic of transfemoral prosthetic gait (see Figure 5-17C). A failure to limit dorsiflexion in a single-axis foot at this juncture will have a destabilizing effect on the prosthetic knee joint during TSt. Without an appropriately placed dorsiflexion stop, nothing will dampen the forward progression of the tibia, and the tibial section may continue its anterior progression to the point of knee collapse.

Preswing

During PSw in transfemoral gait, the vertical force of the sound side is abnormally high and greater than that of the prosthetic side.[146] Abrupt reversal from hip extension to hip flexion occurs because some hip extension is required for knee stability until the moment when the prosthetic knee has to flex to initiate swing. In normal gait, half the knee flexion required for swing phase is obtained passively during PSw.

During prosthetic PSw, inadequate forefoot support can lead to costly compensations in the double limb support period.[146] PSw is characterized by a rapid transfer of body weight to the contralateral limb. In normal gait this transfer begins at 50% of the gait cycle and continues until the end of stance phase (approximately 62% of the gait cycle).

Individuals with transfemoral amputation often have a shortened sound side step length. This may be aggravated by insufficient socket flexion because the individual with transfemoral amputation uses any and all available lumbar lordosis to advance the sound limb. Failure to place the socket in flexion limits the availability of lumbar lordosis and prohibits a sound side step length that is at least somewhat close to normal. Even in an optimal prosthetic gait, typical sound side step length is reduced compared with the prosthetic side or the normal side.

Swing Phase

Gait characteristics during swing phase when wearing a transfemoral prosthesis can be profoundly influenced by prosthetic alignment and design variations. The most challenging factor in achieving a functional swing phase is the lack of active dorsiflexion in most prosthetic designs. The Stewart-Vicars knee developed in 1947 and the more recent Hydracadence knee couple knee flexion with ankle dorsiflexion. However, this design concept has been largely ignored in recent years. With the prosthetic incorporation of active dorsiflexion in early swing, many costly postural substitutions, including vaulting and abducted or circumducted gait, could be minimized.

The swing velocity of the prosthetic limb is often slower than that of the sound limb.[144] The presence or lack of fluid control mechanisms variations in alignment stability, extension assist, and joint friction alignment mechanisms can all influence swing phase timing. During MSw, the individual with transfemoral amputation demonstrates exaggerated hip elevation of the prosthetic side to enable swing clearance. In TSw, prosthetic swing time is much greater than sound limb swing time or normal swing time.[151] Excessive prosthetic swing flexion is one of the commonly reported transfemoral prosthetic gait deviations.[151] Zuniga,[148] however, reports that prosthetic knee flexion reaches a mean of only 45 degrees. This contradiction in results can easily be attributed to the wide variety of prosthetic dampening and extension assist designs as well as other variations in prosthetic adjustment.

James and colleagues[144] and Murray[151] performed gait laboratory investigations of transfemoral stride parameters and their relation to knee flexion/extension angles at various cadences. They confirmed stance and swing phase asymmetry between the prosthetic and sound side, regardless of the speed of walking. Zuniga[148] used electrogoniometers attached to the knee and foot to document asymmetry during stance and swing phases, comparing prosthetic and sound limbs. A lack of symmetrical cadence response on the prosthetic side is seen as partially responsible. Most prosthetic designs permit only one walking speed. No matter how fast the patient walks, the prosthetic wearer must wait for the leg to return from the normal 65 degrees of swing phase flexion to full extension before safely loading the prosthesis for weight bearing in stance.

Common Gait Deviations in Transfemoral Prosthetic Gait

Our understanding of transfemoral prosthetic gait deviations and the dynamic alignment process has evolved over many decades. The important early work of Inman,[6] described previously, served as a basis for subsequent development. In 1951, New York University published a method for observing amputee gait and described eight commonly seen gait deviations.[152] Years later, Hangar and associates[14] at Northwestern University, under a grant from the Veterans Administration, developed an educational film that incorporated the eight deviations defined by NYU and expanded upon these. A brief description of each of these transfemoral gait deviations is given in Table 5-2.[13]

TABLE 5-2 *Common Deviations in Transfemoral Prosthetic Gait*

Deviation	Description
Foot slap	Rapid, uncosmetic plantar flexion movement at heel contact. Most commonly caused by insufficient plantar flexion resistance.
Knee instability	Uncontrollable knee flexion at LR. May be caused by anteriorly placed knee unit, excessive durometer of cushion heel or plantar flexion bumper, or weakness of hip extensors.
Delayed progression	Hesitation or delay in rollover of prosthetic forefoot between MSt and TSt. May be the result of a long toe lever, a plantarflexed prosthetic foot, or shoes with low heel.
Unequal step length	Sound side step length is visibly shorter than the prosthetic step length. May be caused by inadequate preflexion of socket, hip flexion contracture. Associated with excessive lumbar lordosis and low back pain.
External rotation	Foot externally rotates at heel contact. May be caused by excessively firm heel cushion or a tight prosthetic socket (especially on a residual limb with extra soft tissue).
Lateral trunk bend	Significant leaning of the body over the hip during prosthetic MSt. Often caused by excessively outset prosthetic foot, distal lateral femoral discomfort, short prosthesis, excessively abducted socket, or gluteus medius weakness.
Abducted gait	Wide walking base throughout the gait cycle, often caused by pressure or discomfort on medial pubic ramus, small socket, or excessively long prosthesis.
Pelvic elevation	"Hip hiking" on prosthetic side from ISw to MSw, associated with increased energy cost of gait. Often caused by long prosthesis or inadequate knee flexion as swing begins.
Knee hyperextension	Seen at MSt to compensate for perceived knee instability. Often caused by short forefoot lever or dorsiflexed prosthetic foot.
Lateral whip	The heel of the prosthetic foot moves in a lateral arc as swing begins, often caused by excessive internal rotation of the knee bolt.
Medial whip	The heel of the prosthetic foot moves in a medial arch as swing begins, often from excessive external rotation of the knee bolt or improper donning of prosthesis.

(Continued)

TABLE 5-2   *Common Deviations in Transfemoral Prosthetic Gait—cont'd*

Deviation	Description
Excessive heel rise	Prosthetic foot rises abnormally upward during ISw, typically a result of inadequate resistance to knee flexion.
Inadequate heel rise	Heel-off is diminished in ISw, usually because of excessive knee flexion resistance.
Circumduction	A wide lateral arch of the prosthetic limb during swing phase. Often the result of inadequate knee flexion, excessive medial brim pressure, or long prosthesis.
Pistoning	A sense that residual limb slips slightly out of the socket in swing and descends into the socket in stance. Often the result of inadequate fit or suspension.
Vaulting	Rising up on the sound forefoot during MSt in an effort to enhance prosthetic swing limb clearance. May result from a long prosthesis, excessive knee friction, or fear of letting the knee flex.
TSw impact	An audible click at the end of TSw as knee unit fully extends with insufficient resistance or by forceful knee extension by the prosthetic wearer.
Reduced velocity	An adaptation typically observed during initial training or with new components, often related to pain, fear, or insecurity.

ISw, initial swing; LR, loading response; Mst, midstance; MSw, midswing; Tst, terminal stance.

CASE EXAMPLE 6

A Patient with a Hemipelvectomy Amputation

L. is a 38-year-old woman with a right hemipelvectomy amputation secondary to osteosarcoma. She has been referred to the gait laboratory for evaluation as a possible candidate for a microprocessor controlled knee unit. For the past several years she has been ambulatory without the use of assistive devices.

Questions to Consider

- Considering L.'s level of amputation what types of difficulties or deviations might you expect during the course of level over ground ambulation?
- What quantitative measures would serve as indicators of the likely gait deviations?

Examination and Evaluation

L. was fitted with reflective markers and underwent three-dimensional kinetic and kinematic testing. This testing was performed at her self-selected walking speed and she was given a suitable amount of time to become acclimated to the testing environment before data collection. Observational assessment indicates a significant amount of vaulting and excessive pelvic movement, but no indication of circumduction.

The temporal data shows that she walks at a rate of 92 steps per minute and a velocity of 0.96 m/sec. Along with this, her step length on the left side is 0.58 m, while the right side is 0.70 m, even though the total stride length for both sides is 1.24 m. Similarly, the total stride time for both sides was 1.3 seconds; however, the single limb support time was 0.55 seconds on the left side and 0.41 seconds on the right. The step time for the left was 0.59 seconds, while the right was 0.71 seconds. Similarly, toe-off occurred at 68.8% of the gait cycle on the left side, while it occurred at 57.9% on the right.

Kinematic data at the ankle showed a consistent pattern of abnormal plantar-flexion on the left side occurring from approximately 14% of the gait cycle through 60% of the gait cycle. Overall knee flexion on the left side was within the overall expected range, as was hip flexion in swing. The right side knee flexion showed approximately 5 degrees of knee flexion during loading response and a peak average knee flexion of 53 degrees. Exaggerated anterior-posterior pelvic tilt was also documented (Figure 5-21).

Kinetically, the left side consistently showed greater anterior/posterior shear forces compared to the contralateral side, usually twice as much force exerted on the left compared to the right. Along with this there was no clear twin peak maximum in the vertical component of the ground reaction force. Instead, there were multiple maxima over the course of a single stance phase (Figure 5-22).

Questions to Consider

- Based on what is presented here, what possible advantages could a microprocessor controlled knee unit have over a conventional mechanical unit? When considering this bear in mind that the specific microprocessor knee unit she is being evaluated for is designed to allow for adjustments in both flexion and extension resistance based upon the individuals walking velocity.
- What kinematic, kinetic, and temporal changes could you expect to see with a change in knee unit?
- Considering that the potential improvements are not absolute, do the potential benefits warrant the issuance of the device?

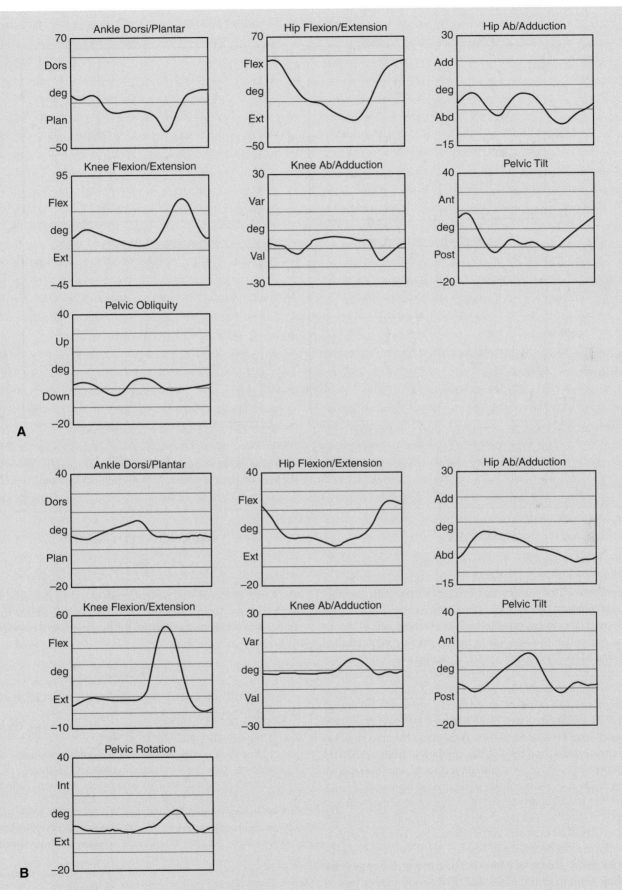

FIGURE 5-21 A patient with right hemipelvectomy amputation: average motion data results for the left (**A**) and right side (**B**). Particularly note the ankle motion on the left side indicating the vaulting pattern.

Continued

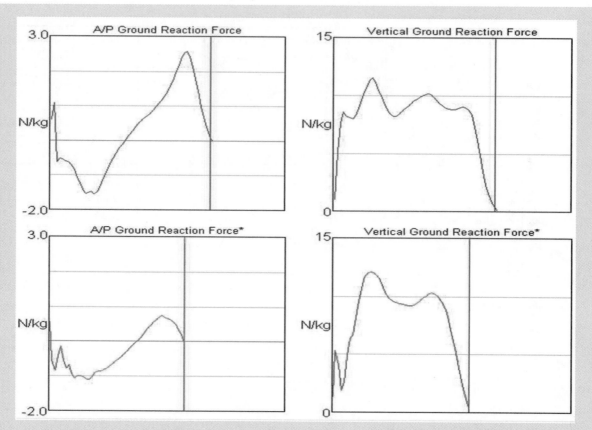

FIGURE 5-22 A patient with right hemipelvectomy amputation: vertical and anterior-posterior ground reaction force data for the left side (**A**) and right side (**B**). Note the difference in the vertical force patterns, especially the lack of two well-defined force peaks on the left side and the difference in magnitudes between the two peak force values on the left.

SUMMARY

The examples of gait deficiencies typical of neuromuscular conditions and in prosthetic gait that we have considered demonstrate the complexity and variety that challenge orthotists, prosthetists, and physical therapists working with individuals with gait problems. Each patient presents unique combinations of pathological and compensatory deficits that require a combination of the essential tools of simple quantitative measure (cadence and velocity, step length, stride length and width, and double support time), systematic qualitative gait analysis (Rancho Los Amigos observational gait assessment protocol), measures of energy cost (PCI), level of assistance (the FAC or FIM), and functional measures (the TUG or GAR-M). These tools help the clinician differentiate primary pathological conditions from secondary compensations, guide orthotic prescription and therapeutic intervention, and assess efficacy of treatment. Instrumented gait assessment is an important part of preoperative assessment and research in orthotic and prosthetic design. In addition, the data collected in gait laboratories are building a database that can provide information necessary to build accurate outcome estimations for many groups of patients. The current challenge is for the clinic team to gain the broadest possible knowledge base in analytical gait assessment and to serve the patient as a team, considering each patient as an individual.

ACKNOWLEDGMENTS

The authors are grateful to Sue Rouleau, PT, and the Physical Therapy Department of Rancho Los Amigos Medical Center for assistance in identifying patient models and to Jacquelin Perry, MD, and Los Amigos Research and Education Institute for permission to duplicate the Rancho full-body gait analysis form.

REFERENCES

1. Shastri JL, ed. *Hymns of the Rig Veda* [Griffith RTH, Trans.]. Varanasi, India: Motilal Banarsidas; 1976:72–80.
2. McMahon TA. *Muscles, Reflexes, and Locomotion.* Princeton, NJ: Princeton University Press; 1984.
3. Finley FR, Cody K, Finizie R. Locomotive patterns in elderly women. *Arch Phys Med Rehabil.* 1969;50(3):140–146.
4. Perry J, Burnfield JM. *Gait Analysis: Normal and Pathological Function.* 2nd ed. Thorofare, NJ: Slack Inc; 2010.
5. Saunders JB, Inman VT, Eberhart HD. The major determinants in normal and pathological gait. *J Bone Joint Surg.* 1953;35A:543–558.
6. Inman V, Ralston HJ, Todd F. *Human Walking.* Baltimore: Williams & Wilkins; 1981.
7. Pathokinesiology Service and Physical Therapy Department. *Observational Gait Analysis.* 4th ed. Downey, CA: Los Amigos Research and Education Institute, Rancho Los Amigos National Rehabilitation Center; 2002.

8. Perry J. Normal and pathological gait. In: Hsu JD, Michael JW, Fisk JR, eds. *AAOS Atlas of Orthoses and Assistive Devices*. 4th ed. Philadelphia: Mosby; 2008:71–80.

9. Epler M. Gait. In: Richardson JK, Iglarsh ZA, eds. *Clinical Orthopaedic Physical Therapy*. Philadelphia: WB Saunders; 1991.

10. Winter DA. Energy generation and absorption at the ankle and knee during fast, natural, and slow cadences. *Clin Ortop*. 1983;174:147–154.

11. Robinson GW. A study of gaits. *J Kans Med Soc*. 1925;25(12): 402–406.

12. Boorstein SW. Abnormal gaits as a guide in diagnosis. *Hebrew Physician*. 1937;1(1):221–227.

13. Northwestern University Prosthetic Orthotic Center. *Gait analysis instructional film*. Chicago: Northwestern University; 1960. (Handbook published by Ideal Picture Co, Chicago).

14. Hangar HB. Personal communication. July 1994.

15. Brunnstrom S. *Movement Therapy in Hemiplegia: Neurophysiological Approach*. New York: Harper & Row; 1970.

16. Perry J. The mechanics of walking: a clinical interpretation. *Phys Ther*. 1967;47(9):777–801.

17. Los Amigos Research and Education Institute. *Observational Gait Analysis*. Downey CA: Los Amigos Research and Education; 2001.

18. Marks AA. *Manual of Artificial Limbs*. New York: AA Marks; 1905.

19. Braun M. *Picturing Time, Work of Etienne-Jules Marey, 1830-1904*. Chicago: University of Chicago Press; 1995.

20. Muybridge E. *Muybridge's Complete Human and Animal Locomotion*. New York: Dover; 1887.

21. Sutherland DH. *Historical perspective of gait analysis (lecture handouts for instructional course)*. Interpretation of Gait Analysis Data. San Diego: Children's Hospital and Health Center; 1994:1–2.

22. Ayyappa E. Gait lab technology: measuring the steps of progress. *Orthot Prosthet Almanac*. 1996;45(2):28–56.

23. Cutlip RG, Mancinelli C, Huber F, et al. Evaluation of an instrumented walkway for measurement of the kinematic parameters of gait. *Gait Posture*. 2000;12(2):134–138.

24. Bilney B, Morris M, Webster K. Concurrent related validity of the GAITRite walkway system for quantification of the spatial and temporal parameters of gait. *Gait Posture*. 2003;17(1):68–74.

25. Wening J, Huskey M, Hasso D, et al. The effect of an ankle-foot orthosis on gait parameters of acute and chronic hemiplegic subjects. AAOP Academy Annual Meeting, Thranhardt Lecture Series Presentation; 2008.

26. Ayyappa E, Craig D, Christensen E, et al. Infusing cutting edge technology into everyday prosthetic and orthotic clinical care. *J Prosthet Orthot*. 2010;22:2–10.

27. Waters RL. Energy expenditure. In: Perry J, ed. *Gait Analysis*. Thorofare, NJ: Slack; 1992:443–489.

28. Torburn L, Perry J, Ayyappa E, et al. Below-knee amputee gait with dynamic elastic response prosthetic feet: a pilot study. *J Rehabil Res Dev*. 1990;27(4):369–384.

29. Houdijk H, Pollman E, Groenewold M, et al. The energy cost for the step-to-step transition in amputee walking. *Gait Posture*. 2009;30:35–40.

30. Schmalz T, Blumentritt S, Jarasch R. Energy expenditure and biomechanical characteristics of lower limb amputee gait: the influence of prosthetic alignment and different prosthetic components. *Gait Posture*. 2002;16:255–263.

31. Winchester PK, Carollo JJ, Parekh RN, et al. A comparison of paraplegic gait performance using two types of reciprocating gait orthoses. *Prosthet Orthot Int*. 1993;17(2):101–106.

32. Kawamura CM, Filho MC, Brreto MM, et al. Comparison between visual and three-dimensional gait analysis in patients with spastic diplegic cerebral palsy. *Gait Posture*. 2007;25:18–24.

33. Kauffman KR, Levine JA, Brey RH, et al. Gait and balance of transfemoral amputees using passive mechanical and microprocessor controlled knees. *Gait Posture*. 2007;26:489–493.

34. McKelvey MW. *Reliability and validity of a golf swing analysis software during a static and a dynamic task*. Proquest Dissertations and Theses, 2007.

35. Raghavan P, Li E. *Mount Sinai School of Medicine's Rehabilitation Department Uses Dartfish in Clinical Laboratory*. Dartfish Case Study. Available at: http://www.dartfish.com/floor/download.cgi?file=/data/document/document/1101.pdf&name; 2009 Accessed 11.12.10.

36. Winter DA. *Biomechanics and motor control of human movement*. Hoboken, NJ: John Wiley & Sons; 2009.

37. Ruhe BL, Gard SA. Effect of prosthetic foot/ankle alignment on balance efficiency while standing on sloped Surfaces in persons with transfemoral amputations. In: *Proceedings of The 35th Annual Meeting and Scientific Symposium of the American Academy of Orthotists and Prosthetists*. Atlanta, GA; 2009.

38. Cavanaugh PR, Ulbrecht JS, Caputo GM, et al. Gait analysis and diabetic footwear prescriptions: is there a marriage on the horizon? *Biomechanics Magazine Annual Desk Reference*. 1996.

39. Biswas A, Lemaire ED, Kofman J. Dynamic gait stability index based on plantar pressures and fuzzy logic. *J Biomech*. 2008;41:1574–1581.

40. Mohamed O, Cerny K, Jones W, et al. The effect of terrain on foot pressures during walking. *Ankle Foot Int*. 2005;26:859–869.

41. Burnfield J, Few CD, Mohamed O, et al. The influence of walking speed and footwear on plantar pressures in older adults. *Clin Biomech (Bristol, Avon)*. 2004;(19):78–84.

42. Holden MK, Maureen K, Gill KM, et al. Gait assessment for neurologically impaired patients; standards for outcome assessment. *Phys Ther*. 1986;66(10):1530–1539.

43. Brandstater M, deBruin H, Gowland C. Hemiplegic gait: analysis of temporal values. *Arch Phys Med Rehabil*. 1983;64(12):583–587.

44. Wall JC, Ashburn A. Assessment of gait disabilities in hemiplegics: hemiplegic gait. *Scand J Rehabil Med*. 1979;11(3):95–103.

45. Olney SJ, Richards C. Hemiparetic gait following stroke. Part 1: characteristics. *Gait Posture*. 1996;4(1):136–148.

46. Corcoran PJ, Jebsen RH, Brengelmann GL. Effects of plastic and metal leg braces on the speed and energy cost of hemiparetic ambulation. *Arch Phys Med Rehabil*. 1970;51(2):69–77.

47. Lehmann JF, Condon SM, Price R, et al. Gait abnormalities in hemiplegia: their correction by ankle-foot orthoses. *Arch Phys Med Rehabil*. 1987;68(11):763–771.

48. Lee K, Johnston R. Effect of below-knee bracing on knee movement: biomechanical analysis. *Arch Phys Med Rehabil*. 1974;55(4):179–182.

49. Mattsson E. Energy cost of level walking. *Scand J Rehabil Med Suppl*. 1989;23:1–48.

50. Waters RL, Lunsford BR, Perry J, et al. Energy-speed relationship of walking: standard tables. *J Orthop Res*. 1988;6(2):215–222.

51. van Iersel MB, Hoefsloot W, Munneke M, et al. Systematic review of quantitative clinical gait analysis in patients with dementia. *Z Gerontol Geriatr*. 2004;37(1):27–32.

52. Perry J, Garrett M, Gronley JK, et al. Classification of walking handicap in the stroke population. *Stroke.* 1995;26(6):982–989.

53. Montero-Odasso M, Schapira M, et al. Gait velocity as a single predictor of adverse events in healthy seniors aged 75 years and older. *J Gerontol A Biol Sci Med Sci.* 2005;60(10):1304–1309.

54. Studenski S, Perera S, Wallace D, et al. Physical performance measures in the clinical setting. *J Am Geriatr Soc.* 2003;51:314–322.

55. Rabadi MH, Blau A. Admission ambulation velocity predicts length of stay and discharge disposition following stroke in an acute rehabilitation hospital. *Neurorehabil Neural Repair.* 2005;19(1):20–26.

56. Salbach NM, Mayo NE, et al. Responsiveness and predictability of gait speed and other disability measures in acute stroke. *Arch Phys Med Rehabil.* 2001;82(9):1204–1212.

57. Hardy SE, Perera S, et al. Improvement in usual gait speed predicts better survival in older adults. *J Am Geriatr Soc.* 2007;55(11):1727–1734.

58. NIH Toolbox. *Assessment of Neurological and Behavioral Function.* http://neuroscienceblueprint.nih.gov/NIH_Toolbox.htm; 2010 Accessed 20.03.11.

59. Fritz S, Lusardi M. White paper: walking speed the sixth vital sign. *J Geriatr Phys Ther.* 2009;32(2):2–5.

60. Waters RL, Hilsop HJ, Perry J, et al. Energetics: application of the study and management of locomotor disabilities. *Orthop Clin North Am.* 1978;9:351.

61. Holden MK, Gill KM, Magliozzi MR. Clinical gait assessment in the neurologically impaired: reliability and meaningfulness. *Phys Ther.* 1984;64(1):35–40.

62. Nilsson L. Walking training of patients with hemiparesis at an early stage after stroke: a comparison of walking training on a treadmill with body weight support and walking training on the ground. *Clin Rehabil.* 2001;15(5):515–527.

63. Sanchez-Blanco I. Predictive model of functional independence in stroke patients admitted to a rehabilitation program. *Clin Rehabil.* 1999;13(6):464–475.

64. Stevenson TJ. Using impairment inventory scores to determine ambulation status in individuals with stroke. *Physiother Can.* 1999;51(3):168–174.

65. Brock KA. Evaluating the effectiveness of stroke rehabilitation: choosing a discriminative measure. *Arch Phys Med Rehabil.* 2002;83(1):92–99.

66. Simondson J, Goldie P, Greenwood KM. The mobility scale for acute stroke patients: concurrent validity. *Clin Rehabil.* 2003;17(5):558–563.

67. Roth EJ. The time logger communicator gait monitor: recording temporal gait parameters using a portable computerized device. *Int Disabil Stud.* 1990;12(1):10–16.

68. Functional Independence Measure. Uniform Data System for Medical Rehabilitation. Buffalo, NY: Research Foundation of SUNY; 1990.

69. Mendelsohn ME. Specificity of functional mobility measures in older adults after hip fracture: a pilot study. *Am J Phys Med Rehabil.* 2003;82(10):766–774.

70. Hannan EL. Mortality and locomotion 6 months after hospitalization for hip fracture: risk factors and risk-adjusted hospital outcomes. *JAMA.* 2001;285(21):2736–2742, 2793–2794.

71. Stratford PW. Validation of the LEFS on patients with total joint arthroplasty. *Physiother Can.* 2000;52(2):97–105.

72. Bahlberg A. Functional independence in persons with spinal cord injury in Helsinki. *J Rehabil Med.* 2003;35(5):217–220.

73. Grey N. The Functional Independence Measure: a comparative study of clinician and self-ratings. *Paraplegia.* 1993;31(7):457–461.

74. MiKinley WO. Rehabilitation outcomes of individuals with nontraumatic myelopathy resulting from spinal stenosis. *J Spinal Cord Med.* 1998;21(2):131–136.

75. Hamilton BB. Disability outcomes following inpatient rehabilitation for stroke. *Phys Ther.* 1994;74(5):494–503.

76. Ziviani J. Concurrent validity of the Functional Independence Measure for children (WeeFIM) and the Pediatric Evaluation of Disability Inventory in children with developmental disabilities and acquired brain injury. *J Phys Occup Ther Pediatr.* 2001;21(2/3):91–101.

77. Azuali M. Measuring functional status and family support in older school aged children with cerebral palsy: comparison of three instruments. *Arch Phys Med Rehabil.* 2000;81(3):307–311.

78. Ottenbacher KJ. Interrater agreement and stability of the Functional Independence Measure for Children (WeeFIM): use in children with developmental disabilities. *Arch Phys Med Rehabil.* 1997;78(12):1309–1315.

79. Ottenbacher KJ. The stability and equivalence reliability of the functional independence measure for children. *Dev Med Child Neurol.* 1996;38(10):907–916.

80. Bohannon RW. Scoring transfer and locomotion independence of home care patients: Barthel Index versus Functional Independence Measure. *Int J Rehabil Res.* 1999;22(1):65–66.

81. Pollack N. Reliability and validity of the FIM for persons aged 80 and above from a multilevel continuing care retirement community. *Arch Phys Med Rehabil.* 1996;77(10):1056–1061.

82. Granger CV. Performance profiles of the functional independence measure. *Am J Phys Med Rehabil.* 1993;72(2):84–89.

83. Daving Y. Reliability of an interview approach to the Functional Independence Measure. *Clin Rehabil.* 2001;15(3):301–310.

84. Wolfson L, Whipple R, Amerman R, et al. Gait assessment in the elderly: a gait abnormality rating scale and its relation to falls. *J Gerontol.* 1990;45(1):M12–M19.

85. VanSwearingen JM, Paschal KA, Bonino P, et al. The modified gait abnormalities rating scale and recognizing recurrent fall risk of community-dwelling frail older veterans. *Phys Ther.* 1996;76(9):994–1002.

86. Huang WN, VanSwearingen JM, Brach JS. Gait variability in older adults: observational rating validated by comparison with a computerized walkway gold standard. *Phys Ther.* 2008;88(10):1146–1153.

87. VanSwearingen JM, Paschal KA, Bonino P, et al. Assessing recurrent fall risk of community dwelling frail veterans using specific tests of mobility and the Physical Performance Test of Function. *J Gerontol.* 1998;53:M457–M464.

88. Mathias S, Nayak US, Isaacs B. Balance in elderly patients: the "timed get-up and go" test. *Arch Phys Med Rehabil.* 1986;6(67):387–389.

89. Posdiadlo D, Richardson S. The "timed up and go"; a test of functional mobility for frail elderly persons. *J Am Geriatr Soc.* 2000;48(1):104–105.

90. Steffen TM, Hacker TA, Mollinger L. Age- and gender-related test performance in community dwelling elderly people: six minute walk test, Berg Balance Scale, Timed up and Go, and gait speed. *Phys Ther.* 2002;82(2):128–137.

91. Biscoff HA. Identifying a cut-of point of normal mobility; a comparison of the timed up and go testing in community dwelling and institutionalized elderly women. *Age Ageing.* 2003;32(3):315–320.

92. Vereeck L, Wuyts F, Truijen S, et al. Clinical assessment of balance: normative data, and gender and age effects. *Int J Audiol.* 2008;47(2):67–75.

93. Pondal M, del Ser T. Normative data and determinants for the Timed "Up and Go" Test in a population-based sample of elderly individuals without gait disturbances. *J Geriatr Phys Ther.* 2008;31:57–63.

94. Bohannon RW. Reference values for the Timed Up and Go Test: a descriptive meta-analysis. *J Geriatr Phys Ther.* 2006;29(2):64–68.

95. Marchetti GF, Whitney SL, Blatt PJ, et al. Temporal and spatial characteristics of gait during performance of the dynamic gait index in people with and people without balance or vestibular disorders. *Phys Ther.* 2008;88:640–651.

96. Thomas SG. Physical activity and its relationship to physical performance in patients with end stage knee osteoarthritis. *J Orthop Sports Phys Ther.* 2003;33(12):745–754.

97. Thompson M. Performance of community dwelling elderly on the timed up and go test. *Phys Occup Ther Geriatr.* 1995;13(3):17–30.

98. Medley A. The effect of assistive devices on the performance of community dwelling elderly on the time up and go test. *Issues Aging.* 1997;20(1):3–7.

99. Matjacic Z. Dynamic balance training during standing in people with transtibial amputation; a pilot study. *Prosthet Orthot Int.* 2003;27(3):214–220.

100. Schoppen T. Physical, mental, and social predictors of functional outcome in unilateral lower limb amputees. *Arch Phys Med Rehabil.* 2003;84(6):803–811.

101. Ingemarsson AH. Walking ability and activity level after hip fracture in the elderly—a follow-up. *J Rehabil Med.* 2003;35(2):76–83.

102. Crotty M. Patient and caregiver outcomes 12 months after home-based therapy for hip fracture: a randomized controlled trial. *Arch Phys Med Rehabil.* 2003;84(8):1237–1239.

103. Campbell CM. The effect of cognitive demand on timed up and go performance in older adults with and without Parkinson disease. *Neurol Rep.* 2003;27(1):2–7.

104. Morris S, Morris ME. Reliability of measurements obtained with the timed up and go test in people with Parkinson disease. *Phys Ther.* 2001;81(2):810–818.

105. Shumway-Cook A, Baldwin M, Polissar N, et al. Predicting the probability for falls in community-dwelling older adults. *Phys Ther.* 1997;77:812–819.

106. McConvey J, Bennett SE. Reliability of the Dynamic Gait Index in individuals with multiple sclerosis. *Arch Phys Med Rehabil.* 2005;86:130–133.

107. Hall CD, Schubert MC, Herdman SJ. Prediction of fall risk reduction as measured by Dynamic Gait Index in individuals with unilateral vestibular hypofunction. *Otol Neurotol.* 2004;25:746–751.

108. Whitney S, Wrisley D, Furman J. Concurrent validity of the Berg Balance Scale and the Dynamic Gait Index in people with vestibular dysfunction. *Physiother Res Int.* 2003;8:178–186.

109. Wrisley DM, Marchetti GF, Kuharsky DK, et al. Reliability, internal consistency, and validity of data obtained with the functional gait assessment. *Phys Ther.* 2004;84:906–918.

110. Von Schroeder HP, Coutts RD, Lyden PD, et al. Gait parameters following stroke: a practical assessment. *J Rehabil Res Dev.* 1995;32(1):25–31.

111. Burdett RG, Borello-France D, Blatchly C, et al. Gait comparison of subjects with hemiplegia walking unbraced, with ankle foot orthosis, and with air-stirrup brace. *Phys Ther.* 1988;68(8):1197–1203.

112. Wade DT, Wood VA, Helleer A, et al. Walking after stroke: measurement and recovery over the first 3 months. *Scand J Rehabil Med.* 1987;19(1):25–30.

113. Ashworth B. Preliminary trial of carisoprodol in multiple sclerosis. *Practitioner.* 1964;192(4):540–542.

114. Lehmann JF, Warren CG, Hertling D, et al. Craig-Scott orthosis: a biomechanical and functional evaluation. *Arch Phys Med Rehabil.* 1976;57(9):438–442.

115. Hirschberg GG, Nathanson K. Electromyographic recording of muscular activity in normal and spastic gaits. *Arch Phys Med Rehabil.* 1952;33(4):217–225.

116. Perry J. Lower extremity bracing in hemiplegia. *Clin Orthop.* 1969;63(4):32–38.

117. Bobath K. The facilitation of normal postural reactions and movements in the treatment of cerebral palsy. *Physiotherapy.* 1964;30(1):246–262.

118. Gage JR. *Gait Analysis in Cerebral Palsy.* New York: Cambridge University Press; 1991.

119. Ounpuu S, Muik E, Davis RB, et al. Rectus femoris surgery in children with cerebral palsy. Part 1: the effect of rectus femoris transfer location on knee motion. *J Pediatr Orthop.* 1993;13(3):325–330.

120. Rodda J, Graham HK. Classification of gait patterns in spastic hemiplegia and spastic diplegia: a basis for a management algorithm. *Eur J Neurol.* 2001;8(5):98–108.

121. Sutherland DH. Common gait abnormalities of the knee in cerebral palsy. *Clin Ortop.* 1993;(288):139–147.

122. Knutsson E, Richards C. Different types of disturbed motor control in gait of hemiparetic patients. *Brain.* 1979;102(2):405–430.

123. Mazur JM, Sienko-Thomas S, Wright N, et al. Swing-through versus reciprocating gait patterns in patients with thoracic-level spina bifida. *Z Kinderchir.* 1990;1(12):23–25.

124. Radcliffe CW. Functional considerations in the fitting of Trans-Femoral prostheses. In: *Selected Articles from Artificial Limbs.* Huntington, NY: Krieger Publishing; 1970:5–30.

125. Eberhart H, Elfman H, Inman V. The locomotor mechanism of the amputee. In: Klopsteg P, Wilson P, eds. *Human Limbs and Their Substitutes.* New York: Hafner; 1968:472–480.

126. Wilson AB. Recent advances in artificial limbs. *Artif Limbs.* 1969;13(2):1–12.

127. Radcliffe CW, Foort J. *The Patellar Tendon Bearing Below Knee Prosthesis.* Berkeley, CA: University of California Biomechanics Laboratory; 1961.

128. Wilson AB. The prosthetic and orthotic program. *Artif Limbs.* 1970;14(2):1–8.

129. Ayyappa E. *Prosthetics Desk Reference: Physiatry Prosthetic Program Manual.* Irvine, CA: University California; 2004.

130. Foort J. The patellar tendon bearing prosthesis for below-knee amputees: a critical review of technique and criteria. In: *Committee on Prosthetic Research and Development, Selected articles from Artificial Limbs (1/54-2/66).* Huntington, NY: Krieger; 1970:353–362.

131. Hannah RE, Morrison JB. Prostheses alignment: effect on gait of persons with below-knee amputation. *Arch Phys Med Rehabil.* 1984;65(4):159–162.

132. Zahedi MS, Spence WD, Solomonidis SE, et al. Alignment of lower-limb prostheses. *J Rehabil Res Dev.* 1986;23(2):2–19.

133. Goh JCH, Solomonidis SE, Spence WD, et al. Biomechanical evaluation of SACH and uniaxial feet. *Prosthet Orthot Int.* 1984;8(3):147–154.

134. Doane NE, Holt LE. A comparison of the SACH and single axis foot in the gait of unilateral below-knee amputees. *Prosthet Orthot Int.* 1983;7:33–36.

135. Culham EG, Peat M, Nowell E. Below-knee amputation: A comparison of the effects of the SACH foot and the single axis foot on electromyographic patterns during locomotion. *Prosthet Orthot Int.* 1986;10(1):15–22.

136. Burgess EM, Hittenberger DA, Forsgren SM, et al. The Seattle prosthetic foot—a design for active sports: preliminary studies. *Orthot Prosthet.* 1983;37(1):25–31.

137. Waters RL, Antonelli D, Hislop H. Energy cost of walking of amputees: the influence of level of amputation. *J Bone Joint Surg.* 1976;58(1):42–46.

138. Wagner EM, Sienko S, Supan T, et al. Motion analysis of SACH vs. Flexfoot in moderately active below-knee amputees. *Clin Prosthet Orthot.* 1987;11:55–62.

139. Torburn L, Perry J, Ayyappa E. Below knee amputee gait with dynamic elastic response prosthetic feet: a pilot study. *J Rehabil Res Dev.* 1990;27(4):369–384.

140. Barth D, Schumacher L, Sienko TS. Gait analysis and energy cost of below-knee amputees wearing six different prosthetic feet. *J Prosthet Orthot.* 1992;4(2):63–75.

141. Gitter A, Czerniecki JM, DeGroot DM. Biomechanical analysis of the influence of prosthetic feet on below-knee amputee walking. *Am J Phys Med Rehabil.* 1990;70:142–148.

142. Powers CM, Torburn L, Perry J, et al. Influence of prosthetic foot design on sound limb loading in adults with uni-lateral below-knee amputations. *Arch Phys Med Rehabil.* 1994;75:825–829.

143. Farivar S, Ayyappa E. Time-distance parameters of trans-femoral amputees. *Proceedings of the 23rd Annual Meeting and Scientific Symposium, American Academy of Orthotists and Prosthetists.* 1996 Orlando.

144. James U, Oberg K. Prosthetic gait patterns in unilateral above-knee amputees. *Scand J Rehabil Med.* 1973;5(1):35–50.

145. Murray MP, Mollinger LA, Sepic SB, et al. Gait patterns in above-knee amputee patients: hydraulic swing control vs. constant-friction knee components. *Arch Phys Med Rehabil.* 1983;64(8):339–345.

146. Suzuki K. Force plate study on artificial limb gait. *J Jap Orthop Assoc.* 1972;46:503–516.

147. Thiele B, James U, Stalberg E. Neurophysiological studies on muscle function in the stump of transfemoral amputees. *Scand J Rehabil Med.* 1983;l5:67–70.

148. Zuniga EN, Leavitt LA, Calvert JC, et al. Gait patterns in trans-femoral amputees. *Arch Phys Med Rehabil.* 1972;53:373–382.

149. Ayyappa E. *Gait and Limb Technology: Microprocessor Knees, Capabilities.* vol. II, no 2. Chicago: Northwestern University; 2002.

150. Kaufman K. Instrumented Comparison Between Mauch SNS Hydraulic Knee and the Otto Bock C-Leg. In: *Proceedings of 4th Annual National VA Conference on Prosthetic & Orthotic Rehabilitation.* Long Beach, CA; 2004.

151. Murray MP, Sepic SB, Gardner GM, et al. Gait patterns of Trans-Femoral amputees using constant-friction knee components. *Bull Prosthet Res.* 1980;13(2):35–45.

152. *Evaluation of Gait of Unilateral AK Individuals with Amputation.* New York: NYU College of Engineering; 1951.

6

Materials and Technology

Géza F. Kogler

LEARNING OBJECTIVES

On completion of this chapter, the reader will be able to:

1. Compare and contrast the materials most often used in current orthoses and prostheses.
2. Describe how the basic mechanical properties of commonly used materials determine how they will be used in orthotic and prosthetic devices.
3. Describe the process of, and measures used in, the formulation of a biomechanically appropriate orthotic or prosthetic prescription that will address a patient's functional deficits.
4. Describe how a prosthetist or orthotist determines the appropriate prosthetic or orthotic controls needed for the management of a patient's impairments or functional limitations.
5. Delineate the steps in the fabrication or production of a custom orthosis or prosthesis.
6. Discuss the use of computer-aided design/computer-aided manufacture (CAD/CAM) in the measurement for and fabrication of orthoses and prostheses.
7. Describe the factors influencing the development of central fabrication centers and the manufacture of prefabricated components, orthoses, and prostheses.

A fundamental concept and common goal within the professions of orthotics, prosthetics, and rehabilitation is the restoration of normal form and function after injury or disease. To accept this challenge, the fields of orthotics and prosthetics have evolved into uniquely specialized professions. In addition to training in the basic biological and medical sciences, orthotists and prosthetists have an understanding of biomechanics, kinesiology, and the material sciences complemented by highly developed technical skills. Knowledge of the physical properties of materials and the techniques to manipulate and use them is essential to the design and fabrication of orthoses and prostheses. The topic is presented here as a general overview so that the rehabilitation clinician can develop a basic understanding of current design and fabrication processes used by orthotists and prosthetists.

ORTHOTICS AND PROSTHETICS IN THE TWENTIETH CENTURY

Orthotics and prosthetics have a rich history of research and development. Many innovative devices have been designed to restore function and provide relief from various medical ailments. Although progress can be documented throughout human history, the most significant contributions to orthotics and prosthetics were made in the twentieth century, stimulated by the aftermath of the world wars. Injured veterans who returned home from battle with musculoskeletal and neuromuscular impairments or traumatic amputation dramatically increased the demand for orthotic and prosthetic services. Although World War I stimulated some clinical progress in the two disciplines, notable scientific advancements did not occur until World War II. To improve the quality and performance of assistive devices at the end of World War II, particularly for veterans with amputation, the U.S. government sponsored a series of research and development projects under the auspices of the National Academy of Sciences (NAS) that would forever change the manner in which orthotics and prosthetics would be practiced.[1]

An extensive research effort was initiated by the NAS in late 1945, when a consensus conference revealed that few modern scientific principles or developments had been introduced in prosthetics.[2] Research and educational committees were formed between 1945 and 1976 to advise and work with the research groups. Universities, the Veterans Administration, private industry, and other military research units were subcontracted to conduct various prosthetic research projects. In summarizing the most notable achievements in prosthetics during this period, Wilson[3] cites the development of the total contact transfemoral socket; the quadrilateral socket design and hydraulic swing-phase knee-control units for the transfemoral prosthesis; the patellar tendon-bearing (PTB) transtibial prosthesis; the solid-ankle, cushioned-heel prosthetic foot; several new designs for the Syme's prosthesis; and the Canadian hip-disarticulation prosthesis. He also notes the implementation of immediate postsurgical and early fitting as having a significant impact on the rehabilitation process for persons with lower extremity amputation. The most notable improvements in upper extremity prosthetics were the lyre-shaped three-jaw chuck terminal device and more efficient harnessing systems. In addition, modular components and advances in bioengineering have permitted increased use and availability of the myoelectric prosthesis since it was first proposed in 1950.[4]

Of the wealth of scientific advances made during this intensive research period, the most important is the greater attention paid to the biomechanics of prosthetic alignment and socket design.[5] According to Wilson,[2] "The introduction of socket designs based on sound biomechanical analyses to take full advantage of the functions and properties of the stump in conjunction with the rationale for alignment undoubtedly represents the greatest achievement in prosthetics since World War II."

Although the focus of the NAS Artificial Limb Program was in prosthetics, it was anticipated that these efforts would also benefit orthotics. A formal research directive in orthotics did not begin until 1960. Biomechanical principles developed for the PTB prosthesis were immediately introduced in orthotics at the Veterans Administration Prosthetic Center, with the PTB orthosis to unload the foot-ankle complex axially.[6] The concept of fracture bracing or cast bracing began at approximately the same time and is now common practice for orthopedic management of fractures.[7,8] Clinical aspects of orthotic practice were also considered; a systematic approach to prescription formulation was established with the development of the technical analysis forms. Nomenclature to describe orthoses and their functions was standardized to identify the body segments they encompassed with the desired biomechanical control mechanisms.[9]

The introduction of new materials led to further advances in the field shortly after World War II. The use of thermosetting plastics in prosthetics permitted the development of the suction socket suspension system.[10] Transparent plastics offered a new approach to diagnostic and fitting evaluation techniques, such as the transparent prosthetic socket (test socket) and the transparent face mask for patients with thermal injuries. In orthotics, the addition of thermoplastics led to numerous innovative designs of ankle-foot orthoses (AFOs) in the 1960s and 1970s. The custom plastic AFO was an important technological advance in lower extremity orthotics. The physical characteristics of thermoformable plastics allowed biomechanical controls to match the prescription for improved function. The mechanical properties of an orthosis could be controlled by the layout of the trimlines of a device or structural reinforcements through specially placed corrugations that could be incorporated into its surface geometry. Advances have been steady in the area of material engineering and continue to have an impact on orthotics and prosthetics. Numerous prosthetic feet have been introduced as elite athletes demand increased performance capabilities from their prosthetic components. Innovative designs for some prosthetic feet have been possible in part because of the diversity of carbon composite technology complemented by sound engineering design.

The development of computer-aided design/computer-aided manufacture (CAD/CAM) systems for orthotics and prosthetics, which began in the 1970s, was another major technological advance, considering the long tradition of custom hand-crafted devices in the profession. In the late 1980s and early 1990s, as computers became more economical, facilities began to integrate CAD/CAM systems into their practices. CAD/CAM systems have now been designed for most orthotic and prosthetic applications, often with specialized digitizers, scanners, and milling equipment to accommodate the unique needs of a particular device. The current trend within the profession is that orthotists and prosthetists use the CAD portion to digitize and manipulate the data, then subcontract the production of a device from a central fabrication company for the CAM portion. The art and workmanship that have distinguished the orthotists and prosthetists from other health professionals for most of the twentieth century continue to evolve as CAD/CAM technologies improve the design, manufacture, and diagnostic aspects of the field.

Orthotics and prosthetics have played an important historical role in the development of medical and surgical orthopedics and rehabilitation. Fundamental concepts that evolved from orthotic and prosthetic advancements are now basic principles in rehabilitation. Orthotics and prosthetics have evolved as sister professions because the technical skills and knowledge base to prescribe, fabricate, and fit the respective mechanical devices are similar. Because of this, material and technological advancements have been shared between these two rehabilitation specialties.

MATERIALS

In the first part of the twentieth century, orthoses were constructed primarily of metal, leather, and fabric, and prostheses were manufactured from wood and leather. In the last 60 years, however, tremendous technological advancements have been made in the material sciences. The demand for strong and lightweight components in the aerospace and marine industries has produced a variety of new materials that possess mechanical properties suitable for use in the construction of orthoses and prostheses. New plastics have led to revolutionary advancements in the profession, permitting increased durability and strength and significant cosmetic improvements. Although a multitude of materials are now available, traditional ones are still in wide use; material selection depends in part on the individual needs of each patient. In a rehabilitation team setting, the orthotist and prosthetist are responsible for choosing the appropriate materials and components for fabrication because their experience and training are specialized in this area.

This chapter presents an overview of the general types of materials used in orthotics and prosthetics for rehabilitation professionals. Publications by the American Society for Testing and Materials contain specific technical information.[11] Industry standards established by the International Organization for Standardization for consumer and patient protection give the strength requirements for orthotic and prosthetic components.[12]

The types of materials used most commonly in current orthotic and prosthetic practice include leather, metal, wood, thermoplastic and thermosetting materials, foamed plastics, and viscoelastic polymers. In deciding which materials are most appropriate for a patient, the orthotist or prosthetist considers the five important characteristics of materials: strength, stiffness, durability, density, and corrosion resistance.[13]

A material's strength is determined by the maximum external load that the material can support or sustain. Strength is especially important in lower limb devices, in which loading forces associated with gait can be very high, or when heavy use of the orthotic or prosthetic device is anticipated.

Stiffness is the amount of bending or compression that occurs when a material is loaded (stress/strain or force/displacement ratios). The stiffer a material, the less flexible it is and the less likely that deformation will occur during wear. When significant external stability is desirable (e.g., in a fracture brace or a rigid prosthetic frame), a stiff material is often chosen. When conformation to body segments is necessary (e.g., in a posterior leaf-spring AFO or a flexible transfemoral prosthetic socket), a more flexible material is used.

Durability (fatigue resistance) of a material is determined by its ability to withstand repeated cycles of loading or unloading during functional activities. Repeated loading compromises the material's strength and increases risk of failure or fracture of the material. Fatigue resistance is especially problematic in the interface of materials with different characteristics.

Density is the material's weight per unit of volume, a prime determinant of energy cost during functional activities while a patient wears a prosthetic or orthotic device. Although the goal is to provide as lightweight a device as possible, strength, durability, and fatigue resistance needs may necessitate a denser material.

Corrosion resistance is the degree to which the material is susceptible to chemical degradation. Many of the materials used for orthoses or prostheses retain heat, making perspiration a problem. For some patients who require lower extremity devices, incontinence may also be a concern. Materials that are impervious to moisture are easier to clean than porous materials.

The ease of fabrication is another important consideration for materials. Certain materials can be easily molded or adjusted for a custom fit; others require special equipment or techniques to shape the material.

Leather

Leather is manufactured from the skin and hides of various animals. Tanning methods and the type of hide determine the final characteristics of the leather. As an interface material for an orthosis or a prosthesis, vegetable-tanned leather is used to protect the skin from irritation. Chrome-tanned leather is used for supportive purposes when strength and resiliency are needed. Additional chemical processes can be incorporated during manufacturing to produce leathers that are waterproof, porous, flexible, or stiff. Useful qualities of leather include its dimensional stability, porosity, and water vapor permeability.[14] These features have made leather a frequently used material within orthopedics, and it continues to be a material of choice in many current devices. Today, leather is used for supportive components such as suspension straps, belts, and limb cuffs. Leather is also used to cover metallic structures such as pelvic, thigh, and calf bands. For foot orthoses and shoe modifications, leather is often preferred over synthetic substitutes because of its superior "breathability" characteristics.

Another important attribute of leather is its moldability. Although numerous techniques are available to mold leather, the most common one in orthotics and prosthetics is to stretch it over a plaster cast after it has been mulled (dampened or soaked) in water. When the water evaporates from the molded leather, its dried shape is maintained, and the leather can be trimmed to the desired dimensions. To increase strength and durability, leather can be reinforced by lamination with plastics or other leathers. Similarly, if padding is desired over bony regions of the body, foamed plastics or felt can be sandwiched between layers of leather for comfort or to distribute applied forces over a larger surface area. Three basic skills are required for crafting orthotic or prosthetic components of leather: cutting, sewing, and molding. A technique specific to leather work is that of skiving, or thinning the edge on the flesh side of the hide. Finishing methods such as these contribute to the final appearance of the leather work and the device.

Metals

The types of metal used in the fabrication of orthoses and prostheses can be categorized into three groups: steel and its alloys, aluminum, and titanium or magnesium alloys. These metals may or may not share similar characteristics. If metals are incorporated into an orthosis or prosthesis, the choice of metal is determined by the needs and preferences of the particular patient.

Steel

The general term *steel* refers to any iron-based alloy material. Carbon alloys have carbon added to the composition of steel. The term *alloy steel* is used when other materials are included in the material manufacture. Alloy steels are further defined as low-alloy or high-alloy steels. Steels are strong, rigid, ductile, and durable, but their high density (weight) and susceptibility to corrosion are major disadvantages. Many different types of steel are available to meet various engineering needs. To assist in identifying the composition and type of material, the American Iron Steel Institute–Society of Automotive Engineers has established a four-digit numbering system. The first two digits in the number indicate the type of steel, and the last two digits identify the carbon content. For alloy steels, the first digit identifies the major alloy and the second digit indicates the percentage of the major alloying element.

The carbon content of steel is the major determinant of its ductility and yield strength characteristics. Yield strength is an offset measure in a stress-strain curve in which strain occurs without an increase in stress. Ductility is the property of a material to deform in the inelastic or plastic range. Low carbon content (0.05% to 0.10%) produces high ductility and a low yield strength.[15] As the carbon concentration increases, yield strength increases and ductility is reduced. Heat treatments can alter the properties of carbon steel by increasing yield strength and reducing ductility. The mechanical properties of low-alloy steels fall between those of carbon steels and high-alloy steels. High strength/weight ratios are possible with the high-alloy steels, an important characteristic for repetitive loading situations. These types of steels are used for some orthotic and prosthetic joint components. High-alloy steels are not very resistant to corrosion and are often more difficult to fabricate.

Stainless steel is a steel alloy that contains 12% or more of chromium, a material that increases resistance to corrosion and oxidation. Chromium produces a light oxide film on the surface that deters deterioration of the base metal. Because durability and protection from corrosion are highly desirable, stainless steels are used extensively within orthotics and prosthetics to enhance longevity of devices. Two types of stainless steel, martensitic steel and ferretic steel, have chromium as the predominant alloying element, but martensitic steel is the only one used in orthotics and prosthetics because it can be hardened by heat treatment. Stainless steel is used for orthotic and prosthetic joints, support uprights, and band material.

Aluminum

Aluminum alloys are well suited for orthotics and prosthetics because of their high strength/weight ratio and resistance to corrosion. As with steels, the properties of aluminum depend on alloying compositions, heat treatments, and cold working. *Wrought* and *cast* are terms used to describe the two major types of aluminum alloys. Alloys are further subdivided into those that are heat treatable and those that are not. The low ductility and low strength of cast aluminum are ideal for prefabricated prosthetic components and in some assemblies for moving parts.

Wrought aluminum alloys are used in orthotics and prosthetics for structural purposes such as prosthetic pylons, orthotic uprights, and upper extremity devices. The high-compression bending stresses of lower extremity prosthetics are well suited to the use of wrought aluminum alloys.

Although aluminum alloys are very resistant to atmospheric and some chemical corrosion, the acids and alkalis in urine, perspiration, and other bodily fluids deteriorate the natural protective oxides on the material's surface, making the aluminum susceptible to corrosion. To deter corrosion in aluminum and to resist abrasive wear, various hard coatings, such as anodic or oxide finishes, can be applied. Mechanical finishes, such as polishing, buffing, and sandblasting, offer attractive cosmetic appearances for devices.

Titanium and Magnesium

Components made of titanium alloys have become more prevalent in prosthetics but are rarely used in orthotics. Although titanium alloys are stronger than those of aluminum and have comparable strength to some steels, their density is 60% that of steel.[16] Because prosthetic components made of titanium are lighter in weight than steel counterparts, they require less energy expenditure by the patient during use. Titanium alloys are also more resistant to corrosion than are aluminum and steel. It is important to note, however, that titanium alloys are often more difficult to machine and fabricate. Consequently, titanium is most often used in prefabricated prosthetic components, when strength and light weight are of concern. Titanium is also more expensive than aluminum and steel, which has been a limiting factor for its use.

Magnesium alloys are lighter than those of aluminum and titanium, are corrosion resistant, and have a lower modulus of elasticity than does aluminum. The modulus of elasticity (Young's modulus) is defined as the ratio of unit stress to unit strain in a stress-strain curve's elastic range; materials with low modulus values are associated with lower rates of fatigue under conditions of repeated stress. Although some of these features are promising, magnesium alloys have not yet been widely used in orthoses and prostheses.

Wood

Wood possesses many desirable characteristics for use in prosthetics. Its wide availability, strength, light weight, and ability to be shaped easily have continued to be of benefit in prosthetic socket and component construction, even with the introduction of thermoplastics. The wood used in prosthetics must be properly cured, free of knots, and relatively strong. Yellow poplar, willow, basswood (linden), and balsa are most commonly used. Hardwoods have been reserved for prosthetic applications in which structural strength is essential, most often in certain types of prosthetic feet or as reinforcement for knee units. The keel prosthetic foot is fabricated of maple and hickory. The solid-ankle, cushioned-heel prosthetic foot has a hardwood keel that is bolted to the prosthetic shank, creating a solid structural unit for standing and ambulation.

Plastics and Composites

One of the most important production-related characteristics of an orthotic or prosthetic material is its ability to be molded over a positive model. Because plastics can be readily formed, they are a very popular, widely used material for orthoses and prostheses. Plastics are grouped into two categories: thermoplastics and thermosetting materials.[17-19]

Thermoplastics

Thermoplastic materials are formable when they are heated but become rigid after they have cooled. Thermoplastics are classified as either low-temperature or high-temperature materials, depending on the temperature range at which they become malleable. Low-temperature thermoplastics become moldable at temperatures less than 149°C and can often be molded directly on the patient's limb, whereas high-temperature materials require heating to much higher temperatures and must be molded over a positive model of the patient's limb.[18] One advantage of thermoplastic materials is that they can be reheated and shaped multiple times, making possible minor adjustments of an orthosis or prosthesis during fittings. Thermoplastics are the material of choice for "shell" designs in which structural strength is required. Some of the more popular materials used are acrylic, copolymer, polyethylene, polypropylene, polystyrene, and a variety of vinyls.

Certain low-temperature thermoplastics, those moldable at temperatures less than 80°C, can be applied and shaped directly to the body. Some of the most commonly available materials include Kydex (Kleerdex, Aiken, S.C.), Orthoplast (Johnson & Johnson, Raynham, Mass.), and Polysar (Bayer, Pittsburgh, Pa.). These materials are most often reserved for orthotic devices that are designed to provide temporary support and protection. Their susceptibility to repetitive stress, high loads, and temperature changes usually limits their use to spinal and upper extremity orthoses. Because these devices are molded directly on the patient, no casting is necessary, and the time required from measurement to finished product is greatly reduced. Another important convenience of low-temperature thermoplastic materials is that no special equipment is required; hot water heated in an electric frying pan, a heat gun, and sharp scissors are all that are necessary to produce a functional splint or orthosis.

High-temperature plastics are frequently used in the production of orthotics and prosthetics. The most commonly used materials include polyethylene, polypropylene, polycarbonate, acrylic, acrylonitrile butadiene styrene, acrylics, polyvinyl acetate, polyvinyl chloride, and polyvinyl alcohol.

Polypropylene is a rigid plastic material that is relatively inexpensive, lightweight, and easy to thermoform. Polypropylenes, which can be further characterized as homopolymers or copolymers, are one of the most widely used plastics in orthotics. The material has a white, opaque color and is available in sheets of various thicknesses, from 1 mm to 1 cm. Polypropylene is impact resistant and can endure several million cycles of repetitive flexes. This attribute has been extremely useful in orthotics for hinge joints and spring assists in AFOs. The material is, however, susceptible to ultraviolet light and extreme cold and is sensitive to scratches and nicks. In prosthetics, the light weight of polypropylene makes it ideal for components such as sockets, pelvic bands, hip joints, or knee joints. Polypropylene is commonly used for prefabricated AFOs and preformed modular orthotic systems.

The long fatigue life of polyethylene during repeated loading situations makes this material suitable for a number of orthotic and prosthetic applications. Prosthetic sockets, orthotic hinge joint components, and compression shells for clamshell design orthoses are common uses of polyethylene plastics. Several densities of polyethylene are available from various manufacturers. Low-density polyethylene is used for upper extremity and spinal orthoses under the trade names Vitrathene (Stanley Smith & Co, Ltd, Isleworth, U.K.) and Streifen (FG Streifeneder KG, Munich, Germany). High-density polyethylene, Subortholen (Wilhelm Julius Teufel GmbH, Stuttgart, Germany), is used for spinal and lower extremity orthoses. The ultra-high-density polyethylenes such as Ortholen (Wilhelm Julius Teufel) are used principally for lower extremity orthoses.

Thermoforming

Thermoforming is one of the most common techniques used in orthotic and prosthetic laboratories to fabricate the "user" interface components of a device (e.g., prosthetic socket, AFO). The process of thermoforming entails heating a sheet of thermoplastic material in an oven until it has reached its "plastic" state (i.e., ability to distort) and then forcing the material over a prescribed shape (i.e., positive mold) under pressure until it has cooled. Negative air pressure or vacuum is the typical method used to apply pressure and form the plastic over the mold, hence the terms "vacuum-form" are also used to describe the process. Once the plastic has cooled

and returned to its solid state, the perimeter of the formed components is determined and trimmed out. The edges of the plastic are then finished on specialized grinding machines that have a diverse set of abrasive sanding and buffing cone options that are used to achieve a high-polish smoothed edge.

Thermosetting Materials

Thermosets are plastics that are applied over a positive model in liquid form and then chemically "cured" to solidify and maintain a desired shape. To enhance their structural properties, thermosets are often impregnated into various fabrics by a process of lamination. Although this group of plastics has inherent structural stability, their rigidity precludes modification by heat molding; their shape can only be changed by grinding. Thermosetting plastics cannot be reheated without destroying their physical properties. Some of the most common thermoset resins used to produce rigid orthoses are acrylic, polyester, and epoxy. Because acrylic resins are strong, lightweight, and somewhat pliable, they offer a different set of characteristics than those of polyester resins. With lamination, acrylic resin can create a thin but strong structural wall for a prosthetic socket or component of an orthosis. If frequent adjustments are anticipated, however, thermoforming plastics are chosen instead because thermoset cannot be heated to make adjustments to their shape.

Composites

Composites are the combination of two or more materials with distinctly different physical or chemical properties that together produce a material with enhanced performance characteristics relative to their material properties as a single substance. Numerous types of composites exist under this broad descriptive term, ranging from natural materials such as wood to manmade materials such as concrete. This chapter focuses on the combination of fibers and matrices associated with thermosetting plastics.

Fiber-reinforced plastics (FRPs), also referred to as *composites*, have revolutionized orthotics and prosthetics, primarily because they can be engineered to have mechanical properties with strength characteristics optimized for specific types of loading situations, thereby greatly improving the functionality of many types of orthoses and prostheses. The mechanical properties of reinforcement fibers, for the most part, dictate the mechanical properties of a composite through the orientation and position of the fibers. In general, FRPs offer high strength and stiffness qualities yet are also capable of incurring compressive or flexural stresses. Plastics can also be reinforced with other fillers, particulates, and short or chopped fibers, but FRPs are most widely used. This section focuses on fiber reinforcement for thermosets.

Polymer composites are made of a binder material (i.e., resin), referred to as the *matrix*, which is reinforced with fibers to improve strength and stiffness. The matrix of a composite encapsulates the fibers to maintain their desired orientation and position and ensure that load sharing of fibers is well distributed through the material. The volume fraction of resin-to-fiber is an important determinant of the mechanical properties of a composite and its performance. In general, the volume of fiber should be higher than the volume of resin matrix. A fiber volume fraction that approaches 90.7% with a matrix volume fraction of 9.3% is considered an ideal ratio.[20]

By comparison, the fibers in composite materials are stronger than the matrix material and can handle stresses applied to them better than the weaker matrix material. Typical fiber reinforcements used in polymer composites are fiberglass, carbon/graphite, and Kevlar aramid fibers (DuPont, Wilmington, Del.). Grades of different fiberglass include E, C, and S glass, which stand for electrical (E), chemical (C), and strength (S), respectively. S glass has a higher tensile strength than E and C glass. Carbon fiber is widely used in orthoses and prostheses having strength properties greater than steel while also being lightweight and very stiff. Carbon fiber has superior stiffness properties in both compression and tension but, because it has relatively low impact strength, it is often combined with other reinforcement fibers like fiberglass or Kevlar to improve its performance. Aramid fibers (e.g., Kevlar) have tensile strength properties that are five times greater than steel for the same weight.

Laminar composites or laminates are fabricated out of "continuous fibers" that may extend the length of a given part and are one of the most common FRPs used in orthotics and prosthetics. Continuous fiber reinforcements can be woven into the form of a fabric in many different weave patterns. By combining different types of fiber fabrics (e.g., carbon graphite, Kevlar) and stacking these plies into layers, the resultant laminate can possess properties for particular modes of loading. When engineering laminates for orthoses and prostheses, the practitioner or technician must understand the manner in which loads will be transmitted through a device so that appropriate layering and orientation of plies will be incorporated into the composite to meet its functional performance duties. A laminate code system is used to describe the direction and ply layer with the longer dimension of the laminate serving as the x-axis and the width serving as the y-axis. A fiber orientation angle is used to describe the orientation of plies with respect to the x-axis, which is designated as 0°. A laminate code describes the sequencing of each layer from top to bottom. An example of a laminate code where the top ply is 0° followed by subsequent plies oriented respectively at 45°, 90°, 45°, with the bottom ply at 0° would be written as follows: $[0/45/90]_2$. Brackets define the code's beginning and end, and the subscript indicates the adjacent plies are oriented the same, which is essentially one half of the ply description. The purpose of having a variety of different fiber orientation angles in composite laminates is that the load can be carried through the fibers in a number of different positions. For example, if the fibers were only oriented in one direction, then structural loading of the material at a different angle could result in a failure. Therefore multidirectional laminates have the capacity to endure loads in an orthotic and prosthetic device in variety of positions.

Processing Technologies and Composite Fabrication

Orthotic and prosthetic devices often are a compilation of custom-molded interface shell components combined with additional premanufactured parts (e.g., prosthetic foot, pylon).

Practitioners and their technical staff have the capability to fabricate the human interface portions of a device within their laboratories, although the processes and equipment in their labs are limited to only a few techniques. Manufacturers on the other hand have the capacity to consider a much wider variety of processing techniques for mass producing composite parts and thus take advantage of processing technologies that can maximize the performance potential of the material.

The most common method for processing FPR composites in orthotic prosthetic laboratories is a contact molding technique called a "vacuum bag" lamination. The technique is relatively simple and does not require any specialized equipment. A flexible membrane bag of plastic is tightly stretched over the positive mold part and sealed; then negative air pressure (i.e., vacuum) is applied between the bag and the mold, drawing the bag tightly to the surface of the mold. A hand layup of fiber cloth is placed on the mold in a predetermined manner with regard to the orientation and position of the fibers with an understanding of how loads will be transmitted through the structure when it is incorporated into a device. After the desired layup of fiber and cloth is achieved, a second flexible membrane bag is pulled over the mold, creating an enclosure that can accommodate the wet liquid resin (matrix) part of the composite. After the resin is poured into an opening of the second bag and sealed, vacuum inside the enclosure draws the outer bag toward the mold, pressing the resin through the fiber in a uniform manner to create a thin-walled structure of composite that has a high fiber-to-resin ratio. If the atmospheric pressure that presses on the outside bag is not adequate to achieve the desired fiber-to-resin ratio, then the vacuum bag mold construct can be placed into an autoclave to create higher pressures on the external bag. Because most orthotic prosthetic laboratories do not have autoclaves for such procedures, central fabrication laboratories equipped with such equipment are being used to a greater extent to maximize the benefits of pressure processing in composites.

Foamed Plastics

Foamed plastics can be used as a protective interface between the orthotic or prosthetic and the skin, especially over areas that are vulnerable to pressure, such as bony prominences. Foamed plastics are grouped into two classes: open and closed cell. Cells are created in rubber or polymers in a high-pressure gassing process.[18] The microcell structure allows the foamed plastic material to be displaced in several planes, which is an ideal physical property for the reduction of shear forces. In an open-cell foam, the cells are interrelated (as in a kitchen sponge); in a closed-cell foam, the cells are separate from each other. Because closed-cell foams are impervious to liquids, they are less likely to absorb body fluids such as perspiration or urine; however, they do act as insulators and can be hot when worn for extended periods.

An orthopedic grade of polyethylene foam was introduced in the 1960s by a British subsidiary of the Union Carbide Company.[21] These closed-cell foams are available in a wide array of durometer hardness. (*Durometer* refers to a spring indenture post instrument that is used to measure the resistance to the compression/hardness of a material.) Polyethylene foams are commercially available under trade names such as Plastazote (Hackettstown, N.J.), Pe-Lite, Evazote (Bakelite Xylonite Ltd., Croydon, U.K.), and Aliplast (Alimed Inc., Dedham, Mass.). Various polyethylene foams are used in the manufacture of soft and rigid orthoses, depending on the density of the material. Plastazote is a low-temperature, heat-formable foam that has been used successfully in the treatment and prevention of neuropathic foot lesions.[22-25] Its light weight and forgiving quality to bony prominences make it a desirable interface for the insensate foot. See Hertzman[22] for a complete review of the use of Plastazote in lower limb orthotics and prosthetics.

Closed-cell foams are also made with synthetic rubber or polychloroprene. Neoprene is available in various densities, making the low-durometer versions suitable as liners for orthoses, whereas the firmer materials are used for posts or soling for shoes. Spenco (Spenco Medical Corp., Waco, Texas) is a microcellular neoprene foam that reduces shear forces to the foot's plantar surface and the occurrence of foot blisters in athletes.[26] The nylon (polyamide)-covered neoprene acts as a shock absorber while also reducing friction on the foot's plantar surface.[21] Although few of these materials are heat moldable, most can be conformed without difficulty to the shallow contours of foot orthoses. Lynco (Apex Foot Health Industries, Teaneck, N.J.) is an open-cell neoprene foam that dissipates heat more efficiently than its closed-cell cousin; however, it does not attenuate shock as well as Spenco.[21]

Polyurethane open-cell foams are alternatives for top covers for foot orthoses. They provide good shock absorption and dissipate heat well. Some of the commercially available open-cell polyurethane foams include Poron (Rogers Corporation, Rogers, Conn.), PPT (Professional Protective Technology, Deer Park, N.Y.), and Vylite (Steins Foot Specialties, Newark, N.J.).

Several studies that compare materials used to fabricate orthoses have been conducted.[27-33] In 1982, Campbell and colleagues[27] conducted compression tests on 31 materials to determine their suitability for insoles in shoes. Materials were classified according to stiffness into the categories "very stiff," "moderately deformable," and "highly deformable." The moderately deformable group of plastics, which included 19 of the tested foamed plastics, was deemed the most beneficial as an insole material. Campbell and colleagues[27] concluded that these materials could relieve stress from bony prominences and transfer the loads to the adjacent soft tissues more effectively than could the very stiff or highly deformable materials. Studies evaluating shoe insole materials also report them to be effective at attenuating shock during walking in various ways.[33]

Viscoelastic Polymers

A viscoelastic solid is a material that possesses the characteristics of stress relaxation and creep. Stress relaxation occurs when a material that is subjected to a constant deformation requires a decreasing load with time to maintain a steady state.[34] Creep refers to the increase in deformation with time to a steady state as a constant load is applied.[34] Sorbothane (Sorbothane, Inc., Kent, Ohio), widely used as an insole material, is made

of a noncellular polyurethane derivative that possesses good shock-attenuating characteristics.[34] Viscolas (Viscolas Corp., Soddy Daisy, Tenn.), another type of viscoelastic solid, has been found to attenuate skeletal shock at heel strike in the tibia to half the normal load.[15,35] Two other viscoelastic polymers used to fabricate orthotic prosthetic components are Viscolite (Polymer Dynamics, Inc., Allentown, Pa.) and PQ (Riecken's Orthotic Laboratories, Evansville, Ind.).

PRESCRIPTION GUIDELINES

The formulation of a prescription for an orthosis or prosthesis greatly influences the potential functional outcome for the patient. It is critical that rehabilitation objectives and design criteria be carefully considered. Physicians, therapists, orthotists, and prosthetists who are involved in developing a prescription for an orthotic or prosthetic device must have a sound understanding of orthotics and prosthetics to be successful in effectively treating patients with these devices.

Assessment of functional deficit includes a thorough evaluation of the patient's present physical status, including muscle strength testing, range of motion measures, and documentation of other physical impairments that would affect the fit or performance of the device. Equally important to the physical examination is the consideration of any individual needs of the patient and an understanding of how the treatment will affect daily activities. To increase the success of treatment, the patient and other rehabilitation team members must reach a consensus on the type of device and the associated training and education required for optimal functional outcome.

Orthotic Prescription

The Committee on Prosthetics and Orthotics of the American Academy of Orthopaedic Surgeons developed a technical analysis form to standardize the process of patient evaluation. This evaluation protocol documents the biomechanical deficits of the patient and provides the basic information needed for orthotic prescription formulation. This systematic approach has two major objectives: to define the anatomical segments that the orthosis will encompass and to accurately describe the biomechanical controls needed for treatment. The underlying principle of this assessment is that orthoses should be designed to control only those movements considered abnormal while permitting free motion in anatomical segments that are not impaired.

Technical analysis forms were developed for three general regions of the body: the upper limb, lower limb, and spine. The forms are four pages long with the same basic approach for formulating an orthotic prescription. The first page has sections for recording general patient information and noting major physical impairments (Figure 6-1). The major impairment section characterizes any functional limitations, such as skeletal structure, sensation, or joint contracture. This information provides an overview of the patient's clinical presentation.

The second and third pages of the technical analysis form (Figure 6-2) contain diagrams of the respective anatomical (limb or trunk) segments for which an orthotic prescription is

Technical Analysis Form	Lower Limb	Revised March 1973

Name _____ No. _____ Age _____ Sex _____

Date of onset _____ Cause _____

Occupation _____ Present lower-limb equipment _____

Diagnosis _____

_____

_____

Ambulatory ☐   Nonambulatory ☐

Major impairments:

A.   Skeletal
1.   Bone and joints: Normal ☐   Abnormal _____
2.   Ligaments: Normal ☐   Abnormal ☐   Knee: AC ☐   PC ☐   MC ☐   LC ☐
                                                    Ankle: MC ☐   LC ☐

3.   Extremity shortening: None ☐   Left ☐   Right ☐
     Amount of discrepancy: ASIS-Heel _____   ASIS-MTP _____   MTP-Heel _____

B.   Sensation: Normal ☐   Abnormal ☐
1.   Anesthesia ☐   Hypesthesia ☐   Location: _____
     Protective sensation: Retained ☐   Lost ☐
2.   Pain ☐   Location: _____

C.   Skin: Normal ☐   Abnormal: _____

D.   Vascular: Normal ☐   Abnormal ☐   Right ☐   Left ☐

E.   Balance: Normal ☐   Impaired ☐   Support: _____

F.   Gait deviations: _____

_____

G.   Other impairments: _____

────────────────────────── **Legend** ──────────────────────────

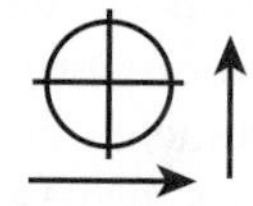

⊕↑ = Direction of translatory motion

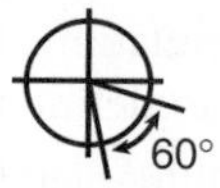

Volitional force (V)
N = Normal
G = Good
F = Fair
P = Poor
T = Trace
Z = Zero

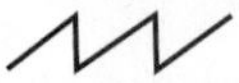

Proprioception (P)
N = Normal
I = Impaired
A = Absent

⊕ 60° = Abnormal degree of rotary motion

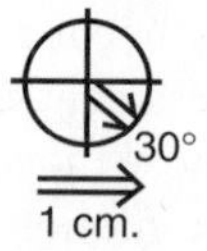

⊕ 30° = Fixed position

1 cm.

D = Local distension or enlargement

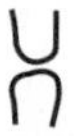

Hypertonic muscle (H)
N = Normal
M = Mild
Mo = Moderate
S = Severe

= Pseudarthrosis

〜〜 = Fracture

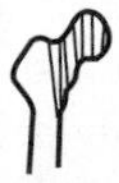

= Absence of segment

FIGURE 6-1 The technical analysis form provides a systematic method of data collection for the development of prescriptions for lower extremity orthoses. The first page of the form is used to record the patient's history and current impairments. AC, Anterior cruciate ligament; ASIS, anterior superior iliac spine; LC, lateral collateral ligament; MC, medial collateral ligament; MTP, medial tibial plateau; PC, posterior cruciate ligament. (From Committee on Prosthetics Research and Development. Report of the Seventh Workshop Panel on Lower Extremity Orthoses of the Subcommittee on Design and Development. Washington, DC: National Research Council–National Academy of Sciences, 1970; and McCollough NC III. Biomechanical analysis systems for orthotic prescription. In American Academy of Orthopaedic Surgeons, *Atlas of Orthotics: Biomechanical Principles and Application*, 2nd ed. St. Louis: Mosby, 1985. pp. 35-75.)

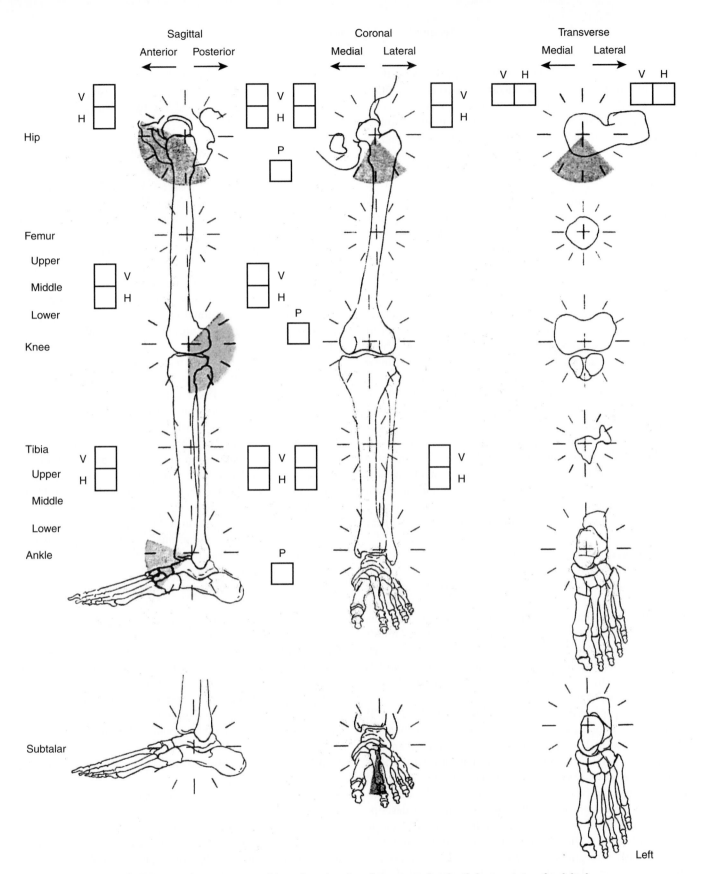

FIGURE 6-2 Subsequent pages of the technical analysis form are used to detail characteristics of each limb or body segment for which the orthosis or prosthesis will be made. Information recorded on these pages includes existing deformity, proprioceptive capacity (P), restriction or hypermobility of joint rotary and translatory range of motion in all three planes of movement, volitional strength (V), and the level of hypertonicity (H). (From Committee on Prosthetics Research and Development. Report of the Seventh Workshop Panel on Lower Extremity Orthoses of the Subcommittee on Design and Development. Washington, DC: National Research Council–National Academy of Sciences, 1970; and McCollough NC III. Biomechanical analysis systems for orthotic prescription. In American Academy of Orthopaedic Surgeons, *Atlas of Orthotics: Biomechanical Principles and Application*, 2nd ed. St. Louis: Mosby, 1985. pp. 35-75.)

being considered. Each skeletal region is represented in three planes of motion: coronal, sagittal, and transverse. On either side of the figures, square boxes at the level of the joints are used to note volitional force, hypertonicity, proprioception, and range of motion. The fourth page consists of a summary of the functional disability, treatment objectives, orthotic recommendation, and a key for the biomechanical controls of function.

Voluntary movements of muscles are assessed by conventional muscle testing techniques. Muscle strength can be recorded with either the standard descriptive or numeric muscle grading systems, depending on regional preferences.

Two types of joint (limb) motion are recorded on the forms: rotary and translatory. According to McCollough,[36] all points of the distal segment move in the same direction, following the same path shape and distance during translatory motion. During rotary motion, one point of the distal segment (or its imaginary extension) remains fixed while other points move in an arc around it. Translatory motion is recorded with linear arrows in the direction of the distal segment's movement relative to its proximal counterpart. The linear arrows are placed below the circle (representing the joint axis) for translatory motion. If translatory force acts in the vertical axis, the linear arrow is placed to the side of the circle. Rotary motion and the related degree of range of motion are documented by an arrow within a protractor-type arrangement for each joint. The established normal range of motion for each joint is shaded on the form for comparative reference. If a fixed contracture or fusion of the joint is present, a double linear arrow is used.

Hypertonicity of muscle groups in each of the body segments is described by a functionally based letter scale.[36] A designation of mild tonicity is given when any hypertonus that is present is thought to be functionally insignificant. Moderate tonicity indicates that tone might have some functional value, such as assisting the patient in holding an item during minor tasks. A designation of severe tonicity indicates that normal function is not possible. The patient's proprioceptive ability is described in a similar way, as absent, impaired, or normal for each of the body segments of interest.

The final page of the technical analysis form (Figure 6-3) contains space for an overview of functional impairments, a checklist of the orthotic treatment objectives, and a chart that details the orthotic recommendation. The desired orthotic control for each body segment is indicated by a specific letter; as many as seven types of orthotic controls can be incorporated into the design of an orthosis. The terms and descriptions of these controls are indicated in the key. If the orthotic recommendation section is completed correctly, the chart will indicate the body segments that the device will encompass and the desired biomechanical control of function needed. Any comments on the specific design requirements or materials, or both, can be detailed in the remarks section of the form.

For the orthotist, the prescription is the blueprint from which the design of a device is based. It specifies the force system requirements needed to achieve the treatment objectives independent of material selection or production processes.

Although an in-depth biomechanical assessment may not always be necessary, a system based on these principles is a logical and objective method for formulating an orthotic prescription.

Prosthetic Prescription

The formulation of a prosthetic prescription requires a different evaluative process. Prosthetic prescription depends on an in-depth understanding of components and materials as well as their indications and contraindications for use. Ideally, prosthetic prescription begins before amputation surgery, so the residual limb is of appropriate length and healing is adequate for optimal prosthetic use. Factors such as vascular supply, anticipated activity level, intelligence, vocation, and age are also important to consider. Range of motion, flexible and fixed contracture, functional strength, skin condition, girth measurements, pain, and sensation of the residual limb and the intact limb are evaluated.

An important part of prosthetic prescription is component selection. The diversity of prosthetic foot-ankle units and knee mechanisms for lower extremity prosthetics, and the variety of terminal devices for the upper extremity, can present difficult decisions for those who are unfamiliar with their intended application. Therefore, prosthetists are often relied on for recommendations on components because they are usually most familiar with the specifications and limitations. Many prosthetic teams have developed data collection forms to standardize the prosthetic prescription process. Redhead[37] suggests that the prescription for a prosthesis consider each of the major "prescription options." Examples of the specifications delineated by Redhead for a transfemoral prosthesis are type of limb, socket material and design, suspension, knee joints, knee controls, ankle joints, feet, and cosmesis.

FABRICATION PROCESS

Once a prescription for a custom orthosis or prosthesis has been created, the fabrication process begins. The traditional fabrication process is composed of six steps:

Step 1: Taking accurate measurements of the limb
Step 2: Making a negative impression (cast)
Step 3: Creating a three-dimensional positive model of the limb or body segment
Step 4: Modifying the positive model to incorporate the desired controls
Step 5: Fabricating the orthosis or prosthetic socket around the positive model
Step 6: Fitting of the device to the patient

In some instances, further modification or adjustment is necessary to achieve optimal fit and function of the device.

Measurement

Measurements are most often referenced from readily palpable bony landmarks. Important measurements include the length, successive circumferences, and mediolateral and anteroposterior dimensions of the body segment for which the orthotic or prosthetic device is being created. Although

Summary of functional disability _____

_____

_____

_____

_____

Treatment objectives:

Prevent/correct deformity ☐	Improve ambulation ☐
Reduce axial load ☐	Fracture treatment ☐
Protect joint ☐	Other _____

Orthotic Recommendation

Lower limb			Flex	Ext	Abd	Add	Rotation		Axial load
							Int	Ext	
HKAO	Hip								
KAO	Thigh								
	Knee								
AFO	Leg								
	Ankle		(Dorsi)	(Plantar)					
		Subtalar					(Inver)	(Ever)	
FO Foot		Midtarsal							
		Met-phal							

Remarks:

_____   _____

Signature   Date

Key: Use the following symbols to indicate desired control of designated function:

F = Free   Free motion
A = Assist   Application of an external force for the purpose of increasing the range, velocity, or force of a motion
R = Resist   Application of an external force for the purpose of decreasing the velocity or force of a motion
S = Stop   Inclusion of a static unit to deter an undesired motion in one direction
v = Variable A unit that can be adjusted without making a structural change
H = Hold   Elimination of all motion in prescribed plane (verify position)
L = Lock   Device includes an optional lock

FIGURE 6-3 The final page of the technical analysis form details the goals for the orthosis and the specific prescription for the desired device. Once the prescription is developed, the form serves as a guideline for fabricating and fitting the orthosis. FO, Foot orthosis; HKAO, hip-knee-ankle orthosis; V, volitional force. (From Committee on Prosthetics Research and Development. Report of the Seventh Workshop Panel on Lower Extremity Orthoses of the Subcommittee on Design and Development. Washington, DC: National Research Council–National Academy of Sciences, 1970; and McCollough NC III. Biomechanical analysis systems for orthotic prescription. In American Academy of Orthopaedic Surgeons, *Atlas of Orthotics: Biomechanical Principles and Application*, 2nd ed. St. Louis: Mosby, 1985. pp. 35-75.)

many measurements can be obtained with simple tools such as a tape measure, specialized measurement devices such as electronic scanning devices have been developed to enhance accuracy and reproducibility. Measurements are recorded on forms that are specific to the body segment being treated, such as the technical analysis form previously described. These measurements are used in two ways: as a reference when modifications to the positive cast are needed and as the way to determine the placement of the perimeter trimlines of the device.

Negative Mold

A negative impression is a mold taken of an actual body part that is used to create the three-dimensional positive cast or model necessary for fabrication of the orthosis or prosthesis. This negative impression is most often taken with a plaster of Paris bandage or fiber resin tape, although in some instances direct impressions are used as an alternative. Creation of a negative impression has four steps. First, a layer of tubular stockinet or a stocking is placed over the skin to create a protective interface and control the position of soft tissue structures within the cast (Figure 6-4). Tubular stockinettes are available in sizes that range from small diameter for the pediatric limb to large diameter for the adult torso. When a direct impression technique is being performed, a topical separator such as petroleum jelly can be used as an interface to minimize the risk of capturing cuticle hair in the impression. Second, bony prominences or other important guiding landmarks are marked on the body segment with indelible ink. These marks transfer to the inside of the negative mold and from there to the surface of the positive model.

Once the limb or body segment has been prepared, a thin layer of plaster of Paris or fiber resin tape is applied (see Figure 6-4B). This procedure differs from that of fracture casts in one important way: the goal is to achieve an "intimate" fit that captures the actual contours of the limb or body segment so that no protective padding is required. Rolls of elasticized plaster can be wrapped circumferentially in no more than two or three layers. Alternatively, strips of the material can be laid along the length of the limb or body segment. Most impression casting materials are readily available in roll form, although special versions have been produced for specific types of impression procedures, such as the fiber resin sock for an AFO. As the molding material is applied, the clinician smoothes the surface, following the normal shape of the limb. While the mold hardens, the clinician supports the limb or segment in the desired position, sometimes applying a light corrective force. As an example, the desired limb position of an orthosis incorporating the ankle joint might be in subtalar and talocrural neutral. If a PTB socket design is desired for a transtibial prosthesis, an extra force applied just distal to the patella marks its desired location on the resulting positive mold.

Once the cast is hardened sufficiently, it is carefully removed from the limb segment, preserving its shape and contours, and checked for alignment (see Figure 6-4C and D). It is essential that the clinician who takes the negative impression has a

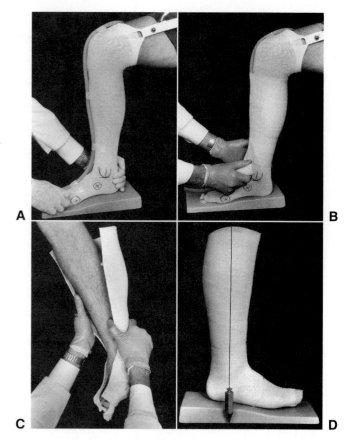

FIGURE 6-4 The procedure for taking a conventional negative impression begins with placing a layer of cotton stockinette over the limb and marking bony prominences with an indelible water-soluble transfer pencil (**A**). Surgical tubing is positioned on the anterior aspect of the limb to serve as a guideline for cast removal and to protect the shin. The limb is positioned on a shoe "last" impression in preparation for circumferential application of a plaster of Paris bandage or fiber resin casting tape (**B**). The impression board allows the foot to assume the contours of a shoe during molding for an optimal foot/shoe/AFO interface. Once the cast is "set," a cast saw is used to open the front of the cast (**C**), and the negative impression is carefully removed from the limb. The anterior edges are closed, and the ankle-foot alignment of the negative impression is verified with a plumb line (**D**).

thorough understanding of the forces that will be applied to the anatomical segments involved to ensure optimal fit and function of the orthosis or prosthesis. Estimates of soft tissue compression and skeletal alignment changes need to be carefully considered during the negative impression procedure. A skilled and experienced professional uses clinical judgment to create a negative impression, not only to capture the shape of the anatomical segment but also to apply an efficient force system to improve or maximize function. Basic design decisions must be made before the impression procedures so that any special accommodations required for the desired functional outcome can be incorporated.

Special negative impression techniques have been developed for specific purposes. Polystyrene foam impression blocks are one of the common methods of acquiring an impression of the plantar surface of the foot.[38] For patients who are recovering from facial burns, fabrication of a facial orthotic designed to deliver even, steady pressure during the period of scar maturation requires a highly detailed mold of the face. Alginate impressions, also referred to as *moulage techniques*, similar to those used in dentistry, are often used.

Fabricating and Modifying the Positive Model

Conventional methods for creating a positive cast are well established. The negative impression is prepared by sealing the mold so that it can accept liquid plaster of Paris. A separator material (e.g., silicone, soap) is added to the inner walls of the mold before the plaster of Paris is poured so that it can be removed more easily once the positive model has set. Once the cast has solidified, the negative impression is stripped away and discarded. The anatomical landmarks and reference points marked on the limb or body segment with indelible pencil and transferred from the patient to the negative impression are again transferred to the positive model. A mandrel (post) is embedded into the setting plaster of the positive model. This mandrel is used to hold the model for cast rectification and the rest of the production processes.

Model rectifications remove artifacts produced during the molding or impression process and bring the cast to specification of the measured values taken from the patient. Once the positive model has been rectified, further modifications can be made on the basis of the design of the orthosis or prosthesis being fabricated. During the negative impression procedure, soft tissue may have been manipulated for specific applications of force or pressure to be incorporated into the final orthosis or prosthesis. Although the positive model represents a three-dimensional shape of a respective body segment, it cannot relay information about the density of the tissue that it will interface. In general, additional plaster is added where relief of pressure is desired (e.g., over bony prominences) (Figure 6-5) or is removed where additional forces are to be applied. When the orthosis or prosthesis is formed over the model, an area of relief for a more intimate fit is achieved. Although some guidelines have been established regarding the amount of material to be removed or added to the positive model, the clinical experience of the prosthetist or orthotist is essential in this stage of the process. The positive model can also be modified to reconfigure surface geometry to improve the strength of the finished product.

Once design changes have been incorporated into the model, its surface is prepared for component production. This involves removing any surface imperfections with abrasive tools and abrasive sanding screen to ensure that the surface in contact with skin will be smooth. The positive cast is then ready to be used as a form from which different materials can be shaped to produce an interface component.

Fabricating the Orthosis or Prosthetic Socket

The fabrication process used with the positive model depends on the material selected for the device. Thermoforming is a common production method used in orthotics and prosthetics. Thermoplastic sheet material is heated in an oven until

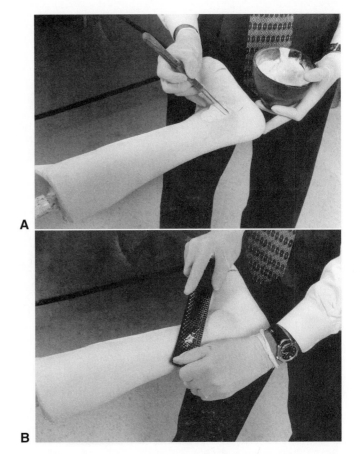

A

B

FIGURE 6-5 In the rectification of a positive model, plaster of Paris added over pressure-sensitive areas, such as the lateral malleolus (**A**), results in a "relief" in the finished orthosis. Modification of the positive model by removal of material with a plaster rasp over pressure-tolerant areas (**B**) increases intimacy of fit for better loading or stabilizing of the limb.

it has reached its "plastic" state, then shaped over a positive model by changing the air pressure difference across its surface (vacuum forming) (Figure 6-6). Once the plastic has cooled and returned to its solid state, trimlines aredelineated on the formed plastic before the edges are finished and smoothed.

CAD/CAM

In the 1960s, an alternative method of prosthetic fabrication that used computers was first introduced. Early CAD/CAM methods used stereophotography and digitization to create a numerical model, which guided a milling machine in the creation of a positive model of the residual limb.[2] A more complete concept of fabrication and manufacture of a prosthesis was developed at the University College London in the late 1970s and early 1980s.[39] After establishing a system for automated production of a prosthesis called Rapidform, the London research group conceived a completely automated fabrication process that used appropriate prosthetic alignment data.[40]

In the United States, the Veterans Administration began funding research projects in the 1980s to investigate

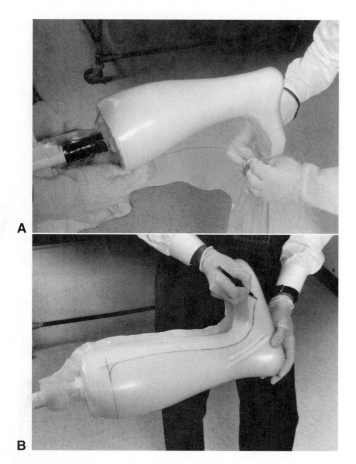

FIGURE 6-6 Once a sheet of thermoplastic material has been heated, it is dropped over the rectified positive model (**A**) and the edges of the thermoplastic are sealed. Negative pressure created by a vacuum pump removes any trapped air and draws the polypropylene to the surface of the positive model. When the material has cooled, trimlines are drawn on the formed plastic (**B**) by using measurements taken during the initial evaluation and bony landmarks as guides. Note the corrugations incorporated to strengthen the orthosis at the ankle.

the potential of CAD/CAM in orthotics and prosthetics. Advances were also made in private industry as the availability of personal computers became widespread. Beginning in the late 1980s, manufacturers have designed a multitude of CAD/CAM systems for various applications in orthotics and prosthetics. Advances in computer hardware, processors, and software have made CAD/CAM systems fast and efficient as well as an economical alternative for fabrication of devices for many orthotic and prosthetic practices.

Today, most CAD systems use a scanning device to record digital information of a body segment for CAM. The primary components of a CAD/CAM system consist of a digitizing device, computer, and milling machine. Surface contours of the anatomical segment are recorded with various digitization devices: optical-laser scanners, surface-contacting stylus, and pneumatically operated mechanical posts. Digital information acquired from a scan of a body segment is processed by the computer and translated into a triordinate data point file. This file is used by the computer to create a graphic image in the form of a surface contour plot.[41] The data are then

relayed to a milling unit to carve an orthosis or prosthesis for a positive model.

Data Acquisition

Each of the many digitizers used for data acquisition is designed for a specific task or to handle certain anatomical regions. Noncontact laser digitizers capable of circumferential scanning are well suited for measurement of cylindrical shapes such as those found in limb prosthetics or spinal orthotics. An optical-laser camera mechanism images the surface topography of the body segment and records the measured data points in a computer. Special holding fixtures and bars to aid in patient comfort and safety are part of each system. An apparatus designed to scan the torso for a spinal orthosis usually requires a different setup than that of a limb prosthesis. Some scanners are capable of digitizing directly from the patient's body segment, whereas other systems take measurements from a negative impression or mold of the segment (Figure 6-7). Compact, handheld contact digitizers have been introduced by several CAD/CAM manufacturers. These units allow the clinician to digitize a body segment by direct contact with the skin. Handheld contact digitizers are described

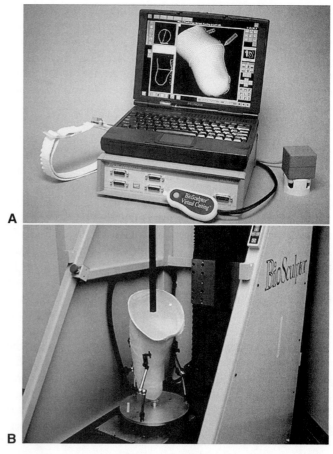

FIGURE 6-7 Examples of CAD/CAM data acquisition systems. A digital model of the residual limb (**A**) can be captured by a laptop computer, appropriate signal processor components, and a handheld digitizer. Laser digitization (**B**) can be used to capture accurately the contours of a conventional negative impression of a residual limb. (Courtesy BioSculptor Corporation, Hialeah, Fla.)

as a wand, pen, stylus, or pointer. Contact digitizers often have special attachments to scan certain shapes or measurement tools, such as calipers, for acquiring anteroposterior or mediolateral dimensions. Their versatility permits data acquisition of complex shapes. In some systems, handheld digitizers can be used in conjunction with a laser scan.

The use of digitizers in the production of foot orthoses is also becoming more common. Several systems based on differences in technique and philosophy in foot orthosis design have been developed for data acquisition of the foot. For full weight-bearing or partial weight-bearing techniques, pneumatically operated mechanical posts are used to digitize the foot's plantar surface (Amfit Corp, Vancouver, Wash.). Orthotic contoured shapes such as metatarsal domes can be evaluated during the digitization procedure to determine optimal position and comfort before fabrication. An optical-laser scanner situated under an acrylic platform has also been used for scanning the foot when a weight-bearing technique is desired (Bergmann Orthotics Lab, Northfield, Ill.). Because this system is also capable of scanning the foot with non–weight-bearing methods without the platform, it is quite versatile in clinical practice.

In many instances, orthotists and prosthetists are restricted to surface geometry and palpation of underlying anatomical structures to interpret the position of skeletal and soft tissue structures of the body segment. Magnetic resonance imaging and computed tomography have been used to create a three-dimensional computer model and assist in making design decisions for a mechanical device (Figure 6-8). Data from these scans are converted to a working format for specific graphic and modeling programs. Although this capability may not be practical for all applications, it may offer insight into areas of further research and development in the field.

Shape-Manipulation Software

The ability to modify the three-dimensional model of a patient's body segment permits the clinician to incorporate the desired biomechanical controls into an orthosis or prosthesis. The amount of force applied to a specific area depends in part on manipulation of the digital three-dimensional model. Software packages are now available to assist orthotists and prosthetists in designing the most appropriate modifications for a given patient. Generic modification templates or custom-designed templates can be used to make a wide range of revisions to the data. The clinician can incorporate reliefs for bony prominences of the limb or trunk or can change the geometry of the shape to enhance structural strength characteristics in the final orthosis or prosthesis. Trimlines can be delineated so that technicians who are involved in the assembly of components can complete a device without further instruction.

Milling and Production

Once the digital model is in place, the milling apparatus creates the actual orthotic or prosthetic device. Because each type of orthosis or prosthesis usually has specific milling parameters, a different setup may be required for each. For instance, the long, rounded shape of a transtibial or transfemoral

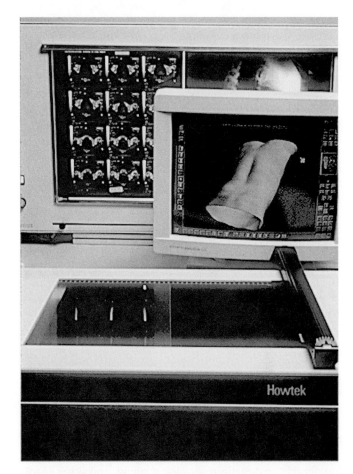

FIGURE 6-8 Computed tomographic or magnetic resonance images can be used to create a digitized computer model of a body segment for various orthotic or prosthetic CAD/CAM applications. The components of this type of system include an image scanner (foreground), a computer monitor for display of digitized images (e.g., the torso; center right), and the computed tomographic or magnetic resonance images being used (background). (Courtesy BioSculptor Corporation, Hialeah, Fla.)

socket is often manufactured with a lathe-type milling machine (Figure 6-9). In contrast, foot orthoses are manufactured by an end mill setup because their platelike structure and production processes create different finishing needs. The production laboratory needs to be large enough to have separate milling stations for each type of orthosis or prosthesis. This manufacturing limitation has led to the establishment of laboratory production companies that mill the positive models and manufacture the orthoses or prostheses from computer data transmitted by modem. Computer production networks can often reduce fabrication time and decrease production times, making the use of CAD/CAM economically feasible even for small orthotic/prosthetic facilities. Special production equipment is available that partially automates the thermoforming processes of some components. In the thermoforming machine for prosthetic sockets, a preformed polypropylene shell travels upward on a mechanical platform to an oven that heats the plastic to its formable temperature. The heated shell is then lowered over the positive model of the residual limb and vacuum formed for an intimate fit.

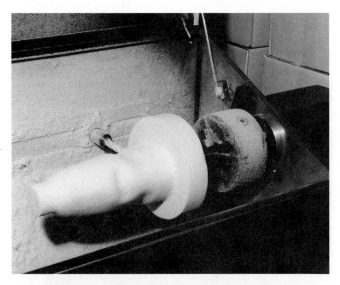

FIGURE 6-9 A positive model for a transtibial prosthetic socket being carved on a computer-controlled milling/lathe machine. (Courtesy Prosthetic Design, Inc., Clayton, Ohio.)

CAD/CAM in orthotics and prosthetics will play an important role in clinical and research settings. Although the development of CAD/CAM in orthotics and prosthetics has a history that spans more than two decades, only since the 1990s has it become an integral part of some clinical practices. Systems that have been designed for virtually all prosthetic and orthotic applications can be integrated with computed tomography, magnetic resonance imaging, and other medical imaging technologies. The technological advancements of CAD/CAM offer orthotists and prosthetists an additional clinical fabrication and research tool. Although this sophisticated equipment can contribute greatly to certain clinical and manufacturing tasks, successful fitting of a device depends on proper data input and prescription formulation.

CENTRAL FABRICATION AND MASS PRODUCTION

The techniques and processes associated with the fabrication of orthoses and prostheses described in this chapter can be relatively labor intensive and expensive. As managed care and insurance companies strive to reduce medical costs, the profession is under greater pressure to remain competitive by finding alternative production methods that are cost effective. One option is to maximize the clinical productivity of orthotists and prosthetists and limit their technical responsibilities. Central fabrication operations allow practitioners to develop clinical practices that do not require large technical facilities and space. Depending on the size of the practice, outsourcing the production portion of the business can be a more economical way to run an orthotic/prosthetic clinic. Some practitioners do not want to manage in-house technical operations that include additional technical staff, specialized equipment, and increased space requirements. Another advantage is that central fabrication may offer improvements in consistency and quality of devices.

Central Fabrication Facilities for Custom Devices

Central fabrication facilities typically specialize in the manufacture of custom orthoses and prostheses, often serving a large number of orthotic and prosthetic practices. These manufacturing services are available to produce almost every kind of orthosis and prosthesis, with many companies specializing in a specific area (e.g., spinal orthoses, knee orthoses, transtibial prosthetics). Some central fabrication operations offer the advantage of producing a device without the need for a negative impression, an additional cost savings in time and materials. A series of conventional measurements of patients combined with height and weight data is entered into a computer to generate a milled positive model for production. Orthotic systems in particular have been refined to produce excellent fitting devices that are comparable in function to custom-molded orthoses produced from a patient model. Although there will always be a need for custom-molded devices, technological advancements in human factors, ergonomics, and computer modeling will improve generic sizing and contoured interface systems, permitting a larger portion of the population to be fit with prefabricated devices and components. Modular components of varying material properties are already a part of general practice in prosthetics.

Mass Production

Mass-produced, prefabricated orthoses outnumber custom-molded orthoses fitted to patients for rehabilitative purposes. Orthopedic companies continue to develop orthotic and prosthetic products whose fit and performance approach that of custom-molded devices through diverse sizing systems and modular components. In the future, prefabricated modular component systems may bridge the gap between prefabricated and custom-molded devices by improving performance outcomes with custom-fitted systems and expanding their use in clinical practice. Although these advances in fit and function are possible for some problems, certain deformities and pathological conditions will almost always require custom-molded or measured orthoses and prostheses made by traditional or CAD/CAM methods of production.

MAINTENANCE OF ORTHOSES AND PROSTHESES

Routine care and maintenance of orthoses and prostheses are important for proper function and long-term use of a device. An orthotic or prosthetic maintenance program usually includes servicing by the orthotist or prosthetist and the patient. The service schedule depends on the specific orthosis or prosthesis, the materials from which it is made, the durability of the components, and the knowledge and ability of the patient and caregivers. Patient instructions for the daily care of an orthosis or prosthesis should include cleaning and inspection. Proper patient education of basic fitting criteria and instructions on donning and doffing a device allow the patient to evaluate the fit of a device during routine use.

Orthoses and prostheses should be inspected weekly for any defects, stress risers (nicks, scratches), loose screws, or weakened rivets. Any device that has mechanical components and moving parts and is subjected to repetitive loading requires periodic servicing; it is less expensive to recognize and fix early signs of a problem than it is to replace a device that has failed because of a lack of proper maintenance. Informing patients of potential problems associated with the use of their orthoses or prostheses and how to resolve these problems can prevent serious problems from arising.

Most plastic components should be cleaned with a mild antibacterial soap and rinsed thoroughly with cold water. Extra moisture should be absorbed with a towel and the orthosis or prosthesis air dried. Heat can distort some plastics; patients should be warned not to use electric hairdryers to dry their devices. Similarly, devices should not be left near direct heat sources, such as radiators, wood stoves, or any appliance that generates heat when running. They must also be protected from intense direct sunlight.

Leather liners and covers are cleaned weekly with a leather "saddle" soap. Leather softeners should not be used unless directed by the orthotist because they can compromise function of some straps and cuffs. Water-repellent treatments and protectants for leather often contain skin irritants and should not be used on leather components that have direct contact with the body.

Most orthoses and prostheses are designed to apply a corrective or stabilizing force to a body segment during wear. For some patients, especially those with fragile skin or scarring, this pressure may increase the risk of skin irritation or damage. The risk of skin problems differs from device to device and depends on the general health and skin condition of the individual who is wearing the orthosis or prosthesis. To minimize problems with skin intolerance of these extra forces, most new orthotic or prosthetic users begin with an intermittent wearing schedule. A treatment plan that incorporates a gradual buildup of orthotic or prosthetic use can avert complications such as excessive redness, chafing, and blisters. For a patient with a high risk for or a history of skin problems, a variety of preventive measures (e.g., foam or silicone interface liners) can be incorporated into the orthotic or prosthetic system.

Most custom orthoses or prostheses are designed to achieve a very intimate fit with the body segments that they encompass. Changes in the physical condition of a patient can significantly alter the fit and function of a device. Compromised fit occurs most often when the patient has had significant growth, weight gain or loss, muscle atrophy, edema, structural degeneration, or trauma. Periodic evaluations are necessary to ensure that fit and function are maintained in the months and years after the initial fitting. Semiannual or annual checkups should be part of the treatment plans for definitive orthotic and prosthetic devices.

To maintain proper function of a lower extremity prosthesis, special attention is needed in several areas. The alignment of a prosthesis is usually based on a specific heel height; variation from the prescribed heel height (when footwear is changed) often leads to functional problems during gait. In the same way, moderate to excessive wear of the shoe at the heel also compromises performance. The condition of footwear must be carefully and frequently monitored. The prosthesis should be free of dirt, sand, and other debris to ensure that joint mechanisms and their movements are not inhibited. Socket attachment and suspension systems need daily attention because they are usually prone to accumulation of lint, dirt, and other debris. If the prosthesis or any of its components are subjected to water, the device should be thoroughly dried to prevent permanent damage. Rubber bumpers in prosthetic feet deteriorate over time and with use and must be replaced regularly. The prosthetist can advise patients on specific parts that require regular maintenance.

The socket portion of a prosthesis should be faithfully cared for to avoid potential skin problems, especially infection, on the residual limb. When a special liner is used with a prosthesis, specific instructions for cleaning are necessary because materials used vary greatly. For patients who are fitted with suction sockets or special socket attachment mechanisms, the joining components or threads should be cleaned with a soft brush or rag to remove debris.

SUMMARY

This chapter explores the materials and methods most commonly used in the prescription, measurement, and production of orthoses and prostheses. The type of design, materials, and components are selected to best facilitate the functional goals of the patient. The foundation for effectiveness of the orthosis or prosthesis is careful measurement of the body segment (by casting or by CAD/CAM) and careful modification of the resulting model for optimal fit. For an individual who is being fit for his or her initial orthosis or prosthesis, shared decision making of the rehabilitation team, including the patient and caregivers, is essential. An orthosis or prosthesis that is difficult to don or is uncomfortable to wear is more likely to be found standing in a closet or pushed under a bed than on the patient for daily use.

REFERENCES

1. Committee on Artificial Limbs. *Terminal Research Reports on Artificial Limbs (Covering the Period from April 1, 1945 through June 30, 1947)*. Washington, DC: National Research Council; 1947.
2. Wilson AB. History of amputation surgery and prosthetics. In: Bowker JH, Michael JW, eds. *Atlas of Limb Prosthetics: Surgical, Prosthetic, and Rehabilitation Principles*. 2nd ed. St. Louis: Mosby; 1992:3–15.
3. Wilson AB. Prosthetics and orthotics research in the U.S.A. *International Conference on Prosthetics and Orthotics*. Cairo: S.O.P. Press; 1972:268–273.
4. Rang M, Thompson GH. History of amputations and prostheses. In: Kostuik JP, Gillespie R, eds. *Amputation Surgery and Rehabilitation: The Toronto Experience*. New York: Churchill Livingstone; 1981:1–12.
5. Eberhart HD, Inman VT, Dec JB, et al. *Fundamental Studies of Human Locomotion and Other Information Relating to the Design of Artificial Limbs. A Report to the National Research Council*. Berkeley, CA: University of California; 1947.

6. Kay HW. Clinical applications of the Veterans Administration Prosthetic Center patellar tendon-bearing brace. *Artif Limbs.* 1971;15(1):46–67.

7. Mooney V, Nickel VL, Harvey JP, et al. Cast-brace treatment for fractures of the distal part of the femur. *J Bone Joint Surg Am.* 1970;52A(8):1563–1578.

8. Sarmiento A, Sinclair WF. *Tibial and Femoral Fractures—Bracing Management.* Miami: University of Miami; 1972.

9. Committee on Prosthetics Research and Development. *Report of the Seventh Workshop Panel on Lower Extremity Orthoses of the Subcommittee on Design and Development.* Washington, DC: National Research Council–National Academy of Sciences; 1970.

10. Eberhart HD, McKennon JC. Suction-socket suspension of the above-knee prosthesis. In: Klopsteg PE, Wilson PD, eds. *Human Limbs and Their Substitutes.* New York: McGraw-Hill; 1954.

11. American Society of Testing and Materials (ASTM). *Standards.* Philadelphia: ASTM; 2001.

12. International Organization for Standardization (ISO). *Prosthetics-Orthotics.* Paramus, NJ: ILI Infodisk; 2000.

13. Shurr DG, Michael JW. Methods, materials, and mechanics. *Prosthetics and Orthotics.* 2nd ed. Norwalk, CT: Appleton & Lange; 2002: 2137.

14. O'Flaherty F. Leather. In: American Academy of Orthopaedic Surgeons, eds. *Orthopaedic Appliances Atlas.* Ann Arbor, MI: JW Edwards; 1952:17–28.

15. Redford II JB. *Orthotics Etcetera.* 3rd ed. Baltimore: Williams & Wilkins; 1986.

16. Murphy EF, Burnstein AH. Physical properties of materials including solid mechanics. In: American Academy of Orthopaedic Surgeons, eds. *Atlas of Orthotics: Biomechanical Principles and Application.* 2nd ed. St. Louis: Mosby; 1985:6–33.

17. Compton J, Edelstein JE. New plastics for forming directly on the patient. *Prosthet Orthot Int.* 1978;2(1):43–47.

18. Lockard MA. Foot orthoses. *Phys Ther.* 1988;68(12):1866–1873.

19. Peppard A, O'Donnell M. A review of orthotic plastics. *Athletic Training.* 1983;18(1):77–80.

20. Manganon PL. The *Principles of materials Selection for Engineering Design.* Prentice Hall; 1999.

21. Levitz SJ, Whiteside LS, Fitzgerald TA. Biomechanical foot therapy. *Clin Podiatr Med Surg.* 1988;5(3):721–736.

22. Hertzman CA. Use of Plastizote in foot disabilities. *Am J Phys Med.* 1973;52(6):289–303.

23. Jopling UH. Observation on the use of Plastizote insoles in England. *Lepr Rev.* 1969;40:175–176.

24. Mondl AM, Gardiner J, Bisset J. The use of Plastizote in footwear for leprosy patients. A preliminary report. *Lepr Rev.* 1969;40(3):177–181.

25. Tuck UH. The use of Plastizote to accommodate foot deformities in Hansen's disease. *Lepr Rev.* 1969;40(3):171–173.

26. Spence WR, Shields MN. Insole to reduce shearing forces on the soles of the feet. *Arch Phys Med Rehabil.* 1968;49(8):476–479.

27. Campbell G, Newell E, McLure M. Compression testing of foamed plastics and rubbers for use as orthotic shoe insoles. *Prosthet Orthot Int.* 1982;6(1):48–52.

28. Campbell G, McLure M, Newell EN. Compressive behavior after simulated service conditions of some foamed materials intended as orthotic shoe insoles. *J Rehab Res.* 1984;21(2):57–65.

29. Leber C, Evanski PM. A comparison of shoe insole material in pressure relief. *Prosthet Orthot Int.* 1986;10(3):135.

30. Pratt DJ, Rees PH, Rodgers C. Assessment of some shock absorbing insoles. *Prosthet Orthot Int.* 1986;10(1):43.

31. Rome K. Behavior of orthotic materials in chiropody. *J Am Podiatry Assoc.* 1990;80(9):471–478.

32. Foto JG, Birke JA. Evaluation of multidensity orthotic materials used in footwear for patients with diabetes. *Foot Ankle Int.* 1999;20(2):143.

33. Gillespie KA, Dickey JP. Determination of the effectiveness of materials in attenuating high frequency shock during gait using filter bank analysis. *Clin Biomech (Bristol, Avon).* 2003;18(1):50–59.

34. Cinats J, Reid DC, Haddow JB. A biomechanical evaluation of sorbothane. *Clin Orthop Relat Res.* 1987;Sep(222):281–288.

35. MacLellan GE, Bybyan B. Management of pain beneath the heel and Achilles tendonitis with visco-elastic heel insert. *Br J Sports Med.* 1981;15(2):117.

36. McCollough III NC. Biomechanical analysis systems for orthotic prescription. In: American Academy of Orthopaedic Surgeons, eds. *Atlas of Orthotics: Biomechanical Principles and Application.* 2nd ed. St. Louis: Mosby; 1985:35–75.

37. Redhead RG. Prescription criteria, fitting, check-out procedures and walking training for the above-knee amputee. In: Murdoch G, Donovan RG, eds. *Amputation Surgery and Lower Limb Prosthetics.* Oxford: Blackwell Scientific; 1988.

38. Schuster RO. Neutral plantar impression cast: methods and rationale. *J Am Podiatry Assoc.* 1976;6(66):422–426.

39. Davies RM, Lawrence RB, Routledge PE, et al. The Rapidform process for automated thermoplastic production. *Prosthet Orthot Int.* 1985;9(1):27–30.

40. Davies RM. Computer aided socket design: the UCL system. In: Davies RM, ed. *Annual Report of the Bioengineering Centre.* Roehampton, England: The Bioengineering Centre; 1986: 9–12.

41. Davis FM. In-office computerized fabrication of custom foot supports. The AMFIT system. *Clin Podiatr Med Surg.* 1993;10(3):393–401.

7

Footwear: Foundation for Lower Extremity Orthoses

Jennifer M. Bottomley

LEARNING OBJECTIVES

On completion of this chapter, the reader will be able to:
1. Determine the proper fit of standard footwear on the basis of necessary function of the foot during gait and the contour and alignment of a patient's foot.
2. Recommend appropriate footwear styles and characteristics for patients with foot deformity and for patients who wear orthoses or prostheses.
3. Describe the shoe modifications and accommodative orthoses that can be used to address musculoskeletal problems affecting the foot and lower limb.
4. Describe the effect of selected problems and deformity of the forefoot, midfoot, or rearfoot on weight bearing and efficiency of the gait cycle, and suggest appropriate footwear or orthotic interventions to reduce pain and improve function.
5. Identify special footwear needs for individuals with arthritis, gout, diabetes, peripheral vascular disease, hemiplegia, and amputation or congenital deformity of the foot and leg.

The most essential element of clothing in any person's wardrobe is the shoe. No other article of clothing is designed to fit so precisely. Continuous pressure from tight shoes can produce ulceration and deformities. Ill-fitting shoes can create shear forces that lead to skin breakdown, create and facilitate toe and foot deformities, and lead to falls.[1] Shoes perform the vital functions of transferring body weight to the floor during walking and of protecting the wearer from any hazards in the environment. A well-designed shoe is the necessary foundation for many lower extremity orthotics and for prosthetic alignment and an energy-efficient gait. This chapter discusses the components and characteristics of shoes, ensuring proper fit, and choosing appropriate footwear for patients with foot dysfunction and deformity.

COMPONENTS OF A GOOD SHOE

A suitable pair of shoes minimizes stress on all portions of the feet, provides support, and acts as a shock absorber of ground reaction forces.[2] The basic parts of a shoe are the sole, upper, heel, and last. Each of these parts is further divided into component parts or areas that are required for proper shoe design (Figure 7-1). Each component is crucial to the prescription of appropriate shoes for the person's individual needs.

Sole

The sole protects the plantar surface of the foot. The traditional sole consists of two pieces of leather sewn together with a layer of compressible cork between. An additional layer, the insole, is situated next to the foot in most shoes. A heavy thick sole protects the foot against walking surface irregularities. The rigidity or stiffness of the sole is also important. Although it needs to be durable, the sole must not be so rigid as to interfere with the toe rocker of the metatarsophalangeal (MTP) hyperextension during terminal stance and preswing phases of gait.

Various areas of the sole are identified by location. The *welt* is the inside piece of the external sole; the *outsole* is the portion that is most external. The area that lies between the heel and the ball of the shoe, the *shank,* is commonly fabricated to provide reinforcement and shape using materials such as spring steel, steel and leatherboard, or wood strips between the welt and the outsole. The purpose of the shank is to prevent collapse of the material between the heel and the ball of the foot and to provide extra support. In most athletic shoes, the sole is rubber to provide maximal traction. Rubber soles absorb shock, thereby minimizing heel impact forces.

Upper

The upper of the shoe—divided into the *vamp, tongue,* and *rear quarters*—covers the dorsum of the foot. The vamp extends from the insole forward. The tongue is an extension of the vamp in a blucher-style closure, but in the bal-type oxford, the tongue is separate (Figure 7-2). The blucher-style closure can be opened slightly more than the bal oxford closure to allow the foot into the shoe. The toe of the vamp is often covered with a separate piece of leather called the *tip.* The rearward line of the tip may be straight or winged. The vamp is joined to the quarters, which make up the sides and back of the upper. The two quarters are joined at a back seam. The design of the shoe dictates the shape and size of the quarters. For the oxford shoe, the outside quarter is cut lower than the inside to avoid contact with the malleoli. In the bal oxford, the back edges of the vamp cover the forward edges of the quarter.

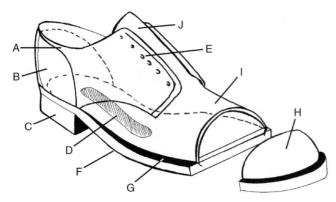

FIGURE 7-1 Basic parts of a shoe. The upper is made up of the quarter (**A**) and its reinforcing counter (**B**), which stabilize the rearfoot within the shoe; the closure (**E**) and the tongue (**J**) across the midfoot; and the shaft (vamp; **I**) and toe box (**H**), which enclose the forefoot. The exterior outsole (**F**) is often reinforced with a steel shank (**D**) and is attached to the upper at the welt (**G**). The standard heel (**C**) is ¾-inch high.

The forward edges of the quarters are on the top of the vamp in the blucher style of shoe.

For individuals wearing orthoses and those with foot deformity, the blucher closure is preferable to the bal-style closure because of its construction. The blucher closure has a separation between the distal margins of the lace stays, thus offering a wide inlet, making the shoes easier to don and doff and having a readily adjustable circumference. High shoes, which encase the malleoli, provide additional mediolateral stability.

Heel

The heel is located beneath the outer sole under the anatomical heel. The heel base is usually rigid rubber, plastic, or wood with a resilient plantar surface. As heel height increases, the ankle range of motion necessary to lower the forefoot to the floor increases. Weight-bearing pressures (vertical forces) on the forefoot and hallux also increase in midstance to late stance.[3] The individual with limited ankle motion may benefit from a compressible heel base to absorb shock and achieve plantar flexion during the early stance phase. A broad, low heel maximizes stability and minimizes stress on the metatarsal heads. Most lower extremity orthoses and prosthetic feet are designed for a specific heel height; efficacy of the orthosis or quality of the prosthetic gait can be significantly compromised if used with shoes that have higher or lower heels.

Reinforcements

Strategic shoe reinforcements contribute to foot protection. Toe boxing at the distal vamp shields the toes and prevents the anterior portion of the vamp from losing its shape. The toe box can also be increased in depth to protect and accommodate any toe deformities. The heel counter reinforces the quarters to help secure the shoe to the anatomical heel. The medial counter helps support the medial arch of the shoe, and the heel counter aids in controlling the rearfoot. The convex shank piece stiffens the sole between the distal border of the shoe heel and the MTP joints and aids in supporting the longitudinal arch.

Lasts

Shoes are constructed over a model of the foot, called a *last*, which is styled from wood, plaster, or plastic. Manufacturers are now converting to computer-aided last designs. Regardless of the origin of the last, it determines the fit, walking ease, and appearance of the shoe. Commercial shoes are made over many different lasts in thousands of size combinations. Most shoes are made with a medial last, which means that the toe box is directed inward from the heel (Figure 7-3). Shoes can also be made from conventional lasts, straight lasts, inflared or medial lasts, or outflared or lateral lasts.

FASHION VERSUS FUNCTION

A revolution to create comfortable and "healthy" shoes has occurred within the shoe industry in response to an epidemic of footwear-related health problems, the result of long-term wearing of improperly fitting shoes, which accounts for more than $3 billion annually in surgery-related costs.[4,5] Even the most savvy, health-conscious women sometimes buy shoes for looks, not fit. A survey of 356 women concluded that almost 90% of women wore shoes that were one to two sizes too small.[6] This trend contributes significantly to the development of bunions, hammertoes, claw toes,

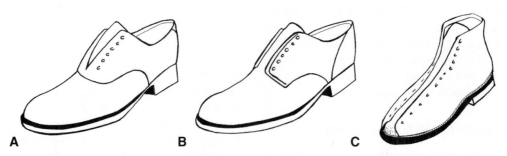

FIGURE 7-2 Three types of shoe closures. **A,** In the bal oxford style, the tongue is a separate piece sewn to the vamp and anterior edges of the quarters. **B,** In the blucher style, the tongue is an extension of the vamp and can be opened slightly wider. **C,** For patients with rigid ankle orthoses, fixed deformity, or fragile neuropathic feet, the lace-to-toe (surgical) style may be necessary.

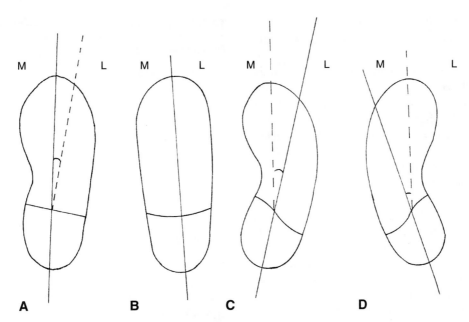

FIGURE 7-3 The last determines the shape of the shoe. **A,** In a conventional last, the forefoot is directly slightly lateral (L) to the midline. **B,** A straight last is symmetrical around the midline. **C,** An inflared last directs the forefoot medially. **D,** An outflared last directs it more laterally than a conventional last. M, medial.

mallet deformities, corns and calluses, and other disabling foot problems in midlife and later life.[7]

Enhancing Function

Foot stability is critical to minimizing ankle injury, excessive pronation, and slipping of the heel during the gait cycle. A well-designed shoe provides a broad heel base, ankle collar, and close-fitting heel counter. A keystone of a good shoe is its ability to absorb shock. The construction of and materials used for the insole, midsole, and outer sole determine the amount of shock absorption that the shoe will provide.

A good shoe must be flexible and provide stability with each step. Flexible construction is especially important in the sole to enhance the toe rocker in late stance phase. The sole should also provide adequate traction as it contacts the ground, especially in early stance as body weight is transferred onto the foot. A coefficient of friction that is sufficient to minimize slips and near slips is vital. Heel height can create stress on the forefoot during gait. Heels of more than 1½ inches exponentially increase weight-bearing forces on the metatarsal heads.[7]

The ability of a shoe to handle moisture is also an important consideration. For optimal foot health and comfort, perspiration must be wicked away and, at the same time, external moisture must be kept out.

The upper should be soft and pliable. Modern tanning techniques can create strong but supple uppers that surround the feet supportively and protectively without rubbing and chafing, while allowing the foot to breathe.

Orthotic-Related Function

A molded insole contributes to foot stability, shock absorption, and a transfer of shear forces away from problem areas. Orthoses can enhance the function of the shoes. Chapter 8 presents the principles and practices of orthotic prescription in commonly occurring conditions of the foot.

PROPER FITTING OF A SHOE: "IF THE SHOE FITS"

The two primary determinants of proper shoe fit are shoe shape and shoe size. *Shoe shape* refers to the shape of the sole and the upper. Proper fit is achieved when shoe shape is matched to foot shape. *Shoe size* is determined by arch length, not by overall foot length.[8] The proper shoe size is the one that accommodates the first metatarsal joint in the widest part of the shoe. Properly fitting shoes are important in avoiding foot discomfort and deformity and are absolutely essential in individuals with arthritis, diabetes, and other foot disorders.

Great variability is found in human foot size and shape. Mass-produced shoes, however, are formed over fairly standard lasts that give a shoe its special size and shape. In the well-fit shoe, the shape determined by the last approximates the human foot. The design and construction of the shoe should allow for a roomy toe box; it should be wide enough for normal toe alignment and be ½ inch longer than the longest toe. Proper fit of the forefoot in the shoe can be a critical factor in reducing the incidence of bunions, hammertoes, and other forefoot deformities. In general, the shoe should be wide enough to accommodate the widest part of the forefoot. A tracing of the foot (standing) should fit within an outline of the shoe bottom.

Proper fit presupposes proper design, shape, and construction and is fundamentally wedded to availability in widths as well as lengths. It is important that the clinician cultivate a consumer mindset that realizes the medical importance of modifying the old cliché "if the shoe fits, wear it" to "if the shoe fits, wear it, and if it doesn't, order it in the correct size."

Determining Measurements

The average shoe salesperson does not offer to measure the foot, instead relying on the consumer to know his or her foot size. However, because foot size changes over time, periodic measurement of both feet for length and width is important. Many shoe styles that are available in retail shoe stores do not appropriately match the shape of an individual's foot. As a result, comfort and protection are compromised in the name of "style." This is especially problematic in the presence of foot deformity. Hallux valgus is a foot deformity that is aggravated by wearing shoes too narrow across the metatarsal heads and triangularly shaped in the toe box. Shoes should be wide enough to allow the material of the upper that surrounds the widest region of the forefoot (i.e., the metatarsal heads) to be compressed at least $\frac{1}{16}$ inch before bony contact is made. Likewise, there should be at least a $\frac{1}{2}$ inch between the tip of the longest toe and the front of the toe box in weight bearing (generally the width of the thumb).

In the United States, 12 standard shoe widths are manufactured. They range from the very narrow AAAAA to the very wide EEEE—that is, AAAAA, AAAA, AAA, AA, A, B, C, D, E, EE, EEE, EEEE. Because most retail stores stock shoes of midrange widths (A-E), patients with narrow or wide feet often have difficulty finding shoes of the optimal width.

Standard shoe sizes are available in half-size increments, from an infant's size 0 to a man's size 16 in U.S. sizes. The difference in length between half sizes is $\frac{1}{16}$ inch. Standard shoe-sizing classifications are made by groups and lasts: infants' sizes 0 to 2; boys' sizes 2½ to 6; girls' sizes 2½ to 9; women's sizes 3 to 10; and men's sizes 6 to 12. Sizes larger than women's size 10 and men's size 12 must often be specially ordered. A U.S. women's shoe size is usually three half sizes smaller than the corresponding men's size (e.g., women's size 9 is the same as a men's size 7½).

European and U.K. manufacturers use a different numbering system. The comparison of European and U.K. women's to men's sizes is based on centimeters (e.g., women's size 38 EUR/5 UK is the same as men's size 40 EUR/5 UK). Table 7-1 compares the standard sizes for U.S., European, and U.K. shoe manufacturers and lists the measures for each size.

Foot Contour

Foot contour changes throughout the life cycle. Aging, pregnancy, obesity, and everyday stresses on the foot cause it to widen. Deformities such as bunions increase the width and shape of the foot, and splaying of the metatarsal heads creates a collapse of the transverse arch, further increasing the width of the forefoot.[9] Forefoot height may increase in the presence of toe deformities. Deformities such as pes planus (foot flattening) or pes cavus (high arches) change the contour of the midfoot. The shape of the foot must be considered and accommodated when an individual is measured for shoes. Often a "combined last" (where the last in the toe box is different from the rearfoot counter) is required to accommodate the contour of the foot. The relationship of the forefoot to the rearfoot is an important consideration in determining if the shoe shape, provided by the last, corresponds to the shape of

TABLE 7-1   *Comparison of Standardized Shoe Sizes*

United States	Europe	United Kingdom	Centimeters
WOMEN'S SIZES			
3	34	1	20
3½	34.5	1.5	20.5
4	35	2	21
4½	35.5	2.5	21.5
5	36	3	22
5½	36.5	3.5	22.5
6	37	4	23
6½	37.5	4.5	23.5
7	38	5	24
7½	38.5	5.5	24.5
8	39	6	25
8½	39.5	6.5	25.5
9	40	7	26
9½	40.5	7.5	26.5
10	41	8	27
MEN'S SIZES			
6	40	5	24
6½	40.5	5.5	24.5
7	41	6	25
7½	41.5	6.5	25.5
8	42	7	26
8½	42.5	7.5	26.5
9	43	8	27
9½	43.5	8.5	27.5
10	44	9	28
10½	44.5	9.5	28.5
11	45	10	29
11½	45.5	10.5	29.5
12	46	11	30

the foot. Shoes with medial, straight, or lateral lasts can be ordered to best meet patient needs.

Obesity and Edema

The additional mechanical stress of carrying excess weight takes its toll on the feet, often resulting in problems such as plantar fasciitis, arthritis and bursitis, heel pain, neuroma, and gait changes.[10] Frey and associates[10] found that a weight gain of as little as 9 lb over a 5-year period increased foot size by one full size. Obesity has been shown to increase the length and the width of the foot. The Frey study also revealed that although women tended to adjust for length increases by purchasing a longer shoe, they rarely increased shoe width. The net result over the 5-year study period included increased incidence of calluses, corns, bunions, hammertoes, ingrown toenails, and neuromas.

Obesity also has an impact on gait patterns. Obese persons demonstrate increased step width, increased ankle dorsiflexion with reduced plantar flexion, increased Q angles at the knee, increased hip abduction angles, increased abducted foot angles, greater out-toeing, a tendency for flat-footed weight acceptance early in the gait cycle, increased touchdown angles, more eversion at the subtalar joint, and a faster maximum eversion velocity. These gait changes may be an

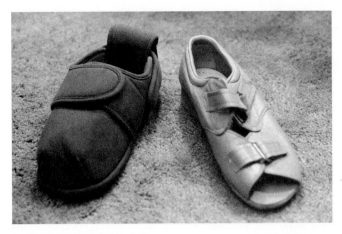

FIGURE 7-4 Thermold (P. W. Minor Shoes, Batavia, N.Y.) Velcro closure shoe/sandal. Adjustable Velcro closures are recommended to accommodate edematous feet and prevent tissue damage due to high pressure.

attempt to increase stability during gait. The net effect, however, is an increased incidence of overuse injuries as a result of everyday activities.[10]

Proper shoe fitting is essential for preventing secondary foot problems that stem from ill-fitting shoes. Overweight individuals should be encouraged to have their feet measured regularly, particularly if they have had a significant weight gain. It is often helpful to shop for shoes at the end of the day, when feet are largest, and the shoe fitting should be done with the person standing to ensure that ½ inch is between the end of the longest toe and the edge of the toe box. The shoes should be comfortable the moment they are worn.

Fluctuation in foot size in individuals with edema (e.g., those with kidney dysfunction or congestive heart failure or any patient who is taking diuretic medication) creates a challenge when fitting shoes. The contour of the foot is constantly changing. For someone with severe edema, a Thermold (P. W. Minor Shoes, Batavia, N.Y.) Velcro closure shoe/sandal (Figure 7-4) is recommended to accommodate and support the foot and prevent the undue pressures imposed by a shoe that becomes too small during the course of the day.

CONSEQUENCES OF THE ILL-FITTING SHOE

The national obsession with beauty has created some not-so-beautiful feet problems, such as bunions, hammertoes, and neuromas. These are particular problems for women, who often select poorly fitting shoes in an attempt to have the foot appear to be smaller, daintier, and narrower than it actually is. In Frey and associates' study,[6] 90% of women surveyed wore shoes that were too small by one or two width and length sizes, and 80% of these women had foot problems. Snow and associates[11] report that 90% of 795,000 surgeries for bunions, hammertoes/claw toes/mallet toes, neuromas, and Taylor bunions could be directly attributed to wearing ill-fitting shoes. Foot problems including bunions, lesser toe deformities, and neuromas are the primary consequences

of wearing ill-fitting shoes. Clearly, many of these problems would be prevented by habitual use of properly fitting shoes.

SPECIAL CONSIDERATIONS

Feet come in many shapes, sizes, and conditions of health. The biomechanical and functional characteristics of feet change over an individual's lifetime and must also be reflected in shoe choice. An infant's foot must adapt to weight bearing, especially as walking becomes functional. The foot of a child continues to adapt as normal growth changes alignment of pelvis, femur, and tibia. The influence of hormones during pregnancy also affects the structure and function of the foot. Finally, the combined influence of the aging process, obesity, and diseases that are common in later life can create special footwear needs for older adults.

Pediatric Foot

Many pediatric and lower extremity foot disorders are minimally symptomatic and do not require treatment, whereas others require more aggressive management. An understanding of the natural history of many of these disorders is important in establishing the appropriate footwear for toddlers and children as they begin to walk and run.[12-14]

In-toeing is a problem caused by positional factors in utero and during sleep, muscle imbalances due to paralytic disorders, and decreased range of motion in the lower kinetic chain. It may also be due to metatarsus adductus, internal tibia torsion, or internal femoral torsion.

Metatarsus adductus is characterized by a bean-shaped foot that results from adduction of the forefoot. In most children (approximately 85%), this disorder resolves itself spontaneously.[15] If it does not improve over the first 6 to 12 weeks of life, the treatment of choice is an outflared shoe. The bones of the foot are soft and can be corrected with positioning in the outflared shoe (reverse last) or Bebax shoe (Camp Healthcare, Jackson, Mich.).

Internal tibial torsion is a twist between the knee and the ankle. Generally, this torsion disappears by 5 years of age. Torsion can be exacerbated by abnormal sitting and sleep postures with the foot turned inward. (Some of the best athletes are in-toers.) The Dennis Browne bar or the counterrotation splint is used in combination with a reverse last shoe to remodel the bones during growth. Persistent severe toeing created by internal tibial torsion requires a derotational osteotomy of the tibia/fibula in the supramalleolar region.

Internal femoral torsion can also be the cause of in-toeing with a twist between the knee and hip. Neither splints nor shoes are effective in treatment of torsion. Habitual sitting in the "W" position (e.g., when a child is watching television or playing games on the floor) can aggravate the problem. Children with internal femoral torsion should be encouraged to sit "X" legged as an alternative.

Out-toeing occurs in children who sleep in the frog position and have soft tissue contractures around the hip. This is usually a hip or a long bone torsion problem and is not affected by footwear.

Toe walking can be the result of an in utero shortening or a congenital shortening of the Achilles tendon but can also be an early sign of cerebral palsy, muscular dystrophy, or Charcot-Marie-Tooth disease.[15] Until 4 years of age, the ability to stretch the tendon is well preserved, and conservative treatment includes stretching, casting, ankle-foot orthoses, and/or a night splint. Z-plasty lengthening is performed if conservative interventions fail. Shoe prescription objectives follow the same principles as those in the older adult with Achilles tendinitis (see Achilles Tendinitis, Bursitis, and Haglund's Deformity).

Flexible flatfoot appears to reflect generalized hereditary ligamentous laxity.[16] Treatment for flatfootedness in children has changed over time. Currently, the shoe used to treat flatfoot is designed to correct heel valgus, support the arch, and pronate the forefoot in relation to the rearfoot. Forefoot pronation is achieved by using a lateral shoe wedge combined with a medial heel wedge. A scaphoid pad supports the arch, and a strong medial counter prevents medial rollover. A Thomas heel is often used to provide additional support for the arch.

Calcaneovalgus is a congenital positional deformity. The heel is in severe valgus, and the foot is dorsiflexed so much that it rests against the anterolateral aspect of the tibia. Calcaneovalgus is usually secondary to intrauterine position. Most cases correct spontaneously. Treatment of the severe cases includes stretching and serial casting. A few severe cases, if left untreated, persist into adolescence as pes planus.

An *accessory navicular bone* is a small ossicle at the medial tuberosity of the navicular. Individuals with an accessory navicular bone often complain of pressure and discomfort when wearing shoes. Often, placement of a prefabricated arch support in the shoe lifts the arch just enough to minimize rubbing on the shoe.

Hallux valgus (bunions) is most often the consequence of rearfoot valgus, leading to varus of the first metatarsal. The conservative approaches to treating this condition in children are orthoses and comfortable shoes, with a good heel counter to maintain the heel in subtalar neutral.

Curly toes involve the congenital shortening of the flexor tendons. Treated conservatively, flexors are stretched, and a rocker-like insole is used in the shoe to support the toes in extension. Shoes must have extra depth with plenty of room in the toe box.

Shoe prescription for these biomechanical problems of the foot and lower extremity in childhood is as valuable as a conservative corrective intervention. Overall, if a child's foot is developing normally and does not exhibit any signs of an abnormality, a soft-soled shoe is appropriate.[17,18] If some degree of abnormality exists, a more supportive, rigid shoe is indicated for toddlers. In general, the stiffer the heel counter, the more effective the intervention.

The most common prescription shoe for young children is a straight last shoe. This type of shoe is roomy enough to accommodate pads or wedges. In addition, a straight last shoe does not generate any abnormal forces against the child's foot.

Foot During Pregnancy

During pregnancy, women may experience problems in lower extremities, including edema, leg cramps, restless legs syndrome, joint laxity, and low back pain. As a result, foot pain is a common problem in pregnant women.[19] An important consideration is the provision of shoes with maximum shock absorption. Gel-cushioned running shoes are recommended, especially if women continue to jog or walk for exercise. Expectant mothers are also advised to exercise on soft surfaces to prevent problems caused by repetitive pounding on unforgiving surfaces.

High-heeled shoes exaggerate the lordotic curve and are inadvisable during pregnancy. As weight distribution shifts with advancing pregnancy, especially if edema occurs, many women choose to wear shoes with laces or a Velcro closure. Athletic and walking shoes provide good support, excellent cushioning, and a solid heel counter. If a heel is desired for special occasions, a 1-inch or lower heeled shoe should be recommended. Even low but tiny tapered heels cause women to wobble as they walk.

Many women find that their feet have "grown" during pregnancy; after having returned to prepregnancy weight and clothing, their shoes no longer fit. Measurements often reflect an increase in shoe length of a half to a full size. The stress of extra body weight coupled with ligamentous laxity can reduce arch height, adding length to feet. This process is a normal age-related change in foot structure, associated with wear and tear of the body over time, which is hastened during pregnancy. The hormonally induced tissue laxity of pregnancy leads to a broader forefoot as the metatarsal heads separate and the distal transverse arch flattens and to a longer foot as the longitudinal arch is less efficiently supported by soft tissue structures. For this reason, pregnant women are advised to wear a larger shoe size, with a square or deeper toe box, or both, especially if edema is also a problem.

Garbalosa and McClure[20] found that almost 80% of the general population has a forefoot varum deformity. This foot deformity displaces the center of gravity forward, which can increase stress on the back during pregnancy. Forefoot varum deformity produces instability whenever the center of gravity is moved anteriorly over the forefoot in weight bearing, forcing the foot into exaggerated pronation.[21] The net effect of the hormonal changes, pregnancy-induced forward displacement of the center of gravity, and the presence of forefoot varum is increased strain on the axial skeleton and reduced efficiency of gait. An orthosis to support the metatarsal heads and medial longitudinal arch, placed in shoes with good shock absorption ability, can help decrease foot discomfort and prevent injury to the low back during pregnancy.

Foot in Later Life

Foot problems are one of the most common complaints of older adults. The foot is also the most frequently neglected area of evaluation by most health care practitioners. In a study of patients who resided in a long-term care facility, 40% did not own properly fitting shoes. A subsequent survey indicated that the majority of community elders preferred to wear slippers and did not own adequate footwear.[22]

Gait disorders are a major cause of morbidity and mortality in older adults, significantly contributing to the risk of disabling injury.[23] Gait changes, poor health, and impaired vision are the major predictors for falls.[24] Many older persons attribute their problems with walking to pain or a sense of unsteadiness, stiffness, dizziness, numbness, weakness, or impaired proprioception.[24]

Physical therapists work with patients to maximize their functional abilities and mobility. Treating foot pain and dysfunction can be a fundamental contributor to becoming functional in ambulation. As Helfand so eloquently stated, "Ambulation is many times the key or the catalyst between an individual retaining dignity and remaining in a normal living environment or being institutionalized."[25]

Gait and foot problems in older adults are associated with diseases that are common in later life and with the aging process itself. Examples of conditions that can compromise gait and foot function include the residuals of congenital deformities, ventricular enlargement, spinal cord diseases, joint deformities, muscle contractures, peripheral nerve injuries, peripheral vascular disease, cerebrovascular accidents, trauma, ulcers, arthritis, diabetes, inactivity, and degenerative and chronic diseases.[23] The anatomical and biomechanical considerations of podogeriatrics focus on the interrelationships of the rearfoot, midfoot, and forefoot, established by osseous, muscle, and connective tissue structures. Movement of one joint influences movement of other joints in the foot and ankle. Soft tissue structures establish an interdependency of the foot and ankle to the entire lower limb. As tissues age, they become stiffer, less compliant, weaker, and more vulnerable to breakdown.

Foot contour alters with aging; the foot gets wider, and bunions and splaying occur from collapse of the transverse arch.[26] Forefoot height increases in the presence of toe deformities. Fat pads under the metatarsal joints atrophy and shift position distally, whereas the calcaneal fat pad atrophies and shifts laterally. These changes leave bony prominences that are vulnerable to breakdown.

In the diabetic patient, development of Charcot's joint (neuropathic arthropathy) is a relatively painless, progressive, and degenerative destruction of the tarsometatarsal or MTP joints.[27-30] With the sensory losses that are common in diabetes, these joints are subjected to extreme stresses without the benefits of normal protective mechanisms. Capsular and ligamentous stretching, joint laxity, distention, subluxation, dislocation, cartilage fibrillation, osteochondral fragmentation, and fracture occur.[31,32] Hyperemia increases the blood supply, which promotes resorption of bone debris with resorption of normal bone as well. The foot often fuses in a deformed rocker bottom shape, vulnerable to pseudoarthrosis, instability, abnormal weight-bearing surfaces, ulcerations, and infections.[33,34]

The majority of foot problems in geriatric patients can be managed with proper shoe fitting and minimal shoe modifications. The most inexpensive footwear for this patient population is running or walking shoes. These are less expensive and fit within a fixed-income budget.[35] They provide good foot support and can be purchased with Velcro straps for closure if hand function or foot edema is a problem. The Thermold shoe is also a blessing for all the pathological and structural deformities with which the older patient must deal.

CHOOSING APPROPRIATE FOOTWEAR AND SOCKS

A vast and somewhat bewildering variety of "off-the-shelf" footwear is available to consumers. Many shoes are designed with certain types of activities in mind. Understanding the design and construction, as well as ensuring proper fit, enhances foot health and minimizes the risk of foot dysfunction, injury, and pain.

Athletic Shoe Gear

Many people jump into fitness activities "feet first" and develop blisters, calluses, and other foot injuries because of inappropriate footwear. A well-fit, activity-appropriate athletic shoe enhances enjoyment of the activity by protecting and supporting the foot and minimizing injury. Athletic shoes are designed for specific activities. A running shoe is designed with a high-force heel impact and forward foot movement in mind; the various shoe models have specific features that are designed for different surface conditions and distances in running. Basketball shoes do not provide as much cushioning as do running shoes but instead focus on foot support during quick lateral movement. Aerobic shoes are also designed for lateral movement but provide more cushioning for the impact anticipated on the ball of the foot. Shoe soles are also designed for the surface on which the activity is performed. Some shoes are manufactured as cross-training shoes so that they can go from the workout in the gym to jogging but are not designed for high-mileage runners.

Determining the foot type is important in prescribing the best shoe. For individuals with a flat, low-arched foot, a shoe that provides maximum stability to prevent the foot from rolling in with each step is required. High-arched feet demand a shoe that is more flexible. "Normal" feet do best in a shoe that combines the last to accommodate the heel and the forefoot and that has forefoot flexibility. The size and shape of the toe box must also be considered. Enough room should be available in the toe box to prevent blisters, ulcers, and chafing of the toes. Shoes made from materials that "breathe" so that perspiration can escape are desirable. Athletic shoes are best used only for their intended activity and should be replaced at regular intervals to maximize their effectiveness.

Most athletic footwear is available in medium widths, although a few manufacturers provide shoes in several widths. Children's athletic footwear is available in narrow, medium, and wide widths. Women's athletic footwear may be available in AA, B, and D widths. Men's athletic footwear may be available in B, D, EE, and EEE widths. The key element in proper fit of athletic shoes is comfort from the moment the shoe is put on, with no break-in period needed. The shoe should also provide adequate support and shock absorption for the sport or activity that is being pursued.

Walking Shoes

A well-designed walking shoe provides stable rearfoot control, ample forefoot room, and a shock absorption heel and sole. This type of footwear may be specifically designed by an athletic footwear manufacturer or even by an orthopedic footwear manufacturer. Walking shoes are available in various widths and in several different lasts. Long medial counters, Thomas heels, and crepe soles can be used to modify this type of shoe gear to meet specific patient needs.

Dress Shoes

Despite the fashionable preference for shoes with narrow or pointed toes and slim high heels, the most foot-friendly dress shoe for women is a rounded-toe Mary Jane style with boxy heels. A good dress shoe approximates the shape of the individual's foot and provides flexibility and sufficient shock absorption. Prerequisites of a good dress shoe include a roomy toe box, low stable heel, proper width in the ball of the foot area, flexible outsole with skid-proof bottoms, and arch support.[36]

Triangular toe boxes and high heels, no matter how dainty, are best avoided because they can and do cause deformity. For a high-heeled shoe to stay on the foot, it must fit closely around the toes, resulting in no room for anything but the foot. The foot is virtually unsupported at the distal end of the shank, and extreme high pressure is present under the metatarsal heads. Heels higher than 2 inches make any kind of orthosis ineffectual.[37] Because the angle of the foot causes the heel of the orthosis to lift up, high heels can transform an orthosis into a catapult. Although orthoses can help relieve metatarsal and heel pain and provide arch support, they cannot offer any corrective features in a shoe that is designed so unnaturally for the human foot.[11]

Socks

The sock is often overlooked when shoes of any kind are prescribed. Socks can aid in shock absorption, shield the skin from abrasion by the shoe stitching and lining, and prevent skin irritation from shoe dyes and synthetic leather materials. Additionally, clean, freshly laundered socks are integral to a sanitary foot environment. Unbleached, white cotton socks are ideal because they lack dyes, are hypoallergenic, and absorb perspiration readily. Cotton socks also provide ample toe room, unlike socks that are made from stretchable fabric, which can crowd the toes.

The size and style of socks also influence foot health. Socks that are too short crowd the toes; those that are too long wrinkle within the shoe, creating potential shear pressure points. If knee-high socks are worn, the proximal band must not be unduly restrictive; similarly, the use of circumferential garters to hold socks can impede circulation to the foot. Any holes worn into the sock also potentially create shear pressures and should be discarded. Mended holes in socks, because of the

difference in thickness and materials, can irritate delicate or insensate soft tissue. An open hole at the toes pinches and constricts the digits, with excessive friction at the edges of the hole.

The Thor-lo sock (Thor-lo Inc., Statesville, N.C.) is specially designed to support and cushion the insensitive foot or athletic/military foot that is exposed to repetitive frictional forces. Use of these specially designed socks not only reduces the frictional shearing forces but also significantly decreases vertical ground reaction pressure forces, preventing blistering and ulceration.[38-43] Extra high-density padding functions as a natural fat pad, reducing the deteriorating effects of shearing forces and the pressure and friction in the toe area. The Thor-lo concept of stockings is beneficial for patients with insensitive feet. It has also been used for individuals involved in aerobic exercise, baseball, basketball, cycling, golf, hiking, trekking and climbing, skiing, tennis, walking, and running.

PRESCRIPTION FOOTWEAR, CUSTOM-MOLDED SHOES, ACCOMMODATIVE MOLDED ORTHOSES, AND SHOE MODIFICATIONS

Alteration of foot function and alignment can be accomplished with one or more of the following strategies: foot orthoses of the appropriate materials, prescription shoes, and modifications of shoes themselves.[44-46] These strategies are used to relieve pain and improve balance and function during standing and locomotion. These alternatives are indicated when a transfer of forces from sensitive to pressure-tolerant areas is needed to reduce friction, shock, and shear forces; to modify weight transfer patterns; to correct flexible foot deformities; to accommodate for fixed foot deformities; and to limit motion in painful, inflamed, or unstable joints.

When special protective or prescription footwear is being considered, the functional objectives must be clearly stated so that the appropriate specific prescription can be developed. Careful examination of the foot helps the clinician identify pathology or mechanical factors, or both, that must be addressed and choose the appropriate materials and footwear styles to meet the patient's specific needs.

Moldable Leathers

Thermold is an example of prescription footwear that can be used to protect feet that are vulnerable due to vascular insufficiency, neuropathy, or deformity (Figure 7-5). It is a cross-linked, closed-cell polyethylene foam laminated to the leather upper of the footwear that can be heat molded directly to the foot. This makes modification for foot deformity easily managed and far less expensive than custom molding. Thermold shoes are also available in extra-depth styles, with a removable ¼-inch insole. Extra-depth shoes enable adequate room for custom-made insoles or orthoses to become an intricate adjunct to the footwear. In some instances, the Thermold can be used as an alternative to the custom-molded footwear.

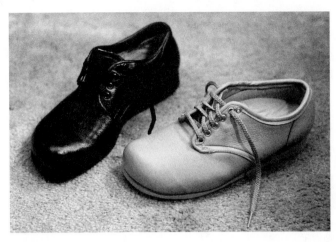

FIGURE 7-5 Thermold shoes (P. W. Minor Shoes, Batavia, N.Y.). These shoes allow for easy modification to accommodate foot deformities.

Custom-Molded Shoes

Some foot problems cannot be accommodated in conventional footwear, and the best solution is custom-molded footwear. This footwear is molded directly over a plaster reproduction of the foot rather than a standard last. Special modifications, such as toe fillers, Plastazote (Zoteforms, Inc., Hackettstown, N.J.), rocker bars, and elevations, can be added during manufacturing to meet the specific requirements of each foot. Because of this process, custom-molded shoes are made to conform to the foot shape in all respects (Figure 7-6). Custom orthopedic shoes represent the ultimate combination of function and aesthetics. Incorporating biomechanics and craftsmanship, shoes can redistribute weight, restrict joint motion, facilitate ambulation, and decrease the probability of neuropathic ulceration.[47,48]

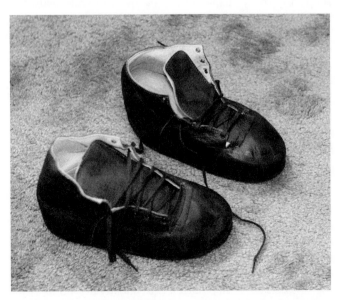

FIGURE 7-6 Examples of custom-molded shoes. These shoes are prescribed when foot deformities are too severe for accommodation in a conventional shoe.

Plastazote Shoe or Sandal

For patients with insensitive or ulcerated feet, a "healing sandal" or Plastazote shoe is often prescribed. This custom shoe is fabricated using a plaster cast of the individual's foot for construction.[49] Temporary protective footwear, such as a Plastazote boot or shoe or a healing sandal, is often used during neuropathic ulcer wound healing to allow for ambulation without pressure on the healing area, especially for patients who are unable to walk or noncompliant with non–weight-bearing ambulation.

Shoe Modifications

Various shoe modifications can be used to address functional and anatomical deformities of the foot and leg. Clearly stated objectives, based on careful evaluation, ensure that the appropriate shoe modifications are chosen.

Lifts for Leg-Length Discrepancy

For patients with leg-length discrepancy of ⅜ inch or more, a full-length external lift can be mounted to the sole of the shoe on the shorter limb to equalize leg length and reduce proximal stresses at the hips and spine. If the length difference is less than ⅜ inch, the discrepancy can usually be accommodated with an orthotic heel wedge worn inside the shoe. If the discrepancy is a result of a unilateral equinus deformity, a heel wedge can be attached to the external surface of the shoe. Leg length discrepancy is a common result of a hip fracture, congenital anomaly, or biomechanical imbalance such as pelvic rotation, hip anteversion or retroversion, or unilateral foot pronation. The level of the pelvis and absolute and relative measures of leg length should be part of a comprehensive gait evaluation.

Heel Wedging

Wedging is used to alter lines of stress to facilitate a more normal gait pattern. The most effective wedges range from ⅛ to ¼ inches in thickness at their apex. Larger wedges tend to cause the foot to slide away from the wedge toward the opposite side of the shoe, drastically reducing the effectiveness of the modification. Wedging is useful for children with a rotational problem, such as tibial torsion. In adults, wedges are used for accommodation in conditions such as a fixed valgus deformity of the calcaneus (Figure 7-7).

A medial heel wedge is used when flexible valgus of the calcaneus is present (Figure 7-8A). As the wedge elevates the

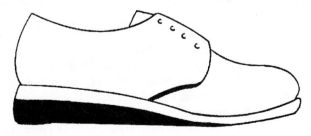

FIGURE 7-7 A heel wedge provides elevation of the heel for equinus deformity.

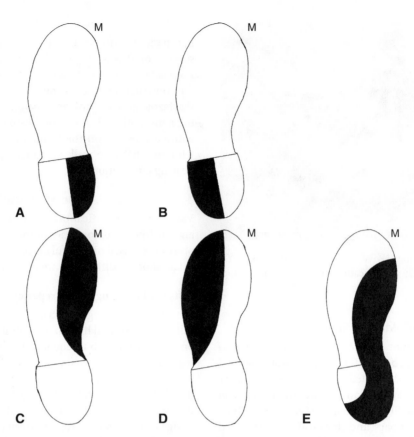

FIGURE 7-8 Examples of heel and sole wedge modifications. A medial (M) heel wedge (**A**) is used when flexible valgus of the calcaneus is present; a lateral heel wedge (**B**) is used for flexible varus of the calcaneus. Medial sole wedges (**C**) create an inversion effect of the forefoot, whereas lateral sole wedges (**D**) create an eversion effect. A Barton wedge (**E**) supports the navicular bone and helps invert the calcaneus, shifting the body weight laterally.

medial heel, a resultant varus tilt acts on the calcaneus, preventing excessive pronation of the foot. A lateral heel wedge is used when flexible varus of the calcaneus is present (see Figure 7-8B). Elevation of the lateral heel decreases the medial drive on floor contact at heel strike, tipping the calcaneus into valgus. A full heel wedge is sometimes used in the presence of fixed or functional equinus deformity. The goal of wedging is to obtain a subtalar neutral position during the stance phase of gait.

Sole Wedging

Wedging can also be used to modify midfoot and forefoot positions. A medial sole wedge produces an inversion effect on the forefoot. This wedge is positioned along the medial aspect of the footwear, from a point just proximal of the first metatarsal head to the midline of the footwear (see Figure 7-8C). Conversely, a lateral sole wedge creates an eversion effect at the forefoot. This wedge is placed proximal to the fifth metatarsal head to the midline of the footwear. The apex of this wedge is the fifth metatarsal head (see Figure 7-8D).

A Barton wedge (see Figure 7-8E) is used in the presence of severe, flexible pronation deformities, such as those seen in pes planus, when control of the midfoot is the goal. The Barton wedge, usually made with 3/16-inch leather, extends

along the medial side of the foot to the midtarsal joint and tapers laterally just anterior to the cuboid bone. It provides support to the navicular and helps invert the calcaneus. It is used when it is necessary to shift body weight laterally. When a Barton wedge is used, the shoe must have a firm medial counter. The Barton wedge can be incorporated in an internally placed lateral heel wedge for patients with fixed calcaneal varus or clubfoot deformity. Because an internal wedge is closer to the target deformity, it creates a positive force of greater magnitude than is possible with the external Barton wedge. Instead of tilting the footgear, the wedge tilts the calcaneus into the desired position.

Steel Spring

The steel spring, an external shoe modification, is a piece of flexible metal that is 1/16 inch in depth and 1 inch in width, extending along the length of the footwear. It is usually placed between the insole and outsole of the shoe to restrict flexion of the sole. The need to enhance the strength of the shoe shank is often required to control the foot when lower extremity bracing is necessary. A steel spring is frequently helpful in assisting an individual who has hemiplegia with forward propulsion during the vertical pathway of the foot, from initial contact through midstance and into push-off/terminal stance.

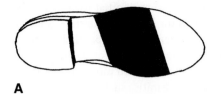 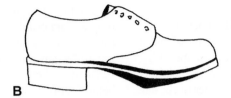 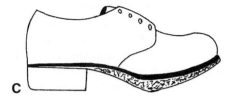

FIGURE 7-9 Examples of rocker bottom soles. A metatarsal bar (**A**) prevents undue pressure at the metatarsal heads during push-off in late stance. A rigid leather rocker sole (**B**) or an extended crepe rocker bar (**C**) redistributes body weight over the entire plantar surface, facilitating a smoother and more normal gait pattern while reducing stress and trauma in the forefoot.

Metatarsal Bars and Rocker Bottoms

A metatarsal bar is a block of material (usually stacked pieces of leather or rubber) that is attached to the sole of the shoe. Its placement proximal to the metatarsal heads significantly reduces pressure at the metatarsal heads during the push-off phase of the gait cycle.[50] The curved distal edge of the metatarsal bar is designed to follow the curve of the metatarsal heads. It is commonly used to adapt shoes worn by patients with transmetatarsal amputations, fixed arthritic deformities, diabetes, forefoot deformities such as hallux rigidus, and neuromas. The placement of a metatarsal bar or rocker facilitates push-off by simulating forward propulsion in the absence of metatarsal flexibility.

Rocker bottoms are made of either lightweight crepe or leather (Figure 7-9). These modifications are flush with the heel and toe, in an arch with an apex of ½ to ⅝ inch. The rocker bar redistributes body forces over the entire plantar surface of the foot while in weight bearing. It facilitates a smooth roll during the stance phase of gait, while reducing sheer stress and trauma to the midfoot and forefoot. It is often used to modify shoes worn by patients with partial foot amputations, arthritis, and diabetes. It is also used for patients who have any lower extremity orthosis that limits forward progression of the tibia over the foot and toes during mid- and late-stance phases. For patients with diabetes, a rigid rocker sole (a steel-spring heel-to-toe with the toes extended and a rocking axis near the center of the foot) can be used to help distribute body weight and compel knee flexion at toe-off, reducing the length of stride and sheer stress on the metatarsal heads.

Thomas Heels

The Thomas heel is designed to improve foot balance and relieve excessive pressure on the shank portion of the footwear. Applied as either a lateral or a medial flare of the heel, its goal is to increase stability during gait by assimilating subtalar neutral. A laterally flared heel is used with a rearfoot varus to decrease the incidence of inversion injuries. A medially flared heel is used with a rearfoot valgus to decrease the incidence of eversion injuries (Figure 7-10). For instance, a medial flare from the heel to the sustentaculum tali prevents excessive pronation of the foot during gait.

Offset Heels and Shoe Counters

The offset heel is a modification used to help correct valgus or varus deformities. It offers a broad support base, especially at the superior surface of the heel, where the broad buildup

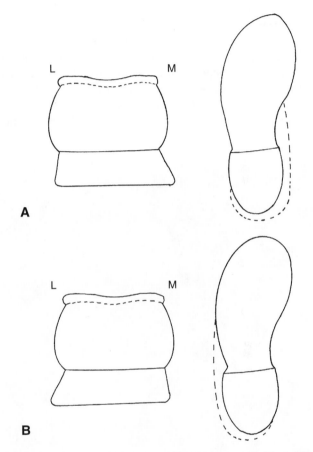

FIGURE 7-10 Examples of Thomas heels. **A,** A medial (M) flared heel provides a broader base of support and prevents eversion of the ankle. **B,** A lateral (L) flared heel prevents inversion of the ankle.

against the shoe's counter provides reinforcement either medially or laterally. A heel counter is an extension along the medial or lateral borders of the shoe from the heel to the proximal border of the fifth or the first metatarsal head. This shoe modification strengthens the shank portion of the footwear for better control of the hind foot. The heel counter is often used in combination with the appropriate Thomas heel. A counter can also be placed medially or laterally in the midfoot region. A patient whose gait exhibits excessive pronation, such as is common in rheumatoid arthritis, may require a firm medial counter to prevent the shoe from collapsing medially and to assist in realigning the foot into a neutral position.

Attachments for Orthoses

For some patients with neuromuscular dysfunction (e.g., hemiplegia, paraplegia, multiple sclerosis), a traditional metal double-upright lower-extremity orthosis can be prescribed. If so, the shoe must be modified: a U-shaped orthotic bracket (stirrup) is attached to the shoe by means of three copper rivets, one on the heel and two in the shank. The metal is riveted through the outsole to the insole. To accomplish this, the heel is removed and the plate of the stirrup is attached. The groove is then cut through the heel, and the heel is reattached. The appropriate orthotic ankle joint is then attached to uprights of the stirrup.

Shoe Stretching

Shoes with leather uppers can be stretched almost one full width. Although a shoe cannot be truly lengthened, it can be made to feel longer with a toe box stretcher device that looks like the shape of the foot and is inserted into the shoe to expand it (Figure 7-11). After the leather is moistened or softened, this device effectively raises and slightly rounds

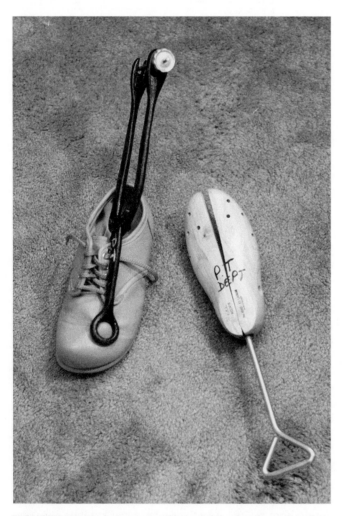

FIGURE 7-11 Tools that are used to stretch leather shoes. Stretching often provides adequate accommodation for deformities in conventional shoes. The toe box stretcher (right) can increase width by one size. The ball-and-socket device (left) is used to stretch specific points that correspond to the forefoot and toe deformity.

the toe box. Frequently, the pressure of a flat toe box on the toes is more problematic than the length of the shoe. Specific points in the shoe can be softened and expanded by placing an "expansion knob" on the toe-box stretcher or using a ball-and-socket device. Site-specific stretching is particularly helpful for patients with toe deformities such as hallux valgus, hammertoe, mallet toe, claw toe, overlapping toes, and Taylor bunion deformity.

Blowout Patches and Gussets

Patients with foot deformities who prefer conventional shoes to Thermold shoes may find temporary pain relief if a blowout patch or gusset is applied to their shoe. The shoe leather around the area of deformity is cut away and replaced with a softer blowout patch or gusset of moleskin, soft leather, or suede.

FOOTWEAR FOR COMMON FOOT DEFORMITIES AND PROBLEMS

Conservative management of common forefoot, midfoot, and rearfoot deformities often involves modification of shoes or prescription footwear, or both. Specific footwear strategies for several common foot problems are described in the following section.

Problems in the Forefoot

The most common footwear variation used for abnormalities in the forefoot is a high toe box. High toe boxes are available in various footgear, including athletic sneakers, comfort shoes, Thermolds, and prescription footwear. To accommodate forefoot deformity optimally, the maximum height of the abnormal toes must be measured in a weight-bearing position. Tables of manufactured shoes by toe box space are available to guide the clinician in recommending shoes that most closely match patient needs.[51]

Metatarsalgia

Metatarsalgia is pain around the metatarsal heads that results from compression of the plantar digital nerve as it courses between the metatarsal heads. Excessive weight bearing with atrophy of the metatarsal fat pad can result in irritation of the nerves and potentially lead to development of a neuroma. The three major objectives in shoe prescription for patients with metatarsalgia are to (1) transfer pressure from painful, sensitive areas to more pressure-tolerant areas, (2) reduce friction by stabilizing the MTP joint, and (3) stabilize the rearfoot and midfoot to reduce pressure on the metatarsal heads.[52] Characteristics of the shoe that will accomplish these goals include wide width to reduce pressure on the transverse metatarsal arch, long fitting to eliminate plantar-flexed MTP joints, cushion soles to enhance shock absorption, and a high toe box to allow forefoot flexion and extension. Additionally, the shoe should include a long medial counter to stabilize the rearfoot, a lower heel to minimize pressure at the metatarsal heads, and preferably thermoldable leather to accommodate deformities. Shoe modifications often include a transverse metatarsal bar to redistribute pressure from metatarsal heads to metatarsal shafts and shorten stride and a rocker sole to reduce motion of painful joints.

Sesamoiditis

Sesamoiditis is an inflammation around the sesamoid bones under the first metatarsal head. It often results from a loss of soft tissue padding under the first metatarsal head and from toe deformities such as hallux valgus and hallux rigidus. The objective of shoe prescription for patients with sesamoiditis is to redistribute weight-bearing forces from the first MTP joint and its sesamoids to the long medial arch and shafts of the lesser metatarsals. A transverse metatarsal bar is used to redistribute pressure from metatarsal heads to metatarsal shafts and to shorten stride. A rocker sole can be used to reduce motion of the painful hallux joint.

Morton's Syndrome

With repetitive irritation of the plantar digital nerve between the first and second metatarsal heads, a neuroma is likely to develop.[53] This condition is known as *Morton's syndrome.* The three major objectives in shoe prescription for patients with Morton's syndrome are to (1) redistribute weight from the lesser metatarsals (especially the second and third) to the proximal phalanx of the hallux, (2) stabilize the rearfoot by maintaining subtalar joint neutral, and (3) accommodate forefoot varus as well as a possibly dorsiflexed first metatarsal. Shoe prescription includes a long medial counter for rearfoot support and stability; a straight or flared last to accommodate foot shape; a high, wide toe box to reduce compression across the transverse metatarsal arch; a large enough shoe size to accommodate the long second toe; and a Thomas heel or wedge sole to support the medial longitudinal arch. A medial heel and medial sole wedge may be necessary when symptoms are severe.

Morton's (Interdigital) Neuroma

Overstretching of the digital nerves in extreme toe extension at the proximal phalanx can also result in the development of a neuroma. Two objectives should be considered for patients with Morton's neuroma. First, the patient must obtain relief from the pain and burning, especially in the third interspace of the MTP joint. Second, compression of the digital nerve as it passes between the heads of the third and fourth metatarsals needs to be reduced. To achieve these goals, the shoe should be wide enough to eliminate transverse compression and have enough length to reduce plantar flexion of the MTP joints. A long medial counter can help reduce pronation; a cushioned sole increases shock absorption, and a low heel unloads pressure on the metatarsals. Elastic laces may be helpful in allowing expansion of the forefoot. Shoe modifications for Morton's neuroma might include a metatarsal bar to elevate the metatarsals and redistribute weight, or a metatarsal rocker bar to immobilize the metatarsals, or a combination of both.

Metatarsalgia of the Fifth Metatarsophalangeal Joint

Like the metatarsalgia described previously, metatarsalgia of the fifth MTP joint results in plantar digital nerve irritation at the interdigital space of the fourth and fifth metatarsal heads. When metatarsalgia of the fifth MTP joint is present, the goals of intervention are to redistribute weight forces to the fifth metatarsal shaft and to provide a broad base of support along the lateral border of the foot. The optimal shoe has a last with enough lateral flare to accommodate the lateral aspect of the foot and fifth metatarsal shaft, a firm lateral counter, and a firm leather or rubber sole. Possible shoe modifications include a lateral heel and sole flare ending proximal to the fifth metatarsal head to provide a broader base of support. Lateral heel and sole wedges may be useful for patients with flexible feet.

Hallux Rigidus (Limitus)

Degenerative joint disease of the first MTP joint causes pain, loss of mobility, and eventually fusion of the joint. Osteophyte formation on the dorsal aspects of the metatarsal head and base of the proximal phalanx can be quite painful and result in a loss of extension. For patients with hallux rigidus or limitus, the goals are to limit motion of the hallux and first MTP joint and to reduce pressure on the dorsal and plantar aspects of the hallux and first MTP joint.[54] To accomplish this, the shoe should have a high and wide toe box and Thermold or soft leather uppers. When significant deformity is present, a steel shank from heel to phalanx of the hallux and a rigid rocker sole with compensating heel elevation may be necessary.

Hallux Valgus (Bunions)

A prominent bony formation on the medial aspect of the first MTP joint can result from lateral deviation of the hallux and from foot pronation.[55] This deformity is often associated with long-term wearing of shoes with a triangular toe box. Five objectives should be considered in the prescription of shoes for patients with hallux valgus: (1) to reduce friction and pressure to the first MTP joint, (2) to eliminate abnormal pressure from narrow-fitting shoes, (3) to reduce pronation of the foot from heel strike to midstance, (4) to correct eversion, and (5) to relieve posterior tibial tendon and ligamentous strain. Patients with hallux valgus benefit from shoes with high, wide toe boxes and Thermold or soft leather uppers. A combined last with increased last width in the toe box and a smaller heel for better control of the subtalar joint may also be indicated. Additionally, the choice of a shoe that is longer and wider helps to accommodate deformity; a lower heel to reduce forefoot pressure and a reinforced medial counter help prevent pronation.

Hammertoes, Claw Toes, and Mallet Toes

Hammertoe deformity is characterized by hyperextension of the MTP joint, flexion of the proximal interphalangeal (PIP) joint, and extension of the distal interphalangeal (DIP) joint. This results in high load during weight bearing at the plantar metatarsal heads and at the plantar surface of the distal phalanx. Claw toe deformity features hyperflexion of the PIP and DIP joints, although the MTP joint can be hyperextended or hyperflexed. Mallet toe deformity results from hyperextension of the MTP joint, flexion of the PIP, and a neutral position of the DIP, so that weight bearing is on the tip of the distal phalanx. Deformities of the lesser toes can be problematic, especially for patients with compromised circulation and neuropathy. For these individuals, there are two major footwear goals: (1) to transfer pressure away from the metatarsal heads, the PIP joints, and the distal phalanx joints, and (2) to encourage flexion of the MTP joints and extension of the PIP joints.[56] Patients with lesser toe deformities should wear shoes with a high, wide toe box made of Thermold or soft leather to reduce the likelihood of microtrauma over the bony prominences. The shoe should also be long enough to allow flexion of MTP joints and extension of PIP joints rather than cramping the toes. Finally, a soft cushion outsole and low heel further reduce pressure on the metatarsal heads. Commonly used shoe modifications for lesser toe deformities include metatarsal bars to reduce pressure to metatarsal heads and shift weight bearing to metatarsal shafts, as well as a rocker bar or rocker sole to accommodate rollover on fixed deformity.

Problems in the Midfoot

Shoe prescriptions or modifications, or both, are also helpful in managing midfoot dysfunction and deformity. The most commonly encountered problems include pes planus, pes equinus, pes cavus, and plantar fasciitis.

Pes Planus

Pes planus is pronation of the midfoot that results in a failure of the foot to supinate during midstance. The longitudinal arch flattens, causing a splaying of the forefoot and lateral deviation of the metatarsals. This deformity can be either flexible or fixed (rigid).

For patients with a flexible pes planus, the goals of intervention are to reduce pronation from heel strike to midstance, correct eversion, relieve tension on the posterior tibial tendonitis, and relieve ligamentous strain. To do these things, the shoe should offer a long medial heel counter, a Thomas heel (medial extension) or a firm wedge sole, and a straight last. A custom shoe is recommended for severe cases. Shoe modifications may include a medial heel wedge to correct eversion and reduce pronation or a medial heel and sole flare in extreme cases.

Because of the fixed nature of a rigid pes planus, the goals are somewhat different: to relieve ligamentous strain, to relieve arch pain, and to correct eversion of the foot. The optimal shoe should offer a broad shank (extra wide midfoot), a straight last, and a long medial counter. Additionally, a wedge sole is applied to reduce the load on the metatarsal heads, stabilize the intertarsal joint, and provide a dorsiflexion assist.

Pes Equinus

In *pes equinus*, the plantar flexor muscles and Achilles tendon are tightened, which limits dorsiflexion of the ankle and results in a plantar flexion deformity. For patients with a flexible pes equinus, the footwear prescribed attempts to reduce ankle plantar flexion, reduce the load on the metatarsal heads, and stabilize the subtalar joint. This can be accomplished in a shoe with a low heel. A rocker bottom can be applied to the sole to provide a dorsiflexion assist and further reduce load on the metatarsal heads.

When the pes equinus deformity is rigid or fixed, the goals of footwear intervention change. Instead of trying to reduce plantar flexion, a posterior platform supports the rearfoot from heel strike to midstance and mimics the dorsiflexion needed at toe-off. It is important to contain the entire foot in the shoe, reducing the load on the metatarsal heads. For patients with unilateral deformity, it is also important to equalize the relative leg length difference between the normal foot and the equinus foot through all phases of gait. Shoe prescription for patients with a fixed equinus deformity includes a Cuban (elevated) heel to provide a platform and deep quarter or high-top shoes. If modifications are necessary, they might include posterior heel elevation on the equinus side, as well as on the contralateral limb, to facilitate swing of the involved limb and reduce pelvic obliquity.

Pes Cavus

Pes cavus is an exaggerated longitudinal arch that can lead to a plantar flexed forefoot with retraction of the toes and severe weight-bearing stresses on the metatarsal heads and heel. Patients with pes cavus benefit from shoes that provide a broad platform for stability; reduce loading at the heels, lateral borders, and metatarsal heads; and accommodate the deformed foot within the shoe. The shoe should also have a firm heel counter to maintain rearfoot stability and a modified, curved last to accommodate foot shape. Custom-molded shoes are recommended in severe cases. Possible shoe modifications for patients with pes cavus include a lateral flare to provide a platform for greater stability, a cushion sole to absorb shock on the heel and metatarsal heads, and a metatarsal bar to shift weight from the metatarsal heads.

Plantar Fasciitis

Plantar fasciitis is inflammation of the plantar fascia at its insertion to the medial aspect of the calcaneus. This inflammatory process can lead to the development of calcification at that insertion, commonly referred to as a *heel spur*. Plantar fasciitis is often a consequence of loss of the longitudinal arch in conditions such as pes planus or of undo stresses created in the forefoot with tightness of the gastrocnemius and soleus muscles or an elevated longitudinal arch. To reduce the painful signs and symptoms of plantar fasciitis, the goals of intervention are to transfer weight-bearing pressure from painful to more tolerant areas, to reduce tension on the plantar fascia and Achilles tendon, to control pronation from heel strike to midstance, and to maintain the subtalar joint in a neutral position. The shoe prescribed for plantar fasciitis has a long medial heel counter to limit heel valgus, a high heel to reduce tension on the plantar fascia and Achilles tendon, and adequate length to minimize compression and promote supination from midstance to toe-off. The types of shoe modifications that may be useful include a posterior heel elevation to reduce tension on the plantar fascia and Achilles tendon.

Problems in the Rearfoot

The most common dysfunctions and deformities of the rearfoot that can be addressed by footwear prescription or modification include arthrodesis, Achilles tendinitis or bursitis, and Haglund's deformity (pump bump).

Arthrodesis

Arthrodesis is a loss of mobility at the ankle mortise, the junction of the talus with the tibia and fibula. This deformity prevents motion at the ankle in all planes and alters progression through the stance phase of gait, and it may also compromise limb clearance in swing phase. When arthrodesis of the ankle is present, the major objectives are to provide effective shock absorption and controlled lowering of the forefoot at loading response, to improve comfort and efficiency of push-off, and to accommodate any shortening or residual equinus. Shoes that address the problems of arthrodesis have a reinforced counter and may have a medial or a lateral flared heel (or a combination of both) to provide greater stability. Some patients benefit from a high-top shoe as well. Modifications that protect the foot and facilitate a more normal gait pattern include application of a cushioned heel to absorb shock and simulate plantar flexion after heel strike and a rocker sole to mimic the dorsiflexion needed in the late stance phase.

Achilles Tendinitis, Bursitis, and Haglund's Deformity

Undue stresses of the Achilles tendon, direct pressure of a too-short shoe, and/or tightness of the gastrocnemius and soleus muscles can result in tendinitis or bursitis. *Haglund's deformity* is an osseous formation at the insertion of the Achilles tendon at the calcaneus. The goals of shoe prescription for patients with Achilles tendinitis, bursitis, and/or Haglund's deformity (pump bump) are similar: (1) to reduce tension on the Achilles tendon, (2) to provide dorsiflexion assist at heel strike and at toe-off, (3) to reduce abnormal pronation, and (4) to reduce pressure and friction (shear) at the insertion of the calcaneus. Patients with these problems require a slightly higher heel to reduce dorsiflexion, a long medial counter to limit subtalar motion, a longer shoe size to reduce compression pressure, and a backless shoe to prevent irritation of the pump bump. The types of shoe modifications that may be helpful include a posterior heel elevation to reduce tension on the Achilles tendon or a foam-filled posterior heel counter.

DIAGNOSIS-RELATED CONSIDERATIONS IN SHOE PRESCRIPTION

Prescription footwear and shoe modifications are also extremely useful tools to protect joints, prevent skin problems, and enhance normal function of patients who are coping with arthritis and gout or diabetes and peripheral vascular disease. Adaptations to footwear may also be helpful for patients with hemiplegia, partial foot amputations, or congenital deformities.

Arthritis

Arthritis, whether degenerative, rheumatoid, or traumatic, leads to destruction of joints. In working with patients with foot arthritis, the goals of intervention are to prevent or limit abnormal motion, accommodate for arthritic deformities, and cushion impact loading and reduce microtrauma within the joint.[57] A reinforced counter can help limit subtalar motion; a high-top design shoe can also help limit ankle motion. Extra-depth shoes may be needed to accommodate deformities of the midfoot and forefoot. Thermoldable leather is preferable if deformities need further accommodation. The application of a rocker bottom helps to improve push-off by shortening the distance between the heel and the MTP joint. It also reduces the total ankle motion required for push-off. Shock-absorbing accommodative orthoses can be placed inside the shoe, and a cushion heel can be added to absorb even more force at heel strike and limit ankle and subtalar motion.[58] A flared heel can reduce medial and lateral movement at the subtalar joint.

Gout

For patients with gout, the treatment objectives are similar to those for patients with arthritis—preventing or limiting motion of painful or inflamed joints, accommodating foot deformities, and cushioning the impact of loading on the involved joints. A reinforced counter to limit subtalar motion or a high-top design to limit overall ankle motion should be considered. An extra-depth shoe of thermoldable leather is best able to accommodate deformities without creating pain and discomfort over sensitive joints. A rocker bottom can be applied to assist push-off, prevent pedal joint movement, and reduce ankle motion required for push-off. Shock-absorbing accommodative orthoses and cushion heels provide even more comfort and protection of inflamed joints during gait.

Diabetes

The loss of protective sensation in patients with diabetic neuropathy creates significant vulnerability to injury from repetitive microtrauma. Protection of the plantar surface of the diabetic foot from microtrauma is of paramount importance. Patients with diabetic neuropathy often have significant weakness of intrinsic muscles. Forefoot deformities develop, including claw toes, which are susceptible to breakdown in areas of excessive shoe pressures. The risk of nonhealing, infection, and subsequent amputation is quite high; prevention is the most effective treatment strategy. Total-contact full-foot orthoses using soft, shock-absorbing materials helps distribute weight-bearing pressures over the entire plantar surface of the foot away from the vulnerable bony prominences. A Thermold leather shoe is recommended for the insensitive diabetic foot.

Peripheral Vascular Disease

Because the ability to heal is compromised in patients with peripheral vascular disease, any irritation or ulceration exponentially increases the risk of infection and subsequent amputation. Here, too, prevention of skin breakdown and protection of the vulnerable foot are the primary goals.

The ability to fit and protect the foot effectively is further challenged by fluctuating edema. A Thermold sandal with Velcro closure is often recommended for patients with peripheral vascular disease-related edema as a safe and effective alternative to standard shoes. If edema is not a problem, a soft Thermold shoe protects the plantar surface of the foot from repetitive pressures and accommodates deformities that are at risk for shoe pressure–related trauma. Because hypersensitivity is often a problem with circulatory pathologies in the lower extremities, a shoe that cushions the foot may be helpful. Elastic shoelaces allow expansion of the shoe for patients with minimal edema-related fluctuations in foot size.

Hemiplegia

The patient with hemiplegia after a cerebrovascular accident (e.g., stroke, may have inadequate or excessive tone of the lower extremity. Many of these patients need orthotic intervention to control the foot and ankle in some or all phases of gait, to accommodate for any fixed deformities and to cushion impact loading at initial contact. Footwear is selected to enhance orthotic function or, in some instances, to directly impact mild dysfunction. A reinforced heel counter helps to limit subtalar motion and stabilize the foot on heel strike. A flared heel or high-top shoe may be recommended to enhance foot placement and stance stability. A rigid shoe shank may be required for some types of lower extremity orthoses. In the presence of an equinus deformity, a heel lift on the shoe provides total contact during weight bearing and facilitates stability. In severe deformities of the ankle, a custom-molded shoe may be the only alternative.

The most common ankle-foot orthoses used in hemiplegia tend to increase shoe length, width, and depth by a half to a whole size. Often the insole can be replaced with an insert foundation, to garner a little more room for the orthosis within the shoe. Extra-depth shoes are particularly helpful for patients who are faced with difficulty in donning their orthosis and shoe because of upper extremity dysfunction in hemiplegia.

Amputation and Congenital Deformity

The foot that is shortened surgically or is congenitally deformed is a management challenge because the weight-bearing surface is reduced or altered, increasing the likelihood of tissue breakdown with repeated loading in gait. The type of protective footwear used can range from an over-the-counter extra-depth shoe for a mild deformity to a custom-molded shoe for a severe deformity. When the feet are of unequal size, it is more

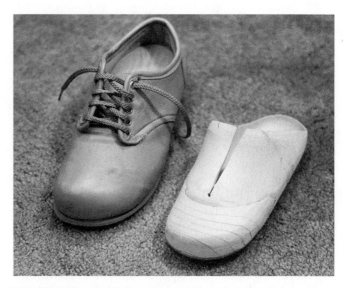

FIGURE 7-12 A toe filler can be used on a foot that has been shortened by amputation or congenital deformity.

difficult to fit them without buying two pairs of shoes or having custom footwear made. If the difference between the feet is no more than one size in length, the larger size can be used with toe padding for the shorter deformed or amputated foot or with an orthosis to accommodate the deformity (Figure 7-12). Frequently, the shorter foot is also wider and must be accommodated by the appropriate orthosis custom molded to the shoe. A toe filler prevents the shortened foot from sliding within the shoe during gait but also increases the risk of skin breakdown. It is crucial that the first MTP joint be aligned with the "toe break" point in the shoe. If the foot falls posterior to the toe break, stress is concentrated at the distal end of the foot, increasing the chance of pressure imposition by the "filler."

READING THE WEAR ON SHOES

For the clinician who is faced with decisions about modifying, repairing, or replacing footwear, examination of patterns of wear and erosion provides important information. Deterioration of the shoe itself impairs tactile sensibility and position sense judgment.[59] Shoes that have outlasted their purpose often create abnormal forces and shearing that increase the risk of repetitive microtrauma to the skin and joints of the foot and ankle. Analysis of the wear and erosion of the shoe is a prescriptive tool in advising, prescribing, and modifying a shoe to fit individual needs.

CASE EXAMPLE 1

A Patient with Diabetes Who Is Homeless and Has a Neuropathic Foot Ulcer

---

J. H. is a 71-year-old homeless, Hispanic man with a 22-year history of type 2 diabetes mellitus treated with glibenclamide 2.5 mg three times daily. He presents with a large ulcer (6.552 cm²) of the plantar surface of the midfoot with significant arch deformity of the right foot, subsequent to

an episode of Charcot arthropathy several years ago. J. H. reports that the ulcer has been present for more than 1 year. He has complications resulting from diabetes, including retinopathy, peripheral neuropathy, and history of numerous neuropathic ulcerations involving both feet. He also has a 24-year history of arterial hypertension and a documented myocardial infarction. He is currently managed with angiotensin-converting enzyme inhibitors and calcium antagonists. It is unclear how regularly he has taken his medications, although they are available at no cost through the shelter's clinic. J. H. has been homeless for 7 years.

J. H. is referred to the health clinic at the homeless shelter for diabetic and hypertensive assessment and conservative treatment of the foot ulceration.

Questions to Consider

- What tests and measures might the foot clinic team use to assess current status and changes in J. H.'s neuropathic wound, the deformity of his feet, the circulation and sensory status of his limbs, and his functional status and gait? What is the evidence of reliability and validity of these measures?
- What does the team need to understand about his current health status and diabetic control? How will they gather this information?
- What are the immediate needs, in terms of footwear, for J. H.? How might his needs change over time as his wound heals?
- Given his current health status and lifestyle, what factors will likely affect (both positively and negatively) clinical decision making about footwear, wound care, diabetic management, and follow-up care? How might the team prioritize goals and possible interventions?
- How would the team assess efficacy of their interventions?

Initial Results

Satisfactory metabolic control and blood pressure values are achieved during the initial week of medical management at the shelter clinic. J. H. is referred to Boston City Hospital (BCH) for a series of tests and measures on an outpatient basis. Although J. H. is found to have bilateral diabetic retinopathy (*fundus oculi*), there is no evidence of diabetic nephropathy. Echocardiogram evidences a left ventricular hypertrophy with a normal regional kinesis and an ejection fraction of 50%.

Electromyography shows normal conduction velocity and slight abnormalities of sensory action potentials in the nerves of both lower extremities. An elevated threshold of 40 V to biothesiometer and a partial loss of sensitivity (nine of nine areas tested are insensitive bilaterally) to Semmes-Weinstein 5.07 monofilament are recorded. The transcutaneous oxygen tension is 30 mm Hg at the dorsum of the involved foot (right) and 15 mm Hg at the perilesional site. In the ulcerated limb, the ankle-brachial index measured with Doppler technique is 0.8. Duplex scanning shows widespread atheromasic lesions in the carotids and in the lower limb arteries without hemodynamically significant stenoses and no significant alterations in the venous district of the lower limbs.

J. H.'s ulcer on the right foot appears superficial and is graded as a Wagner grade II ulcer. The ulcer is covered by a fibrinous exudate with keratotic margins. The microbiological cultures are negative. A surgical debridement is performed at BCH and the patient/client is sent back to the shelter with instructions for local treatment before and after daily sharps debridement consisting of the daily application of sterile paraffin gauze and for "evaluation and conservative treatment" by a physical therapist.

Questions to Consider

- How might the team interpret the results of the tests performed at BCH? How will this information influence or inform wound care and recommendations for footwear for this gentleman?
- What additional information will the physical therapist and foot care clinic team need to gather?
- What are the primary goals of physical therapy/foot care intervention? What is the prognosis and anticipated outcome? What is the anticipated duration of this episode of care? How frequently might J. H. receive care?
- What interventions would be most appropriate to address the goals of wound healing and prevention of future recurrence of neuropathic ulcers?

Physical Therapy Examination, Evaluation and Intervention

J. H. is examined at the shelter by a physical therapist on the Foot Clinic Team. He arrives at the clinic ambulating independently, without any assistive devices. The ulcer on the plantar surface of his midfoot measures 6.552 cm^2, in the Charcot joint deformity region of the right foot. The ulcer is determined to be secondary to repetitive trauma to this region in shoes that had a large hole in the midsection of the sole.

A total contact cast is applied. Selective padding of the cast includes foam padding over the toes and an ulcerated area of the foot; felt pads over the malleoli and navicular prominence; and cotton cast padding around the proximal and anterior lower leg, heel, sides, and dorsum of the foot. A rubber heel mount is applied to the cast for ambulation. Fiberglass casting material is used to decrease the effects of the elements (weather) on a plaster cast in this homeless individual who spends much time outdoors. The cast is also bifurcated to allow high galvanic electrical stimulation to be used as a local treatment modality to the wound and to provide access for daily debridement, application of dressings, and monitoring for secondary lesions. The cast is secured using Velcro strapping. The patient is allowed to walk freely and is highly compliant, wearing the cast continuously.

The ulcer responds favorably to a combination of periodic surgical debridement, local wound care and daily sharps debridement, a modified total contact casting protocol, and high galvanic electrical stimulation. After 6 weeks, the ulcer is completely closed and J. H.'s condition remains stable. He is subsequently fitted with a total contact foot orthosis bilaterally and provided with a pair of Reebok walking sneakers with an extra width to accommodate the Charcot foot deformity bilaterally.

(Continued)

With proper intervention and attention to J. H.'s social situation, it is determined that the prognosis for preventing recurrence of neuropathic foot ulcer wound is good and that he can be integrated into appropriate home, community, and work environments within the context of his disability. J. H. is placed in a permanent shelter-housing residence and assumes part-time employment as a guide at the Boston Museum of Science.

Discussion

For individuals with neuropathic wounds, total contact casting allows ambulation with protection from external stress and trauma. In addition, because the cast is well molded and minimal padding is applied, pressure is distributed evenly and maintained as long as the cast is worn. This total-contact cast also counteracts lymphatic congestion, which compromises the healing process. For J. H., the cast was bifurcated to allow for daily wound care while providing consistent pressure relief and foot protection.

The major objectives of treatment after J. H.'s diabetic neuropathic wound healed were to protect the plantar surface from repetitive microtrauma and accommodate deformities that could be traumatized by excessive shoe pressures, which could result in ulceration and subsequent injury. A total-contact, full-foot orthosis using soft shock-absorbing materials helps distribute weight-bearing pressures over the entire plantar surface of the foot away from the vulnerable bony prominences. A Thermold leather shoe or good walking sneaker is recommended for the insensitive diabetic foot.

Accommodative devices are insoles that are placed in shoes to balance the feet, allowing pressures to be evenly distributed and permitting support and shock absorption of the foot. An orthosis, in contrast, supports and also controls the foot by neutralizing pronatory forces. Following wound healing, a total-contact orthosis (Plastazote with a layer of ⅜-inch PPT) was fabricated for J. H. and placed in a pair of extra-depth Reebok walking shoes.

Accommodating shoe gear should be used by patients with diabetes, and walking barefooted should not be permitted. The shoe's upper should be soft, so as not to irritate any prominence or developing deformity. The accommodative

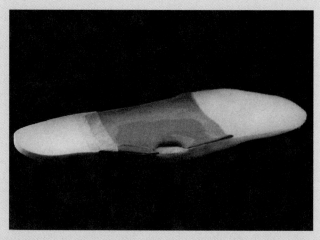

FIGURE 7-13 An example of an accommodative orthosis for a patient with diabetic neuropathy and Charcot deformity of the left midfoot. Note the "cutout" to reduce weight-bearing pressure on the most prominent area of bony deformity and the use of materials to "fill" space around the deformity and distribute weight-bearing pressures over the entire plantar surface of the foot.

insole that is used should be adaptable to changes as well. A combination of an expanded polyethylene such as Plastazote, which can be heat molded to provide total contact, mounted on a shock-absorbing material such as PPT, or covered with a neoprene, such as Spenco, which is soft and retains its shape, makes an excellent accommodative insole. This type of accommodative orthosis protects the foot from trauma to prominent areas and redistributes the forces to provide even weight bearing through total contact upon the plantar surface (Figure 7-13). When accommodative orthoses are used, the shoe must have adequate depth to accommodate it. Extra-depth shoes such as Thermold shoes or extra-depth sneakers allow not only the room needed for the accommodative insole but also modification of the upper through heat molding to accommodate lesser toe deformities. A rigid-sole rocker-bottom shoe might also be recommended to reduce pressures under the metatarsal heads during push-off. The apex of the rocker is positioned just proximal to the metatarsal heads, allowing for the shoe itself to provide forward propulsion of the foot.

SUMMARY

The shoe is an essential interface between the foot and the ground. It protects the foot from trauma and supports the structures of the foot as an individual walks, runs, and changes direction. Fashionable footwear, especially for women, often compromises, rather than enhances, foot function. Foot function and footwear needs have a developmental aspect as well; an understanding of how the foot changes over the life span and of the special needs of children, pregnant women, and older adults is essential. Knowledge about the components of shoes and their variations, the criteria for proper fitting, and the relationship

between shoe design and activity-related demands is an important tool for clinical practice. Physical therapists are often called on to recommend footwear for patients with special needs. A baseline knowledge of shoe characteristics and modifications for certain types of deformities or diagnoses enhances this ability.

REFERENCES

1. Finlay OE. Footwear management in the elderly care programme. *Physiotherapy.* 1986;72(4):171–178.
2. Fuller EA. A review of the biomechanics of shoes. *Clin Podiatr Med Surg.* 1994;11(2):241–258.

3. Mandato MG, Nester E. The effects of heel height on forefoot peak pressure. *J Am Podiatr Med Assoc.* 1999;89(2):75–80.

4. Black E, Black E. Comfort shoes: the long overdue revolution. *Biomechanics.* 1995;2(10):27–33.

5. Frey C. If the shoe fits…. *Biomechanics.* 1995;2(4):26–28.

6. Frey C, Thompson F, Smith J, et al. American Orthopaedic Foot and Ankle Society Women's Shoe Survey. *Foot Ankle.* 1993;14(2):78–81.

7. Coughlin MJ. Lesser toe abnormalities. Oregon Health Science University. *Instr Course Lect.* 2003;52:421–444.

8. Janisse DJ. The art and science of fitting shoes. *Foot Ankle.* 1992;13(5):257–262.

9. Herman HH, Bottomley JB. Anatomical and biomechanical considerations of the elder foot. *Top Geriatr Rehabil.* 1992;7(3):1–13.

10. Frey C, Chan C, Carrasco N. Obesity: do weight gains lead to lower extremity pain? *Biomechanics.* 1996;3(1):30–35.

11. Snow RE, Williams KR, Holmes GB. The effects of wearing high heeled shoes on pedal pressures in women. *Foot Ankle.* 1992;13(2):85–92.

12. Sass P, Hassan G. Lower extremity abnormalities in children. *Am Fam Physician.* 2003;68(3):417–419.

13. Charrette M. Foot care: do children need corrective footwear? *Dynamic Chiropract.* 2003;21(12):28–33.

14. Hein NM. [Inserts and shoes for foot deformities]. *Orthopade.* 2003;32(2):119–132.

15. Shapiro S. Pediatrics: a reasoned approach to common lower limb disorders. *Biomechanics.* 1995;2(5):18–21.

16. Rao UB, Joseph B. The influence of footwear on the prevalence of flat foot: a survey of 2300 children. *J Bone Joint Surg.* 1992;74(4):630–631.

17. Valmassy RL. Pediatric biomechanics. *Podiatry Today.* 1989; May:86–92.

18. Valmassy RL. The use of gait plates for in-toed and out-toed deformities. *Clin Podiatr Med Surg.* 1994;11(2):211–217.

19. Black E, Cooke Anastasi S. Pregnancy and the lower extremities. *Biomechanics.* 1995;2(4):22–25, 68–69.

20. Garbalosa JC, McClure MH. The frontal plane relationship of the forefoot to the rearfoot in an asymptomatic population. *J Sports Phys Ther.* 1994;20(4):200–206.

21. Rothbart BA, Hansen KH, Yerratt MK. Resolving chronic low back pain: the foot connection. *Am J Podiatry Med.* 1995;5(3):84–90.

22. Karpman R. Geriatric prefab. *Biomechanics.* 1995;2(5):53–58.

23. Sudarsky L, Ronthal M. Gait disorders among elderly patients. *Arch Neurol.* 1993;40(2):740–743.

24. Hough JC, McHenry MP, Kammer LM. Gait disorders in the elderly. *Assoc Prescription Footwear.* 1987;35(6):191–196.

25. Helfand AE. Common foot problems in the aged and rehabilitative management. In: Williams TF, ed. *Rehabilitation in the Aging.* New York: Raven; 1984:291–303.

26. Edelstein JE. Foot care for the aging. *Phys Ther.* 1988; 68(12):1882–1886.

27. Pinzur MS. Charcot's foot. *Foot Ankle Clin.* 2000;5(4):897–912.

28. Pinzur MS, Shields N, Trepman E, et al. Current practice patterns in the treatment of Charcot foot. *Foot Ankle Int.* 2000;21(11):916–920.

29. Frykerg RG, Kozak GP. The diabetic Charcot foot. In: Kozak GP, Hoar CS, Rowbotham JL, et al., eds. *Management of Diabetic Foot Problems.* Philadelphia: Saunders; 1984:103–112.

30. Frykerg RG. Podiatric problems in diabetes. In: Kozak GP, Hoar CS, Rowbotham JL, et al., eds. *Management of Diabetic Foot Problems.* Philadelphia: Saunders; 1984:45–67.

31. Prior T, Gardiner A, Thomas A, Maitland P. Footwear requirements of patients with diabetes mellitus. *Diabet Foot.* 2000;3(1):24–28.

32. Ramuglia VJ, Palmarozzo PM, Rzonca EC. Biomechanical concepts in the treatment of ulcers in the diabetic foot. *Clin Podiatr Med Surg.* 1988;5(3):613–626.

33. Bailey TS, Yu HM, Rayfield EJ. Patterns of foot examination in a diabetes clinic. *Am J Med.* 1985;78(3):371–374.

34. Pinzur MS. Benchmark analysis of diabetic patients with neuropathic (Charcot) foot deformity. *Foot Ankle Int.* 1999;20(9):564–567.

35. Bottomley JB, Herman H. Making simple, inexpensive changes for the management of foot problems in the aged. *Top Geriatr Rehabil.* 1992;7(3):62–77.

36. Seale KS. Women and their shoes: unrealistic expectations? American College of Podiatry. *Instr Course Lect.* 1995;44: 379–384.

37. Corrigan JP, Moore DP, Stephens MM. Effect of heel height on forefoot loading. *Foot Ankle.* 1993;14(3):148–152.

38. Herring KM, Richie DH. Friction blisters and sock fiber composition: a double-blind study. *J Am Podiatr Med Assoc.* 1990;80(2):3–7.

39. Richie DH, Herring KM. Friction blisters and sock construction. Presented at the annual meeting of the American Academy of Podiatric Sports Medicine, Miami, May 29, 1990.

40. Herring KM, Richie DH. Friction blisters and sock fiber composition: a single-blind study. Part 2. Presented at 75th annual meeting of the American Podiatric Medical Association, Las Vegas, August 15, 1990.

41. Murray HJ, Veves A, Young MJ, et al. Role of experimental socks in the care of the high-risk diabetic foot. *Diabetes Care.* 1993;16(8):1190–1192.

42. Veves A, Masson E, Fernando D, Boulton AJM. Use of experimental padded hosiery to reduce abnormal foot pressures in diabetic neuropathy. *Diabetes Care.* 1989;12(9):16–19.

43. Veves A, Masson E, Fernando D, Boulton AJM. Studies of experimental hosiery in diabetic neuropathic patients with high foot pressures. *Diabet Med.* 1990;7(3):324–326.

44. Lord M, Hosein R. Pressure redistribution by molded inserts in diabetic footwear. *J Rehabil Res Dev.* 1994;31(3):214–222.

45. Shrader JA. Nonsurgical management of the foot and ankle affected by rheumatoid arthritis. *J Orthop Sports Phys Ther.* 1999;29(12):703–717.

46. Egan M, Brosseau L, Farmer M, et al. Splints and orthosis for treating rheumatoid arthritis. *Cochrane Database Syst Rev.* 2003;(1):CD004018.

47. White J. Custom shoe therapy. Current concepts, designs, and special considerations. *Clin Podiatr Med Surg.* 1994;11(2): 259–270.

48. Reiber GE, Smith DG, Wallace C, et al. Effect of therapeutic footwear on foot reulceration in patients with diabetes: a randomized controlled trial. *JAMA.* 2002;287(19):2552–2558.

49. Breuer U. Diabetic patient's compliance with bespoke footwear after healing of neuropathic foot ulcers. *Diabetes Metab.* 1994;20(4):415–419.

50. Brown D, Wertsch JJ, Harris GF, et al. The effect of rocker soles on plantar pressure. *Arch Phys Med Rehabil.* 2004;85(1):81–86.

51. Kaye RA. The extra-depth toe box: a rational approach. *Foot Ankle Int.* 1994;15(3):146–150.

52. Kelly A, Winson I. Use of ready made insoles in the treatment of lesser metatarsalgia: a prospective randomized controlled clinical trial. *Foot Ankle Int.* 1998;19(4):217–220.

53. Childs SG. Diagnosis and treatment of interdigital perineuronal fibroma (a.k.a. Morton's syndrome). *Orthop Nurs.* 2002;21(6):32–34.

54. Shrader JA, Siegel KL. Non-operative management of functional hallux limitus in a patient with rheumatoid arthritis. *Phys Ther.* 2003;83(10):831–844.

55. Caselli MA. Foot deformities: biomechanical and pathomechanical changes associated with aging. *Clin Podiatr Med Surg.* 2003;20(3):487–509.

56. Hurwitz S. Hammer toe in adults: recognition and clinical management. *J Musculoskel Med.* 1999;16(8):460–465.

57. Michelson J, Easley M, Wigley FM, Hellmann D. Foot and ankle problems in rheumatoid arthritis. *Foot Ankle Int.* 1994;15(11):608–613.

58. Li CY, Imaishi K, Shiba SJ, et al. Biomechanical evaluation of foot pressure and loading force during gait in rheumatoid arthritic patients with and without foot orthosis. *Kurume Med J.* 2000;47(3):211–217.

59. Robbins S, Waked E, McClaran J. Proprioception and stability: foot position awareness as a function of age and footwear. *Age Ageing.* 1995;24(1):67–72.

II

Orthoses in Rehabilitation

8

Foot Orthoses

ROBERTA NOLE, DONALD S. KOWALSKY, JUAN C. GARBALOSA,
ELICIA POLLARD, AND JOHN THOMPSON

LEARNING OBJECTIVES

On completion of this chapter, the reader will be able to do the following:

1. Describe the major anatomical structures of the foot as well as the basic biomechanical principles associated with these structures.
2. Describe effects of extrinsic and intrinsic deformities and of abnormal pronation on the function of the foot during the various phases of gait.
3. Explain strategies used to examine and evaluate intrinsic foot deformities.
4. Describe abnormal pronation and the pathological conditions that contribute to abnormal pronation in gait.
5. Describe components of a foot orthosis, goals of orthotic intervention, and specific purposes of the most common orthotic interventions.
6. Discuss controversy related to traditional orthotic theory.
7. Review literature related to the efficacy of foot orthoses for the management of common disorders.

HISTORY OF THE FUNCTIONAL FOOT ORTHOSIS

The use of foot orthoses as an effective treatment tool for biomechanical dysfunction of the feet evolved during the twentieth century and continues to be the subject of research and technology. Early on, foot orthoses were used to redistribute plantar surface foot forces to alleviate discomfort in pressure-sensitive areas of the foot. Little consideration was given to the specific foot abnormality that led to the pathological condition.[1] In the early 1900s metal foot braces began to be used to control motion at specific joints of the foot and prevent pathological conditions.[2] These devices, although functional, were often not well tolerated because of the rigidity of the materials and the mismatch between brace design and foot pathokinesiology. In 1948, Schreber and Weineman first identified forefoot invertus (varus) and evertus (valgus) as primary foot deformities that required correction by an orthosis.[3] In the 1960s, Merton Root developed neutral impression casting techniques, positive cast modifications, and posting (mechanical correction) techniques.[4] The standards that Root established have enhanced orthotic comfort and function. Since then, functional foot orthosis use has increased considerably to address lower limb muscle activation pathology of the mechanics of the foot and ankle in musculoskeletal disorders and neurological disorders.[5-11]

TRIPLANAR STRUCTURE OF THE FOOT

The foot is a complex of bones interconnected by a series of multiplanar articulations supported by soft tissue structures. It is subdivided into three functional components: the rearfoot, the midfoot, and the forefoot.

Several important articulations of the foot (talocrural, subtalar, midtarsal, first and fifth rays) are triplanar; the axis of rotation in these joints is not perpendicular to any of the cardinal planes (sagittal, horizontal, frontal) of the human body. As a result, motion about triplanar joints leads to simultaneous movement in all three of these cardinal planes.[4] The amount of motion evident in any single plane is related to the pitch (inclination) of the triplanar axis from the respective cardinal plane. Triplanar motion occurs in three-dimensional space; the breakdown of triplanar motion into its three constituent cardinal plane movements is artificial.

Because motion about a triplanar axis is three dimensional, motion occurs simultaneously in the three cardinal planes. Blocking any one component of triplanar motion in a single cardinal plane prevents movement in the other two planes as well. This "all-or-nothing" rule is the premise for orthotic posting or wedging.[4] Theoretically, the addition of a post or wedge to an orthosis blocks the frontal plane component of triplanar motion, which in turn blocks or limits the triplanar motion of pronation. The design principles of foot orthoses are founded on knowledge of the functional anatomy of the foot.

Talocrural Joint

The talocrural joint (TCJ) (articulation between tibia, fibula, and talus, connecting the foot to the lower leg) has a triplanar axis of rotation. In neutral position, the TCJ axis passes through the tips of the medial and lateral malleoli, pitched 10 degrees from the transverse plane and 20 to 30 degrees from the frontal plane (Figure 8-1).[12-14] Although sagittal plane plantarflexion and dorsiflexion are primary motions at this joint, the slight inclination of the TCJ axis of rotation leads to concomitant transverse and frontal plane motion. During plantarflexion, the foot adducts and inverts; with dorsiflexion it abducts and everts. Normal range of motion (ROM) of the TCJ is between 12 and 20 degrees of dorsiflexion and 50 and 56 degrees of plantarflexion.[15] The medial (deltoid) and lateral collateral ligaments stabilize and limit motion that occurs at the TCJ.[16]

Rearfoot

The osseous structures of the rearfoot are the calcaneus (inferior) and the talus (superior) (Figure 8-2). The articulation between the calcaneus and talus is the subtalar joint (STJ).

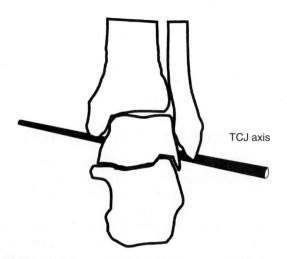

FIGURE 8-1 Posterior view of the osseous components and axis of the talocrural joint. The osseous components of the talocrural joint are the tibia medially and superiorly, the fibula laterally, and the talus inferiorly. The axis of the joint passes in a posterolateral to anteromedial direction through the tips of the lateral and medial malleoli. (Courtesy Juan C. Garbalosa, University of Hartford, West Hartford, Conn.)

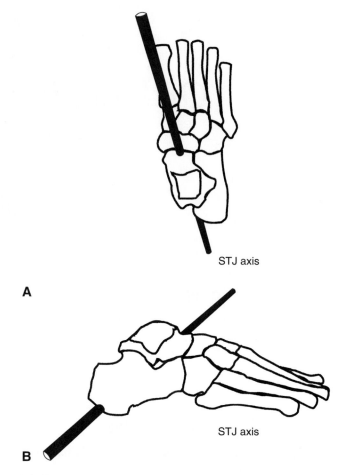

FIGURE 8-2 Superior (**A**) and lateral (**B**) views of the osseous structures in the rearfoot: the superior talus and inferior calcaneus. Also pictured is the triplanar axis of the subtalar joint. Note the inclination of the axis from all three cardinal planes of the body. (Courtesy Juan C. Garbalosa, University of Hartford, West Hartford, Conn.)

Three joint surfaces are present in this articulation: posterior, anterior, and middle. The posterior joint surface has a concave talar and convex calcaneal portion, whereas the anterior and middle joint surfaces have convex talar and concave calcaneal arrangements. This structurally based articular geometry, along with the interosseous talocalcaneal ligament, limits the amount and type of motion occurring at the STJ.[17,18] The medial and lateral collateral ligaments and the posterior and lateral talocalcaneal ligaments also offer support to the STJ.[19]

At the STJ, the triplanar axis of rotation is oriented in an anterosuperior to posteroinferior direction, pitched approximately 42 degrees from the transverse plane, 48 degrees from the frontal plane, and 16 degrees from the sagittal plane (see Figure 8-2). The location of the STJ axis in the human foot varies greatly. Manter[20] reported that the inclination from the transverse and sagittal planes varies from 29 degrees to 47 degrees and from 8 degrees to 24 degrees, respectively.

The triplanar motions at the STJ are supination and pronation. Supination of the weight-bearing foot leads to dorsiflexion and abduction of the talus with simultaneous inversion of the calcaneus. Pronation of the weight-bearing foot results in plantarflexion and adduction of the talus and eversion of the calcaneus.[4] Because of the variability in location of the axis of rotation of the STJ, the component motions of supination and pronation vary as well. As the axis becomes more perpendicular to a particular cardinal plane, the motion occurring in that plane becomes more pronounced, whereas the other motions become less prominent.[21,22] This variability affects coupled motion between the joints of the foot and the lower leg. During pronation and supination of the rearfoot, the tibia and fibula rotate internally and externally in the transverse plane.[4,23,24] An increase in the frontal plane motion of the rearfoot could cause a simultaneous increase in the transverse plane motion of the lower leg.

Midfoot

The midfoot is composed of two bones: the cuboid and the navicular. The talonavicular and calcaneocuboid articulations between the midfoot and rearfoot form an important composite joint: the midtarsal joint (MTJ) or transverse tarsal joint. The articular surfaces of the talonavicular joint are convex-concave, whereas the surfaces of the calcaneocuboid joint are sellar shaped.[13,20] MTJ movement is supported and restricted by the bifurcate, short and long plantar, and plantar calcaneonavicular (spring) ligaments. The short and long plantar ligaments and the plantar calcaneonavicular ligaments also support the longitudinal and transverse plantar arches of the foot.[25]

Because the MTJ is a composite joint, motion occurs about two separate triplanar joint axes: a longitudinal and an oblique axis (Figure 8-3). Movement of the forefoot about each joint axis can occur independently of the other. Manter[20] reported that the longitudinal axis is inclined superiorly 15 degrees from the transverse plane and medially 9 degrees from the sagittal plane, whereas the oblique axis is pitched superiorly 52 degrees from the transverse plane and medially 57 degrees from the sagittal plane. The predominant motion about the longitudinal axis is frontal plane inversion and eversion. Because of the slight deviation of the longitudinal axis from the three cardinal planes, small amounts of forefoot plantarflexion and dorsiflexion and adduction and abduction occur during inversion and eversion. Plantarflexion and dorsiflexion and abduction and adduction are the predominant movements around the oblique MTJ axis, with little concomitant inversion and eversion.[4,18]

These two joint axes produce the combined motion of supination and pronation of the MTJ. During supination and pronation, the forefoot inverts and everts about the longitudinal axis. The motion around the oblique axis is plantarflexion with adduction and dorsiflexion with abduction. The amount of motion possible at these MTJ axes is determined by the position of the STJ. In STJ supination, the two joint axes are nearly perpendicular so that MTJ mobility is restricted. This mechanism helps convert the forefoot into a rigid structure for propulsion during the push-off phase of gait (from heel rise through toe-off).[20,26] When the STJ is pronated, the joint axes are more parallel, allowing a greater degree of MTJ mobility.

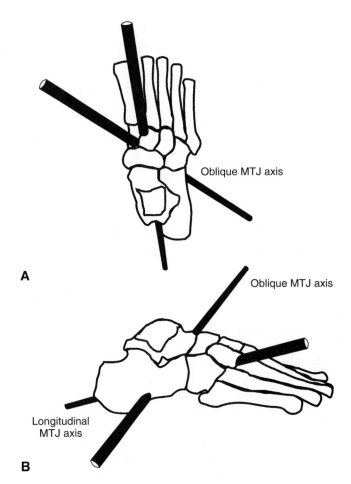

FIGURE 8-3 A superior **(A)** and lateral **(B)** view of the osseous components of the midtarsal joint (MTJ). The anterior portion of the MTJ is composed of the navicular and cuboid bones, whereas the posterior portion is composed of the calcaneus and talus. The two axes of the MTJ, the oblique and longitudinal axes, are also depicted. Like the subtalar joing, both axes of the MTJ are triplanar. (Courtesy Juan C. Garbalosa, University of Hartford, West Hartford, Conn.)

Forefoot

The forefoot includes all structures distal to the navicular and cuboid bones; it is subdivided into five rays and toes. The first through third rays consist of a cuneiform and its associated metatarsal bone; the fourth and fifth rays consist only of a metatarsal. The tarsometatarsal joints, the primary joints of the ray complexes, have two opposing planar surfaces.[4,25] The hallux, or first toe, has two bones (a proximal and distal phalanx) and two corresponding joints (metatarsophalangeal [MTP] and interphalangeal [IP]). The lesser toes have three bones (proximal, middle, and distal phalanges) and three associated joints. The proximal articular surfaces of the MTP and IP joints are convex, and the distal articular surface is concave.[4] Numerous soft tissue structures support these joints.[27,28]

Although each ray has its own axis of motion, the first and fifth rays are of particular interest. The triplanar axes of rotation of these two joints are nearly perpendicular. The axis of the first ray is pitched at a 45-degree angle from the sagittal and frontal planes; the primary motions possible are plantarflexion with eversion and dorsiflexion with inversion.

Because the axis of the first ray is minimally pitched from the transverse plane, insignificant transverse motion occurs.[4] In contrast, the axis of rotation of the fifth ray is oriented at a 20-degree angle from the transverse plane and a 35-degree angle from the sagittal plane. The resulting motions combine inversion with plantarflexion and eversion with dorsiflexion. Less motion is present about the axis of rotation of the fifth ray than of the first ray.[4] MTP joints have two separate axes of rotation: the vertical axis (abduction and adduction) and the transverse axis (plantarflexion and dorsiflexion).[4,13,25] Little frontal plane motion at MTP joints is normal; frontal plane motion leads to subluxation.[4]

Plantar Fascia and Arches of the Foot

The plantar aponeurosis, one of the most functionally important soft tissue structures of the foot, is a sheath of fascia spanning most of the foot's plantar surface. Arising from the medial process of the calcanean tuberosity, it passes distally along the plantar aspect of the foot, then divides into five slips for its distal attachment at the base of the proximal phalanges by the plantar pads.[29] This fascial sheath plays an extremely important role in providing the stability needed by the foot during the toe-off phase of stance during gait and in supporting the longitudinal arch of the foot.

The medial longitudinal and transverse arches are formed by the ligamentous and osseous structures of a "normal" foot.[30] The medial longitudinal arch (MLA) extends from the calcaneus (posterior) to the first metatarsal head (anterior) and is supported by the plantar aponeurosis, short and long plantar ligaments, and the spring ligament. During weight bearing, the height of the arch is reduced as the supporting ligamentous structures are elongated. The transverse arch reaches across the foot from medial to lateral borders. The height of the arch varies along the length of the foot: Its maximum height occurs at the cuboid-cuneiform bones of the midfoot, and its lowest point is at the metatarsal heads.

FUNCTION OF THE FOOT IN GAIT

The foot and ankle complex has three major functions in the gait cycle: attenuating the impact forces, maintaining equilibrium, and transmitting propulsive forces. For optimal biomechanical and energy-efficient performance, the joints of the foot and ankle must work in harmony. In early stance, the foot-ankle complex absorbs energy generated at initial contact and decreases forces transmitted to proximal structures during loading. The foot and ankle must also adapt to surface conditions encountered by the foot as stance begins. In late stance, the foot and lower leg transmit propulsive forces generated by muscles of the lower extremity onto the ground. The ability of the foot and lower leg to accomplish these functions depends on the integrity of the various structures of the foot. Gait abnormalities occur when the foot and ankle complex is unable to compensate for deficits in motion or structure.

The kinematic, kinetic, and neuromuscular events of the normal human gait cycle have been described in many ways.[4,31,32] Most focus on five distinct events: initial contact

(IC) or heel strike, loading response (LR) or foot flat, midstance (MSt), terminal stance (TSt) or heel-off, and preswing (PSw) or toe-off. See Chapter 5 for a more detailed description of the gait cycle.

Shock Absorption

Musculoskeletal structures of the lower limb act from IC to MSt to attenuate impact forces.[4,31,33] Force plate recording of ground reaction forces (GRFs) estimates the foot's ability to absorb energy and decelerate the lower leg. The push of the foot against the floor creates a GRF with three components: vertical, medial and lateral, and fore and aft forces. The vertical component of a typical GRF record has a bimodal shape (Figure 8-4). The brief first peak results from the impact of the heel with the ground. Some of the vertical GRF is attributed to acceleration of the centers of mass of the foot and shank of the leg.

In early stance, from IC to LR, the STJ moves into pronation as the TCJ is plantarflexing.[4,31,34,35] The fibula and tibia internally rotate with respect to the foot.[22,23] Pronation of the STJ is controlled by eccentric contraction of the tibialis anterior, posterior tibialis, flexor hallucis longus, and flexor digitorum longus muscles.[4,31,36] Plantarflex of the foot is controlled primarily by eccentric action of the tibialis anterior.[4,35] The combined muscle activity decelerates plantarflex and pronation motion of the TCJ, STJ, and MTJ, slowing vertical and anterior movement of the center of mass of the foot and shank and decreasing impact forces encountered at IC.

The viscoelastic plantar fat pad absorbs some of the energy generated between IC and LR.[37] Pronation of the STJ flattens the arches of the foot, elongating plantar connective tissue structures. Because these tissues are viscoelastic, they also absorb some of the energy generated from IC to LR.

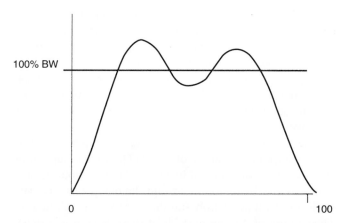

FIGURE 8-4 Typical vertical ground reaction pattern during walking. Note the bimodal shape of the ground reaction force. The first peak occurs at initial contact, and the second peak occurs during the toe-off phase of gait. The recorded ground reaction force represents the whole body center of mass acceleration. BW, Body weight. (From Valiant GA. Transmission and attenuation of heelstrike accelerations. In Cavanagh PR [ed], *Biomechanics of Distance Running.* Champaign, Ill: Human Kinetics, 1990. pp. 225-249.)

Adaptation to Surfaces

In everyday walking, the foot must be able to adapt quickly to many types of terrains and uneven surfaces. The key contributor to surface adaptation is STJ pronation, which unlocks the MTJ, permitting the joints of the foot to function in loose-packed positions and enabling the osseous elements to shift their relative positions.

At IC, the forefoot is in a supinatory twist (inverted) about the longitudinal MTJ axis. Eccentric action of the anterior tibialis decelerates plantarflex of the forefoot, lowering it to the ground. The MTJ becomes fully supinated at LR, as a result of eversion of the STJ and GRFs acting upward on the foot's medial border. Contraction of the extensor digitorum longus and peroneus tertius abducts and dorsiflexes (pronates) the forefoot, locking it about the oblique MTJ axis and preparing the forefoot to receive the loading forces encountered at MSt.[4]

Propulsion

During MSt (LR to PSw), the STJ is maximally pronated and begins to resupinate. At this time, the GRF maintains the MTJ in a pronated position about its oblique axis. At the same time, a pronatory twist is initiated at the longitudinal axis by concentric action of the peroneals. The MTJ locks in a fully pronated position around the longitudinal axis just before heel rise, as the STJ reaches its neutral position. The MTJ must remain locked in this position throughout propulsion, as the peroneals contract to lift the lateral side of the foot from the ground and transfer weight medially to the other foot. As the heel is raised from the ground, the rearfoot continues to supinate (talus abducts and dorsiflexes) as the lower limb rotates externally. This coupled motion necessitates supination of the MTJ about the oblique axis to maximize joint stability and convert the foot into a rigid lever for propulsion.

Supination of the STJ occurs with concentric action of the tibialis posterior, flexor hallucis longus, and flexor digitorum longus and soleus, as well as the antagonistic functioning of the peroneus brevis.[4,31] The concentric activity of the gastrocnemius and soleus muscles causes vertical acceleration of the foot and lower leg. Propulsive forces generated by the foot and lower leg are transmitted to the floor.[4,31,35] The second peak of a GRF curve corresponds to propulsion in late stance phase (see Figure 8-4).

Supination of the STJ and locking of the MTJ about the longitudinal axis place the foot in a closed-packed position, transforming the foot into a rigid lever.[4,14,23,31] This transformation is aided by the action of the plantar aponeurosis as it wraps around the metatarsal heads. During TSt, the MTP joints extend (dorsiflex), creating a "windlass effect." This action compresses joints of the midfoot and forefoot, facilitating the transition from flexibility to rigidity required for effective push-off.

BIOMECHANICAL EXAMINATION

The biomechanical examination of the foot and ankle has three components: a non–weight-bearing assessment, a static weight-bearing assessment, and a dynamic gait analysis (Figure 8-5).

Five common intrinsic foot deformities are identified in the biomechanical examination: rearfoot varus, forefoot varus, forefoot valgus, equinus deformity, and plantar flexed first ray.

The theoretical model of biomechanical foot and ankle examination is based on the work of Root and colleagues.[4] Debate continues about the validity of Root's criteria for normalcy and the assumption that the STJ is in neutral position from MSt to TSt of the gait cycle. Reliability of the measurement techniques used to determine STJ neutral position has also been questioned.[38-40] Although controversial, Root's theory and his biomechanical evaluation and treatment techniques are used by many clinicians.

Root describes deviations from normal foot alignment as "intrinsic" foot deformities, which can lead to aberrant lower extremity function and musculoskeletal pathological conditions.[4,41] To prescribe an appropriate biomechanical foot orthosis, the source of the pathological condition or deformity must be determined by a detailed patient history and a comprehensive biomechanical examination.[42] This helps the clinician identify resultant pathomechanical abnormalities and determine the benefits of orthotic intervention.

NON–WEIGHT-BEARING OPEN CHAIN EXAMINATION

During the non–weight-bearing open chain examination, the basic architecture of the foot and ankle is assessed. Any bony deformities or prominence of the joints, rays (toes), and callosities are noted. The examiner uses a goniometer to locate the subtalar neutral (STN) position and identify any intrinsic foot deformities.

The non–weight-bearing goniometric examination is performed with the patient in the prone position, with the targeted lower extremity positioned with extended knee, and the foot 6 to 8 inches off the treatment table. Placing the contralateral lower extremity in a figure-four position orients the ipsilateral lower extremity in the frontal plane, reducing the influence of proximal rotational limb disorders on measurement.[43]

Examination of the Rearfoot

Goniometric measurements of the non–weight-bearing examination assess the rearfoot with respect to STN position, as well as STJ mobility, based on calcaneal positioning in the frontal plane. Calcaneal frontal plane motion is the most readily examined component of triplanar STJ motion. To perform the examination, the stationary arm of a goniometer is aligned with an imagined bisection of the lower third of the limb (tibiofibular complex), the mobile arm is aligned with an imaginary bisection of the posterior surface of the calcaneus, and the axis of the goniometer is aligned at the STJ axis, just above the superior border of the calcaneus but beneath the level of the medial and lateral malleoli (Figure 8-6).[43,44]

Subtalar Neutral Position

STN position can be manually estimated by palpation or by using a mathematical model developed by Root. If using palpation, the examiner identifies the anteromedial and

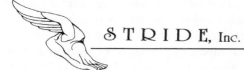

$\mathcal{S}\,T\,R\,I\,D\,E$, Inc.

Physical Therapy and Pedorthic Services
530 Middlebury Road • Suite 102 • Middlebury, CT 06762
TEL.: (203) 598-0070 • FAX: (203) 598-0075

BIOMECHANICAL FOOT EVALUATION

Patient: _____   Phone: _____

Address: _____

Age: _____   Height: _____   Weight: _____   Shoe size: _____   Shoe Style: _____

Occupation: _____   Activity level: _____   Sports: _____

Referring Practitioner: _____   Date of Evaluation: _____

Diagnosis: _____

I. NON-WEIGHTBEARING EVALUATION

	Left	**Right**

Rearfoot:

STN position _____ varus _____ varus

calcaneal inversion _____ degrees _____ degrees

calcaneal eversion _____ degrees _____ degrees

rearfoot dorsiflexion _____ degrees _____ degrees

Forefoot:

STN position _____ varus/valgus _____ varus/valgus

locking mechanism

poor   fair   normal   rigid   poor   fair   normal   rigid

MTJ dorsiflexion _____ degrees _____ degrees

First Ray:

STN position and mobility

hallux dorsiflexion _____ degrees _____ degrees

Arch Position:

low   med   high   low   med   high

Toe Position/Deformities: _____   _____

Lesions/Shoe Wear: **Calluses:**   L   R

R   L   L   R

FIGURE 8-5 Biomechanical examination form outlining components of the non–weight-bearing and weight-bearing assessment. *Ante,* Femoral anteversion; *ASIS,* anterior superior iliac spine; *DLS,* double-limb stance; *Gastroc,* gastrocnemius; *G.T.,* greater trochanter; *ITB,* iliotibial band; *M.M.,* medial malleolus; *PSIS,* posterior inferior iliac spine; *Retro,* femoral retroversion; *SLS,* single-limb stance; *T.T.,* tibial tubercle; *VAR,* varus; *VAL,* valgus. (Courtesy Stride, Inc., Middlebury, Conn.) Biomechanical examination form outlining components of the weight-bearing assessment.

II. WEIGHTBEARING EVALUATION

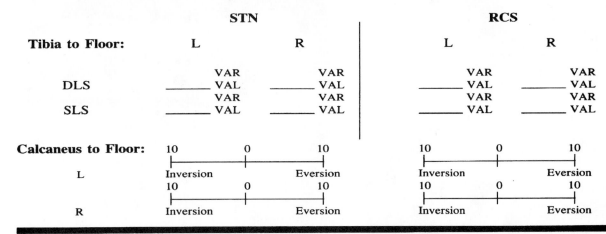

	STN			RCS	
Tibia to Floor:	L	R		L	R
DLS	_____ VAR / VAL	_____ VAR / VAL		_____ VAR / VAL	_____ VAR / VAL
SLS	_____ VAR / VAL	_____ VAR / VAL		_____ VAR / VAL	_____ VAR / VAL

Calcaneus to Floor:

L: 10 — 0 — 10 | Inversion — Eversion   10 — 0 — 10 | Inversion — Eversion

R: 10 — 0 — 10 | Inversion — Eversion   10 — 0 — 10 | Inversion — Eversion

III. SOFT TISSUE RESTRICTIONS

	L	R			L	R
Iliopsoas	_____	_____		**Hip Rotation (Hips 90°, Knees 90°)**		
Rectus Femoris	_____	_____		Internal	_____	_____
ITB	_____	_____		External	_____	_____
Hamstring	_____	_____		**Hip Rotation (Hips 0°, Knees 90°)**		
Gastroc	_____	_____		Internal	_____	_____
Soleus	_____	_____		External	_____	_____

IV. POSTURAL OBSERVATIONS

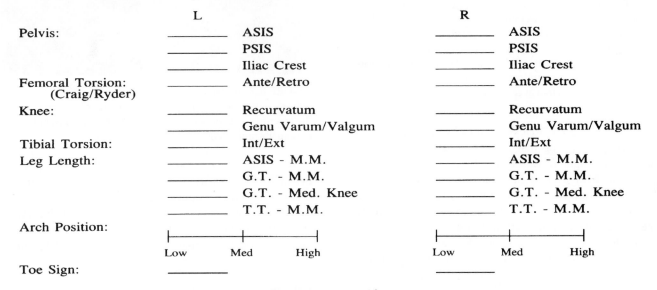

	L		R	
Pelvis:	_____	ASIS	_____	ASIS
	_____	PSIS	_____	PSIS
	_____	Iliac Crest	_____	Iliac Crest
Femoral Torsion: (Craig/Ryder)	_____	Ante/Retro	_____	Ante/Retro
Knee:	_____	Recurvatum	_____	Recurvatum
	_____	Genu Varum/Valgum	_____	Genu Varum/Valgum
Tibial Torsion:	_____	Int/Ext	_____	Int/Ext
Leg Length:	_____	ASIS - M.M.	_____	ASIS - M.M.
	_____	G.T. - M.M.	_____	G.T. - M.M.
	_____	G.T. - Med. Knee	_____	G.T. - Med. Knee
	_____	T.T. - M.M.	_____	T.T. - M.M.
Arch Position:	Low — Med — High		Low — Med — High	
Toe Sign:	_____		_____	

FIGURE 8-5—cont'd

anterolateral aspects of the talar head with the thumb and index fingers of the hand closest to the patient's midline, placing the thumb just proximal to the navicular tuberosity, approximately 1 inch below and 1 inch distal to the medial malleolus (Figure 8-7). In STJ pronation, the anteromedial talar head is most prominent beneath the thumb, and an anterolateral sulcus (the sinus tarsi) is apparent. The index finger is placed in this sulcus, where the talar head is found to protrude when the foot is fully supinated. The thumb and index finger of the other hand grasp the fourth and fifth metatarsal heads, moving the foot in an arc of adduction and inversion (supination) and abduction and eversion (pronation). STN is the point where the talar head is equally prominent anteromedially and anterolaterally.[41,43,44]

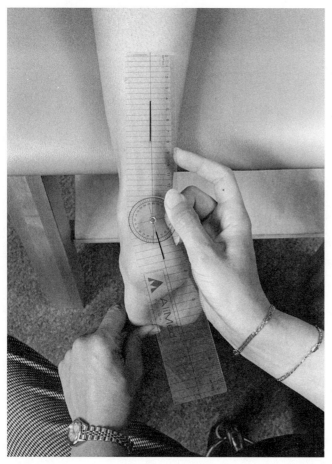

FIGURE 8-6 Non–weight-bearing goniometric technique. A loading force applied by the examiner over the fourth and fifth metatarsal heads locks the forefoot on the rearfoot while the examiner's opposite hand operates the goniometer to measure subtalar neutral position and calcaneal range of motion. The examiner is seated at the distal end of the treatment table, with chair height adjusted to position the patient's foot at chest level.

The examiner then "loads" the foot by applying a dorsally directed pressure against the fourth and fifth metatarsal heads until slight resistance is felt. The loading procedure locks the MTJ against the rearfoot, mimicking GRFs of MSt.[4,45] The angular relation between the bisection of the calcaneus and the bisection of the lower third of the leg is measured with a goniometer (see Figure 8-6), recorded on the evaluation form as rearfoot STN position.

Root's mathematical model for determining STN position uses a quantitative goniometric formula.[4,41] First, end ROM calcaneal inversion and eversion are determined by goniometric measurement. Total calcaneal ROM is the sum of the inversion and eversion values. The STN position is determined as the calcaneus is moved into inversion at one third of the total calcaneal ROM. If end-range calcaneal inversion is 25 degrees and end-range calcaneal eversion is +5 degrees, total calcaneal ROM would be 30 degrees. STN position is calculated to be at 5 degrees calcaneal inversion, one third of the distance from its fully everted position.

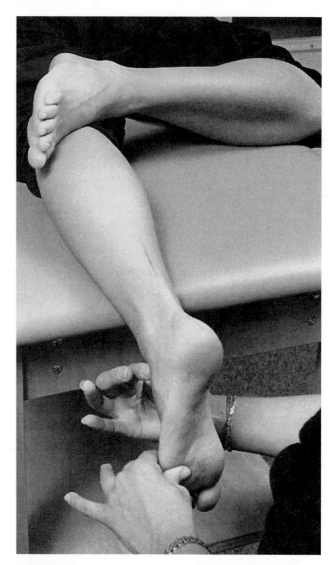

FIGURE 8-7 To determine subtalar neutral position, the examiner moves the forefoot slowly between supination and pronation until the anteromedial and anterolateral surfaces of the head of the talus are equally prominent.

Reliability and clinical validity of both models have been debated.[40,41,43,46-48] Although acceptable reliability is possible, it is influenced by examiner experience. Palpation to determine STN position is efficient in terms of time but requires more advanced manual skills and experience than the mathematical model. The mathematical model may be more reliable for the entry-level practitioner.

Calcaneal Range of Motion

Calcaneal inversion and eversion occur primarily at the STJ, with lesser contributions from the TCJ. Calcaneal ROM is assessed with the patient in the prone position with the same anatomical landmarks and lines of bisection as for STN assessment. The examiner grasps the calcaneus in one hand, fully inverts it in the frontal plane until end ROM is achieved, and then takes a goniometric measurement.[48] The procedure is repeated for calcaneal eversion. The TCJ must be maintained in a neutral to slightly dorsiflexed position while measuring to lock it in a closed-packed position and better isolate STJ motion.[49] Normative values of 20 degrees for calcaneal inversion and 10 degrees beyond vertical for eversion have been reported.[4]

Because values of calcaneal eversion are larger when assessed in a full weight-bearing position, some clinicians suggest that this position is more clinically valid.[38,48] Assessment of calcaneal eversion in the weight-bearing position represents a total "functional" pronation and eversion that is the summation of motion occurring at the STJ and compensatory motion occurring extrinsic to the STJ (e.g., TCJ, MTJ). Passive assessment of calcaneal eversion in non–weight bearing remains the most accurate method to determine the degree of composite pronation acquired from the STJ itself.

Talocrural Joint Range of Motion

In normal walking, the TCJ is maximally dorsiflexed just before heel rise when the knee is fully extended and the STJ is in a nearly neutral position.[4,50] When and whether an actual STN position ever occurs during gait is disputed.[38] The use of a standard position of knee extension and STN, however, offers a consistent point of reference when assessing TCJ dorsiflexion. According to most sources, a minimum of 10 degrees TCJ dorsiflexion is required for normal gait; anything less is classified as an equinus deformity.[4,50-53] A minimum of 20 degrees of plantarflex is also required for normal gait.[4]

Ankle dorsiflexion is measured in a non–weight-bearing position with the STJ held in the neutral position and the knee extended. The examiner forcefully dorsiflexes the ankle with active assistance from the patient. Active assistance encourages reciprocal inhibition of the calf muscle group and is essential for accurate measurement.[50] The proximal arm of the goniometer is positioned along the lateral aspect of the fibula, the distal arm along the lateral border of the fifth metatarsal, and the axis distal to the lateral malleolus.[54] An alternative placement of the distal arm of the goniometer along the inferolateral border of the calcaneus may more effectively isolate true TCJ dorsiflexion (Figure 8-8). This value is recorded as rearfoot dorsiflexion. Forefoot dorsiflexion is measured by repositioning the distal arm along the lateral aspect of the fifth metatarsal. This method allows the examiner to identify contributions or restrictions in sagittal plane motion from the oblique axis of the MTJ.

If ankle dorsiflexion is less than 10 degrees when measured with the knee extended, remeasurement with the knee flexed may rule out soft tissue restriction of the gastrocnemius-soleus complex.[4,50] If dorsiflexion values are consistent in both positions, the limitation is likely a result of osseous equinus formation of the ankle.

During gait, ankle dorsiflexion occurs in a closed kinetic chain as the tibia and fibula rotate forward over a fixed foot. On the basis of this, some have suggested that assessing ankle dorsiflexion may be more accurate with the patient in a weight-bearing position.[38,52] The weight-bearing technique measures the angle between the tibia and the floor as the patient leans forward with the foot flat on the floor. Unwanted compensations are often difficult to control during

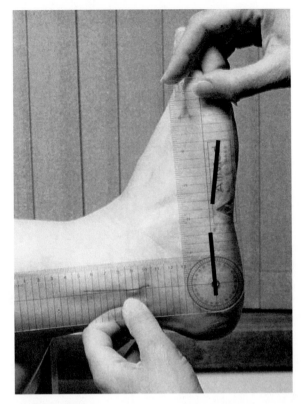

FIGURE 8-8 Alignment of the distal arm of the goniometer along the inferior-lateral border of the calcaneus may provide a more accurate measure of talocrural joint dorsiflexion than the traditional alignment along the shaft of the fifth metatarsal used to measure overall ankle dorsiflexion.

weight bearing and may mask true TCJ limitations. The non–eight-bearing technique allows the examiner to assess end feel and joint play, as well as mechanical blocks or joint laxity, providing additional information not accessible in the weight-bearing examination.

Rearfoot Deformities

Normal rearfoot position is one in which STN is 1 to 4 degrees of varus.[39,40,47,48] Values of more than 4 degrees are described as a rearfoot varus deformity. This deformity may be the result of ontogenetic failure of the calcaneus to derotate sufficiently during early childhood development.[4,45,55] Because this deformity is a torsional structural malalignment of the calcaneus, not a joint-related problem, the TCJ and STJ lines remain congruent when observed in the non–weight-bearing STN position. As a structural deformity, it cannot be corrected or reduced by joint mobilization or a strengthening program. Instead, it is managed with a functional foot orthosis that partially supports the calcaneus in its inverted alignment while preventing excessive STJ pronation.

Assessment of calcaneal ROM predicts quality of motion and the integrity of the STJ. Measuring calcaneal motion into eversion allows the examiner to determine whether a rearfoot deformity is compensated or uncompensated (Figure 8-9).

In a compensated rearfoot varus deformity, the calcaneus fully everts to vertical or beyond in weight bearing

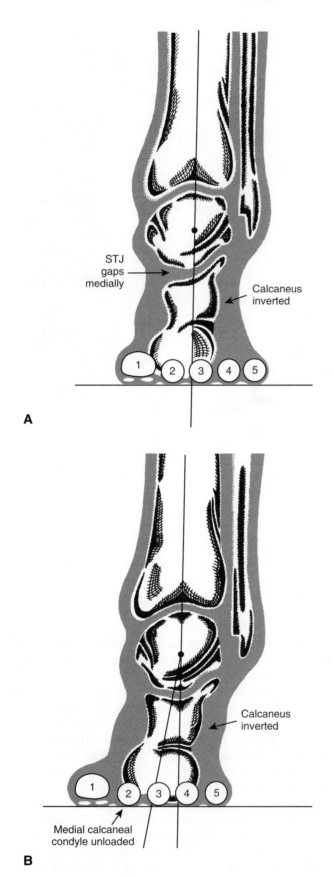

A

STJ
gaps
medially

Calcaneus
inverted

1 2 3 4 5

B

Calcaneus
inverted

1 2 3 4 5

Medial calcaneal
condyle unloaded

FIGURE 8-9 A, In relaxed calcaneal stance, compensation for a rearfoot varus is normally subtalar joint pronation. **B,** In an uncompensated rearfoot varus, the subtalar joint cannot pronate and instead may develop compensatory midtarsal joint pronation about the longitudinal joint axis. (Courtesy Stride, Inc., Middlebury, Conn.)

because the STJ possesses an adequate amount of pronatory motion to compensate for the deformity. A compensated rearfoot varus deformity of 10 degrees (STN position) requires that the STJ pronate or evert at least 10 degrees to enable the medial condyle of the calcaneus to achieve ground contact in weight bearing. Such excessive pronatory motion causes medial gapping and lateral constriction at the STJ line and a medial bulge of the talus as it moves into adduction and plantarflex.

In an uncompensated rearfoot varus deformity, the calcaneus remains fixed in its inverted STN position with no eversion motion at the STJ. A partially compensated rearfoot varus deformity allows for partial STJ eversion so that the medial condyle of the calcaneus does not make complete contact with the ground on weight bearing. Alternative compensatory motion, extrinsic to the STJ, is necessary to achieve weight bearing on the medial aspect of the foot. One common compensation is an acquired soft tissue (valgus) deformity of the forefoot caused by a plantar flexed first ray. Other sources of compensatory motion can occur at the MTJ or proximally at the knee, hip, or sacroiliac joints.

An equinus deformity occurs when fewer than 10 degrees of ankle dorsiflexion are available as a result of osseous or muscular problems.[51,53,56,57] Clubfoot (talipes equinovarus) is a congenital osseous deformity that includes varus deformity of both rearfoot and forefoot, rearfoot equinus, and an inverted and adducted forefoot.[58,59] The angular relation between the body and the head and neck of the talus is decreased, and the navicular is shifted medially. Muscular forms of equinus include congenital or acquired soft tissue shortening or muscle spasm.[53] Tissue contracture or shortening occurs in both contractile tissues (gastrocnemius, soleus, and plantaris) and noncontractile tissues (teno-Achilles and plantar fascia).[51,53]

Compensation for an equinus deformity occurs at the foot through pronation, perpetuating soft tissue contractures. The STJ is forced to pronate maximally to gain as much sagittal plane dorsiflexion as possible. Although foot pronation allows some dorsiflexion from the STJ, the amount is often inadequate. Pronation of the STJ unlocks the MTJ, creating an unstable midfoot while allowing further dorsiflexion and forefoot abduction from the oblique axis of the MTJ.[53] Other compensatory strategies for equinus deformity include knee flexion (especially in individuals with cerebral palsy), early heel rise, toe walking, shortened stride length of the contralateral lower limb, and toe-out walking.[31,41,53] Clinical consequences of long-term ankle equinus include many conditions normally associated with the excessively pronated foot: plantar fasciitis, heel spurs, bunions, and capsulitis.[53]

Examination of the Forefoot

Forefoot position is assessed with the STJ in neutral position. Because the first and fifth rays have independent axes of motion, forefoot orientation is defined by the planar relation of the second, third, and fourth rays to the bisection line of the calcaneus.

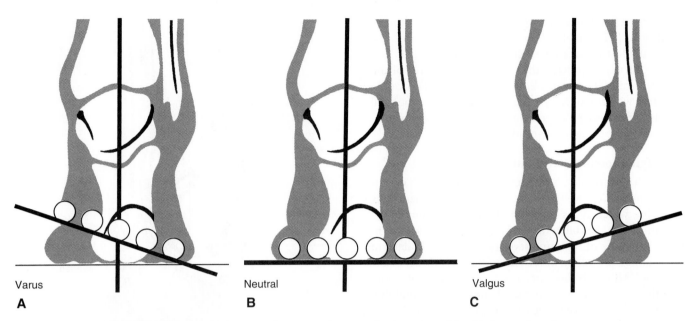

Varus
A

Neutral
B

Valgus
C

FIGURE 8-10 In subtalar neutral position, the normal orientation of the forefoot to the calcaneus (**B**) is perpendicular. Excessive supination and inversion of the forefoot in subtalar neutral position indicates a forefoot varus (**A**), whereas excessive pronation and eversion of the forefoot indicates a forefoot valgus (**C**). (Courtesy Stride, Inc., Middlebury, Conn.)

Neutral Forefoot Position

If the forefoot is properly balanced, the plane of the three central metatarsals is perpendicular to the bisection of the calcaneus when in STN (Figure 8-10). In a forefoot varus deformity, the forefoot is excessively supinated or inverted, whereas in a forefoot valgus the forefoot is excessively pronated or everted.

Mobility Testing: Locking Mechanism

To isolate STN position in the non–weight-bearing examination, the examiner attempts to lock the MTJ by applying a dorsally directed loading pressure with the thumb and index fingers over the fourth and fifth metatarsal heads of the patient's foot (see Figures 8-6 and 8-7). Loading force must be gently applied over the fourth and fifth metatarsal heads until tissue slack is taken up from the normally plantar flexed resting position of the ankle.[4,55] Overload of the forefoot leads to dorsiflexion and abduction of the foot, placing the forefoot in an excessively pronated position and giving a false valgus orientation.

Although many forefoot measurement devices are available, forefoot orientation can be accurately assessed with a standard goniometer.[60] To assess the forefoot to rearfoot relation, the proximal arm of the goniometer is aligned along the bisection of the calcaneus, with the axis just below its distal border. The distal arm is positioned in the plane of the three central metatarsal heads (Figure 8-11). The angular displacement is recorded on the evaluation form under STN position for the forefoot assessment (see Figure 8-5).

In normal walking, the MTJ locks as heel rise begins so that the foot is converted into a rigid lever for propulsion. This lock requires that the STJ be in the neutral position. Clinical assessment of MTJ mobility and the locking mechanism is an advanced manual skill. Observations made during weight-bearing assessment (e.g., toe sign, navicular

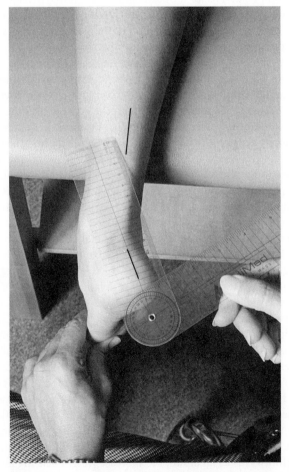

FIGURE 8-11 Measurement of forefoot orientation in subtalar neutral position with a standard goniometer. The proximal arm of the goniometer is aligned with the bisection of the posterior surface of the calcaneus, and the distal arm parallels the plane of the metatarsal heads. The axis lies beneath the distal aspect of the calcaneus.

drop test, talar bulge) provide an elementary method to identify an MTJ unable to lock.

An ineffective locking mechanism at the MTJ is often more clinically significant than the absolute degree of forefoot deformity. For example, a forefoot varus deformity of 3 degrees with a poor MTJ locking mechanism may be symptomatic, whereas an 8-degree forefoot varus deformity with a normal MTJ locking mechanism may not be.

Identifying Forefoot Deformities

Although the prevalence of forefoot deformity, with or without symptoms, is well documented, less agreement exists regarding which types of deformity are most common.[47,61] If an individual has bilateral forefoot deformity, the deformities may not be of the same severity or type. MTJ deformities change the location of the lock of the forefoot against the rearfoot.[4] Although these osseous frontal plane deformities alter the direction of motion, they do not limit the total ROM of the MTJ.[4] In forefoot varus, locking of the forefoot occurs in an inverted position relative to the rearfoot.[4] Forefoot varus results from ontogenetic failure of the normal valgus rotation of the head and neck of the talus in relation to its body during early childhood development.[4,45,55]

Compensations for foot deformities are viewed in a relaxed weight-bearing position referred to as relaxed calcaneal stance (RCS). When excessive pronation of the STJ compensates for the deformity on weight bearing, the condition is called a compensated forefoot varus (Figure 8-12A). When the STJ cannot adequately pronate to accommodate an inverted forefoot, an uncompensated forefoot varus is present. The medial forefoot does not make contact with the ground, and the lateral forefoot is subjected to excessive pressure. Thick callus develops beneath the head of the fifth metatarsal, and the risk of stress fracture is increased. Plantarflex of the first ray and pronation at the MTJ are common compensations that allow the medial forefoot to make contact with the ground (see Figure 8-12B). Persistent MTJ stress may lead to joint damage and excessive forefoot abduction and eversion.

Forefoot valgus occurs in the frontal plane deformity, locking the forefoot in eversion relative to the rearfoot.[4] Root suggests that this deformity results from ontogenetic overrotation of the talar head and neck in relation to its body during early childhood development.[4,45,55] Forefoot valgus can be a rigid or flexible deformity. In rigid forefoot valgus, the compensatory weight-bearing mechanism occurs at the STJ as excessive supination or calcaneal inversion. It is a result of excessive premature GRFs at the first metatarsal head, causing rapid STJ inversion and increasing loading forces beneath the fifth metatarsal head. Thick callosities are often present beneath the first and fifth metatarsal heads. In contrast, flexible forefoot valgus is usually an acquired soft tissue condition. It most often occurs as a consequence of uncompensated rearfoot varus as an attempt to increase weight bearing along the medial foot. Because this deformity is flexible, no compensatory mechanism is necessary. Contact force beneath the first metatarsal head simply pushes it up out of the way, and the foot functions as if this condition were not present.

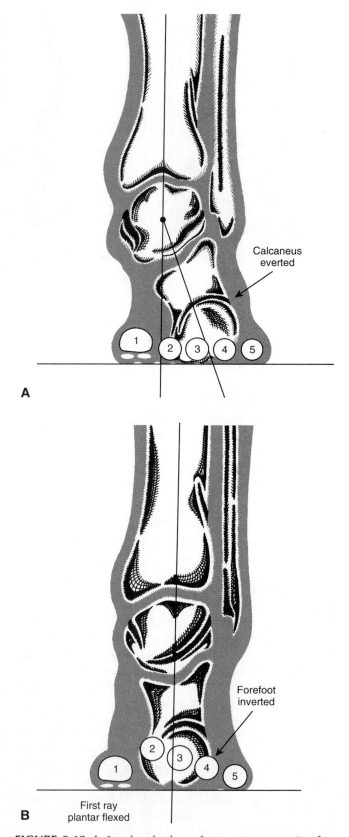

FIGURE 8-12 A, In relaxed calcaneal stance, compensation for a forefoot varus deformity is normally subtalar joint pronation, resulting in an everted calcaneus. **B,** In an uncompensated forefoot varus, the subtalar joint is unable to compensate. Instead, the first ray plantarflexes to achieve weight bearing medially on the foot. (Courtesy Stride, Inc., Middlebury, Conn.)

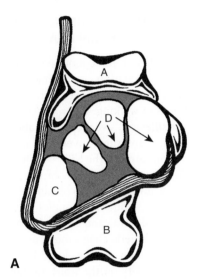 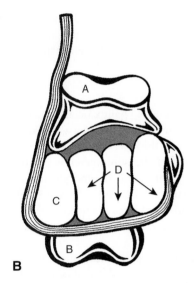

FIGURE 8-13 A, Cuboid pulley mechanism in a normal foot. **B,** In an abnormally pronated foot, the mechanical advantage of the peroneals is impaired. *A,* Talus; *B,* calcaneus; *C,* cuboid; *D,* the cuneiforms. (Courtesy Stride, Inc., Middlebury, Conn.)

The First Ray

Assessment of first ray position is also carried out in STN position. Ideally, the first ray lies within the common transverse plane of the lesser metatarsal heads. To examine mobility of the first ray, the examiner holds the first metatarsal head between the thumb and index finger and performs a dorsal and plantar glide while stabilizing the lesser metatarsal heads with the other hand. Normally, first ray movement is at least one thumb width above and below the plane of the other metatarsal heads.[4]

As stance phase is completed, activity of the peroneus longus creates a pronatory twist of the forefoot, stabilizing the medial column of the foot on the ground, locking the MTJ about its longitudinal axis, and converting the foot to a rigid lever for propulsion. Adequate plantarflex of the first ray must be present for conversion from flexible forefoot to a rigid lever. Three factors determine how much first ray plantarflex must occur: amount of inversion of the foot at propulsion, width of the foot, and length of the second metatarsal.[4] The more the foot inverts during propulsion, the further the first ray must plantarflex to make ground contact. Elevation of the medial forefoot is related to foot width; wide feet require more first ray plantarflex. An excessively long second metatarsal also increases the distance that the first ray must plantarflex to make ground contact.

In some instances, the first ray is inappropriately dorsiflexed above the plane of the other metatarsals, resulting in restriction of plantarflex and impeding normal propulsion. The first ray may also be plantar flexed below the plane of the other metatarsals. In uncompensated rearfoot varus, for example, the eversion motion of the calcaneus is insufficient, the medial condyle fails to make contact with the ground, and excessive weight bearing is present on the lateral border of the foot. The peroneus longus contracts to pull the first metatarsal head toward the ground in an attempt to load the medial side of the foot. This action is possible because of the cuboid pulley system (Figure 8-13).[4] When the STJ remains abnormally pronated in late stance phase, orientation of the cuboid tunnel is altered and the mechanical advantage of the peroneus longus is lost. The MTJ cannot lock, and the foot is unstable throughout propulsion.

The presence of a rigid plantar flexed first ray sometimes results in a functional forefoot valgus (Figure 8-14).

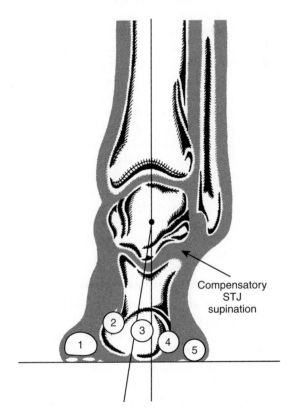

FIGURE 8-14 Plantarflexed first ray deformity in relaxed calcaneal stance. Compensation occurs at the subtalar joint, with lateral gapping and medial compression. (Courtesy Stride, Inc., Middlebury, Conn.)

The compensatory mechanism for this condition is similar to that for rigid forefoot valgus: STJ supination or calcaneal inversion on weight bearing to lower the lateral aspect of the foot to the ground.

The Hallux

In normal gait, dorsiflexion of the hallux occurs during the late propulsive phase as the body moves forward over the foot. Sagittal plane motion of the hallux is assessed as passive ROM. The stationary arm of the goniometer is positioned along the medial first metatarsal and the mobile arm along the medial proximal phalanx of the hallux. The axis is medial to the first MTP joint.[54] Sufficient force is applied to bring the hallux to its end ROM. Normal range of hallux dorsiflexion is between 70 and 90 degrees.[4,54]

In hallux limitus deformity, pathomechanical functioning of the first MTP joint prevents the hallux from moving through its full range of dorsiflexion during propulsion. Repetitive trauma to the first MTP joint can lead to ankylosis, or hallux rigidus. Functional hallux limitus is a condition in which full first MTP ROM is present when non–weight bearing, but a functional restriction of hallux dorsiflexion occurs during gait. Functional hallux limitus disrupts the normal windlass mechanism previously described.[62,63]

Limitation of hallux dorsiflexion prohibits the normal progression of the foot and interferes with propulsion of the body over the hallux. Several gait compensations can overcome this limitation.[62,63] An abducted or toe-out gait pattern shifts propulsion to the medial border of the hallux. A pinched callus then develops from friction between the hallux and shoe during propulsion. Alternatively, the IP joint of the hallux may hyperextend, causing a callus in the sulcus of the IP joint.

Hallux abductovalgus (HAV) is a progressive, acquired deformity of the first MTP joint that eventually results in a valgus subluxation of the hallux.[4,45] This deformity is caused by abnormal STJ pronation with hypermobility of the first ray.[4] A common misconception is that HAV is hereditary. Although the congenital osseous abnormalities that lead to aberrant STJ pronation are hereditary, HAV occurs to compensate for these other deformities. Another misconception is that HAV is caused by restrictive footwear. Although inappropriate or restrictive footwear can accentuate or speed the progression of HAV deformity when present, the deformity is frequently observed in populations that do not typically wear shoes.[4,45]

Additional Observations

Several other important observations are made as the non–weight-bearing examination is completed. Non–weight-bearing arch height is observed for later comparison to weight-bearing arch height as a composite estimate of foot pronation. Toes are inspected for positional deformities such as hammertoe, claw toe, crossover deformity, and the presence of bunions or bunionettes. The plantar foot is checked for callus, plantar warts, or other signs of excessive pressure. The shoes are inspected for excessive or uneven wear patterns.

STATIC WEIGHT-BEARING CLOSED KINETIC CHAIN EXAMINATION

The open chain kinetic motion evaluated in the non–weight-bearing examination is dramatically different from the functional sequence of events in the closed kinetic chain of standing and walking. Open kinetic chain pronation (calcaneal dorsiflexion, eversion, and abduction) and supination (calcaneal plantarflex, inversion, and adduction) are triplanar motions around the STJ.[4,13,29] During closed kinetic chain pronation, internal rotation of the leg is coupled with talar adduction and calcaneal plantarflex and eversion. Closed kinetic chain supination couples external rotation of the leg with talar abduction and calcaneal dorsiflexion and inversion. In the open kinetic chain, movement is initiated in the distal segment (the foot). In the closed kinetic chain, motion is initiated proximally (at the tibia and talus). A thorough closed kinetic chain examination includes static postural observations, dynamic motion testing, and gait assessment.

Compensatory mechanisms that result from intrinsic deformities are assessed as the foot is subjected to GRFs during the static weight-bearing examination. This provides valuable insight regarding how the body compensates for the intrinsic foot deformities or impairments of normal foot joint function identified in the non–weight-bearing examination. Improper foot functioning can lead to a complex series of compensations that influence the mobility patterns of the foot and lower leg, as well as the knee, hip, pelvis, and spine.

The patient stands in a relaxed, weight-bearing posture (RCS). The examiner observes the patient's preferred stance, noting postural alignment and foot placement angle. The patient then adjusts the stance position, if necessary, to assume equal weight-bearing double-limb support, with feet 5 to 10 cm apart and oriented in neutral toe-in and toe-out foot placement angle. This adjusted posture, with neutral foot placement angle, offers a better frame of reference for assessing planar alignment and enhances the reliability and consistency of the measurement.[41] Postural alignment or body symmetry of the patient is evaluated in the frontal, sagittal, and transverse planes.

Frontal Plane

Static weight-bearing examination in the frontal plane focuses on the angular relation of the calcaneus and the tibia and fibula with respect to the floor and the relation between the pelvis and the lower leg.

Calcaneal Alignment to the Floor

With the patient in double-limb stance posture, a line bisecting the posterior surface of the calcaneus is visualized and the angular relation between the line and the floor taken. Because the infracalcaneal fat pad often migrates (related to prolonged weight bearing), care must be taken to avoid errors in visual assessment (Figure 8-15). Palpation of the osseous medial, lateral, and inferior borders of the calcaneus helps factor out fat pad migration and improve measurement accuracy. Calcaneal alignment can also be quantified with a protractor to measure the degree of calcaneal tilt relative to vertical.[64]

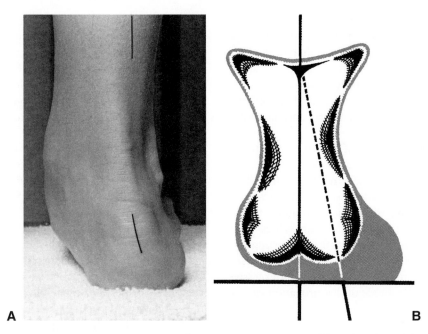

A   B

FIGURE 8-15 A, Calcaneal alignment to floor. **B,** Lateral migration of the infracalcaneal fat pad can give the illusion of an everted calcaneal to floor alignment. (Courtesy Stride, Inc., Middlebury, Conn.)

The key question to answer is whether the calcaneus is inverted, vertical, or everted relative to the floor during stance; the actual angular degree is not as important as the relative orientation of the calcaneus. This component of the examination assesses the ability of the STJ to provide enough pronation to compensate for its neutral position. In the normal closed chain STN position, the calcaneus is in 1 to 4 degrees of varus (inversion). The STJ must have an equal amount of compensatory pronation to lower the medial condyle to the ground for a vertical calcaneus. If a patient has uncompensated rearfoot varus of 10 degrees in STN as well as restricted calcaneal motion (−4 degrees) eversion, the STJ would not be able to achieve sufficient pronation or eversion in stance for normal calcaneal alignment. Instead, the calcaneus would be in an inverted alignment relative to the floor. Inverted calcaneal position also occurs when a rigid forefoot valgus or rigid plantarflexed first ray deformity is present. STJ supination is a compensatory mechanism for both deformities.

In contrast, forefoot varus deformity requires excessive compensatory STJ pronation; calcaneal eversion occurs in weight bearing. The position of the calcaneus with respect to the floor provides insight into the type of STJ compensation present and can be correlated with the biomechanical findings of the non–weight-bearing examination. If the STJ is unable to pronate enough to compensate completely for a deformity, additional pronatory motion occurs at the MTJ or by eversion tilting of the talus within the ankle mortise.[4,41,48] The functional rearfoot unit (calcaneus and talus) may assume a valgus (everted) position relative to the floor, even if calcaneal eversion is restricted.

Tibiofibular Alignment

Proximal structural malalignments, such as tibial varum or valgum, contribute to abnormal foot pronation and overuse injuries. In osseous congenital tibial varum, the distal third of the tibia is angled medially in the frontal plane, whereas in tibial valgum, the distal tibia inclines away from the midline.[41]

Tibial alignment can be measured with either a standard goniometer (Figure 8-16) or a bubble inclinometer; both assess the angular relation between the bisection of the distal third of the lower leg relative to the supporting surface.[41,65] Radiographic measurement of lower leg position is better correlated with clinically assessed tibiofibular position values than with isolated tibial position. Radiographic measurement may be the most accurate method to isolate true tibial varum.[66]

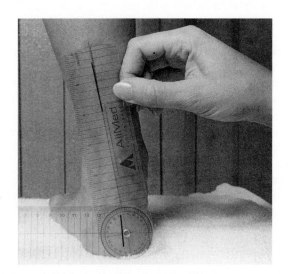

FIGURE 8-16 Goniometric assessment of tibiofibular varum. The proximal arm of the goniometer is aligned with the bisection of the distal third of the tibiofibular complex, and the distal arm is level with the floor. The axis of measurement shifts with the degree of varum or valgum deformity and may not always fall directly behind the calcaneus.

Test position is critical because variation in STJ alignment greatly influences tibiofibular varum measurement values. Tibiofibular varum values are larger in RCS than in the STN position because of the combined effects of osseous malalignment and varus leg alignment associated with compensatory STJ pronation in stance.[65-67] The incidence of tibiofibular varum appears to be high, although no clear normative values have been established.

The alignment of the distal third of the leg relative to the floor more accurately represents tibiofibular position than tibial position. Values assessed in STN reflect neutral tibiofibular alignment, whereas values assessed in RCS represent compensatory tibiofibular repositioning in response to STJ and MTJ pronation. High tibiofibular varum values measured in STN elevate the medial foot from the supporting surface, requiring excessive compensatory foot pronation during gait. High tibiofibular varum values in RCS suggest excessive foot pronation, although the source of that pronation cannot be isolated.

Alignment of the Pelvis and Lower Leg

The final component of the frontal plane assessment evaluates symmetry of the anterosuperior iliac spines, iliac crests, greater trochanters, gluteal folds, popliteal creases, genu varum or valgum deformities, fibular heads, patellae, and malleolar levels. Asymmetry often indicates sacroiliac joint dysfunction or leg length discrepancy, influencing foot position and function in the closed kinetic chain.

Sagittal Plane

The second component of the weight-bearing examination considers function in the sagittal plane. The examiner looks for evidence of genu recurvatum or excessive knee flexion, navicular drop, talar bulge, and inadequate or excessive height of the longitudinal arch.

Knee Position

Viewing the patient's stance from the side, the examiner observes the verticality of the tibia. In genu recurvatum, the proximal tibia is aligned behind the axis of the TCJ, resulting in hyperextension of the knee and plantarflex of the TCJ with relative shortening of the limb. Genu recurvatum also occurs as a compensation for equinus deformity at the ankle. When true leg-length discrepancy is present, two types of compensation are possible. If limb length difference is small, genu recurvatum may adequately shorten the longer limb. For larger limb length differences, knee flexion of the longer limb is often used to minimize asymmetry.

Navicular Drop

The position of the navicular is examined by using the navicular drop test, a composite measure of foot pronation focusing on displacement of the navicular tuberosity as a patient moves from closed kinetic chain STN to RCS position.[68] Excessive navicular displacement is associated with collapse of the MLA and may be correlated with midfoot pain or other symptoms of excessive foot pronation.[41] Subotnick[69]

established an interdependency between MTJ and STJ function based on articulation of the navicular and cuboid with the talus and calcaneus. Brody[68] suggested that the navicular drop test is a valid assessment of STJ function in the closed kinetic chain. Although navicular drop occurs with STJ pronation that stems from intrinsic foot deformity, it can also be the result of muscle insufficiency or ligamentous laxity.[41]

To measure navicular drop, an index card is held perpendicular to the medial foot, the level of the navicular tuberosity is marked in STN position and RCS, and the distance between the marks is calculated.[38] Normative studies report a mean navicular drop of between 7.3 and 9 mm.[39,70] A navicular drop of more than 10 mm is considered abnormal.[70]

Talar Bulge and Arch Height

When excessive STJ pronation is present in stance, the talus moves into adduction and plantarflex. Displacement of the talar head causes an observable medial bulge in the region of the talonavicular joint.[71] The height of the MLA normally decreases moderately in weight bearing as a result of normal STJ pronation. Pes planus deformity (flatfootedness) is characterized by excessive collapse of the MLA. In hereditary rigid flatfoot, the MLA is low or absent in non–weight-bearing and weight-bearing positions. In flexible flatfoot, the height of the MLA is normal in non–weight bearing but drops excessively in weight bearing because of abnormal STJ pronation. In normal foot alignment, the medial malleolus, navicular tuberosity, and first metatarsal head fall along the Feiss line.[71] In a severely pronated foot, the navicular tuberosity lies below the Feiss line. In extreme cases the tuberosity may even rest on the floor.[71,72]

Transverse Plane

The final component of the static weight-bearing examination considers foot function in the transverse plane. The examiner looks for signs of excessive pronation or forefoot adduction and torsional deformities of the lower extremities.

Toe Sign

A positive toe sign indicates excessive pronation or abduction of the foot in the transverse plane (Figure 8-17). The sign is determined by the number of toes that can be seen, in a posterior view, when the patient is standing in RCS with a neutral foot placement angle.[63] Normally no more than 1.5 toes are visible beyond the lateral border of the foot. If more toes can be seen, abnormal pronation may be present, causing excessive transverse plane motion or abduction of the foot. A false-positive toe sign can occur in the presence of a relative toe-out foot placement angle associated with lateral rotational deformities (e.g., femoral retroversion) or muscle imbalances that limit internal rotation of the hip (e.g., tight piriformis). Ensuring that the patient's patellae are oriented in the frontal plane before assessing toe sign reduces the risk of false-positive findings.

Torsional Deformities

Transverse plane abnormalities of the femur and tibia also adversely affect normal foot functioning. The femoral shaft normally has 12 degrees of medial rotation relative to the

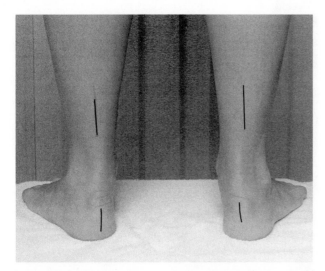

FIGURE 8-17 Toe sign, demonstrating excessive transverse plane motion as evidenced by the abducted position of the forefoot.

femoral head and neck (Figure 8-18). In femoral anteversion more than 12 degrees of rotation are present, whereas in retroversion, fewer than the expected 12 degrees of medial rotation are present.[71] In normal transverse plane tibial alignment, the fibular malleolus is situated posterior to the tibial malleolus, for 20 to 30 degrees of lateral rotation.[71] Internal tibial torsion or femoral anteversion increase medial rotational forces, leading to abnormal foot pronation. Excessive external tibial rotation or femoral retroversion increases lateral rotational forces, leading to abnormal foot supination.

To assess femoral torsion, the patient lies in the prone position with the knee in 90 degrees of flexion.[41] The examiner palpates the greater trochanter as the lower limb is passively moved laterally (representing hip internal rotation) and medially (representing hip external rotation). Femoral torsion is measured at the point where the greater trochanter is most prominent (Figure 8-19). When there is "normal"

anteversion of 12 degrees, tibial position will indicate slight internal rotation of the hip. A vertical tibia indicates femoral retroversion.

Tibial torsion is assessed with the patient in the supine position, with 90 degrees of ankle dorsiflexion and the leg placed neutrally in the frontal plane (Figure 8-20). The examiner holds the stationary arm of the goniometer parallel to the table surface while the mobile arm is aligned with the TCJ axis as it passes through the medial and lateral malleoli. This angular displacement represents tibial torsion. Normally, 20 degrees of external tibial torsion are present.

DYNAMIC GAIT ASSESSMENT

The final component of the clinical evaluation is observation of foot function during walking. During the dynamic gait assessment, extrinsic factors that affect foot function (e.g., muscle imbalances or weaknesses, proximal structural deformities, kinesthetic or proprioceptive losses) are observed. Videotaping the individual while he or she is walking on a runway or treadmill may enhance the accuracy of the assessment. The function of the rearfoot, midfoot, and forefoot is examined at each of the subphases of the gait cycle, with special attention to compensatory gait mechanisms.

FUNCTIONAL FOOT ORTHOSES

Although 4 to 6 degrees of triplanar STJ pronation are necessary to provide adequate shock absorption and accommodation to uneven ground terrain, persistent or recurrent abnormal pronation disrupts normal temporal sequencing of the gait cycle. This disruption creates an unstable osseous and arthrokinematic situation that contributes to pathological musculoskeletal conditions.[4,44]

Compensatory motion occurs in the primary plane of a given deformity. In frontal plane deformities (e.g., rearfoot varus or

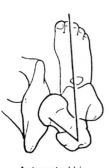
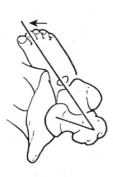
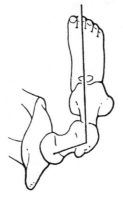
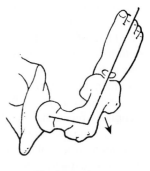

Anteverted hip

"Toeing in" due to anteverted hip

Retroverted hip

"Toeing out" due to retroverted hip

A   **B**

FIGURE 8-18 A, With excessive femoral anteversion, the limb appears to be internally rotated when the head of the femur is well seated in the acetabulum. **B,** With femoral retroversion, the limb appears to be externally rotated when the femur is well seated in the acetabulum. (From Magee DJ. *Orthopedic Physical Assessment*, 3rd ed. Philadelphia: Saunders, 1997. p. 475.)

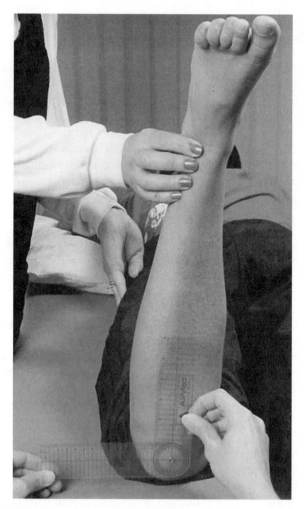

FIGURE 8-19 Assessment of femoral torsion in prone position with a standard goniometer. The examiner palpates the greater trochanter and rotates the lower leg. Femoral torsion is measured at the point of greatest prominence of the greater trochanter.

forefoot varus), the typical compensatory motion is eversion at the STJ. In transverse plane deformities (e.g., torsional deformities of the hip, femur, or tibia), the typical compensatory motion is adduction at the STJ. In sagittal plane deformities (e.g., ankle equinus), the typical compensatory motion is dorsiflexion at the STJ. Root's model suggests that single-plane compensatory motion is beneficial, allowing adequate accommodation for a deformity.[4] Because the STJ is a triplanar structure, however, movement in one plane leads to movement in the others as well. The associated motion of the other planes has the potential to become dysfunctional and destructive.[4]

A functional foot orthosis is an orthopedic device designed to promote structural integrity of the joints of the foot and lower limb by resisting the GRFs that cause abnormal skeletal motion during the stance phase of gait.[45] A functional foot orthosis attempts to control abnormal foot functioning during stance by controlling excessive STJ and MTJ motion, decelerating pronation, and allowing the STJ to function closer to its neutral position at MSt.[73-76] In contrast, an accommodative foot orthosis is used to distribute pressures over the plantar surface for individuals with fixed deformity or vulnerable neuropathic feet.

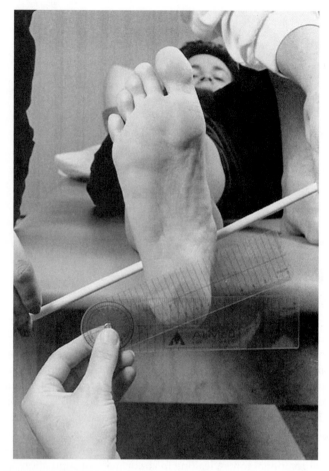

FIGURE 8-20 Tibial torsion is measured as the angle between horizontal and the plane of the axis of the talocrural joint.

Criteria for Abnormal Pronation

Five criteria are used to determine whether pronation is abnormal. Pronation is considered an abnormal mechanical condition when the following conditions are present:

1. STJ pronation is more than the normal 4 to 6 degrees.[4,27,36,75]
2. The foot pronates at the wrong time, disrupting the normal sequencing of events during closed kinetic chain motion.
3. Pronation is recurrent, with each step contributing to repetitive microtrauma to musculoskeletal structures.
4. Pronation happens at a location other than the STJ (e.g., when MTJ pronation compensates for limited STJ motion).
5. Unnecessary destructive compensatory motion occurs in the other planes of motion of the STJ.[4]

Causes of Abnormal Foot Mechanics

Three pathological situations contribute to abnormal foot mechanics: structural malalignment, muscle weakness or imbalance, and loss of structural integrity.

Structural Malalignment

Structural malalignment can be intrinsic or extrinsic to the foot or caused by abnormal mechanical forces.[4] Rearfoot and forefoot varus and valgus, ankle equinus, and deformities of the rays are examples of intrinsic deformities. Congenital and developmental conditions, such as tibial varum or valgum, torsional deformities of the tibia or femur, and other conditions that occur above the foot and ankle are extrinsic deformities. The types of abnormal mechanical forces that might contribute to pathomechanical foot function include obesity, leg length discrepancies, and genu valgum or varum. Orthotic management for structural malalignment is preventive; control of aberrant or excessive STJ and MTJ motion forestalls the sequence of mechanical events associated with abnormal pronation or supination, minimizing the consequences of painful foot conditions.

Muscle Weakness or Imbalance

A variety of upper and lower motor neuron diseases result in muscular weakness, abnormal muscle tone, or paralysis of the foot, with resultant instability of foot structure and reduced mechanical efficiency during gait.[42] In Charcot-Marie-Tooth disease (hereditary sensory motor neuropathy), for example, weakness of intrinsic, peroneal, and anterior tibial muscles contributes to development of a "cavus" foot, with claw toes, metatarsus adductus, or other deformities of the rays.[42] When muscle weakness or imbalance is present, the examiner must identify its origin and extent, the specific soft tissue structures involved, the resultant mechanical foot deformities, and the potential to reduce them. An effective foot orthosis for a patient with muscular weakness deters the pathomechanical sequelae that result from such induced structural foot deformities.

Compromised Joint Integrity

Compromised joint integrity and mechanical instability can also be caused by pathological musculoskeletal conditions of the foot or ankle, including arthritis, acute trauma, or chronic repetitive injury. In rheumatoid arthritis, for example, joint deformity results from synovitis and pannus formation. Autodestruction of connective tissue weakens tendons, contributes to muscle spasm and shortening, and erodes cartilaginous surfaces. Eventually, joint dislocations occur.[77]

The loss of protective sensation associated with peripheral neuropathy also contributes to compromised joint integrity. Patients with diabetes mellitus, chronic alcoholism, or Hansen's disease (leprosy) are particularly vulnerable. Inability to perceive microtrauma because of sensory compromise, weakness of intrinsic muscles of the foot, compromised autonomic control of the distal blood flow, and the poor nutritional and metabolic state of soft tissues combine to increase the risk of plantar foot ulceration. If neuropathic osteoarthropathy (Charcot-Marie-Tooth disease) occurs, significant bone and joint destruction, collapse of the midfoot, and a fixed rocker bottom deformity can result.[78] Plantar ulceration at the apex of the collapsed cuneiforms or cuboid is common.[79] Whenever mechanical instability is present, normal joint orientation is altered, and gait compensation shifts weight-bearing forces. A foot orthosis can be used to reduce pain, reduce weight-bearing stresses, control abnormal or excessive joint motion, or compensate for restricted motion.

GOALS OF ORTHOTIC INTERVENTION

A functional foot orthosis attempts to improve foot mechanics during walking, regardless of the cause of foot dysfunction, by the following actions:

- Controlling velocity of pronation
- Redistributing plantar pressures
- Supporting abnormal structural forefoot positions that lead to abnormal rearfoot function in stance
- Supporting abnormal rearfoot deformities that lead to excessive STJ pronation
- Resisting extrinsic forces of the leg that lead to aberrant pronation and supination of the foot
- Improving calcaneal positioning at IC
- Repositioning the STJ in neutral position just before heel rise
- Fully pronating the MTJ, when the STJ is in the neutral position, to lock and stabilize the foot, converting it into a rigid lever for propulsion
- Allowing normal plantarflex of the first ray and stabilizing the forefoot in response to the retrograde GRFs sustained during propulsion
- Providing a normal degree of shock absorption during LR

A functional foot orthosis does not support the MLA of the foot; STJ pronation is controlled by the pressure of the rearfoot post on the calcaneus at the sustentaculum tali. The ultimate goal is to stop, reduce, or slow abnormal compensatory motion of the joints of the foot as the foot and leg interact with the GRFs.

MEASUREMENT AND FABRICATION

The information gathered in the non–weight-bearing and static weight-bearing examinations and in gait analysis provides direction for orthotic prescription. A simple plaster cast is used to make an accurate negative impression of the patient's foot in the STN position. A positive model based on this impression is then prepared. Thermoplastic materials are heat molded over the model to form an orthotic shell. Accommodative padding, soft tissue supplements, and covering materials are added to address the patient's functional foot problem. The orthosis is fitted to the patient, and its effect on foot function during gait is evaluated. An early wearing schedule is devised, and an appointment for a recheck visit is scheduled.

Negative Impression

If a foot orthosis is to control abnormal pronation and supination effectively and minimize painful symptoms in gait, the negative foot impression must precisely duplicate the existing foot structure, including any intrinsic deformities. The goal of the foot impression is to capture the patient's STN position during the MSt phase of the gait cycle.

Comparison of Negative Casting Techniques Used for Fabrication of Foot Orthotics

Multiple strategies can be used to take negative impressions, including suspension techniques, modified suspension techniques, direct pressure techniques, foam impression systems, digital casting, and in-shoe vacuum casts. The negative impression techniques may be applied with the patient in semi–weight-bearing, weight-bearing, or non–weight-bearing positions. Foot measurements are greatly influenced by the technique used to obtain the impression.[80]

The foam box technique (Figure 8-21) captures a negative impression of the foot with the patient in semi–weight-bearing. Typically, the patient is seated on a firm surface and the practitioner directs the foot to the foam box. After the foot makes contact with the foam and the desired position is established, the practitioner applies a downward pressure along the tibial axis moving the heel into the foam followed by the forefoot. The foot is then removed from the box leaving a negative impression in the foam. The foam box technique requires less technical skills and is more time efficient than plaster negative casting. It might be used when the goal is to fabricate an accommodative (soft) foot orthosis.[81,82]

Digital casting technique produces a digital foot impression and allows for a variety of positions depending on the scanning device, which might include an optic laser, digitizer, pressure mat system, or digital photography.[83,84] Computerized images of the foot can be viewed by the practitioner from multiple angles and some software allows the practitioner to modify the images (Figure 8-22). The CAD/CAM system uses a milling apparatus to create the actual orthosis.

Plaster casting has traditionally been the gold standard for obtaining negative cast impressions.[85] Because maintenance of the STN position and correct loading of the forefoot are difficult to control in weight-bearing impression techniques, suspension and direct pressure non–weight-bearing techniques appear to be the most reliable methods for making accurate negative impressions. The direct pressure technique, one of the easiest procedures to learn, captures the STN position by loading the fourth and fifth metatarsal heads to mimic GRFs during MSt (Figure 8-23). Alternative casting procedures are also available.[86,87]

Direct Pressure Impression Technique

The patient is placed in the prone position, in the figure-of-four position used for goniometric measurement. Two double-layer thickness wraps of 5-inch plaster bandage are used to make the negative cast. The first wrap is cut to surround the foot from just distal to the fifth metatarsal head, around the posterior heel, to just beyond the first metatarsal head. The second wrap is cut so that, when draped over the plantar surface of the forefoot, it overlaps the first wrap at the metatarsals.

The first wrap is thoroughly moistened with tepid water and any wrinkles in the mesh are smoothed. The top edge of the plaster splint is folded 0.5 inch, providing reinforcement to prevent distortion when the cast is later removed. The first wrap is draped over the heel, just below the malleoli, and along the borders of the foot to just beyond the first and fifth metatarsal heads. Because total contact with the sole of the foot is essential, the plaster is carefully smoothed along the sides of the foot, across its plantar surface, and around the curves of the malleoli. The second wrap is moistened and draped

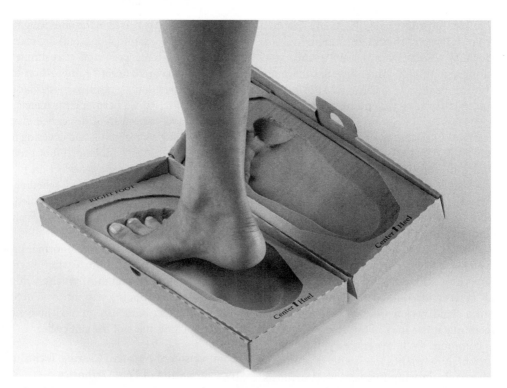

FIGURE 8-21 Negative cast impression using the foam box technique. (Courtesy of Amfit, Inc., Vancouver, Wash.)

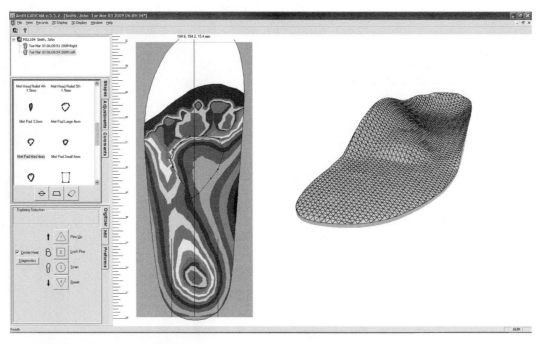

FIGURE 8-22 Example of a negative cast impression using the digital casting technique. (Courtesy of Amfit, Inc., Vancouver, Wash.)

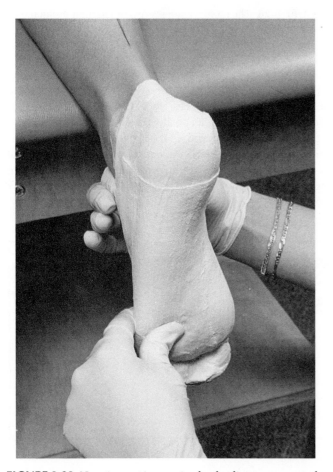

FIGURE 8-23 Negative cast impression by the direct pressure technique. The foot is maintained in STN position while the plaster hardens.

around the forefoot, overlapping the distal edges of the first layer. Any excess bandage is folded into the sulcus of the toes. This layer should also have a wrinkle-free total contact with the foot and toes.

Once both wraps are in place, the foot is positioned in the STN position by maintaining appropriate forefoot loading pressure at the fourth and fifth metatarsal heads. The plaster splint is sufficiently hardened when an audible click is produced when it is tapped. The negative cast is then carefully removed. The skin is gently pulled around the reinforced top edge to loosen contact from the cast. A downward force over the superior border of the heel cup is exerted to free the heel from the cast. A gentle forward force is then provided to free the forefoot and remove the cast from the foot.

Errors in Negative Casting

Accuracy in the negative impression is the key to an effective orthotic. Although the casting procedure is simple, three types of errors during the process can compromise the efficacy of orthotic design.

First, the foot may be inadvertently supinated at the longitudinal MTJ axis as a result of contraction of the anterior tibialis while the patient "helps" hold the foot still. Alternatively, the loading force may be applied too far medially at the forefoot, creating a false forefoot varus. An orthosis manufactured from such a cast can cause excessive pressure plantar to the distal aspect of the first metatarsal shaft. It can also lead to lateral ankle instability or the development of a functional hallux limitus or HAV deformities.[88]

The second common casting error occurs when the foot is excessively supinated at the oblique MTJ axis. Improper loading at the fourth and fifth metatarsal heads results in insufficient dorsiflexion of the forefoot. When this happens, transverse skin folds can be seen inside the negative cast at the MTJ. An orthosis manufactured from this cast creates an excessive sagittal plane angulation plantar to the calcaneocuboid joint (lateral longitudinal arch), with pain and irritation on weight bearing.[88]

The third error occurs when the STJ is excessively pronated during casting, placing the foot in a false forefoot valgus position. An orthosis manufactured from this cast does not capture the STN position and is ineffective in controlling the symptoms of abnormal pronation.[88]

Positive Cast Modifications

Once a satisfactory negative impression of the patient's foot has been obtained, a positive cast is made and then modified. The hardened negative impression is filled with liquid plaster and allowed to dry. The negative cast is peeled away, leaving a positive mold of the foot (Figure 8-24). Modifications to the positive cast ensure an effective correction in foot alignment and function by redirecting forces through the foot. Those made to enhance comfort include plaster additions to relieve pressure-sensitive regions of the forefoot and MLA. Because the negative cast is taken in a non–weight-bearing position, it is also modified to allow for the elongation of the foot and expansion of the soft tissues in weight bearing. The cast is also modified to allow for normal plantarflex of the first metatarsal during propulsion.[45,89] Intrinsic or extrinsic posts can be added for further correction of forefoot or rearfoot deformities.

Forefoot Posting

Two techniques can be used to provide orthotic correction for forefoot deformity. Both are based on modification of the positive cast impression. The first, a traditional Root functional orthosis, uses an intrinsic correction. A plaster platform is applied to the positive cast at the level of the MTP

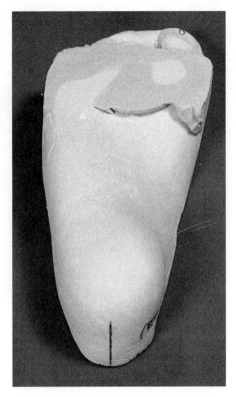

FIGURE 8-24 The modification process of forefront position on a positive cast.

joints to balance the abnormal forefoot to rearfoot relation (Figure 8-25). A lateral platform corrects forefoot valgus, and a medial platform corrects forefoot varus.[45] When the shell is pressed over the modified positive mold, it creates a convexity at the distal anterior border of the orthosis. This posting technique achieves correction by effectively realigning the skeletal structure of the foot.[89] The intrinsic posting technique is often selected when shoe volume is limited, as in some women's footwear.

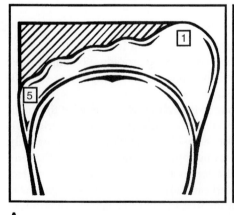 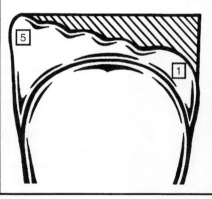 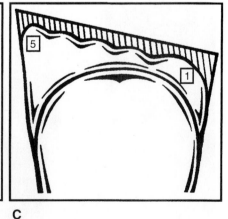

A   B   C

FIGURE 8-25 Cross section at the level of the metatarsophalangeal joints, with first and fifth metatarsals labeled, demonstrating intrinsic modifications to the positive mold. **A,** A lateral platform corrects forefoot valgus. **B,** A medial platform corrects forefoot varus. **C,** A neutral balancing platform maintains forefoot alignment and serves as a base for extrinsic posts. (Courtesy Stride, Inc., Middlebury, Conn.)

A second forefoot posting technique involves a variation of Root's original design, referred to as a standard biomechanical orthosis. In this technique, a neutral platform is formed on the positive mold, but the existing valgus or varus position of the forefoot is maintained. An extrinsic forefoot post or wedge is attached to the bottom of the orthotic shell to support the forefoot in its position of deformity. Unwanted compensatory motion is prevented by stabilizing the distal border of the orthosis (Figure 8-26). Although an orthosis with an extrinsic correction takes up more space inside the shoe than an intrinsically corrected orthosis, it can more easily be modified if the individual has difficulty tolerating the original posting prescription.

Rearfoot Posting

As the foot makes contact with the ground and moves through stance during gait, GRFs act on the joints of the foot. An orthosis acts as an interface between the ground and the foot, creating its own orthosis reactive force. In a foot that pronates excessively, the foot orthosis is designed to decrease STJ pronation during weight bearing by creating a supination moment acting medial to the STJ axis.[2] This can be accomplished by adding an extrinsic rearfoot post or wedge to the inferior surface of the heel cup or by modifying the plaster mold to incorporate an intrinsic rearfoot post to the heel cup of the orthosis. A rearfoot post effectively reduces rearfoot pronation (eversion) during the contact phase of gait as well as the angular velocity of eversion.[2,90,91]

Extrinsic rearfoot posts are attached to the bottom of the orthosis shell beneath the heel (see Figure 8-26B). A medial wedge or rearfoot post increases orthosis reactive forces at the sustentaculum tali (medial to the STJ axis) to reduce abnormal STJ pronation. It also promotes stability of the heel by increasing the contact surface of the orthosis beneath the heel.[89,90] An intrinsic rearfoot post can be made with a medial heel skive technique. A plaster modification is performed on the medial aspect of the heel of the positive mold to increase the amount of varus (medial) sloping within the heel cup of the orthosis in an effort to control pronation.[2] An intrinsic rearfoot post

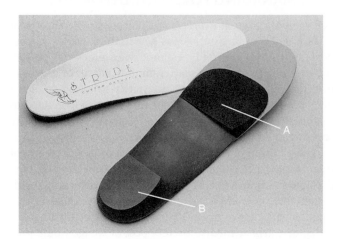

FIGURE 8-26 Standard biomechanical orthosis with an extrinsic forefoot post **(A)** and an extrinsic rearfoot post **(B).**

reduces overall bulk of the orthosis for optimal fit within a shoe. A combination of intrinsic and extrinsic rearfoot posting permits more correction than possible with either method independently.

The Orthotic Shell

To be effective, a functional orthosis must be made on the basis of a neutral position model of the patient's foot. Prefabricated foot supports do not offer adequate control of foot motion or resistance to GRFs and cannot fulfill all criteria of functional foot orthoses. A custom orthosis, made of rigid or semirigid materials, can offer maximal resistance to weight-bearing forces and optimal realignment of foot structure. Accommodative orthoses, made of softer materials, support the arches of the foot and provide relief to pressure-sensitive areas while offering minimal control of STJ motion.[92,93] A semifunctional orthosis is a hybrid of functional and accommodative orthoses that combines the motion effectiveness of a semirigid shell with soft posting and accommodative material to cushion the foot.

Many studies have evaluated the effectiveness of the different types of orthotic materials in controlling rearfoot mechanics and clinical symptoms.[92-96] Some suggest that orthotic materials be classified by degree of rigidity (soft, semirigid, rigid), but standards for the classification of materials are not well established.[1]

A rigid orthosis achieves maximal motion control and biomechanical correction of a foot deformity, is lightweight, and takes up the least space within the shoe. Some clinicians are concerned that orthoses made of rigid materials are uncomfortable to the wearer. Anthony[45] suggested, however, that those "who propose rigid devices to be patient intolerant are generally less acquainted with the theory of podiatric biomechanics and the correct diagnostics and prescription formularies that are critical for the provision of a truly functional foot orthosis."

Semirigid materials, such as polypropylene and TL-2100 (Performance Materials Corp., Camarillo, Calif.), are attractive alternatives to rigid orthotic shells. Polypropylene is a flexible olefin polymer that resists breakage. TL-2100 is a thermoplastic composite of resin and fiber that is harder and more rigid than polypropylene.[1]

Soft orthoses are often made of closed-cell foams manufactured from heat-expanded polyethylene. Examples of such foams include Aliplast and Nickleplast (Alimed, Inc., Dedham, Mass.) and Plastazote (Bakelite Xylonite Ltd, Croydon, United Kingdom), cross-linked polyethylene expanded foams available in many densities. Pelite (Fillauer, Inc., Chattanooga, Tenn.) is a cross-linked, closed-cell foam that can be heat molded in the fabrication of semiflexible foot orthoses. Various rubberized or thermoplastic cork materials are also used.[1] Lightweight and available in different densities, these materials are effective in orthotics for which accommodation and shock absorption are desirable. These same features limit the durability and the useful life of the orthosis, however, because these materials are prone to rapid and permanent shape deformation.[1]

TABLE 8-1   *Accommodative Padding and Soft Tissue Supplements for Functional Foot Orthotics*

Supplement	Description
Metatarsal mound	A dome-shaped addition in the form of a teardrop positioned with the apex just proximal to the metatarsal heads to support a collapsed transverse metatarsal arch. Often used to control symptoms of neuroma by reducing shearing of the metatarsals during contact phase. Reduction of the shearing eliminates irritation to the interdigital nerves of the forefoot.
2-5 bar	A pad of uniform thickness placed beneath the second through fifth metatarsal heads relieves pressure beneath the first metatarsal head during propulsion. Used when a rigid plantar flexed first ray is present.
Metatarsal head cutout	A U-shaped pad positioned beneath a rigid plantar flexed metatarsal head to relieve pressure from a painful callosity. Often used for hammertoe deformity.
Morton's extension	An extension of the plastic shell, or the addition of an inlay made of dense material, beneath the shaft of the first metatarsal to the sulcus of the hallux. Often used for a dorsiflexed first ray or Morton's toe.
Heel cushion	Placed in the heel cup of the orthosis to enhance heel cushioning and shock absorption. Often made of the soft tissue–supplementing material Poron (Rodgers Co., Rogers, Conn.) or a viscoelastic polymer. Used when irritation or atrophy of the infracalcaneal fat pad is present or for calcaneal stress fracture.
Forefoot extension	A soft tissue–supplementing material such as Poron is added to the distal end of the orthotic shell to cushion the metatarsal heads or as a base for other forefoot inlays.
Scaphoid pad	A material of soft to medium density placed beneath the medial longitudinal arch to decelerate pronatory forces.

For some individuals, extrinsic accommodative modifications are necessary to address a particular deformity. Examples of accommodative supplements are listed in Table 8-1.

Covering Materials

Once appropriate posts and supportive materials are attached to the shell of the orthosis, a covering material is applied to provide an interface with the skin of the foot. Vinyl is a commonly used orthosis-covering material. Spenco (Spenco Medical Corporation, Waco, Texas) and various other fabric-covered neoprene materials are resistant to shearing and enhance shock absorption. They are often chosen as covering materials for certain sport orthoses when shear forces are expected to be high or for occupational situations that demand prolonged standing on hard surfaces.

MANAGING REARFOOT DEFORMITY

In a well-aligned foot, 4 to 6 degrees of STJ pronation occur during the stance phase of gait. In rearfoot varus, more than 6 degrees of STJ pronation are present. A fully compensated rearfoot varus deformity of 10 degrees pronates at the STJ 10 degrees during gait to lower the medial condyle of the calcaneus to the ground, but only 6 degrees of this pronation are considered excessive.

The appropriate orthotic design for rearfoot varus is a medial post or medial wedge. Complete orthotic correction is difficult to achieve and quite uncomfortable for the individual wearing the orthosis. Because of this, the initial goal is often to create an orthosis that provides 50% correction of a rearfoot deformity. To correct the excessive 6 degrees of pronation, for example, a medial rearfoot post or wedge of 3 degrees would be applied to the orthosis.

If an individual with a rearfoot varus deformity of 10 degrees is uncompensated to −5 degrees of calcaneal eversion, a medial or varus wedge of 3 degrees is not effective because the STJ would reach its end-range eversion motion (−5 degrees) before the orthosis provided support. To manage uncompensated rearfoot deformity effectively, the varus wedge must be large enough to prevent the STJ from reaching its end ROM. In this example, a larger medial rearfoot varus post or wedge of at least 5 degrees is necessary. When the rearfoot is aggressively posted (more than 3 or 4 degrees of varus posting), the distal medial aspect of the orthosis shell loses contact with the ground, as if a forefoot varus deformity were present. In these circumstances, a medial forefoot post is used to counteract the induced apparent forefoot varus.

MANAGING FOREFOOT DEFORMITY

For forefoot varus deformities, a medial (varus) wedge or post is indicated. For forefoot valgus deformities, lateral (valgus) posts or wedges are used. Forefoot deformities can be corrected through intrinsic plaster modifications or extrinsic posting. For an orthosis to be accurately balanced so that it does not wobble, a forefoot deformity must be corrected to its fullest extent (e.g., an 8-degree forefoot varus deformity requires an 8-degree medial wedge or post).

The addition of a large extrinsic post to the distal end of the orthotic shell often creates problems with shoe fit. One possible solution is to correct large forefoot deformities with a combination of intrinsic and extrinsic techniques. In this example, a 4-degree medial intrinsic plaster platform and a 4-degree extrinsic medial forefoot post or wedge would provide the desired correction without bulkiness. For individuals with a forefoot varus deformity of 10 degrees or more, a semipronated or pronated negative cast can reduce the forefoot deformity to a more manageable degree.[86]

Plantarflex of the first ray is managed according to the level of flexibility of the deformity. A fully flexible plantar flexed first ray deformity does not require orthotic intervention. A semirigid or rigid plantar flexed first ray deformity requires the addition of a metatarsal (second through fifth) bar inlay. The thickness of the inlay is determined by how far below the first metatarsal head lies relative to the plane of the remaining metatarsal heads. The orthotic intervention for patients with a rigid plantar flexed first ray and forefoot varus is an extended medial forefoot wedge. The forefoot post is modified with a cutout to accommodate the dropped first metatarsal head position. In some cases, a small forefoot varus deformity combined with a large, rigidly plantar flexed first ray deformity results in a functional forefoot valgus (see Figure 8-14).

ORTHOTIC CHECKOUT AND TROUBLESHOOTING

Delivery of an orthosis includes evaluation of its fit, comfort, and mechanical alignment. The orthotic shell should end just proximal to the metatarsal heads. The width is evaluated to ensure that normal first ray plantarflex and propulsion are not compromised. The position of the orthosis within the shoe is also evaluated; its volume, impact on heel height, points of excessive pressure, and tendency to cause pistoning during gait are considered. On initial fitting, many individuals report that the orthosis feels slightly strange or unusual. The orthosis should not, however, cause undue discomfort. Fit and mechanical functioning of the orthosis are evaluated in standing and walking.

Patient education in appropriate break-in protocols and wearing schedules is an important component of orthotic delivery. A new orthosis is usually worn for 2 hours on day 1, 4 hours on day 2, 6 hours on day 3, and so forth, until the individual is able to wear the orthosis comfortably all day. A follow-up visit is scheduled after the orthosis has been worn for at least 2 weeks. By this time, the patient should feel comfortable with the orthosis for normal activities of daily living. Thereafter, progressively increased use of the orthosis for all activities, including sport and occupational use, should be well tolerated. Adjustments are occasionally necessary to optimize patient comfort and mechanical alignment.

CONTROVERSY WITH ROOT'S PARADIGM

Much discussion on the basic components of Root's theory has occurred in the past decade.[50,97-104] Root's theory is founded on "normal" foot structure and the concept of the STN position: the point of maximal congruence in the articulation of the talus and navicular.[4,13,29,60] STN position supposedly (1) minimizes stress to the surrounding joints and ligaments, (2) is the most efficient position regarding muscle function and attenuation of the impact forces at IC, and (3) represents the point at which the foot converts from a mobile adapter to a rigid lever.[4,41,60] According to Root's traditional theory, normal foot alignment occurs just before TSt during gait, when the STJ is in the neutral position and the MTJ is fully locked.[4]

The major criticisms of Root's paradigm raise concerns about reliability of measurement of the STN position, the position of STN position during the gait cycle, and criteria for "normal" foot alignment.[38,61,99,103]

Reliability of Measurement

When considering available evidence about reliability of foot measurements and the STN position, although acceptable levels of intrarater reliability exist,[39,40,46,48,105,106] interrater reliability of foot measurements and the STN position is low.[38,97,99,103] Diamond and colleagues[107] and Cook and colleagues[106] found that interrater reliability can be improved with training. McPoil and Hunt[38] noted that considerable confusion exists regarding the definition and measurement of STN position. They suggested that Root's STN position may misinterpret the of work by Wright and colleagues,[108] who referenced relaxed standing position, not STN neutral, as the basis of their work. To further add to the confusion, the definition of STN position used in some reliability studies was not identical to Root's methods.[103] Based on the review of reliability studies, McPoil and Hunt[38] suggested that physical therapists are not able to agree on position and motion of the STJ.

Subtalar Position in Stance

According to Root, ideal foot alignment occurs just before TSt during gait, when the STJ is in the neutral position and the MTJ is fully locked.[4,109] In a study of rearfoot motion of 51 healthy adults, McPoil and Cornwall[110] marked patients' lower leg and calcaneus with bisection lines and then filmed relative calcaneal and lower leg position while walking, while standing in a double-support relaxed standing, and while in STN position. Their findings did not support Root's paradigm. They found that (1) the rearfoot is slightly inverted before IC, (2) maximal rearfoot pronation was reached at the 37.9% point of stance phase, and (3) the neutral position of the rearfoot for the typical pattern of rearfoot motion should be the resting standing foot posture rather than STN position.[108] As a result, they suggested that the relaxed standing foot position rather than the STN position should be used during casting.[108]

Pierrynowski and Smith[111] used three-dimensional analysis and six experienced raters to study the pattern of rearfoot motion throughout the gait cycle relative to the STN position. The right lower extremities of nine patients were evaluated by each rater six to seven times, and the STN position was recorded. Patients then walked on a treadmill and were recorded for 30 seconds to allow the capture of approximately 25 walking cycles. For most patients, the rearfoot was everted throughout stance, with maximal eversion occurring at 44% of the gait cycle.[111] They found that STN position occurs at 64% and 74% of the gait cycle, with the rearfoot inverted between these points. The rearfoot was everting from 0% to 44%, inverting from 44% to 70%, everting from 70% to 90%, and inverting from 90% to 100% of the gait cycle.[109]

The authors concluded that the manufacture of foot orthoses should not be associated with the STN position.[111]

Criteria for Normal Alignment

Root described deviations from normal foot alignment as intrinsic foot deformities, which can lead to aberrant lower extremity function and musculoskeletal pathological conditions.[4,60] Root and colleagues[109] defined three criteria for normal foot and ankle alignment in the loaded STN position: (1) a bisection of the lower leg being in parallel to the bisection of the calcaneus, (2) the plane of the metatarsal heads being perpendicular to the bisection of the calcaneus, and (3) the distal third of the lower leg being perpendicular to the floor. McPoil and colleagues[38,97] examined 116 feet in 58 asymptomatic individuals, finding 8.6% with forefoot varus, 44.8% with forefoot valgus, 14.7% with a plantar flexed first ray, 83.6% with subtalar varus, and 98.3% with tibiofibular varum. Only 17% (116 feet) of the 58 individuals evaluated demonstrated normal criteria.[38] In an examination of forefoot to rearfoot relations of 120 healthy asymptomatic individuals, Garbalosa and colleagues[47] found that only 4.58% of the 234 feet studied exhibited normal criteria, 86.67% had forefoot varus, and 7.75% had forefoot valgus. Astrom and Arvidson[112] performed standardized clinical assessments on 121 healthy individuals, finding that none demonstrated an ideal foot position; most had a valgus position in the STN position (mean, 2 degrees), forefoot in varus (mean, 6 degrees), calcaneal valgus in stance valgus (mean, 7 degrees), and 6 degrees of tibial varus with respect to vertical. The evidence from these studies suggests that an "ideal" foot may be based on a questionable theoretical concept.

FOOT TYPE AND LOWER EXTREMITY BIOMECHANICS

A question that has been the focus of recent research focuses on the relation between various foot types and the amount of pronation during gait. Recent reviews of the literature suggest this question might not have a simple answer. Dicharry and colleagues[113] compared static and dynamic measures of navicular drop in 72 healthy adults. Although the participants had significantly different static measures of various foot types, they only displayed small or no differences during running and walking. The findings suggest that features other than foot type affect dynamic joint function. According to Razeghi and Batt,[114] foot type alone cannot explain ankle and foot kinematics because of the interrelated function of the subtalar, talocrural, and knee joints. Ball and Afheldt[103] suggested that attempts to justify static classification of foot type schemes as a means of predicting dynamic joint function have had mixed results.

FOOT TYPE AND LOWER EXTREMITY OVERUSE INJURIES

Many researchers have reported an association between abnormal alignment of the foot and lower extremity and occurrence of lower extremity injuries. Dahle and colleagues[115] studied the relation between foot type (classified in standing as supinated, pronated, or neutral) and occurrence of ankle sprain and knee pain in 55 athletes during the football and cross country seasons. Although the relation between foot type and subsequent ankle sprain was not supported, foot type was strongly related to knee pain; 48% of those with pronated feet and 50% of those with supinated feet had significant knee pain compared with 21% of those classified with neutral alignment. Gross and colleagues[116] examined the relationship between forefoot and rearfoot varus alignment to hip conditions in 385 older adults. Older adults with more forefoot varus were 1.8 times more likely to have ipsilateral hip pain, 1.9 times more likely to have hip pain or tenderness, and 5.1 times more likely to have undergone total hip replacement when compared to older adults with less forefoot varus. There was not a significant relationship between older adults with rearfoot varus and hip conditions. Powers and colleagues[117] compared prone STN rearfoot position of 15 patients diagnosed with patellofemoral pain with 15 control subjects, reporting a statistically significant difference in rearfoot varus found in the patellofemoral group (8.9%) compared with control subjects (6.8%). In a retrospective study of the relation between foot posture and incidence of medial tibial stress syndrome, Sommer and Vallentyne[118] measured foot angle in 14 standing limbs with medial tibial stress syndrome (MTSS) and 36 control limbs. They reported mean foot angle of 137 degrees in symptomatic limbs compared with 145 degrees in asymptomatic limbs. They also reported that a standing foot angle of less than 140 degrees and a varus alignment of the rearfoot or forefoot, measured qualitatively in STN position, were predictive of a previous history of MTSS.

Some reports do not support the relation between foot type and lower extremity injury. Donatelli and colleagues[119] reported no statistically significant relations among static or dynamic foot posture and injury status in professional baseball players. Razeghi and Batt[114] suggested that arch height may not influence injury occurrence. Similarly, Cowan and colleagues[120,121] found that individuals in the U.S. Army with low arches might be less likely to have lower extremity injury. Considering the variety of reports in the literature, Razeghi and Batt[114] surmised that "the effect of foot type on the occurrence of lower extremity injuries has not been the subject of well-controlled studies and few, if any, causal correlations have been demonstrated."

ORTHOSES AND LOWER EXTREMITY FUNCTION

Overpronation has been implicated as a cause of many overuse injuries. Traditionally a foot orthosis is used to help control abnormal foot functioning during the stance phase by controlling excessive STJ motion, decelerating pronation, and allowing the STJ to function closer to its neutral position during stance.[74-76] Literature about efficacy of foot orthoses in controlling lower extremity and foot biomechanics is growing.[7,122] A systematic review and metaanalysis conducted by Richter and colleagues[120] reported there is evidence for the use of foot orthoses to prevent lower limb overuse conditions.

Effect on Rearfoot Biomechanics

The use of foot orthoses is based on the premise that control of frontal plane rearfoot motion in stance provides a means of controlling pronation of the foot. Novick and Kelley[123] investigated the effects of medially posted rigid orthoses in 20 asymptomatic individuals during the LR phase of the gait cycle. They report a significant decrease in calcaneal angle (angle between the sagittal plane and bisected posterior tubercle of the calcaneus), calcaneal eversion angle (mathematical sum of the tibia vara angle plus the calcaneal angle), angular velocities and angular accelerations, as well as a shift medially in the center of pressure relative to the ankle joint. These findings that an orthosis is able to reposition the rearfoot concur with earlier studies examining the effects of orthoses on rearfoot mechanics.[93,96,124,125] McClean and colleagues[126] examined the impact of custom foot orthoses on lower extremity mechanics of 15 female runners. The runners performed five running trials with and without the orthoses. The runners displayed significant reduction in maximum rearfoot eversion angle (2 degrees) and rearfoot eversion velocity while wearing the orthoses.

Johanson and colleagues[127] examined the effects of three different orthotic posting methods on subtalar pronation during ambulation in 22 individuals with a forefoot varus deformity of at least 8 degrees. Individuals ambulated in running shoes with (1) unposted prefabricated shells with a polyurethane arch support and (2) individualized shells posted at the rearfoot, (3) at the forefoot, and (4) at both the rearfoot and forefoot. Forefoot posts were approximately 50% of the measured forefoot varus deformity, and the rearfoot posts were 80% of the forefoot post. Running shoes without shells were used as the control. Measurements of calf to calcaneus and calcaneus to vertical were recorded for each situation. Shells with and without posting decreased calcaneal angles compared with running shoes alone. Concurrent posts of rearfoot and forefoot decreased calcaneal angles similar to rearfoot posting alone; both decreased the angle more than forefoot posting alone. Similarly, Genova and Gross[128] found significant reduction in calcaneal eversion during static stance with shoes alone and shoes with orthoses, compared with the barefoot condition, in 13 individuals with barefoot standing calcaneal eversion angles of at least 10 degrees. The condition of the shoes and the orthoses was not statistically different in controlling eversion in static standing. Individuals demonstrated lower angles for maximal calcaneal eversion during stance and for calcaneal eversion at heel rise for the shoe with an orthosis compared with the shoe alone during fast walking on a treadmill. Branthwaite and colleagues[129] investigated the biomechanical effects of simple orthotic designs at rearfoot in 9 individuals with varus deformities of the feet by using biplanar orthoses (medial wedging at the heel) or cobra pads (medial wedging and an arch support). A decrease in calcaneal eversion occurred with the biplanar orthosis compared with no insole, but no difference occurred with cobra insoles. Neither condition produced significant changes in the maximal eversion velocity.

The difficulty in predicting the biomechanical effects of orthoses on the rearfoot was demonstrated by Brown and colleagues,[130] who compared shoes only, over-the-counter arch supports, and custom-made semirigid orthoses to control rearfoot pronation in 24 patients with a forefoot varus deformity. Custom-made orthoses were posted at both the rearfoot and forefoot, with forefoot posts at 60% of the forefoot deformity and rearfoot posts at 50% of the forefoot deformity. Although a difference was found in the total pronation among the three groups, the authors suggest additional research is warranted to identify orthotic factors responsible for the biomechanical effects associated with the clinical successes of foot orthotics. Butler and colleagues[131] found that rigid or soft orthoses posted 6 degrees at rearfoot were unable to control calcaneal eversion excursion, peak eversion, and eversion velocity during running in individuals with normal foot alignment.

Miller and colleagues[132] suggested that mechanisms by which orthoses control rearfoot motions are not as clear as might be expected. The examination of GRFs during ambulation of 25 individuals with pes planus with or without a rearfoot device found no significant change in the mediolateral GRFs during the stance phase of gait. Significant differences were found, however, in the vertical and anterior posterior GRFs during various percentages of the stance phase.

Several variables that must considered in interpreting these disparate findings, including the materials used, whether individuals are running or walking, foot alignment and biomechanics, and posting methods. Although rearfoot mechanics appear to be altered by foot orthoses, further investigation into the mechanisms responsible for these effects is needed.

Effect on Lower Limb Biomechanics

Foot orthoses influence lower extremity kinematics and kinetics as well as rearfoot mechanics. Eng and Pierrynowski[95] examined the three-dimensional effects of soft foot orthoses during the contact, MSt, and propulsion phases of walking and running on the talocrural and subtalar joints and knee joints in 10 women with a history of patellofemoral joint pain and forefoot varus or calcaneal valgus greater than 6 degrees. Soft orthoses produced a modest decrease in frontal and transverse plane motion in the talocrural and subtalar joints and knee joint during walking and running. Knee joint motion in the frontal plane decreased during the early and MSt phases of walking but increased during the contact and MSt phases of running. This work demonstrates the complex coupling of lower extremity kinematics with motions of the STJ; reductions in subtalar motion in the frontal plane have an impact on knee function in both the frontal and transverse planes during walking.

McPoil and Cornwall[133] also studied the effects of soft and rigid orthoses on tibial rotation. Ten individuals with documented rearfoot or forefoot deformity ambulated with unposted, premolded, soft orthoses and rigid polyethylene orthoses posted according to the individual's deformity. Both orthoses decreased the rate and amount of tibial internal rotation during walking. Stacoff and colleagues[134] observed the effects of medially posted cork orthoses on calcaneal and tibial motions in five runners. Three-dimensional tibiocalcaneal rotations were assessed after inserting intracortical bone pins into the calcaneus and tibia. Although the effects on eversion and tibial rotation were small and variable, a statistically significant orthotic effect was present for total tibial rotation. The authors, noting that the differences were unsystematic across conditions and were specific to each individual, speculated that the effects of orthoses might be proprioceptive as well as mechanical.

Joseph and colleagues[135] studied the relationship between ankle pronation/eversion with excessive knee valgus and risk of anterior cruciate ligament injury in female athletes during drop jumps. Ten female athletes performed drop jump landings with and without a medially posted orthosis. A three-dimensional kinematics of the knee and ankle were measured during the jump. The authors reported a significant decrease in ankle pronation/eversion and knee valgus at initial contact when the athletes had a medial post in their shoes. Their findings support medial orthotic posts for potentially decreasing the risk of anterior cruciate ligament injury. Tillman and colleagues[136] evaluated the impact of orthotic posting on the tibial rotation induced by jumping from a 43-cm-high platform in seven women without foot malalignments by using three conditions (shoes only, shoes with orthoses posted 8 degrees medially, and shoes with orthoses posted 8 degrees laterally). Tibial internal rotation increased by 2.6 degrees with laterally posted inserts and decreased by 3.1 degrees with medially posted inserts. Nester and colleagues[137] examined the effects of medially and laterally wedged orthoses on the kinematics of the rearfoot, knee, hip, and pelvis during walking, reporting main effects on the rearfoot, with minimal effects at knee, hip, or pelvis. Laterally wedged orthoses increased pronation and decreased laterally directed ground forces, whereas medially wedged orthoses decreased pronation and increased the laterally directed ground forces.

Williams and colleagues[138] examined the effects of graphite "inverted" orthoses (orthoses used to provide more aggressive control of pronation by using an inverted position as opposed to a more vertical orientation), standard graphite orthoses posted with a 4-degree medial wedge, or shoes alone in 11 runners who had been initially fitted with the standard orthoses for various lower extremity injuries. Surprisingly, the three conditions produced no significant differences in the peak rearfoot eversion or rearfoot eversion excursion.

A significant decrease in the rearfoot inversion moment and work with the inverted orthosis suggests this orthotic design might decrease demand on the structures controlling eversion. However, increased internal tibial rotation as well as an adduction moment at the knee occurred with the inverted orthosis, raising concern that potential for lateral stress increases with this aggressive orthotic approach.

Kuhn and colleagues[139] examined quadriceps femoris Q-angle in 40 men with bilateral pes planus or hyperpronation syndrome before and after the insertion of foot orthotics. Thirty-nine of the 40 men had significant decrease in bilateral Q-angle in the direction of correction after insertion of full-length flexible orthotics. Men with asymmetrical Q-angle measurements showed significantly greater symmetry of Q-angle measures after orthotic placement.

Kuhn and colleagues[134] noted that hyperpronation can cause the tibia to internally rotate, leading to femur internal rotation and resulting in lateral tracking of the patella. They concluded that insertion of full-length flexible orthotics in men with hyperpronation significantly improves quadriceps femoris Q-angle.

Stackhouse and colleagues[140] studied biomechanics during running in 15 individuals with normal alignment. Individuals ran with both rearfoot and forefoot strike patterns and with and without semirigid orthoses with 6 degrees of rearfoot posting. The orthoses did not change rearfoot motion in either strike pattern but did reduce internal rotation and genu valgum by approximately 2 degrees through most of the stance phase. Although no statistically significant reduction occurred in the inversion moment and inversion work, the authors believed that the reductions they found were clinically relevant and might explain the reduction of injuries seen when orthoses are used.

Although evidence supports the fact that foot orthoses can and do influence lower extremity kinematics and kinetics, the variability of individual responses makes it difficult to determine exactly which biomechanical effects will occur. This variability also makes it difficult to forecast who is likely to benefit from orthotic intervention. Efficacy of foot orthoses is not solely the result of altered rearfoot kinematics, as proposed by Root. The contribution of the neuromuscular system to the effect of orthotic intervention is now being considered.

Effect of the Neuromuscular System

Nigg and colleagues,[141] citing problems in previous studies (e.g., small skeletal changes produced by orthotic use, minimal decrease in impact forces, and nonsystematic effects caused by individual variability), proposed that mechanisms involving the neuromuscular system contribute to the way that foot orthoses alter lower extremity function. They were especially interested in sensitivity of the foot and pressure distribution on the foot surface, noting that (1) the foot has many sensory receptors to detect forces and deformations acting on it, (2) the sensors detected input signals into the foot with patient-specific thresholds, and (3) individuals with similar sensitivity thresholds seem to respond to their movement patterns in a similar way. They suggested that force signals from the floor were filtered by the shoe, the orthosis, and finally by the plantar surface of the foot, which then transferred the filtered information to the central nervous system. The central nervous system, in turn, prompted dynamic responses in the lower extremity on the basis of patient-specific conditions. Comfort of the orthosis is an important consideration; a comfortable orthosis is likely to minimize muscular work during walking. According to Nigg and colleagues,[136] an optimal orthosis would reduce muscle activity, feel comfortable, and improve musculoskeletal and neuromuscular performance in walking.

Based on his analysis of the role of impact forces on foot function in gait, Nigg[142] proposed a new paradigm focusing on locomotor systems and strategies for impact and movement control. The dynamical systems model of motor control suggests that locomotor systems keep general kinematic and kinetic situations similar for any given task. Nigg suggests that a muscle tuning reaction occurs to cause forces that affect muscle activation before ground contact, and that muscle adaptation (to ensure constant joint movement pattern) affects muscle activation during ground contact. The interplay of realignment of the skeleton and locomotor system muscle tuning affects joint and tendon loading and, in turn, fatigue, comfort, work, and performance.

Electromyographic and Imaging Evidence

Mundermann and colleagues[143] studied 21 recreational runners who used a flat shoe insert, posting alone, custom-molded orthoses, and custom-molded orthoses and posting. They analyzed the effects of each condition on lower extremity kinematics, kinetics, and electromyographic data as well as comfort during use. Thirty-five percent of differences in comfort were explained by changes in 15 kinematic, kinetic, and electromyographic variables, and these 15 variables correctly classified the corresponding orthotic condition in 75% of cases. Mundermann and colleagues[144] suggested that comfort not only reflected subjective perceptions but was also related to biomechanical variables. In an extension of their work, Mundermann and colleagues[144] observed that the effects of molding were more important than posting on change in kinematic and kinetic variables.

Hertel and colleagues[145] examined electromyographic activity of the vastus medialis, vastus lateralis, and gluteus medius during functional activities in 30 individuals with different foot types, comparing electromyographic activity in four conditions: no orthotic, 7 degrees medial rearfoot post, 4 degrees lateral rearfoot post, and neutral rearfoot post. Surface electromyographic activity data of the muscles was collected while the individuals performed single-leg squatting, lateral stepdown, and maximum vertical jump. During single-leg squat and lateral stepdown, higher vastus medialis and gluteus medius activity was noted with all orthotic conditions. During the vertical jump, less vastus lateralis was noted with all orthotic conditions. Foot type did not influence the outcome in any of the activities.

Kulig and colleagues[146] studied the influence of foot orthoses on tibialis posterior activation in six adults with pes planus. Exercises consisting of resisted foot adduction and plantarflex were performed barefoot and then with foot orthoses and shoes a week later. Magnetic resonance images of tibialis posterior, tibialis anterior, peroneus longus, medial gastrocnemius, and soleus were obtained pre- and postexercise. When wearing foot orthoses and shoes, only the tibialis posterior was activated. When barefoot, the magnetic resonance image signal intensity of the tibialis posterior was lower and five of the six participants activated the tibialis posterior and additional muscles. The researchers concluded that selective activation of the tibialis posterior can be improved in people with pes planus by wearing foot orthoses with shoes.[142]

Bird and colleagues[147] considered electromyographic activity of lumbar erector spinae and gluteus medius muscles with prefabricated foot wedges (a 5-degree lateral wedge, a 5-degree medial wedge, or a 2-cm heel wedge). Although no change in amplitude of electromyographic signal occurred, wedging at the heel and lateral forefoot led to earlier electromyographic activity of the erector spinae. Gluteus muscle activity was delayed with bilateral heel wedges, as was ipsilateral gluteus activity when a unilateral heel wedge was used. Although changes of onset for the erector spinae and gluteus medius averaged only 4% and 2% of the gait cycle, respectively, the researchers suggested that these changes are likely to be clinically significant over the course of a day.

Vanicek and colleagues[148] considered how foot orthoses affected the ability of six healthy alpine skiers to hold a skier's squat position and on the duration of fatigue of the vastus lateralis. Individuals were examined under three conditions: no orthoses, high-volume orthoses, and low-volume orthoses (based on the amount of foam incorporated into the orthosis). A decrease in median firing frequencies toward the end of contraction suggested that high-volume orthoses reduced myoelectric fatigue. However, no significant differences in the ability to sustain a squat occurred under the three conditions.

Postural Control

If neuromuscular systems play a role in the effectiveness of orthoses, changes in balance and posture control would be anticipated with their use. Guskiewicz and Perrin[149] examined the effects of custom orthoses in 13 patients with acute ankle inversion sprains and in 12 noninjured patients. As anticipated, orthoses reduced postural sway in the medial and lateral and inversion and eversion directions, with a larger effect in patients who had the injury. The researchers propose that, by restricting undesirable motions, the orthoses enhanced the ability of joint mechanoreceptors to detect movement. In contrast, Hertel and colleagues[150] found that six different orthotic interventions (shoe only; molded Aquaplast orthoses [Aquaplast Thermoplastics, Wyckoff, NJ]; orthoses in the neutral, medially posted, and laterally posted positions; and a prefabricated, rigid, laterally posted heel wedge) did not influence postural sway in 15 patients with unilateral ankle sprains while they performed unilateral standing. None of the orthotic conditions decreased frontal or sagittal postural sway compared with shoes alone. Hertel and colleagues[151] also studied 15 healthy patients with normally aligned feet under the same six conditions, focusing on center of pressure length and velocity in both the frontal and sagittal planes during unilateral stance. In this study, sagittal plane motion was not different among the various conditions; however, medially posted orthoses reduced frontal plane motion more than the other conditions. Frontal plane center of pressure excursion increased with a prefabricated, rigid, laterally posted heel wedge compared with medially and neutrally posted conditions. Frontal plane velocity was lower with medial posting compared with a prefabricated, rigid, laterally posted heel wedge and neutral orthoses. The prefabricated, rigid, laterally posted heel wedge, however, produced significantly greater frontal plane velocities than the medially or laterally posted conditions.

Percy and Menz[152] found that orthoses did not affect postural stability in 30 professional soccer players in bipedal, dominant leg, and tandem stance. Sway was assessed under four conditions: barefoot, soccer shoes only, soccer shoes with soft insoles, and soccer shoes with rigid orthoses. The researchers concluded that orthoses had no beneficial or detrimental effects in the elite athletes studied. In contrast, Olmsted and Hertel[153] found that foot orthoses differentially benefit those with various foot types. They assessed static and dynamic postural control in 30 patients grouped by rectus, planus, or cavus foot type. Patients wore custom-molded, semirigid foot orthoses for 2 weeks between baseline and posttest measurement. Improvement in reach occurred in three of eight directions on the Star Excursion Balance Test in those with cavus foot type. Patients with cavus foot type also demonstrated a decreased center of pressure velocity in static stance.

Rome and Brown[154] examined postural sway in 50 patients identified as pronators (per the Foot Posture Index) in a randomized clinical trial. Patients were assigned either to a control or orthotic group. The orthotic group wore prefabricated, high-density ethyl vinyl acetate orthoses with low-density ethyl vinyl acetate rearfoot wedging for 4 weeks. At 4 weeks, medial-lateral sway decreased in the orthotic group; however, no differences in anterior-posterior sway or mean balance occurred between the groups.

Collectively, these studies suggest that orthoses do affect electromyographic activity, balance, and postural control. Health professionals may be better able to identify those most likely to benefit from orthotic intervention if measures of postural control and neuromuscular function are incorporated along with the assessment of lower extremity and foot skeletal alignment.

MANAGEMENT OF OVERUSE INJURIES

Although the specific biomechanical and neurological effects of foot orthoses on walking and running are not completely understood, orthoses can and do reduce symptoms and improve function. Although current evidence does not include many randomized, controlled clinical trials, the available evidence does support efficacy of orthotic intervention in the management of lower extremity injuries.

Pain Associated with Foot Deformity

Burns and colleagues[155] examined the effect of custom foot orthoses on foot pain (and other factors) in individuals with cavus foot type. The study consisted of 154 individuals with 75 randomly selected to the custom foot orthoses group and 79 to the control group. At 3 months' follow-up,[153] individuals reported data with mean foot pain improvement of 31.2 points with custom foot orthosis and 20.3 points with the control. Individuals with the custom foot orthoses improved pain scores by 74% compared with 43% with the control group. D'Ambrosia[156] reported on 200 individuals who had used orthoses to manage a variety of running injuries, including posterior tibial syndrome, pes plano valgum, metatarsalgia, plantar fasciitis, and iliotibial band tendonitis. Almost all had severe pronation with forefoot varus before prescription of an orthosis. Rates of reported improvement were quite high: 73% in posterior tibial syndrome, 90% in pes plano valgum, 86% in metatarsalgia, 82% in plantar fasciitis, and 66% in iliotibial band syndrome. Of those with cavus foot type, only 25% showed improvement with orthotic use.

Donatelli and colleagues[157] received follow-up surveys from 53 (65%) of 81 individuals who had previously been fitted with custom-molded, semirigid orthoses for pes planus and chondromalacia, with 95% having a forefoot varus deformity. All respondents had a 6 to 8 week trial of temporary orthoses modified according to alterations in pain before receiving custom-molded, semirigid orthoses. Respondents were asked to describe or rate pain relief with orthoses, orthotic satisfaction, continued use of orthoses, and ability to return to previous level of activity. Ninety-six percent of respondents reported pain relief, 91% were satisfied with their orthoses, 94% were still wearing their orthoses (length of time with orthoses varied from 3 months to 2 years from time surveyed), and 70% were able to return to their previous level of activity.

Moraros and Hodge[158] surveyed 525 individuals who used custom-fitted orthoses provided by podiatric physicians to determine effectiveness and patient satisfaction. Of the 453 records completed in useable form (89% response rate), the chief symptom was fully resolved in 62.5%, partially resolved in 32.8%, and unresolved in 4.7%. Overall satisfaction for fit and quality was 83.1%. Although limitations are inherent in survey research, the relatively high response rate and sample support the usefulness of orthoses in relieving painful foot symptoms.

Patellofemoral Pain Syndrome

The role of foot orthoses on patellofemoral pain has been the subject of several studies that have provided research data for a systematic review on the efficacy of foot orthoses in the treatment of patellofemoral pain.[6] Barton and colleagues found evidence to support the use of foot orthoses for treatment of patellofemoral pain.[6] Johnston and Gross[159] assessed the effect of foot orthoses on pain, stiffness, and function in sixteen individuals with patellofemoral pain and excessive foot pronation. Following baseline assessments, the individuals were fitted with custom foot orthoses. Statistically significant improvements in pain and stiffness were found 2 weeks following the foot orthotic intervention and improvements in physical function were noted at the 3-month follow-up.

Barton and colleagues[160] used a variety of weight-bearing measurements to compare foot and ankle characteristics of individuals with patellofemoral pain syndrome to those without the syndrome. In relaxed stance, individuals with patellofemoral pain syndrome had signifcantly greater pronated foot posture than the control group when determined by longitudinal arch angle and posture index measurements. The patellofemoral pain syndrome group also demonstrated greater ranges of motion when subtalor joint neutral was used as a reference posture.

In a single subject design, Way[161] investigated the use of a custom-molded thermoplastic foot orthosis on PFPS in a 19-year-old collegiate softball player with a mild forefoot varus bilaterally and increased midfoot pronation during MSt and TSt. Intervention included pain-free stretching and strengthening exercises, modalities, and nonsteroidal antiinflammatory medication. The study design involved a 13-day baseline phase, a 17-day intervention phase (after which the patient removed orthoses for an 11-day withdrawal phase), and a second intervention phase in which orthoses were reintroduced for the last 32 days of the study. Pain was rated by a visual analog scale, and function was evaluated with the Functional Index Questionnaire. Pain decreased in each consecutive phase; function improved between phases for seven of the nine functional activities assessed in the Functional Index Questionnaire. On the basis of these findings, Way[161] suggested that orthotic intervention is appropriate for PFPS.

Saxena and Haddad[162] retrospectively reviewed 102 outcomes of interventions in individuals with chondromalacia patella, retropatellar dysplasia, or PFPS. Multiple interventions were noted, including semiflexible orthotics. Overall, 76.5% of patients demonstrated a reduction in pain and improved function, and 2% were asymptomatic after a 2- to 4-week intervention period.

Sutlive and colleagues[163] sought to identify characteristics of patients with PFPS likely to improve with a combination of orthoses and modified activity. They examined 50 patients in active military duty who had symptoms of PFPS during a partial squat or when ascending stairs. Measures included (1) rearfoot alignment in STN, (2) forefoot to rearfoot alignment, (3) navicular drop, (4) RCS, (5) Q angle, (6) tibial varum or valgum, (7) tibial torsion, (8) leg length, and (9) standard goniometric and postural test positions to determine ROM and tissue tightness. Patients wore unposted, premolded, full-length insoles with full arch support and heel cushioning for 21 days while concurrently limiting various activities. All completed a visual analog scale and a Global Rating of Change Questionnaire at baseline and at the end of the intervention period. Thirty-three of 50 patients completed the study, with a total of 78 knees with PFPS (many had bilateral symptoms). Data from 27 patients who demonstrated 50% or more improvement in visual analog scale scores were examined to determine which patient characteristics could predict orthotic success. Likelihood ratios identified several predictors of successful outcome: forefoot valgus of 2 degrees or more, great toe extension of 78 degrees or less, and navicular drop of 3 mm or less. Of those with PFPS, the patients with these three characteristics were more likely to respond to orthotic intervention.

Plantar Fasciitis

The use of foot orthoses in the management of plantar fasciitis has also been examined. A 12-month study by Landorf and colleagues[164] compared the effectiveness of sham, prefabricated and custom orthoses on pain and function in 136 individuals with plantar fasciitis. Participants were allocated to one of the three groups (sham, prefabricated, or custom) by a computer-generated random assignment and no other treatments were allowed during the 12-month trial. The prefabricated and customized groups experienced greater improvements in function and pain as compared to the sham group at 3 months but only the orthotic effects on function were statistically significant. Compared to the sham, the mean pain score for the prefabricated and custom orthosis was 8.7 and 7.4 points better and the mean function score was 8.4 and 7.5 points better respectively. All three groups improved with function and pain compared with baseline status at 3 months and 12 months, and there were only slight differences between the groups at 12 months.

Gross and colleagues[165] studied 15 individuals with plantar fasciitis for at least 1 month. Eight patients had excessively

pronated feet, and seven had a cavus foot type. Eleven of 15 had unsuccessfully used noncustom arch supports before enrollment in the study. At baseline, patients completed the pain and disability index of the Foot Function Index, were timed during a 100-m walk, and rated pain experienced during the walk with the visual analog scale. They received custom-fabricated, posted, multilayer orthoses with a thermoplastic core and were reevaluated after 12 to 17 days of orthotic use. Although no differences in preintervention and postintervention walk times occurred, visual analog scale pain ratings after the walk were lower than baseline, with only one patient demonstrating increased pain after the walk test. The scores on the subsections of the Foot Function Index also improved after orthotic use, with improvement of 66% in the pain subscale and 75% in the disability subscale. All patients continued to wear their orthoses at a follow-up phone call made 2 to 6 months after testing.

Seligman and Dawson[166] retrospectively evaluated 10 older individuals (mean age, 71 years) with heel pain from plantar fasciitis who used a heel pad made of Sorbothane (Sorbothane, Inc., Kent, Ohio) attached to a custom-molded, medium-density Plastazote insert reinforced with cork in the medial longitudinal arch. Duration of pain ranged from 6 months to several years; 5 of 10 patients previously tried other interventions. Pain was rated by a 10-point Likert pain rating scale. A significant difference occurred between baseline pain ratings (5.7/10) and postintervention pain ratings (1.85/10).

Morton's Neuroma

Kilmartin and Wallace[167] found that orthotic intervention did not improve symptoms of Morton's neuroma. Twenty-three individuals with pain of the third and fourth intermetatarsal space, aggravated by exercise and relieved by rest, were randomly assigned to two groups, with no consideration of foot type. Those in the supination group wore a Cobra orthosis with a thicker medial heel and arch filler. Those in the pronation group wore a reverse Cobra orthosis with a thicker lateral heel. Pain was measured by a visual analog scale. Sensory impairment and pain were objectively measured by tests that elicit neuroma pain. Function was assessed with the McMaster-Toronto Arthritis Patient Function Preference Questionnaire patient-specific measure of maximal function. No differences in pain or function occurred between the supination and pronation groups. Neither orthosis produced additional symptoms in the lower extremity.

The authors suggested that prescribing a custom orthosis based on foot type would have provided greater relief of symptoms.

Low Back Pain

Dananberg and Guiliano[168] examined the effects of orthotic intervention in 32 patients with chronic low pain. Patients completed the Quebec Back Pain Disability Scale at baseline after wearing foot orthoses for 1 month and after wearing orthoses for at least 6 months. The Quebec Scale provided a back pain score and a disability score. Permanent orthoses were fabricated on the basis of the results of temporary orthoses with modifications specific to each patient, in-shoe pressure analysis, gait video analysis, and clinical examination. At 1 month, significant reduction was observed in the mean pain and disability scores. Twenty-three of the original 32 patients were contacted at 6-month follow-up and reported significant improvement in function and reduction in pain. In comparing their outcomes to previous work by Kopec and colleagues,[169] who used the Quebec Back Pain Disability Scale to evaluate improvement in 178 patients undergoing standard back care interventions, the authors suggested that the use of foot orthoses enhanced outcomes over traditional back care. Of note, the protocol for evaluating patients for permanent orthoses was extensive.[169]

Although few randomized, controlled clinical studies have been undertaken, and most have been done with a small sample size in specific patient populations, current evidence supports that foot orthoses reduce symptoms of pain and improve function in individuals with overuse injury. Foot structure and type, orthotic materials, posting methods, and fabrication methods must be considered in determining who is likely to respond to orthotic intervention and comparing the effectiveness of various orthotic interventions.

SUMMARY

Although many components of Root's theory have been questioned, little doubt is present concerning the importance of his work in the field of foot biomechanics and orthotic intervention. Root's work provides a foundation for most of the research performed to gain a better understanding of the influence of the foot on lower extremity biomechanics and overuse injuries. Although research has provided some answers about mechanisms underlying efficacy of orthotic intervention, many more questions have also been raised. Additional research is necessary before clinicians will be able to prescribe orthoses confidently based on likely outcomes.

The effectiveness of biomechanical foot orthoses depends on a number of factors. An understanding of causes and effects of aberrant foot motion on pathological conditions of the foot is essential in determining the appropriate orthosis prescription and plan of care. Clinicians who do not carefully consider biomechanical principles and other factors that contribute to clinical signs and symptoms are likely to prescribe an ineffective or inappropriate orthosis. Information gathered from all three components of the biomechanical examination (non–weight-bearing, static weight-bearing, and dynamic gait assessment) is critical for orthotic design and prescription.

Historically, the principles and design of the Root functional orthosis and the biomechanical foot orthosis have had consistently effective clinical results. Root's model demands a keen understanding of foot biomechanics, careful prescription, and advanced fabrication skills. With this understanding and attention to detail, the end result may be a lightweight, durable, cost-effective foot orthosis that substantially reduces the detrimental effects of aberrant foot motion.

CASE EXAMPLE 1

Individual with Rearfoot and Forefoot Dysfunction

M. L. is an active 50-year-old woman who recently began to train for a local 10-km race. She is referred by her family physician for evaluation and intervention because of thickened and painful plantar callus under the second and fourth metatarsal heads and on the lateral surface of the hallux in both feet. The discomfort has increased to a point that she is unable to complete the distances she needs to run to prepare for the upcoming race.

M. L. is 5 feet, 5 inches tall and weighs 132 lb. In relaxed standing, no leg-length discrepancy is apparent, although both patellae are rotated inward, slight hyperextension and recurvatum at the knee is present (left more than right), and both feet are markedly pronated.

The following values are recorded in the non–weight-bearing and weight-bearing examinations:

Non–Weight-Bearing Examination Component	Left	Right
Rearfoot STN position	6 degrees varus	7 degrees varus
Calcaneus inversion	18 degrees	22 degrees
Calcaneus eversion	12 degrees	14 degrees
Ankle dorsiflexion	9 degrees	7 degrees
Rearfoot dorsiflexion	2 degrees	0 degrees
Forefoot STN position	Mild valgus	Moderate valgus
Locking mechanism	Fair	Poor
First ray	Slightly plantar flexed	Slightly plantar flexed
Hallux dorsiflexion	75 degrees	80 degrees
Medial longitudinal arch	Medium height	Medium height

Weight-Bearing Examination Component	Left	Right
Calcaneal/floor alignment	Eversion	Eversion
Tibiofibular position	40 degrees	37 degrees
Navicular drop (STN to relaxed calcaneal stance)	10 mm	12 mm
Navicular position (Feiss)	Slightly below	Moderately below
Toe sign	2.5 toes visible	3 toes visible
Femoral torsion	14 degrees	16 degrees
Tibial torsion	25 degrees	27 degrees

STN, Subtalar neutral.

Questions to Consider

- What are the normative values for non–weight-bearing range of motion in the rearfoot (STN position, calcaneal inversion and eversion, dorsiflexion) and forefoot (STN position, midtarsal joint dorsiflexion, first ray position, and mobility)?
- What rearfoot and forefoot deformities do M. L.'s examination findings suggest?
- What are normal findings for the closed chain static weight-bearing examination?
- How should the findings for M. L.'s weight-bearing examination be interpreted?
- How do the findings of M. L.'s non–weighting-bearing and weight-bearing examinations relate to each other? What deformities are compensated versus uncompensated?

CASE EXAMPLE 2

Individual with Rearfoot and Forefoot Dysfunction

M. L. wants to continue training for her upcoming race without increasing her pain and further damaging soft tissue in her feet. An appropriate prescription is being created for M. L. on the basis of the findings of her examination and the principles of orthotic design.

Examination Findings

Relaxed standing: no apparent leg-length discrepancy, both patella rotated inward, slight hyperextension and recurvatum at the knee (left more than right), marked pronation of both feet.

Non–Weight-Bearing Examination Component	Left	Right
Rearfoot STN position	6 degrees varus	7 degrees varus
Calcaneus inversion	18 degrees	22 degrees
Calcaneus eversion	12 degrees	14 degrees
Ankle dorsiflexion	9 degrees	7 degrees
Rearfoot dorsiflexion	2 degrees	0 degrees
Forefoot STN position	Mild valgus	Moderate valgus
Locking mechanism	Fair	Poor
First ray	Slightly plantar flexed	Slightly plantar flexed
Hallux dorsiflexion	75 degrees	80 degrees
Medial longitudinal arch	Medium height	Medium height

Weight-Bearing Examination Component	Left	Right
Calcaneal/floor alignment	Eversion	Eversion
Tibiofibular position	40 degrees	37 degrees
Navicular drop (STN to relaxed calcaneal stance)	10 mm	12 mm
Navicular position (Feiss)	Slightly below	Moderately below
Toe sign	2.5 toes visible	3 toes visible
Femoral torsion	14 degrees	16 degrees
Tibial torsion	25 degrees	27 degrees

STN, Subtalar neutral.

Continued

Questions to Consider

- What are the primary short-term and long-term goals of orthotic intervention for M. L.? Are the therapeutic goals for orthotic intervention similar to or different from M. L.'s goals? How quickly will the orthosis have an impact on level of pain and function?
- What options should be considered in addressing her forefoot deformity in each foot? What type of posting (intrinsic versus extrinsic, medial versus lateral) is most appropriate? How much of a wedge or post should be recommended? Why? How might the recommendations for each foot be similar or different?
- What options should be considered in addressing the rearfoot deformity in each foot? What type of posting (intrinsic versus extrinsic, medial versus lateral) would

be most appropriate? How much of a wedge or post should be recommended? Why? How might the recommendations for each foot be similar or different?
- What type of materials would be most appropriate to use in her orthosis? Why?
- Is fabricating orthoses for both her running shoes and her usual daily footwear advisable? Why or why not?
- What type of wearing schedule should be recommended? Should she alter her training schedule or expectations about participating in the upcoming race? Why or why not?
- How frequently should M. L. be followed up during this episode of care? How should the outcomes of orthotic intervention be assessed?

REFERENCES

1. Olson WR. Orthotic materials. In: Valmassy RL, ed. *Clinical Biomechanics of the Lower Extremities.* St. Louis: Mosby–Year Book; 1996:307–326.
2. Kirby KA. The medial heel skive technique. Improving pronation control in foot orthoses. *J Am Podiatr Med Assoc.* 1992;82(4):177–188.
3. Shuster RO. A history of orthopaedics in podiatry. *J Am Podiatry Assoc.* 1974;64(5):322.
4. Root ML, Orien WP, Weed JH. *Normal and Abnormal Function of the Foot.* vol 2. Los Angeles: Clinical Biomechanics Corporation; 1977.
5. Hatton AL, Dixon J, Rome K, Martin D. Effect of foot orthoses on lower limb muscle activation: a critical review. *Phys Ther Rev.* 2008;13(4):280–293.
6. Hume P, Hopkins W, Rome K, et al. Effectiveness of foot orthoses for treatment and prevention of lower limb injuries. *Sports Med.* 2008;38(9):759–779.
7. Barton CJ, Munteanu SE, Menz HB, et al. The efficacy of foot orthoses in the treatment of individuals with patellofemoral pain syndrome-a systematic review. *Sports Med.* 2010;40(5):377–395.
8. Collins N, Bisset L, McPoil T, et al. Foot orthoses in lower limb overuse conditions: a systematic review and meta-analysis. *Foot Ankle Int.* 2007;28(3):396–412.
9. Burns J, Wegener C, Begg L, et al. Randomized trial of custom orthosis and footwear on foot pain and plantar pressure in diabetic peripheral arterial disease. *Diabet Med.* 2009;86:893–899.
10. Erel S, Uygur F, Simsek IE, Yakut Y. The effects of dynamic ankle-foot orthoses in chronic stroke patients at three-month follow-up: a randomized controlled trial. *Clin Rehabil.* 2011;25(6):515–523.
11. Ramdharry GM, Marsden JF, Day BL, Thompson AJ. De-stabilizing and training effects of foot orthoses in multiple sclerosis. *Mult Scler.* 2006;12:219–226.
12. Barnett CH, Napier JR. The axis of rotation at the ankle joint in man. Its influence upon the form of the talus and the mobility of the fibula. *J Anat (Lond).* 1952;86:1–9.
13. Hicks JH. The mechanics of the foot. Part I: the joints. *J Anat.* 1953;87:345–347.
14. Morris JM. Biomechanics of the foot and ankle. *Clin Orthop.* 1977;122(1):10–17.
15. American Orthopedics Association. *Manual of Orthopedic Surgery.* Chicago: American Orthopedics Association; 1972.
16. Rasmussen O, Tovberg-Jevsen I. Mobility of the ankle joint. *Acta Orthop Scand.* 1982;53(1):155–160.
17. Norkin CC, Levangie PK. The ankle foot complex. In: Levangie PK, Edd CC, Norkin PT, eds. *Joint Structure and Function: A Comprehensive Analysis.* 2nd ed. Philadelphia: F.A. Davis; 1992:379–419.
18. Lapidius PW. Kinesiology and mechanics of the tarsal joints. *Clin Orthop.* 1963;30:20–35.
19. Kjaergaard-Andersen P, Wethelund J, Nielsen S. Lateral talo-calcaneal instability following section of the calcaneofibular ligament: a kinesiologic study. *Foot Ankle.* 1987;7(6):355–361.
20. Manter JT. Movements of the subtalar and transverse tarsal joints. *Anat Rec.* 1941;80:397–410.
21. Phillips RD, Christeck R, Phillips RL. Clinical measurement of the axis of the subtalar joint. *J Am Podiatry Assoc.* 1985;75(3):119–131.
22. Green DR, Carol A. Planal dominance. *J Am Podiatr Med Assoc.* 1984;74(2):98–103.
23. Perry J. Anatomy and biomechanics of the hindfoot. *Clin Orthop.* 1983;177(1):9–15.
24. Olerud C, Rosendahl Y. Torsion-transmitting properties of the hindfoot. *Clin Orthop.* 1987;(214):285–294.
25. Warwick R, Williams PL, eds. *Gray's Anatomy.* 35th ed. Philadelphia: Saunders; 1973:373–385, 460–471, 571–585.
26. Elftman H. The transverse tarsal joint and its control. *Clin Orthop.* 1960;16:41–45.
27. Sarrafian SK. *Anatomy of the Foot and Ankle: Descriptive, Topographic, and Functional.* Philadelphia: JB Lippincott; 1983.
28. Moore KL. *Clinically Oriented Anatomy.* Baltimore: Williams & Wilkins; 1980.
29. Hicks JH. The mechanics of the foot. Part II: the plantar aponeurosis and the arch. *J Anat.* 1954;88:25–31.
30. Sarafian SK. Functional characteristics of the foot and plantar aponeurosis under tibiotalar loading. *Foot Ankle.* 1987;8(1):1–4.
31. Perry J. *Gait Analysis: Normal and Pathological Function.* Thorofare, NJ: Slack; 1992.
32. Vaughn CL, Davis DL, O'Connor JC. *Dynamics of Human Gait.* Champaign, Ill: Human Kinetics; 1992.

33. James SL, Jones DC. Biomechanical aspects of distance running injuries. In: Cavanagh PR, ed. *Biomechanics of Distance Running.* Champaign, Ill: Human Kinetics; 1990:249–271.

34. Wright DG, Desai M, Henderson WH. Action of the subtalar and ankle-joint complex during the stance phase of walking. *J Bone Joint Surg.* 1964;46A(2):361–382.

35. Perry J, Hislop HJ. *Principles of Lower Extremity Bracing.* Washington, DC: American Physical Therapy Association; 1967.

36. Close JR, Todd FN. The phasic activity of the muscles of the lower extremity and the effect of tendon transfer. *J Bone Joint Surg.* 1959;41A(2):189–208.

37. Valiant GA. Transmission and attenuation of heelstrike accelerations. In: Cavanagh PR, ed. *Biomechanics of Distance Running.* Champaign, IL: Human Kinetics; 1990:225–249.

38. McPoil TG, Hunt GC. Evaluation and management of foot and ankle disorders. Present problems and future directions. *J Occup Sports Phys Ther.* 1995;21(6):381–388.

39. Picciano AM, Rowlands MS, Worrell T. Reliability of open and closed kinetic chain subtalar joint neutral positions and navicular drop test. *J Occup Sports Phys Ther.* 1993;18(4):553–558.

40. Smith-Oricchio K, Harris BE. Interrater reliability of subtalar neutral, calcaneal inversion and eversion. *J Occup Sports Phys Ther.* 1990;12(1):10–15.

41. Gross MT. Lower quarter screening for skeletal malalignment. Suggestions for orthotics and shoewear. *J Occup Sports Phys Ther.* 1995;21(6):389–405.

42. Pratt D, Tollafield D, Johnson G, et al. Foot orthoses. In: Wallace WA, ed. *Biomechanical Basis of Orthotic Management.* Oxford: Butterworth-Heinemann; 1993:70–98.

43. Wooden MJ. Biomechanical evaluation for functional orthotics. In: Donatelli RA, ed. *The Biomechanics of the Foot and Ankle.* 2nd ed. Philadelphia: F.A. Davis; 1996:168–183.

44. McPoil TG, Brocato RS. The foot and ankle. In: Gould JA, Davis GJ, eds. *Orthopaedics and Sports Physical Therapy.* St. Louis: Mosby; 1985:322–325.

45. Anthony RJ. *The Manufacture and Use of the Functional Foot Orthosis.* Basel, Switzerland: Karger; 1991.

46. Elveru RA, Rothstein JM, Lamb RC. Goniometric reliability in a clinical setting. Subtalar and ankle joint measurements. *Phys Ther.* 1988;68(5):672–677.

47. Garbalosa JC, McClure MH, Catlin PA, et al. The frontal plane relationship of the forefoot to the rearfoot in an asymptomatic population. *J Occup Sports Phys Ther.* 1994;20(4):200–206.

48. Lattanza L, Gray GW, Kantner RM. Closed versus open kinematic chain measurements of subtalar joint eversion. Implications for clinical practice. *J Occup Sports Phys Ther.* 1988;9(9):310–314.

49. Vitasalo JT, Kvist M. Some biomechanical aspects of the foot and ankle in athletes with and without shin splints. *Am J Sports Med.* 1983;2(3):125–130.

50. Tiberio D. Evaluation of functional ankle dorsiflexion using subtalar neutral position. *Phys Ther.* 1987;67(6):955–957.

51. Baggett BD, Young G. Ankle joint dorsiflexion. Establishment of a normal range. *J Am Podiatr Med Assoc.* 1993;83(5):251–254.

52. Hillstrom HJ, Perlberg G, Sieglers S, et al. Objective identification of ankle equinus deformity and resulting contracture. *J Am Podiatr Med Assoc.* 1991;81(10):519–524.

53. Hill RS. Ankle equinus: prevalence and linkage to common foot pathology. *J Am Podiatry Assoc.* 1995;85(6):295–300.

54. Hoppenfeld S. *Physical Examination of the Spine and Extremities.* Norwalk, Conn: Appleton-Century-Crofts; 1976.

55. Tachdjian MO. *The Child's Foot.* Philadelphia: Saunders; 1985.

56. McGlamry ED, Kitting RW. Equinus foot. An analysis of the etiology, pathology, and treatment techniques. *J Am Podiatry Assoc.* 1973;63:165.

57. Whitney AK, Green DR. Pseudo equinus. *J Am Podiatry Assoc.* 1982;72:365.

58. Davidson RS. Deformities of the child's foot. In: Sammarco JG, ed. *Foot and Ankle Manual.* Philadelphia: Lea & Febiger; 1991:296.

59. Donatelli RA. Abnormal biomechanics. In: Donatelli RA, ed. *The Biomechanics of the Foot and Ankle.* Philadelphia: F.A. Davis; 1990:32–65.

60. D'Ambrosia RD. Orthotic devices in running injuries. *Clin Sports Med.* 1985;4(4):611–619.

61. McPoil TG, Knecht HG, Schuit D. A survey of foot types in normal females between the ages of 18 and 30 years. *J Occup Sports Phys Ther.* 1988;9(12):346–349.

62. Dananberg HJ. Gait style as an etiology to chronic postural pain. Part I: functional hallux limitus. *J Am Podiatr Med Assoc.* 1993;83(8):433–441.

63. Dananberg HJ. Gait style as an etiology to chronic postural pain. Part II: postural compensatory process. *J Am Podiatr Med Assoc.* 1993;83(11):615–624.

64. Gastwirth BW. Biomechanical examination of the foot and lower extremity. In: Valmassy RL, ed. *Clinical Biomechanics of the Lower Extremities.* St. Louis: Mosby–Year Book; 1996:132–147.

65. Tomaro J. Measurement of tibiofibular varum in subjects with unilateral overuse symptoms. *J Occup Sports Phys Ther.* 1995;21(2):86–89.

66. McPoil TG, Schuit D, Knecht HG. A comparison of three positions used to evaluate tibial varum. *J Am Podiatr Med Assoc.* 1988;78(1):22–28.

67. Lohmann KN, Rayhel HE, Schneiderwind P, et al. Static measurement of tibial vara. Reliability and effect of lower extremity position. *Phys Ther.* 1987;67(2):196–200.

68. Brody D. Techniques in evaluation and treatment of the injured runner. *Orthop Clin North Am.* 1982;13(3):541–558.

69. Subotnick SI. Biomechanics of the subtalar and midtarsal joints. *J Am Podiatry Assoc.* 1975;65(8):756–764.

70. Mueller MJ, Host JV, Norton BJ. Navicular drop as a composite measure of excessive pronation. *J Am Podiatr Med Assoc.* 1993;83(4):198–202.

71. Norkin C, Levangie P. *Joint Structure and Function: A Comprehensive Analysis.* Philadelphia: F.A. Davis; 1983.

72. Dahle LK, Mueller M, Delitto A, et al. Visual assessment of foot type and relationship of foot type to lower extremity injury. *J Occup Sports Phys Ther.* 1991;14(2):70–74.

73. Close JR, Inman VT, Poor PM, et al. The function of the subtalar joint. *Clin Orthop.* 1967;50(1–2):159–179.

74. Donatelli R, Hurlbert C, Conaway D, et al. Biomechanical foot orthotics. A retrospective study. *J Occup Sports Phys Ther.* 1988;10(6):205–212.

75. Inman VT, Rolston HJ, Todd F. *Human Walking.* Baltimore: Williams & Wilkins; 1981.

76. Johnson MA, Donatelli R, Wooden M, et al. Effects of three different posting methods on controlling abnormal subtalar pronation. *Phys Ther.* 1994;74(2):149–161.

77. Schumacher HR. *Primer of the Rheumatoid Diseases.* 10th ed. Atlanta: The Arthritis Foundation; 1993.

78. Harper MC. Failed treatment and residual deformity of the midfoot and hindfoot. In: Sammarco JG, ed. *Foot and Ankle Manual.* Philadelphia: Lea & Febiger; 1991:212–213.

79. Boulton A. Diabetic neuropathy. In: Frykberg RG, ed. *The High Risk Foot in Diabetes Mellitus*. New York: Churchill Livingstone; 1991:49–59.

80. Laughton C, Davis IM, Williams DS. A comparision of four methods of obtaining a negative impression of the foot. *J Am Podiatr Med Assoc*. 2002;92:261–268.

81. Redford J. *Orthotics: Clinical Practice and Rehabilitation Technology*. Philadelphia: Churchill Livingston; 1995.

82. DiGiovanni CW, Greisberg J. *Foot and Ankle: Core Knowledge in Orthopedics*. Philadelphia: Mosby; 2007.

83. Carroll M, Annabell M, Rome K. Reliability of capturing foot parameters using digital scanning and the neutral suspension casting technique. *J Foot Ankle Res*. 2011;4:1–7.

84. Schrank ES, Stanhope SJ. Dimensional accuracy of ankle-foot orthoses constructed by rapid customization and manufacturing framework. *J Rehabil Res Dev*. 2011;48:31–42.

85. Trotter LC, Pierrynowski MR. Ability of foot care professionals to cast feet using the nonweightbearing plaster and gait referenced foam casting techniques. *J Am Podiatr Med Assoc*. 2008;98:14–18.

86. Valmassy RL. Advantages and disadvantages of various casting techniques. *J Am Podiatry Assoc*. 1979;69(12):707–712.

87. McPoil TG, Schuit D, Knecht HG. Comparison of three methods used to obtain a neutral plaster foot impression. *Phys Ther*. 1989;69(6):448–450.

88. Kirby KA. Troubleshooting functional foot orthoses. In: Valmassy RL, ed. *Clinical Biomechanics of the Lower Extremities*. St. Louis: Mosby–Year Book; 1996:327–348.

89. Philips JW. *The Functional Foot Orthosis*. Edinburgh: Churchill Livingstone; 1995.

90. Blake RL, Ferguson H. Extrinsic rearfoot posts. *J Am Podiatr Med Assoc*. 1992;82(4):202–207.

91. Blake RL, Ferguson HJ. Effect of extrinsic rearfoot posts on rearfoot position. *J Am Podiatr Med Assoc*. 1993;83(8):202.

92. Brown GP, Donatelli R, Catlin PA, et al. The effects of two types of foot orthoses on rearfoot mechanics. *J Occup Sports Phys Ther*. 1995;21(5):258–267.

93. Smith LS, Clarke TE, Hamill CL, et al. The effects of soft and semi-rigid orthoses upon movement in running. *J Am Podiatr Med Assoc*. 1986;76(4):227–233.

94. Eng JJ, Pierrynowski MR. The effects of soft foot orthotics on three-dimensional lower-limb kinematics during walking and running. *Phys Ther*. 1994;74(9):836–844.

95. Eng JJ, Pierrynowski MR. Evaluation of soft foot orthotics in the treatment of patellofemoral pain syndrome. *Phys Ther*. 1993;73(2):62–70.

96. Rodgers MM, Leveau BF. Effectiveness of foot orthotic devices used to modify pronation in runners. *J Occup Sports Phys Ther*. 1982;4(2):86–90.

97. McPoil TG, Hunt GC. *An Evaluation and Treatment Paradigm for the Future in Physical Therapy of the Foot and Ankle*. 2nd ed. Philadelphia: Churchill Livingstone; 1995: 1–10.

98. Sobel E, Levitz SJ. Reappraisal of the negative impressioncast and subtalar joint neutral position. *J Am Podiatr Med Assoc*. 1997;8(1):32–33.

99. Payne CB. The past present and future of podiatric biomechanics. *J Am Podiatr Med Assoc*. 1998;88(2):53–63.

100. Payne C, Chuter V. The clash between theory and science of kinematic effectiveness of foot orthoses. *Clin Podiatr Med Surg*. 2001;18(4):705–713.

101. Lee WE. Podiatric biomechanics. A historical appraisal and discussion of the Root model as a clinical system of approach in the present context of theoretical uncertainty. *Clin Podiatr Med Surg*. 2001;18(4):555–684.

102. Ball KA, Afheldt MJ. Evolution of foot orthotics-part 1: coherent theory or coherent practice. *J Manipulative Physiol Ther*. 2002;25(2):116–124.

103. Ball KA, Afheldt MJ. Evolution of foot orthotics-part 2: research reshapes long-standing theory. *J Manipulative Physiol Ther*. 2002;25(2):125–134.

104. Payne CB, Bird AR. Teaching clinical biomechanics in the context of uncertainty. *J Am Podiatr Med Assoc*. 1999; 89(10):525–530.

105. Pierrynowski MR, Smith SB, Mlynarczyk JH. Proficiency of foot care specialists to place the rearfoot at subtalar neutral. *J Am Podiatr Med Assoc*. 1996;86:217–223.

106. Cook A, Gorman I, Morris J. Evaluation of the neutral position of the subtalar joint. *J Am Podiatr Med Assoc*. 1988;78:449–451.

107. Diamond JE, Mueller MJ, Delitto A, et al. Reliability of a diabetic foot evaluation. *Phys Ther*. 1989;69:797–802.

108. Wright DG, Desai SM, Henderson WH. Action of the subtalar joint and ankle joint complex during the stance phase of walking. *J Bone Joint Surg Am*. 1964;46A:361–382.

109. Root ML, Orien WP, Weed JH, et al. *Biomechanical Examination of the Foot, vol 1*. Los Angeles: Clinical Biomechanics; 1971.

110. McPoil TG, Cornwall MW. Relationship between neutral subtalar joint position and pattern of rearfoot motion during walking. *Foot Ankle Int*. 1996;15:141–145.

111. Pierrynowski MR, Smith SB. Rear foot inversion/eversion during gait relative to the subtalar joint neutral position. *Foot Ankle Int*. 1996;17(7):406–412.

112. Astrom M, Arvidson T. Alignment and joint motion in the normal foot. *J Orthop Sports Phys Ther*. 1995;22(5):216–222.

113. Dicharry JM, Franz JR, Croce UD, et al. Differences in static and dynamic measures in evaluation of talonavicular mobility in gait. *J Orthop Sports Phys Ther*. 2009;39(8):628–634.

114. Razeghi M, Batt ME. Biomechanical analysis of the effect of orthotic shoe inserts; review of the literature. *Sports Med*. 2000;29(6):425–438.

115. Dahle LK, Mueller M, Delitto A, et al. Visual assessment of foot types and relationship of foot type to lower extremity injury. *J Orthop Sports Phys Ther*. 1991;14(2):70–74.

116. Gross KD, Niu J, Zhang YQ, et al. Varus foot alignment and hip conditions in older adults. *Arthritis Rheum*. 2007;56(9):2993–2998.

117. Powers CM, Maffucci R, Hampton S. Rearfoot posture in subjects with patellofemoral pain. *J Orthop Sports Phys Ther*. 1995;22(4):155–160.

118. Sommer HM, Vallentyne SW. Effect of foot posture on the incidence of medial tibial stress. *Med Sci Sports Exerc*. 1995;27(6):800–805.

119. Donatelli R, Wooden M, Ekedahl SR, et al. Relationship between static and dynamic foot postures in professional baseball players. *J Orthop Sports Phys Ther*. 1999;29(6):316–330.

120. Cowan DN, Jones BH, Robinson JR. Medial longitudinal arch height and risk of training-associated injury. *Med Sci Sports Exerc*. 1989;21(suppl):S60.

121. Cowan DN, Jones BH, Robinson JR. Foot morphology and alignment and risk of exercise-related injury in runners. *Arch Fam Med*. 1993;2:273–277.

122. Richter RR, Austin TM, Reinking MF. Foot orthoses in lower limb overuse conditions: a systematic review and meta-analysis-critcal appraisal and commentary. *J Athl Train*. 2011;46(1):103–106.

123. Novick A, Kelley D. Position and movement changes of the foot with orthotic intervention during the loading response of gait. *J Orthop Sports Phys Ther.* 1990;11(7):301–312.

124. Bates BT, Osternig LR, Mason B, et al. Foot orthotic devices to modify selected aspects of lower extremity mechanics. *Am J Sports Med.* 1979;7:338–342.

125. Clark TE, Fredrick EC, Hlavac HF. Effects of a soft orthotic device on rearfoot movements in running. *Podiatr Sports Med.* 1983;1(1):26–33.

126. MacLean C, Davis IM, Hamill J. Influence of a custom foot orthotic intervention on lower extremity dynamics in healthy runners. *Clin Biomech (Bristol, Avon).* 2006;21(6):623–630.

127. Johanson MA, Donatelli R, Woodon MJ, et al. Effects of three different posting methods on controlling abnormal subtalar pronation. *Phys Ther.* 1994;74(2):149–161.

128. Genova JM, Gross MT. Effect of foot orthotics on calcaneal eversion during standing and treadmill walking for subjects with abnormal pronation. *J Orthop Sports Phys Ther.* 2000;30(11):664–675.

129. Branthwaite HR, Payton CJ, Chockalingam N. The effect of simple insoles on three-dimensional foot motion during normal walking. *Clin Biomech (Bristol, Avon).* 2004;19(9):972–977.

130. Brown GP, Donatelli R, Catlin PA, et al. The effect of two types of foot orthoses on rearfoot mechanics. *J Orthop Sports Phys Ther.* 1995;21(5):258–267.

131. Butler RJ, Davis IM, Laughton CM, et al. Dual-function foot orthosis: effect on shock and control of rearfoot motion. *Foot Ankle Int.* 2003;24(5):410–414.

132. Miller CD, Laskowski ER, Suman VJ. Effect of corrective rearfoot orthotic devices on ground reaction forces during ambulation. *Mayo Clin Proc.* 1996;71(8):757–762.

133. McPoil TG, Cornwall MW. The effect of foot orthoses on transverse tibial rotation during walking. *J Am Podiatr Med Assoc.* 2000;90(1):2–11.

134. Stacoff A, Reinschmidt C, Nigg BM, et al. Effects of foot orthotics on skeletal motion during running. *Clin Biomech (Bristol, Avon).* 2000;15:54–64.

135. Joseph M, Tiberio D, Baird JL, et al. Knee valgus during drop jumps in National Collegiate Athletic Association Division I female athletes: the effect of a medical post. *Am J Sports Med.* 2008;36(2):285–289.

136. Tillman MD, Chiumento AB, Trimble MH, et al. Tibiofemoral rotation in landing: the influence of medially and laterally posted orthotics. *Phys Ther Sport.* 2003;4(1):34–39.

137. Nester CJ, van der Linden ML, Bowker P. Effect of foot orthoses on the kinematics and kinetics of normal walking gait. *Gait Posture.* 2003;17(2):180–187.

138. Williams DS, Davis IM, Baitch SP. Effect of inverted orthosis on lower extremity mechanics in runners. *Med Sci Sports Exerc.* 2003;35(12):2960–2968.

139. Kuhn RD, Yochum TR, Cherry AR, et al. Immediate change in the quadriceps femoris angle after insertion of an orthotic device. *J Manipulative Physiol Ther.* 2002;25(70):465–470.

140. Stackhouse CL, Davis IM, Hamill J. Orthotic intervention in forefoot and rearfoot strike running patterns. *Clin Biomech (Bristol, Avon).* 2004;19(1):64–70.

141. Nigg BM, Nurse MA, Stefanyshyn DJ. Shoe inserts and orthotics for sport and physical activities. *Med Sci Sports Exerc.* 1999;31(suppl 7):S421–S428.

142. Nigg BM. The role of impact forces and foot pronation: a new paradigm. *Clin J Sport Med.* 2001;11(1):2–9.

143. Mundermann A, Nigg BM, Humble RN, et al. Orthotic comfort is related to kinematics, kinetics, and EMG in recreational runners. *Med Sci Sports Exerc.* 2003;35(10):1710–1719.

144. Mundermann A, Nigg BM, Humble RN, et al. Foot orthotics affect lower extremity kinematics and kinetics during running. *Clin Biomech (Bristol, Avon).* 2003;18(3):254–262.

145. Hertel J, Sloss BR, Earl JE. Effect of foot orthotics on quadriceps and gluteus mediuselectromyographic activity during selected exercises. *Arch Phys Med Rehabil.* 2005;86(1):26–30.

146. Kulig K, Burnfield JM, Reishchl S, et al. Effect of foot orthoses on tibialis posterior activation in persons with pes planus. *Med Sci Sports Exerc.* 2005;37(1):24–29.

147. Bird AR, Bendrups AP, Payne CB. The effect of foot wedging on electromyographic activity in the erector spinae and gluteus medius muscles during walking. *Gait Posture.* 2003;18(2):81–91.

148. Vanicek KN, Kingman J, Hencken C. The effect of foot orthotics on myoelectric fatigue in the vastus lateralis during a simulated skiers squat. *J Electromyogr Kinesiol.* 2004;14(6):693–698.

149. Guskiewicz KM, Perrin DH. Effect of orthotics on postural sway following inversion ankle sprain. *J Orthop Sports Phys Ther.* 1996;23(5):326–331.

150. Hertel J, Denegar CR, Buckley WE, et al. Effect of rearfoot orthotics on postural control in healthy subjects. *J Sports Rehabil.* 2001;100:36–47.

151. Hertel J, Denegar CR, Buckley WE, et al. Effect of rearfoot orthotics on postural sway after lateral ankle sprain. *Arch Phys Med Rehabil.* 2001;82(7):1000–1003.

152. Percy ML, Menz HB. Effects of prefabricated foot orthoses and soft insoles on postural stability in professional soccer players. *J Am Podiatr Med Assoc.* 2001;91(4):194–202.

153. Olmsted LC, Hertel J. Influence of foot type and orthotics on static and dynamic postural control. *J Sports Rehabil.* 2004;13(1):54–66.

154. Rome K, Brown CL. Randomized clinical trial into the impact of rigid foot orthoses on balance parameters in excessively pronated feet. *Clin Rehabil.* 2004;18(6):624–630.

155. Burns J, Crosbie J, Ouvrier R, et al. Effective orthotic therapy for the painful cavus foot. *J Am Podiatr Med Assoc.* 2006;96(3):205–211.

156. D'Ambrosia RD. Orthotic devices in running injuries. *Clin Sports Med.* 1985;4(4):611–619.

157. Donatelli R, Hulbert C, Conaway D, et al. Biomechanical foot orthotics: a retrospective study. *J Orthop Sports Phys Ther.* 1988;10(6):205–212.

158. Moraros J, Hodge W. Orthotic survey preliminary results. *J Am Podiatr Med Assoc.* 1993;83(3):139–148.

159. Johnston LB, Gross MT. Effects of foot orthoses on quality of life for individuals with patellofemoral pain syndrome. *J Orthop Sports Phys Ther.* 2004;34(8):440–448.

160. Barton CJ, Bonanno D, Levinger P, et al. Foot and ankle characteristics in patellofemoral pain syndrome: A case control and reliability study. *J Orthop Sports Phys Ther.* 2010;40(5):286–296.

161. Way MC. Effects of a thermoplastic foot orthosis on patellofemoral pain in a collegiate athlete: a single subject design. *J Orthop Sports Phys Ther.* 1999;29(6):331–338.

162. Saxena A, Haddad J. The effect of foot orthoses on patellofemoral pain syndrome. *J Am Podiatr Med Assoc.* 2003;93(4):264–271.

163. Sutlive TG, Mitchell SD, Maxfield SN, et al. Identification of individuals with patellofemoral pain whose symptoms improved after a combined program of foot orthosis use and modified activity: a preliminary investigation. *Phys Ther.* 2004;84(1):49–61.

164. Landorf KB, Keenan A, Herbert RD. Effectiveness of foot orthoses to treat plantar fasciitis. *Arch Intern Med.* 2006; 166(12):1305–1310.

165. Gross MT, Byers JM, Krafft JL, et al. The impact of custom semi-rigid foot orthotics on pain and disability for individuals with plantar fasciitis. *J Orthop Sports Phys Ther.* 2002;32(4):149–157.

166. Seligman DA, Dawson DR. Customized heel pads and soft orthotics to treat heel pain and plantar fasciitis. *Arch Phys Med Rehabil.* 2003;84(10):1564–1567.

167. Kilmartin TE, Wallace WA. Effect of pronation and supination orthosis on Morton's neuroma and lower extremity function. *Foot Ankle Int.* 1994;15(5):256–262.

168. Dananberg HJ, Guiliano M. Chronic low-back pain and its response to custom made foot orthoses. *J Am Podiatr Med Assoc.* 1999;89(3):109–117.

169. Kopec JA, Esdaile JM, Abrahamowicz M, et al. The Quebec Back Pain Disability Scale: measurement properties. *Spine.* 1995;20(3):341–352.

9

Principles of Lower Extremity Orthoses

MICHELLE M. LUSARDI

LEARNING OBJECTIVES

On completion of this chapter, the reader will be able to:

1. Define the functional objectives (reasons) that an ankle foot orthosis (AFO), knee ankle foot orthosis (KAFO), or hip knee ankle foot orthosis (HKAFO) would be prescribed for persons with mobility dysfunction.

2. Explain the evaluative process used to determine appropriate prescription for individuals requiring a lower extremity orthosis.

3. Describe the biomechanical control systems for foot, ankle, knee, and/or hip designed into an AFO, KAFO, or HKAFO.

4. Describe how each type of lower extremity orthosis is designed to enhance achievement of stance phase stability, swing limb clearance, limb prepositioning, adequate step length, and efficiency of gait.

5. Describe how each of the most commonly prescribed AFO, KAFO, and HKAFO designs affect transition through the rockers of stance and swing phase of gait.

6. Compare and contrast the indications and limitations of prefabricated, custom fit, and custom molded lower extremity orthoses.

7. Apply knowledge of normal and pathological gait, assessment of impairment, and functional potential in the selection of an appropriate lower extremity orthosis for patients with neuromuscular impairments.

8. Identify effective strategies for donning/doffing the orthosis, gait and mobility training, and orthotic maintenance for children and adults using lower extremity orthoses.

9. Select appropriate outcome measures to evaluate effectiveness of orthotic intervention and gait training for persons using lower extremity orthoses.

There are many factors to consider when selecting a lower extremity orthosis for individuals with musculoskeletal or neuromuscular dysfunction who have difficulty with mobility and walking. An orthosis may be designed to substitute for impaired muscle performance in the presence of weakness to improve foot clearance in the swing phase of gait.[1] An orthosis may be used to provide stance phase stability and support to enhance alignment of limb segments when there is structural instability of one or more lower extremity joints.[2] An orthosis may be designed to limit joint motion or unload forces during weight bearing to allow healing after surgery or prevent injury to vulnerable joints.[3] For persons with impaired motor control and abnormal tone, orthoses may enhance mobility by minimizing the impact of abnormal movement associated with hypertonicity by positioning limb segments for optimal function.[4,5] Alternatively, an orthosis may be used to minimize the risk of development of bony deformity and contracture associated with longstanding hypertonicity, especially in growing children.[6] Given the many different reasons that an orthosis might be prescribed, there is no "one size fits all" option: Health professionals must clearly define what they want an orthosis to accomplish, consider its practicality and cost, and sort through the many options available to select the design and components that will best meet the patient's needs and goals.

This chapter systematically reviews the design, and the pros and cons of ankle-foot orthoses (AFOs), knee-ankle-foot orthoses (KAFOs), and hip-knee-ankle-foot orthoses (HKAFOs) as a means to improve mobility and function for children and adults with neuromuscular dysfunction. We will start with a quick review of the gait cycle and its "rockers" as a foundation for understanding how an orthosis can provide stance phase stability or enhance swing phase mobility. Then we will compare and contrast the various AFO designs, discuss contemporary KAFO components and design, explore traditional HKAFOs and their uses, investigate the clinical use of the parapodium and standing frames, and finally consider orthotic options for reciprocal gait for patients with significant neuromuscular disease or disability. We will apply our growing understanding of lower extremity orthoses in problem-based cases for children and adults with cerebral palsy, hemiplegia following stroke, postpolio syndrome, and spinal cord injury (SCI).

WHAT TYPE OF ORTHOSIS IS BEST?

When an individual with neuromuscular or musculoskeletal dysfunction has difficulty with mobility and walking, decisions about orthotic options are best made by collaborative interaction within the framework of an interdisciplinary team.[7] Members of this team include the person who will be using the orthosis, their family members or caregivers, any physicians involved in his or her care (e.g., a neurologist, orthopedist, or physiatrist), the physical and occupational therapists who are likely to be involved in functional training, and the orthotist who will design, fabricate, deliver, and maintain the orthosis. The combined knowledge and skills of all members of the team ensure that the prescription will best match orthotic design to the patient's functional needs (Table 9-1).[8] If the team is not able to gather in one place as decisions are being made, there must be effective strategies for communication in place so that each team member can

contribute his or her unique perspective about why an orthosis is indicated and how the orthosis will facilitate the individual's functional ability.

Physical therapists examine the patient to provide information about muscle performance and motor control, range of motion, alignment of the limbs, information about the gait cycle with attention to both primary impairments and the compensation strategies the individual uses while walking, as well as how the orthosis might impact biomechanically

TABLE 9-1   *Components of the Preorthotic Prescription Examination Organized by ICF Categories*

ICF Category	Domain		Concerns
Body structure and function	Joint integrity and stability		Ligamentous instability, joint deformity
	Range of motion		Soft tissue contracture, joint deformity
	Limb length and alignment		Rotational deformity, unequal limb length
	Muscle length		Fixed versus modifiable contracture
	Overall flexibility		Ability to don/doff; impact of orthosis on trunk, back
	Motor control		Quality of voluntary motion
	Muscle tone		Flaccidity, hypotonicity, hypertonicity, fluctuating tone
	Muscle performance		Strength, power, endurance
	Involuntary movement		Impact on tolerance of orthosis
	Coordination		Ability to don/doff
	Somatosensory function		Ability to detect skin irritation/damage
	Perceptual function		Ability to don/doff
	Upper extremity function		Ability to don/doff
	Postural control, balance		Ability to don/doff
	Visual function		Ability to perform skin checks, donning/doffing
	Cognitive function		Understanding of how to use orthosis
	Cardiovascular endurance		Ability to functionally use orthosis
Activity level	Gait analysis	Observational	Primary gait problems and compensations
		Kinematic	Primary gait problems and compensations
		Kinetic	Impact of orthosis on moment throughout gait cycle
		Energetics	Impact of orthosis on physical work of walking
		Assistive device	Safe function with orthosis and assistive device
		Various surfaces	Impact of resistance, unstable surface on gait
	Transitions	Sit to/from stand	Preparing to walk and returning to seated position
		To/from floor	Activities on the floor (especially for children/play)
		Managing falls	How to protect self and recover from fall
		Inclines/stairs	Degree of mobility in home and public environment
	Activities of daily living	Donning/doffing	Will assistance be necessary? Who will provide help?
		Self care	How will orthosis impact on self-care ability?
		Toileting	Will orthosis need to be removed to use the bathroom?
		Dressing	Ability to manage clothes and shoes
Participation level	Home		Ability to take part in family activities, roles
	School		Mobility in classroom, hallways, outside play areas
	Work		Mobility in entrance, workspace, common areas
	Leisure		Mobility over surfaces, use of tools/devices
	Transportation		Ability to drive, use public transportation

ICF, The World Health Organization's International Classification of Functioning, Disability and Health.

on other daily motor tasks (e.g., a child's ability to get up and down from the floor).[9] Physicians bring to the team an understanding of the specific disease or disorder that the patient is dealing with, including the condition's natural history and likely prognosis, types of secondary musculoskeletal problems that are commonly encountered, and any cognitive, developmental or multisystem involvement that may be associated with the disease.[10] Family members and the individual needing the orthosis are concerned with practical issues, such as who will be responsible for applying (donning) or removing (doffing) the device and the ease with which this can be accomplished, as well as information about the types of activities that the individual wants to be involved in while using the orthosis (lifestyle and leisure activities).[11] The orthotist uses knowledge of materials and biomechanics, information provided by team and family members, and results of the individual's physical examination to design and fabricate the orthosis that will best address the mobility problem that needs to be solved.[9]

The team must not overlook the significant contribution of the individual and caregiver in the prescription process. The use of an orthosis enhances as well as constrains lower limb function; as such, it requires considerable adjustment on the part of the person who will be wearing the orthosis. An understanding of the individual's or the caregiver's expectations about what the orthosis will accomplish is a key component of orthotic prescription and training. Discussion and education about what an orthosis will and will not do for the wearer can minimize potential mismatch of expectation versus actual outcome. Acceptance and functional use of the orthosis depends on just how well it meets identified needs and goals, as well as the cost of its use in terms of inconvenience and disruption of lifestyle.[12]

Careful consideration of the individual's diagnosis is also critical when selecting materials and designing the orthosis.[13] Questions that the team should consider during the decision making process include: Can we reasonably expect that an individual's musculoskeletal or neuromuscular status is stable and likely to remain the same over time? Does the disease typically have a progressive course, such that decline in function is anticipated over time? Or, as in the case of traumatic injury, will the person's condition and functional ability improve with time as healing occurs? What can be expected in terms of muscle function and strength, range of motion and joint function, and functional mobility and gait over time? How might growth and developmental status influence future orthotic needs? All of these must be accounted for in the design of the orthosis.

The selection of any orthotic device must include careful consideration of four factors:

1. The *advantages* or positive outcomes expected when using the orthosis (i.e., how it will improve mobility and gait, influence tone, or protect a limb or body segment).
2. Any disadvantages or *tradeoffs* that may be associated with its use (i.e., the ways in which it may complicate daily activity, mobility, or preferred activities; the energy cost of associated with its use; the relative expense of the device).
3. The *indications* that the orthosis may be useful to the individual (i.e., the match between the person's characteristics and needs, and what the orthosis will provide).
4. The circumstances or characteristics of the individual that make use of the device detrimental or *contraindicated*.

Consideration of these four factors guide clinical decision making when comparing and contrasting the various options for lower extremity orthoses. Characteristics of an ideal orthosis are summarized in Box 9-1.

To help an individual use the orthosis most effectively, the physical therapist must understand how the orthosis should fit with respect to its design (i.e., what are the optimal trim lines?) and force control systems (how does it act on the limb segments?) (Box 9-2). Every orthosis uses force applied to the

---

BOX 9-2 *Principles Underlying Control Systems in Orthotic Design*

1. Pressure = Force/Area
2. Torque = Force × distance
3. Control direction of primary force direction of counter-forces
4. Equilibrium $\Sigma_{forces} = 0$

BOX 9-1 *Characteristics of an 'Ideal' Orthosis*

FUNCTION
- Meets the individuals mobility needs and goals
- Maximizes stance phase stability
- Minimizes abnormal alignment
- Minimally compromises swing clearance
- Effectively pre-positions the limb for initial contact
- Is energy efficient with the individual's preferred assistive device

COMFORT
- Can be worn for long periods without damaging skin or causing pain
- Can be easily donned and doffed (e.g., considering clothing, footwear, toileting)

COSMESIS
- Meets the individual's need to fit in with peers

FABRICATION
- Can be made in the shortest period of time
- Uses a minimally complex design
- Has some degree of adjustability to enhance initial fitting
- For children, responds to growth or change over time
- Is durable: stands up to stresses/strains of daily activity

COST
- Can be made with minimal initial cost, and minimal cost for maintenance

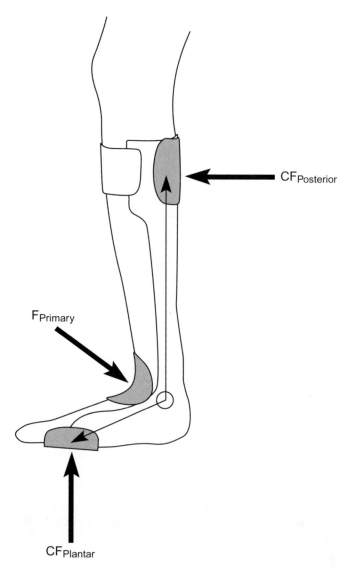

CF_{Posterior}

F_{Primary}

CF_{Plantar}

FIGURE 9-1 Principles underlying the plantarflexion control system acting during swing phase in a rigid/solid ankle-foot orthosis (SAFO). The large primary force ($F_{Primary}$) is applied in a posterior-inferior direction over a large surface area (stippled area) anterior to the axis of the ankle joint, usually by the shoe's closure or reinforced by webbing across the anterior ankle. The two counterforces, applied in an upward ($CF_{Plantar}$) and anterior ($CF_{Posterior}$) direction, also over a large surface area, far from the axis of the ankle joint, create an effective moment arm so that less force is required to achieve the desired stabilization. The sum of the primary *(large arrow)* and two opposing counterforces *(small arrows)* is zero in a well-balanced orthosis.

limb to accomplish the goals of its design. An orthosis is most comfortable and effective when (Figure 9-1):

1. The forces are distributed over large surface areas to minimize pressure on skin and soft tissue.
2. The forces are applied in such a way that a large moment arm reduces the amount of force needed to control the joint.
3. The sum of the primary force and opposing counterforces of each control system equals zero.

DETERMINANTS OF FUNCTIONAL GAIT

There are five factors that influence how well an individual is able to walk.[14] The first is *stance phase stability*: The limb in contact with the ground must be stable enough to support body weight and respond to the ground reaction forces (GRF) as the individual moves through stance phase. The second is *clearance in swing*: The advancing limb must clear the ground adequately during swing phase to minimize risk of stumbling and trips. Swing limb clearance is influenced by the ability to maintain a level pelvis by stance limb abductor muscle as well as by action of the hip, knee flexors, and dorsiflexors of the swing limb as they relatively shorten the length of the swinging limb. The third is *swing phase pre-positioning*: By the end of swing, the foot about to contact the ground must be positioned for an effective initial contact and loading response as stance begins. The fourth is *adequate step length*: There must be adequate motor control and range of motion at the hip, knee, ankle, and forefoot of both limbs so that optimal step length can occur. The fifth is *energy conservation*: If there are problems with timing, muscle performance, coordination, or postural control during the gait cycle, the energy cost of walking rises substantially, and efficiency of ambulation is compromised.

If neuromuscular or musculoskeletal dysfunction substantially interferes with these determinants, functional ambulation may be an unrealistic goal without an appropriate orthosis. Refer to Chapter 5 for greater detail about characteristics of the normal and pathological gait cycle.

THE ROCKERS OF STANCE PHASE

Orthotists describe three transitional periods, or rockers, during stance phase of walking as the body progresses forward over the foot (Figure 9-2).[15] During the *first (heel) rocker*, there is a controlled lowering of the foot from neutral ankle position at initial contact to a plantarflexed foot flat, as well as acceptance of body weight on the limb during loading response. When motor control and muscle performance is efficient, eccentric contraction of the quadriceps and anterior tibialis prevents "foot slap" and protects the knee as GRF is translated upward toward the knee. In the *second (ankle) rocker*, the tibia begins to rotate over the weight-bearing foot, from its initial 10 degrees of plantarflexion at the end of loading response, then through vertical into dorsiflexion as midstance is completed. Eccentric contraction of the gastrocnemius and soleus muscles "puts on the brakes" to control the speed of the forward progression of the tibia over the fixed foot throughout midstance. At the start of the *third (toe) rocker*, the forefoot has converted from its mobile adaptor function of early stance to a rigid lever for an effective late stance, and the heel rises off the ground so that body weight has to roll over the first metatarsophalangeal joint through push-off in terminal stance. During fast walking and running, acceleration occurs as active contraction of the gastrocnemius-soleus complex propels the foot and leg into swing phase.

All lower extremity orthoses provide some degree of external stability to foot and ankle joints; as a result, the smooth transition through the rockers of stance phase is often compromised.[16]

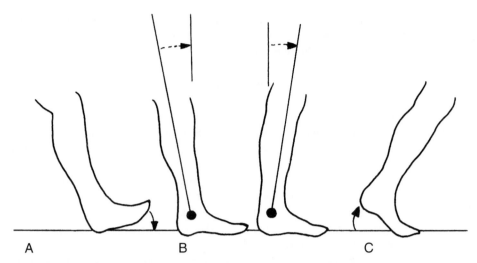

FIGURE 9-2 Three transitional rocker periods occur as the body moves forward over the foot during stance. **A,** During first rocker, the transition from swing into early stance, controlled lowering of the fore-foot occurs, with a fulcrum at the heel. **B,** During second rocker, controlled forward progression of the tibia over the foot occurs, with motion of the talocrural joint of the ankle. **C,** In the third rocker, transition from stance toward swing occurs as the heel rises, with dorsiflexion of the metatarsophalangeal joints.

Disruption of forward progression during stance negatively impacts step length, cadence, and single limb support time.[15] The optimal orthotic prescription must balance the need to provide external support with the possible compromise on forward progression and mobility: The orthotist strives to select an orthotic design that provides minimum necessary stability so that mobility will be the least compromised.[16] In many instances, modifications of footwear, such as the addition of a cushion heel (which simulates controlled lowering of the foot in loading response) or a rocker bottom sole (which simulates forward progression of the tibia over the foot throughout midstance), can substitute to some degree for the mobility lost when external control is necessary.[17] The rehabilitation team must weigh the impact of stability provided by an orthosis on progression through stance and its impact on a patient's functional status: At times compromise is unavoidable if the patient's functional deficits are to be addressed effectively.

PREFAB, CUSTOM FIT, OR CUSTOM MOLDED?

How does the team determine whether an individual would benefit from a relatively less expensive prefabricated orthosis versus a more costly (in both time and money) custom-molded orthosis designed specifically for the person? There are a number of factors to consider in making this decision.

The effectiveness of an AFO is determined by to the intimacy and consistency of its fit. Thermoplastic AFOs can be very effective in controlling a wide range of orthopedic deformities; however, this requires a total contact, intimate fit in all three planes of motion. Intimacy of contact between limb and orthosis is best achieved in custom molded designs.

Mass manufactured, prefabricated orthoses are available in a wide spectrum of orthotic designs, by shoe size, and made of a number different of materials. The degree to which they can be modified or adjusted to fit an individual varies; this may be problematic for persons with foot deformity, extremely wide or narrow feet, or large calf muscles. They are attractive to payers because they are significantly less expensive that custom-fit or custom-molded orthoses. Many rehabilitation professionals, however, are not satisfied with the ability of a prefabricated orthosis to provide optimal external support and control of motion over time: Durability is directly related to the quality of material used and by the lack of intimate fit to an individual's limb. Even a minimal amount of pistoning or heel elevation within the orthosis during walking can lead to skin irritation or breakdown, and in the presence of hypertonicity, increase of underlying abnormal extensor tone. Therapists may opt to use a trial run with prefabricated orthoses as an evaluative tool to determine which orthotic design might best meet the patient's needs during the time that a custom orthotic is being prepared or when the patient's condition requires use of an orthosis for only a short time period.[18] Because prefabricated orthoses do not fit the foot intimately, they should be used with extreme caution in persons with neuropathic foot conditions whose ability to perceive soft tissue irritation and damage is compromised.[19]

Another alternative is an orthosis that begins as a manufactured "blank" that is then custom fit using heating or relieving techniques or the application of additional materials to obtain as close a fit to the individual's foot and limb as possible. While custom-fit orthoses provide better control than similar prefabricated versions, they are not as effective in terms of fit and function as a custom-molded orthosis.[20] Custom-fit orthoses may be appropriate when change in functional status (either improvement or deterioration) is anticipated, such that the orthosis will need to be replaced or adjusted frequently.

Custom-molded orthoses provide the optimal control of the limb and, because of their intimate fit, are especially important for patients with impaired sensation, significant hypertonicity, or risk of progressive deformity associated with their condition. The orthotist constructs the orthosis around a rectified model of the person's limb, ensuring adequate pressure relief over vulnerable areas (i.e., bony prominences) and building in the desired stabilizing forces based on the orthotic prescription.[21] Refer to Chapter 6 for more details about the process of fabrication.

The only true contraindication of a custom-molded thermoplastic design is significantly fluctuating limb size, associated with conditions that lead to edema of the braced extremity.[22] When limb size fluctuates, intimacy of custom molded fit is lost: When the limb is at its lowest volume, excessive movement of the limb within the orthosis occurs, compromising orthotic control and increasing risk of skin irritation and damage. When the limb is significantly edematous, the AFO may become constricting, leading to pressure-related problems. For persons with congestive heart failure, advanced kidney disease on dialysis, or other conditions associated with unpredictable fluctuation in limb volume, the total contact of a custom-molded orthosis may be inappropriate, and a conventional double upright orthotic design should be considered.

APPROPRIATE FOOTWEAR

Whether the decision is to use a prefabricated, custom-fit, or custom-molded orthosis, the ultimate ability of the AFO to meet its therapeutic goals depends on the type and condition of the individual's footwear.[17] Refer to Chapter 7 for more information about key characteristics of shoes worn with an orthosis. Recognition of the need to consider footwear is not always intuitive to the individual, caregivers, or health professionals working on improving the ability to ambulate. It may be necessary for the individual to wear a shoe that is one-half to a whole size larger to accommodate an orthosis; a shoe that is too short or too tight can interfere with the biomechanical function of the orthosis. Shoe closure of an oxford style or athletic shoe (whether tied with laces or closed with Velcro) often provides the diagonally directed force that stabilizes the calcaneus in the heel cup of the orthosis; if the calcaneus moves out of position during walking, the effectiveness of orthotic control is compromised. Loafer type shoes and most sandals do not provide adequate stabilizing forces during the stance phase of gait. While most thermoplastic AFO designs allow individuals to alternate among several pairs of shoes, changing heel heights dramatically alters the biomechanical function of the orthosis. The orthotist and therapist share responsibility for patient and family education about appropriate footwear, monitoring shoe condition to assess impact of wear and tear on its construction and stability, as well as ongoing evaluation of the effectiveness of the orthosis in meeting the individual's functional needs over time.

ANKLE-FOOT ORTHOSES

AFOs are, by far, the most frequently prescribed device used to control the lower extremity during each phase of the gait cycle for individuals with neuromuscular or musculoskeletal impairments that make walking difficult. It is important to note that the acronyms used to name lower extremity orthoses describe joints that are positioned within the orthosis. In reality, AFOs also effectively address stability of the knee joint (proximal to the orthosis) during stance.[23]

AFOs fall into two categories: *static orthoses* that prohibit motion in any plane at the ankle (e.g., solid ankle AFO, anterior floor reaction AFO, patellar tendon–bearing/weight-relieving AFO). In contrast, *dynamic orthoses* allow some degree of sagittal plane motion at the ankle (e.g., posterior leaf spring or spiral AFOs, articulating ankle AFOs). Whether static or dynamic, the primary goal of an AFO is to provide just enough external support for stability in stance and clearance in swing with minimal compromise of forward progression through the heel, ankle, and toe rockers of gait.[16] The actions, indications, and contraindications for the various AFO designs are summarized in Table 9-2.

Biomechanical Principles

The biomechanical principles of AFOs are founded on the functional anatomy of the ankle-foot complex. Dorsiflexion and plantarflexion of the ankle are multiplanar (i.e., movement occurs in all three planes of motion) as the talus rotates through the mortise of the ankle in both open chain movement, and when the mortise moves over a relatively fixed (weight-bearing) talus in a closed chain movement.[24] The proximal surface of the mortise is shaped by the syndesmosis (fibrous articulation) between the distal tibia and fibula. The medial wall of the talocrural joint is formed by the medial malleolus, a downward extension of the tibia. The lateral wall, formed by the lateral malleolus of the fibula, is both longer and shifted posteriorly. Because of the shape of the articular surfaces of the talus in its mortise and the offset position of the malleoli, the axis of the ankle joint is slightly oblique, running in an anteromedial to posterolateral direction. As a result, dorsiflexion is accompanied by some degree of forefoot pronation and abduction along with hind foot valgus. Plantarflexion is accompanied by forefoot supination with adduction and hind foot varus. Note that during stance, movement occurs in closed chain situation because the foot is fixed on the ground by weight-bearing forces, so that the mortise rolls over the head of the talus.

If an AFO has mechanical ankle joints, the axis of the mechanical joints should be aligned as closely as possible to the obliquely oriented anatomical axis of motion (Figure 9-3). The mechanical joint heads are placed at approximately midline of the malleoli in the sagittal plane. This strategy reduces likelihood of abnormal torque and shearing between the orthosis and limb as the individual wearing the orthosis walks. When there is incongruence between the anatomical and mechanical axes, excessive motion of the limb within the orthoses is likely, and action of the mechanical ankle joint is compromised.

TABLE 9-2 *Summary of Indications for, Impact on Gait of, and Contraindications for Commonly Prescribed Lower Extremity Orthoses*

Type of Orthosis	Category	Actions	Indications	Contraindications	Options
UCBL orthosis	Static	Stabilize subtalar and tarsal joints in stance	Rearfoot valgus/varus Flexible pes planus	Rigid foot deformity	Thermoplastic Gillette modification
DAFO	Dynamic	Stabilize subtalar and tarsal joints in stance	Flexible pes planus Mild to moderate spastic diplegic or hemiplegic CP Hypotonic CP	Rigid foot deformity	Thermoplastic
Supramalleolar	Dynamic	Stabilize subtalar and tarsal joints in stance Preposition foot for IC by heel	Flexible pes planus Mild to moderate spastic diplegic or hemiplegic CP Hypotonic CP	Significant equinovarus hypertonicity	Thermoplastic
Posterior Leaf Spring	Dynamic	Assist limb clearance in swing Preposition foot for IC by heel	Dorsiflexion weakness, impaired motor control, LMN flaccid paralysis of dorsiflexors	Moderate to severe hypertonicity	Thermoplastic
Carbon Graphite AFO	Dynamic	Assist limb clearance in swing pre-position foot for IC by heel	Paralysis or impaired muscle performance of dorsiflexors	Moderate to severe hypertonicity	Custom or prefabricated
Neuro-orthoses	Dynamic	Assist limb clearance in swing Preposition foot for IC by heel	Dorsiflexion weakness or low tone	Flaccid paralysis Patient intolerance of electrical stimulation	Functional electrical stimulation
Articulating ankle	Dynamic	Assist limb clearance in swing Preposition foot for IC by heel Permit advancement of tibia (2nd rocker) in stance	Impaired motor control of ankle musculature Potential for recovery of neuromotor function	LMN paralysis (flaccidity) or hypotonicity as primary problem	Thermoplastic or metal double-upright Dorsiflexion assist Plantarflexion stop Adjustable range into dorsiflexion can be incorporated Often requires shoe with cushion heel

(Continued)

TABLE 9-2   *Summary of Indications for, Impact on Gait of, and Contraindications for Commonly Prescribed Lower Extremity Orthoses—cont'd*

Type of Orthosis	Category	Actions	Indications	Contraindications	Options
Solid-ankle AFO	Static	Control ankle position throughout stance Provide stance phase stability via ankle-knee coupling Assist limb clearance in swing Pre-position foot for IC by heel Distal trim line behind metatarsal heads or extended toe-plate	Significant hypertonicity with seriously impaired motor control at ankle and knee	LMN paralysis (flaccidity) or hypotonicity as primary problem	Thermoplastic Basis for KAFO and HKAFO Requires cushion heel and rocker bottom shoe
Tone-inhibiting AFO	Static	Control ankle position throughout stance Provide stance phase stability via ankle-knee coupling Typically extended toeplate	Significant hypertonicity with seriously impaired motor control	LMN paralysis (flaccidity) or hypotonicity as primary problem	Thermoplastic, Basis for KAFO and HKAFO Requires cushion heel and rocker bottom shoe
Anterior floor reaction AFO	Static	Provide stability in stance via ankle-knee coupling Control ankle position throughout stance	Weakness or impaired motor control at knee and ankle	Ligamentous insufficiency at the knee Genu recurvatum	Thermoplastic or carbon composite Custom-made or custom-fit
Weight-relieving AFO	Static	Protect lower leg and foot during stance by reducing weight bearing forces.	Healing soft tissue, ligamentous, or bone injuries of the lower leg, ankle, or foot	Mechanical instability of the knee, or injury to proximal tibia Patient intolerance of PTB weight-bearing forces (rare)	Thermoplastic and metal hybrid Custom or prefabricated

AFO, ankle-foot orthosis; CP, cerebral palsy; DAFO, dynamic ankle foot orthosis; IC, initial contact; HKAFO, hip-knee-ankle-foot orthosis; KAFO, knee-ankle-foot orthosis; LMN, lower motor neuron ; PTB, patellar tendon bearing ; UCBL, University of California Biomechanics Laboratory orthosis .

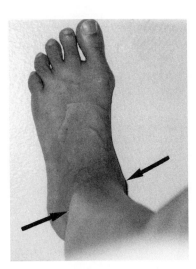

FIGURE 9-3 Alignment of the mechanical ankle joint axes must reflect the degree of external rotation/tibial torsion that is present in the transverse plane.

STATIC ANKLE-FOOT ORTHOSES

Static AFOs are the most aggressive of the AFO designs in providing external support. They restrict ankle and foot motion is all three planes to provide significant stance phase stability and swing limb clearance. Because of their rigidity, however, these orthoses greatly compromise transitions through the first (heel), second (ankle), and to a lesser degree third (toe) rockers of stance phase. Individuals using static AFOs do better functionally wearing a shoe with a cushion heel and rocker bottom to simulate these key transitions. The decision to recommend a static AFO should be made carefully, weighing the benefit of greater stability against the cost of lost mobility.

Solid Ankle-Foot Orthoses

The solid-ankle AFO (SAFO), also known as a rigid AFO, is typically fabricated from relatively thick thermoplastic and aims to hold the ankle and foot in as close to biomechanically neutral position (zero degrees of ankle dorsiflexion, subtalar and calcaneal neutral, with a balanced forefoot) as possible given the individual's functional anatomy.[25] The anteroposterior trim line of the SAFO falls at or near the midline of the medial and lateral malleolus (Figure 9-4). Medial and lateral corrugations may be incorporated into the shell of the orthosis to provide additional strength when hypertonicity or excessive weight creates loading forces that require a stronger orthosis. The proximal border is typically trimmed to fall 1.5 inches below the apex of the head of the fibula. The footplate it either trimmed just short of the plantar metatarsal heads or can be lengthened beyond the metatarsal distally into a toe plate if hypertonicity is a concern.[26] Some orthotists recommend the addition of a tone-inhibiting bar if hypertonicity is severe.[27] There is a tradeoff to consider if the footplate is lengthened: It is much easier to fit into and put on shoes with a shorter footplate; assistance may be necessary to don shoes when the SAFO has a full toeplate.

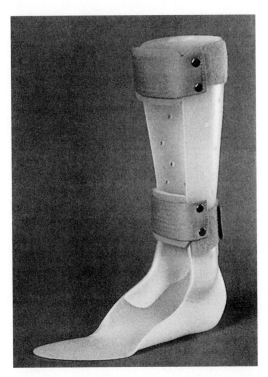

FIGURE 9-4 Custom-molded, solid-ankle ankle-foot orthosis holds the ankle in as close to optimal static alignment as possible for a given patient. Mediolateral ankle stability is a result of trim lines at the midline of the malleoli. Note the high medial border at the foot and the slight flaring just proximal to the medial malleolus. This strategy is used to counteract an abnormal, flexible subtalar valgus. The crossed Velcro strap anterior to the ankle helps position the rear foot appropriately within the heel section of the orthosis. (Reprinted with permission from Zablotny CM. Use of orthoses for the adult with neurological involvement. In Nawoczenski DA, Epler ME [eds], *Orthotics in Functional Rehabilitation of the Lower Limb.* Philadelphia: WB Saunders, 1997. p. 223)

SAFO Control Systems

There are four distinct control systems incorporated into the SAFO design (Figure 9-5). To resist plantarflexion during swing phase, there is a fulcrum force applied at the anterior ankle (by strapping or by the shoe's laces or Velcro closure) opposed by a distal counterforce upward under the metatarsal heads and a proximal counterforce at the posterior proximal surface of the AFO. To resist dorsiflexion during stance phase, there is an upward and inward compressive force at the posterior heel, opposed by a distal downward counterforce delivered by the shoe, and a proximal force applied by the anterior closure straps just below the knee. It is important to note that the locked ankle created by an AFO generates an extensor moment at the knee during stance. In this way, a SAFO can substitute for impaired motor control or muscle performance of knee extensors for persons with stroke, cerebral palsy, or other neuromotor dysfunction.

To resist varus and inversion of the foot, a medially directed force is applied just above and below the lateral malleolus with laterally directed counterforces at the proximal medial tibia and the medial foot. To resist valgus and eversion of the foot, there is a laterally directed force applied above and

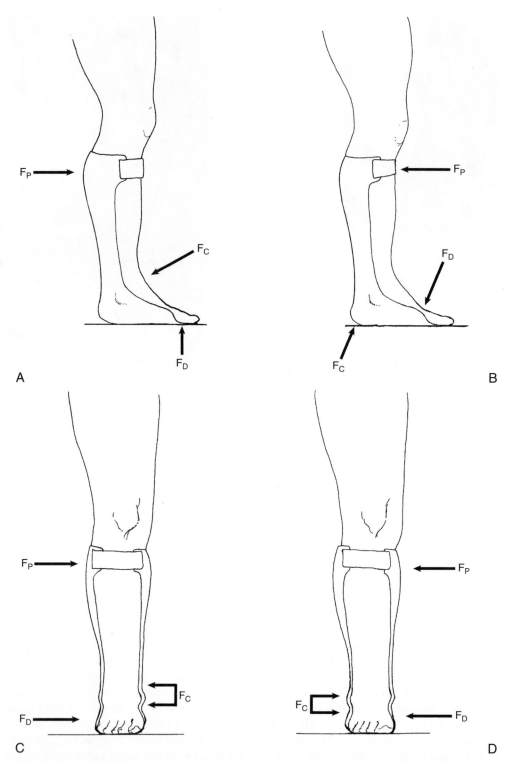

FIGURE 9-5 The four force systems in a molded thermoplastic solid-ankle ankle-foot orthosis design. **A,** Plantarflexion is controlled during swing phase by a proximal force (F_p) at the posterior calf band and a distal force at the metatarsal heads (F_d) that counter a centrally located stabilizing force (F_c) applied at the ankle by shoe closure. **B,** For control of dorsiflexion during stance phase (i.e., forward progression of the tibia over the foot), F_p is applied at the proximal tibia by the anterior closure, F_d at the ventral metatarsal heads by the toe box of the shoe, and counterforce F_c at the heel, snugly fit in the orthosis. **C,** The force system for eversion (valgus) locates F_d along the fifth metatarsal, F_p at the proximal lateral calf band, and F_c on either side of the malleolus. **D,** To control inversion (varus) of the foot and ankle, F_d is applied by the distal medial wall of the orthosis against the first metatarsal, F_p at the proximal medial calf band, and F_c at the distal lateral tibia and calcaneus/talus on either side of the lateral malleolus.

below the medial malleolus, with medially directed counterforces just below the fibular head proximally and at the lateral foot distally.

The degree of control for the foot is also influenced by the position of the trim lines of the foot section. When there is midtarsal joint deformity with forefoot abduction or adduction to contend with, trim lines are adjusted to capture the shafts of the first and fifth metatarsals. If there is too much subtalar valgus, the height of the medial wall is increased, and a flange might be placed proximal to the medial malleolus. These strategies provide greater surface area for distribution of corrective forces applied by the orthosis, so that the patient is more comfortable with the external stability it provides. If knee hyperextension at midstance is a problem for individuals with impaired motor control, the orthotist might fabricate the SAFO set in just a couple of degrees of ankle dorsiflexion, rather than neutral, to minimize excessive extension moment and preserve knee joint health over time. A Gillette modification can be added to the outer medial or lateral surface of the heel cup to influence excessive valgus or varus moment at the knee joint during stance. A medial or lateral post (similar to those used in a biomechanical foot orthosis) can be incorporated into the foot section to equalize forefoot to rearfoot relationships or to enhance biomechanical effects on the knee.

Progression Through Stance Phase

The SAFO biomechanically interferes with transitions through all three rockers of gait in stance phase because of the fixed ankle position inherent in the design.

The orthosis prevents the controlled lowering of the foot that usually occurs in the ankle/first rocker during loading response. If the shoe does not have a compressive cushion heel to mimic controlled lowering, the orthosis propels the tibia rapidly to achieve foot-flat position. The individual wearing the orthosis needs some eccentric ability of the quadriceps to counteract the rapid knee flexion moment that accompanies the SAFOs propulsive force acting on the tibia. This is especially true if the SAFO has been set in a few degrees of dorsiflexion to minimize risk of knee hyperextension in early stance.

The proximal anterior strapping used to hold the limb in the upper part of the SAFO acts with the fixed ankle position to prevent forward progression of the tibia over the weight-bearing foot during the second/ankle rocker that typically occurs during midstance. If the individual's shoe does not have rocker bottom characteristics, this check of forward momentum compromises effective preparation for push-off and transition from stance into swing phase and necessarily shortens stride length achieved by the swinging limb.

In nonpathological gait, there is 60 degrees of extension at the hallux during the third, or toe rocker of gait. For persons wearing a SAFO with a footplate that extends into a stiff toeplate, the third/toe rocker of the foot will certainly be limited. A shoe with rocker bottom characteristics can assist a smoother rollover when extension of the hallux is limited.

Indications for SAFO

The SAFO design is often selected for individuals with moderate to severe hypertonicity where equinovarus significantly impairs the ability to walk.[26,28,29] It may also be used for persons with unpredictable fluctuating muscle tone (athetosis) to provide external stability that makes ambulation possible in the presence of unpredictable variation in antigravity tone.[30] While the SAFO has been used in persons with multiple sclerosis with tremor and ataxia, the evidence of its efficacy for improved coordination during walking is limited.[31] It may be recommended for persons with significant generalized lower extremity weakness or significant hypotonicity, providing external support as a substitute for impaired muscle performance that would otherwise prevent ambulation.[32,33] In both of these circumstances the SAFO is a substitute for severely impaired muscle activity. A custom-molded SAFO has also been used to protect the foot and ankle in the management of persons who need stabilization after foot or ankle surgery, or for those with ankle instability and pain secondary to rheumatoid arthritis.[34,35]

The Anterior Floor Reaction Ankle-Foot Orthosis

All static AFO designs use moments that result from the GRF to provide stability during stance. An orthosis that has evolved from the basic SAFO design to better address impaired motor control of the knee and weakness of the quadriceps is the anterior floor reaction orthosis (FRO)[36,37] (Figure 9-6). The FRO is fabricated to hold the ankle in a few degrees of plantarflexion. This restricts the ability of the tibia to roll forward over the foot in the second/ankle rocker of gait, creating an extensor moment that stabilizes the knee during stance (Figure 9-7). If stability is also needed in late stance phase, a stiff toeplate can be added to reinforce the extension moment at the knee. The FRO and SAFO use the same force systems to control foot and ankle position. Whether the FRO is fabricated in a single piece (see Figure 9-7A) or as a SAFO with the addition of a thermoplastic anterior shell (see Figure 9-7B), padding is added where the FRO contacts the proximal surfaces of the tibia to make the extra extension force delivered by the orthosis more tolerable to the wearer.

The FRO is often used for children with cerebral palsy who demonstrate "crouch gait," or for children with myelomeningocele and persons with postpolio syndrome who have paralysis or weakness at the knee and ankle.[36-38] To be efficacious, the FRO relies on a GRF vector that passes anterior to the anatomical knee joint. As knee and hip flexion contractures approach or exceed 10 degrees, the GRF vector nears or passes posterior to the anatomical knee joint, and the FRO is less effective in stabilizing the knee during stance.[36] The FRO is contraindicated for persons with notable recurvatum during stance as well as those with cruciate ligament insufficiency; in these circumstances, the extra knee extension moment can further damage joint structure. While the rigid control of ankle and knee enhances mechanical stability in stance, these external restrictions imposed by the FRO may compromise efficacy of postural responses. In those with

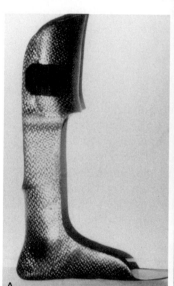
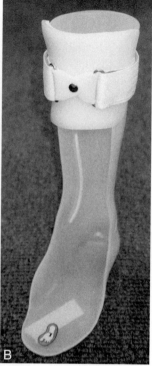

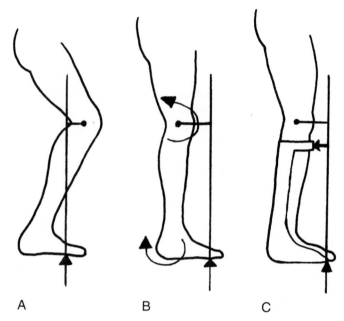

A   B   C

FIGURE 9-7 **A,** When a patient walks in a "crouch gait" pattern, the ground reaction force vector passes behind the knee at midstance, creating a flexion moment at the knee, which must be counteracted to maintain upright position. **B,** In normal gait, knee stability at midstance is assisted by a ground reaction moment as the body moves over the foot, and the ground reaction force vector passes anterior to the knee. **C,** The solid-ankle ankle-foot orthosis and the floor reaction orthotic designs use a fixed ankle position to harness the ground reaction force, creating a large extension moment at the knee.

FIGURE 9-6 A, This floor reaction orthosis (FRO) was fabricated using carbon graphite and fiberglass in a thermosetting process because of the desire to provide maximum stiffness. The combination of a solid-ankle design and an anterior wall produces a knee extension moment at midstance and enhances stance phase stability. **B,** This FRO has a posterior shell much like a solid-ankle ankle-foot orthosis. The combination of slight plantarflexion at the ankle and a stiff, long toeplate creates a plantarflexion–knee extension couple that acts in mid to late stance. The padded anterior shell more comfortably captures the resultant extension moment, stabilizing the knee. Note also the corrugation incorporated in the medial and lateral walls of the ankle-foot orthosis to provide additional rigidity to the orthosis.

balance impairment, an ambulatory assistive device (e.g., a cane, Lofstrand crutches, or rolling walker) may be needed for safety, especially if FROs are worn on both limbs.

Weight-Relieving Ankle-Foot Orthoses

The weight-relieving AFO, also known as a patellar tendon–bearing AFO (PTB-AFO), incorporates the intimate fit and load-bearing characteristics of a PTB prosthetic socket into a SAFO or traditional metal double upright AFO (discussed later) as a means of offloading or unloading weight-bearing forces during stance phase for individuals with painful, unstable, or recently repaired ankle or foot (Figure 9-8).[39-42] The anterior shell of the AFO is modified to accept weight-bearing forces via the medial tibial flare and patellar tendon bar, along with total contact around the upper calf. As with a PTB prosthetic socket, the proximal portion of the PTB-AFO is set in approximately 10 degrees of knee flexion (with respect to vertical) to load some of the body weight onto the anterior shell at the medial tibial flare and patellar tendon bar during stance. This axial force is then transmitted to the ground through the medial and lateral

walls of the thermoplastic orthosis, which may be reinforced with metal uprights or through the medial and lateral uprights of a traditional double upright AFO. This strategy effectively reduces axial loading of the ankle and foot during gait.

The weight-relieving AFO is used for persons with Charcot arthropathy, plantar neuropathic ulcers, slowly healing fractures, severe rheumatoid or osteoarthritis of the ankle, surgically repaired ankles after fracture, synovial debridement in hemophilia, and other circumstances that require protection of the foot and ankle when non–weight bearing is not possible. A tibial fracture orthosis and the Charcot restraint orthotic walker (CROW) are adaptations of the weight-relieving AFO; both encase the entire lower limb to provide maximal reduction of axial loading while healing takes place.[43,44] Individuals wearing a weight-relieving AFO must have normal anatomical structure of the knee, adequate muscle performance and motor control of the quadriceps muscles for stability in early stance, and sufficient skin integrity to tolerate the loading forces applied by this orthotic design.

DYNAMIC ANKLE FOOT ORTHOSES

Dynamic orthoses allow some degree of sagittal plane motion at the ankle; many permit dorsiflexion during stance phase to facilitate the second/ankle rocker of gait, but restrict plantarflexion during swing phase to facilitate swing limb

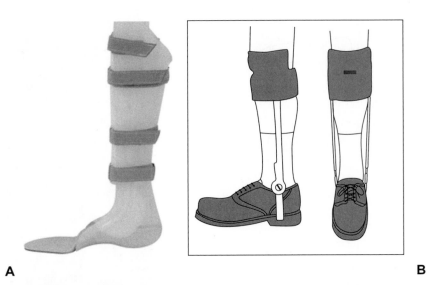

A   **B**

FIGURE 9-8 Lateral views of the PTB AFO (weight relieving orthosis) loads weight bearing onto the orthosis during stance, offloading the tibia and fibula, carrying some or all of body weight through the solid-ankle ankle-foot orthosis shell (**A**) or double uprights (**B**) to the floor. (**A,** Courtesy Elite Orthotics, Zelienople, Penn. **B,** Reprinted with permission from Edelstein JE, Bruckner J. *Orthotics: A Comprehensive Clinical Approach*, Fig. 3-27a. Thorofare, N.J.: Slack Inc., 2007. p. 50.)

clearance, incorporating some type of orthotic ankle joint. These dynamic orthoses are available in both thermoplastic and more traditional metal double-upright designs. These are reviewed in order from least restrictive to most supportive designs.

The UCBL Orthosis

In the 1970s, researchers at the University of California Biomechanics Laboratory developed a custom-molded shoe insert, now known as the *UCBL orthosis*, as an orthotic intervention for subtalar joint instability (Figure 9-9).[45] The UCBL controls flexible calcaneal deformities (rearfoot valgus or varus) as well as transverse plane deformities of the midtarsal joints (forefoot abduction or adduction) by "grabbing" the calcaneus and supporting the midfoot with high medial and lateral trim lines; it realigns the calcaneus, improving the angle of pull of the Achilles tendon, providing a more stable foundation for the articular surfaces of the talus, navicular, and cuboid bones.[46] The UCBL is also used to improve functional alignment of children and adolescents with flexible pes planus, a longitudinal arch deformity.[47] The *Gillette modification*, an external post positioned either on the medial or lateral border of the heel cup, can be used to apply additional rotatory moments to the calcaneus during weight bearing. In addition to being useful when there is flexible structural malalignment of the rear and midfoot, the UCBL shoe insert may improve foot performance during stance for persons with hypotonicity. It is important to recognize that the UCBL orthosis acts primarily at subtalar and midfoot tarsal joints during weight bearing; it would not be appropriate for persons with swing phase clearance issues, which require the trim line of the orthosis placed above the ankle joint.

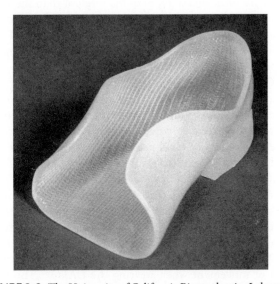

FIGURE 9-9 The University of California Biomechanics Laboratory orthosis is designed to position the calcaneus optimally for effective subtalar joint function. The deep heel cup, with its high medial and lateral trim lines, snugly holds the calcaneus. The orthosis also encompasses the joints of the midfoot, providing support for the longitudinal arch. In this example, a medial post (Gillette modification) has been added.

Dynamic Ankle Foot Orthosis

The dynamic ankle-foot orthosis (DAFO), also known as a flexible supramalleolar orthosis (SMO), is a custom-molded orthosis that has evolved from the UCBL shoe insert to better address sagittal plane control of the ankle and foot during stance and to facilitate foot clearance in swing.[48] Custom-molded from relatively thin thermoplastic, its proximal trim lines are just superior to the ankle joint, and its

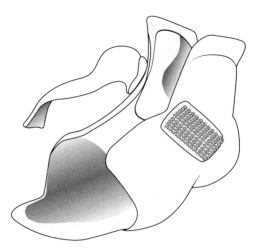

FIGURE 9-10 The dynamic ankle-foot orthosis (DAFO) is a flexible polypropylene brace designed to optimize subtalar joint alignment through its supramalleolar design. (Reprinted with permission from Zablotny CM. Use of orthoses for the adult with neurological involvement. In Nawoczenski DA, Epler ME [eds], *Orthotics in Functional Rehabilitation of the Lower Limb.* Philadelphia: WB Saunders, 1997. p. 229.)

distal trim lines encase more of the forefoot than the UCBL (Figure 9-10). By limiting movement of the midfoot and forefoot and by holding the foot in functional position, the DAFO provides a stable base for more effective motor performance and postural control during standing and ambulation.[49,50] The DAFO is designed to redistribute plantar pressures of spastic equinovarus from the anterior foot to the heel, perhaps by reducing overall stimulation of reflexes that would otherwise reinforce extensor hypertonicity in children with mild to moderate diplegic cerebral palsy.[51] By providing a stable base during stance phase, the DAFO improves swing limb clearance, stride length, cadence, and self-selected walking speed of children with diplegic cerebral palsy, nearly to that of age-matched peers without neuromotor impairment.[50,52] Parents of children using DAFOs report improved upright posture as well as enhanced ability of their children to participate in play activities, based on perceived changes in stability, agility, and speed of movement when wearing the DAFO.[49] The major complaint about the DAFO was that there was a need to frequently change socks because confinement of the foot within the plastic DAFO shell and shoe contributed to sweaty feet.

Posterior Leaf Spring Ankle-Foot Orthosis

The Posterior Leaf Spring (PLS) AFO is a dynamic thermoplastic AFO designed to accomplish two things[53]:

- Support the weight of the foot during swing phase as a means of enhancing swing limb clearance
- Assist with controlled lowering of the foot during loading response in stance as part of the first/heel rocker

The PLS is one of the group of AFOs that provide dorsiflexion assistance. In contrast to the SAFO, medial and lateral trim lines are located well posterior to the midline of both malleoli so that the orthosis is flexible at the anatomical ankle joint (Figure 9-11).[54] The degree of flexibility is determined by the thickness of the thermoplastic material used to construct the

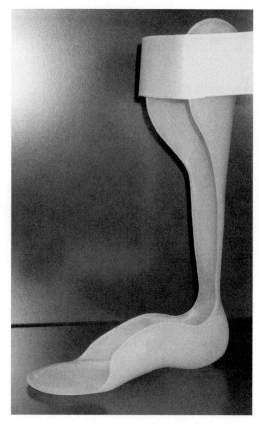

FIGURE 9-11 The posterior position and arc of the trim lines at the ankle, as well as the thickness of thermoplastic material used, determine the degree of flexibility of the posterior leaf spring ankle-foot orthosis. This design approximates the first and second rockers of stance phase and assists clearance and pre-positioning of the foot during swing.

orthosis and width of the posterior upright in the distal third of the orthosis.[54] In custom-molded PLS orthosis, the orthotist tailors the stiffness of the orthosis using the trim line pattern that will best support the weight of the foot during swing as well as the individual's needs for stability in stance.[54]

Once the heel contacts the ground at initial contact and loading response begins, the flexible plastic of the PLS serves as a proxy for impaired or absent eccentric activity of the tibialis anterior muscle, slowing but not stopping the foot's descent toward the ground.[53] As stance phase continues, the flexible PSL allows the tibia to roll forward over the weight-bearing foot to accomplish a smooth second/ankle rocker of midstance to terminal stance. As the foot leaves the ground in initial swing, the PLS is able to hold the ankle at the desired neutral 90-degree position, which assists swing clearance and keeps the toes elevated so that next initial contact will be made at the heel. Compared to the stiffness of the SAFO, which makes walking up and down inclines even more challenging than walking on level surfaces, the flexibility inherent in the PLS provides a notable functional advantage.[55–57]

Owing to its narrow posterior upright and relatively shallow heel cup, a PSL is not as effective in stabilizing the calcaneus and talus during stance as are the SAFO, DAFO, or UCBL designs. This makes it less effective in controlling mediolateral foot position, especially for persons with flexible deformities of the forefoot, midfoot, or rearfoot.[58] In these circumstances, the orthotist may opt to place medial and lateral trim lines somewhere between the mid-malleolar position of a SAFO and the narrower PLS to provide additional stability. This modification is sometimes referred to as a *semisolid AFO*. The modification provides better control of ankle motion, but at the cost of limiting mobility during the second/ankle rocker of gait.[59] Note that the flexibility of a PLS and a semisolid AFO make them inappropriate for individuals with significant equinovarus or spasticity of the lower extremity: A high level of abnormal tone will overpower the control systems in these designs.

Additional Dorsiflexion Assist Options

There are a number of commercially available prefabricated as well as custom-molded AFO designs available as alternatives for individuals whose primary need is for dorsiflexion assistance as a substitution for weakness and/or impaired motor control at the ankle. Three of the more frequently used options are reviewed here: (1) Dual Carbon Fiber Spring Orthosis, (2) wearable functional neuromuscular electrical stimulation units, and (3) novel commercially available alternative designs.

Carbon Fiber Spring Orthoses

The Dual Carbon Fiber Spring orthosis (CFO), developed and tested primarily in Germany, is a modification of the traditional PLS design that cuts the PLS into a foot and calf section, then attaches overlapping carbon fiber springs (carbon fiber and Kevlar fibers impregnated with epoxy resin) between the sections (Figure 9-12A).[60] Spring resistance is selected based on the individual's weight. This design aims

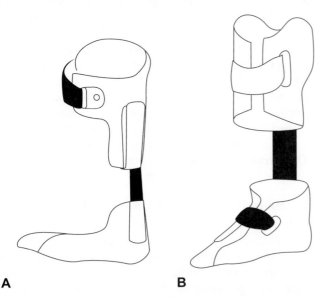

A   **B**

FIGURE 9-12 A, Note the carbon fiber springs inserted posteriorly between the foot and calf component of this carbon-fiber orthosis. The springs provide dorsiflexion assistance for clearance in swing and pre-positioning of the foot for initial contract, as well as preservation of the second and third rockers of stance phase. **B,** The Dual Carbon Fiber Spring orthosis (CFO) designed to provide assistance with plantarflexion/push-off for the transition from stance to swing for persons with weakness or paralysis of calf muscles/plantarflexors.

not only to substitute for impaired or absent anterior compartment muscle activity, but also to enhance the third/toe rocker of stance phase that is typically compromised by thermoplastic AFOs.[60] A more powerful push-off is attributed to loading of the spring during early and midstance as the tibia moves forward over the foot, and release of the spring in transition from terminal swing to preswing.[61]

The CFO design has been adapted to enhance walking ability of children with myelomeningocele and other neuromuscular conditions that contribute to impaired or absent plantarflexor muscle performance.[62,63] In this version, the carbon fiber spring is L-shaped (see Figure 9-12B) with its attachment to the foot component (a stiffer version of a supramalleolar DAFO) on the plantar surface rather than posterior heel. The slight distance between the spring and posterior foot section acts as a dorsiflexion stop during stance, allowing some dorsiflexion for second/ankle rocker until the two surfaces come into contact. The proximal carbon fiber spring is fit into a slot in the posterior of a custom-molded section that resembles the upper half of a total contact prosthetic socket. A vertical slot drilled into the proximal spring allows it to slide up and down for several centimeters during stance phase to minimize potential skin friction. This CFO appears to enhance transition through both second/ankle and third/toe rockers of gait, and to provide assistance for push-off. This design has also been incorporated into a knee-anklefoot orthosis for children who require additional support or control at the knee and hip.[64]

Both versions of the CFO may require a larger size shoe to accommodate the orthosis in the shoe.

Functional Neuromuscular Electrical Stimulation

For persons with impaired motor control resulting from disease or trauma of the central nervous system, several commercially available, wearable functional electrical stimulation units, also called *neuroprostheses,* are available (e.g., WalkAide, Hanger Orthopedic Group, Austin, Texas; Odstock Dropped Foot Stimulator, Salisbury, UK; NESS L300 Foot Drop System, Bioness Inc. Valencia, Calif.). The individual wears a cuff that is positioned snugly just below the knee, rather than an orthosis that must fit into the shoe (Figure 9-13). The cuff holds a small stimulator medially with electrodes positioned laterally over motor end points of the peroneal nerve.[65] Depending on the model, appropriate timing of the functional electrical stimulation for dorsiflexion activity is determined by a switch worn in the shoe, an inclinometer, or an accelerometer. Most use surface electrodes to deliver the stimulus for muscle contraction although cuffless versions with surgically implantable electrodes are available. Studies evaluating the device have demonstrated improved spatial and temporal characteristics and safety of walking in persons with acute and chronic stroke when worn as an orthosis alone or when integrated with rehabilitation interventions.[66-68] Similar findings support its use for persons with traumatic brain injury, multiple sclerosis, and Parkinson's disease.[69-72]

Each of these devices must be adjusted to the individual's typical gait pattern by an orthotist trained to fine-tune

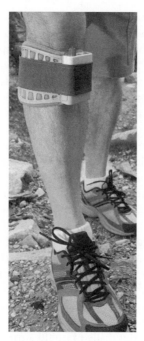

FIGURE 9-13 The Hanger WalkAide System, as an example of a wearable functional electrical stimulation unit, is used to trigger muscle contraction of dorsiflexors during appropriate points in the gait cycle. (Courtesy Hanger Orthopedics, Austin, Texas.)

the device. To be effective, all of these devices require an intact and healthy peroneal nerve. They would not be appropriate for persons with peripheral nerve injury or neuropathy (e.g., traumatic or compressive dysfunction of the peroneal nerve, Guillain-Barré syndrome, longstanding radiculopathy, lower motor neuron SCI, polio, or postpolio syndrome).

Manufacturers note that such devices are contraindicated in individuals with demand pacemakers or defibrillators, healing fractures, metal implants in the limb, or history of phlebitis; the unit should be used with caution in persons with varicose veins, inflammation in or around the knee, or sensory impairment. While most devices are resistant to splashes, immersion in water during bathing or swimming, or saturation while shoveling snow, for example, will damage the unit, rendering it nonfunctional.

Commercially Available Dorsiflexion-Assist Designs

A number of manufacturers have developed carbon fiber orthoses to provide dorsiflexion assistance at the appropriate times in the gait cycle (e.g., Camp ToeOFF series, Allard USA, Rockaway, N.J.; AFO Dynamic, Ossur Americas, Foothill Ranch, Calif.; Matrix and Matrix Max, Prolaborthotics USA, Napa, Calif.). In contrast to thermoplastic designs, many of these orthoses use a cushioned anterior shin or medial shank piece, held in place by strapping, that transitions into a medial upright and continues into a full footplate (Figure 9-14). These orthoses are designed to preposition the foot for heel strike at initial contact, substitute for impaired anterior compartment to allow controlled lowering of the foot into foot flat position during the first/heel

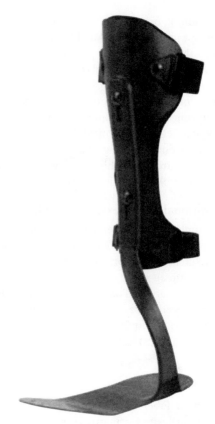

FIGURE 9-14 An example of a carbon fiber composite dorsiflexion assist ankle-foot orthosis used to substitute for activity of anterior compartment muscles of the lower leg. (Courtesy Trulife USA, Jackson, Miss.)

rocker of loading response, provide some medial-lateral stability during stance while allowing forward progression of the tibial during the second/ankle rocker of stance phase, contribute to push-off in the transition from stance to swing, and support the weight of the foot for effective swing limb clearance.[73] Although there is some evidence that these dorsiflexion-assist designs have a positive impact on both the kinematics and energy cost of walking, there have been few published studies that directly compare them with traditional PLS orthoses, or with articulating (hinged) thermoplastic AFOs or traditional metal double upright AFOs with dorsiflexion-assist orthotic ankle joints.[73]

Hinged Thermoplastic Ankle-Foot Orthosis

The thermoplastic hinged (articulating) ankle-foot orthosis (HAFO) allows sagittal plane motion at the ankle by incorporating a mechanical ankle joint between the foot and calf sections of the orthosis. This variation of the SAFO was designed primarily to allow the tibia to roll over the weight-bearing foot during stance, for a smooth second/ankle rocker, at the same time holding the foot in optimal alignment to control the impact of tone-related equinovarus forces throughout the gait cycle (Figure 9-15). In children with cerebral palsy and in adults after stroke, these orthoses reduce energy cost of walking (compared to barefoot), as well as improve stride length, cadence, and walking speed.[74-76]

As compared with the SAFO, the HAFO also improves mobility in many functional activities, such as rising from the floor (an important component of play for children), ascending and descending stairs, and walking up or down inclines.[56–58] There is some indication that HAFOs lessen the magnitude of abnormal muscle activation associated with spasticity in children with cerebral palsy.[77] HAFOs appear to reduce risk of falls in adults with longstanding hemiplegia after stroke, improve static postural control, and have less negative impact on dynamic postural control in standing than SAFOs.[78,79] For some children with moderate to severe spastic diplegic cerebral palsy, however, the mobility provided by a HAFO compromises stability in early stance, reinforcing crouch gait pattern, reducing walking speed, and increasing energy cost as compared to a SAFO.[74] Multiple perspectives on function, as well as the desired impact on quality of gait, must be considered when deciding which orthosis is best.

The shape, dimensions, and force control systems of the HAFO are almost exactly the same as those of a SAFO, except it has two separate pieces linked by an orthotic ankle joint rather than being a single, solid piece. The HAFO has a larger width at the ankle than the SAFO to accommodate the mechanical ankle joint; this may require larger or wider shoe size to accommodate the orthosis.

Hinged AFOs can be fabricated to allow free motion at the ankle, to allow limited range of motion (i.e., allow dorsiflexion and stop plantarflexion, or the inverse), or to provide some assistance to dorsiflexion, depending on what orthotic ankle joint option motion best meets the individual's needs and maximizes the resources they bring to the task of walking. A variety of mechanical thermoplastic joints are commercially available (Figure 9-16). Those with true articulations (e.g., the Oklahoma joint) have a single axis of motion that should be aligned as closely as possible to the anatomic ankle joint; other orthotic joints (e.g., the Gillette joint) are flexible and nonarticulating.

Traditional metal orthotic ankle joints have been incorporated into thermoplastic HAFOs as well; These designs are referred to as *hybrid orthoses*. Simple single axis joints provide mediolateral stability without restriction of available dorsiflexion or plantarflexion; a motion stop can be

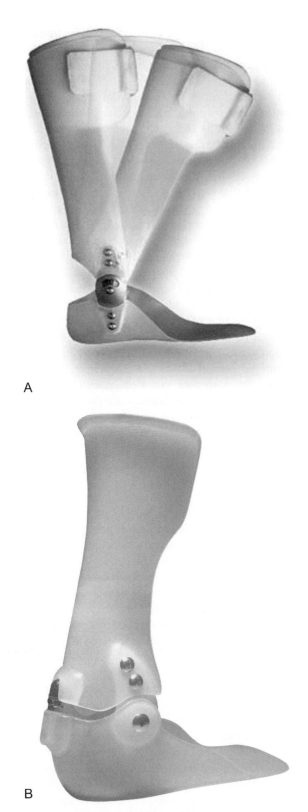

A

B

FIGURE 9-15 A, This hinged ankle-foot orthosis (AFO), with Camber Axis Hinges as the orthotic ankle joint, allows forward motion of the tibia through the second/ankle rocker of stance phase. **B,** This hinged AFO, with Oklahoma orthotic ankle joints, has a built-in plantarflexion stop (when the posterior edges of the foot and calf section come into contact) and posterior strapping that can be adjusted to limit the amount of dorsiflexion available, based on the wearer's motor control and need for stability in stance. (**A,** Courtesy Becker Orthopedic, Troy, Mich.)

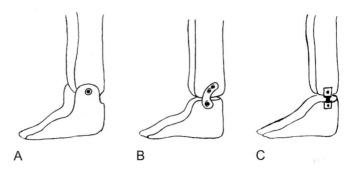

A   **B**   **C**

FIGURE 9-16 Examples of thermoplastic ankle joints used in hinged ankle foot orthosis. The overlap joint (**A**) and Oklahoma joint (**B**) are single axis joints, whereas the flexible Gillette mechanism (**C**) allows movement into dorsiflexion and plantarflexion without an actual articulation.

incorporated if there is need to limit plantarflexion beyond neutral (for stability in early stance) or dorsiflexion (to limit weight bearing on the forefoot in later stance) as the individual's needs dictate. A bi-channel adjustable ankle joint (also referred to as a *double action ankle joint* or a *double Klenzak joint*) (Figure 9-17) can be used to provide assistance and/or limit motion based on an individual's capabilities and needs for support. If motion assistance is desired, a coil spring is placed in the channel, and a screw is used to adjust compression until the desired level of assistance is achieved. If motion is to be blocked, a solid steel pin is inserted instead of the spring, to stop motion beyond a particular point in the range of motion. Because of its versatility and adjustability, the double action ankle joint is

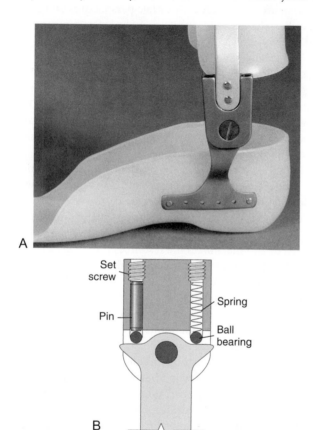

FIGURE 9-17 A, The double-action joint can be used in a conventional double-upright, metal ankle-foot orthosis and a thermoplastic-metal hybrid ankle-foot orthosis. Motion is assisted if a spring is compressed within the channel or can be blocked by placement of a steel pin within the channel. **B,** The internal anatomy of the double adjustable ankle joint. Ankle joint mobility restrictions (e.g., plantarflexion stop) result from the locations of the pins in the anterior and posterior channels of the orthotic joint. A spring may occupy one of the channels, as depicted here, to assist motion (e.g., dorsiflexion assistance). The ball bearings allow the brace uprights to pivot with ease over the brace stirrup. The set screw can be adjusted to change the relative positions of the rods in each of the channels. (**B,** From Zablotny CM. Use of orthoses for the adult with neurological involvement. In Nawoczenski DA, Epler ME [eds], *Orthotics in Functional Rehabilitation of the Lower Limb.* Philadelphia: WB Saunders, 1997. p. 227.)

often chosen when change in a patient's functional status (improvement or deterioration) is anticipated. Orthotic ankle joints such as the Camber Axis Hinge® allow the orthotist to adjust the available range of motion from none (as in a SAFO) through an array of limited anteroposterior stop settings. This would be an advantage when motor control around the ankle and knee is expected to improve over time, for example, in individuals who are recovering from an acute stroke.

For many adults with stroke and for some children with cerebral palsy, the HAFO allows free dorsiflexion; however, when motor control is compromised, such that additional support is needed during stance, the orthotist may choose to incorporate a mechanism, such as a check strap, to adjust the amount of dorsiflexion allowed (see Figure 9-16B). If the check strap is maximally tightened, the orthosis functions like a solid-ankle AFO. The check strap can be loosened, lengthened, or elasticized as neuromotor control improves, thus allowing only as much forward progression of the tibia in the second rocker as is safe and functional for the individual. This adaptation makes the HAFO versatile and useful when return of neuromotor control or function is anticipated.

It is important to note that a prerequisite for using this orthosis is at least 5 degrees of true ankle dorsiflexion, accomplished without compromise of subtalar or midtarsal joint position; for this reason, a HAFO may not be an appropriate choice for persons with severe spasticity that limits ankle motion or those with significant instability or malalignment of the midfoot.

Conventional Dorsiflexion-Assist Ankle Foot Orthosis

The conventional double upright counterpart to the PLS uses a spring mechanism incorporated into the mechanical ankle joints of the orthosis (Figure 9-18). The uprights are connected to the distal stirrup at the mechanical ankle joint, and the stirrup is fixed between the heel and sole of the shoe. A coiled spring and small ball bearing are placed in a channel in the distal uprights that runs toward the posterior edge of the stirrup. When the spring is compressed at initial contact and early loading response, it resists plantarflexion, allowing a controlled lowering of the foot to the floor, substituting for the second/heel rocker of early stance. Recoil of the spring when the foot is unloaded in preswing and initial swing assists dorsiflexion for swing phase toe clearance.[74] The amount of dorsiflexion assist provided is determined by adjustment of a screw placed in the top of the channel to compress or decompress the spring further. Another option is the dual channel (*double Klenzak*) orthotic ankle joint (see Figure 9-17); by placing a spring in one channel and a rod in the other, this mechanical ankle joint can provide adjustable dorsiflexion assistance and plantarflexion stop (in persons with impaired dorsiflexion muscle performance) or plantarflexion assistance and dorsiflexion stop (for those with motor control or muscle performance impairment of the gastrocsoleus complex).

Traditional or conventional double upright orthoses are typically used when the individual who needs dorsiflexion assistance and plantarflexion control has a comorbid condition

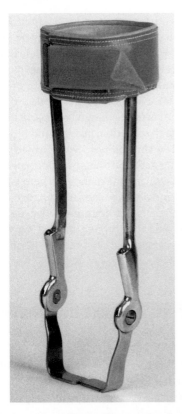

FIGURE 9-18 Conventional double-upright dorsiflexion assist ankle-foot orthosis, with a single-channel orthotic ankle joint. Tightening the screw at the top of the channel compresses a spring to increase the amount of dorsiflexion assistance provided. This split stirrup would be fit into a shoeplate positioned between the sole and heel, making it possible for the patient to use the ankle-foot orthosis with more than one shoe.

that causes fluctuation in limb size (edema), such as congestive heart failure or the need for kidney dialysis, that would compromise the intimate fit of a thermoplastic orthosis. The downside of the double upright AFO is its less effective control of abnormal foot position and risk of skin irritation as the foot moves within the shoe. For persons with neuropathic foot conditions who are unable to directly perceive abnormal pressures and the discomfort of tissue stress, a custom-molded AFO that is intimately fit for the individual's foot would be the orthosis of choice unless significant fluctuating edema precludes this choice.

AFO Designs, Tone, and Postural Control

Although some AFOs are described as having tone-reducing (TR-AFO) or tone inhibiting (TI-AFO) effects and are prescribed for persons with hypertonicity (spasticity) from upper motor neuron diseases (stroke, cerebral palsy, traumatic brain injury), the evidence of this effect is primarily based on cross-sectional studies and case reports, rather than randomized controlled clinical trials.[80] Historically, such AFO designs have their roots in the principles of serial casting, which sought to lessen the impact of tonic plantar reflexes that reinforce extensor tone of the lower extremity in children with cerebral palsy.[81,82] An early review of how these

principles were applied to AFO designs suggested that the orthosis incorporate the following[83]:
- A metatarsal bar or dome to alter loading on metatarsal heads
- A mechanism to encourage toe extension
- Additional loading on either side of the distal point of attachment of the Achilles tendon
- An ankle held in neutral subtalar and dorsiflexion position

Tone-reducing principles have been applied to SAFO, DAFO, and HAFO designs, and studied in children with cerebral palsy and in adults with stroke or traumatic brain injury. This variation makes comparison of efficacy across studies challenging.[80] The impact of TR- and TI-AFO use on kinematic measures of gait (e.g., speed, stride length, cadence) and on posture is similar to, rather than consistently superior to, other AFO designs.[52] The forecasted positive influence of TR-AFO on abnormal muscle activity of the gastrocnemius muscle (as measured by EMG and Hoffman reflex amplitude) during walking, while challenging to measure, has not been well supported in children with cerebral palsy or adults with stroke or spinal cord injury.[52,84,85]

How does this evidence affect the decision making of the team about whether to incorporate tone reducing characteristics into an AFO? At this point, it appears that TR- and TI-AFOs are equivalent in effect on function in children with cerebral palsy and perhaps in adults with stroke. We do not understand the effect of TR-AFOs on muscle tone. Current evidence does not support a positive neurophysiological consequence, and there is no alternative means to *quantify* muscle tone (the modified Ashworth Scale is a categorical measure, rather than a continuous measure).[86] Consensus statements of the International Society for Prosthetics and Orthotics suggest that the terms *tone-reducing* or *tone-inhibiting* should not be used to describe AFOs until stronger evidence of their efficacy for specific patient groups become available based on randomized controlled trials.[87,88]

While all AFO designs have a positive impact on quality and efficiency of walking (speed, stride, joint kinematics, kinetics, and energy cost), they vary in their impact on efficacy of postural responses, and balance during functional activities while walking, standing, or moving between sitting and standing.[89,90] Because many individuals whose walking would improve if they used AFOs also have deficits in motor control that impact the efficacy of balance and postural responses, and because risk for falling is high, it is important to consider the interaction of the orthosis with the individual's own movement resources.[91] A key question to consider is how the orthosis influences an individual's ability to dynamically control the body's center of mass within his or her base of support in standing, and while transitioning and walking. Does the orthosis constrain, maintain, or improve the individual's limits of stability during functional tasks that are meaningful and important for that person? For some persons with motor control dysfunction, the limitation of ankle motion may enhance stability in stance enough to improve ability to perform functional tasks while standing. For others, the same AFO design may impair the ability to respond effectively to both internally generated and external perturbations that shift the center of mass toward the edges of the individual's limits of stability.

Studies evaluating the impact of AFOs on static and dynamic postural control are challenging to interpret because of variation in the AFO designs being evaluated, the outcome measures used to assess balance, and the patient groups included in the sample.[89] In general, the SAFO and semisolid AFOs positively impact on static balance but appear to delay or impair response to perturbations.[92-94] For persons with stroke using a PLS orthosis, evidence is relatively convincing that both static and dynamic postural control improve with use of the orthosis (when compared to no orthosis or to SAFO) as measured by Timed Up-and-Go times, Berg Balance Scale score, and limits of stability testing.[95-97] There is little evidence about the impact of HAFOs and DAFOs on balance: The few available studies suggest a modest improvement in both static and dynamic postural control.[98]

How does this evidence impact clinical decision making when selecting an orthotic design for a particular patient? The team must weigh the potential positive and negative influences of the orthosis on the ability to walk, as well as on postural control during all activities that are important to the individual who will be wearing the orthosis. There is not a clear best or worst AFO; instead the team must match the pros of the orthosis with the person's neuromuscular resources, physical characteristics, and abilities and desired activities, tempered by the prognosis associated with the condition or diagnosis.

CASE EXAMPLE 1

A Child with Spastic Diplegia/Cerebral Palsy

P. M. is a 7-year-old child with a primary diagnosis of spastic diplegic cerebral palsy. He is anxious to keep up with his nonimpaired peers at school, but his moderate "crouch gait" (despite using Lofstrand crutches as assistive devices) limits his mobility and endurance. He is referred by his neurologist for evaluation in the interdisciplinary "brace clinic" at the local children's medical center.

On physical examination, P. M. is found to have moderate tightness and soft tissue shortening of his plantarflexors, distal hamstrings, adductors, and hip flexors. While he exhibits moderate extensor-pattern spasticity in both lower extremities, sagittal and coronal plane motions of his hip, knee, and ankle are within 10 degrees of normal. Structurally, he exhibits 25 degrees of femoral anteversion and 15 degrees of internal tibial torsion. Upon barefoot weight bearing, however, his foot progression angles appear to be normal, at approximately 10 degrees external (outward) angle.

Questions to Consider
- What are the most likely gait problems in each subphase of gait that might be effectively addressed by an AFO?
- What musculoskeletal (alignment and flexibility) and neuromuscular (control) impairments or characteristics, as well as developmental issues will have to be considered by the team as they sort through orthotic options for this child?
- Which of the orthotic options (static vs. dynamic) might you choose for this child? What are the possible benefits and trade-offs of each?
- How might you assess if the orthosis chosen is accomplishing the desired outcomes?

Recommendations of the Team
Given the finding of dynamic pes planus and valgus deformity, and the boy's propensity to crouch during stance, the team recommends bilateral polypropylene solid ankle AFO be custom molded for P. M. When P. M. receives his AFOs, he attends several sessions of outpatient gait training. His gait pattern demonstrates improved plantarflexion–knee extension couples, with virtually all of the preorthosis knee persistent knee flexion eliminated. Subtalar joint alignment is also improved, with an effective support of the medial longitudinal arch.

Follow-up Care
Three weeks later, the patient's mother schedules a follow-up visit because she observes, "The AFO is causing P. M.'s feet to turn in." On this return visit, observational gait assessment reveals an apparent 30-degree internal (inward) foot progression bilaterally. This is causing difficulty with clearance of the advancing limb during swing phase. Examination of the fit and alignment of the AFOs reveal appropriate design and fit, with effective subtalar neutral position.

The team recommends computerized gait analysis to be performed to determine the underlying factors leading to this significant change in foot progression angle despite appropriately fit and designed SAFO. The team suspects that this altered foot progression angle is most likely the result of underlying musculoskeletal deformities (tibial torsion and femoral anteversion) unmasked when compensatory motion of the subtalar and midtarsal joints during stance is restricted by the AFOs. In effect, when foot alignment is well supported by the AFO, the effect of excessive tibial torsion and femoral anteversion during gait become more evident.

It is not possible for an AFO to effectively address or control gait problems arising from existing underlying transverse plane (rotational) deformity. The team and family begin to consider the possibility of femoral/tibial derotation osteotomy as a solution to the gait problems that have emerged.

An Adult with Recent Stroke

Mrs. O is a 74-year-old woman who has just been admitted to an inpatient rehabilitation facility following a 4-day hospitalization for a thromboischemic stroke of one of the penetrating branches of the right middle cerebral artery. MRI indicated most of the damage involved the right internal capsule and fibers to and from the motor cortex in the frontal lobe. Mrs. O presents with left hemiplegia, positive Babinski reflex of the left foot, and several beats of clonus at the left Achilles tendon on reflex testing. Movement of the left lower extremity (LLE) occurs in a generalized extensor synergy pattern. She is unable to isolate ankle or knee motion in the LLE at the present time. Spatial perception appears to be grossly intact at proximal and mid-extremity joints of the LLE. She is able to mimic hip and knee position with her right lower extremity when her LLE is passively positioned but does not accurately mimic ankle and foot position. Static postural control in unsupported sitting on firm surfaces is intact; however, when sitting at the edge of the bed, reach distances are less than 10 inches in both directions. She comes to standing with moderate assistance of one person. Once standing, she is able to maintain the position with contact guard. In standing, Mrs. O can reach forward and to the right 6 inches, but is very reluctant to reach to the left. In the parallel bars, she demonstrates a step-to gait pattern, requiring minimal assistance to advance

LLE. Her relevant past medical history includes a right total hip arthroplasty 2 years ago and recent diagnosis of type 2 diabetes controlled by oral hypoglycemic medication. She lives (with her golden retriever) in a ranch style home with four steps to enter and hopes to eventually return to independent living. Before her stroke she was an avid walker, participating in an informal walking group that trekked in various local and state parks twice a week.

Questions to Consider

- What are the most likely gait problems, in each subphase of gait, that you expect to observe in Mrs. O as she begins her rehabilitation program?
- How will these gait problems change as she recovers from her stroke?
- What musculoskeletal (alignment and flexibility) and neuromuscular (control) impairments or characteristics will have to be considered by the team as they sort through orthotic options for Mrs. O?
- Which of the options for AFOs (static vs. dynamic) might you choose for Mrs. O? Why have you selected the particular design or components you are recommending?
- What are the possible benefits and trade-offs of each?
- How might you assess whether the orthosis chosen is accomplishing the desired outcomes?

WHEN SHOULD A KAFO BE CONSIDERED?

The rehabilitation team considers a knee ankle-foot orthoses (KAFOs) only when stability during stance cannot be effectively provided by one of the AFO options.[99,100] KAFOs are often prescribed when in addition to impairment of ankle control there is the presence of (1) hyperextension or recurvatum that jeopardize structural integrity of the knee joint, and/or (2) abnormal or excessive varus or valgus angulation that occurs during weight bearing in stance phase.[101] If not recognized and addressed appropriately, both threaten joint function and structure during walking and, with repeated abnormal loading, increase risk of permanent damage to supporting structures within the knee and development of degenerative joint disease. KAFOs can be used unilaterally (e.g., for individuals with polio affecting one limb) or bilaterally (e.g., for those with SCI or myelomeningocele).

The KAFO metal and leather design was used during the 1950s to make ambulation possible for those recovering for polio.[16] The weight of the orthosis, however, increased energy cost of ambulation significantly, and ultimately made use of a wheelchair the preferred method of mobility for those requiring bilateral KAFOs to walk.[102] The development of the lighter weight Craig Scott orthosis in the 1970s, the advent of thermoplastic custom-fit or custom-molded components in the 1980s, and emergence of stance control orthotic knee joints since 2000 have contributed to reduction in energy cost of ambulation with

KAFOs; walking while wearing these orthoses has became more reasonable.[100] Even now, however, many individuals decide that walking with bilateral KAFOs is too slow and requires too much effort to be truly functional for daily use.

Many KAFO designs use a SAFO or HAFO as the distal component, one or more thermoplastic thigh bars or cuffs as proximal components, with metal uprights with a variety of orthotic knee joints to interconnect them.[101]

Challenges to KAFO Use

The key issues that must be addressed for safe ambulation with KAFOs are the same as those discussed earlier in the chapter for AFOs[102]:

- To provide stance phase stability with minimal disruption of forward progression (especially through the second/ankle rocker of stance)
- To minimize disruption of swing limb clearance
- To prepare for an effective initial contact by holding the ankle in a neutral position

Once the knee joint is encased in an orthosis, however, meeting these goals can be challenging, especially for persons who require bilateral KAFOs. These individuals typically have more proximal deficits in muscle performance, motor control, and postural control than those whose need for stability in stance and mobility in swing are addressed by any of the AFO designs.[103]

The movement of transitioning from sitting to standing while wearing bilateral KAFOs is a complex and demanding motor task. The stability provided by KAFOs may constrain dynamic anticipatory and reactionary postural responses during activities in standing, especially on uneven, high resistance, or slippery surfaces. Many persons who use KAFOs for ambulation also need to use an ambulatory assistive device (e.g., crutches, walkers). Fear of falling and fall-related injury while walking with the KAFOs may be an important concern for those who use them, as well as for their caregivers. Primary and comorbid conditions that limit cardiovascular fitness and effectiveness of exercise response may further reduce endurance, making true functional ambulation with KAFOs unlikely. The combination of fewer resources that the individual has to use for walking, an orthosis that may be challenging to don and wear (given disease-related impact on activities of daily living and self-care), and the energy cost of walking even with the current lighter weight KAFO designs can contribute to an individual's abandonment of walking with his or her KAFOs after an effort-filled trial period.[104,105] This becomes a consideration when the cost of fitting, fabrication, and training for KAFO use is factored in.

Knee Function and Alignment

In early stance, under normal gait conditions, the GRF passes through the ankle, behind the knee, and through the hip, creating an external flexion moment at the knee (Figure 9-19). To counteract this GRF-related flexion moment, the quadriceps muscles contract to prevent the knee from collapsing into further flexion, the hamstrings and hip abductors contract to stabilize hip position and maintain a level pelvis, and the gastrocnemius prepares to eccentrically control forward progression of the tibia.[14] This combination of muscle activity provides an internally generated knee extension moment that balances the external flexion moment at the knee generated by the GRF.[14] When musculoskeletal or neuromuscular impairment alters limb position or muscle activity at any lower extremity joint, the internal/external force system is no longer in equilibrium, and efficiency of walking and stability in stance will be compromised.[106] The magnitude of disruption of the equilibrium between externally and internally generated moments determines whether the individual will be able to use his or her own resources (often in compensatory patterns or deviations) to address the imbalance, or if an AFO or KAFO is necessary for functional walking. Consideration of the magnitude of disruption of this equilibrium helps the team determine whether an AFO can effectively influence the position of the GRF as it crosses the knee, or if instead a KAFO is needed to restore equilibrium. If there is evidence of ligamentous instability that threatens anteroposterior or medial lateral stability at the knee, or markedly abnormal varus or valgus of the knee, a KAFO would clearly be indicated.

As when collecting data during the clinical examination, when an AFO is being considered, the evaluation process for KAFOs includes documentation of the individual's height and weight, the status of circulation and sensation in lower

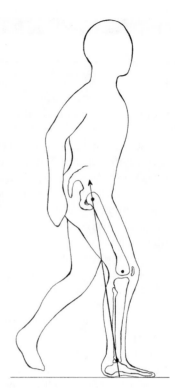

FIGURE 9-19 The ground reaction force passes through the ankle, behind the knee, and through the hip as loading response moves toward midstance, creating an external flexion moment at the knee. To achieve stability, muscle activity of the quadriceps, hamstrings, and gastrocnemius/soleus combine to create an internal extension moment to counterbalance the flexion moment of the ground reaction force.

extremities, the condition and integrity of the skin, soft tissue density and bony prominences, and living, school, working, and leisure environments, in which the KAFO is likely to be used. Specific attention is given to determination of available range of motion, ligamentous activity, fixed contractures, muscle performance, muscle and antigravity tone, leg length, and limb girth. The use of observational gait analysis, walking speed, other kinematic parameters, and if appropriate kinetic analysis is used to document preorthotic gait pattern. The team synthesizes this information to make a recommendation. The orthotist selects appropriate materials and components, then fabricates and fits the orthosis, making adjustments as necessary.[103] The physical therapist and individual using the orthosis begin the process of gait training, initially concentrating on walking, but eventually adding transitions and management of falls.[105]

KAFO DESIGN OPTIONS

KAFOs, much like the AFOs that form their distal component, can be made of primarily metal materials (e.g., steel, aluminum, titanium alloys, carbon fiber), primarily thermoplastics, or as a hybrid combining both types of materials. Historically, the orthotic knee joints of a KAFO were locking or free swinging; the development of stance-control (SC) knee units in the early 2000s have significantly changed function and energy cost for individuals who use SC-KAFO for function or for exercise.[107] While a KAFO does not directly control hip motion, if the individual wearing bilateral KAFOs is trained to stand with a forward pelvis, lumbar lordosis, and an extended trunk, the GRF at midstance will pass anterior to the knee and posterior to the hip, creating an extensor moment that will enhance stability. In this position, the Y ligaments of the hip are elongated, contributing an internal stabilizing force at the hips as well.[108] It is important to recognize that this strategy to achieve stable stance is not appropriate for children, however, until musculoskeletal maturity is reached.[109] Use of this strategy may, if used frequently over a long period of time, contribute to the development of degenerative joint disease of the lumbar spine and chronic low back pain.

Like any orthosis, KAFOs can both facilitate and challenge function. What works for one person may be inappropriate for another who has different physical or emotional characteristics or a different medical condition. For persons who want to walk using a KAFO, the orthotist must be even more thoughtful about durability and weight, matching the alignment of anatomical and orthotic joints, the impact of the forces used in each of the control system across all planes of motion, the ease of donning and doffing the device, the adjustability of the orthosis, the need for maintenance or replacement of worn-out components, as well as whether the orthosis will be comfortable and cosmetically acceptable to the person who will wear it.[103] The decision to prescribe a conventional or thermoplastic KAFO is founded on the needs and characteristics of the individual.

Conventional KAFOs

During the early 1900s until the 1980s, most KAFOs were fabricated using a pair of uprights (stainless steel, titanium alloy, aluminum, or carbon composite) as a frame, with leather-covered posterior thigh and calf cuffs that buckled across the anterior thigh and leg to secure the orthosis on the limb, a pair of single-axis locking orthotic knee joints, a pair of single-axis dorsiflexion assistance orthotic ankle joints with a plantarflexion stop, and metal stirrups that attached between the heel and sole of the shoe (Figure 9-20). At times, a leather anterior knee pad was added as an additional contact point for force application to stabilize the knee. These KAFOs were often worn over clothing during gait training and could later be worn under clothing if the individual so desired.

In most KAFO designs, a three-point pressure system is used to stabilize the knee in the sagittal plane to control flexion/extension: There is a single posteriorly directed force (applied by the anterior kneepad or by anterior thigh and calf straps, or both) and two anteriorly directed counterforces (applied by the posterior thigh band proximally and the shoe and posterior calf band distally) that keep the knee extended in stance. There are two additional force systems acting in the frontal plane: one to control valgus and one to control varus at the knee. Given the less-than-intimate fit of a conventional KAFO at the knee, the efficacy of the varus and valgus systems is likely to be less than optimal. The advantages of conventional KAFOs include their durability and adjustability;

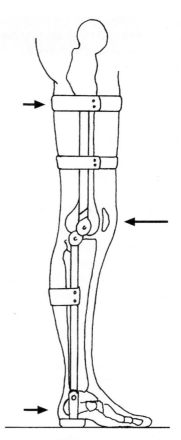

FIGURE 9-20 Schematic diagram of the components and sagittal plane force system acting at the knee in a conventional knee-ankle-foot orthosis. The posteriorly directed force at the knee is counterbalanced by a pair of anteriorly directed forces at the posterior proximal thigh and posterior distal ankle.

however, they tend to be heavier and less cosmetically pleasing than thermoplastic versions. Additionally, if porous leather is used to cover thigh cuffs, the absorption of sweat or urine (note that many who require KAFOs for ambulation have conditions that also impair continence) may render their KAFO malodorous over time. The advantages and disadvantages and the indications and contraindications of conventional KAFOs are summarized in Box 9-3.

The Craig-Scott orthosis, also known as a *double-bar hip-stabilizing orthosis* (Figure 9-21), is a lightweight variation of a traditional KAFO designed for persons with paraplegia after SCI.[99] The goal of this KAFO design is to maximize stability in stance with the minimal amount of bracing possible. A single thigh band and anterior strap are positioned just below the ischial tuberosity at the level of the greater trochanter; a single calf band and support are positioned just below the knee. Persons without active hip control are stable in standing with hip hyperextension, exaggerated lumbar lordosis and a backward leaning trunk; stability is augmented by the orthosis' dorsiflexion-assist ankle joints and offset locking knee joints. With this combination of orthotic design and exaggerated posture, the GRF passes just anterior to the knee and posterior to the hip, so that little or no muscular activity to provide internally generated counterforce is necessary. While a reciprocal gait pattern with Lofstrand crutches typically requires the ability

---

BOX 9-3   *Advantages and Disadvantages of Conventional Knee-Ankle-Foot Orthoses*

ADVANTAGES
- Strong
- Most durable
- Easily adjusted

DISADVANTAGES
- Heavy
- Must be attached to shoe or shoe insert
- Less cosmetic
- Fewer contact points reduce control

INDICATIONS
- When maximum strength and durability are needed
- For individuals with significant obesity
- For individuals with uncontrolled or fluctuating edema (e.g., congestive heart failure, dialysis)

CONTRAINDICATIONS
- When issues of energy expenditure make weight of the orthosis a factor
- When control of transverse plane motion is important

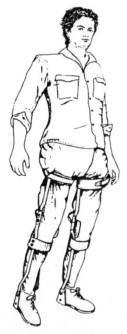

FIGURE 9-21 The Craig-Scott orthosis is a modified version of a conventional knee-ankle-foot orthosis, designed to be as lightweight as possible and to capitalize on alignment stability to enhance ambulation and upright activities in patients with low thoracic and lumbar spinal cord injury. Note that the individual wearing the orthosis stands with hyperextended hips, exaggerated lumbar lordosis, and backward lean of the trunk, "hanging" on his Y ligaments to maintain upright position. (Reprinted with permission from DG Shurr, TM Cook. Prosthetics and Orthotics. Norwalk, Conn: Appleton & Lange, 1990. p. 141.)

to volitionally activate hip flexions and quadratus lumborum (hip hikers) to initiate a step, persons with thoracic level SCI can use Craig-Scott orthoses and Lofstrand crutches using a two-point swing-through gait pattern.[108]

Conventional KAFOs are frequently used to preserve upright mobility for children with Duchenne muscular dystrophy (DMD).[110] While initially perceived as a sign of disease-related decline, parents and children often come to appreciate the continued mobility that KAFOs allow.[111] Use of a KAFO may provide limited household or community ambulation ability for boys with DMD for 2 or more years. Fitting for KAFOs may be challenging because of the primary and compensatory deformities that develop as children with DMD strive to remain upright as their disease progresses.[112] A lightweight modular system that allows the orthotist to adjust the length of the uprights and quickly replace outgrown thigh or calf supports has been developed specifically for children with DMD.[113]

Thermoplastic KAFOs

A *molded thermoplastic* KAFO (also known as a hybrid thermoplastic and metal orthosis) is designed to have an intimate fit so that it can be worn under clothing and fits within the patient's shoe (Figure 9-22). The distal component (a SAFO or HAFO, depending on the individual's needs) and the proximal thigh component are vacuum formed over a rectified positive model of the patient's limb. The proximal component often encases the thigh from greater trochanter to femoral condyles, and is closed with a pair of anterior Velcro straps. Orthotic knee joints and metal uprights (sidebars) connect the proximal and distal shells. The intimate total contact fit of molded thermoplastic allows significantly more effective control of the limb. The forces necessary for stabilization of the limb are distributed over a large surface area, reducing the possibility of discomfort or skin irritation. Such problems would arise only if the fit of the orthosis allows pistoning of the limb within the components while walking, or if growth, weight gain, or edema makes the fit too snug, such that tissue is compressed and damaged while walking.

This design also controls the limb using a series of overlapping three-point force systems. Flexion/extension control in the sagittal plane is the same one used in a conventional KAFO, except that the posterior counterforces are distributed over a wider surface area. The intimate fit provides more precise control in both the frontal and transverse planes; this is particularly important when dealing with segmental deviations arising from transverse plane rotation related to abnormal tone or longitudinal rotational deformity.[114]

Because any movement of the knee joint occurs in multiple planes of motion, any varus or valgus problems at the knee will necessarily have a rotatory component. Control of rotation is better accomplished with the intimate fit, total contact thermoplastic KAFO as compared to the double upright system of conventional KAFOs. This intimate fit, however, is problematic for persons with medical conditions associated with fluctuating edema and changing limb volume

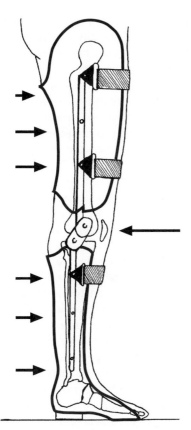

FIGURE 9-22 Schematic diagram of the components and sagittal plane force systems that are necessary to control knee flexion/extension. Because the point of force application is distributed over the entire posterior surface of the intimately fitting orthotic shell, more precise and more comfortable control of the limb is possible.

(e.g., congestive heart failure, kidney dialysis), as well as those who cyclically gain and lose weight.

Similar to most thermoplastic AFOs, the use different pairs of shoes (as long as heel height is constant) can also occur with thermoplastic KAFOs. One of the downsides of using thermoplastics, however, is keeping cool while wearing them. As lightweight as they are, the large contact area inherent in thermoplastic KAFOs compromises dissipation of body heat; they may be uncomfortably warm for wearers who are very active or who live in hot climates. Advantages and disadvantages of thermoplastic KAFOs are summarized in Box 9-4.

Carbon Composite KAFOs

Recently, carbon composite materials have begun to be used in place of thermoplastics in KAFOs for persons with residual impairment following polio (postpolio syndrome) for whom fatigue is a major concern (Figure 9-23).[115] On average, because CC-KAFOs are as much as 30% lighter in weight than other materials, the energy cost of walking with CC-KAFOs may be up to 10% less (as measured by VO_2 max and physiological cost index).[116,117] In addition, CC-KAFOs have been deemed to be cosmetic by users, persevered or increased walking speed, improved kinetic characteristics of walking, and demonstrated exceptional

BOX 9-4 *Advantages and Disadvantages of Thermoplastic Knee-Ankle-Foot Orthoses*

ADVANTAGES
- Lightweight
- Interchangeability of shoes
- Greater cosmesis worn under clothing

DISADVANTAGES
- Can be hot to wear

INDICATIONS
- Intimate/total contact fit makes maximum limb control possible
- When energy expenditure makes weight of the orthosis an issue
- When control of transverse plane motion is needed

CONTRAINDICATIONS
- Intimacy of fit is difficult when the individual is significantly obese
- Intimacy of fit is compromised when the individual has uncontrolled or fluctuating edema

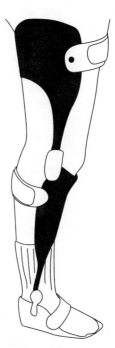

FIGURE 9-23 This carbon composite knee-ankle-foot orthosis (CC-KAFO) has a posterior proximal shell, uses a stance control knee unit, an anterior tibial shell, and a foot component similar to that of a hinged AFO. Because CC-KAFOs are much lighter than thermoplastic and conventional KAFO designs, they are well suited for individuals with post-polio syndrome, reducing energy cost of gait by improve most gait parameters. They are, however, much more expensive to fabricate.

durability.[116,117] It is important to note, however, that the cost of CC-KAFOs may be nearly double that of a custom-molded thermoplastic KAFO.[116,117]

Controlling the Ankle

The ankle joints used in KAFOs are the same as those that are available for AFOs: either nonarticulating solid (rigid) designs that hold the ankle in a fixed position (i.e., SAFO) or hinged orthotic joints that allow dorsiflexion (for forward progression of the tibia over the foot in stance) block plantarflexion, provide dorsiflexion assistance (to enhance swing phase clearance), or allow free dorsiflexion and plantarflexion within a specific range of motion.

The key question to consider in deciding which ankle control system is appropriate for a given individual is how orthotic control at the ankle and the GRF will impact knee function and forward progression during stance phase. If a locked ankle is necessary, the orthotist may opt to set the orthosis in several degrees of dorsiflexion to minimize compromise of forward progression and to allow the individual to achieve the stable hips-forward trunk-back stance position quickly (i.e., to achieve stability with the GRF passing anterior to the knee and posterior to the hip as soon as possible during stance) (see Figure 9-21). When ankle motion must be constrained to protect the joint, to control the impact of abnormal tone, or because of fixed deformity, the orthotist may use a rocker sole on the patient's shoe to simulate the normal rockers of gait. This strategy facilitates forward progression during stance by reducing the toe lever of the orthosis, improving the smoothness of the patient's gait and reducing the likelihood of compensatory gait deviations.

An articulating or hinged orthotic ankle joint that allows some plantarflexion enhances the transition from initial contact to loading response (although the locked knee may compromise the shock absorption function of loading response). Similarly, a hinged orthotic ankle joint that permits movement into dorsiflexion during stance enhances forward progression of the body over the foot during stance, especially when the orthotic knee is also locked.

Controlling the Knee

Historically, if a patient with motor control or muscle performance impairment was unable to keep the knee stable in stance by using their quadriceps or alignment of limb segments (i.e., hanging on the Y ligament at the hip), and an AFO was not able to provide the necessary stability, the only option was a KAFO with knee joints that remained locked at all times while walking.[118,119] This created a challenge for limb advancement in swing, and often resulted in compensatory patterns such as circumduction or lateral leaning to the opposite side in an effort to clear the swinging leg. While compensatory strategies accomplished the goal of limb clearance, they also markedly increased the energy cost of walking. Those who had functional motor control and muscle performance who required a KAFO to protect a mechanically unstable knee from extreme valgus or varus may be able to use unlocked single axis orthotic knee joints.

There are a number of options for orthotic knee joints that provide mechanical stability. The recent development of various SC-KAFO knee joints that allow free knee motion in swing but lock into extension during stance has had significant impact of KAFO prescription and use.[120,121] A brief overview of the mechanical joints is provided, and the impact of SC-KAFOs is considered in more detail. See Table 9-3 for a set of general guidelines for choosing the conventional orthotic knee joints, based on the knee control they provide.

Single-Axis Knee Joints

The single-axis knee orthotic knee joint *(straight knee joint without drop lock or a free knee)* is, essentially, a simple hinge that allows full flexion and extension to neutral in the sagittal plane (most designs prevent hyperextension) while providing mediolateral stability (Figure 9-24A). It is important that the medial and lateral orthotic joints be positioned at the approximate axis of the anatomical knee joint. Given the polycentric structure of the anatomical knee versus the single axis structure of the orthotic knee joint, a small torque is likely, even if the single axis orthotic joints are correctly positioned. For the majority of persons using the orthosis, this is not problematic. This knee joint is appropriate for those who have sufficient muscle performance resource to achieve knee stability in stance but need a KAFO to minimize or prevent recurvatum, protect a structural (mediolateral) unstable knee, or prevent excessive varus or valgus in stance.[121]

Single-Axis Locking Knee

When a locking mechanism is added to maintain knee extension, the KAFO with a single-axis knee joint becomes rigidly stable in all planes. A locked knee has traditionally been used for those whose motor control or muscle performance deficits make them unable to control the knee effectively during stance phase, such that they need additional external stability to prevent knee flexion as body weight is transferred onto the limb during stance.[118]

The most commonly used locking mechanism is a simple ring or drop that captures the halves of the orthotic joint when fully extended, blocking subsequent movement into flexion or hyperextension (see Figure 9-24B). A small ball bearing in the upright holds the drop lock in position until the individual or caregiver purposefully unlocks the orthosis. Optimally, there is a drop lock on both the medial and lateral uprights of the orthosis. Note that the knee must be fully extended for the lock to be engaged or disengaged; this can be challenging when transitioning between standing and sitting, especially for persons with limited hand function, significant lower extremity spasticity, or dependence on assistive devices when standing.

An alternative lock that may be considered is a spring-loaded bail lock (also known as pawl or Swiss lock) (Figure 9-25). The posterior bail connects the medial and lateral locks so that they can be locked or unlocked simultaneously. To unlock the KAFO when returning to sitting, the individual backs up against the edge of a seating surface (e.g., wheelchair, mat table, kitchen, or desk chair) and

TABLE 9-3 *Indications and Contraindications for Orthotic Knee Joint Designs*

Desired Knee Control	Orthotic Knee Design				
	Single Axis Unlocked	Single Axis Locked	Offset Unlocked	Offset Locked	Variable Position Locked
Stabilization of flail knee with knee extension moment and free knee joint motion	Contraindicated	Contraindicated	**Indicated**	Contraindicated	Contraindicated
Stabilization of flail knee without use of knee extension moment and free knee joint motion	Contraindicated	**Indicated**	Contraindicated	**Indicated**	Unnecessary
Control of genu recurvatum	Contraindicated	**Indicated** if orthosis will only be locked when ambulating	**Indicated**	**Indicated** when individual will lock knee intermittently	Contraindicated
Reduction of knee flexion contracture	Contraindicated	Lacks adjustability	Contraindicated	Lacks adjustability	**Indicated**
Control of genu valgum	**Indicated**	**Indicated** Use of lock optional	**Indicated**	**Indicated** Use of lock optional	Unnecessary
Control of genu varum	**Indicated**	**Indicated** Use of lock optional	**Indicated**	**Indicated** Use of lock optional	Unnecessary

Modified from Short Course in Orthotics and Prosthetics—Course Manual. Dallas, Texas: University of Texas, Southwestern Medical Center, 1993. pp. 8-22.

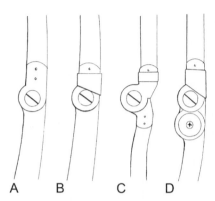

FIGURE 9-24 Orthotic knee joints historically used in conventional and thermoplastic knee-ankle-foot orthoses. **A,** A single-axis, or free, knee allows full flexion and extension while providing mediolateral and rotational stability to the knee joint. **B,** A drop lock holds the knee in extension in standing, providing stability in all planes. It must be unlocked for knee flexion to occur when returning to sitting position. **C,** Because the axis of the offset orthotic knee joint is positioned behind the anatomical knee axis, biomechanical stability of the orthosis is enhanced. It is available with and without a locking mechanism. **D,** A variable position, or adjustable, orthotic knee joint permits the orthotist to accommodate for changing range of motion or for fixed contracture at the knee.

pushes the posterior bar into the seat to disengage the lock. This option is best used for persons with enough upper body strength and coordination to control the descent into sitting. There is a risk that the lock will disengage if the bail behind the knee is inadvertently bumped, and a fall will occur.

Offset Knee Joint

The offset knee joint (also known as a *posteriorly offset, free knee)* is aligned with its axis posterior to the axis of the anatomic knee (see Figure 9-24C). In early stance, during double support, the ground reaction passes nearer to the axis of the orthotic joint, reducing the magnitude of the external flexion moment that is acting to flex the limb. With forward progression toward midstance, the GRF moves anterior to the orthotic joint, creating an extensor force that mechanically augments stance phase stability during single limb support. To be effective, however, the alignment between ankle and knee must be finely tuned. Transitions between sitting and standing become less problematic if the knee does not have to be unlocked. A drop lock or other locking mechanism can be added, however, to stabilize the knee when the individual using the orthosis will be standing for long periods of time or when additional stability is advisable (e.g., when the patient is walking on uneven ground). An offset knee joint is often most suitable for those with lower motor neuron disease (e.g., poliomyelitis) or low thoracic upper lumbar SCI.[118,121]

Variable Position Orthotic Knee Joint

The variable position locking orthotic knee joint (*dial lock, adjustable locking knee joint, serrated knee lock*) (see Figure 9-24D) is used for those who are unable to fully

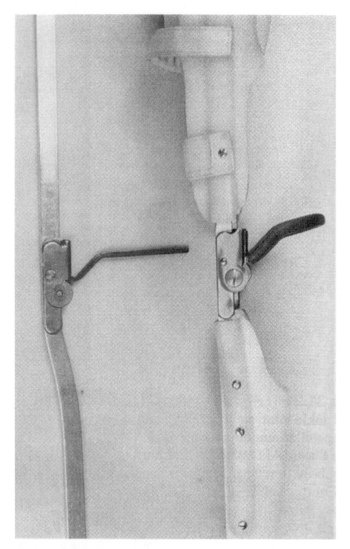

FIGURE 9-25 A pawl and bail-locking mechanism allows the medial and lateral locks to be disengaged at the same time by a posterior pressure, as against the edge of the seating surface. This mechanism is often used for patients with paraplegia who must maintain bilateral upper extremity support via crutches for stability. (Reprinted with permission from O'Sullivan S, Schmitz TJ [eds]. *Physical Rehabilitation*, 5th ed. Philadelphia: FA Davis, 2007. p. 1224.)

extend the knee during stance because of knee flexion contracture. When there is a knee flexion contracture of more than 10 degrees, the GRF remains posterior to the anatomic knee joint during all of stance phase, and it becomes significantly more difficult for those with weakness or motor control impairment to generate the necessary muscle force for stance stability. For these individuals, the variable position knee joint is locked in the most extended position possible, providing an external mechanical stability.[16,118]

Stance Control Orthotic Knee Joints

The initial SC options for KAFO orthotic knee joints were intended for individuals with a history of poliomyelitis who were coping with ineffective quadriceps activity as well as postpolio syndrome.[122-124] Use of SC-KAFO

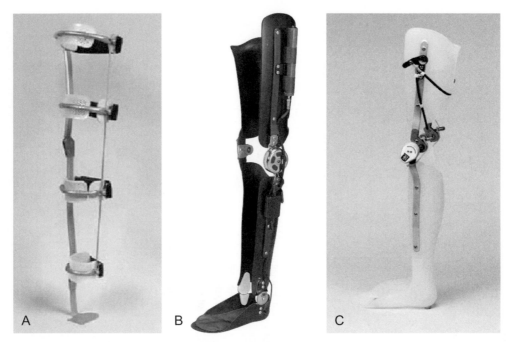

FIGURE 9-26 A, The Becker UTX is a mechanical stance-control knee-ankle-foot orthosis (SC-KAFO): The knee unit contains a cable-driven ratchet that locks the knee as it extends in terminal swing in preparation for stance phase, and unlocks it at terminal stance to allow knee flexion necessary for limb clearance during swing phase. Note the lightweight lateral upright, medial cable, anterior padded cuffs, and Velcro-closing posterior straps. **B,** The Becker E-knee is an example of a microchip-controlled and battery-powered SC-KAFO. A pressure-sensing footplate signals the microprocessor to lock the knee joint when the limb is loaded (regardless of knee position), and unlock the unit when unloaded in late stance. **C,** The Becker Load Response SC-KAFO also contains a torsional spring that mimics controlled knee flexion for shock absorption in loading response. (Reprinted with permission from Becker Orthopedic, Troy, Mich.)

has been extended to persons with stroke, brain tumor, acquired brain injury, incomplete SCI, spinal degenerative diseases, muscular dystrophy, multiple sclerosis, myopathy, radicular and peripheral nerve injury, and polyneuropathy.[125-127] A variety of mechanisms (i.e., mechanical, hydraulic, or computer microchip electronic joints) are available (Figure 9-26).[128-130] All are designed to lock the orthotic knee joint in extension at initial contract and during most of stance, while unlocking the knee on heel rise during the third rocker, in the transition from terminal stance to preswing.[131] Hydraulic and electronic SC orthotic joints add resistance to knee flexion when the limb is loaded in less than a fully extended position, which potentially improves function when the wearer is ascending stairs or walking on uneven surfaces. Most SC orthotic knee joints are placed on the lateral upright of the KAFO. Pneumatic orthotic knee joints to assist with knee extension during swing are also available, added onto the media or lateral uprights of the KAFO.[126] Many of the SC knee units can be incorporated into KAFOs based on metal uprights, thermoplastic thigh and AFO components, or laminated designs. Characteristics of some of the commercially available SC and swing assist knee units are summarized in Table 9-4.

Most prescription guidelines for SC-KAFO indicate that the individual must demonstrate muscle strength of at least 3/5 on manual muscle testing at hip extensors and flexors, and full extension of the anatomical knee joint.[125-127] Contraindications for SC-KAFO use include fixed hip or knee flexion contracture, fixed plantarflexion contracture, significant spasticity, leg length discrepancy greater than 3 inches (8 cm), valgus or varus deformity greater than 10 degrees, and excessive body weight (above 220 to 265 pounds).[125-127] Persons with cognitive impairment may not be able to comprehend how to safely use or maintain a SC-KAFO; SC options must be used with caution when cognitive ability and judgment are impaired.

The positive impact of SC knee joints on kinematics of walking is well documented. In addition to improving self-selected walking speed, cadence, and stride length, use of these orthotic knee joint improves symmetry of gait, reduces compensatory movement, and allows safer management of inclines and obstacles when compared with KAFOs with locked knees.[120,122-124,128] Persons who have used traditional KAFOs with locked knees for long periods before adopting SC designs benefit from additional functional training to be able to take full advantage of the mobility that a SC-KAFO provides.[132] The few studies that have examined wearers' experience with SC-KAFOs indicate better acceptance and general satisfaction with the devices in terms of effectiveness in improving mobility, dependability, and performance of the device and

TABLE 9-4   *Stance-Control Knee-Ankle-Foot Orthosis Characteristics*

Name	Manufacturer	Control System	Orthotic Components	Other Characteristics
Stance-control orthosis	Horton Little Rock, Ark.	Mechanical	Pushrod and cam system Thermoplastic stirrup at ankle causes pushrod to engage cam into friction ring to lock knee at initial contact unloading in late stance Pushrod re-positions Pushrod to disengage cam from friction ring, allowing free knee flexion during swing	Dual uprights Three settings: locked, automatic, unlocked Lightweight, but bulky May require larger shoe size to accommodate nested thermoplastic stirrup and AFO Most effective at constant walking speed and consistent stride length (not cadence responsive)
Free Walk	Otto Bock Healthcare Duderstadt, Germany	Mechanical	Cable driven pawl lock system Spring-loaded pawl locks the knee when in full extension during stance	Single lateral upright with medial cable Very light weight
UTX	Becker Orthopedic	Mechanical	Unit unlocks with dorsiflexion of ankle in late stance to allow free knee flexion during swing	Requires full knee extension to engage the lock, although uprights can be contoured to accommodate up to 10 degrees of knee flexion contracture Requires at least 5 degrees of mobility at ankle Requires at least ⅔ hip flexion and extension strength for safe and effective use Not appropriate for those with varus > 10 degrees
Swing Phase Lock 2	Fillauer Chattanooga, Tenn.	Mechanical	Gravity-activated pendulum system with weighted pawl lock Weighted pawl causes knee to lock when hip flexion in late swing Moves thigh anterior to body in preparation for initial contact in late stance, when thigh is posterior to body, weight pawl moves to unlocking position	Dual-upright, with SC gravity system in lateral upright Swing control spring to control/assist knee extension during swing phase can be incorporated into medial knee unit No cables or pushrods Not effective on stairs, inclines, uneven ground Four settings controlled by a remote push button switch: manual lock, manual unlock, automatic, or free swing
E-Knee	Becker	Microchip	Electromechanical system with pressure sensitive footplate that feeds information to micro processor to engage/disengage locking mechanism	Dual-uprights Can be used with thermoplastic and laminated materials Lithium battery must be charged daily Provides locking in increments of 8 degrees at any angle of knee flexion at initial contract No minimum strength or ROM requirements
Load Response	Becker	Mechanical	Spiral torsional spring designed to mimic shock absorption during loading response	Locking mechanism responsive for 0 to 18 degrees of knee flexion at initial contract Not effective for persons with fixed knee flexion contracture or valgus > 15 degrees

GX-Knee	Becker	Mechanical and pneumatic	Pneumatic spring on lateral joint provides assistance with knee extension during swing phase	Does not provide mechanical stability in stance phase Requires ⅔ hip flexion and extension strength for safe use
Full Stride	Becker	Mechanical	Cable-driven system	Requires full-knee extension to engage lock, although uprights can be contoured to accommodate knee flexion contracture <10 degrees Requires 5 degrees of ankle motion to achieve necessary cable excursion to operate locking mechanism
Safety Stride	Becker Orthopedic	Mechanical	Cable-driven system	Resists knee flexion in stance regardless of knee angle No minimum strength or ROM requirements GX swing assist system can be incorporated
Sensor Walk	Otto Bock Healthcare	Electromechanical	Unidirectional wrap-spring clutch-actuated by pressure sensors in heel and forefoot and motion sensor at knee	Heavy-duty custom KAFO accommodates up to 15 degrees of knee flexion contracture Powered by lithium-ion battery Locks knee joint when footplate indicates a stumble

AFO, ankle-foot orthosis; KAFO, knee-ankle-foot orthosis; ROM, range of motion; SC, stance control.

Adapted from Operating instructions for the E-Mag and Free Walk orthosis, Ottobock Germany. Available at: http://www.ottobock.com/cps/rde/xbcr/ob_com_en/im_646a214_gb_free_walk.pdf; Stance Control Overview Guide II, Becker Orthopedic Troy, Mich. Available at: http://www.beckerorthopedic.com/assets/pdf/stance:control.pdf; MO25-SPL Manual, Fillauer, Chattanooga Tenn. Available at: http://www.fillauer.com/Orthotics/SPL2.html; Yakimovich T, Lemaire ED, Kofman J. Engineering design review of stance-control knee-ankle-foot orthoses. *J Rehabil Res Dev.* 2009;46(2):257-267.

enhancing the wearer's sense of well-being.[133,134] The major concerns raised by wearers include ease of donning and doffing, weight of the orthosis, and cosmesis.[133,134]

Medially Linked Bilateral KAFO Designs

For persons with mid to low thoracic and lumbar SCI, several options have been developed to link a pair of conventional KAFOs in an effort to allow reciprocal gait without having to brace about the hip in a conventional HKAFO (Figure 9-27). The Walkabout Orthosis, and the Moorling Medial Linkage Orthosis, both of which use a single axis hinge between the two medial uprights of the KAFOs, are most effective for individuals with some residual volitional hip flexion who have sufficient thoracolumbar spinal mobility, especially into lateral flexion.[135-137] In both of these systems, the linkage system limits abnormal abduction of the limbs during gait. Preparation for swing limb advancement begins with an exaggerated lateral lean for weight shift onto the stance limb; the wearer then initiates swing using residual hip hiking or hip flexion ability. When compared with reciprocal gait HKAFO (see later), medially linked KAFOs provided better ability (less assistance required) to accomplish sit to stand transitions, but walking speed tended to be slower, management of inclines more problematic, and performance on measures of balance somewhat less effective.[138,139] In addition, persons with SCI who wore both devices over a 3-month period reported that both were useful for standing and there was no functional advantage of medially linked KAFOs over reciprocal gait HKAFOs in terms of mobility.[140] Hybrid systems, consisting of medially linked KAFOs and functional electrical stimulation (FES), have also been used as an approach to improve the ability to walk for persons with SCI.[141]

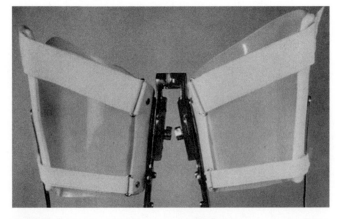

FIGURE 9-27 The Walkabout Orthosis connects a pair of conventional thermoplastic knee-ankle-foot orthoses with a single axis joint attached to the proximal edge of the medial uprights. (Reprinted with permission from Middleton JW, Yeo JD, Blanch L, Vare V, Peterson K, Brigden K. Clinical evaluation of a new orthosis, the 'Walkabout,' for restoration of functional standing and short distance mobility in spinal paralysed individual. *Spinal Cord.* 1997;35:574-579.)

KAFO DELIVERY AND FUNCTIONAL TRAINING

Once fabrication is completed, the orthotist inspects the KAFO to ensure that selected components work as intended, that finish work of plastic edges and metal components are effective, that the placement and contours are appropriate to the individual's limbs, and that orientation of the axis of the orthotic ankle and knee match anatomical joint axis. This initial fitting process not only identifies the fit of the orthosis in its intended functional upright and weight-bearing positions but also closely examines potential for soft tissue irritation in vulnerable areas of the person's skin. Length of the uprights as well as position and alignment of components are carefully inspected. The goal is a comfortable standing position, with no discomfort or skin irritation. If minor problems are identified, the orthotist often makes simple adjustments of fit and alignment before functional training. The team then evaluates the ability of the orthosis to meet the functional goals of the orthotic prescription.

If the team determines that fit is acceptable and that orthotic goals (a combination of joint protection, structural stability, especially in stance, and functional mobility) have been met, functional training then begins. In most cases, especially if a patient is new to the use of an orthosis, a wearing schedule is developed, tailored to the patient's specific needs and physical condition, in which the patient gradually increases to full-time wear.

Whether the orthosis is of conventional KAFO design or is a SC-KAFO, physical therapy programs should include:

- exercises to strengthen muscle groups that control hip, knee, and core (trunk) (concentric, eccentric, and holding contractions) to maximize ability to use the device;
- practice donning/doffing the device;
- rising to standing and returning to sitting;
- activities to facilitate anticipatory and reactionary postural control and balance;
- gait training in parallel bars (emphasizing weight acceptance in early stance, single limb stability in midstance, and swing limb clearance), progressing to over-ground activities, and (for SC-KAFO) on treadmill training to improve gait speed and other gait kinematics;
- practice on stairs, uneven surfaces, and inclines;
- functional activities in open environments where the individual is called upon to adjust speed and avoid obstacles in relation to others who are moving around within the same space.

Walking speed would be an appropriate and powerful outcome indicator for physical therapy intervention.

Training should also focus on developing a clear understanding of the fit of the orthosis on the limb, proper adjustment of stabilizing straps, education about appropriate footwear, and management of the locking mechanisms and function of the knee unit. Wearers and their caregivers must understand the care and maintenance of the orthosis, which is a mechanical device with moving parts that requires regular cleaning and occasional lubrication of its mechanical parts.

An Individual with Poliomyelitis-Related Impairment

T. C., a 63-year-old man who survived acute poliomyelitis as a 7-year-old, has been living with longstanding atrophy and weakness of his right lower extremity since that time. Until recently, he used a conventional KAFO with drop locks to maintain knee stability in stance. He used a combination of circumduction of the right lower extremity and vaulting on the left lower extremity to achieve right swing limb clearance. In his home, on level surfaces, he is able to ambulate without assistive device, touching furniture or wall surfaces to occasionally provide additional stability. Until recently, when he began to have difficulty with back pain, he had been using either a straight cane or single forearm (Lofstrand) crutch for mobility outside and for long distances. He recently read about SC-KAFOs and made an appointment at the orthotic clinic of a nearby rehabilitation center to determine whether this would be an appropriate option. He has two goals: (1) improve his mobility (both quality and distance) and (2) reduce the intensity of his back pain when walking.

Examination reveals a fairly fit and active man with marked atrophy of anterior thigh and calf muscles. There is a 5-degree hip flexion contracture noted bilaterally using Thomas test, and slightly exaggerated lumbar lordosis is noted in stance. There is no restriction in knee range of motion, and all knee ligaments are intact, although there is mild valgus noted, along with moderate knee hyperextension passively and in stance. No rotational or torsional deformities are apparent. Ankle dorsiflexion (0 to 7 degrees) and plantarflexion (0 to 10 degrees) are limited by longstanding soft tissue tightness.

Right lower extremity muscle performance per MMT is as follows:

Hip flexion and rotation: 3+/5
Hip extension and abduction: 4/5
Knee extension (quadriceps): 2/5
Knee flexion (hamstrings): 4/5
Dorsiflexion: 3+/5
Plantarflexion: 2+/5
Sensation: exteroception and kinesthesia (vibration) appear to be intact

Questions to Consider

- What are the major benefits and tradeoffs associated with a conventional locked-knee KAFO versus a SC-KAFO?
- What are the minimum requirements for muscle strength, range of motion, and limb alignment that an individual must have to use the various SC-KAFO designs currently available?
- Is T. C. a suitable candidate for a SC-KAFO? Why or why not? Which of the SC joints would be most appropriate for him? Why would you recommend this particular orthotic option?
- Given that T. C. has used a conventional KAFO with a locked knee for most of his life, what challenges do you expect him to encounter as he learns to use a SC-KAFO and its improved mobility? How might you structure a physical therapy exercise and functional training intervention to help him quickly learn to trust and effectively use his new orthosis?

An Individual with L1 Traumatic Spinal Cord Injury

K. G. is a 19-year-old woman who sustained traumatic complete SCI in a motor vehicle accident 3 months ago. She underwent surgical fusion of T10 to L2 spinal vertebrae and wore a thoracolumbar orthosis for 8 weeks. She has completed her inpatient rehabilitation, is no longer required to wear the spinal orthosis, and functions independently indoors in a solid frame wheelchair, needing minimal assistance for ramps and curbs. Her rehabilitation continues on an outpatient basis, and she wants to "give walking a try." She is referred to the Gait & Orthotics Clinic at the rehabilitation center for evaluation.

At present, K. G. presents with 3/5 hip flexion strength on the right and 2/5 hip flexion strength on the left. Reflexes at the knee and ankle are "0" with flaccid paralysis and complete sensory loss below the L1 neurological level. She has hip and knee flexion contractures of 10 degrees bilaterally. Skin is intact at the moment, although a grade 3 sacral decubitus ulcer has recently healed. Upper extremity and upper body strength and flexibility are sufficient for ambulation with an appropriate assistive device.

Questions to Consider

- What additional information is important for the clinic team to gather as they prepare to make recommendations about orthotic options for K. G.? What additional tests and measures might be important to use?
- Given her current level of function, as well as her lower motor neuron SCI, what orthotic options are the team likely to consider for K. G.?
- If the team opts for a KAFO, which design would you recommend using: conventional thermoplastic KAFO, with or without FES, a pair of SC-KAFOs, a pair of Craig-Scott orthoses, a set of linked orthoses such as the Walkabout, conventional HKAFOs, a parawalker, or hip guidance orthosis? What are the benefits or tradeoffs of each? Why have your chosen the orthosis that you are recommending?
- In addition to learning to ambulate with the orthoses, what additional motor tasks will K. G. have to master to use them functionally?
- How will the team evaluate the effectiveness and efficiency of K. G.'s ability to walk with the orthoses as she becomes more adept at using them?

WHEN IS AN HKAFO INDICATED?

There is much less evidence available in the clinical research literature to guide prescription and selection of HKAFOs than for selecting AFOs and KAFOs. Because HKAFO encompass the hip, pelvis, and sometimes the trunk, they tend to be much more cumbersome to use, more challenging to don and doff, more expensive to fabricate, and require more maintenance than AFOs and KAFOs. HKAFOs only partially restore functional mobility, often with high energy cost. The additional control of joint motion achieved by moving proximally with a hip joint and pelvic band or an attached lumbosacral orthosis must be balanced against the practical challenges that the wearer will face when using the device.

Persons who use HKAFOs for standing and the limited mobility that they provide typically have much more neuromotor system impairment that those who use AFOs and KAFOs. These orthoses are most often prescribed for children with myelomeningocele and individuals with SCI but may also be appropriate for those with progressive neuromuscular disorders; in effect for any person for whom the ability to stand may not only enhance function for some functional tasks, but also contribute to bone health, skin integrity, efficacy of digestion, urinary and bowel health, respiratory capacity, cardiovascular fitness and exercise response, and the psychological benefit that that comes from being upright when interacting with peers.[142] Children, with their lower center of mass, may not be quite as concerned about the consequences of a fall, but for adults, upright standing in HKAFOs may be made more challenging by concerns about the potential to fall, the risk of being injured, or the thought of being stranded on the ground due to inability to get back up.[143]

HKAFO DESIGN OPTIONS

As in the case of AFOs and KAFOs, HKAFOs can be fabricated with many different materials (e.g., metals, thermoplastics, carbon composites) and orthotic ankle, knee, and hip components. Historically, during the years immediately following the polio epidemic until the mid to late 1980s, orthotists fabricated HKAFOs by adding a hip joint and pelvic band to conventional KAFOs. To better meet the developmental and educational needs of children with myelomeningocele (spina bifida), conventional HKAFO designs evolved into standing frames, parapodiums, and swivel walkers. Building on this, a number of HKAFOs specifically designed to mechanically facilitate reciprocal gait were developed to meet the needs of persons with SCI.

Conventional HKAFOs

Figure 9-28 illustrates the configuration of conventional HKAFOs. These devices are designed to hold both lower extremities in a stable extended position for upright standing; persons wearing this orthosis use either a hop-to gait with walkers or a swing-through gait with a pair of crutches for ambulation. On rare occasions, a single HKAFO might be used for persons with neuromuscular or musculoskeletal

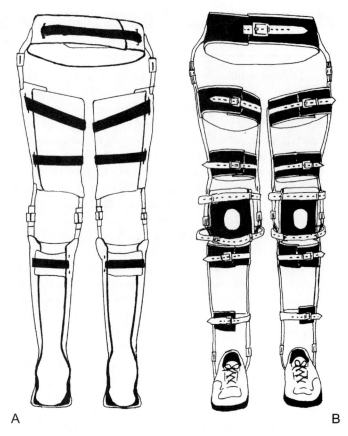

A   B

FIGURE 9-28 A, Example of a traditional metal and leather hip-knee-ankle-foot orthosis (HKAFO), with its pelvic band, orthotic hip joints and locks, proximal and distal thigh bands, orthotic knee joints and stabilization pads, proximal and distal calf bands, ankle joints, and stirrups. **B,** Themoplastic HKAFOs, typically lighter in weight than conventional HKAFOs, also have a pelvic band and orthotic hip and knee joints. Because they distribute forces over a wider thigh and calf band, an anterior knee stabilization pad may not be necessary. Many incorporate a solid-ankle or articulating ankle ankle-foot orthosis design, fitting inside the shoe rather than in an external stirrup.

impairment affecting one lower extremity. Even after the incorporation of lightweight thermoplastic or carbon composite materials, the energy cost of ambulation with conventional HKAFOs is significant and often functionally prohibitive. With rare exception, HKAFOs are used in the parallel bars, or on level surfaces with bilateral crutches or solid frame or reciprocal (nonrolling) walker.

The most distal component of the HKAFO is usually a solid ankle or dorsiflexion assist articulating ankle AFO. These are typically set in a few degrees of dorsiflexion to direct the tibia forward enough that the individual's weight line falls anterior to the knee and posterior to the hip in when in tripod standing position with crutches or a walker. Traditionally, the orthotic knee joint is locked into extension, although for persons with incomplete SCI capable of reciprocal gait, a stance control knee joint might be considered. Thermoplastic thigh cuffs are effective in resisting torsional forces that would otherwise act on the limb in standing. A variety of commercially available orthotic hip

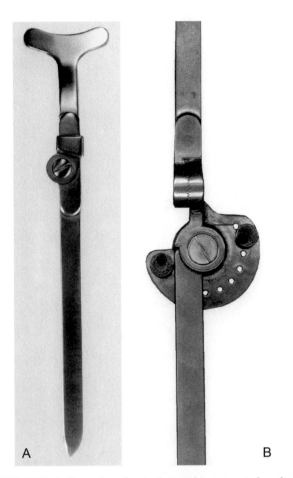

FIGURE 9-29 A, Examples of a single-axis hip joint. A drop lock holds the hip in extension in standing, but when pulled upward to disengage, allows free hip flexion for sitting. **B,** This hip joint allows controlled flexion and extension within a limited range of motion while limiting abduction/adduction and rotation.

joints include various single axis designs that can be used in locked position, allow free motion when unlocked, or allow motion only within a limited range (Figure 9-29). The axis of motion (center) of the orthotic hip joint must be positioned just proximal and anterior to the greater trochanter to best match the anatomical axis of motion of the hip. Because orthotic hip joints are fixed to the pelvic band and to lateral uprights of the thigh section, they effectively restrict abduction/adduction and rotation of the limb as well. Single axis hip joints meet the needs of most individuals who require HKAFOs to stand and to ambulate. There are also several types of dual-axis hip joints with separate mechanical control systems for flexion/extension and for abduction/adduction. The proximal pelvic band is positioned between the trochanter and iliac crest. The pelvic band provides solid support from a position slightly medial to the anterior superior iliac spines (ASIS) and around the posterior pelvis. The pelvic band can be fabricated from metal, laminated components, or thick thermoplastic, and is typically closed anteriorly by a belt or webbing with Velcro fastener.

For stability in standing, the individual typically stands in a tripod position, with crutch tips diagonally 12 to 18 inches forward and a slightly exaggerated lumbar lordosis.

This position ensures that the individual's center of gravity (weight line) falls posterior to the hip joint, creating an extension moment at the hip, achieving stability by alignment. To achieve forward motion, the individual uses the "head-hips" principle with shoulder joints a pivot point. (Figure 9-30) A quick forceful "pike" (chin tuck and forward inclination of the trunk) while pushing downward through the handles of the assistive device elevates the lower extremities from the ground. This is immediately followed by head, neck, and back extension to "throw" the lower extremities forward for the next initial contact. As soon as the feet contact the ground, the individual quickly advances the crutches to once again reach the stable "tripod" position.

To effectively use HKAFOs, hip and knee joints of the lower extremity must be flexible enough to be positioned in extension. Although exaggerated lumbar lordosis may compensate for mild hip flexion contracture in achieving upright position, over time and with repeated forceful loading of swing through gait, this lordosis will likely contribute to development of disabling low back pain. Prevention of flexion contracture or deformity of the hips and knees is a key component of physical therapy intervention, especially for growing children with myelomeningocele

Parapodiums, Standing Frames, and Swivel Walkers

This group of HKAFOs emerged to meet the developmental needs of children with myelomeningocele and cerebral palsy. As a group, these devices allow a young child to maintain upright standing posture and provide limited mobility for home and classroom use. Many include components to address alignment and control thoracic spine. Most can be used without an ambulatory assistive device (i.e., walker or crutches), allowing individuals to use their hands during activity. Cost may be lower than for conventional HKAFOs, because many can be fabricated from commercially available components and kits.

The simplest in this group of orthoses are *standing frames.* Prone standers primarily support the anterior surface of the body and can be positioned against a counter or table work surface so that the child can use the upper extremities for functional activities (Figure 9-31A). Some versions of prone standers incorporate wheels that children can use to propel themselves from place to place. Fully upright standing frames (see Figure 9-31, B) have restraining straps anterior to the knee and posterior to the pelvis, and provide circumferential support for the trunk. A lever is used to unlock the orthotic knee and hip joints of the device so the individual can move from standing to sitting.

Standers are used for children who are not developmentally ready to walk and for those with impairments so significant that the ability to walk is unlikely. Standing frames are most often prescribed to allow children with significant mobility impairment to participate in activities typically done in standing position in school and home settings.[144] Some children may fear falling and be reluctant to use full upright standers. Routine use of standing frames appears to limit severity of knee and hip flexion contracture, as

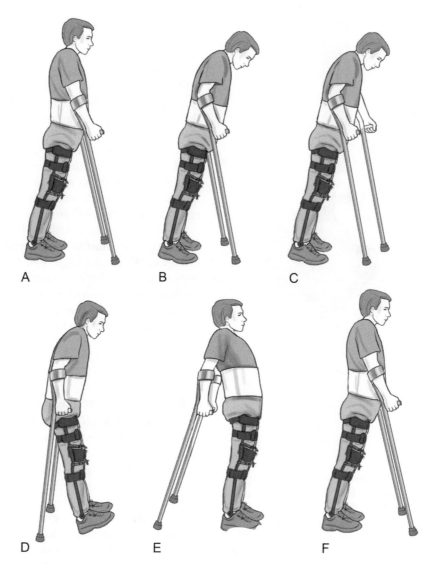

FIGURE 9-30 Illustration of the head-hips principle in swing through gait using bilateral KAFOs and lofstrand crutches, with shoulder joints acting as the fulcrum for movement. **A,** Resting position is a stable hips forward, shoulders back posture, with a tripod formed by the individuals feet and the tips of the crutches. **B,** Mobility is initaited with a quick and forceful chin tuck that **C,** is combined with downard pressure through the crutches to unweight the feet. **D,** A backward head movement then propels the lower body forward until **E,** the hips are forward and shoulders back to once again assume a stable inverted tripod position. Finally **F,** the individual quickly propels off of the crutches to move them anteriorly to the stable starting position. (From Sisto SA, et al. *Spinal Cord Injuries: Management and Rehabilitation.* St. Louis: Mosby, 2009, p. 388.)

well as decrease level of assistance needed and/or difficulty performing transfers and activities of daily living.[145] Standing frames provide an opportunity for children with mobility impairment to interact with peers at eye level, empowering them to participate more fully in academic and social activities.

Standing frames have also been adapted and developed for adults with neuromuscular impairments such as SCI, severe stroke, traumatic brain injury, and other diseases that compromise motor control such that independent standing is no longer possible. The benefits for adult users are the same as for children: better physiological function of many body structures and systems, enhanced ability to perform tasks usually performed in standing position, and the psychological benefits of being upright at one's full height.[146-148] Some specialized wheelchairs (both manual and powered versions) may have a built-in standing function.[149]

There are constraints to consider, however, when deciding if standing frames would be appropriate: (1) getting into and out of a standing frame may require considerable assistance; (2) the frame may not be easily mobile such that it should be pre-positioned before donning, (3) the frame may need adjustment or replacement as the child grows, and (4) the frame may require maintenance, mechanical hydraulic components, or replacement of worn straps and locking mechanisms.

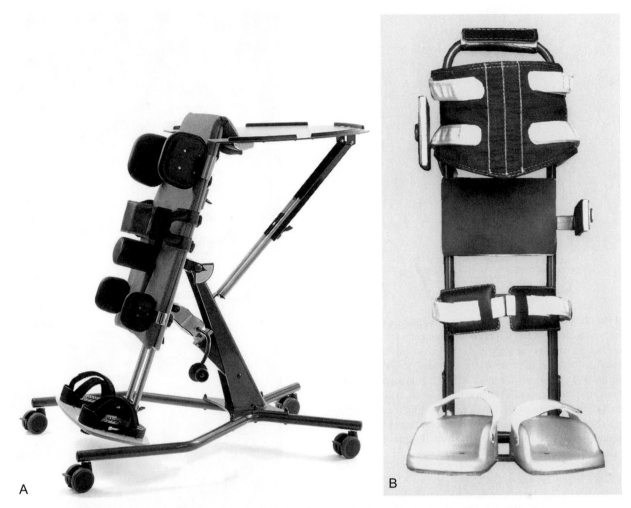

A

B

FIGURE 9-31 A, Example of a prone standing frame with adjustable angle of inclination. This device supports the anterior surface of the body to allow a child to work at a counter or table. Safety straps hold the pelvis and thighs against the anterior supports. **B,** Standing frame orthosis developed at Gillette Children's Hospital. The tubular frame has hip and knee joints, allowing the child to transfer into the device and then raise into standing. The fulcrum of the three-force system used to ensure hip extension is the broad posterior pelvic pad (at the center, without Velcro straps), with counterforces delivered by the anterior thoracic corset and the anterior kneepads. (A, Courtesy Rifton Equipment, Rifton, N.Y.)

The Parapodium (Ontario Crippled Children's Center in Toronto) and the Swivel Walker (Orthotic Research and Locomotor Assessment Unit, Oswestry, England), first introduced in the 1980s, are essentially standing frames with mobile attachment to a solid base (Figure 9-32).[150-152] Limited mobility is achieved by a combination of weight shifting and arm swing. While both are also available in adult sizes, they are primarily used for young children with myelomeningocele and cerebral palsy as an early aid to standing and mobility.[153,154]

HKAFOs for Reciprocal Gait

A number of lumbosacral-HKAFO systems have been developed for persons with high level (above T10 neurological level) spinal cord dysfunction (congenital and traumatic) who do not have motor function at the hip or higher. All use a lateral weight shift from one limb to the other as the basis for orthotic-assisted reciprocal gait. The hip guidance orthosis (HGO) was developed for children with myelomeningocele at the Orthotic Research and Locomotor Assessment Unit, Edinburgh, Scotland.[155,156] The ORLAU Parawalker uses similar principles to enable ambulation for adults with SCI.[157] The reciprocating (reciprocation, reciprocal) gait orthosis (RGO), developed at Louisiana State University assists walking using a dual cable-driven orthotic system.[158] The Advance Reciprocating Gait Orthosis (ARGO) with its simplified cable system was introduced in the 1990s.[159,160] The underlying goal for all of these orthoses was to achieve mobility with a lower energy cost than expended in a typical swing through gait pattern.[161] Many persons fitted with these devices use them primarily for exercise or activities in standing, finding that wheelchairs are more efficient for mobility tasks.[162] The complexity of these systems contribute to relatively frequent need for adjustment and repair

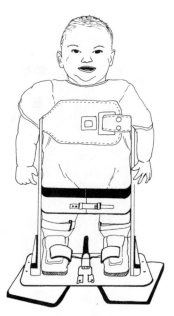

FIGURE 9-32 A young child with myelomeningocele, upright in an Orthotic Research and Locomotor Assessment Unit (ORLAU) swivel walker. The ankles are stabilized in a neutral position against the footplate, with knees in extension by a padded anterior bar, hips in extension by a broad pelvic band, and the trunk supported by a broad chest strap. Some versions have orthotic joints at the knee and hip that allow the child to sit but lock when the child is assisted into standing. The child learns to use reciprocal movement of the arms to shift weight from side to side, alternately advancing one of the swivel pads under the footplate.

with consistent use. Individuals who used the devices at least several times a week over long periods of time were less likely to develop serious decubitus ulcers or sustain fractures than their peers who discontinued use of this type of orthosis.[163,164]

Hip Guidance Orthosis and Parawalker

The HGO and the ORLEAU Parawalker allow individuals with impaired muscle performance (those unable to accomplish the lifting of body weight needed for swing through gait pattern with crutches) to "walk" with crutches with a lateral weight shift (Figure 9-33). The HGO and Parawalker require the use of an ambulatory assistive device; training usually begins in the parallel bars and progresses to over ground level surfaces using a rolling walker or bilateral Lofstrand crutches. The HGO's orthotic hip joint is stable when weight is borne through the lower extremity during stance but allows a pendular swing of the unweighted extremity for swing clearance. This occurs because of the rigid support that the HGO provides during single limb stance, keeping the limbs parallel in the coronal plane, which enhances swing limb clearance as the opposite limb advances.[165,166] In the original evaluation of the HGO prescribed for children with myelomeningocele, the ability to sit unsupported (hands free) for extended periods was the best predictor of successful use of the HGO.[156] The Parawalker, similar in design, provides more proximal

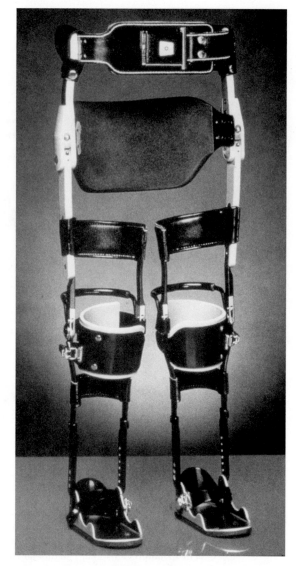

FIGURE 9-33 The hip guidance orthosis, usually worn over clothing, provides a rigid support system for the stance limb. Advancement of the swing limb occurs with its unweighting when the patient leans or shifts laterally onto the stable stance limb.

support to the thorax and trunk (making it even more rigid) and uses a smaller orthotic hip joint. Because of its higher proximal trim line, the Parawalker can be used for standing and limited mobility (i.e., therapeutic walking) for persons with SCI at upper thoracic levels.[167-169]

Reciprocal Gait Orthoses

The LSU RGO, originally designed for children with myelomeningocele and now used for adults with traumatic SCI, extends a pair of thermoplastic KAFOs upward to include a pelvis and thoracic bands (Figure 9-34); providing rigid stability for stance, it uses a cable-coupling system to provide hip joint motion for swing phase.[170,171] Its dual cable system operates by reinforcing extension of the stance limb as the swing limb flexes forward when unloaded by lateral weight shift. This reciprocal dual cable also reduces risk of "jack-knifing" during ambulation by preventing

ulcers, and/or scoliosis) than those with similar conditions who do not.[158]

Hybrid Orthoses: Functional Electrical Stimulation

The most recent investigations of reciprocal orthoses for persons with upper motor neuron SCI have added FES to HGO/Parawalker and RGO/ARGO designs.[175,176] SC orthotic knee joints (described in the section on KAFOs) have also been incorporated in hybrid RGO-FES systems, to afford a more natural pattern of swing limb advancement.[177] The major benefit of hybrid RGO-FES systems appears to be in greater distance covered, lower energy cost (as measured by physiological cost index), and somewhat faster walking speed.[174-176] It is important to note that, while such hybrid systems are promising, they do not fully restore the ability to walk at preinjury levels. Walking speeds with hybrid devices have been reported to be between 0.20 and 0.45 m/sec, while limited community walking becomes possible when walking speed is above 0.6 m/sec, and usual waking speed for healthy adults ranges from 1.0 to 1.3 m/sec, depending on height.[176-178]

IMPLICATIONS FOR REHABILITATION

When the rehabilitation team considers whether an orthosis that would facilitate therapeutic reciprocal walking would be appropriate for an individual with paralysis, the costs and benefits need to be weighed carefully. The individual and/or their caregivers must clearly understand that these devices cannot fully restore the ability to walk at what would be considered community level. They must explore and embrace the goals of therapeutic walking: enhancement of bone health, cardiovascular conditioning, digestive and urinary health, among others. For many individuals, gaining the motor skills necessary for safe use of the device may require substantial time and effort; training times reported in the literature range from 45 to 80 hours over a period of weeks to months. They must be ready to adhere to stretching protocols to ensure sufficient range of motion at hip, knee, and ankle so that the device will both fit and operate optimally. They must be prepared to work to improve muscle performance and postural control of trunk and upper extremities so that they can use the orthosis most effectively. They must be willing to maintain a stable weight so that the orthosis will fit over many months or years. They must have the postural control necessary to (eventually) don and doff the orthosis without substantial assistance. They must understand the design of the orthosis and the function of its components enough to recognize when maintenance, adjustment, or repair is necessary. This is quite a bit to commit to; it is often wise to have the person interested in pursuing use of such an orthosis interact with someone else who has successfully used one to get a clear sense of what is required and what the potential outcomes are.

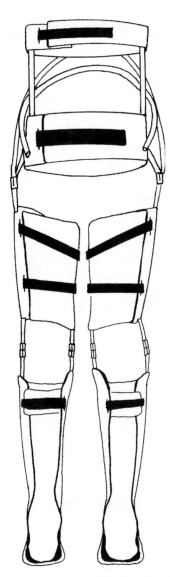

FIGURE 9-34 The reciprocal gait orthosis uses a dual cable system to couple flexion of one hip with extension of the other. This coupling assists forward progression of the swing limb while ensuring stability of the stance limb.

both hips from flexing at the same time. Like the HGO and Parawalker, the RGO requires the person to use an assistive device (rolling walker, bilateral Lofstrand crutches, bilateral canes), relying on upper extremity motor control and muscle performance to a large degree to operate the system. The ARGO is an adaptation of the design, using a single cable, and engineered to allow standing with unilateral or no upper extremity support.[172,173] A prototype for an adjustable AGRO has been described; this would provide opportunity for a trial of ambulation with ARGO during rehabilitation to assist decision making about capacity to use the device before a custom ARGO is fabricated.[174] There is some evidence that persons with neuromuscular conditions who consistently use an RGO or ARGO for therapeutic walking are less likely to develop significant secondary complications (i.e., contractures, decubitus

CASE EXAMPLE 5

A Young Child with Myelomeningocele

J. B. is an 18-month-old girl with myelomeningocele at L1 neurological level. Her spinal defect was surgically repaired the day after her birth. A ventriculoperitoneal shunt was placed to control hydrocephalus when she was 2 months old. She has attended a spinal bifida clinic at a regional children's hospital, 2 hours from her home, and participated in a home-based "birth to three" program since birth.

Currently, there is no active contraction of muscle in either lower extremity and no evidence of withdrawal response to painful stimuli at or below the L1 dermatome or myotome. J. B. has consistently worn night splints to prevent plantarflexion contractures at the ankle. At 14 months of age, she sustained a midfemoral fracture while playing on the floor with her brothers; the fracture was managed by immobilization in a spica cast for 6 weeks. She has developed soft tissue tightness such that her lower extremities are in a somewhat abducted and externally rotated position at the hip. Knee range of motion is sufficient for sitting and supported standing.

J. B.'s primary means of mobility is by an upper extremity powered commando crawl when playing with her brothers and similar-aged peers. For longer distances, she is wheeled in a stroller by a family member. Recently, her behavior suggests she is frustrated by her inability to pull into standing and

her limited mobility. Her family and therapists have returned to the spina bifida clinic for evaluation of her readiness for orthotic intervention that would allow her to stand and walk.

Questions to Consider

- What additional information would be important for the clinic team to gather as they prepare to make recommendations about orthotic options for J. B.? What additional tests and measures might be important to use?
- Given her current level of function and her lower motor neuron deficit, what orthotic option is the team likely to consider: KAFO or HKAFO? Why?
- If the team opts for an HKAFO, which design would you recommend: a thermoplastic HKAFO, standing frame, parapodium, swivel walker, or HKAFO designed for reciprocal gait? What are the benefits and tradeoffs of each? Why have you chosen the one you are recommending for J. B.?
- In addition to learning to stand and perhaps to ambulate with her HKAFO, what other motor tasks will J. B. and her family have to master to use the HKAFO functionally?

CASE EXAMPLE 6

An Adult with Traumatic Spinal Cord Injury

L. F. is a 20-year-old man who sustained multiple gunshot wounds to his abdomen during an armed robbery of the convenience store where he worked. He was airlifted to a regional level 1 trauma center for initial evaluation. He underwent several surgeries to repair internal organs, remove his spleen, and stabilize burst fractures of T-9 to T-11 vertebral bodies with fusion. Once stable, L. F. was transferred to a rehabilitation center wearing a TLSO for a 4-week stay. He is now living at home and the TLSO has been discontinued. L. F. has continued his rehabilitation on an outpatient basis for the past 3 months. He is independent in wheelchair mobility on level surface, ramps, and curbs. He has been actively involved in an FES program using the ERGYS cycle ergometer for the past 2 months. He has expressed interest in walking for cardiovascular fitness exercise, perhaps combining an orthosis with FES.

At present, there is no apparent neuromuscular or sensory function below the level of T-9. Deep tendon reflexes are +3 at knee and +4 at ankle, with occasional spasm of lower extremities, typically a sign of bladder infection or skin irritation. Range of motion is within normal limits at ankle and knee, but there are hip flexion contractures of 10 degrees bilaterally.

Questions to Consider

- What additional information would be important for the clinic team to gather as they prepare to make recommendations about orthotic options for L. F.? What additional tests and measures might be important to use?
- Given L. F.'s current level of function and his upper motor neuron deficit, what orthotic options are the team members likely to consider: KAFO or HKAFO? Why?
- If the team opts for an HKAFO, which design would you recommend they use: a conventional thermoplastic HKAFO with locked hip and knees or an HKAFO that would allow reciprocal gait? What are the benefits and tradeoffs of each? Why have you chosen the one that you are recommending?
- In addition to learning to stand and ambulate with his new HKAFO, what other motor tasks must L. F. master to use his orthosis functionally?
- How will the team evaluate the effectiveness and efficiency of the orthosis as L. F. becomes more adept at using it?

OUTCOME MEASURES IN ORTHOTIC REHABILITATION

How do the health care team, the individual using an orthosis and their caregivers, and the payers of the health care system determine successful use of a lower extremity orthosis, whether it be as simple as a UCBL insert for a child with mild diplegic cerebral palsy, an adult using an articulating AFO, a person with postpolio syndrome using a SC-KAFO, or a person with SCI using an ARGO? Initial criteria to consider might include:

- Can the person don and doff the orthosis independently?
- Does the person understand how the orthosis should fit on the limb, and can the person recognize signs that fit may not be appropriate (especially for growing children and for adults with peripheral or central sensory impairment)?
- Can the person transition from sitting to standing and back to sitting safely, independently, and with reasonable effort?
- Does the person have sufficient postural control to use the device not only on level nonresistant surfaces (e.g., tile or wood floors) but also on other surfaces (e.g., carpet, grass, inclines, stairs), which are likely to be encountered in the course of daily life?
- Children often play on the floor, and adults are often quite concerned about being stranded on the floor if they fall. Can the person transition from the floor to standing safely, independently, and with reasonable effort? If not, can the person direct those who would offer assistance?
- Does the person know how to manage his or her body and assistive devices in case of a fall?
- Does the person understand the care and maintenance requirements of the device?

These questions, while ensuring that the individual is able to use the orthosis safely, do not sufficiently address the efficacy of the orthosis in enhancing the individual's ability to walk. While observational gait analysis might allow the orthotist and physical therapist to evaluate changes an orthosis effects at each subphase of the gait cycle, this description of the quality of walking is not enough evidence to justify orthotic intervention. The ceiling effects and poor ecological validity of the distance criteria for independent locomotion of measures such as Functional Independence Measure are likewise insufficient.[179] A variety of outcome measures must be used to address efficacy of an orthosis and the physical therapy intervention that facilitates its use.

Walking Speed

Probably the most robust indicator of the ability to walk is walking (gait) speed. Although technology such as motion analysis and the GAITRite system provide precise data about gait velocity, walking speed can be quickly and easily captured using a stopwatch over a known distance.[178,180] There is clear evidence for validity, reliability, and responsiveness of walking speed (measured over 10 m or over 4-m distances), as well as information about typical walking performance values, and criteria for limited versus full community ambulation ability for most of the medical diagnoses in which a lower extremity

orthosis may be prescribed (stroke, SCI, cerebral palsy, traumatic brain injury, among others).[181-189] Documenting comfortable and maximum walking speed at intervals without and with the orthosis at time of delivery, and change in walking speed over the course of physical therapy intervention, along with discussion of the change in walking speed with respect to age-base and disease-reference norms provide powerful information about efficacy of intervention.

Endurance During Walking

The ability to sustain walking over a period of time is also a key outcome of orthotic and physical therapy intervention. The most frequently used measure of endurance while walking is the 6-minute walk test (6MW), in which the distance that an individual walks (with rests as needed) during a 6-minute period is measured. Originally developed for persons unable to perform treadmill or cycle ergometer stress tests because of congestive heart failure, the 6MW has been used for many of the groups of patients who would benefit from orthoses.[190] Clinometric properties of the 6MW have been evaluated for persons with stroke, SCI, cerebral palsy, traumatic brain injury, myelomeningocele, and chronic poliomyelitis.[191-196]

A self-report indicator of effort of physical activity that has also been used extensively in the clinical research literature is Rating of Perceived Exertion (RPE). In his original work, Borg presented a scale ranging from 6 (no effort) to 20 (maximum effort)[197]; a modified version, which uses a 1 to 10 scale (for adults) or color-coded schematic pictures of the face (for children and those with cognitive dysfunction) may be more interpretable for patients.[198,199] The question that use of RPE scale addresses is, "Does the orthosis reduce the perceived work (effort) of walking?" RPE scales have been used to assess efficacy of therapeutic intervention for persons with stroke, brain injury, SCI, and cerebral palsy.[176,200-202]

Mobility and Balance While Walking

The ability to change direction and transition between surfaces (i.e., sit to stand) is also a key aspect of successful use of a lower extremity orthosis. During the Timed Up-and-Go (TUG) test, an individual must rise from a seated position, walk forward over a 10-m distance, turn around, walk back to the chair, and return to sitting, either at a usual pace or as quickly as safely able.[203] Because most lower extremity orthoses constrain joint movement, and many of those who use them have neuromuscular impairments that place them at risk for falling, the TUG may provide a snapshot of dynamic postural control during walking with an orthosis. The TUG has been successfully used to assess functional status and predict outcomes in persons with stroke, in children with cerebral palsy, brain injury, and myelomeningocele, and in persons with SCI.[193,204-209]

SUMMARY

This chapter explores the biomechanical design and component options of lower extremity orthoses used to facilitate the ability to walk for persons with a variety of neuromuscular impairments, and at various ages and developmental stages of the life span. We have discovered that no orthosis can make walking "normal," although an appropriate orthosis can make walking more functional and less energy costly. We now can evaluate how an orthosis will impact each of the rockers of stance phase, as well as the ability to clear the limb during swing phase. We now have ideas about how footwear, such as an athletic shoe that provides a cushion heel and a rocker bottom, may compensate if an orthosis limits forward progression over the foot during stance. We have discovered that the selection of an appropriate orthosis involves input from many members of the rehabilitation team, not the least being the person who will wear the orthosis and his or her caregivers. We certainly have gained an appreciation that there is no "one size fits all" when it comes to choosing an orthosis, but that orthotic prescription requires thoughtful deliberation about both the functional benefits and tradeoffs, as well as the financial cost of the device. We have learned that using an orthosis effectively requires much more than simply putting it on; there must be adequate time filled with appropriately challenging activities so that motor practice can build skill, postural control, and endurance necessary for functional walking. Finally, we have begun to consider strategies to assess outcomes of orthotic and physical therapy interventions for persons who require an AFO, KAFO, or HKAFO to accomplish their mobility goals.

ACKNOWLEDGMENTS

The author would like to recognize professional colleagues Robert S. Lin, CPO (Director of Pediatric Clinical Services and Academic Programs, Hanger Orthopedic Group at the Connecticut Children's Medical Center, Hartford, Conn.), Thomas V. DiBello, BS, CO (President, Dynamic Orthotics and Prosthetics, Inc., Houston, Texas), and James H. Campbell, PhD, CO (Director of Research and Development, Engineering and Technical Services, Becker Orthopedic, Troy Mich.), whose excellent chapters on ankle-foot orthoses, knee-ankle-foot orthoses, and hip-knee-ankle-foot orthoses in the previous editions of this text provided a solid foundation for the this integrative chapter.

REFERENCES

1. Sheffler LR, Bailey SN, Chae J. Spatiotemporal and kinematic effect of peroneal nerve stimulation versus an ankle-foot orthosis in patients with multiple sclerosis: a case series. *Phys Med Rehabil.* 2009;1(7):604–611.
2. Rosenbloom KB. Pathology-designed custom molded foot orthoses. *Clin Podiatr Med Surg.* 2011;28(1):171–187.
3. Trepman E, Donnelly P. Patellar tendon-bearing, patten-bottom caliper suspension orthosis in active Ankle Charcot arthropathy: crutch-free ambulation with no weight bearing in the foot. *Foot Int.* 2002;23(4):335–339.
4. Lin SS, Sabharwal S, Bibbo C. Orthotic and bracing principles in neuromuscular foot and ankle problems. *Foot Ankle Clin.* 2000;5(2):235–264.
5. Pavlik AJ. The effect of long-term ankle-foot orthosis use on gait in the poststroke population. *J Prosthet Orthot.* 2008;20(2):49–52.
6. Woo R. Spasticity: orthopedic perspective. *J Child Neurol.* 2001;16(1):47–53.
7. Lemaire E, Necsulescu L, Greene G. Service delivery trends for a physical rehabilitation outreach program. *Disabil Rehabil.* 2006;28(21):1349–1359.
8. Morris C, Newdick H, Johnson A. Variations in the orthotic management of cerebral palsy. *Child Care Health Dev.* 2002;28(2):139–147.
9. Bedotto RA. Biomechanical assessment and treatment in lower extremity prosthetics and orthotics: a clinical perspective. *Phys Med Rehabil Clin N Am.* 2006;17(1):203–243.
10. Davids JR, Rowan F, Davis RB. Indications for orthoses to improve gait in children with cerebral palsy. *J Am Acad Orthop Surg.* 2007;15(3):178–188.
11. Capjon H, Bjørk IT. Rehabilitation after multilevel surgery in ambulant spastic children with cerebral palsy: children and parent experiences. *Dev Neurorehabil.* 2010;13(3):182–191.
12. Basford JR, Johnson SJ. Form may be as important as function in orthotic acceptance: a case report. *Arch Phys Med Rehabil.* 2002;83(3):433–435.
13. Chang MW, Cardenas DD. Ankle-foot orthoses: clinical implications. *Phys Med Rehabil..* 2000;14(3):435–554.
14. Perry J, Burnfield JM. Basic Functions. In: Perry J, Burnfield JM, eds. Gait Analysis: Normal and Pathological Function. 2nd ed. Thorofare, NJ: Slack; 2010:19–47.
15. Perry J. Normal and pathological gait. In: Hsu HD, Michael JW, Fisk JR, eds. Atlas of Orthoses and Assistive Devices. 4th ed. Philadelphia: Mosby; 2008:61–81.
16. Michael JW. Lower limb orthoses. In: Hsu HD, Michael JW, Fisk JR, eds. Atlas of Orthoses and Assistive Devices. 4th ed. Philadelphia: Mosby Elsevier; 2008:343–356.
17. Janisse DJ. Shoes and shoe modifications. In: Hsu HD, Michael JW, Fisk JR, eds. Atlas of Orthoses and Assistive Devices. 4th ed. Philadelphia: Mosby; 2008:325–334.
18. McHugh B. Analysis of body-device interface forces in the sagittal plane for patients wearing ankle-foot orthoses. *Prosthet Orthot Int.* 1999;23(1):75–81.
19. Chambers RB, Elftman N, Bowker JH. Orthotic management of the neuropathic and dysvascular patient. In: Hsu HD, Michael JW, Fisk JR, eds. Atlas of Orthoses and Assistive Devices. 4th ed. Philadelphia: Mosby; 2008:391–410.
20. Mavroidis C, Ranky RG, Sivak ML, et al. Patient specific ankle-foot orthoses using rapid prototyping. *J Neuroeng Rehabil.* 2011;8(1). Available at: http://www.jneuroengrehab.com/content/pdf/1743-0003-8-1.pdf.
21. Brncick M. Computer automated design and computer automated manufacture. *Phys Med Rehabil Clin N Am.* 2000; 11(3):701–713.
22. Edelstein JE, Bruckner J. Ankle foot orthoses. In: Edelstein EJ, Bruckner J, eds. Orthotics: A Comprehensive Clinical Approach. Thorofare, NJ: Slack; 2002:39–57.
23. Franceschini M, Massucci M, Ferrari L, Agosti A, Paroli C. Effects of an ankle foot orthosis on spatiotemporal parameters and energy cost of human gait. *Clin Rehabil.* 2003;17: 368–372.
24. Meadows B, Bowers RJ, Owen E. Biomechanics of the hip, knee and ankle. In: Hsu HD, Michael JW, Fisk JR, eds. Atlas of Orthoses and Assistive Devices. 4th ed. Philadelphia: Mosby; 2008:299–310.

25. Hanna D, Harvey RL. Review of preorthotic biomechanical considerations. *Top Stroke Rehabil.* 2001;7(4):29–37.

26. Lin SS, Sabharwal S, Bibbo C. Orthotic and bracing principles in neuromuscular foot and ankle problems. *Foot Ankle Clin.* 2000;5(2):235–264.

27. Iwata M, Kondo I, Sato Y, Satoh K, Soma M, Tsushima E. An ankle-foot orthosis with inhibitor bar: effect on hemiplegic gait. *Arch Phys Med Rehabil.* 2003;84(6):924–927.

28. Maeda N, Kato J, Azuma Y, et al. Energy expenditure and walking ability in stroke patients: their improvement by ankle-foot orthoses. *Isokinetics Ex Sci.* 2009;17(2):57–62.

29. Buckon CE, Thomas SS, Jakobson-Huston S, et al. Comparison of three ankle foot orthosis configurations for children with spastic diplegia. *Dev Med Child Neurol.* 2004;46(9):590–598.

30. Brophy LS. Gait in cerebral palsy. *Ortho Phys Ther Clin N Am.* 2001;10(1):55–76.

31. Koch M, Mostert J, Heersema D, Keyser J. Tremor in multiple sclerosis. *J Neurol.* 2007;254(2):133–145.

32. Khan F. Rehabilitation in Guillain-Barre syndrome. *Aust Fam Physician.* 2004;33(12):1013–1017.

33. Morris C. A review of the efficacy of lower limb orthoses used for cerebral palsy. *Dev Med Child Neurol.* 2002;44(3):205–211.

34. Fröberg A, Komi P, Ishikawa M, Movin T, Arndt A. Force in the Achilles tendon during walking with ankle foot orthosis. *Am J Sports Med.* 2009;37(6):1200–1207.

35. Belt EA, Mäenpää H, Lehto MU. Outcome of ankle arthrodesis performed by dowel technique in patients with rheumatic disease. *Foot Ankle Int.* 2001;22(8):666–669.

36. Rogozinski BM, Davids JR, Davis RB, Jameson GG, Blackhurst DW. The efficacy of the floor-reaction ankle-foot orthosis in children with cerebral palsy. *J Bone Joint Surg Am.* 2009; 91(10):2440–2447.

37. Polliack AA, Elliot S, Caves C, McNeal DR, Landsberger SE. Lower extremity orthoses for children with myelomeningocele: user and orthotist perspectives. *J Prosthet Orthot.* 2001; 13(4):123–129.

38. Kelley C, DiBello TV. Orthotic assessment for individuals with postpolio syndrome: a classification system. *J Prosthet Orthot.* 2007;19(4):109–113.

39. Luc M, Bensoussan L, Viton J, et al. Gait recovery in a distal spinal muscular atrophy patient wearing a patellar tendon-bearing orthosis and orthopaedic shoes. *Stiftelsen Rehabilitering-sinformation.* 2007;39(2):181–184.

40. Khaira HS, Coddington T, Drew A, Roberts PN, Imray CH. Patellar tendon bearing orthosis—application as adjunctive treatment in healing of lower-limb tissue loss. *Eur J Vasc Endovasc Surg.* 1998;16(6):485–488.

41. Rodriguez-Merchan EC. Ankle surgery in haemophilia with special emphasis on arthroscopic debridement. *Haemophilia.* 2008;14(5):913–919.

42. Sella EJ, Barrette C. Staging of Charcot neuroarthropathy along the medial column of the foot in the diabetic patient. *J Foot Ankle Surg.* 1999;38(1):34–40 86–87, 89.

43. Sarmiento A. A functional below-the-knee brace for tibial fractures: a report on its use in one hundred thirty-five cases. *J Bone Joint Surg Am.* 2007;89(Suppl 2, Part 2):157–169.

44. Koller A, Meissner SA, Podella M, Fiedler R. Orthotic management of Charcot feet after external fixation surgery. *Clin Podiatr Med Surg.* 2007;24(3):583–599.

45. Inman VT. Dual axis ankle control systems and the UCBL shoe insert: biomechanical considerations. *Bull Prosthet Res.* 1969;(10–11):130–146.

46. Carlson J, Berglund C. An effective orthotic design for controlling the unstable subtalar joint. *Orthot Prosthet.* 1979; 33(1):39–49.

47. Leung AK, Mak AF, Evans JH. Biomedical gait evaluation of the immediate effect of orthotic treatment for flexible flat foot. *Prosthet Orthot Int.* 1998;22(1):25–34.

48. Hylton N. Postural and functional impact of dynamic AFOs and FOs in a pediatric population. *J Prothstet Orthot.* 1989;2(1):40–53.

49. Naslund A, Tamm M, Ericsson A, vonWendt L. Dynamic ankle foot orthoses as a part of treatment in children with spastic diplegia. *Physiother Res Int.* 2003;8(2):59–68.

50. Romkes J, Brunner R. Comparison of a dynamic and a hinged ankle-foot orthosis by gait analysis in patients with hemiplegic cerebral palsy. *Gait Posture.* 2002;15(1):18–24.

51. Radtka SA, Skinner SR, Dixon DM, Johanson ME. A comparison of gait with solid, dynamic and no ankle foot orthoses in children with spastic cerebral palsy. *Phys Ther.* 1997; 77(4):395–409.

52. Lam WK, Leong JCY, Li YH, Hu Y, Lu WW. Biomechanical and electromyographic evaluation of ankle foot orthosis and dynamic ankle foot orthosis in spastic cerebral palsy. *Gait Posture.* 2005;22(3):189–197.

53. Ounpuu S, Bell KJ, Davis RB, DeLuca PA. An evaluation of the posterior leaf spring orthosis using joint kinematics and kinetics. *J Pediatr Orthop.* 1996;16(3):378–384.

54. Sumiya T, Suzuki Y, Kasahara T. Stiffness control in posterior-type plastic ankle-foot orthoses: effect of ankle trimline. Part 2: Orthosis characteristics and orthosis/patient matching. *Prosthet Orthot Int.* 1996;20(2):132–137.

55. Lewallen J, Miedaner J, Amyx S, Sherman J. Effect of three styles of custom ankle foot orthoses on the gait of stroke patients while walking on level and inclined surfaces. *J Prosthet Orthot.* 2010;22(2):78–83.

56. Sienko-Thomas S, Buckon SE, Jakobson-Huston S, Sussman MD, Aiona MD. Stair locomotion in children with spastic hemiplegia: the impact of three different ankle foot orthosis configurations. *Gait Posture.* 2002;16(3):180–187.

57. Radtka SA, Oliveira GB, Lindstrom KE, Borders MD. The kinematic and kinetic effects of solid, hinged, and no ankle–foot orthoses on stair locomotion in healthy adults. *Gait Posture.* 2006;24(2):211–218.

58. Buckon CE, Sienko-Thomas S, Jakobson-Huston S, Moor M, Sussman M, Aiona M. Comparison of three anklefoot orthosis configurations for children with spastic diplegia. *Dev Med Child Neurol.* 2004;46(9):590–598.

59. Bielby SA, Warrick TJ, Benson D, et al. Trimline severity significantly affects rotational stiffness of ankle-foot orthosis. *J Prosthet Orthot.* 2010;22(4):204–210.

60. Desloovere K, Molenaers G, Van Gestel L, et al. How can push off be preserved during use of an ankle foot orthosis in children with hemiplegia? A prospective controlled study. *Gait Posture.* 2006;24:142–151.

61. Van Gestel L, Molenaers G, Huenaerts C, Seyler J, Desloovere K. Effect of dynamic orthoses on gait: a retrospective control study in children with hemiplegia. *Dev Med Child Neurol.* 2008;50(1):63–67.

62. Bartonek A, Eriksson M, Guitierrez-Farewik EM. A new carbon fibre spring orthosis for children with plantarflexor weakness. *Gait Posture.* 2007;25(4):652–656.

63. Wolf SI, Alimusaj M, Rettig O, Doderlein L. Dynamic assist by carbon fiber spring AFOs for patients with myelomeningocele. *Gait Posture.* 2008;28(1):175–177.

64. Bartonek A, Erisson M, Gutierrez-Farewik EM. Effects of carbon fibre spring orthoses on gait in ambulatory children with motor disorders and plantarflexion weakness. *Dev Med Child Neurol.* 2007;49(8):615–620.

65. Stein RB, Chong S, Everaert DG. A multicenter trial of a foot-drop stimulator controlled by a tilt sensor. *Neurorehabil Neural Repair.* 2006;20(3):371–379.

66. Dunning K, Black K, Harrison A, McBride K, Israel S. Neuroprosthesis peroneal functional electrical stimulation in the acute inpatient rehabilitation setting: a case series. *Phys Ther.* 2009;89(5):499–506.

67. Sheffler LR, Hennessey MT, Naples GG, Chae J. Peroneal nerve stimulation versus an ankle foot orthosis for correction of foot-drop in stroke: impact on functional ambulation. *Neurorehabil Neural Repair.* 2006;20(3):355–360.

68. Sabut SK, Sikdar C, Mondal R, Kumar R, Mahadevappa M. Restoration of gait and motor recovery by functional electrical stimulation therapy in persons with stroke. *Disabil Rehabil.* 2010;32(19):1594–1603.

69. Ring H, Treger I, Gruendlinger L, Hausdorff JM. Neuroprosthesis for footdrop compared with an ankle-foot orthosis: effects on postural control during walking. *J Stroke Cerebrovasc Dis.* 2009;18(1):41–47.

70. Sheffler LR, Bailey SN, Chae J. Spatiotemporal and kinematic effect of peroneal nerve stimulation versus an ankle-foot orthosis in patients with multiple sclerosis: a case series. *Phys Med Rehabil.* 2009;1(7):604–611.

71. Barrett CL, Mann GE, Taylor PN, Strike P. A randomized trial to investigate the effects of functional electrical stimulation and therapeutic exercise on walking performance for people with multiple sclerosis. *Multiple Sclerosis.* 2009;15(4):493–504.

72. Mann GE, Finn SM, Taylor PN. A pilot study to investigate the feasibility of electrical stimulation to assist gait in Parkinson's disease. *Neuromodulation.* 2008;11(2):143–149.

73. Danielsson A, Sunnerhagen KS. Energy expenditure in stroke subjects walking with a carbon composite ankle foot orthosis. *J Rehabil Med.* 2004;36(4):165–168.

74. Brehm MA, Harlaar J, Schwartz M. Effect of ankle-foot orthoses on walking efficiency and gait in children with cerebral palsy. *J Rehabil Med.* 2008;40(7):529–534.

75. Fatone S, Gard SA, Malas BS. Effect of ankle-foot orthosis alignment and foot-plate length on the gait of adults with post-stroke hemiplegia. *Arch Phys Med Rehabil.* 2009;90(5):810–818.

76. Lewallen J, Miedaner J, Amyx S, Sherman J. Effect of three styles of custom ankle foot orthoses on the gait of stroke patients while walking on level and inclined surfaces. *J Prosthet Orthot.* 2010;22(2):78–83.

77. Romkes J, Hell AK, Brunner R. Changes in muscle activity in children with hemiplegic cerebral palsy while walking with and without ankle–foot orthoses. *Gait Posture.* 2006; 24(4):467–474.

78. Cakar E, Durmus O, Tekin L, Dincer U, Kiralp MZ. The ankle-foot orthosis improves balance and reduces fall risk of chronic spastic hemiparetic patients. *Eur J Phys Rehabil Med.* 2010;46(3):363–368.

79. Cattaneo D, Marazzini F, Crippa A, Cardini R. Do static or dynamic AFOs improve balance? *Clin Rehabil.* 2002; 16(8):894–899.

80. Kobayashi T, Leung AKL, Hutchins SW. Design and effect of ankle-foot orthoses proposed to influence muscle tone. *J Prosthet Orthot.* 2011;23(2):52–57.

81. Duncan WR, Mott DH. Foot reflexes and the use of "inhibitive cast". *Foot Ankle.* 1983;4(3):145–148.

82. Bertoti DB. Effect of short leg casting on ambulation in children with cerebral palsy. *Phys Ther.* 1986;66(10):1522–1529.

83. Lohman M, Goldstein H. Alternative strategies in tone reducing AFO design. *J Prosthet Orthot.* 1993;5(1):21–24.

84. Ibuki A, Back T, Rogers D, et al. An investigation of the neurophysiological effect of tone-reducing AFOs on reflex excitability in subjects with spasticity following stroke while standing. *Prosthet Orthot Int.* 2010;34(2):154–165.

85. Nash B, Roller JM, Parker MG. The effects of tone-reducing orthotics on walking of an individual after incomplete spinal cord injury. *J Neurol Phys Ther.* 2008;32(1):39–47.

86. Blackburn M, van Vliet P, Mockett SP. Reliability of measurements obtained with the Modified Ashworth Scale in the lower extremities of people with stroke. *Phys Ther.* 2002;82(1):25–34.

87. Morris C, Condie D, eds. Recent Developments in Healthcare for Cerebral Palsy: Implications and Opportunities for Orthotics. Copehangen Denmark: International Society for Prosthetics and Orthotics; 2009.

88. Condie E, ed. Report of a Consensus Conference on the Orthotic Management of Stroke Patients. Copehangen Denmark: International Society for Prosthetics and Orthotics; 2004.

89. Ramstrand N, Ramstrand S. The effect of ankle foot orthoses on balance: a systematic review. *J Prosthet Orthot.* 2010; 22(4 S):4–23.

90. Malas BS. The effect of ankle-foot orthoses on balance: a clinical perspective. *J Prosthet Orthot.* 2010;22(4 S):24–33.

91. Stevens P. Prevalence of balance compromise in commonly treated patient populations: an introduction to the academy's state of the science conference on the effects of ankle-foot orthoses on balance. *J Prosthet Orthot.* 2010;22(4 S):1–3.

92. Cattaneo D, Marazizini F, Crippa A, Cardini R. Do static or dynamic AFOs improve balance? *Clin Rehabil.* 2002;16(8):894–899.

93. Pavlik A. The effect of long term ankle foot orthosis use on gait in the post-stroke population. *J Prosthet Orthot.* 2008;20(2):49–52.

94. Kott KM, Held SL. Effects of orthoses on upright functional skills of children and adolescents with cerebral palsy. *Pediatr Phys Ther.* 2002;14(4):119–207.

95. Buurke JH, Nijlant JMM, et al. The effect of an ankle foot orthosis on walking ability in chronic stroke patients. A randomized controlled trial. *Clin Rehabil.* 2004;18(5):550–557.

96. Wang RY, Yen L, Lee CC, et al. Effects of an ankle-foot orthosis on balance performance in patients with hemiparesis of different durations. *Clin Rehabil.* 2005;19(1):37–44.

97. Wang RY, Lin PY, Lee CC, Yang YR. Gait and balance performance improvements attributable to ankle foot orthoses in subjects with hemiparesis. *Am J Phys Med Rehabil.* 2007; 86(7):556–562.

98. Pohl M, Mehrholz J. Immediate effects of an individually designed functional ankle foot orthosis on stance and gait in hemiparetic patients. *Clin Rehabil.* 2006;20:324–330.

99. Merritt JL, Yoshida MK. Knee-ankle-foot orthoses: indications and practical applications of long leg braces. *Phys Med Rehabil.* 2000;14(3):395–422.

100. Herbert JS. Ambulatory KAFOs: a physiatry perspective. *J Prosthet Orthot.* 2006;18(Proceedings 7):P169–P174.

101. Kenton KR, Irby SE. Ambulatory KAFOs: a biomechanical engineering perspective. *J Prosthet Orthot.* 2006;18(Proceedings 7): P175–P182.

102. Merkel KD, Miller NE, Westbrook PR, Merritt JL. Energy expenditure of paraplegic patients standing and walking with two knee-ankle-foot orthoses. *Arch Phys Med Rehabil.* 1984;65(3):121–124.

103. Michael JW. KAFOs for ambulation: an orthotist's perspective. *J Prosthet Orthot.* 2006;18(Proceedings 7):P187–P191.

104. Hurley EA. Use of KAFOs for patients with cerebral vascular accident, traumatic brain injury, and spinal cord injury. *J Prosthet Orthot.* 2006;18(Proceedings 7):P199–P201.

105. Edelstein JE. Ambulatory KAFOs: a physical therapist's perspective. *J Prosthet Orthot.* 2006;18(Proceedings 7):P183–P186.

106. Perry J, Burnfield JM. Pathological mechanisms. In: Perry J, Burnfield JM, eds. Gait Analysis: Normal and Pathological Function. 2nd ed. Thorofare NJ: Slack; 2010:165–174.

107. Zissimopoulos A, Fatone S, Gard SA. Biomechanical and energetic effects of a stance-control orthotic knee joint. *J Rehabil Res Dev.* 2007;44(4):503–513.

108. Kubota KL, Eberly V, Mulroy SJ. Lower extremity orthotic prescription. In: Field-Foote E, ed. Spinal Cord Injury Rehabilitation. Philadelphia: FA Davis; 2009:191–314.

109. Kermoian R, Johanson ME, Butler EE, Skinnner S. Development of gait. In: Rose J, Gamble JG, eds. Human Walking. 3rd ed. Philadelphia: Lippincott Williams & Wilkins; 2006:119–130.

110. Bakker JP, Groot IJ, Beckerman H, Jong BA, Lankhorst GJ. The effects of knee-ankle-foot orthoses in the treatment of Duchenne muscular dystrophy: review of the literature. *Clin Rehabil.* 2000;14(4):343–359.

111. Garralda ME, Muntoni F, Cunniff A, Caneja AD. Knee-ankle-foot orthosis in children with duchenne muscular dystrophy: user views and adjustment. *Eur J Paediatr Neurol.* 2006;10(4):186–191.

112. Siegel IM. Kinematics of gait in Duchenne muscular dystrophy: implications for orthotic management. *J Neurol Rehabil.* 1997;11(3):169–173.

113. Taktak DM, Bowker P. Lightweight, modular knee-ankle-foot orthosis for Duchenne muscular dystrophy: design, development, and evaluation. *Arch Phys Med Rehabil.* 1995;76(12):1156–1162.

114. Kauffman KR, Irby SE. Ambulatory KAFOs: a biomechanical engineering perspective. *J Prosthet Orthot.* 2006;18 (Proceedings 7):P175–P182.

115. Hachisuka K, Makino K, Wada F, Saeki S, Yoshimoto N, Arai M. Clinical application of carbon fibre reinforced plastic leg orthosis for polio survivors and its advantages and disadvantages. *Prosthet Orthot Int.* 2006;30(2):129–135.

116. Brehm MA, Beelen A, Doorenbosch CA, Harlaar J, Nollet F. Effect of carbon-composite knee-ankle-foot orthoses on walking efficiency and gait in former polio patients. *J Rehabil Med.* 2007;39(8):651–657.

117. Hachisuka K, Makino K, Wada F, Saeki S, Yoshimoto N. Oxygen consumption, oxygen cost and physiological cost index in polio survivors: a comparison of walking without orthosis, with an ordinary or a carbon-fibre reinforced plastic knee-ankle-foot orthosis. *J Rehabil Med.* 2007;39(8):646–650.

118. Nene AV, Hermens HJ, Zivold G. Paraplegic locomotion; a review. *Spinal Cord.* 1995;34(9):507–524.

119. Fatone S. A review of the literature pertaining to KAFOs and HKAFOs for walking. *J Prosthet Orthot.* 2006;18(Proceedings 7):P137–P168.

120. McMillan AG, Kendrick K, Michael JW, Aronson J, Horton GW. Preliminary evidence for effectiveness of a stance control orthosis. *J Prosthet Orthot.* 2004;16(1):6–15.

121. Edelstein JE. Orthotic assessment and management. In: O'Sullivan SB, Schmitz TJ, eds. Physical Rehabilitation: Assessment and Treatment. 5th ed. Philadelphia: Davis; 2007:1213–1248.

122. Hebert JS, Liggins AB. Gait evaluation of an automatic stance-control knee orthosis in a patient with postpoliomyelitis. *Arch Phys Med Rehabil.* 2005;86(8):1676–1680.

123. Yakimovich T, Lemaire ED, Kofman J. Preliminary kinematic evaluation of a new stance-control knee-ankle-foot orthosis. *Clin Biomech.* 2006;21(10):1081–1089.

124. Irby SE, Bernhardt KA, Kaufman KR. Gait of stance control orthosis users: the dynamic knee brace system. *Prosthet Orthot Int.* 2005;29(3):269–282.

125. Operating instructions for the E-Mag and Free Walk orthosis, Ottobock Germany. Available at: http://www.ottobock.com/cps/rde/xbcr/ob_com_en/im_646a214_gb_free_walk.pdf.

126. Stance Control Overview Guide II, Becker Orthopedic Troy, Michigan. Available at: http://www.beckerorthopedic.com/assets/pdf/stance:control.pdf.

127. MO25-SPL Manual, Fillauer, Chattanooga TN. Available at: http://www.fillauer.com/Orthotics/SPL2.html.

128. Davis PC, Bach TM, Pereira DM. The effect of stance control orthoses on gait characteristics and energy expenditure in knee-ankle-foot orthosis users. *Prosthet Orthot Int.* 2010; 34(2):206–215.

129. Lemaire ED, Goudreau L, Yakimovich T, Kofman J. Angular-velocity control approach for stance-control orthoses. *IEEE Trans Neural Syst Rehabil Eng.* 2009;17(5):497–503.

130. Yakimovich T, Kofman J, Lemaire E. Design, construction and evaluation of an electromechanical stance-control knee-ankle-foot orthosis. *Conf Proc IEEE Eng Med Biol Soc.* 2005;7:6934–6941.

131. Yakimovich T, Lemaire ED, Kofman J. Engineering design review of stance-control knee-ankle-foot orthoses. *J Rehabil Res Dev.* 2009;46(2):257–267.

132. Irby SE, Bernhardt KA, Kaufman KR. Gait changes over time in stance control orthosis users. *Prosthet Orthot Int.* 2007;31(4):353–361.

133. Bernhardt KA, Irby SE, Kaufman KR. Consumer opinions of a stance control knee orthosis. *Prosthet Orthot Int.* 2006;30(3):246–256.

134. Peethambaran A. The relationship between performance, satisfaction, and well being for patients using anterior and posterior design knee-ankle-foot-orthosis. *J Prosthet Orthot.* 2000;12(1):33–45.

135. Middleton JW, Yeo JD, Blanch L, Vare V, Peterson K, Brigden K. Clinical evaluation of a new orthosis, the 'walkabout', for restoration of functional standing and short distance mobility in spinal paralysed individuals. *Spinal Cord.* 1997;35(9):574–579.

136. Middleton JW, Fisher W, Davis GM, Smith RM. A medial linkage orthosis to assist ambulation after spinal cord injury. *Prosthet Orthot Int.* 1998;22(3):258–264.

137. Kawashima N, Taguchi D, Nakazawa K, Akai M. Effect of lesion level on the orthotic gait performance in individuals with complete paraplegia. *Spinal Cord.* 2006;44(8):487–494.

138. Harvey LA, Smith MB, Davis GM, Engel S. Functional outcomes attained by T9–12 paraplegic patients with the Walkabout and the Isocentric Reciprocal Gait Orthoses. *Arch Phys Med Rehabil.* 1997;78(7):706–711.

139. Abe K. Comparison of static balance, walking velocity, and energy consumption with knee-ankle-foot orthosis, walkabout orthosis, and reciprocating gait orthosis in thoracic-level paraplegic patients. *J Prosthet Orthot.* 2006;18(3):87–91.

140. Harvey LA, Newton-John T, Davis GM, Smith MB, Engel S. A comparison of the attitude of paraplegic individuals to the walkabout orthosis and the isocentric reciprocal gait orthosis. *Spinal Cord.* 1997;35(9):580–584.

141. Shimada Y, Hatakeyama K, Minato T, et al. Hybrid functional electrical stimulation with medial linkage knee-ankle-foot orthoses in complete paraplegics. *Tohoku J Exp Med.* 2006; 209(2):117–123.

142. Edelstein JE. Orthotic options for standing and walking. *Top Spinal Cord Inj Rehabil.* 2000;5(4):11–23.

143. John LT, Cherian B, Babu A. Postural control and fear of falling in persons with low-level paraplegia. *J Rehabil Res Dev.* 2010;47(5):497–502.

144. Taylor K. Factors affecting prescription and implementation of standing-frame programs by school-based physical therapists for children with impaired mobility. *Pediatr Phys Ther.* 2009;21(3):282–288.

145. Gibson SK, Sprod JA, Maher CA. The use of standing frames for contracture management for nonmobile children with cerebral palsy. *Int J Rehabil Res.* 2009;32(4):316–323.

146. Sprigle S, Maurer C, Soneblum SE. Load redistribution in variable position wheelchairs in people with spinal cord injury. *J Spinal Cord Med.* 2010;33(1):58–64.

147. Alekna V, Tamulaitiene M, Sinevicius T, Juocevicius A. Effect of weight-bearing activities on bone mineral density in spinal cord injured patients during the period of the first two years. *Spinal Cord.* 2008;46(11):727–732.

148. Biering-Sørensen F, Hansen B, Lee BS. Non-pharmacological treatment ad prevention of bone loss after spinal cord injury: a systematic review. *Spinal Cord.* 2009;47(7):508–518.

149. Edlich RF, Nelson KP, Foley ML, Buschbacher RM, Long WB, Ma EK. Technological advances in powered wheelchairs. *J Long Term Eff Med Implants.* 2004;14(2):107–130.

150. Brown JA, Gram M, Kinnen E. Parapodium design with knee and hip locks. *Orthot Prosthet.* 1980;34(2):14–20.

151. Gram M, Kinnen E, Brown JA. Parapodium redesigned for sitting. *Phys Ther.* 1981;61(5):657–660.

152. Mazur JM, Kyle S. Efficacy of bracing the lower limbs and ambulation training in children with myelomeningocele. *Dev Med Child Neurol.* 2004;46(5):352–356.

153. Butler PB, Abist RP, Abist IRF. Use of the ORLAU swivel walker for the severely handicapped patient: experience with five patients. *Physiother.* 1982;68(10):324–346.

154. Seymour RJ, Knapp CF, Anderson TR. Paraplegic use of the Orlau swivel walker: case report. *Arch Phys Med Rehabil.* 1982;63(10):490–494.

155. Rose GK, Sankarankutty M, Stallard J. A clinical review of the orthotic treatment of myelomeningocele patients. *J Bone Joint Surg Br.* 1983;65(3):242–246.

156. Rose GK, Stallard J, Sankarankutty M. Clinical evaluation of spina bifida patients using hip guidance orthosis. *Dev Med Child Neurol.* 1981;23(1):30–40.

157. Summers BN, McClelland MR, el Masri WS. A clinical review of the adult hip guidance orthosis (Para Walker) in traumatic paraplegics. *Paraplegia.* 1988;26(1):19–26.

158. Douglas R, Larson PF, D'Ambrosio R, McCall RE. The LSU reciprocation gait orthosis. *Orthopedics.* 1983;6:834–839.

159. Lissene MA, Peeraer L, Goditiabois F, Lysens R. Advanced reciprocating gait orthosis in paraplegic patients. In: Zupko JK, ed. Proceedings of the 7th World Congress; Chicago: International Society for Prosthetics and Orthotics (ISPO); 1992:3.

160. Massucci M, Brunetti G, Piperno R, Betti L, Franceschini M. Walking with the advanced reciprocating gait orthosis (ARGO) in thoracic paraplegic patients: energy expenditure and cardio-respiratory performance. *Spinal Cord.* 1998;36(4):223–227.

161. Leung AK, Wong AF, Wong EC, Hutchins SW. The Physiological Cost Index of walking with an isocentric reciprocating gait orthosis among patients with T(12) - L(1) spinal cord injury. *Prosthet Orthot Int.* 2009;33(1):61–68.

162. Merati G, Sarchi P, Ferrarin M, Pedotti A, Veocsteomas GA. Paraplegic adaptation to assisted-walking: energy expenditure during wheelchair versus orthosis use. *Spinal Cord.* 2000;38(1):37–44.

163. Stallard J, Major RE, Patrick JH. The use of the Orthotic Research and Locomotor Assessment Unit (ORLAU) ParaWalker by adult myelomeningocele patients: a seven year retrospective study—preliminary results. *Eur J Pediatr Surg.* 1995;5(suppl 1):24–26.

164. Roussos N, Patrick JH, Hodnett C, Stallard J. A long-term review of severely disabled spina bifida patients using a reciprocal walking system. *Disabil Rehabil.* 2001;23(6):239–244.

165. Whittle MW, Cocharne GM. A comparative evaluation of the hip guidance orthosis and reciprocating gait orthosis. Health Equipment Information No. 192 London: National Health Service Procurement Directorate; 1989.

166. Jefferson RJ, Whittle MW. Performance of three walking orthoses for the paralyzed: a case study using gait analysis. *Prosthet Orthot Int.* 1990;14(3):103–110.

167. Stallard J, McLeod N, Woollam PJ, Miller K. Reciprocal walking orthosis with composite material body brace: initial development. *Proc Inst Mech Eng H.* 2003;217(5):385–392.

168. Stallard J, Major RE. The case for lateral stiffness in walking orthoses for paraplegic patients. *Proc Inst Mech Eng H.* 1993;207(1):1–6.

169. Major RE, Stallard J, Farmer SE. A review of 42 patients of 16 years and over using the ORLAU Parawalker. *Prosthet Orthot Int.* 1997;21(2):147–152.

170. Dall PM, Müller B, Stallard I, Edwards J, Granat MH. The functional use of the reciprocal hip mechanism during gait for paraplegic patients walking in the Louisiana State University reciprocating gait. *Prosthet Orthot Int.* 1999;23(2):152–162.

171. Johnson WB, Fatone S, Gard SA, Johnson WB, Fatone S, Gard SA. Walking mechanics of persons who use reciprocating gait orthoses. *J Rehabil Res Dev.* 2009;6(3):435–446.

172. IJzerman MJ, Baardman G, Hermens HJ, Veltink PH, Boom HB, Zilvold G. The influence of the reciprocal cable linkage in the advanced reciprocating gait orthosis on paraplegic gait performance. *Prosthet Orthot Int.* 1997;21(1):52–61.

173. Baardman G, IJzerman MJ, Hermens HJ, Veltink PH, Boom HB, Zilvold G. The influence of the reciprocal hip joint link in the Advanced Reciprocating Gait Orthosis on standing performance in paraplegia. *Prosthet Orthot Int.* 1997;21(3):210–221.

174. Scivoletto G, Mancini M, Fiorelli E, Morganti B, Molinari M. A prototype of an adjustable advanced reciprocating gait orthosis (ARGO) for spinal cord injury. *Spinal Cord.* 2003; 41(3):187–191.

175. Solomonow M, Aguilar E, Reisin E, et al. Reciprocating gait orthosis powered with electrical muscle stimulation (RGO II). Part I: Performance evaluation of 70 paraplegic patients. *Orthopedics.* 1997;20(4):315–324.

176. Marsolais EB, Kobetic R, Polando G, et al. The Case Western Reserve University hybrid gait orthosis. *J Spinal Cord Med.* 2000;23(2):100–108.

177. Stein RB, Hayday F, Chong SL, et al. Speed and efficiency in walking and wheeling with novel stimulation and bracing systems after spinal cord injury: a case study. *Neuromodulation.* 2005;8(4):264–271.

178. Fritz S, Lusardi MM. Walking speed: the sixth vital sign. *J Geriatr Phys Ther.* 2009;32(2):46–49.

179. Williams G, Robertson V, Greenwood K. Measuring high-level mobility after traumatic brain injury. *Am J Phys Med Rehabil.* 2004;83(12):910–920.

180. Turner-Stokes L, Turner-Stokes T. The use of standardized outcome measures in rehabilitation centres in the UK. *Clinical Rehabil.* 1997;11(4):306–313.

181. Carvalho C, Sunnerhagen KS, Willén C. Walking speed and distance in different environments of subjects in the later stage post-stroke. *Physiother Theory Pract.* 2010; 26(8):519–527.

182. Bowden MG, Balasubramanian CK, Behrman AL, Kautz SA. Validation of a speed-based classification system using quantitative measures of walking performance poststroke. *Neurorehabil Neural Repair.* 2008;22(6):672–675.

183. Jackson AB, Carnel CT, Ditunno FJ, et al. Outcome measures for gait and ambulation in the spinal cord injury population. *J Spinal Cord Med.* 2008;31(5):487–499.

184. van Hedel HJA. Gait speed in relation to categories of functional ambulation after spinal cord injury. *Neurorehabil Neural Repair.* 2009;23(4):343–350.

185. van Hedel HJ, Wirz M, Curt A. Improving walking assessment in subjects with an incomplete spinal cord injury: responsiveness. *Spinal Cord.* 2006;44(6):352–356.

186. Martin L, Baker R, Harvey A. A systematic review of common physiotherapy interventions in school-aged children with cerebral palsy. *Phys Occup Ther Pediatr.* 2010;30(4):294–312.

187. Kurz MJ, Stuberg W, DeJong SL. Body weight supported treadmill training improves the regularity of the stepping kinematics in children with cerebral palsy. *Dev Neurorehabil.* 2011;14(2):87–93.

188. van Loo MA, Moseley AM, Bosman JM, de Bie RA, Hassett L. Inter-rater reliability and concurrent validity of walking speed measurement after traumatic brain injury. *Clin Rehabil.* 2003;17(7):775–779.

189. Moseley AM, Lanzarone S, Bosman JM, et al. Ecological validity of walking speed assessment after traumatic brain injury: a pilot study. *J Head Trauma Rehabil.* 2004;19(4):341–348.

190. Pollentier B, Irons SL, Benedetto CM, et al. Examination of the six minute walk test to determine functional capacity in people with chronic heart failure: a systematic review. *Cardiopulm Phys Ther J.* 2010;21(1):13–21.

191. Fulk GD, Echternach JL, Nof L, O'Sullivan S. Clinometric properties of the six-minute walk test in individuals undergoing rehabilitation poststroke. *Physiother Theory Pract.* 2008;24(3):195–204.

192. Ditunno JF, Barbeau H, Dobkin BH, et al. Validity of the walking scale for spinal cord injury and other domains of function in a multicenter clinical trial. *Neurorehabil Neural Repair.* 2007;21(6):539–550.

193. vanHedel HJ, Wirz M, Dietz V. Assessing walking ability in subjects with spinal cord injury: validity and reliability of 3 walking tests. *Arch Phys Med Rehabil.* 2005;86(2):190–196.

194. Thompson P, Beath T, Bell J, et al. Test-retest reliability of the 10-metre fast walk test and 6-minute walk test in ambulatory school-aged children with cerebral palsy. *Dev Med Child Neurol.* 2008;50(5):370–376.

195. Hassan J, van der Net J, Helders PJ, Prakken BJ, Takken T. Six-minute walk test in children with chronic conditions. *Br J Sports Med.* 2010;44(4):270–274.

196. Gylfadottir S, Dallimore M, Dean E. The relation between walking capacity and clinical correlates in survivors of chronic spinal poliomyelitis. *Arch Phys Med Rehabil.* 2006;87(7):944–952.

197. Borg G. Psychophysical bases of perceived exertion. *Med Sci Sports Exerc.* 1982;14(5):377–381.

198. Lamb KL, Eston RG, Corns D. Reliability of ratings of perceived exertion during progressive treadmill exercise. *Br J Sports Med.* 1999;33(5):336–339.

199. Groslambert A, Hintzy F, Hoffman MD, Dugué B, Rouillon JD. Validation of a rating scale of perceived exertion in young children. *Int J Sports Med.* 2001;22(2):116–119.

200. Eng JJ, Chu KS, Dawson AS, Kim CM, Hepburn KE. Functional walk tests in individuals with stroke: relation to perceived exertion and myocardial exertion. *Stroke.* 2002;33(3):756–761.

201. Kelly S. Oxygen cost, walking speed, and perceived exertion in children with cerebral palsy when walking with anterior and posterior walkers. *Pediatr Phys Ther.* 2002;14(3):159–161.

202. Merritta C, Cherian B, Macaden AS, John JA. Measurement of physical performance and objective fatigability in people with mild-to-moderate traumatic brain injury. *Int J Rehabil Res.* 2010;33(2):109–114.

203. Podsiadlo D, Richardson S. The timed 'up and go' a test of basic functional mobility for frail elderly persons. *J Am Geriatr Soc.* 1991;39(2):142–148.

204. Ng SS, Hui-Chan CW. The timed up & go test: its reliability and association with lower-limb impairments and locomotor capacities in people with chronic stroke. *Arch Phys Med Rehabil.* 2005;86(8):1641–1647.

205. Erel S, Uygur F, Engin Simsek I, Yakut Y. The effects of dynamic ankle-foot orthoses in chronic stroke patients at three-month follow-up: a randomized controlled trial. *Clin Rehabil.* 2011; 25(6):515–523.

206. Andersson AG, Kamwendo K, Seiger A, Appelros P. How to identify potential fallers in a stroke unit: validity indexes of four test methods. *J Rehabil Med.* 2006;38(3):186–191.

207. Gan S, Tung L, Tang Y, Wang C. Psychometric properties of functional balance assessment in children with cerebral palsy. *Neurorehabil Neural Repair.* 2008;22(6):745–753.

208. Katz-Leurer M, Rotem H, Keren O, Meyer S. Balance abilities and gait characteristics in post-traumatic brain injury, cerebral palsy and typically developed children. *Dev Neurorehabil.* 2009;12(2):100–105.

209. Williams EN, Carroll SG, Reddihough DS, Phillips BA, Galea MP. Investigation of the timed 'up & go' test in children. *Dev Med Child Neurol.* 2005;47(8):518–524.

10

Orthotic Decision Making in Neurological and Neuromuscular Disease

MICHELLE M. LUSARDI AND DONNA M. BOWERS

LEARNING OBJECTIVES

On completion of this chapter, the reader will be able to:

1. Describe the contribution of the major components of the central nervous system (CNS) and the peripheral nervous system (PNS) to functional, goal- directed movement.

2. Describe the impact of CNS and PNS pathologies commonly encountered in physical therapy and orthotic practice on functional, goal-directed movement.

3. Explain the continuum of muscle tone and of muscle performance and their interactive effect on goal-directed, functional movement.

4. Describe the characteristics of muscle tone in the CNS and PNS pathologies most commonly encountered in physical therapy and orthotic practice and how altered tone impacts on functional movement.

5. Describe the contributions of various CNS and PNS components to, and key determinants of, effective postural control.

6. Describe the contributions of various CNS components to, and key determinants of, mobility and coordination during functional activity.

7. Discuss the roles of orthopedic and neurosurgical procedures, central and peripherally acting pharmacological agents, and various orthotic options for the management of hypertonicity.

8. Describe strategies used by rehabilitation professionals to reduce the risk of developing secondary musculoskeletal impairments in persons with hypertonicity.

9. Plan a strategy for examination and evaluation of persons with CNS and PNS dysfunction to determine the need for an orthosis or adaptive equipment.

10. Describe a strategy for clinical decision making in the selection of an appropriate orthosis for individuals with neurological and neuromuscular pathologies.

MOVEMENT IMPAIRMENT IN NEUROLOGICAL AND NEURNEUROMUSCULAR PATHOLOGY

Pathologies of the neuromuscular system manifest in a sometimes confusing array of clinical signs and symptoms. To select the most appropriate therapeutic intervention, be it exercise to promote neuroplasticity and recovery, functional training, or the use of various orthoses and assistive devices to accommodate for impairment of a body system or structure, the clinician must develop a strategy to "classify" the movement disorder that has produced the observed impairments and functional limitations.[1] The clinician must understand the medical prognosis and potential progression of the disease process, as well as the lifestyles and risk factors that might contribute to secondary impairments that limit function over time (even if the disease is "nonprogressive") and their impact on the individual's growth and development.[1-3]

Health professionals use a number of organizational strategies as frameworks for decision making during rehabilitation of individuals with pathologies leading to neuromuscular dysfunction. Many neurologists use a medical differential diagnosis process to locate the lesion as being within the central nervous system (CNS) or involving structures of the peripheral nervous system (PNS) or the muscle itself.[4] They do this by triangulating evidence gathered by examining tone and deep tendon reflexes, observing patterns of movement and postural control, and looking for specific types of involuntary movement.[5,6] They may also interpret results of special tests such as nerve conduction studies, electromyography (EMG), computed tomography (CT), and magnetic resonance imaging (MRI).[7,8] These tests might pinpoint areas of denervation, ischemia, or demyelinization and help the health professionals arrive at a medical diagnosis.

Rehabilitation professionals are most interested in the functional consequences associated with the various neuromotor conditions. They examine the ways in which abnormal tone (hypertonicity—excessive tone; hypotonicity—insufficient tone; or flaccidity—absence of tone) affects mobility and locomotion, postural control, motor planning and motor control during movement, coordination (error control), and muscle performance during functional activities.[9,10] Rehabilitation professionals are not only concerned about function at the present time but also consider the long-term impact of neuromotor impairment on the person's joints and posture, especially in children who are growing with abnormal tone and postures.[11,12]

This chapter considers the ways that key components of the CNS and PNS contribute to functional movement. We explore the concepts of muscle tone and muscle performance, considering how their interaction influences an individual's ability to move. We investigate how abnormalities of tone resulting from CNS and PNS pathologies are described in clinical practice. We consider the determinants of postural control and of coordination and how CNS and PNS pathologies might lead to impairments of balance and movement. We provide an overview of the ways that commonly encountered CNS pathologies impact muscle tone, muscle performance, postural control, movement, and coordination as a way of understanding how an orthosis or adaptive equipment might help improve an individual's ability to walk and participate in meaningful activities and roles. We consider how the physical therapy examination contributes to the determination of a need for an orthosis or adaptive equipment. We also explore the clinical decision-making process by asking key questions about how an orthosis might help (or hinder) function. Finally, we apply what we have learned using five clinical cases to develop orthotic prescriptions.

DIFFERENTIAL DIAGNOSIS: WHERE IS THE PROBLEM?

Most neurological and neuromuscular diseases affect either the CNS or the PNS; only a few diseases, such as amyotrophic lateral sclerosis, affect both CNS and PNS. Diseases of the CNS and of the PNS may contribute to motor or sensory impairment; however, there are patterns and characteristics of dysfunction that are unique to each. Selection of the appropriate orthosis, seating/wheelchair system, or assistive devices is facilitated when the therapist, orthotist, members of the rehabilitation team, patient, and patient's family understand the normal function and consequences of the disease process of the neurological subsystem that is affected.

The Central Nervous System

The CNS is a complex of dynamic and interactive subsystems that mediates purposeful movement and postural control, vital autonomic vegetative and physiological functions, and learning of all types.[13] Readers are encouraged to refer to a recent neuroanatomy or neuropathology textbook to refresh their understanding of CNS structure and function. Knowledge of the roles of various CSN structures and their interactions (for perception, problem solving, motor planning, and coordination) is foundational for clinical decision making when considering orthoses for individuals with neuromuscular dysfunction.

Some diseases affect a single CNS system or center (e.g., Parkinson's disease affects the function of the basal ganglia in regulating agonist/antagonist muscle activity; a lacunar stroke in the internal capsule may interrupt transmission only within the pyramidal/corticospinal pathway) leading to a specific array of signs/symptoms characteristic of that system or center. Other pathologies disrupt function across several systems: a thromboembolic stroke in the proximal left middle cerebral artery may disrupt volitional movement and sensation of the right side of the body, as well as communication and vision. Several exacerbations of multiple sclerosis (MS) may lead to plaque formation in the cerebral peduncles/pyramidal system, superior cerebellar peduncle/error control system, restiform body/balance system, and fasciculus gracilis/lower extremity sensation; in this case, it can be challenging but imperative to sort through the various types of impairments that may result in order to select the most appropriate therapeutic or orthotic intervention for the individual.

Pyramidal System

The *pyramidal system* is responsible for initiation of volitional movement and plays a major role in the development of skilled and manipulative activities. The cell bodies of pyramidal neurons are located in the postcentral gyrus/primary motor cortex. The motor cortex in the left cerebral hemisphere influences primarily the right side of the body (face, trunk, and extremities); the right cortex influences the left body. The axons of pyramidal neurons form the corticobulbar and corticospinal tracts, projecting toward α motor neurons in cranial nerve nuclei and anterior horn of the spinal cord. To reach their destination, these axons descend through the genu and posterior limb of the internal capsule, the cerebral peduncles, the basilar pons, the pyramids of the medulla, and finally the opposite lateral funiculus of the spinal cord. A lesion at any point in the pyramidal system has the potential to disrupt volitional movement. The degree of disruption varies with the extent and functional salience of the structures that are damaged, manifest on a continuum from mild weakness (paresis) to the inability to voluntarily initiate and direct movement (paralysis).

Immediately following insult or injury of the pyramidal system, during a period of neurogenic shock, there may be substantially diminished muscle tone and sluggish or absent deep tendon reflexes.[14] As inflammation from the initial insult subsides, severely damaged neurons degenerate and are resorbed, while minimally damaged neurons may repair themselves and resume function.[15,16] The more neurons that are destroyed, the greater the likelihood that hypertonicity will develop over time due to the altered balance of descending input of pyramidal and extrapyramidal systems. As the recovery period continues, individuals may begin to move in abnormal synergy patterns whenever volitional movement is attempted.[17,18] When the damage to the system is less extensive, individuals may eventually recover some or all volitional motor control; the more extensive the damage to the system, the more likely there will be residual motor impairment.[15,18]

Extrapyramidal System

The extrapyramidal system is made up of several subcortical subsystems that influence muscle tone, organize patterns of movement from among the many possible movement strategies, and make both feedforward adjustments (in anticipation of movement) and refining feedback adjustments (in response to sensations generated as movement occurs) during performance of functional tasks.[19] The motor planning subsystem is a series of neural loops interconnecting the premotor and accessory motor cortices in the frontal lobes, the nuclei of the functional basal ganglia (caudate, putamen, globus pallidus, substantia nigra, subthalamus), and several nuclei of the thalamus. Damage to the premotor and accessory motor cortex leads to apraxia, the inability to effectively sequence components of a functional task and to understand the nature of a task and the way to use a tool in performance of the task.[20] If there is damage to the caudate and putamen (also called the *corpus striatum*), underlying muscle tone may fluctuate unpredictably (athetosis) and involuntary dancelike movements (chorea) are likely to occur.[21] Damage to the subthalamic nuclei can lead to forceful, often disruptive, involuntary movement of the extremities (ballism) that interrupts purposeful activity.[22] Damage to the substantia nigra characteristically leads to resting tremor, rigidity of axial and appendicular musculature (hypertonicity in all directions), and bradykinesia (difficulty initiating movement, slow movement with limited excursion during functional tasks), which are most commonly seen in persons with Parkinson's disease.[23] Motor impairments resulting from damage to the ventral anterior nucleus and related thalamic nuclei are less well understood but may contribute to less efficient motor planning, especially when the individual is learning or performing novel tasks.[24]

Extrapyramidal structures influence muscle tone and readiness to move via a network of interconnections among motor centers in the brainstem. The reticulospinal tracts, originating in the lower pons and medulla, are thought to influence tone by acting on γ motor neurons and their associated muscle spindles. They play a major role in balancing the stiffness required for antigravity position and the flexibility necessary for movement of the limbs through space during functional activity and are likely the effectors for tonic hindbrain reflexes.[19,25] The vestibulospinal tracts, also originating from the pons and medulla, influence anticipatory postural adjustment in preparation for movement and reactionary postural adjustments as movement occurs. These tracts are thought to be the "effectors" for postural control and balance.[19,26] The tectospinal tracts, originating in the collicular nuclei of the dorsal midbrain, influence linkages between the head and extremities (especially arms and hands) so that the visual and auditory systems can be used effectively to orient the head and body during tasks that require visual (eye-hand) and auditory (ear-hand) guidance.[16,27]

Coordination Systems

The error control, or coordination subsystem, has several interactive components.[28] Feedforward information (how movement is likely to occur) from the forebrain's motor cortex is relayed through the thalamus to the deep nuclei of the cerebellum via the middle cerebellar peduncle (brachium pontis). Feedback information generated by movement travels from the muscle spindle and anterior horn of the spinal cord via the inferior cerebellar peduncle (restiform body), as does sensory information from static and dynamic vestibular receptors (head position and movement in space) and

the vestibular nuclei in the brainstem. Through interaction of Purkinje cells in the cerebellar cortex and neurons in the deep cerebellar nuclei, the cerebellum judges how "in sync" these various types of information are (essentially asking the questions, "Did the movement occur as planned? Was the outcome of the movement as intended?") and suggests refinements for more precise and coordinated movement.[29] These adjustments are relayed to the red nucleus in the midbrain via the superior cerebellar peduncle (brachium conjunctiva) and are forwarded back to the thalamus and the motor cortex, as well as to the spinal cord via the rubrospinal tract. The rubrospinal tract is thought to be essential for refinement and correction of direction and control of movement as it occurs.[29]

Somatosensory and Perceptual Systems

The somatosensory system is composed of a set of ascending pathways, each carrying a specific sensory modality from the spinal cord and brainstem to the thalamus and postcentral gyrus of the cerebral cortex, reticular formation, or cerebellum. The anterolateral (spinothalamic) system carries exteroceptive information from mechanoreceptors that monitor protective senses (e.g., pain, temperature, irritation to skin and soft tissue).[30] This tract originates in the dorsal horn (substantia gelatinosa) of the spinal cord and the spinal trigeminal nucleus, crosses the midline of the neuraxis to ascend in the lateral funiculus of the spinal cord to the contralateral ventral posterior thalamus, and then continues to the postcentral gyrus. The dorsal column/medial lemniscus carries information from encapsulated receptors that serve as internal monitors of body condition and motion.[31] This tract ascends from the spinal cord to reach the nuclei gracilis and cuneatus in the medulla of the brainstem, then crosses midline to ascend to the contralateral ventral posterior thalamus and on to the posterior central gyrus. The postcentral gyrus (somatosensory cortex) is organized as a homunculus, with each region of the body represented in a specific area.[32] Sensation from the lower extremities (lumbosacral spinal cord) is located at the top of the gyrus near the sagittal fissure. Moving downward toward the lateral fissure, the next area represented is the trunk (thoracic spinal cord), followed by upper extremities and head (cervical spinal cord), and finally face, mouth, and esophagus (trigeminal nuclei) just above the lateral fissure. A lesion such as an MS plaque in one of the ascending pathways may result in a discrete area of loss of exteroception or of conscious proprioception in one area of the body; a lesion on the somatosensory cortex can lead to a more profound, multimodality impairment on the opposite side of the body.

Although sensory information is logged in at the postcentral gyrus, the location of the somatosensory cortex, interpretation and integration of this information occurs in the somatoperceptual system in the parietal association areas, with specialization in the right hemisphere.[32] These association areas give meaning to the sensations that are generated as people move and function in their environments. This is where people understand the relationships among their various extremities and trunk (body schema), as well as their relationship to and position within our physical environment. Damage to the parietal lobes leads to problems ranging from left-right confusion to the inability to recognize and monitor the condition of a body part (neglect, agnosia), depending on how much of the association area is involved.[33,34]

Visual and Visual-Perceptual Systems

The visual system begins with processing of information gathered by the rods and cones in the multiple layers of specialized neurons in the retina, located in the posterior chamber of the eye. Axons from retinal ganglion cells are gathered into the optic nerve, which carries information from that eye toward the brain. At the optic chiasm there is reorganization of visual information, such that all information from the left visual field (from both eyes) continues in the right optic tract and that from the right field continues in the left tract. This information is relayed, through the lateral geniculate body of the thalamus, via the optic radiations, to the primary visual cortex on either side of the calcarine fissure of the midsagittal occipital lobe.[35] Damage to the retina or optic nerve results in loss of vision from that eye. Damage to the optic chiasm typically leads to a narrowing of the peripheral visual field (bitemporal hemianopsia); a lesion of one of the optic tracts or radiations leads to loss of part or all of the opposite visual field (homonymous hemianopsia). Damage to the visual cortex can result in cortical blindness, in which visual reflexes may be intact but vision is impaired.[36]

Visual information is interpreted in the visual association areas in the remainder of the occipital lobe.[37] The visual association areas in the left hemisphere are particularly important to interpretation of symbolic and communication information, while spatial relationships are of more interest in the right hemisphere. Specific details about the environment, especially about speed and direction of moving objects with respect to the self and of the individual with respect to a relatively stationary environment, are important contributors to functional movement and to the development of skilled abilities.[38] Interconnections between the parietal and occipital association areas serve to integrate visual and somatic/kinesthetic perception and provide important input to motor planning and motor learning systems.[39]

Effective visual information processing is founded on three interactive dimensions: visual spatial orientation, visual analysis skills, and visual motor skills.[40] Developmentally, visual spatial orientation includes spatial concepts used to understand the environment, the body, and the interaction between the body and environment that are part of functional activity (e.g., determining location or direction with respect to self, as well as respect to other objects or persons encountered as people act in their environment). Visual analysis skills allow people to discriminate and analyze visually presented information, identify and focus on key characteristics or features of what people see, use mental imagery and visual recall, and respond or perceive a whole when presented with representative parts. The visual motor system links what is seen to how the eyes, head, and body move, allowing one to use visual information processing skills during skilled, purposeful activities. This also provides the foundation for fine manipulative skills requiring eye-hand coordination.[37]

Executive Function and Motivation

The ability to problem solve, consider alternatives, plan and organize, understand conceptual relationships, multitask, set priorities, and delay gratification, as well as the initial components of learning are functions of the frontal association areas of the forebrain.[41,42] These dimensions of cognitive function are often described by the phrase *higher executive function*. Quantitative and other analytical skills are thought to be primarily housed in the frontal association areas of the left hemisphere, while intuitive understanding and creativity may be more concentrated in the right hemisphere. Most people tap the resources available in both hemispheres (via interconnections through the corpus callosum) during daily life, although some may fall toward one end or another of the analytical-intuitive continuum. Individuals with acquired brain injury involving frontal lobes often exhibit subtle deficits that have a significant impact on their ability to function in complex environments, as well as under conditions of high task demand; difficulty in these areas certainly compromises functional efficiency and quality of life.[43,44]

The neuroanatomical structures that contribute to the motivational system include the nuclei and tracts of the limbic system, prefrontal cortex, and temporal lobes; all play major roles in managing emotions, concentration, learning, and memory.[45] The motivational system not only has an important impact on emotional aspects of behavior but also influences autonomic/physiological function, efficacy of learning, interpretation of sensations, and preparation for movement (Figure 10-1).[46] Dimensions of limbic function that influence motivation and the ability to manage challenges and frustration include body image, self-concept, and self-worth as related to social roles and expectations, as well as the perceived relevance or importance (based on reward or on threat) of an activity or situation.[47,48] *Central set* is a phrase used to describe the limbic system's role as a motivator and repository of memory on readiness to move or act.[46] Central set helps people predict movement needs relevant to a given situation or circumstance (considering both the physical and affective dimensions of the environment in which they are acting) from past experience.[49]

Consciousness and Homeostasis

The ability to be alert and oriented when functioning in a complex environment is the purview of the consciousness system and is a function of interaction of the brainstem's reticular formation, the filtering system of thalamic nuclei, and the thought and problem solving that occur in the association areas of the telencephalon, especially in the frontal lobes.[50] The reticular activating system, found in the inferior mesencephalon and upper pons of the brainstem, is the locus of sleep-wake and level of alertness.[51] The thalamus and the reticular formation help people habituate to repetitive sensory stimuli while they focus on the type of sensory information that is most germane to the task at hand.[52] The frontal

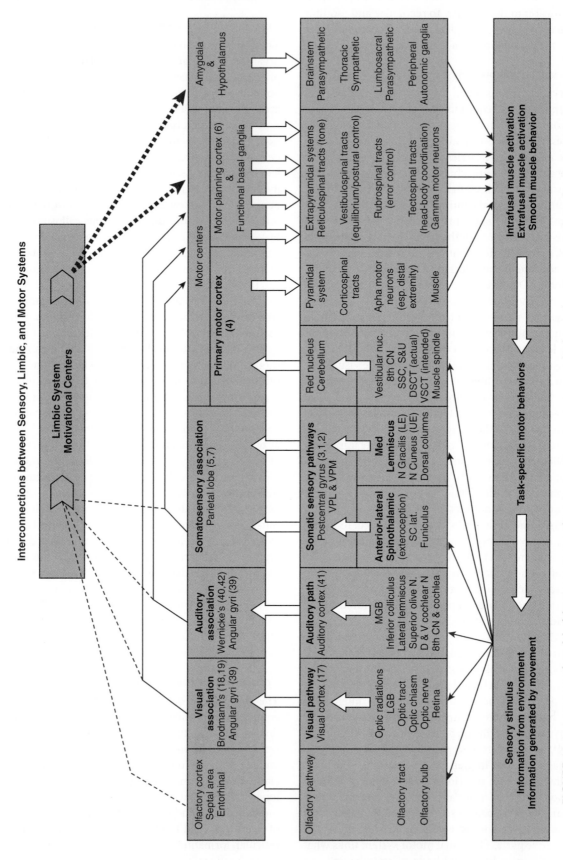

FIGURE 10-1 A conceptual model of the interactions and interconnections among sensory, limbic, and motor systems that influence functional movement.

association areas add content to one's consciousness: the ability to reason and to adapt to challenges encountered as one moves through daily life.[53] Alteration in quality and level of consciousness and behavior are indicators of evolving problems within the CNS.[54] Increasing intracranial pressure, the result of an expanding mass or inflammatory response following trauma or ischemia, may be initially manifest by confusion or agitation; progression into a state of lethargy, stupor, or unresponsiveness (coma) indicates deteriorating compromise of the CNS structures.[55]

Homeostasis and the ability to respond to physiological stressors are functions of the components of the autonomic nervous system.[56] The nuclei of the hypothalamus serve as the command center for parasympathetic and sympathetic nervous system activity via projections to parasympathetic cranial nerve nuclei in the brainstem, the sympathetic centers of the intermediate horn in the thoracic spinal cord, and the parasympathetic centers in the lumbosacral spinal cord. The hypothalamus has extensive interconnections with the limbic system, bridging physiological and emotional/psychological aspects of behavior and activity.[57] The hypothalamus also integrates neural-endocrine function through interconnections with the pituitary gland.[58] Clearly, this relatively small area of forebrain plays a substantial integrative role in physiological function of the human body. Damage or dysfunction to this area therefore has significant impact on physiological stability and stress response.

Peripheral Nervous System

The PNS serves two primary functions: to collect information about the body and the environment and to activate muscles during functional activities. Afferent neurons collect data from the various sensory receptors distributed throughout the body and transport this information to the spinal cord and brainstem (sensory cranial nerves) for initial interpretation and distribution to CNS centers and structures that use sensory information in the performance of their various specialized roles.[33] The interpretation process can have a direct impact on motor behavior at the spinal cord level (e.g., deep tendon reflex) or along any synapse point in the subsequent ascending pathway (e.g., righting and equilibrium responses) as sensory information is transported toward its final destination within the CNS.[59] Efferent neurons (also described as lower motor neurons or, more specifically, α and γ motor neurons) carry signals from the pyramidal (voluntary motor) and extrapyramidal (supportive motor) systems to extrafusal/striated and intrafusal (within muscle spindle) muscle fibers that direct functional movement by enacting the CNS's motor plan.[26,60,61]

The cell bodies of these α and γ motor neurons live in the anterior horn of the spinal cord and in cranial nerve somatic motor nuclei. In the spinal cord, α and γ axons project through the ventral root, are gathered into the motor component of a spinal nerve, and (in cervical and lumbosacral segments) are reorganized in a plexus before continuing toward the targeted muscle as part of a peripheral nerve. In the brainstem, α and γ axons project to target muscles via motor cranial nerves (oculomotor, III; trochlear, IV; motor trigeminal, V; abducens, VI; facial, VII; glossopharyngeal, IX; spinal accessory, XI; hypoglossal, XII).[62] When α and γ axons reach their target set of muscle fibers (motor unit), a specialized synapse—the neuromuscular junction—triggers muscular contraction.[63]

Pathologies of the PNS can be classified by considering two factors: the modalities affected (only sensory, only motor, or a combination of both) and the anatomical location of the problem (at the level of the sensory receptor, along the neuron itself, in the dorsal root ganglion, in the anterior horn, at the neuromuscular junction, or in the muscle itself).[64,65] Poliomyelitis is the classic example of an anterior horn cell disease; Guillain-Barré syndrome is a demyelinating infectious-autoimmune neuropathy that impairs transmission of electrical impulses over the length of motor and sensory nerves. The polyneuropathy of diabetes (affecting motor, sensory, and autonomic fibers) is the classic example of a metabolic neuropathy. Radiculopathies (e.g., sciatica) result from compression or irritation at the level of the nerve root, while entrapment syndromes (e.g., carpal tunnel) are examples of compression neuropathies over the more distal peripheral nerve. Myasthenia gravis, tetanus, and botulism alter function at the level of the neuromuscular junction. Myopathies and muscular dystrophies are examples of primary muscle diseases.[65]

DETERMINANTS OF EFFECTIVE MOVEMENT

Regardless of the underlying neurological or neuromuscular disease, rehabilitation professionals seek to understand the impact of the condition on an individual's underlying muscle tone and motor control (ability to initiate, guide, sustain, and terminate movement), muscle performance (strength, power, endurance, speed, accuracy, fluidity), and postural control and balance (ability to stay upright, to anticipate how to make postural adjustment during movement, and to respond to unexpected perturbations) in order to move effectively during goal-directed, functional movement necessary for daily life.

Muscle Tone and Muscle Performance

Effectiveness of movement is determined by the interaction of underlying muscle tone and muscle performance. *Muscle tone* can be conceptualized as the interplay of compliance and stiffness of muscle, as influenced by the CNS. Ideally the CNS can set the neuromotor system to be stiff enough to align and support the body in functional antigravity positions (e.g., provide sufficient baseline postural tone) but compliant enough in the limbs and trunk to carry out smooth and coordinated functional movement and effectively respond to changing environmental conditions or demands as daily tasks are carried out.[66,67] At the center of the tone continuum, the interplay of stiffness and compliance is optimal, such that motor performance is well supported (Figure 10-2, horizontal continuum). At the low-tone end of the continuum, where there is low stiffness and high compliance, individuals are challenged by inadequate postural control and inability to support antigravity movement. At the high tone end of the continuum,

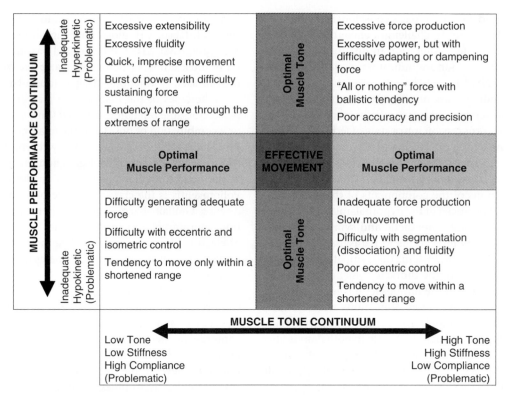

FIGURE 10-2 A conceptual model of the interrelationship of muscle tone and muscle performance as they interact to influence functional abilities. The muscle tone ranges from excessively compliant (easily extensible on passive movement) to excessively stiff (resistant to passive movement). The muscle performance continuum ranges from hypokinetic (exhibiting minimal movement during task activity) to hyperkinetic (exhibiting excessive and poorly controlled movement during task activity). Movement is most effective at the intersection of optimal muscle tone and optimal muscle performance.

where there is high stiffness and low compliance, freedom and flexibility of movement are compromised. Among individuals, postural tone varies with level of consciousness, level of energy or fatigue, and perceived importance (salience) of the tasks they are involved with at the time.[68,69]

Effective movement occurs when *muscle performance* meets the demands of the task. The components of muscle performance are the ability to (1) generate sufficient force (strength); (2) at the rate of contraction required for the task at hand (speed and power); (3) to sustain the concentric, holding/isometric, or eccentric contraction necessary to meet task demands (muscle endurance); (4) to ramp up or dampen force production in response to task demands (accuracy); and (5) coordinate mobility and stability of body segments to complete the task (fluidity). Muscle performance can also be conceptualized as having a continuum with optimal control of its components around the center and inadequate control on either side: hypokinesis (little movement) at one extreme and hyperkinesis (excessive movement) at the other (see Figure 10-2, vertical continuum).

While muscle tone and muscle performance are distinct contributors to movement, they are certainly interactive.[70,71] Movement is most effective and efficient if an individual's resources fall at the center of each continuum. A problem with muscle tone, or with muscle performance, or a combination of both leads to abnormal and less efficient movement. Consider what will happen if there is a combination of low

tone and inadequate hypokinetic muscle performance: individuals will have difficulty with force production and power, as well as with eccentric and isometric control, such that movement tends to occur in shortened ranges. For example, an infant with Down syndrome (with low tone) struggles to sustain an upright head in prone on elbows position in order to visually interact or reach for a toy (hypokinesis).

In the presence of low tone and hyperkinetic muscle performance, movement is fast but imprecise, with bursts of power that cannot be sustained. For example, a toddler with Down syndrome (with low tone) who is beginning to walk takes rapid and inconsistent steps (hyperkinesis). In contrast, the presence of high tone and hypokinetic muscle performance, movement is slow and stiff, with inadequate force production, compromised segmentation, impaired eccentric control (difficulty letting go), and constrained range. For example, an individual with Parkinson's disease takes short steps and has little reciprocal arm swing when walking.

In the presence of high-tone and hyperkinetic muscle performance, there tends to be "all or nothing" force production, with somewhat ballistic and inaccurate movement occurring between the extremes of ranges. For example, a child with spastic quadriplegic cerebral palsy (CP) rising from sitting to standing often employs rapid mass extension (lower extremity and trunk), compromising his or her ability to move toward flexion in order to effectively rise; the child would also have difficulty lowering back into sitting without collapsing.

Although muscle performance, especially the ability to generate force, does tend to decline with aging, the impact of inactivity is even more profound; all aspects of muscle performance can improve with appropriate training, even in the very old.[72-74]

Traditionally, an individual's muscle tone has been described clinically as hypertonic or spastic, rigid, hypotonic or low, flaccid, or fluctuating.

Hypertonus

Hypertonus is a term used to describe muscles that are influenced to be too stiff or are excessively biased toward supporting antigravity function. Spasticity is a type of hypertonus that typically occurs when there is damage to one or more CNS structures of the pyramidal motor system and is encountered as a component of many neuromuscular pathologies.[75-79] Decrements in underlying tone and muscle performance, in bipedal humans with impairment of the pyramidal system, most often occurs in a *decorticate* pattern: The upper extremity is typically biased toward flexion, such that the limb can be easily moved into flexion but not into extension (decreased compliance of flexors). The lower extremity is biased toward extension, such that the impaired compliance of extensors makes movement into flexion difficult (Figure 10-3).[80] In persons with severe acquired brain injury the entire body may be biased toward extension, a condition or posture described as *decerebrate* pattern spasticity (Sherrington originally described this phenomenon as decerebrate rigidity).[80] Both decorticate and decerebrate conditions are unidirectional in nature; there is an increase of muscle stiffness and resistance

to passive elongation (impaired compliance) in one group of muscles (agonists) with relatively normal functioning of opposing muscle groups (antagonists).

Spasticity is a velocity-dependent phenomenon. Under conditions of rapid passive elongation, spastic muscle groups "fight back" with increased stiffness, a result of a hypersensitive deep tendon reflex loop (Figure 10-4). This has been described as *clasp-knife spasticity*, in which the spastic limb "gives" after an initial period of resisting passive movement in the way that a pocket knife initially resists opening when near its initially closed position but then becomes more compliant once moved past a threshold position as it is opened. Growing evidence indicates that the stiffness encountered during passive movement has both neurological (spasticity) and musculoskeletal (changes in muscle and associated soft tissue) components that combine to increase the risk of contracture development.[81,82]

Given the unidirectional nature of severe hypertonus, it is common for persons with severe hypertonus to develop chronic abnormal postures. The limb or body segment assumes an end-range position that the limb would not normally be able to assume (e.g., extreme equinovarus with marked supination in an individual with severe acquired brain injury, equinovalgus with marked pronation in a child with CP).[80,81] If persistent, these fixed postures are associated with a significant likelihood of secondary contracture development.[83]

Hypertonicity is also associated with deficits in muscle performance, most notably diminished strength, diminished ability to produce power (generate force quickly), diminished ability to effectively isolate limb and body segments, diminished excursions of movements within joints (i.e., moving within a limited range of motion [ROM]), and inefficiency with altering force production or timing of contractions to meet changing (fluid) demands of tasks.[84-86] Muscle performance deficits can contribute to an imbalance of forces around a joint that leads to habitual abnormal patterns of movement. These habitual patterns are often biomechanically inefficient and, over time, contribute to the development of secondary musculoskeletal impairments such as adaptive shortening or lengthening of muscles and malalignment of joints.[83] Strengthening exercises can have a positive impact on function, even in the presence of hypertonicity.[85-87]

Rigidity

Individuals with Parkinson's disease and related neurological disorders often demonstrate varying levels of rigidity: a bidirectional, co-contracting hypertonicity in which there is resistance to passive movement of both agonistic and antagonistic muscle groups.[88] Co-contraction of flexor and extensor muscles of the limbs and trunk creates a bidirectional stiffness that interferes with functional movement. Rigidity is often accompanied by slowness in initiating movement (bradykinesia), decreased excursion of active ROM, and altered resting postures of the limbs and trunk (Figure 10-5). The rigidity of Parkinson's disease can be overridden under certain environmental conditions: Persons with moderate to

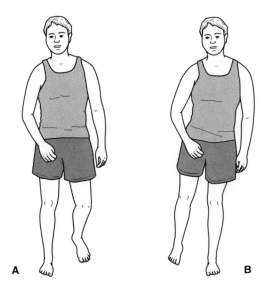

FIGURE 10-3 Decorticate pattern hypertonicity following cerebrovascular accident. **A,** The affected upper extremity is held in a flexed posture, while the extensor bias in the lower extremity provides stability at midstance and permits swing limb advancement of the less-involved extremity. **B,** The extensor pattern hypertonus in the affected lower extremity precludes swing-limb shortening normally accomplished by hip and knee flexion; instead, the individual uses an abnormal strategy such as pelvic retraction and hip hiking to advance the involved limb.

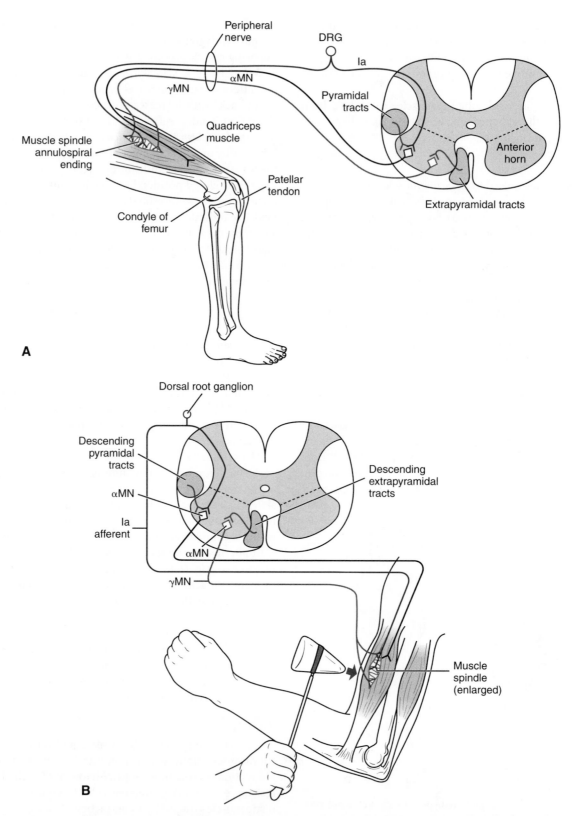

FIGURE 10-4 Diagram of the deep tendon reflex loop: stimulation of the annulospiral receptor within muscle spindle of the quadriceps (**A**) and biceps brachii (**B**) (via "tap" on the patellar tendon with a reflex hammer) activates 1a afferent neurons, which in turn assist motor neurons in the anterior horn of the spinal cord. These motor neurons project to extrafusal muscle fibers in the quadriceps, which contract, predictably, as a reflex response. Sensitivity of muscle spindle (threshold for stimulation) is influenced by extrapyramidal input, reaching γ motor neurons in the anterior horn, which project to intrafusal muscle fibers within the muscle spindle itself.

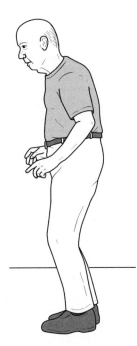

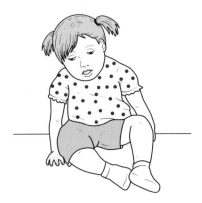

FIGURE 10-6 Postural control is often inefficient in children (and adults) with hypotonicity or low tone. This 10-month-old child has insufficient muscle tone to maintain her head and trunk in an upright position and uses her upper extremities to reach or manipulate, visually track objects in her environment, or safely transition into and out of a sitting position. (Modified from Stokes M. *Physical Management in Neurological Rehabilitation.* Edinburgh: Mosby, 2004. p. 322.)

FIGURE 10-5 Typical standing posture in individuals with Parkinson's disease, with a forward head, kyphotic and forward flexed trunk, and flexion at hip and knees. Upper extremities are often held in protracted and flexed position. The altered position of the body's center of mass, when combined with rigidity and bradykinesia, significantly decreases the efficacy of anticipatory postural responses during ambulation, as well a response to perturbation.

severe disease can suddenly run reciprocally if they perceive danger to themselves or a loved one; once this initial limbic response has dissipated, they will resume a stooped and rigid posture, with difficulty initiating voluntary movement, limited active ROM, and bradykinesia. Because rigidity creates a situation of excessive stability of the trunk and limbs, orthoses are not typically a component in the plan of care for persons with Parkinson's disease.[89]

Hypotonus

Hypotonus (low muscle tone) describes a reduced stiffness of muscle that does not effectively support upright posture against gravity or to generate force during contraction; as a result, hypotonic muscles are more compliant than they are stiff.[90] In children, hypotonia can arise from abnormal function within the CNS (approximately 75%) or from problems with peripheral structures (peripheral nerve and motor units, neuromuscular junction, the muscle itself, or unknown etiology).[91] Hypotonia can be congenital (seen as "floppy" infants), transient (e.g., in preterm infants), part of the clinical presentation of CP, Down syndrome and other genetic disorders, as well as Autism spectrum disorders.[91-96]

Hypotonic muscles are considerably more compliant on rapid passive elongation (i.e., less resistant to passive stretch) than muscles with typical tone, as well as those with hypertonus/spasticity. Because their postural muscles are less stiff, individuals with hypotonicity often have difficulty when assuming and sustaining antigravity positions.[97] To compensate for their reduced postural tone, persons with

hypotonicity may maintain postural alignment by relying on ligaments and connective tissue within joint capsule and muscle to sustain upright posture (Figure 10-6). With overreliance on ligaments in extreme ends of range, further degradation to joint structures often occurs.

In addition to postural control dysfunction, individuals with hypotonia often have difficulty with coordination of movements. This may be due to the decreased efficacy of afferent information collected by a lax muscle spindle during movement execution.[98] Children with hypotonia often have impaired control of movements at midrange of muscle length, suggesting that kinesthetic information is not being used efficiently to guide movement or that the ability to regulate force production throughout movements is compromised. In either case, muscle performance is notably less efficient, especially in activities that require eccentric control (e.g., controlled lowering of the body from a standing position to sitting on the floor).[97] Individuals with hypotonia have difficulty regulating force production and collaboration between agonists and antagonists is not well coordinated.[97]

Immediately after an acute CNS insult or injury there is often a period of neurogenic shock in which the motor system appears to shut down temporarily, with apparent loss of voluntary movement (paralysis) and markedly diminished or absent deep tendon reflex responses.[98-100] This phenomenon is observed following cervical or thoracic spinal cord injury and early on following significant stroke. During this period, individuals with extreme levels of hypotonus are sometimes (erroneously) described as having flaccid paralysis. Most individuals with acute CNS dysfunction will, within days to weeks, begin to show some evidence of returning muscle tone; over time, many develop hyperactive responses to deep tendon reflex testing and other signs of hypertonicity.[99] If they continue to have difficulty activating muscles voluntarily for efficient functional movement, these individuals are described as demonstrating spastic paralysis.

Flaccidity

The term *flaccidity* is best used to describe muscles that cannot be activated because of interruption of transmission or connection between lower motor neurons and the muscles they innervate.[101] True flaccidity is accompanied by significant atrophy of muscle tissue, well beyond the loss of muscle mass associated with inactivity; this is the result of loss of tonic influence of lower motor neurons on which muscle health is based.[102]

The flaccid paralysis seen in persons with myelomeningocele (spina bifida) occurs because incomplete closure of the neural tube during the early embryonic period (soon after conception) prevents interconnection between the primitive spinal cord and neighboring somites that will eventually develop into muscles of the extremities.[103] The flaccid paralysis observed in persons with cauda equina level spinal cord injury is the result of damage to axons of α and γ motor neurons as they travel together as ventral roots to their respective spinal foramina to exit the spinal column as a spinal nerve.[104] After acute poliomyelitis, the loss of a portion of a muscle's lower motor neurons will lead to marked weakness; the loss of the majority of a muscle's lower motor neurons will lead to flaccid paralysis.[65] In Guillain-Barré syndrome, the increasing weakness and flaccid paralysis seen in the early stages of the disease are the result of demyelination of the neuron's axons as they travel toward the muscle in a peripheral nerve.[105] After injection with botulinum toxin, muscle tone and strength are compromised because of the toxin's interference with transmitter release from the presynaptic component of the neuromuscular junction.[106]

Fluctuating Tone: Athetosis and Chorea

Athetosis is the descriptor used when an individual's underlying muscle tone fluctuates unpredictably.[107] Athetosis is characterized by random changes in postural tone, with variations from hypertonus to hypotonus. Athetosis, although less common than spastic CP, can have as significant (and often more pronounced) an impact on daily function.[108] Although etiology of athetosis is not well understood, it is most frequently described as a type of basal ganglia or thalamic dysfunction associated with bilirubin toxicity or significant perinatal anoxia.[107] Persons with athetosis typically demonstrate truncal hypotonia, with fluctuating levels of hypertonus in antigravity musculature and the extremities. In some individuals, movements appear to have a writhing dancelike quality (choreoathetosis) in addition to the tonal influences. Others may compensate for postural instability by assuming end-range positions, relying on mechanical stability of joints during functional activity. Although persons with athetosis are less likely to develop joint contracture than those with long-standing hypertonicity, they are more likely to develop secondary musculoskeletal complications that compromise stability of joints, a result of extreme posturing, imbalance of forces across joint structures, and the need to stabilize in habitual postural alignment patterns for function.[109]

Postural Control

Postural control has three key dimensions: (1) *Static postural control* is defined as the ability to hold antigravity postures at rest; (2) *dynamic anticipatory postural control* is the ability to sustain a posture during movement tasks that shift (internally perturb) the center of mass; and (3) *dynamic reactionary postural control* is the ability to be able to withstand or recover from externally derived perturbations without loss of balance.[110] One has functional postural control if the center of mass (COM) can be maintained within one's base of support (BOS) under a wide range of task demands and environmental conditions. This requires some level of ability across the triad of static, anticipatory, and reactionary control.

The key interactive CNS systems involved in postural control include extrapyramidal and pyramidal motor systems, visual and visual-perceptual systems, conscious (dorsal column/medial lemniscal) and unconscious (spinocerebellar) somatosensory systems, the vestibular system, and the cerebellar feedback/feedforward systems.[111,112] Clinical measures used to assess efficacy of static postural control include timing of sitting or standing activities and measures of center of pressure excursion in quiet standing.[113] The Clinical Test of Sensory Interaction and Balance sorts out the contribution of visual, vestibular, and proprioceptive systems' contribution to balance, as well as the individual's ability to select the most relevant sensory input when there is conflicting information collected among these systems.[114]

Measures of anticipatory postural control consider how far the individual is willing to shift his or her center of mass toward the edge of his or her sway envelope.[115,116] Clinically, anticipatory postural control is often quantified by measuring reaching distance in various postures.[117-119] Measures of dynamic reactionary postural control consider the individual's response to unexpected perturbations (e.g., when pushed or displaced by an external force, when tripping/slipping in conditions of high environmental demand).[120,121] Although these three dimensions of postural control are interrelated, competence in one does not necessarily ensure effective responses in the others.[122]

Many individuals with neuromuscular disorders demonstrate inefficiency or disruption of one or more of the CNS subsystems necessary for effective postural control and balance.[123] An individual with mild to moderate hypertonicity or spasticity often has difficulty with anticipatory and reactionary postural control, especially in high task demand situations within a complex or unpredictable open environment.[124] Difficulty with muscle performance, such as impairment of control of force production or the imbalance of forces acting across a joint, might constrain anticipatory postural control in preparation for functional tasks such as reaching or stepping. Impairment of the ability to segment trunk from limb or to individually control joints within a limb may affect the individual's ability to react to perturbations in a timely or consistent manner.[125]

Persons with hypotonicity, on the other hand, often have difficulty with sustaining effective postural alignment in antigravity positions such as sitting and standing. They are likely to demonstrate patterns of postural malalignment such as excessive lumbar lordosis and thoracic kyphosis.[97] Because of difficulty with muscle force production (especially in midrange of movement), individuals with hypotonia also have difficulty with anticipatory postural control.[90] A lack of on-demand motor control contributes to difficulty moving within one's postural sway envelope; this may be observed as a tendency to stay in one posture for long periods of time, with infrequent alterations in position during tasks.[94] Reactionary control may also be altered, particularly with respect to the use of equilibrium reactions and the reliability of protective responses. Individuals with hypotonia have difficulty when a task requires them to absorb small-amplitude perturbations; they must use equilibrium or balance strategies more frequently than persons with adequate muscle tone.[90] Additionally, a lack of stability in joints, from both tonal and ligamentous laxity, contributes to an inability to safely stop an accelerating body part as it comes into contact with a surface during a loss of balance episode.[94]

Movement and Coordination

Many functional activities require us to move or transport the entire body (e.g., mobility or locomotion) or a segment of the body (e.g., using one's upper extremity to bring a cup toward the mouth to take a drink) through space.[126,127] The locomotion task that receives much attention in rehabilitation settings is bipedal ambulation—the ability to walk. For full functional ability, individuals must be able to manage a variety of additional locomotion tasks: running, skipping, jumping, and hopping.[128] To fully understand an individual's functional ability, therapists and orthotists must also consider the environmental context in which ambulation is occurring.[129] What are the physical characteristics of the surface on which the individual needs to be able to walk or traverse? Is it level, unpredictably uneven, slippery or frictional, or structurally unstable? Is the ambulation task occurring where lighting is adequate for visual data collection about environmental conditions? Does it involve manipulation of some type of object (e.g., an ambulatory assistive device, a school backpack, shopping bags, suitcases)? Is it occurring in a familiar and predictable environment (e.g., at home) or in a more unpredictable and challenging open environment such as a busy school, supermarket, mall, or other public space? The task demands of locomotion in complex and challenging environments create more demand on the CNS structures involved in motor control (perceptual-motor function, motor planning, cerebellar error control), as well as on the musculoskeletal effectors (muscles and tendons, joints, ligaments, and bones) that enact the motor plan necessary for successful completion of the task that relies on body transport. Individuals with neurological and neuromuscular system problems related to muscle tone, muscle performance, and postural control are typically less efficient, less adaptable, and more prone to fall when walking, especially if there are competing task demands and the environment is complex and challenging.[130]

The use of a limb segment can also be defined by the nature of the task and the circumstances in which the movement is performed. Upper extremity functional tasks can involve one or more components: reaching, grasping, releasing, manipulating, or any combination of these four purposes.[126] Upper extremity tasks can also be defined by considering the function to be accomplished by the movement: grooming, dressing, meal preparation, self-care, or writing. Many upper extremity mobility tasks are founded on effective postural control (e.g., making appropriate anticipatory postural adjustments as the COM shifts while throwing, lifting, lowering, or catching an object).[126] Complex mobility tasks require simultaneous locomotion and segmented use of extremities (e.g., reaching for the doorknob while ascending the steps toward the front door, throwing or catching a ball while running during a football or baseball game). For individuals with neurological and neuromuscular system dysfunction, the ability to safely and efficiently perform complex mobility tasks is often compromised due to abnormal muscle tone, impaired muscle performance, and poor postural control.[130]

Coordination can be thought of as the efficacy of execution of the movement necessary to complete a task. A well-coordinated movement requires effective simultaneous control of many different dimensions of movement: the accuracy of a movement's direction and trajectory; the timing, sequencing, and precision of muscle activation; the rate and amplitude of force production; the interaction of agonistic and antagonistic muscle groups; the ability to select and manage the type of contraction (concentric, holding, or eccentric) necessary for the task; and the ability to anticipate and respond to environmental demands during movement.[131] Coordination can be examined by considering the individual's ability to initiate movement, sustain movement during the task or activity, and terminate movement according to task demands.[132]

For movement and coordination to be functional, one must have muscle performance that is flexible/adaptable to varying demands.[133] Mobility or transport tasks cannot be performed independently (safely) unless the individual is able to (1) transition into and out of precursor positions (e.g., getting up from the floor into a standing position, rising from a chair), (2) initiate or begin the activity (e.g., take the first step), (3) sustain the activity (control forward progression with repeated steps), (4) change direction as environmental conditions demand (e.g., step over or avoid an obstacle), (5) modulate speed as environmental conditions demand (e.g., increase gait speed when crossing the street), and (6) safely and effectively stop or terminate the motion, returning to a precursor condition or position (quiet standing, return to sitting).[133]

For individuals with neuromuscular disorders who have difficulty with muscle performance, abnormal underlying tone, or poor postural control, coordination of functional movement can be compromised in several ways. In order to approach and complete a movement task, the individual might rely on abnormal patterns of movement with additional effort and energy cost.[134] Many individuals with hypertonicity initiate movement with strong bursts of muscle contractions but have difficulty sustaining muscle activity and force of contraction through the full

ROM necessary to perform a functional movement.[98,108] Deficits in timing and sequencing of muscle contractions, as well as difficulty with dissociation of limb and body segments, also contribute to difficulty with performance of functional tasks.[135] An adult with hemiplegia following a cerebrovascular accident may be able to initiate a reach toward an object but not be able to bring the arm all the way to the target.[136] The same individual may have difficulty with timing and segmentation, leading to inability to open the hand before reaching the target in preparation for grasping the object.[137,138] The muscle performance of many children with CP is compromised by inappropriate sequencing of muscle contractions when activation of synergists and antago-

nists happens simultaneously.[108] Conversely, an individual with hypotonus who has difficulty with stabilization often moves quickly with diminished accuracy and coordination.[90]

The following tables provide an overview of incidence/prevalence, etiology and risk factors, clinical presentation, and impact on muscle tone, muscle performance, postural control, and movement for of the most common pathologies that might include use of an orthosis: stroke (Table 10-1), CP (Table 10-2), spina bifida (Table 10-3), MS (Table 10-4), and spinal cord injury (Table 10-5).

When considering an upper or lower extremity orthosis or a seating system to support the trunk for individuals with

TABLE 10-1   *Stroke*

Also known as	Brain attack, cerebrovascular accident (CVA)
Incidence	Approximately 610,000 per year in the U.S.*
Prevalence	2.6% of total US population have had stroke* 8.1% of US population over age 65 have had stroke*
ETIOLOGY AND RISK FACTORS **Ischemic Stroke (88%)**	
Thrombus	Hypertension, hypercholesterolemia, diabetes and metabolic syndrome, overweight and obesity, smoking, sedentary lifestyle*
Embolism	Atrial fibrillation, atherosclerosis in carotid/vertebral arterial systems; previous embolic stroke
Hemorrhagic Stroke (12%) Intracranial hemorrhage	Uncontrolled hypertension, ruptured aneurysm
STROKE SYNDROMES (BY ARTERY) Middle cerebral (most common)	Contralateral hemiparesis/hemiplegia, lower face, UE > LE Contralateral sensory loss of lower face, UE > LE Contralateral homonymous hemianopia (optic tract) Possible dysarthria and dysphagia R hemisphere: visual-spatial or somatic perceptual impairment L hemisphere: communication impairment (various aphasias)
Lenticulo-striate (lacunar MCA)	Contralateral hemiparesis/hemiplegia, lower face, UE = LE Cortical functions (perception, communication) intact
Anterior cerebral	Contralateral hemiparesis/hemiplegia LE > UE Sensation often intact or only mildly impaired (contralateral) Incontinence "Alien hand" syndrome (involuntary/unintended movement) Motor (nonfluent/Broca's) aphasia may occur
Posterior cerebral	Contralateral homonymous hemianopsia (optic radiations) Visual inattention L hemisphere: alexia (unable to read), with ability to write preserved
Thalamogeniculate (lacunar PCA)	Contralateral sensory loss, often severe Sensory ataxia (uncoordinated movement due to lack of proprioception) Thalamic pain and hyperpathia syndrome
Basilar (complete)	Loss of consciousness, coma High mortality
Superior cerebellar	Ipsilateral ataxia, falling to side of lesion Intention tremor Contralateral loss of pain temperature sensation from body Contralateral loss of proprioception Ipsilateral Horner's syndrome (meiosis, ptosis, anhydrosis)

TABLE 10-1   *Stroke—cont'd*

Anterior-inferior cerebellar	Ipsilateral facial paralysis (both upper and lower face) Ipsilateral loss of pain and temperature of entire face Contralateral loss of pain and temperature from body Loss of taste sensation, loss of corneal reflex, ipsilateral hearing loss, nystagmus, vertigo, nausea Ataxia and incoordination of limb movement Ipsilateral Horner's syndrome (meiosis, ptosis, anhydrosis)
Vertebral	Contralateral loss of pain, temperature sensation from body
Posterior-inferior cerebellar (Wallenberg's syndrome) (lateral medullary syndrome)	Ipsilateral loss of pain and temperature sensation from face Ipsilateral Horner's syndrome (meiosis, ptosis, anhydrosis) Dysphonia, dysphagia, dysarthria, diminished gag reflex Nystagmus, diplopia, vertigo, nausea Ipsiversive falling (toward side of lesion), incoordination, ataxia
PROGNOSIS	Ischemic: severity depends on site of occlusion within arterial tree and the size of the area that is without blood flow Embolic: risk of recurrence is higher than in thrombosis; risk of hemorrhage at site of embolism Hemorrhagic: highest morbidity and mortality Static event, with evolving symptoms in weeks/months following initial damage, due to initial inflammatory response and subsequent tissue remodeling/healing.
MUSCLE TONE	Initial hypotonus (sometimes appearing to be flaccid) due to neurogenic shock. Some individuals remain hypotonic, most develop various levels of hypertonus in weeks/months following event. Hyperactive deep tendon reflexes evolve over time.
MUSCLE PERFORMANCE	Upper extremity often biased toward flexion, with lower extremity biased toward extension. Impaired force production, speed and power, eccentric/isometric control, accuracy, and fluidity.
POSTURAL CONTROL	Frequently impaired, especially if lesion included gray matter of R hemisphere, with perceptual dysfunction.
MOBILITY AND COORDINATION	Asymmetry in ability to use trunk, limbs during functional .activity; tendency to move in abnormal "synergy" (flexion UE, extension LE). Frequently require AFO and ambulatory device.

AFO, ankle-foot-orthosis; *L*, left; *LE*, lower extremity; *MCA*, middle cerebral artery ; *PCA* posterior cerebral artery, ; *R*, right; *UE*, upper extremity.
*American Heart Association Risk Factors for Stroke. Available at: http://www.heart.org/HEARTORG/General/Risk-Factors_UCM_319118_Article.jsp; accessed 8/9/11.

neurological or neuromuscular dysfunction, the therapist and orthotist must clearly define what they hope the orthosis will accomplish (e.g., management of abnormal tone, provision of stability for a limb segment in the presence of impaired muscle performance or motor control, or enhancing positioning to allow more efficient function and movement). They must also consider the impact of the orthosis on postural control, overall mobility, and ability to adapt to environmental demands. There is no perfect orthosis that will address all dimensions of movement dysfunction; there are always trade-offs that must be taken into account.

MANAGEMENT OF NEUROMUSCULAR IMPAIRMENTS

Effective care of persons with movement dysfunction secondary to neurological and neuromuscular pathologies requires collaboration of health professionals from many disciplines: neurologists, orthopedist, physiatrists, physical and occupational therapists, and orthotists, among others.[139-141]

Physicians and surgeons manage spasticity and correct orthopedic deformity with medication and surgery. Nurses are involved in wellness care, as well as medical and surgical management. Rehabilitation professionals facilitate return of function after an acute event and provide functional training and postoperative rehabilitation for individuals across the spectrum of neurological and neuromuscular pathologies. Orthotists contribute their knowledge of orthotic options to improve gait and function. The multidisciplinary approach leads to greater satisfaction with care and less risk of abandonment of orthoses and assistive devices by the person they were made for.[142]

Medical and Surgical Care

Medical management of CNS dysfunction often includes prescription of pharmacological agents. Physicians can select from a range of centrally acting tone-inhibiting medications (e.g., baclofen [Lioresal]) or pharmacological interventions that target lower motor neurons, peripheral nerves, or muscle (e.g., botulinum toxin injection, intrathecal baclofen) for

TABLE 10-2   *Cerebral Palsy*

Incidence	Approximately 11,500 new cases diagnosed per year*
Prevalence	764,000 children and adults in the U.S.; 3.3 per 1000*
Etiology	Unknown in most instances
Risk factors	Prematurity, high-risk pregnancy, low birth weight, perinatal or neonatal respiratory distress/anoxia, mother's substance abuse while pregnant

TYPES OF CEREBRAL PALSY

Spastic (85%-93%)*,†	Quadriplegia/tetraplegia: global impact on both gray and white matter structures in forebrain. Some individuals have concomitant cognitive impairment and seizure disorders. Diplegia: usually due to damage of white matter of internal capsule/corona radiate, impacting on motor and sensory systems more than perceptual. Hemiplegia: may be due to intracerebral hemorrhage or ischemia affecting one hemisphere.
Dyskinetic (5%-10%)*,† (choreoathetoid)	May be related to perinatal damage of basal ganglia Unpredictably fluctuating tone of head/neck, trunk, and extremities; may be associated with perinatal bilirubin toxicity
Ataxic/cerebellar (5%)	May be related to perinatal damage of cerebellar cortex, nuclei, or peduncles
PROGNOSIS	Static event occurring at or around the time of birth. Signs and symptoms become apparent over first 2 years of life as motor developmental delay. High risk of secondary musculoskeletal deformity due to impact of abnormal tone during periods of growth and repetitive impact of muscle imbalance on movement. Level of disability often becomes more pronounced as child moves into middle childhood, adolescence, and young adulthood due to increasing body size and weight.

MUSCLE TONE

Spastic	Initial hypotonus in premature and low-birth-weight infants common. Hypertonus develops over time; severity of hypertonus varies depending on extent of central nervous system damage. Hypertonus may increase in times of growth, or in times of excitement and stress. Hyperactive deep tendon reflexes, as well as abnormal tonic developmental reflexes.
Dyskinetic	Unpredictable fluctuation of muscle tone (from very low tone to significant hypertonus), affecting muscles of limbs, axial skeleton, respiration, and phonation. Often appears as writhing motions of trunk and extremity. Response to tendon reflexes varies due to changing tone.
Ataxic	Frequently hypotonic with hyperflexible joints in both appendicular and axial skeleton. At risk for secondary overuse injury with habitual and long-term hyperflexibility during movement and in static postures. Often pendular deep tendon reflexes.

MUSCLE PERFORMANCE

Spastic	May be hypokinetic (small excursion of movement) or hyperkinetic (large excursion of movement) with difficulty modulating force; force production can be great (strong forceful unrelenting contraction) or small (inability to sustain contraction for functional movements); difficulty with eccentric and isometric control, poor accuracy and precision of movement.
Dyskinetic	May be hypokinetic (slow and minimal movement) or hyperkinetic (movements can be random and/or repetitive with minimal purpose); force production, speed, and timing of contractions do not match task demands; poor accuracy.
Ataxic	May be hypokinetic or hyperkinetic; tasks demanding greater accuracy lead to faster and greater excursions, with worsening accuracy; tasks demanding less accuracy lead to slower and lesser excursions with some accuracy. Timing of agonist and antagonist sequencing is impaired.

POSTURAL CONTROL

Spastic	Often impaired, due to influence of persistent tonic reflexes, and less efficient development of righting and equilibrium responses in trunk and affected limbs.
Dyskinetic	May be significantly impaired; fluctuating tone challenges ability to attain and hold positions or move dynamically through space.

TABLE 10-2 *Cerebral Palsy—cont'd*

Ataxic	Sitting and standing postures may be "floppy," as child relies on soft tissue structures of the musculoskeletal system to support upright position because of inadequate antigravity postural control.

MOBILITY AND COORDINATION

Spastic	Frequently employ movement strategies based on atypical and less variable patterns/synergies; over time may develop rotational deformity of lower extremity as well as joint contracture due to combination of preferred abnormal positions/patterns of movement and hypertonus. Often require ankle-foot-orthosis, assistive devices, or wheelchair for locomotion. Those with significant trunk and upper extremity involvement may require adaptive equipment for feeding, communication, and activities of daily living. Orthoses or resting splints may be used as a means of managing abnormal tone, minimizing risk of musculoskeletal deformity, or after orthopedic surgery to correct deformity.
Dyskinetic	Often depend on external support for stability during functional tasks and locomotion. May benefit from use of ambulatory device, adaptive equipment, seating systems, or upper and lower extremity orthoses.
Ataxic	Depending on severity of impairment, may have difficulty with trunk stability during functional tasks using upper extremity (activities of daily living), and lower extremity (walking). May use ankle-foot orthosis to provide external support/positioning during functional task.

*Centers for Disease Control and Prevention: Cerebral Palsy http://www.cdc.gov/ncbddd. Accessed 8/11/11.
†Kirby RS, Wingate MS, Van Naarden Braun K. Prevalence and functioning of children with cerebral palsy in four areas of the United States in 2006: a report from the Autism and Developmental Disabilities Monitoring Network. *Res Dev Disabil.* 2011;32(2):462-469.

TABLE 10-3 *Spina Bifida*

Incidence	.05 per 1000 live births; approximately 3000 per year in the U.S.[*†‡]
Prevalence	1.9 to 3.1 per 10,000 children 0-19 years in the U.S.[a,b,c]
Etiology	Unknown
Risk factors[§¶]	Folate deficiency Advanced maternal age Genetic tendency/previous pregnancy or family member with spina bifida Taking valproic acid or carbamazepine for seizures Having high temperatures early in pregnancy

TYPES OF SPINA BIFIDA[ǁ]

Occulta	Abnormal formation of lumbar or sacral vertebrae, with intact spinal cord and spinal nerves, and full skin coverage. May be a progressive deterioration of function in late childhood into adulthood.
Meningocele	Vertebral defect such that meninges and cerebrospinal fluid protrude but spinal cord, cauda equina, and spinal nerves remain within the spinal column. Vertebral defect may or may not be covered by skin. Often associated with minor to mild impairment of motor and sensory function.
Myelomeningocele	Defect such that meninges and incompletely closed spinal cord protrude; associated with lower motor neuron dysfunction (flaccid paralysis) and complete sensory loss below level of lesion; may have spasticity of muscles innervated by spinal nerves just proximal to level of lesion. Urinary and fecal incontinence common, risk of neuropathic wounds high; risk of osteoporosis of lower extremities high.
PROGNOSIS	Incomplete closure of neural tube soon after conception; leading to flaccid paralysis and total sensory impairment of all structures innervated at and below level of lesion. May be concurrent with hydrocephalus, often managed by ventriculoperitoneal shunt. Static, nonprogressive condition; however level of disability often becomes more pronounced as child moves into middle childhood, adolescence, and young adulthood due to increasing body size and weight. High risk of secondary musculoskeletal deformity (e.g., osteoporosis, fracture, contracture) due to combination of motor and sensory impairment. Depending on level of lesion, voluntary bladder and bowel control may also be impaired or absent.

(Continued)

TABLE 10-3   *Spina Bifida—cont'd*

MUSCLE TONE	Typically flaccid paralysis with absent deep tendon reflexes. May have spotty hypertonicity of muscle innervated by nerve roots proximal to level of lesion.
MUSCLE PERFORMANCE	No muscle activity below level of lesion
POSTURAL CONTROL	Normal righting reactions and equilibrium responses above level of lesion; with absence of righting and equilibrium responses in trunk and limbs below level of lesion. Postural control in sitting influenced by how much of trunk and pelvis is innervated. At risk of developing hypermobility of spinal column around level of lesion.
MOBILITY AND COORDINATION	Impairment and functional limitation proportional to level of lesion. Those with sacral or low lumbar level lesions may be able to ambulate with ankle-foot orthosis, with or without assistive devices. Those with mid to high lumbar lesions may use knee-ankle-foot orthosis or hip-knee-ankle-foot orthosis for limited mobility. Many individuals with lumbar and higher levels opt, over time, to use seating and wheelchair systems for functional mobility. Orthoses and splints may be used after orthopedic surgeries to repair fracture or correct deformity.

*Shin M, Besser LM, Siffel C, et al. Prevalence of spina bifida among children and adolescents in 10 regions in the United States. *Pediatrics.* 2010;126(2):274-279.

†Boulet SL, Gambrell D, Shin M, Honein MA, Matthews TJ. Racial/ethnic differences in the birth prevalence of spina bifida—United States, 1995-2005. *JAMA.* 2009;301(21):2203-2204.

‡Racial/ethnic differences in the birth prevalence of spina bifida—United States, 1995-2005. *MMWR Morb Mortal Wkly Rep.* 2009;57(53):1409-1413.

§Bowman RM, Boshnjaku V, McLone DG. The changing incidence of myelomeningocele and its impact on pediatric neurosurgery: a review from the Children's Memorial Hospital. *Child Nervous Syst.* 2009;25(7):801-806.

¶http://www.spinabifidaassociation.org/site/c.liKWL7PLLrF/b.2738091/k.9A71/Risk_Factor.

‖http://www.ninds.nih.gov/disorders/spina_bifida/detail_spina_bifida.htm#183133258 Accessed 8/11/11.

TABLE 10-4   *Multiple Sclerosis*

Incidence	10,000 new cases of MS are diagnosed yearly in the U.S.*
Prevalence	between 350,000 and 400,000 people living with MS; 1 in 750 people, 90 per 100,000*†
Etiology	Unknown; CNS demyelinating disease affecting CNS subsystem
Risk factors	May be exposure to slow virus, environmental toxin, possible autoimmune components, risk higher among siblings, more common in women than men, more common among persons in northern latitudes; more common among Caucasians. Most commonly diagnosed in early to mid adulthood.
CLASSIFICATIONS OF MS‡	
Possible MS	an individual experiences a clinically isolated syndrome (CIS): a single neurologic episode that lasts at least 24 hours, and is caused by inflammation/demyelination in one or more sites in the central nervous system, especially if lesions are present on MRI.
Relapsing remitting (85%)	cycle of exacerbations (new signs/symptoms) followed by partial to complete recovery during which there is no apparent worsening of the disease process
Progressive	steadily worsening of symptoms from time of diagnosis, with incomplete recovery between exacerbations.
PROGNOSIS	Unpredictable exacerbations result from inflammation and destruction of myelin around pathways within the CNS.
	Residual impairments are the consequence of slowed transmission of neural impulses across plaques interrupting connections between CNS structures.
	May impact on any subsystem within CNS (voluntary motor, postural control, coordination, memory, perception, sensation).
	Definitive diagnosis made if there have been at least two different episodes of impairment, involving two different neurological subsystems, affecting two different parts of the body, at two different periods of time.
	Variable course, with many different types of impairment accruing over time with repeated exacerbations.
	Typically onset of initial symptoms in young and mid-adulthood. Often diagnosis by exclusion; when neurological signs/symptoms cannot be attributed to other disease processes.

TABLE 10-4   *Multiple Sclerosis—cont'd*

MUSCLE TONE	Varies, depending on location and size of residual plaque. Some individuals may exhibit normal tone and deep tendon reflexes, in the presences of perceptual, postural, or coordination impairment. Others may demonstrate hypertonus and hyperactive reflexes is various muscles. Others may have hypotonus and impaired muscle performance.
MUSCLE PERFORMANCE	Varies, depending on location of MS plaque. If in pyramidal system, may have weakness, impaired muscle endurance, poor eccentric control, among others. If in cerebellar systems, may demonstrate ataxia, intention tremor, among others.
POSTURAL CONTROL	Postural control and equilibrium responses may be impaired due to a combination of pyramidal and/or extrapyramidal motor system impairment, sensory impairment or somatosensory, spinocerebellar, or visual pathways, or damage of major integrative while matter structures such as the corpus callosum, or medial longitudinal fasciculus
MOBILITY AND COORDINATION	Mobility and locomotion may be impaired, along with postural control, depending on location of lesion. Some individuals with impaired muscle performance benefit from AFOs (for support and positioning of lower extremity in gait) associated with weakness or hypertonicity. Many choose to use ambulatory aides and assistive devices for function and safety. Some with significant multisystem impairment benefit from seating and wheeled mobility systems.

AFO, ankle-foot orthosis; CNS, central nervous system; MRI, magnetic resonance imaging; MS, multiple sclerosis.
*Rumrill PD. Multiple sclerosis: medical and psychosocial aspects, etiology, incidence, and prevalence. *J Vocat Rehabil.* 2009;31(2):75-78.
†http://www.clevelandclinicmeded.com/medicalpubs/diseasemanagement/neurology/multiple_sclerosis/#s0015.
‡National MS Society. About MS. Available at: http://www.nationalmssociety.org/about-multiple-sclerosis/index.aspx. Accessed 3/9/12.

TABLE 10-5   *Spinal Cord Injury*

Incidence	11,000 new cases in the U.S. per year,* 4.5 per 100,000†
Prevalence	Nearly 250,000 persons in the U.S. are living with spinal cord injury (SCI)*
Etiology	Usually traumatic, sometimes infectious (e.g., transverse myelitis) or ischemic (e.g., complication of abdominal aortic aneurysm repair)
Risk factors	Young age, male gender, drunk driving, participation in extreme sports, all terrain vehicle accidents, military injury
SCI SYNDROMES	
Complete upper motor neuron (UMN)	Quadriplegia (cervical cord injury) or paraplegia (thoracic cord injury) with spastic paralysis. Consequence of compression, contusion, or ischemia of spinal cord as a result of vertebral fracture or dislocation sustained in fall, collision, diving, gunshot wound, or other high-impact event. Exacerbated by resultant inflammatory process. Spinal cord below level of lesion survives but is unhooked from brain and brainstem, only able to operate reflexively (e.g., neurogenic bladder and bowel function).
Incomplete (>60%)‡	Similar mechanism of injury but with sparing of one or more areas of spinal cord such that there is some volitional motor function and sensation along with more typical UMN (for cervical and thoracic vertebral lesions) or lower motor neurons (LMN) (for lumbosacral vertebral lesions) (e.g., central cord syndrome: upper extremity involvement > lower extremity involvement, often with preserved volitional bladder and bowel function). Becoming more common with advances in emergency care on newly injured persons.
Complete LMN	Paraplegia consequence of compression, contusion of lumbosacral nerve roots (cauda equina) within the lower spinal canal, resulting in flaccid paralysis and sensory loss below the level of lesion.
Prognosis	Improved emergency and acute medical management often results in incomplete lesion, with varying combinations of return of function and spastic paralysis.
MUSCLE TONE	
Complete UMN	Initial hypotonicity during period of neurogenic shock. Many develop significant hypertonicity in the months after injury; some may have muscle spasm needing pharmacological intervention. Sudden increase in resting tone may signal unrecognized skin irritation, bladder distention or infection, or bowel impaction. At risk of secondary musculoskeletal deformity (contracture) due to longstanding abnormal tone and limited mobility.

(Continued)

TABLE 10-5   *Spinal Cord Injury—cont'd*

Incomplete	Also may demonstrate hypotonicity in the days immediately following injury. Some volitional muscle function may be apparent early on; spasticity may develop in other muscles over time. Muscles with spasticity similar to complete UMN injury.
Complete LMN	Considered a lower motor neuron lesion with flaccid paralysis and absence of deep tendon reflexes at and below level of lesion.

MUSCLE PERFORMANCE

Complete UMN	Impaired and inadequate; reflexive function only.
Incomplete	Muscles that remain innervated often initially weak; responsive to interventions to enhance force production, muscle endurance, power.
Complete LMN	No muscle function and areflexic below level of lesion.

POSTURAL CONTROL

Complete UMN	Disconnection of lower motor neuron pool below level of lesion results in loss of volitional movement, as well as automatic postural responses, despite hypertonus. Deep tendon reflexes are often brisk, sometimes resulting in sustained clonus.
Incomplete	Varies from significantly impaired to minimally impaired, depending on location and extent of lesion.
Complete LMN	Postural control of trunk intact, although flaccid paralysis of lower extremities limit stability in standing without external support of orthoses.

MOBILITY AND COORDINATION

All Types	May temporarily use spinal orthosis (CO, CTO, TLSO) until surgical stabilization of damaged vertebrae is well healed. Often require seating and wheelchair systems for mobility.
	Persons with cervical level lesions may require upper extremity splints and adaptive equipment for activities of daily living, or resting splints or orthoses to manage abnormal tone and prevent contracture.
Complete LMN	Persons with low thoracic and lumbosacral lesions may use AFO, KAFO, or HKAFO along with assistive device (rolling walker, crutches) for ambulation, either as part of rehabilitation or of fitness program; energy cost of ambulation for community distances often high enough to be impractical.

AFO, ankle-foot orthosis; CO, cervical orthosis; CTO, cervical thoracic orthosis; TLSO, thoraco-lumbo-sacral orthosis; HKAFO, hip-ankle-foot orthosis; KAFO, knee-ankle-foot orthosis.

*Sipski ML, Richards S. Spinal cord injury rehabilitation. *Am J Phys Med Rehabil.* 2006;85(4):310-342.

†Hirtz D, Thurman DJ, Gwinn-Hardy K, et al. How common are the "common" neurologic disorders? *Neurology.* 2007;68(5):326-337.

‡Wyndaele M, Wyndaele J. Incidence, prevalence and epidemiology of spinal cord injury: what learns a worldwide literature survey? *J Spinal Cord.* 2006;44(9):523-529.

individuals with significant hypertonicity.[143-149] A host of medications have become available to reduce likelihood of exacerbation, delay disease progression, and manage fatigue for persons with MS.[150,151] Many individuals with CNS disorders also must cope with seizure management; many antiepileptic drugs affect tone, arousal, and ability to learn.[152] It is important for physical therapists and orthotists to be aware of the potential impact of neuroactive medications on an individual's ability to concentrate and learn, overall health status, and neuromotor control.[153,154] A summary of pharmacological agents used in the management of hypertonicity resulting from CNS disease, in the management of MS, and for seizure disorders is presented in Table 10-6.

Alternatively, physicians may recommend various neurosurgical procedures and orthopedic surgeries to correct deformity, improve flexibility, or reduce level of abnormal tone, with the goal of enhancing mobility and improving performance of functional tasks. Neurectomy and neurotomy, for example, may be used to manage severe equinovarus and upper extremity spasticity after stroke and for children with CP.[155-159] Selective dorsal rhizotomy effectively reduces problematic hypertonicity for children with CP but does not seem to reduce future risk of developing deformity, which would then require orthopedic surgery.[160-162] Intrathecal baclofen pumps have been used as a strategy to manage severe spasticity in persons with traumatic brain injury, stroke, spinal cord injury, and CP.[163-165]

Despite pharmacological and positioning interventions, musculoskeletal deformities can still develop, particularly in the growing child. Surgical interventions are used to correct musculoskeletal defaults of the spine and limbs, realign joints for better mechanical advantage, improve ease of caregiving and hygiene management, promote cosmesis, or reduce and prevent pain. Tendon lengthenings or transfers are commonly used to correct contractures and provide

TABLE 10-6 *Pharmacological Interventions for Individuals with Neurological and Neuromuscular System Impairments*

Trade Names	Generic Name (class)	Administration	Indications	Adverse Effects
MANAGEMENT OF DYSTONIA AND CENTRAL NERVOUS SYSTEM (CNS)-RELATED SPASM				
NeuroBloc Myobloc	botulinum B toxin (neurotoxin)	Intramuscular	Facial spasm, spasmodic torticollis, blepharospasm	Pain at injection site, ptosis, eye irritation, weakness of neck muscles, dysphagia, dry mouth, heartburn
MANAGEMENT OF HYPERTONICITY, CLONUS, AND TICS				
Botox Dysport	botulinum A toxin (neurotoxin)	Intramuscular or perineural injection, intrathecal	Chronic severe spasticity or dystonia	Pain or bruising at injection site, muscle weakness, tiredness, drowsiness, nausea, anxiety
Catapres	clonidine (antihypertensive)	Oral or transdermal	Spasticity in MS	Dry mouth, gastrointestinal disturbances, fatigue, headache, nervousness, insomnia, skin irritation (transdermal)
Ceberclon Klonopin Rivotril Valpax	clonazepam (benzodiazepine)	Oral	Spasticity in CP, dystonic, chorea, akathisia (also for seizures, panic attacks)	Sedation, dizziness, unsteadiness, incoordination, memory problems, muscle or joint pain, blurred vision, frequent urination
Dantrium	dantrolene sodium (skeletal muscle relaxant)	Oral or injection	Chronic severe spasticity of UMN orgin	Drowsiness, dizziness, generalized weakness, malaise, fatigue, nervousness, headache
Ethanol	ethyl alcohol (neurotoxin)	Intramuscular or perineural injection	Severe spasticity, with serial casting follow-up	Neuritis, hyperesthesia, or parasthesia
Lioresal	baclofen (skeletal muscle relaxant)	Oral, injection, or intrathecal	Chronic severe spasticity for conditions including SCI, ABI, MS; not effective in CP	Sedation, confusion, hypotension, dizziness, ataxia, headache, tremor, nystagmus, paresthesia, diaphoresis, muscular pain or weakness, insomnia, behavioral changes
Neurontin	gabapentin	Oral	Adjunct to other antispasticity medications for SCI and MS	Drowsiness, dizziness, ataxia, fatigue, nystagmus, nervousness, tremor, diplopia, memory impairment
Phenol	phenol	Intramuscular or perineural injection	Severe lower limb spasticity (with serial casting follow-up) pain control	Damage to other neural structures
Robaxin	methocarbamol	Oral or injection	Short-term relief of muscle spasm or spasticity	Sedation, drowsiness, lightheadedness, fatigue, dizziness, nausea, restlessness
Valium	diazepam	Oral or injection	Short-term relief of muscle spasm or spasticity	Sedation, drowsiness, fatigue, ataxia, confusion, depression, diplopia, dysarthria, tremor
Zanaflex Sirdalud	tizanidine (skeletal muscle relaxant)	Oral	Spasticity from MS or SCI	Sedation, drowsiness, fatigue, dizziness, mild weakness, nausea, hypotension, GI irritation

(Continued)

TABLE 10-6   *Pharmacological Interventions for Individuals with Neurological and Neuromuscular System Impairments—cont'd*

Trade Names	Generic Name (class)	Administration	Indications	Adverse Effects
MANAGEMENT OF MULTIPLE SCLEROSIS: ACUTE EXACERBATION				
Aristocort Aristo-Pak Kenacort	triamcinolone (corticosteroid)	Oral	Acute exacerbation	Electrolyte disturbances, CHF, hypokalemia, weakness, myopathy, osteoporosis, seizures, papilledema, vertigo, headache
Decadron Hexadrol Maxidex Mymethasone	dexamethasone (corticosteroid)	Oral, injection, or intravenous	Acute exacerbation	Electrolyte disturbances, weakness, atrophy, osteoporosis, seizure, high ICP, vertigo headache, Cushing's syndrome
Depo-Medrol Solu-Medrol	methylprednisolone dexamethasone (corticosteroid)	Oral, injection, or intravenous	Acute exacerbation	Cushing's syndrome, hypertension, confusion, muscle wasting, insomnia, psychosis, GI irritation, osteoporosis, delayed wound healing
Deltasone	prednisone (corticosteroid)	Oral	Acute exacerbation	Electrolyte imbalance, CHF, weakness, atrophy, Achilles tendon rupture, osteoporosis, papilledema, vertigo, headache
Delta-Cortef	prednisolone	Intravenous	Acute exacerbation	Electrolyte imbalance, CHF, weakness, atrophy, Achilles tendon rupture, osteoporosis, papilledema, vertigo, headache
Decadron Medrol	dexamethasone (corticosteroid)	Oral	Acute exacerbation	GI disturbance, headache, dizziness, insomnia, restlessness, depression or anxiety, easy bruising
MANAGEMENT OF MULTIPLE SCLEROSIS: MANAGE DISEASE PROGRESSION				
Actimmune Avonex Betaseron Extavia Rebif	beta-1a-interferon beta-1b-interferon	Injection, every 2 to 7 days	To reduce frequency and severity of exacerbations for relapsing/remitting MS	Injection site reaction, anxiety, convulsion, seizure
Azasan Imuran	azathioprine (chemotherapeutic)	Oral	To slow disease progression over time when other medications are not effective	Nausea, vomiting, diarrhea, muscle aches, cough, mouth sores, fatigue, loss of appetite, GI disturbance, jaundice, flulike symptoms, blurred vision
Copaxone	glatiramer	Daily injection	To reduce frequency, severity of exacerbations for relapsing/remitting MS	On injection: flushing, chest pain, palpitation, tachycardia, dyspnea After Injection: nausea, edema, syncope, headache, tremor, diaphoresis, hypotonia, arthralgia, seizure
Cytoxan CTX Neosar	cyclophosphamide (chemotherapeutic)	Oral or injection	To slow disease progression over time when other medications are not effective	Loss of appetite or weight gain, changes in skin color, fatigue, dizziness, chills, shortness of breath, edema, nausea, vomiting, GI or urinary bleeding

Drug	Route	Indication	Side Effects
Gengraf Neoral Sandimmune SangCya cyclosporin-modified (immunosuppressant)	Oral	To slow disease progression over time	Headache, GI disturbance, tremor, muscle or joint pain, paresthesia, insomnia, nephrotoxicity, hypertension, exacerbation when discontinued
Gammagard Gammar-P IV Gaminune N Iveegam Panglobulin Sandoglobulin Venoglobulin intravenous immunoglobulin (antibody)	Intravenous	To slow disease progression over time when other medications are not effective	Flulike symptoms immediately following infusion, headache
Gilenya fingolimod (immunosuppressant)	Oral	To reduce frequency, severity of exacerbations for relapsing/remitting MS	Bradycardia, headache, hypertension, weakness, back pain, paresthesias, depression, fatigue, dizziness, chest pain, nausea, vomiting, loss of appetite, jaundice
Leustatin Mylinax 2-CdA cladribine (chemotherapeutic)	Intravenous	To slow disease progression when other medications are not effective	GI disturbance, loss of appetite, muscle or joint pain, headache, insomnia, fatigue
MTX Rheumatrex Trexall methotrexate (chemotherapeutic)	Oral	To slow disease progression over time when other medications are not effective	Dizziness, drowsiness, headache, loss of appetite, blurred vision, seizures, confusion, weakness
Novantrone mitoxantrone (chemotherapeutic)	Intravenous, every 3 months	Severe advanced MS	Ventricular cardiac dysfunction, myelosuppression (risk of leukemia)
Tysabri natalizumab (immunosuppressant)	Monthly, intravenous	To slow disease progression over time when other medications are not effective	Headache, UTI, muscle and joint pain, GI disturbance, fatigue, depression, allergic reactions, liver dysfunction, risk of progressive multifocal leukoencephalopathy
Zovirax acyclovir (antiviral)	Oral	To reduce frequency, severity of exacerbations for relapsing/remitting MS	GI disturbances, dizziness, fatigue, agitation, joint pain, changes in vision

MULTIPLE SCLEROSIS: MANAGEMENT OF DYSESTHESIA/NEUROPATHIC PAIN

Drug	Route	Indication	Side Effects
Carbatrol Epitol Tegretol carbamazepine	Oral	Trigeminal neuralgia, pelvic pain, intense episodic/lancinating/burning pain	See Seizure Medications
Dilantin Neurontin Zonegran Norpramin phenytoin gabapentin zonisamide desipramine (anticonvulsants)		Pins/needles, cramping, dysesthetic extremity pain, tonic spasms, other neurogenic pain, nocturnal spasms	

(Continued)

TABLE 10-6 *Pharmacological Interventions for Individuals with Neurological and Neuromuscular System Impairments—cont'd*

Trade Names	Generic Name (class)	Administration	Indications	Adverse Effects
Adapin Sinequan Triadapin Zonalon	doxepin	Oral	Chronic neurogenic pain (e.g., dysesthetic extremity pain such as burning, tingling)	Drowsiness, blurred vision, dizziness, GI and urinary disturbances, tachycardia, hypotension, weight gain, fatigue, headache
Elavil Imavate Janimine Tofranil	amitriptyline imipramine			
Vivactil	protriptyline (tricyclic antidepressants)			
MULTIPLE SCLEROSIS: MANAGEMENT OF FATIGUE				
Contenton Symmetrel Symadine Topharmin	amantadine (antiviral, Parkinson's)	Oral	To manage fatigue associated with chronic MS, and drug-induced extrapyramidal symptoms	Nervousness, restlessness, tremor, dizziness, seizure, headache, blurred vision, GI disturbance, edema, dry mouth, diaphoresis, tics
Provigil	modafinil (CNS stimulant)	Oral	To manage fatigue associated with chronic MS	Risk of dependence, allergic reaction, depression or anxiety, hallucination, aggressiveness, arrhythmia, dyspnea, back pain, GI disturbances
MANAGEMENT OF SEIZURES				
Amytal	amobarbital (barbiturate)	Intravenous	Status epilepticus	Sedation, nystagmus, ataxia, vitamin K and folate deficiency
Ativan	lorazepam (benzodiazepine)	Intravenous	Status epilepticus	Sedation, ataxia, changes in behavior
Atretol Convline Epitol Macrepan Tegretol	carbamazepine (iminostilbene)	Oral	Complex partial seizures, tonic-clonic seizures, trigeminal neuralgia, bipolar disorder	Ataxia, diplopia, drowsiness, fatigue, dizziness, vertigo, tremor, headache, nausea, dry mouth, anorexia, agitation, rashes photosensitivity, heart failure
Celontin	methsuximide (succinimide)	Oral	Alternative to ethosuximide for absence seizures	Nausea, vomiting, headache, dizziness, fatigue, lethargy, dyskinesia, bradykinesia
Cerebyx	fosphenytoin (hydantoin)	Intravenous	Status epilepticus	GI irritation, confusion, sedation, dizziness, headache, nystagmus, ataxia, dysarthria
Depacon	Sodium valproate (carboxylic acid)	Oral or injection	All types of seizures	Ataxia, tremor, sedation, nausea, vomiting, hyperactivity weakness, incoordination, risk of hepatotoxicity

		Route	Indications	Side effects
Depakene	valproic acid (carboxylic acid)	Oral	Absence seizures, as adjunct for other seizure types	Nausea, sedation, ataxia headache nystagmus, diplopia, asterixis, dysarthria, dizziness, incoordination, depression, hyperactivity, weakness, risk of hepatotoxicity
Depakote	divalproex sodium (carboxylic acid)	Oral	Complex partial seizures, absence seizures, as adjunct for other seizure types	Headache, asthenia, nausea, somnolence, tremor, dizziness diplopia, risk of hepatotoxicity
Diamox	acetazolamide (sulfonamide)	Oral	Absence seizures, myoclonic seizures	Drowsiness, dizziness
Dilantin Diphen Diphentoin Dyantoin Phenytex	phenytoin (hydantoin)	Oral or injection	Status epilepticus, tonic-clonic seizures, simple complex seizures	Ataxia, slurred speech, confusion, insomnia, nervousness, hypotension, nystagmus diplopia, nausea, vomiting
Felbatol	felbamate (2nd generation)	Oral	Partial seizures, absence seizures Used for severe seizure disorders unresponsive to other medications	Aplastic anemia, liver failure, insomnia, headache, dizziness, loss of appetite, nausea, vomiting
Gabitril	tiagabine (2nd generation)	Oral	Partial seizures	Generalized weakness, dizziness, tiredness, nervousness, tremor, distractibility, emotional lability
Keppra	levetiracetam (2nd generation)	Oral	Adjunct for partial seizures in adults	Sedation, dizziness, generalized weakness
Klonopin Rivotril	clonazepam (benzodiazepine)	Oral or injection	Myoclonic seizures, absence seizures, kinetic seizures	Drowsiness, dizziness, ataxia, dyskinesia, irritability, disturbances of coordination, slurred speech, diplopia, nystagmus, thirst
Lamictal	lamotrigine (2nd generation)	Oral	Partial seizures, tonic-clonic seizures	Dizziness, headache, ataxia, drowsiness, incoordination, insomnia, tremors, depression, anxiety, diplopia, blurred vision, GI disturbances, agitation, confusion, rash
Luminol Solfoton	phenobarbital (barbiturate)	Oral or injection	Status epilepticus, all seizure types except absence seizures	Drowsiness, lethargy, agitation, confusion, ataxia, hallucination, bradycardia, hypotension, nausea
Mebaral	mephobarbital (barbiturate)	Oral	Tonic-clonic seizures, simple and complex partial seizures	Drowsiness, sedation, nystagmus, ataxia, folate and vitamin K deficiency
Mesantoin	mephenytoin (hydantoin)	Oral	Partial seizures, tonic-clonic seizures used if Dilantin is not effective	Similar to Dilantin, but more toxic
Milontin	phensuximide (succinimide)	Oral	Alternative to Zarontin for absence seizures	Nausea, vomiting, headache, dizziness, fatigue, lethargy, bradykinesia, dyskinesia

(Continued)

TABLE 10-6   *Pharmacological Interventions for Individuals with Neurological and Neuromuscular System Impairments—cont'd*

Trade Names	Generic Name (class)	Administration	Indications	Adverse Effects
Mysoline	primidone (barbiturate)	Oral	All seizure types except absence seizures, essential tremor	Ataxia, vertigo, drowsiness, depression, inattention, headache, nausea, visual disturbances
Nembutal	pentobarbital (barbiturate)	Intravenous	Tonic-clonic seizures, simple and complex partial seizures	Sedation, nystagmus, ataxia, vitamin K and folate deficiency
Neurontin	gabapentin (2nd generation)	Oral	Partial seizures in adults and children older than 3 years, neuropathic pain	Drowsiness, dizziness, ataxia, fatigue, nystagmus, nervousness, tremor, diplopia, memory impairment
Peganone	ethotoin (hydantion)	Oral	Tonic-clonic seizures; used if Dilantin is not effective	Similar to Dilantin, but more toxic
Seconal	secobarbital (barbiturate)	Intravenous	Tonic-clonic seizures, partial seizures	Sedation, nystagmus, vitamin K and folate deficiency
Topamax	topiramate (2nd generation)	Oral	Partial seizures, adjunct to tonic-clonic seizures	Ataxia, confusion, dizziness, fatigue, paresthesia, emotional lability, confusion, diplopia, nausea
Thosutin Zarontin	ethosuximide (succinimide)	Oral	Absence seizures	Drowsiness, headache, fatigue, dizziness, ataxia, euphoria, depression, myopia, nausea, anorexia
Tranxene	clorazepate (benzodiazepine)	Oral	Adjunct for partial seizures	Sedation, ataxia, changes in behavior
Trileptal	oxcarbazepine (iminostilbene)	Oral	Partial seizures, tonic-clonic seizures	Ataxia, drowsiness, nausea, dizziness, headache, agitation, memory impairment, asthenia, ataxia, confusion, tremor, nystagmus
Valium Valrelease	diazepam (benzodiazepine)	Injection	Status epilepticus, severe recurrent seizures	Drowsiness, fatigue, ataxia, confusion, depression, dysarthria, syncope, tremor, vertigo
Zonegran	zonisamide (2nd generation)	Oral	Adjunct for partial seizures in adults	Sedation, ataxia, loss of appetite, fatigue

ABI, acquired brain injury; CHF, congestive heart failure; CNS, central nervous system; CP, cerebral palsy; GI, gastrointestinal; ICP, intracranial pressure; MS, multiple sclerosis; NMJ, neuromuscular junction; SCI, spinal cord injury; UMN, upper motor neuron; UTI, urinary tract infection.

greater functional ROM to improve the ability to walk in children with CP.[166-169] Derotation osteotomies are another option that have traditionally been used to improve or correct deformity and improve walking ability in children with CP.[170-173] Because children with CP and acquired brain injury who have significant hypertonicity are at risk for developing neuromuscular scoliosis, various spinal surgeries are used to improve spinal alignment and reduce pelvic obliquity, to improve physiological and daily function, and to reduce caregiver burden.[174-176] Rather than subject children with CP to multiple surgeries over time, many centers perform multiple procedures at the same time.[177,178] To achieve maximum benefit, rehabilitation is a necessary component following any of these surgeries.[179-181]

Individuals with significant spasticity are commonly managed with a combination of these strategies to most effectively diminish the impairment, improve functional ability, and help them participate in activities that are important to them.[182-184] Increasingly, instrumented gait analysis is being used to inform clinical decision making in selecting the most appropriate intervention or combination of interventions for ambulatory individuals with functional limitation secondary to neuromuscular pathologies and their associated secondary impairments.[185-188]

Rehabilitation

Rehabilitation professionals use a variety of examination strategies to determine the nature and extent of dysfunction, across systems, associated with a particular pathological condition (Table 10-7).[9] The physical therapist evaluates this information to (1) determine an appropriate movement-related physical therapy diagnosis, (2) predict potential outcomes (prognosis), and (3) structure an appropriate plan of care.[189-191]

Physical therapists use adaptive equipment, orthoses, and seating as key components of an effective plan of care for persons with neuromotor/neurosensory system dysfunction.[192-196] Orthoses are used to:

1. align or position limb segments to enhance voluntary limb movement and improve function (e.g., an ankle-foot orthosis to provide prepositioning of the foot during swing limb advancement and stability during the stance phase of gait);
2. influence abnormal tone (tone-inhibiting designs);
3. provide individuals with a variety of comfortable and safe positions in which they can sleep, eat, travel, work, or play;
4. promote joint alignment and minimize risk of contracture development and other secondary musculoskeletal sequelae (especially in growing children);

TABLE 10-7 *Components of a Physical Therapy Examination and Evaluation in Preparation for Serial Casting or Prescription/Fitting of Appropriate Splint or Orthoses*

Component	Dimension	Examination Strategies
Chief complaint	What is the *MOVEMENT PROBLEM* that brings the individual to physical therapy?	Interview of individual and caregivers
History of current illness, past medical history	How did the *MOVEMENT PROBLEM* develop or evolve: Duration of the presenting problem Previous and concurrent pharmacological management Previous and concurrent orthopedic or neurosurgical management Previous orthotic management Current health status Comorbidities and their management	Review of medical record Interview with individual and caregivers Consultation with clinical colleagues
Biomechanical evaluation	ROM Flexibility (especially of multijoint muscles) End feel Integrity of ligaments and supportive structures Alignment of joints, pelvis, and spine	Goniometric measurement Evaluation of muscle length (e.g., Thomas test, straight leg raise) Gentle overpressure at end of available ROM Various orthopedic special tests appropriate to the joint being examined (e.g., ACL/PCL drawer tests) Radiograph Goniometry Inclinometer
	Torsional/rotational deformity of hip, femur, tibia	Radiograph, various orthopedic special tests
	Postural alignment in sitting and standing	Spatial relationships of head, upper trunk/limb girdle, mid trunk, lower trunk/pelvic girdle, extremity symmetry
	Anthropomorphic characteristics	Height, weight, limb length, limb girth, body mass

(Continued)

TABLE 10-7   *Components of a Physical Therapy Examination and Evaluation in Preparation for Serial Casting, or Prescription/Fitting of Appropriate Splint or Orthoses—cont'd*

Component	Dimension	Examination Strategies
Neuromotor status	Muscle tone (compliance vs stiffness)	Resistance to passive movement at various speeds Palpation tone scales (e.g., modified Ashworth), descriptive category (hypertonic/spastic, rigid, hypotonic, fluctuating, flaccid)
	Tonal response to deep tendon reflex testing	Amplitude of response (absent/0, diminished /+1, normal/+2, brisk/3, clonus/+4, sustained clonus +5) Pattern of response (distal-proximal) Symmetry of response (right-left)
	Tonal response to change in position	Appearance or influence of abnormal developmental reflexes (e.g., ATNR, positive supportive reaction)
	Antigravity stiffness/postural tone	Assessing stiffness to support trunk or body segment in various antigravity positions
	Involuntary movement	Observation at rest and during movement; descriptive category (e.g., chorea, athetosis, tremor, tics)
	Muscle performance	Observation of antigravity movement
	Strength	Manual muscle testing, dynamometer
	Speed/power	Isokinetic testing
	Accuracy	Description: hypokinetic, functional, hyperkinetic
	Timing	
	Fluidity	
	Muscle endurance	
Motor control	Postural control	Static balance tests (e.g., timed single limb stance) Anticipatory balance tests (e.g., reach distances, ability to change direction) Reactionary balance test: perturbation
	Recruitment/adaptation of contractions	Ability to move between concentric, eccentric, and holding contractions during functional activity Ability to initiate, sustain, and terminate contraction and movement
	Ability to isolate limb segments as needed for effective task performance	Observation of motor performance during functional tasks or challenges Influence of abnormal synergy or abnormal developmental reflexes
	Ability to adapt movement strategies to task demands	Observation of ability to generate appropriate force and type of contract at appropriate times
	Ability to adapt movement strategies in different environment	Observation of movement in low light, different floor surfaces, inclines, stairs, closed versus open (distracting, demanding) environments
	Relationship of agonist/antagonist	Ability to alter muscle activity of agonist/antagonist on demand (within the limb, across limb and limb girdle, within trunk) during functional activities
	Dexterity, coordination, agility	Observation of performance during functional activity Special tests Developmental scales and profiles
Functional movement ability	Activities of daily living (ADL)	Observation of movement during task Self-report of individual or caregiver Various ADL scales Ability to don/doff orthosis
	Transitional movements and transfers	Observation during performance
	To/from floor	Movement strategy
	Sit to stand	Assistance required
	Bathroom transfers	Level of difficulty
	Car transfers	Task analysis to identify where in movement difficulty occurs and contributors to difficulty

TABLE 10-7 *Components of a Physical Therapy Examination and Evaluation in Preparation for Serial Casting, or Prescription/Fitting of Appropriate Splint or Orthoses—cont'd*

Component	Dimension	Examination Strategies
	Mobility and locomotion	Observational gait analysis, with and without orthosis
		Gait speed, other kinematic measures
		Use of assistive devices
		Level of assistance required
		Gait lab kinetic measures (moments, torques, and muscle activity via video, force plate, and EMG analysis)
	UE function and use of hands	Observation during various fine and gross UE motor tasks
	Cardiovascular endurance	Heart rate, blood pressure, oxygen saturation during activity
		Ratings of perceived exertion during tasks
		6-Minute walk test
		Fatigue scales
	Environmental assessment (home, work, school, leisure)	Environmental safety checklists
		Interview with individual and caregivers about characteristics of environments in which individual must function
Integumentary integrity	Skin condition	Inspection for neuropathic, dysvascular, or traumatic wounds
		Document callus and scarring
		Document pressure sensitive areas
		Document protective sensation, insensate weight-bearing areas
Sensory organization and processing	Sensory integrity	Adequacy of vision (acuity, peripheral vision, tracking, visual field loss)
		Screening for exteroception, proprioception ability
		Document insensate areas, especially of hands/feet
		Document paresthesia and dysesthesia
	Perceptual function	Observation of movement during functional tasks
	Visual spatial perception	Developmental tests, measures
	Awareness of position in space	Special perceptual tests, measures
	Awareness of body parts	
	Sensory integration	Observation of movement during functional tasks
	Habituation to stimulus	of increasing demand
	Ability to sort through conflicting sensory information	
Cognitive function	Communication	Adequacy of hearing and auditory processing
		Ability to understand language
		Ability to use language
		Oral-motor function (dysarthria)
		Impact of position on voice
	Ability to learn and remember	Reports of teachers, neuropsychological testing
	Ability to problem solve	Observation when presented with challenge
		Results of neuropsychological testing
	Motivation	Observation
		Self-report of individual and caregivers
	Distractiblility/focus	Observation
		Self-report of individual, caregiver, teachers
		Results of neuropsychological testing
	Ability to manage frustration, uncertainty	Observation
		Self-report of individual, caregiver, teachers
Psychosocial factors	Family and caregiver	Availability and capacity with respect to use of orthosis
	School or work-related activities	Typical activities and roles: demands and barriers encountered
	Leisure or play activities	Typical activities and roles: demands and barriers encountered

ACL, anterior collateral ligament of the knee; ATNR, asymmetrical tonic neck reflex; EMG, electromyographic; PCL, posterior collateral ligament of the knee; ROM, range of motion; UE, upper extremity.

5. protect a limb following orthopedic surgery performed to correct deformity or instability;

6. enhance alignment following pharmacological intervention with botulinum toxin; and

7. provide alternative methods for mobility.

The risk for developing secondary musculoskeletal impairments is high in the presence of hypertonicity.[108,197-200] Passive stretching programs alone are generally ineffective as a management strategy for reducing risk for contracture development.[201,202] Prolonged positioning for several hours a day is a critical adjunct to stretching.[203-206] Adaptive equipment can be used to provide structural alignment for prolonged periods of time to maintain extensibility of muscles, decrease the effect of muscle imbalance across joints, and provide postural support. An adaptive seating system, for example, would provide upright postural support for sitting; maintain spinal alignment and pelvic positioning; support optimal hip, knee, and ankle positions; and promote the best position for upper extremity function.[207-210] Positioning devices for supported standing are often used to maintain extensibility of muscles, promote bone mineral density through weight bearing, and promote musculoskeletal development such as acetabular depth in a developing child with hypertonicity (Figure 10-7).[211-213] Other examples of positioning

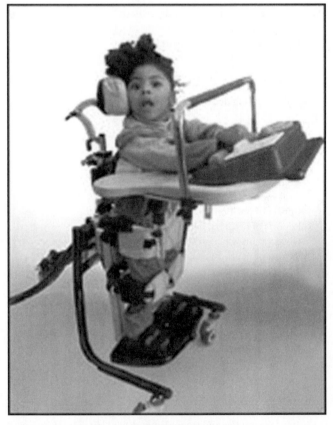

FIGURE 10-7 Example of adaptive equipment (stander) available to assist appropriate alignment and function in the presence of impairment of muscle tone, muscle performance, postural control, or difficulty with movement and coordination. (Used with permission of http://www.rehabpub.com/issues/articles/2008-10_04.aspth.)

devices include prone, supine and sidelyer systems, bathing and toileting seating systems, and a variety of mobility alternatives such as gait trainers.[214-217] Although there are many options for adaptive equipment designed to assist function and caregiving for persons with neurological and neuromuscular dysfunction, knowledge about options and limitations in funding limit access for many who might otherwise benefit from such devices.[218-221]

Serial corrective casts have long been used as a primary intervention for individuals with significant hypertonus to provide a prolonged elongation of soft tissue over a long time period. They increase the length of a contracted muscle and its supportive tissues and reset the threshold for response to stretch reflex.[155-160] Some splints or dynamic orthoses are used primarily at night to provide 8 or more hours of stretch on a regular basis; others can be worn during daily activities to provide a longer period of stretch (Figure 10-8).[222-226] More recently, serial casting and dynamic splinting have been used in conjunction with pharmacological interventions for management of spasticity in both children and adults with severe hypertonicity (Figure 10-9).[227,228] Although the pharmacological agent may reduce the degree of spasticity in hypertonic muscles, concomitant shortening of the muscles and tendons must be addressed while the neurological influence is altered, as should concomitant deficits in other dimensions of muscle performance and motor control.[229-231] A young child with spastic diplegic CP, for example, may receive botulinum injections to the gastrocnemius and soleus muscles to reduce severity of spasticity as an alternative to early orthopedic surgery.[232,233]

Selecting the Appropriate Orthosis

Rehabilitation professionals play an active role in deciding what type of orthosis would be most appropriate for an individual with neuromuscular impairment. A number of factors contribute to the decision-making process; the collective wisdom of physical and occupational therapists, orthotists, physicians, family, and the patient who might benefit from orthotic intervention is necessary for appropriate and effective casting or orthotic intervention.[192,234,235]

The primary goal of orthotic prescription is to select the device and components that will best improve function, given the individual's pathology and prognosis, desired activities, and participation needs, both in the immediate situation and over time. To do this, the cast, splint, or orthosis might provide external support, control or limit ROM, optimally position a limb for function, reduce risk of secondary musculoskeletal complications, or provide a base for adaptive equipment that would make function more efficient. What evidence is available to support clinical decision making with respect to orthotic prescription? Although many professionals rely on expertise gained by working with persons with neuromotor impairment over years of clinical practice, a growing number of articles on orthotic design for particular patient populations in the rehabilitation and orthotic research literature are available to guide decision making, not only for individuals with hypertonicity but also for those with spinal cord injury, myelomeningocele, and muscular dystrophy.[195,234-241]

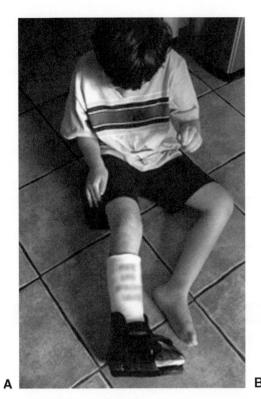
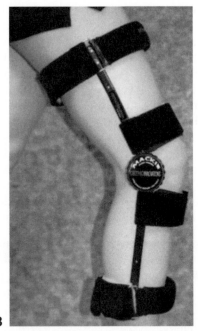
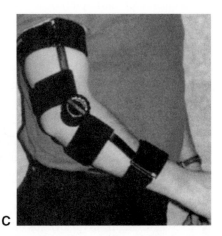

A   **B**   **C**

FIGURE 10-8 Examples of a serial cast (**A**) used to provide sustained stretch to the Achilles tendon and foot in a child with spastic cerebral palsy, and of dynamic orthoses used to provide prolonged stretch to tissues contributing to joint contracture at the knee (**B**) and elbow (**C**). Both serial casts and dynamic orthoses can be used for persons with both musculoskeletal and neuromuscular pathologies that have resulted in joint contracture, and may be used as an adjunct to surgical and pharmacological interventions for persons with hypertonicity. (**B** and **C** Courtesy Ortho Innovations, Rochester, Minn.)

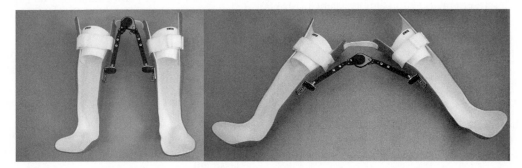

FIGURE 10-9 Example of a custom-molded orthosis, worn in the immediate postoperative period and later during sleep, designed to enhance range of motion following botulinum toxin type A injection. The goal was to reduce hypertonicity and delay corrective orthopedic surgery for a child with spastic cerebral palsy. (Courtesy Ultraflex Systems Inc., Downingtown, Pa.)

If the primary goal of orthotic intervention is to improve safety and functionality during ambulation, it is imperative to identify where in the gait cycle abnormal tone or muscle performance is impaired (refer to Chapter 5 for more information on critical events in each subphase of gait, as well as detailed information about strategies to examine gait). Systematic consideration of a series of questions can help identify where within the gait cycle (considering both stance and swing phases) problems occur.[242–244]

Rehabilitation professions must recognize that no orthosis will normalize gait for persons with neurologically based gait difficulties. Whenever an external device is placed on a limb, it is likely to solve one problem while at the same time creating other constraints on limb function. The therapist, orthotist, and patient collectively problem solve during the orthotic prescription phase to prioritize the difficulties the individual is having during gait and then select the design and components that will allow the person to be most functional while walking, with the least additional constraint on other mobility and functional tasks.

The rehabilitation team at Rancho Los Amigos National Rehabilitation Center has developed an algorithm that is particularly useful in guiding clinical decision making and sorting through possible orthotic options for adults with neuromotor impairment (ROADMAP: Recommendations for Orthotic Assessment, Decision Making, and Prescription).[192] When considering orthotic interventions for persons having difficulty with ambulation, this team suggests asking the following questions:

1. Is there adequate ROM in the lower extremities to appropriately align or position limb segments in each subphase of gait?
2. Does the individual have the motivation and cognitive resources necessary to work toward meeting the goal of ambulation?
3. Does the individual have enough endurance (cardiovascular and cardiopulmonary resources) to be able to functionally ambulate? If endurance is not currently sufficient, might it be improved by a concurrent conditioning program?
4. Does the individual have adequate upper extremity, trunk, and lower extremity strength; power; motor control; and postural control for ambulation (with an appropriate assistive device, if necessary)? If these dimensions of movement are not currently sufficient, might they be improved with concurrent rehabilitation intervention?
5. Is there sufficient awareness of lower limb position (proprioception, kinesthesia) for controlled forward progression in gait? If not, might alternative sensory strategies be learned or used to substitute for limb position sense?

If the answers to most of these questions are "yes," the individual is considered to be a candidate for orthotic intervention. The next determinant is knee control and strength: If the individual has antigravity knee extension with the ability to respond to some resistance (MMT [Manual Muscle Testing] grade of 3+ strength), even if there is impaired proprioception in the involved limb, then an ankle-foot orthosis may be appropriate. If there is impairment of strength or of proprioception (or both), then the team is more likely to recommend a knee-ankle-foot orthosis. Box 10-1 is an example of a decision tree used to guide the selection of components.

BOX 10-1   *Decision Tree for Orthotic Options*

IS A KNEE-ANKLE-FOOT ORTHOSIS (KAFO) INDICATED?
- Is there at least antigravity with some resistance (MMT 3+/5 strength) in quadriceps bilaterally?
- Is proprioception intact bilaterally?
  If yes: continue with the assessment for AFO
  If no: KAFO may improve gait, continue assessment process

WHICH KAFO COMPONENTS ARE THE MOST APPROPRIATE?
- Is there at least antigravity with some resistance (MMT 3+/5 strength) in one lower extremity?
- Is proprioception intact in at least one lower extremity?
  If no: consider trial of bilateral KAFOs or a reciprocal gait orthosis
  If yes: unilateral KAFO may be indicated—continue assessment to determine if knee locking mechanism necessary

CAN THE KNEE BE FULLY EXTENDED, WITHOUT PAIN, DURING STANCE?
If no: consider KAFO with knee lock
  If yes: consider KAFO with variable knee mechanism and continue assessment

IS THERE AT EFFECTIVE ACTIVE CONTROL OF KNEE EXTENSION DURING STANCE?
If no: consider stance control knee mechanism
  If yes: consider free motion knee mechanism
  Continue with ankle-foot orthosis (AFO) decision tree to determine appropriate ankle control strategy

IS AN AFO INDICATED?
- Is there impairment of ankle strength?
- Is there impairment of proprioception?
- Is there hypertonicity of plantar flexors?
- Is there a combination of all of the above?
  If no: may not require lower extremity orthosis
  If yes: lower extremity orthosis may improve gait—continue assessment process

WHICH AFO DESIGN AND COMPONENTS ARE THE BEST OPTION?
- Does impaired strength hamper foot position in stance or swing?
- Does impaired proprioception hamper foot placement in stance or swing?
- Does hypertonicity/spasticity hamper foot position in stance or swing?
  If no: consider adjustable articulating ankle joint (allows full dorsiflexion [DF] and plantar flexion [PF])
  If yes: consider limiting or blocking ankle motion, continue assessment process

IS THERE MORE THAN MINIMAL IMPAIRMENT OF STATIC AND DYNAMIC POSTURAL CONTROL IN STANDING?
- Is there significant spasticity?
- Is proprioception significantly impaired?
  If no: consider adjustable articulating ankle joint that blocks PF beyond neutral ankle position and continue assessment
  If yes: consider solid-ankle AFO or adjustable articulating ankle that is fully locked (consider rocker bottom shoe)
- Is there also plantar flexion strength ≤ MMT 4 in standing?
- Is there also excessive knee flexion and dorsiflexion during stance?
- Is there also excessive plantar flexion with knee hyperextension during stance?
  If no: consider adjustable articulating ankle joint with PF stop, and continue assessment
  If yes: consider adjustable articulating ankle joint with PF stop and limited DF excursion, and continue assessment
- Is there also dorsiflexion strength ≤ 4 in standing?
  If no: consider adjustable articulating ankle with PF stop, limited DF excursion in stance, no DF assist necessary
  If yes: consider adjustable articulating ankle with PF stop, limited DF excursion, and DF assist for effective swing phase

Especially important is that the individual who will use the orthosis and caregivers, as appropriate, are actively involved in the decision-making process. To make an informed decision, the person needing an orthosis must understand both the benefits and constraints associated with the orthotic designs and components being considered. He or she must be able to consider the range of orthotic options, as well as medical/surgical intervention and additional rehabilitation interventions that might affect his or her ability to walk. The entire team must consider what the individual who will be wearing the orthosis wants to accomplish, as well as the preferences he or she might have in terms of ease of donning/doffing, wearing schedule, and cosmesis of the device being recommended. Beginning with a trial orthosis, perhaps a prefabricated or multiadjustable version, is helpful before finalizing the orthotic prescription, especially if it is unclear whether ambulation will eventually be possible. Certainly, most individuals with neuromuscular conditions that compromise their ability to walk benefit from a chance to experience what ambulation with an orthosis requires, given their individual constellation of impairments. Some may decide that using orthoses and an appropriate assistive device for functional ambulation throughout the day meets their mobility needs. Others may opt, because of the energy cost of walking with knee-ankle-foot orthoses or hip-knee-ankle-foot orthoses, to use a wheelchair for primary mobility and reserve the use of orthoses to exercise bouts aimed at building cardiovascular endurance. Finally, some may decide that orthotic intervention will not meet their needs and pursue other avenues to address mobility and endurance issues.

SUMMARY

This chapter reviews the functions and roles of structures and systems in both the central and peripheral nervous systems, the impairments that are likely to occur when particular structures or systems are damaged by injury or disease process, abnormalities of tone and motor control that influence an individual's ability to ambulate and affect the likelihood of developing secondary musculoskeletal impairments, and some of the pharmacological and surgical options that are available to manage hypertonicity and correct deformity that may develop over time. Strategies to determine where in the gait cycle an individual with various neuromotor impairments is likely to have difficulty are explored, as are the orthotic options that might best address the limitations that the individual faces. This chapter provides a strong foundation for physical therapy examination and evaluation. Next, the reader should consider physical therapy interventions that will focus on wearing, using, and caring for the prescribed orthosis, including (1) strategies to enhance motor learning when a new ambulatory aid (orthosis and/or assistive device) is introduced, (2) practice using the device under various environmental conditions (surfaces, obstacles, people moving within the environment), and (3) the ability to use the orthosis and ambulatory assistive device during functional activities beyond walking at comfortable gait speed.

CASE EXAMPLE 1

A Young Child with Spastic Diplegic Cerebral Palsy

T. H. is a 4-year-old child who was born prematurely at 32 weeks of gestation and diagnosed with spastic diplegic CP at 10 months of age. She is being evaluated for potential botulinum A injection as a strategy to manage significant extensor hypertonicity that is increasingly limiting her ability to ambulate as she grows. At present she uses bilateral articulating ankle-foot orthoses with a plantar flexion stop and a posterior rolling walker for locomotion at her preschool program; she prefers creeping in quadruped for mobility at home. Her articulating orthoses allow her to move into some dorsiflexion as she transitions to and from the floor during play. She has difficulty pushing to stand from half-kneel secondary to poor force production of hip and knee extensors. Muscle endurance is impaired, contributing to a crouch gait position, especially as she tires after a full day of activity. She falls frequently when she tries to run. She has been monitored in a CP clinic at the regional children's hospital; the team is concerned that she is developing rotational deformity of the lower extremities, as well as plantar flexion contracture and forefoot deformity due to her longstanding hypertonicity.

Questions to Consider

- In which subphases of the gait cycle is function or safety compromised when T. H. ambulates without her orthoses?
- In what way does T. H.'s hypertonicity contribute to her difficulty with floor mobility and ambulation?
- In what ways does T. H.'s inadequate muscle performance contribute to her difficulty with floor mobility and ambulation? What are the most likely dimensions of muscle performance that are impaired, given her diagnosis of spastic diplegia?
- In what ways does T. H.'s impaired postural control contribute to her difficulty with locomotion/ambulation? What are the most likely dimensions of her impairment in postural control, given her diagnosis of spastic diplegia?
- Are there primary or secondary musculoskeletal impairments that are influencing her function and safety during ambulation? How do her age and future growth influence her risk for developing secondary impairments?
- Given her constellation of impairments, what compensatory strategies is T. H. likely to use to accomplish the task of locomotion?
- Which of T. H.'s anticipated or observed impairments are remediable? Which will require accommodation?
- What orthotic options (design, components) are available to address T. H.'s impairment of locomotion and related functional limitations? What are the pros and cons of each?
- What alternative or concurrent medical (surgical/pharmacological) interventions might assist improvement in safety and function for T. H.?

Continued

- What additional rehabilitation interventions might assist improvement in function and safety for T. H.?
- How do you anticipate T. H.'s orthotic needs might change as she develops and grows?
- What outcome measures can be used to assess efficacy of orthotic, therapeutic, pharmacological, or surgical intervention for T. H.?

CASE EXAMPLE 2

A Child with Spastic Quadriplegic Cerebral Palsy

J. T. is an 11-year-old boy with significant spastic quadriplegic CP who is in the midst of a preadolescent growth spurt. He currently uses a custom seating system in a power wheelchair for self-directed mobility at school and in the community. Recently he has nearly fallen out of his chair when negotiating around sharp corners. At home he divides his time between his chair and rolling/crawling on the floor. J. T.'s mom reports that it is becoming increasingly difficult to assist him in transfers into the family's sport utility vehicle and help him with self-care activities because of upper extremity flexor tightness, increasing hip and knee flexion contractures, and plantar flexion tightness.

In addition, when supine, J. T.'s resting position is becoming more obviously "windswept", with excessive right hip external rotation and excessive left hip internal rotation, causing a pelvic obliquity. He attends physical therapy at school several times each week to help him with functional abilities in the classroom and around campus, with additional outpatient visits focusing on improving postural control and muscle performance. Both of his therapists are becoming concerned about his increasing limitation in ROM, as well as the risk for increasing rotational deformity and hip dysfunction as he grows. His outpatient therapist accompanies J. T. and his mother to the CP orthotics clinic at the regional children's medical center to explore the possibility of functional bracing or dynamic orthoses, or both, to manage the musculoskeletal complications that are developing because of his spasticity. They also have questions about surgical and pharmacological intervention.

Questions to Consider

- In what way does J. T.'s hypertonicity contribute to his difficulty with mobility/locomotion and other functional activities?
- In what ways does J. T.'s impaired muscle performance contribute to his difficulty with functional activities?
- In what ways does J. T.'s impaired postural control contribute to his difficulty with locomotion/ambulation? What are the most likely dimensions of his impairment in postural control, given his diagnosis of spastic quadriplegic cerebral palsy?
- Are any primary or secondary musculoskeletal impairments influencing J. T.'s function and safety during mobility and transfer tasks?

- Given his constellation of impairments, what compensatory strategies is J. T. likely to use to accomplish his functional tasks at school and at home?
- Which of J. T.'s anticipated or observed impairments are remediable? Which will require accommodation?
- What orthotic options (design, components) are available to address J. T.'s impairments and functional limitations? What are the pros and cons of each?
- Given the pelvic obliquity, what secondary musculoskeletal complications need to be monitored as he grows? How might these concerns be addressed by seating?
- What alternative or concurrent medical (surgical/pharmacological) interventions might assist improvement in safety and function for J. T.?
- What additional rehabilitation interventions might assist improvement in function and safety for J. T.?
- How do you anticipate J. T.'s orthotic needs might change as he develops and grows?
- What outcome measures can be used to assess efficacy of orthotic, therapeutic, pharmacological, or surgical intervention for J. T.?

CASE EXAMPLE 3

A Young Adult with Acquired Brain Injury and Decerebrate Pattern Hypertonicity

P. G. is a 17-year-old girl who sustained significant closed-head injury in a motor vehicle accident 3 weeks ago. She was admitted to the brain injury unit at the regional rehabilitation hospital earlier this week. Now functioning at a Rancho Los Amigos Cognitive Level 5 (confused and inappropriate), P. G. exhibits significant decorticate posturing whenever she attempts to move volitionally (right greater than left). She has marked limitations in passive ROM at the elbow and wrist, as well as equinovarus at the ankle, both of which are limiting her ability to stand and effectively propel her wheelchair. While sitting, she falls when she tries to throw a ball to her therapist. Her gait is characterized by large range ballistic extensor thrust throughout stance, which impedes forward progression. She is most focused and responsive to intervention when involved in ambulation-oriented activities. Currently, her hypertonicity is being managed with oral baclofen (Lioresal). However, her therapists are concerned that contracture formation continues. During rehabilitation rounds, the physiatrist, neurologists, and therapists agree that a trial of serial casting should be added to her regimen to enhance her rehabilitation.

Questions to Consider

- In which subphases of the gait cycle is function or safety compromised when G. P. attempts to ambulate?
- In what way does G. P.'s hypertonicity contribute to her difficulty with locomotion/ambulation?

- In what ways does G. P.'s impaired muscle performance contribute to her difficulty with locomotion/ambulation? What are the most likely dimensions of her impairment in muscle performance, given her diagnosis of acquired brain injury?
- In what ways does G. P.'s impaired postural control contribute to her difficulty with locomotion/ambulation? What are the most likely dimensions of her impairment in motor control, given her diagnosis of acquired brain injury?
- Are any primary or secondary musculoskeletal impairments influencing her function and safety during ambulation? What do you think is likely to develop as she recovers from her head injury?
- Given her constellation of impairments, what compensatory strategies is G. P. likely to use to accomplish the task of locomotion?
- Which of G. P.'s anticipated or observed impairments are remediable? Which will require accommodation?
- What orthotic options (design, components) are available to address G. P.'s impairment of locomotion and related functional limitations? What are the pros and cons of each?
- What alternative or concurrent medical (surgical/pharmacological) interventions might assist improvement in safety and function for G. P.?
- What additional rehabilitation interventions might assist improvement in function and safety for G. P.?
- How do you anticipate G. P.'s orthotic needs might change as she recovers over the next year?
- What outcome measures can be used to assess efficacy of orthotic, therapeutic, pharmacological, or surgical intervention for G. P.?

CASE EXAMPLE 4

Two Individuals with Recent Stroke

You work in the short-term rehabilitation unit associated with the regional tertiary care hospital in your area. This week two gentlemen recovering from stroke/brain attack sustained 3 days ago were admitted to the unit for a short stay in preparation for discharge home. Both indicate that their primary goals at this time are to be able to walk functional distances within their homes, manage stairs to enter/leave the house, and get to bedrooms on the second floor. You anticipate that they will receive intensive rehabilitation services for 5 to 8 days, with home care for follow-up after discharge.

M. O., 73 years old with a history of hypertension, mild chronic obstructive pulmonary disease, and an uncomplicated myocardial infarction 2 years ago, has been diagnosed with a lacunar infarct within the left posterior limb of internal capsule. On passive motion, he has been given modified Ashworth scores of 3 in his right upper extremity and 2 in his right lower extremity. When asked to bend his knee (when supine), he demonstrates difficulty initiating flexion, and when he finally begins to move, his ankle, knee, and hip move in a mass-flexion pattern; he is unable to isolate limb segments. When asked to slowly lower his leg to the bed, he "shoots" into a full lower extremity synergy pattern. He rises from sitting to standing with verbal and tactile cueing, somewhat asymmetrically, relying on his left extremities. Once upright, he can shift his center of mass to the midline, holding an effective upright posture, but feels unsteady when shifted beyond midline to the right. With encouragement and facilitation, he can shift weight toward his right in preparation for swing-limb advancement of the left lower extremity, and he is pleased to have taken a few steps, however short, in the parallel bars. Before his infarct, he was an avid golfer and enjoyed bowling. He is fearful that he will never be able to resume these activities.

E. B., 64, is a recently retired car mechanic with an 8-year history of diabetes mellitus previously controlled by diet and oral medications but requiring insulin since his stroke. MRI indicates probable occlusion in the right posteroinferior branch of the middle cerebral artery, with ischemia and resultant inflammation in the parietal lobe. Because E. B. has been afraid of hospitals for most of his life, he resisted seeking medical care as his symptoms began, arriving at the emergency department 12 hours after onset of hemiplegia. He currently displays a heavy, hypotonic, somewhat edematous left upper extremity. He is unusually unconcerned about the fact that he has had a stroke and tells you that he should be able to function "well enough" when he returns home to his familiar environment. On examination, he demonstrates homonymous hemianopsia, especially of the lower left visual field, and impaired kinesthetic awareness of his left extremities. You observe that he appears to be unaware when his lower upper extremity slips off the tray table of his wheelchair and his fingers become entangled in the spokes of the wheel as he propels forward using his right leg. When assisted to standing in the parallel bars, he does not seem to be accurately aware of his upright position, requiring moderate assistance to keep from falling to the left. When asked to try to walk forward a few paces, he repeatedly advances his right lower extremity, even when prompted to consider the position and activity of his lower left extremity.

Questions to Consider

- In what ways are the stroke-related impairments observed in these two gentlemen similar or different? How can you explain these differences?
- In what subphases of the gait cycle is function or safety compromised when each of these gentleman attempts to ambulate?
- In what way does each gentleman's abnormal tone contribute to his difficulty with locomotion/ambulation?
- In what ways does each gentleman's impaired muscle performance contribute to his difficulty with locomotion/

Continued

ambulation? What are the most likely dimensions of each man's impairment in muscle performance, given his etiology and location of stroke?

- In what ways does each gentleman's impaired postural control contribute to his difficulty with locomotion/ambulation? What are the most likely dimensions of each man's impairment in postural control, given the etiology and location of his stroke?
- Are any primary or secondary musculoskeletal impairments influencing each man's function and safety during ambulation? How does each man's age and concomitant medical conditions influence his risk for developing secondary impairments?
- Given each gentleman's constellation of impairments, what compensatory strategies is each likely to use to accomplish the task of locomotion?
- Which of each gentleman's anticipated or observed impairments are remediable? Which will require accommodation?
- What orthotic options are available to address each gentleman's impairment of locomotion and related functional limitations? What are the pros and cons of each?
- What alternative or concurrent medical (surgical/pharmacological) interventions might help improve in safety and function for each individual?
- What additional rehabilitation interventions might help improve in function and safety for M. O. and E. B.?
- How do you anticipate each gentleman's orthotic needs might change as he recovers from CNS damage?
- What outcome measures can be used to assess the efficacy of orthotic, therapeutic, pharmacological, or surgical intervention for each gentleman?

CASE EXAMPLE 5

A Young Adult with Incomplete Spinal Cord Injury

Z. C. is a 23-year-old man who sustained an incomplete C7 spinal cord injury 3 weeks ago when he lost control and crash-landed during a failed acrobatic stunt during a half-pipe snowboard competition at a local ski resort. After being stabilized on site, he was quickly airlifted to a regional spinal cord injury/trauma center. Methylprednisolone was administered within 1.5 hours of injury, and his cervical fractures were repaired by fusion (C5 through T1) the day after injury; he now wears a Miami J cervical orthosis. He was admitted to your rehabilitation center 5 days ago. He demonstrates no activity of triceps brachii bilaterally but reports dysesthesia in the C7 and C8 dermatomes and can point his index finger on the left. He is aware of lower limb position in space and can activate toe flexors and extensors, plantar flexors, knee extensors, and hip flexors and abductors at 2 +/5 levels of strength. Deep tendon reflex at the Achilles heel is brisk bilaterally, while more proximal lower extremity reflexes are diminished. He demonstrates positive

Babinski reflex bilaterally. Biceps and wrist extensor deep tendon reflexes, initially diminished, are now more consistently rated 2+; the triceps reflex, initially diminished, is now quite brisk. He requires moderate assistance of 1 to come to sitting from supine but can hold a static posture in sitting, demonstrating a limited sway envelope when attempting to shift his weight anteriorly, posteriorly, and mediolaterally. He requires moderate assistance of 1 to rise from seated in his wheelchair to standing position in the parallel bars. He is determined to "walk" out of the facility on discharge, anticipated after 3 more weeks of rehabilitation.

Questions to Consider
- Given Z. C.'s history and present point in recovery from spinal cord injury, what is the anticipated prognosis concerning his functional performance and ability to ambulate?
- In what subphases of the gait cycle is function or safety likely to be compromised when Z. C. attempts to ambulate?
- In what way does Z. C.'s abnormal tone contribute to his difficulty with locomotion/ambulation? What strategies would be useful in documenting/assessing the severity and type of his abnormal tone?
- In what ways does Z. C.'s impaired muscle performance contribute to his difficulty with locomotion/ambulation? What are the most likely dimensions of his impairment in muscle performance, given his etiology and level of injury?
- In what ways does Z. C.'s impaired postural control contribute to his difficulty with locomotion/ambulation? What are the most likely dimensions of Z. C.'s impairment in postural control, given his etiology and level of injury?
- Are any primary or secondary musculoskeletal impairments likely to influence Z. C.'s function and safety during ambulation? How do Z. C.'s age and concomitant medical conditions influence his risk for developing secondary impairments?
- Given Z. C.'s constellation of impairments, what compensatory strategies is he likely to use to accomplish the task of locomotion?
- Which of Z. C.'s anticipated or observed impairments are remediable? Which will require accommodation?
- What orthotic options (design, components) are available to address Z. C.'s difficulty with locomotion and related functional limitations? What are the pros and cons of each?
- What alternative or concurrent medical (surgical/pharmacological) interventions might assist improvement in safety and function?
- What additional rehabilitation interventions might assist improvement in function and safety for Z. C.?
- How do you anticipate Z. C.'s orthotic needs might change as he recovers from his spinal cord injury?
- What outcome measures can be used to assess the efficacy of orthotic, therapeutic, pharmacological, or surgical intervention for Z. C.?

REFERENCES

1. *Who are physical therapists? Guide to Physical Therapist Practice.* Alexandria, Va: American Physical Therapy Association. Available at: http://guidetoptpractice.apta.org.

2. Dean E. Physical therapy in the 21st century (part II): evidence-based practice within the context of evidence-informed practice. *Physiother Theory Pract.* 2009;25(5/6):354–368.

3. Sullivan KJ, Hershberg J, Howard R, et al. Neurologic differential diagnosis for physical therapy. *J Neurol Phys Ther.* 2004;28(4):162–168.

4. Lewis SL. An approach to neurological symptoms. In: Weiner WJ, Goetz CG, Shin RK, Lewis SL, eds. *Neurology for the Non Neurologist.* 6th ed. Philadelphia: Lippincott Williams & Wilkins; 2010:20–42.

5. Weiner WJ, Lang KE. *Behavioral Neurology of Movement Disorders.* Philadelphia: Lippincott Williams & Wilkins; 2005.

6. Biller J, Grueer G, Brazis PW. *DeMyer's The Neurological Examination: A Programmed Text.* 6th ed. New York: McGraw Hill; 2010.

7. Azar NJ, Arain AM. *Focus on Clinical Neurophysiology.* Philadelphia: Lippincott Williams & Wilkins; 2009.

8. Osborn AG, Salzman KL, Barkovich AJ, eds. *Diagnostic Imaging: Brain.* 2nd ed. Philadelphia: Lippincott Williams & Wilkins; 2009.

9. American Physical Therapy Association. *What are tests and measures? Guide to Physical Therapist Practice.* Alexandria, VA: American Physical Therapy Association. Available at: http://guidetoptpractice.apta.org.

10. Lazarro RT, Roller M, Umphred DA. Differential diagnosis phase 2: examination and intervention of functional movement activities and system/subsystem impairment. In: Umphred DA, ed. *Neurological Rehabilitation.* 5th ed. St. Louis: Mosby; 2007:163–186.

11. Strax TE, Luciano L, Dunn AM, et al. Aging and developmental disability. *Phys Med Rehabil Clin N Am.* 2010;21(2):419–427.

12. Klingbeil H, Baer HR, Wilson PE. Aging with a disability. *Arch Phys Med Rehabil* 2004;85(7 suppl 3):S68–S75 S85–S86.

13. Shumway-Cook A, Woollacott MH. Physiology of motor control. In: Shumway-Cook A, Woollacott MH, eds. *Motor Control: Translating Research into Clinical Practice.* 4th ed. Philadelphia: Wolters Kluwer/Lippincott Williams & Wilkins; 2012:45–82.

14. Rehme AK, Fink GR, von Cramon DY, et al. The role of the contralesional motor cortex for motor recovery in the early days after stroke assessed with longitudinal FMRI. *Cereb Cortex.* 2011;21(4):756–768.

15. Cramer SC, Riley JD. Neuroplasticity and brain repair after stroke. *Curr Opin Neurol.* 2008;21(1):76–82.

16. Shumway-Cook A, Woollacott MH. Physiological basis of motor learning and recovery of function. In: Shumway-Cook A, Woollacott MH, eds. *Motor Control: Translating Research into Clinical Practice.* 4th ed. Philadelphia: Wolters Kluwer/Lippincott Williams & Wilkins; 2012:83–103.

17. Alarcon F, Zijlmans JC, Duenas G, et al. Post-stroke movement disorders: report of 56 patients. *J Neurol Neurosurg Psychiatry.* 2004;75(11):1568–1574.

18. Ryerson SD. Hemiplegia. In: Umphred DA, ed. *Neurological Rehabilitation.* 5th ed. St. Louis: Mosby; 2007:857–901.

19. Bear MF, Connors BW, Paradiso MA. Brain control of movement. In: Bear MF, Connors BW, Paradiso MA, eds. *Neuroscience: Exploring the Brain.* 3rd ed. Philadelphia: Lippincott Williams & Wilkins; 2006:451–478.

20. Gravenhorst RM, Walter CB. Cognitive mechanisms of visuo-motor transformation in movement imitation: Examining predictions based on models of apraxia and motor control. *Brain Cogn.* 2009;71(2):118–128.

21. Galbreath AD, Goldstein LB. Dysnomia, ataxia, choreoathetosis, sensory impairment, and gait imbalance after lentiform nucleus stroke. *J Stroke Cerebrovasc Dis.* 2009;18(6):494–496.

22. Grandas F. Hemiballismus. *Handbook Clin Neurol.* 2011; 100:249–260.

23. Pahwa R, Lyons KE. *Handbook of Parkinson's Disease.* 4th ed. New York: Informa Healthcare; 2007.

24. Haber SN, Calzavara R. The cortico-basal ganglia integrative network: the role of the thalamus. *Brain Res Bull.* 2009;78(2/3):69–74.

25. Garcia-Rill E, Homma Y, Skinner RD. Arousal mechanisms related to posture and locomotion: 1. Descending modulation. *Prog Brain Res.* 2004;143:281–290.

26. Kiernan JA. Motor systems. In: Kiernan JA, ed. *Barr's The Human Nervous System.* 8th ed. Philadelphia: Lippincott Williams & Wilkins; 2005:374–390.

27. Shinoda Y, Sugiuchi Y, Izawa Y, et al. Long descending motor tract axons and their control of neck and axial muscles. *Prog Brain Res.* 2006;151:527–563.

28. Melnick ME. Clients with cerebellar dysfunction. In: Umphred DA, ed. *Neurological Rehabilitation.* 5th ed. St. Louis: Mosby; 2007:834–856.

29. Stoodley CJ, Schmahmann JD. Evidence for topographic organization in the cerebellum of motor control versus cognitive and affective processing. *Cortex.* 2010;46(7):831–844.

30. Bear MR, Connors BW, Paradiso MA. The somatic sensory system. In: Bear MF, Connors BW, et al., eds. *Neuroscience: Exploring the Brain.* 3rd ed. Philadelphia: Lippincott Williams & Wilkins; 2006:387–422.

31. Marini E, Schoen JH. A reappraisal of the ascending systems in man, with emphasis on the medial lemniscus. In: *Advances in Anatomy, Embryology and Cell Biology.* New York: Springer Verlag; 2005.

32. Kiernan JA. Functional localization in the cerebral cortex. In: Kiernan JA, ed. *Barr's The Human Nervous System, An Anatomical Viewpoint.* 9th ed. Philadelphia: Lippincott Williams & Wilkins; 2008:227–244.

33. Zucker-Levin A. Sensory and perceptual issues related to motor control. In: Montgomery PC, Connolly BH, eds. *Clinical Applications for Motor Control.* Thorofare, NJ: Slack Inc; 2003:207–243.

34. Zoltan B. *Vision, Perceptions and Cognition: A Manual for the Evaluation and Treatment of the Adult with Acquired Brain Injury.* 4th ed. Thorofare, NJ: Slack Inc; 2007.

35. Kiernan JA. The visual system. In: Kiernan JA, ed. *Barr's The Human Nervous System, an Anatomical Viewpoint.* 9th ed. Philadelphia: Lippincott Williams & Wilkins; 2005:303–318.

36. Chaikin LE. Disorders of vision and visual perceptual dysfunction. In: Umphred DA, ed. *Neurological Rehabilitation.* 5th ed. St. Louis: Mosby; 2007:973–1004.

37. Schwartz SH. *Visual Perception: A Clinical Orientation.* New York: McGraw Hill; 2010.

38. Isableu B, Ohlmann T, Cremieux J, et al. Individual differences in the ability to identify, select and use appropriate frames of reference for perceptuo-motor control. *Neuroscience.* 2010;169(3):1199–1215.

39. Medendorp WP. Spatial constancy mechanisms in motor control. *Philos Trans R Soc Lond B Biol Sci.* 2011;366(1564):476–491.

40. Scheiman M. *Understanding and Managing Vision Deficits: A Guide for Occupational Therapists.* 3rd ed. Thorofare, NJ: Slack Inc; 2011.

41. Anderson A, Jacobs R, Anerson P, eds. *Executive Functions and the Frontal Lobe: A Lifespan Perspective.* New York: Taylor & Francis; 2010.

42. Miller BL, Cummings JL, eds. *The Human Frontal Lobe: Functions and Disorders.* 2nd ed. New York: Guilford Press; 2007.

43. Sliver JM, McAllister TW, Yudofsky SC, eds. *Textbook of Traumatic Brain Injury.* 2nd ed. Washington, DC: American Psychiatric Publishing; 2011.

44. Winkler PA. Traumatic brain injury. In: Umphred DA, ed. *Neurological Rehabilitation.* 5th ed. St. Louis: Mosby; 2007: 532–566.

45. Rudy JW. *The Neurobiology of Learning and Memory.* Sunderland, MA: Sinaur; 2008.

46. Umphred DA. The limbic system: influence over motor control and learning. In: Umphred DA, ed. *Neurological Rehabilitation.* 5th ed. St. Louis: Mosby; 2007:71–118.

47. Cunningham WA, Van Bavel JJ, Johnsen IR. Affective flexibility: evaluative processing goals shape amygdala activity. *Psychol Sci.* 2008;19(2):152–160.

48. Reeve JM. *Understanding Motivation and Emotion.* 5th ed. Hoboken, NJ: John Wiley & Sons; 2009.

49. Light KE. Issues of cognition for motor control. In: Montgomery PC, Connolly BH, eds. *Clinical Applications for Motor Control.* Thorofare, NJ: Slack Inc; 2003:245–268.

50. Kiernan JA. Reticular formation. In: Kiernan JA, ed. *Barr's The Human Nervous System: An Anatomical Viewpoint.* 9th ed. Philadelphia: Lippincott Williams & Wilkins; 2009:141–156.

51. Lin JS, Anaclet S, Sergeeva O, et al. The waking brain: an update. *Cell Mol Life Sci.* 2011;68(15):2499–2512.

52. Fernández-Gil MA, Palacios-Bote R, Leo-Barahona M, et al. Anatomy of the brainstem: a gaze into the stem of life. *Semin Ultrasound CT MR.* 2010;31(3):196–219.

53. Laureys S, Tononi G. *The Neurology of Consciousness: Cognitive Neuroscience and Neuropathology.* London: Academic Press; 2009.

54. Liebmann O, Simon B. Evaluating the patient with altered level of consciousness. *Emerg Med.* 2006;38(2):35–36, 39–42.

55. Poster JB, Saper CB, Schiff ND, et al. *Plum and Posner's Diagnosis of Stupor and Coma.* 4th ed. Oxford: New York; 2007.

56. Janig W. *Integrative Action of the Autonomic Nervous System: Neurobiology of Homeostasis.* New York: Cambridge University Press; 2008.

57. Hall JE. Behavioral and motivational mechanisms of the brain: the limbic system and the hypothalamus. In: *Guyton and Hall Textbook of Medical Physiology.* 12th ed. Philadelphia: Saunders; 2011: 711–720.

58. Bear MF, Connors BW, Paradiso MA. Chemical control of the brain and behavior. In: Bear MF, Connors BW, Paradiso MA, eds. *Neuroscience: Exploring the Brain.* 3rd ed. Philadelphia: Lippincott Williams & Wilkins; 2006:481–508.

59. Gescheider GA, Wright JH, Verrillo RT. *Information Processing Channels in the Tactile Sensory System.* New York: Psychology Press/Taylor & Francis Group; 2009.

60. Newton RA. Neural systems underlying motor control. In: Montgomery PT, Connelly BH, eds. *Clinical Applications for Motor Control.* Thorofare, NJ: Slack Inc; 2003:53–77.

61. Schmidt RA, Lee TD. Central contributions to motor control. In: Schmidt RA, Lee TD, eds. *Motor Control and Learning: A Behavioral Emphasis.* 3rd ed. Champaign, IL: Human Kinetics; 2005:131–169.

62. Bear MF, Connors BW, Paradiso MA. Spinal control of movement. In: Bear MF, Connors BW, Paradiso MA, eds. *Neuroscience: Exploring the Brain.* 3rd ed. Philadelphia: Lippincott Williams & Wilkins; 2006:423–478.

63. Keynes RD, Aidley DJ, Huang CL. *Nerve and Muscle.* 4th ed. Cambridge, UK: Cambridge University Press; 2011.

64. Hughes R. Peripheral nerve diseases: the bare essentials. *Practical Neurol.* 2008;8(6):396–405.

65. Cohen JA, Mowchun J, Grudem J. *Peripheral Nerve and Muscle Diseases (What Do I Do Now?).* New York: Oxford University Press; 2009.

66. Shumway-Cook A, Woollacott MH. A conceptual framework for clinical practice. In: Shumway-Cook A, Woollacott MH, eds. *Motor Control: Translating Research into Clinical Practice.* 4th ed. Philadelphia: Wolters Kluwer/Lippincott Williams & Wilkins; 2011:141–158.

67. Gurfinkel V, Cacciatore TW, Cordo P, et al. Postural muscle tone in the body axis of healthy humans. *J Neurophysiol.* 2006;96(5):2678–2687.

68. Fort P, Bassetti CL, Luppi PH. Alternating vigilance states: new insights regarding neuronal networks and mechanisms. *Eur J Neurosci.* 2009;29(9):1741–1753.

69. Takakusaki K. Forebrain control of locomotor behaviors. *Brain Res Rev.* 2008;57(1):192–198.

70. Gardiner PF. *Advanced Neuromuscular Exercise Physiology.* Champaign, Ill: Human Kinetics; 2011.

71. Paterson DH, Jones GR, Rice CL. Ageing and physical activity: evidence to develop exercise recommendations for older adults. *Appl Physiol Nutr Metab.* 2007;32(2E):S69–S108.

72. Marcus RL, Westlen-Boyer K, LaStayo P. Impaired muscle performance. In: Giccione AA, Avers D, Wong RA, eds. *Geriatric Physical Therapy.* 3rd ed. St. Louis: Mosby; 2012:263–271.

73. Hurley BF, Hanson ED, Sheaff AK. Strength training as a countermeasure to aging muscle and chronic disease. *Sports Med.* 2011;41(4):289–306.

74. Hvid L, Aagaard P, Justesen L, et al. Effects of aging on muscle mechanical function and muscle fiber morphology during short-term immobilization and subsequent retraining. *J Appl Physiol.* 2010;109(6):1628–1634.

75. Nielsen JB, Crone C, Hultborn H. The spinal pathophysiology of spasticity—from a basic science point of view. *Acta Physiol (Oxf).* 2007;189(2):171–180.

76. Ryu JS, Lee JW, Lee SI, et al. Factors predictive of spasticity and their effects on motor recovery and functional outcomes in stroke patients. *Top Stroke Rehabil.* 2010;17(5):380–388.

77. Wu YN, Ren Y, Goldsmith A, et al. Characterization of spasticity in cerebral palsy: dependence of catch angle on velocity. *Dev Med Child Neurol.* 2010;52(6):563–569.

78. Hsieh JT, Wolfe DL, Connolly S. Spasticity after spinal cord injury: an evidence-based review of current interventions. *Top Spinal Cord Injury Rehabil.* 2007;13(1):81–97.

79. Sosnoff JJ, Shin S, Motl RW. Multiple sclerosis and postural control: the role of spasticity. *Arch Phys Med Rehabil.* 2010;91(1):93–99.

80. Brashear A, Elovic E, eds. *Spasticity: Diagnosis and Management.* New York: Demos Medical; 2011.

81. Sheean G, McGuire JR. Spastic hypertonia and movement disorders: pathophysiology, clinical presentation, and quantification. *PMR.* 2009;1(9):827–833.

82. Dietz V, Sinkjaer T. Spastic movement disorder: impaired reflex function and altered muscle mechanics. *Lancet Neurol.* 2007;6(8):725–733.

83. Mueller MJ, Kaluf KS. Tissue adaptation to physical stress: a proposed "physical stress theory" to guide physical therapist practice, education and research. *Phys Ther.* 2002;82(4):383–403.

84. Guiliani CA. Spasticity and motor control. In: Montgomery PC, Connolly BH, eds. *Clinical Applications for Motor Control.* Thorofare, NJ: Slack Inc; 2003:309–332.

85. Borges CA, Castao KC, Souto PA, et al. Effect of resisted exercise on muscular strength, spasticity and functionality in chronic hemiparetic subjects: a systematic review. *J Appl Res.* 2009;9(4):147–158.

86. Patten C, Lexell J, Brown HE. Weakness and strength training in persons with poststroke hemiplegia: rationale, method, and efficacy. *J Rehabil Res Dev.* 2004;41(3A):293–312.

87. Pak S, Patten C. Strengthening to promote functional recovery poststroke: an evidence-based review. *Top Stroke Rehabil.* 2008;15(3):177–199.

88. Ahlskog JE. *Parkinson's Disease: Treatment Guide for Physicians.* New York: Oxford University Press; 2009.

89. Ransmayr G. Physical, occupational, speech and swallowing therapies and physical exercise in Parkinson's disease. *J Neural Transm.* 2011;118(5):773–781.

90. Hypes B. *Heads Up on Hypotonia: Understanding Complexities of Hypotonia and Strategies for Treatment.* Brooklyn, NY: Therapeutic Services Inc; 2008.

91. Harris S. Congenital hypotonia: clinical and developmental assessment. *Dev Med Child Neurol.* 2008;50(12):889–892.

92. Stephens BE, Liu J, Lester B. Neurobehavioral assessment predicts motor outcome in preterm infants. *J Pediatr.* 2010;156(3):366–371.

93. Deon LL, Gaebler-Spira D. Assessment and treatment of movement disorders in children with cerebral palsy. *Orthop Clin North Am.* 2010;41(4):507–517.

94. Rigoldi C, Galli M, Mainardi L, et al. Postural control in children, teenagers and adults with Down syndrome. *Res Dev Disabil.* 2011;32(1):170–175.

95. Goldstein S, Reynolds CR. *Handbook of Neurodevelopmental and Genetic Disorders in Children.* 2nd ed. New York: Guilford Press; 2011.

96. Ming X, Brimacombe M, Wagner GC. Prevalence of motor impairment in autism spectrum disorders. *Brain Dev.* 2007;29(9):565–570.

97. Martin K, Inman J, Kirschner A, et al. Characteristics of hypotonia in children: a consensus opinion of pediatric occupational and physical therapists. *Pediatr Phys Ther.* 2005;17(4):275–282.

98. Fitzgerald D, Stokes M. Muscle imbalance in neurological conditions. In: Stokes M, ed. *Physical Management in Neurological Rehabilitation.* 2nd ed. Edinburgh: Mosby; 2004:501–516.

99. Wissel J, Schelosky LE, Scott J, et al. Early development of spasticity following stroke: a prospective, observational trial. *J Neurol.* 2010;257(7):1067–1072.

100. Sheerin F. Spinal cord injury: acute care management. *Emerg Nurse.* 2005;12(10):26–34.

101. Young PA, Yound PH, Tolbert DL. Lower motor neurons; flaccid paralysis. *Clinical Neuroscience.* 2nd ed. Philadelphia: Wolters Kluwer/Lippincott Williams & Wilkins; 2008 47–64.

102. Salmons S, Ashley Z, Sutherland H, et al. Functional electrical stimulation of denervated muscles: basic issues. *Artif Organs.* 2005;29(3):199–202.

103. Krosschell KJ, Pesavento MJ. Congenital spinal cord injury. In: Umphred DA, ed. *Neurological Rehabilitation.* 5th ed. St. Louis: Mosby; 2007:567–604.

104. Atrice MB, Morrison SA, McDowell SL, et al. Traumatic spinal cord injury. In: Umphred DA, ed. *Neurological Rehabilitation.* 5th ed. St. Louis: Mosby; 2007:605–657.

105. Parry GJ, Steinberg MD. *Guillain-Barré Syndrome: From Diagnosis to Recovery.* St. Paul, MN: American Academy of Neurology Press; 2007.

106. Osterbauer PJ. Botulinum neurotoxin. In: Dobbs MR, ed. *Clinical Neurotoxicology: Syndromes, Substances, Environments.* Philadelphia: Saunders; 2009:421–426.

107. Singer HS, Jankovic J, Mink JW, Gilberts DL, eds. *Chorea, athetosis and ballism. In Movement Disorders in Childhood.* Philadelphia: Saunders; 2010:76–95.

108. Wright MJ, Wallman L. Cerebral palsy. In: Campbell SK, Vander Linden DW, Palisano RJ, eds. *Physical Therapy for Children.* 4th ed. St. Louis: Saunders; 2012:577–626.

109. Jensen MP, Molton IR. *Aging With a Disability.* Philadelphia: Saunders; 2010.

110. Shumway-Cook A, Woollacott MH. Normal postural control. In: Shumway-Cook A, Woollacott MH, eds. *Motor Control: Translating Research into Clinical Practice.* 4th ed. Philadelphia: Wolters Kluwer/Lippincott Williams & Wilkins; 2012:161–194.

111. Allison L, Fuller K. Balance and vestibular disorders. In: Umphred DA, ed. *Neurological Rehabilitation.* 5th ed. St. Louis: Mosby; 2007:732–774.

112. Takakusaki K, Okumura T. Neurobiological basis of controlling posture and locomotion. *Adv Robot.* 2008;22(15):1629–1663.

113. Seeger MA. Balance deficits: examination, evaluation and intervention. In: Montgomery PC, Connolly BH, eds. *Clinical Applications for Motor Control.* Thorofare, NJ: Slack Inc; 2003:271–308.

114. Pagnacco G, Oggero E, Carrick FR. Repeatability of posturographic measures of the MCTSIB static balance tests a preliminary investigation. *Biomed Sci Instrum.* 2008;44(1):41–46.

115. Santos MJ, Knekar N, Aruin AS. The role of anticipatory postural adjustments in compensatory control of posture: 1. Electromyographic analysis. *J Electromyogr Kinesiol.* 2010;20(3):388–397.

116. Santos MJ, Kanekar N, Aruin AS. The role of anticipatory postural adjustments in compensatory control of posture: 2. Biomechanical analysis. *J Electromyogr Kinesiol.* 2010;20(3):398–405.

117. Duncan PW, Studenski S, Chandler J, et al. Functional reach: a new clinical measure of balance. *J Gerontol.* 1990;45(6):M192–M197.

118. Newton RA. Validity of the multi-directional reach test: a practical measure for limits of stability in older adults. *J Gerontol.* 2001;56A(4):M248–M252.

119. Bartlett D, Birmingham T. Validity and reliability of a pediatric reach test. *Pediatr Phys Ther.* 2003;15(2):84–92.

120. Washington K, Shumway-Cook A, Price R, et al. Muscle responses to seated perturbations for typically developing infants and those at risk for motor delays. *Dev Med Child Neurol.* 2004;46(10):681–688.

121. Sang IL, Woollacott M. Association between sensorimotor function and functional and reactive balance control in the elderly. *Age Ageing.* 2005;34(4):358–363.

122. Mackey DC, Robinovitch SN. Postural steadiness during quiet stance does not associate with ability to recover balance in older women. *Clin Biomech (Bristol, Avon).* 2005;20(8):776–783.

123. Shumway-Cook A, Woollacott MH. Abnormal postural control. In: Shumway-Cook A, Woollacott MH, eds. *Motor*

Control: Translating Research into Clinical Practice. 4th ed. Philadelphia: Wolters Kluwer/Lippincott Williams & Wilkins; 2012:246–270.

124. Sosnoff JJ, Shin S, Motl RW. Multiple sclerosis and postural control: the role of spasticity. *Arch Phys Med Rehabil.* 2010;91(1):93–99.

125. Westcott SL, Burtner P. Postural control in children: implications for pediatric practice. *Phys Occup Ther Pediatr.* 2004;24(1/2):5–55.

126. Shumway-Cook A, Woollacott MH. Normal reach, grasp and manipulation. In: Shumway-Cook A, Woollacott MH, eds. *Motor Control: Translating Research into Clinical Practice.* 4th ed. Philadelphia: Wolters Kluwer/Lippincott Williams & Wilkins; 2012:477–501.

127. Shumway-Cook A, Woollacott MH. Reach, grasp and manipulation: changes across the lifespan. In: Shumway-Cook A, Woollacott MH, eds. *Motor Control: Translating Research into Clinical Practice.* 4th ed. Philadelphia: Wolters Kluwer/ Lippincott Williams & Wilkins; 2012:502–528.

128. Stout JL. Gait: development and analysis. In: Campbell SK, Vander Linden DW, Palisano RJ, eds. *Physical Therapy for Children.* 4th ed. St. Louis: Mosby; 2012.

129. Corrigan R, McBurney H. Community ambulation: environmental impacts and assessment inadequacies. *Disabil Rehabil.* 2008;30(19):1411–1419.

130. Shumway-Cook A, Woollacott MH. Abnormal mobility. In: Shumway-Cook A, Woollacott MH, eds. *Motor Control: Translating Research into Clinical Practice.* 4th ed. Philadelphia: Wolters Kluwer/Lippincott Williams & Wilkins; 2012:381–415.

131. Schmidt RA, Lee TL. Coordination. In: Schmidt RA, Lee TL, eds. *Motor Control and Learning: A Behavioral Emphasis.* 4th ed. Champaign, IL: Human Kinetics; 2005:243–270.

132. Schmitz TJ. Examination of coordination. In: O'Sullivan SB, Schmitz TJ, eds. *Physical Rehabilitation.* 5th ed. Philadelphia: FA Davis; 2007:193–225.

133. Shumway-Cook A, Woollacott MH. A lifespan perspective of mobility. In: Shumway-Cook A, Woollacott MH, eds. *Motor Control: Translating Research into Clinical Practice.* 4th ed. Philadelphia: Wolters Kluwer/Lippincott Williams & Wilkins; 2012:348–380.

134. Richards CL, Malouin F, Dumas F. Patterns of locomotor recovery after stroke. In: Stein J, Harvey RL, Macko RF, eds. *Stroke Recovery and Rehabilitation.* New York: Demos Medical; 2009:245–268.

135. Smits DW, Gorter JW, Ketelaar M, et al. Relationship between gross motor capacity and daily-life mobility in children with cerebral palsy. *Dev Med Child Neurol.* 2010;52(3):60–66.

136. Shumway-Cook A, Woollacott MH. Abnormal reach grasp and manipulation. In: Shumway-Cook A, Woollacott MH, eds. *Motor Control: Translating Research into Clinical Practice.* 4th ed. Philadelphia: Wolters Kluwer/Lippincott Williams & Wilkins; 2012:529–551.

137. Winstein CJ, Wolf SL. Task-oriented training to promote upper extremity recovery. In: Stein J, Harvey RL, Macko RF, et al., eds. *Stroke Recovery and Rehabilitation.* New York: Demos Medical; 2009:267–290.

138. Zackowski KM, Dromerick AW, Sahrman SA, et al. How do strength, sensation, spasticity, and joint individuation relate to the reaching deficits of people with chronic hemiparesis? *Brain.* 2004;127(5):1035–1046.

139. Lynn AK, Turner M, Chambers HG. Surgical management of spasticity in persons with cerebral palsy. *Phys Med Rehabil.* 2009;1(9):834–838.

140. Miller EL, Murray L, Richards L, et al. Comprehensive overview of nursing and interdisciplinary rehabilitation care of the stroke patient: a scientific statement from the American Heart Association. *Stroke.* 2010;41(10):2402–2448.

141. Stevenson VL, Playford ED. Rehabilitation and MS. *Int MS J.* 2007;14(3):85–92.

142. Verza R, Carvalho ML, Battaglia MA, et al. An interdisciplinary approach to evaluating the need for assistive technology reduces equipment abandonment. *Mult Scler.* 2006;12(1):88–93.

143. Simon O, Yelnik AP. Managing spasticity with drugs. *Eur J Phys Rehabil Med.* 2010;46(3):401–410.

144. Elbasiouny SM, Moroz D, Bakr MM, et al. Management of spasticity after spinal cord injury: current techniques and future directions. *Neurorehabil Neural Repair.* 2010;24(1):23–33.

145. Caty GD, Detrembleur C, Bleyenheuft C, et al. Effect of simultaneous botulinum toxin injections into several muscles on impairment, activity, participation, and quality of life among stroke patients presenting with a stiff knee gait. *Stroke.* 2008;39(10):2803–2808.

146. Damiano DL, Alter KE, Chambers H. New clinical and research trends in lower extremity management for ambulatory children with cerebral palsy. *Phys Med Rehabil Clin N Am.* 2009;20(3):469–491.

147. Love SC, Novak I, Kentish M, et al. Botulinum toxin assessment, intervention and after-care for lower limb spasticity in children with cerebral palsy: international consensus statement. *Eur J Neurol.* 2010;17(suppl 2):9–37.

148. Johnson J, Jarrett L, Porter B, et al. Strategies and challenges in managing spasticity. In: Halper J, ed. *Advanced Concepts in Multiple Sclerosis Nursing Care.* 2nd ed. New York: Demos Medical Publishing; 2007:145–174.

149. Francisco GE, McGuire JR, Stein J, et al. Physiology and management of spasticity after stroke. In: Stein J, Harvey R, Macko E, et al., eds. *Stroke Recovery & Rehabilitation.* New York: Demos Medical Publishing; 2009:413–436.

150. Ryan M. Drug therapies for the treatment of multiple sclerosis. *J Infus Nurs.* 2009;32(3):137–144.

151. Derwenskus J. Current disease-modifying treatment of multiple sclerosis. *Mt Sinai J Med.* 2011;78(2):161–175.

152. Ciccone CD. Antiepileptic drugs. In: Ciccone CD, ed. *Pharmacology in Rehabilitation.* 4th ed. Philadelphia: FA Davis; 2007:105–117.

153. Papavasiliou AS. Management of motor problems in cerebral palsy: a critical update for the clinician. *Eur J Paediatr Neurol.* 2009;13(5):387–396.

154. Burke-Doe A, Runion HI, Smith TJ. Impact of drug therapy on patients receiving neurological rehabilitation. In: Umphred DA, ed. *Neurological Rehabilitation.* 5th ed. St. Louis: Mosby; 2007:1119–1137.

155. Bollens B, Deltombe T, Detrembleur C, et al. Effects of selective tibial nerve neurotomy as a treatment for adults presenting with spastic equinovarus foot: a systematic review. *J Rehabil Med.* 2011;43(4):277–282.

156. Palacio A, Milliez PY, Le Jean T, et al. Direct neurectomy of the motor branches of the tibial nerve in hemiplegic adults: an assessment with a mean follow-up period of 11 years. *Ann Phys Rehabil Med.* 2010;53(6/7):417–433.

157. Maarrawi J, Mertens P, Luaute J, et al. Long-term functional results of selective peripheral neurotomy for the treatment of spastic upper limb: prospective study in 31 patients. *J Neurosurg.* 2006;104(2):215–225.

158. Sindou MP, Simon F, Mertens P, et al. Selective peripheral neurotomy (SPN) for spasticity in childhood. *Child Nerv Syst.* 2007;23(9):957–970.

159. Fitoussi F, Ilharreborde B, Presedo A, et al. Shoulder external rotator selective neurotomy in cerebral palsy: anatomical study and preliminary clinical results. *J Pediatr Orthop.* 2010;19(1):71–76.

160. van Schie PE, Schothorst M, Dallmeijer AJ, et al. Short- and long-term effects of selective dorsal rhizotomy on gross motor function in ambulatory children with spastic diplegia. *J Neurosurg Pediatr.* 2011;7(5):557–562.

161. Tedroff K, Lowing K, Jacobson DN, et al. Does loss of spasticity matter? A 10-year follow-up after selective dorsal rhizotomy in cerebral palsy. *Dev Med Child Neurol.* 2011;53(8):724–729.

162. Langerak NG, Hillier SL, Verkoeijen PP, et al. Level of activity and participation in adults with spastic diplegia 17-26 years after selective dorsal rhizotomy. *J Rehabil Med.* 2011;43(4):330–337.

163. Dvorak EM, Ketchum NC, McGuire JR. The underutilization of intrathecal baclofen in poststroke spasticity. *Top Stroke Rehabil.* 2011;18(3):195–202.

164. Keenan E. Spasticity management, part 3: surgery and the use of intrathecal baclofen. *Br J Neurosci Nurs.* 2010;6(1):12–18.

165. Ward A, Hayden S, Dexter M, et al. Continuous intrathecal baclofen for children with spasticity and/or dystonia: goal attainment and complications associated with treatment. *J Pediatr Child Health.* 2009;45(12):720–726.

166. Rutz E, Baker R, Tirosh O, et al. Tibialis anterior tendon shortening in combination with Achilles tendon lengthening in spastic equinus in cerebral palsy. *Gait Posture.* 2011;33(2):152–157.

167. de Morais Filho MC, Kawamura CM, Kanaji PR, et al. The relation of triceps surae surgical lengthening and crouch gait in patients with cerebral palsy. *J Pediatr Orthop B* 2010;19(3):226–230.

168. Bernthal NM, Gamradt SC, Kay RM, et al. Static and dynamic gait parameters before and after multilevel soft tissue surgery in ambulating children with cerebral palsy. *J Pediatr Orthop.* 2010;30(2):174–179.

169. Paul SM, Siegel KL, Malley J, et al. Evaluating interventions to improve gait in cerebral palsy: a meta-analysis of spatiotemporal measures. *Dev Med Child Neurol.* 2007;49(7):542–549.

170. Yun AG, Severino R, Reinker K. Varus derotational osteotomy for spastic hip instability: the roles of femoral shortening and obturator neurectomy. *Am J Orthop.* 2005;34(2):81–85.

171. Westwell M, Öunpuu S, DeLuca P. Effects of orthopedic intervention in adolescents and young adults with cerebral palsy. *Gait Posture.* 2009;30(2):201–206.

172. Amichai T, Harries N, Dvir Z, et al. The effects of femoral derotation osteotomy in children with cerebral palsy: an evaluation using energy cost and functional mobility. *J Pediatr Orthop.* 2009;29(1):68–72.

173. Novacheck TF, Stout JL, Gage JR, et al. Distal femoral extension osteotomy and patellar tendon advancement to treat persistent crouch gait in cerebral palsy. *J Bone Joint Surg.* 2009;91A (suppl 2):271–286.

174. Imrie MN, Yaszay B. Management of spinal deformity in cerebral palsy. *Orthop Clin North Am.* 2010;41(4):531–547.

175. Auerbach JD, Spiegel DA, Zgonis MH, et al. The correction of pelvic obliquity in patients with cerebral palsy and neuromuscular scoliosis: is there a benefit of anterior release prior to posterior spinal arthrodesis? *Spine.* 2009;34(21):E766–E774.

176. Keeler KA, Lenke LG, Good CR, et al. Spinal fusion for spastic neuromuscular scoliosis: is anterior releasing necessary when intraoperative halo-femoral traction is used? *Spine.* 2010;35(10):E427–E433.

177. Thomason P, Baker R, Dodd K, et al. Single-event multilevel surgery in children with spastic diplegia: a pilot randomized controlled trial. *J Bone Joint Surg Am.* 2011;93(5):451–456.

178. Akerstedt A, Risto O, Odman P, et al. Evaluation of single event multilevel surgery and rehabilitation in children and youth with cerebral palsy—a 2-year follow-up study. *Disabil Rehabil.* 2010;32(7):530–539.

179. Seniorou M, Thompson N, Harrington M, et al. Recovery of muscle strength following multi-level orthopaedic surgery in diplegic cerebral palsy. *Gait Posture.* 2007;26(4):475–481.

180. Kondratek M, McCollum H, Garland A. Long-term physical therapy management following a single-event multiple level surgery. *Pediatr Phys Ther.* 2010;22(4):427–438.

181. Capjon H, Bjork IT. Rehabilitation after multilevel surgery in ambulant spastic children with cerebral palsy: children and parent experiences. *Dev Neurorehabil.* 2010;13(3):182–191.

182. Miller F. Spinal deformity secondary to impaired neurologic control. *J Bone Joint Surg Am.* 2007;80(suppl 1):143–147.

183. Fowler EG, Kolobe TH, Damiano DL, et al. Promotion of physical fitness and prevention of secondary conditions for children with cerebral palsy: section on pediatrics research summit proceedings. *Phys Ther.* 2007;87(11):1495–1510.

184. Tosi LL, Maher N, Moore DW, et al. Adults with cerebral palsy: a workshop to define the challenges of treating and preventing secondary musculoskeletal and neuromuscular complications in this rapidly growing population. *Dev Med Child Neurol.* 2009;51(suppl 4):2–11.

185. Novacheck TF, Gage JR. Orthopedic management of spasticity in cerebral palsy. *Child Nerv Syst.* 2007;23(9):L1015–L1031.

186. Rodda JM, Graham HK, Nattrass GR, et al. Correction of severe crouch gait in patients with spastic diplegia with use of multilevel orthopaedic surgery. *J Bone Joint Surg Am.* 2006;88(12):2653–2664.

187. Novacheck TF, Stout JL, Gage JR, et al. Distal femoral extension osteotomy and patellar tendon advancement to treat persistent crouch gait in cerebral palsy. *J Bone Joint Surg Am.* 2009;19 (suppl 2):271–286.

188. de Vries G, Roy K, Chester V. Using three-dimensional gait data for foot/ankle orthopaedic surgery. *Open Orthop J.* 2009;3:89–95.

189. Westcott SL, Goulet C. Neuromuscular system: structures, functions, diagnoses, and evaluation. In: Effgen SK, ed. *Meeting the Physical Therapy Needs of Children.* Philadelphia: FA Davis; 2005:185–244.

190. Lazaro RT, Roller M, Umphred DA. Differential diagnosis phase 2: examination and evaluation of functional movement activities and system/subsystem impairments. In: Umphred DA, ed. *Neurological Rehabilitation.* 5th ed. St. Louis: Mosby; 2007:163–186.

191. American Physical Therapy Association. *Basics of Patient/Client Management: The Five Elements of Patient/Client Management. Guide to Physical Therapist Practice.* Alexandria VA: American Physical Therapy Association. Available at: http://guidetoptpractice.apta.org.

192. Eberly V, Kubota K, Weiss W. *To brace or not to brace: making evidenced based decisions with our clients with neurological*

impairments. Session handouts, American Physical Therapy Association Combined Sections Meeting, San Diego, February 2 2006.

193. Racette W. Orthotics: evaluation, prognosis, and intervention. In: Umphred DA, ed. *Neurological Rehabilitation*. 5th ed. St. Louis: Mosby; 2007:1086–1118.

194. Effgen SK, McEwen IR. Review of selected physical therapy interventions for school age children with disabilities. *Phys Ther Rev*. 2008;13(5):297–312.

195. Morris C, Bowers R, Ross K, et al. Orthotic management of cerebral palsy: recommendations from a consensus conference. *NeuroRehabilitation*. 2001;28(1):37–46.

196. American Physical Therapy Association. *What Are Interventions? Guide to Physical Therapist Practice*. Alexandria, VA: American Physical Therapy Association. Available at: http://guidetoptpractice.apta.org.

197. Lowes LP, Sveda M, Gajdosik CG, et al. Musculoskeletal development and adaptation. In: Campbell SK, Vander Linden DW, Palisano RJ, eds. *Physical Therapy for Children*. 4th ed. St. Louis: Saunders; 2012:175–204.

198. Malhotra S, Pandyan AD, Rosewilliam S, et al. Spasticity and contractures at the wrist after stroke: time course of development and their association with functional recovery of the upper limb. *Clin Rehabil*. 2011;25(2):184–191.

199. Sullivan KJ, Mulroy S, Kautz SA, et al. Walking recovery and rehabilitation after stroke. In: Stein J, Harvey RL, Macko RF, et al., eds. *Stroke Recovery and Rehabilitation*. New York: Demos Medical; 2009:323–342.

200. Pohl M, Mehrholz J, Rockstroh G, et al. Contractures and involuntary muscle overactivity in severe brain injury. *Brain Inj*. 2007;21(4):421–432.

201. Katalinic OM, Harvey LA, Herbert RD. Effectiveness of stretch for the treatment and prevention of contractures in people with neurological conditions: a systematic review. *Phys Ther*. 2011;91(1):11–24.

202. Swanton R, Kinnear B. There is robust evidence that stretch interventions do not prevent or reverse joint contractures in people with neurological conditions. *Aust Occup Ther J*. 2011;58(2):134–135.

203. Lannin NA, Novak I, Cusick A. A systematic review of upper extremity casting for children and adults with central nervous system motor disorders. *Clin Rehabil*. 2007;21(11):963–976.

204. Harvey LA, Glinsky JA, Katalinic OM, et al. Contracture management for people with spinal cord injuries. *NeuroRehabilitation*. 2011;28(1):17–20.

205. Gao F, Ren Y, Roth EJ, et al. Effects of repeated ankle stretching on calf muscle–tendon and ankle biomechanical properties in stroke survivors. *Clin Biomech (Bristol, Avon)*. 2011;26(5):516–522.

206. Bonutti PM, McGrath MS, Ulrich SD, et al. Static progressive stretch for the treatment of knee stiffness. *Knee*. 2008;15(4):272–276.

207. Redstone F. The importance of postural control for feeding. *Pediatr Nurs*. 2004;30(2):97–100.

208. McDonald R, Surtees R, Wirz S. The International Classification of Functioning, Disability and Health provides a model for adaptive seating interventions for children with cerebral palsy. *Br J Occup Ther*. 2004;67(7):293–302.

209. Hahn ME, Sihemkins SL, Gardner JK, et al. A dynamic seating system for children with cerebral palsy. *J Musculoskel Res*. 2009;12(1):21–30.

210. Stavness C. The effect of positioning for children with cerebral palsy on upper-extremity function: a review of the evidence. *Phys Occup Ther Pediatr*. 2006;26(3):39–53.

211. Gudjonsdottir B, Mercer VS. Effects of a dynamic versus static prone stander on bone mineral density and behavior in four children with severe cerebral palsy. *Pediatr Phys Ther*. 2002;14(1):38–46.

212. Dalén Y, Sääf M, Ringertz H, et al. Effects of standing on bone density and hip dislocation in children with severe cerebral palsy. *Adv Physiother*. 2010;12(4):187–193.

213. Farrell E, Naber E, Geigle P. Description of a multifaceted rehabilitation program including overground gait training for a child with cerebral palsy: a case report. *Physiother Theory Pract*. 2010;26(1):56–61.

214. Peredo DE, Davis BE, Norvell DC, et al. Medical equipment use in children with disabilities: a descriptive survey. *J Pediatr Rehabil Med*. 2010;3(4):259–267.

215. Hong CW. Assessment for and provision of positioning equipment for children with motor impairments. *Int Ther Rehabil*. 2005;12(3):126–131.

216. Jones MA, Gray S. Assistive technology: positioning and mobility. In: Effgen SK, ed. *Meeting the Physical Therapy Needs of Children*. Philadelphia: FA Davis; 2005:455–474.

217. Thorton H, Kilbride C. Physical management of abnormal tone and movement. In: Stokes M, ed. *Physical Management in Neurological Rehabilitation*. 2nd ed. Edinburgh: Mosby; 2004:431–450.

218. Beatty PW, Hagglund KJ, Neri MT, et al. Access to health care services among people with chronic or disabling conditions: patterns and predictors. *Arch Phys Med Rehabil*. 2003;84(10):1417–1425.

219. Bingham SC, Beatty PW. Rates of access to assistive equipment and medical rehabilitation services among people with disabilities. *Disabil Rehabil*. 2003;25(9):487–490.

220. Gulley SP, Rasch EK, Chan L. The complex web of health: relationships among chronic conditions, disability, and health services. *Public Health Rep*. 2011;126(4):495–507.

221. O'Neil ME, Costigan TE, Gracely EJ, et al. Parents' perspectives on access to rehabilitation services for their children with special healthcare needs. *Pediatr Phys Ther*. 2009;21(3):254–260.

222. Westberry DE, Davids JR, Jacobs JM, et al. Effectiveness of serial stretch casting for resistant or recurrent knee flexion contractures following hamstring lengthening in children with cerebral palsy. *J Pediatr Orthop*. 2006;26(1):109–114.

223. Jain S, Mathur M, Joshi JR, et al. Effect of serial casting in spastic cerebral palsy. *Indian J Pediatr*. 2008;75(10):997–1002.

224. McNee AE, Will E, Lin JP. The effect of serial casting on gait in children with cerebral palsy: preliminary results from a crossover trial. *Gait Posture*. 2007;25(3):463–468.

225. Romeiser L. Rehabilitation techniques to maximize spasticity management. *Top Stroke Rehabil*. 2011;18(3):203–211.

226. Marshall S, Teasell R, Bayona N. Motor impairment rehabilitation post acquired brain injury. *Brain Inj*. 2007;21(2):133–160.

227. Yaşar E, Tok F, Safaz I, et al. The efficacy of serial casting after botulinum toxin type A injection in improving equinovarus deformity in patients with chronic stroke. *Brain Inj*. 2010;24(5):736–739.

228. Park ES, Rha DW, Yoo JK, et al. Short-term effects of combined serial casting and botulinum toxin injection for spastic equinus in ambulatory children with cerebral palsy. *Yonsei Med J*. 2010;51(4):579–584.

229. Haslekorn JK, Loomis S. Multiple sclerosis and spasticity. *Phys Med Rehabil Clin N Am*. 2005;16(2):467–481.

230. Morris SL, Dodd KJ, Morris ME. Outcomes of progressive resistance strength training following stroke; a systematic review. *Clin Rehabil.* 2004;18(1):27–39.

231. Foran JR, Steinman S, Barash I, et al. Structural and mechanical alterations in spastic skeletal muscle. *Dev Med Child Neurol.* 2005;47(10):713–717.

232. Hagglund G, Anderson S, Duppe H, et al. Prevention of severe contractures might replace multilevel surgery in cerebral palsy: results of a population-based health care programme and new techniques to reduce spasticity. *J Pediatr Orthop.* 2005;14(4):269–273.

233. Molenaers G, Desloovere K, Fabry G, et al. The effects of quantitative gait assessment and botulinum toxin A on musculoskeletal surgery in children with cerebral palsy. *J Bone Joint Surg.* 2006;88A(1):161–170.

234. Fatone S. Orthotic management in stroke. In: Stein J, Harvey R, Macko R, et al., eds. *Stroke Recovery & Rehabilitation.* New York: Demos Medical Publishing; 2009:515–530.

235. Lannin NA, Ada L. Neurorehabilitation splinting: theory and principles of clinical use. *NeuroRehabilitation.* 2011;28(1):21–88.

236. Webster JB, Miknevich MA, Stevens P, et al. Lower extremity orthotic management in neurologic rehabilitation. *Crit Rev Phys Rehabil Med.* 2009;21(1):1–23.

237. Knutson J, Audu M, Triolo R. Interventions for mobility and manipulation after spinal cord injury: a review of orthotic and neuroprosthetic options. *Top Spinal Cord Injury Rehabil.* 2006;11(4):61–81.

238. Kawashima N, Taguchi D, Nakazawa K, et al. Effect of lesion level on the orthotic gait performance in individuals with complete paraplegia. *Spinal Cord.* 2006;44(8):487–494.

239. Malas BS. What variables influence the ability of an AFO to improve function and when are they indicated? *Clin Orthop Relat Res.* 2011;469(5):1308–1314.

240. Shipley JS, Shipley RW. Orthotic considerations for pediatric pathologies. *J Nurse Life Care Planning.* 2010;10(1):213–217.

241. Stevens PM. Lower limb orthotic management of Duchenne muscular dystrophy: a literature review. *J Prosthet Orthot.* 2006;18(4):111–119.

242. Perry J, Burnfield J. *Gait Analysis: Normal and Pathological Function.* 2nd ed. Thorofare, NJ: Slack Inc; 2010.

243. Gage JR, Schwartz MH, Koop SE, et al. *The Identification and Treatment of Gait Problems in Cerebral Palsy.* 2nd ed. London: MacKeith Press; 2009.

244. *Observational Gait Analysis.* Downey, CA: Pathokinesiology Service & Physical Therapy Department, Rancho Los Amigos Medical Center; 2001.

11

Orthoses for Knee Dysfunction

ANTHONY E. "TOBY" KINNEY AND ELLEN WETHERBEE

LEARNING OBJECTIVES

On completion of this chapter, the reader will be able to:

1. Describe the normal anatomical structure and biomechanical function (kinematic and kinetic) of the human tibiofemoral and patellofemoral joints.
2. Appreciate the anatomical structures of the knee that provide intraarticular stability.
3. Explain the most common mechanism of injury to the knee while understanding the biomechanical implications of pathological changes to the knee and lower extremity mechanics.
4. Describe the various classification systems used to describe knee orthoses.
5. Compare and contrast the purposes, indications, and limitations of rehabilitative, functional, and prophylactic knee orthoses.
6. Identify the force vectors used to control knee motion used in various designs of knee orthoses.
7. Become familiar with current research evidence that will drive clinical decision making in determining rationale for brace intervention.
8. Use evidence of efficacy of various knee orthoses to select the most appropriate device for a given injury to the knee
9. Provide clinical rationale for utilizing bracing as an intervention for impairments at the knee.

Knee braces have been used as a common intervention in the protection and stabilization of the knee joint to decrease a person's pain and improve their functional and recreational activities (Figure 11-1). It has become commonplace for anyone to walk into a pharmacy or drug store and purchase a knee brace such as a neoprene sleeve (Figure 11-2). However, their effectiveness in providing ligamentous stability and optimal patellofemoral tracking has been debated.[1,2]

In 1984, the American Academy of Orthopaedic Surgeons developed a classification system that grouped knee orthotics by their intended function: *prophylactic, rehabilitative,* and *functional* knee braces.[3] Currently, *patellofemoral* braces and *unloader* knee braces are additional classification categories.[4,5] It could be debated that unloader braces are merely functional osteoarthritis (OA) braces. *Prophylactic knee orthoses* are designed to reduce the risk of knee injury for those individuals who are engaged in "high-risk" activities, especially those

individuals who have a history of previous knee dysfunction. *Rehabilitative knee orthoses* are used to protect a knee that has been injured or surgically repaired until adequate tissue healing has occurred. *Functional knee orthoses* (FKOs) attempt to provide biomechanical stability when ligaments are unable to do so during daily activities. *Patellofemoral knee braces* are intended to optimize tracking of the patella and decrease anterior knee pain. *Unloader knee braces* are meant to decrease compressive forces across the tibiofemoral joint and decrease arthritic knee pain. This functional classification system continues to be helpful for health care providers who work with patients who have knee dysfunction.

It is imperative during the clinical decision making process that clinicians use a patient-centered approach while at the same time incorporating the best available scientific research and their own clinical expertise. Patient goals, function, preferences, and impairments should be factors in deciding the type of knee orthosis to use. For instance, a patient who has anterior cruciate ligament (ACL) deficiency will use a different brace than a patient with medial compartment knee OA. In all circumstances, it is important to understand the anatomy and biomechanics of the knee joint and subsequent knee dysfunction when providing a knee orthosis to a patient.

In order for a clinician to select the appropriate knee orthosis for the patient, the clinician needs a mastery of normal knee structure and function. This chapter reviews the anatomy and biomechanical stability of the knee and patellofemoral joints and the physiological and accessory motions of the tibiofemoral and patellofemoral joints. The implications of knee pathology on knee biomechanics are discussed, and the design and functional goals of prefabricated and custom-made knee orthoses are examined. Indications for knee orthoses in the management of common knee injuries and dysfunction are also discussed. Finally, the chapter concludes with discussion about strategies for clinical decision making in choosing an appropriate functional orthosis for active patients and athletes with ligamentous instability of the knee.

ANATOMY OF THE KNEE

The articulations at the tibiofemoral joint and the patellofemoral joint form the knee complex. An understanding of the anatomy and biomechanics of each respective joint is critical in

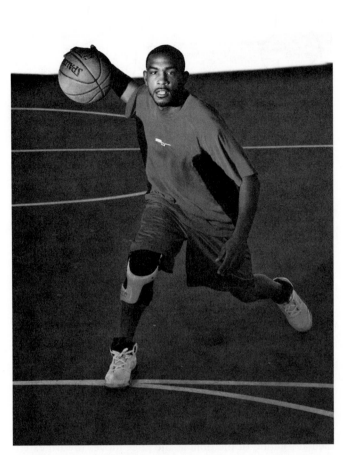

FIGURE 11-1 An example of a basketball player using a knee orthosis during activity. (Reprinted with permission, Hanger Orthopedic Group, Inc., Jacksonville Beach FL)

knowing the potential stresses and implications of knee pathology that can occur at the knee complex.

The Tibiofemoral Joint

The knee joint is a hinge-like articulation between the medial and lateral condyles of the femur and the medial and lateral tibial plateau (Figure 11-3). Because of the shape and asymmetry of the condyles, the instantaneous axis of knee flexion/extension motion changes through the arc of motion. As the knee moves from extension to flexion, the instant center moves posteriorly.[6] In open chain movements (non–weight-bearing activities), the tibia rotates around the femoral condyles. In closed chain movements (weight-bearing activities), an anatomical locking mechanism is present in the final degrees of extension as the longer medial femoral condyle rotates medially on the articular surfaces of the tibia. Consequently, if the instant center of pathway changes, it will alter the optimal joint mechanics and therefore result in abnormal knee stressors. The alignment between an adducted femur and relatively upright tibia creates a vulnerability to valgus stress in many weight-bearing

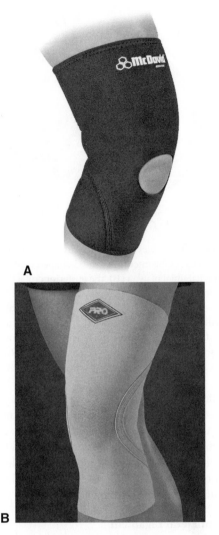

FIGURE 11-2 Examples of neoprene sleeves used for knee pain and protection. **A,** #402 Knee Support, Open Patella from McDavid. **B,** PRO Orthopedic #100 Deluxe Knee Support Sleeve. (**A,** Reprinted with permission from McDavid Inc., Woodridge, IL; **B,** Reprinted with permission, PRO Orthopedic Devices Inc., Tucson, AZ.)

activities. The capsule that encases the knee joint is reinforced by the collagen-rich medial and lateral retinaculum. The medial and lateral menisci rest on the tibial plateau. They are fibrocartilaginous, nearly ring-shaped disks that are flexibly attached around the edges of the tibial plateau (see Figure 11-3). These menisci increase the concavity of the tibial articular surface, enhancing congruency of articulation with the femoral condyles to facilitate normal gliding and distribute weight-bearing forces within the knee during gait and other loading activities.[7] The menisci also play an important role in nutrition and lubrication of the articular surfaces of the knee joint.

Stability to the tibiofemoral joint is provided by sets of ligaments. The medial (tibial) collateral ligament and the lateral (fibular) collateral ligament are extrinsic ligaments. The collateral ligaments counter valgus and varus forces that act on the knee. In addition, two intrinsic ligaments of the tibiofemoral joint, the anterior cruciate and posterior cruciate ligaments check translatory forces that displace the tibia on the femur.

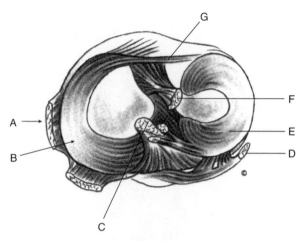

FIGURE 11-3 In this view of the surface of the tibia, we can identify the medial collateral ligament (**A**), the C-shaped medial meniscus on the large medial tibial plateau (**B**), the posterior cruciate ligament with the accessory anterior and posterior meniscofemoral ligaments (**C**), the tendon of the popliteus muscle (**D**), the circular lateral meniscus on the smaller lateral tibial plateau (**E**), the anterior cruciate ligament as it twists toward the inside of the lateral femoral condyle (**F**), and the transverse ligament (**G**). (From Greenfield BH. *Rehabilitation of the Knee: A Problem Solving Approach*. Philadelphia: FA Davis; 1993.)

The location of attachments makes each of these ligaments most effective at particular places in the knee's normal arc of motion.[7] Additionally, contraction of the quadriceps and knee flexor muscle groups produce compressive forces that help stabilize the knee. Muscles of the hip and lower leg also make contributions to the mechanics of the femur and tibia, respectively, which impact the movements of the knee complex.

Medial Collateral Ligament

The medial (tibial) collateral ligament (MCL) is a strong, flat membranous band that overlays the middle portion of the medial joint capsule (Figure 11-4). It is most effective in counteracting valgus stressors when the knee is slightly flexed to fully extended. Approximately 8 to 10 cm in length, it originates at the medial epicondyle of the femur and attaches to the medial surface of the tibial plateau. The MCL can be subdivided into a set of oblique posterior fibers and anterior parallel fibers.

A bundle of meniscotibial fibers, also known as the *posterior oblique ligament*, runs deep to the MCL, from the femur to the midperipheral margin of the medial meniscus and toward the tibia. These fibers connect the medial meniscus to the tibia and help form the semimembranosus corner of the medial knee. Additionally, the medial patellar retinacular fibers play a reinforcing role.[8]

Lateral Collateral Ligament and Iliotibial Band

The lateral (fibular) collateral ligament (LCL) resists varus stressors and lateral rotation of the tibia and is most effective when the knee is slightly flexed. The LCL runs from the lateral femoral condyle (the back part of the outer tuberosity of the femur) to the proximal lateral aspect of the fibular head (see Figure 11-4). The tendon of the popliteus muscle and the external articular vessels and nerves pass beneath this ligament.

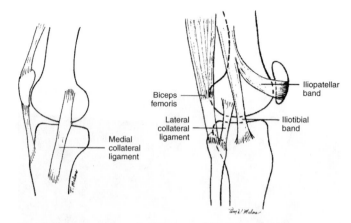

FIGURE 11-4 A, A medial view of the right knee showing structures that provide medial support to the right knee. **B,** A lateral view of the right knee illustrating structures that give lateral support to the knee. (Reprinted with permission from Levangie, PK, Norkin CC. The knee complex. In *Joint Structure and Function: A Comprehensive Analysis*, 3rd ed. Philadelphia: FA DAVIS; 2001.)

Another lateral structure that acts on the knee complex is the iliotibial band (ITB). The ITB is positioned slightly anterior to the LCL and is taut in all ranges of knee motion. Although the position of the ITB allows it to stabilize against varus forces, as does the LCL, the ITB also appears to assist the ACL, preventing posterior displacement of the tibia when the knee is extended.[9]

Anterior Cruciate Ligament

The ACL runs at an oblique angle between the articular surfaces of the knee joint and prevents forward shift and excessive medial rotation of the tibia as the knee moves toward extension (Figure 11-5). The ACL attaches to the tibia in a fossa just anterior and lateral to the anterior tibial spine and to the femur in a fossa on the posteromedial surface of the lateral femoral condyle. The ACL's tibial attachment is somewhat wider and stronger than its femoral attachment. Some authors divide the fasciculi that make up the broad, somewhat flat ACL into two or three distinct bundles. The ligament's anteromedial band, with fibers running from the anteromedial tibia to the proximal femoral attachment, is most taut in flexion and relatively lax in extension. The posterolateral bulk (PLB), which begins at the posterolateral tibial attachment, is most taut in extension and relatively lax in flexion. An intermediate bundle of transitional fibers between the anteromedial band and PLB tends to tighten when the knee moves through the midranges of motion. This arrangement of fibers ensures tension in the ACL throughout the entire range of knee motion. The ACL is most vulnerable to injury when the femur rotates internally on the tibia when the knee is flexed and the foot is fixed on the ground during weight-bearing activities.[10]

Posterior Cruciate Ligament

The posterior cruciate ligament (PCL) restrains posterior displacement of the tibia in its articulation with the femur, especially as the knee moves toward full extension.[7] The PCL is shorter and less oblique in orientation than the ACL; it is the strongest and most resistant ligament of the knee. PCL fibers

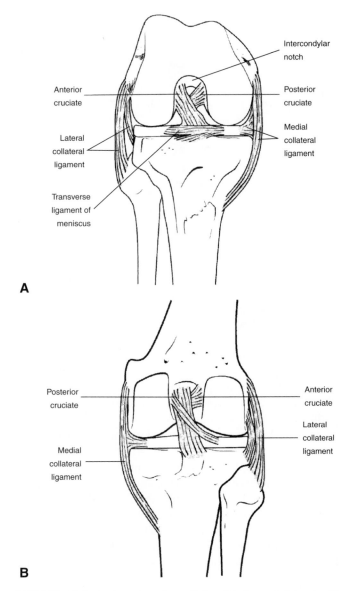

A

B

FIGURE 11-5 **A,** Anterior view of the tibiofemoral joint in 90 degrees of knee flexion showing the menisci and the ligamentous structures that stabilize the knee. **B,** Posterior view of the knee in extension. (Reprinted with permission from Antich TJ. Orthoses for the knee; the tibiofemoral joint. In Nawoczenski DA, Epler ME [eds], *Orthotics in Functional Rehabilitation of the Lower Limb.* Philadelphia: Saunders, 1997. p. 59.)

run from a slight depression between articular surfaces on the posterior tibia to the posterolateral surface of the medial femoral condyle (see Figures 11-3 and 11-5). Like the ACL, the PCL can be divided into anterior and posterior segments. The larger anterior medial band is most taut between 80 and 90 degrees of flexion and is relatively lax in extension. The smaller PLB travels somewhat obliquely across the joint, becoming taut as the knee moves into extension. The PCL plays a role in the locking mechanism of the knee, as tension in the ligament produces lateral (external) rotation of the tibia on the femur in the final degrees of knee extension. The PCL may also assist the collateral ligaments when varus or valgus stressors are applied to the knee.[7]

Coursing along with fibers from the MCL is the meniscofemoral ligament, which stretches between the posterior horn of the lateral meniscus and the lateral surface of the medial femoral condyle. The meniscofemoral ligament has sometimes been described as a third cruciate ligament.[11] The anterior meniscofemoral band (ligament of Humphry) runs along the medial anterior surface of the PCL and may be up to one-third its diameter. The posterior meniscofemoral band (ligament of Wrisberg) lies posterior to the PCL and may be as much as one-half its diameter. The meniscofemoral ligaments pull the lateral meniscus forward during flexion of the weight-bearing knee to maintain as much articular congruency as possible with the lateral femoral condyle.

Posterolateral Corner of the Knee

The lateral meniscus is somewhat more mobile than the medial meniscus because of the anatomy of the posterolateral corner of the knee. The arcuate complex and posterolateral corner run from the styloid process of the fibula, joining the posterior oblique ligament on the posterior aspect of the femur and tibia. The arcuate ligament is firmly attached to the underlying popliteus muscle and tendon. The tendon of the popliteus muscle separates the deep joint capsule from the rim of the lateral meniscus.

Patellofemoral Joint

The *patella,* a sesamoid bone embedded in the tendon of the quadriceps femoris, is an integral part of the extensor mechanism of the knee. The patella functions as an anatomical pulley, increasing the knee extension moment created by contraction of the quadriceps femoris by as much as 50%. It also guides the forces generated by the quadriceps femoris to the patellar ligament, protects deeper knee joint anatomy, protects the quadriceps tendon from frictional forces, and increases the compressive forces to which the extensor mechanisms can be subjected.[12-15]

Although the anterior surface of the patella is convex, the posterior surface has three distinct anatomical areas: a lateral, medial, and odd facet. The lateral and medial facets are separated by a vertical ridge. The odd facet articulates with the medial condyle at the end range of knee extension (Figure 11-6). The posterior patellar surface is covered with hyaline articular cartilage, except for the distal apex, which is roughened for the attachment of the patellar tendon. Pressure between the patella and trochlear groove of the femur increases substantially as the knee flexes. During knee flexion, the patella moves in a complex but consistent three-dimensional pattern of flexion/extension rotation, medial/lateral rotation, medial/lateral tilt (also described as wavering), and a medial/lateral shift relative to the femur.[13,15] These motions occur biomechanically in the X, Y, and Z planes.

The stability of the patella is derived from the patellofemoral joint's static structural characteristics and dynamic (muscular) control. Static stability is a product of the anatomy of the patella, the depth of the intercondylar groove, and the prominent and longer lateral condyle of the femur. The sulcus angle, formed by the sloping edges of the condyles, is

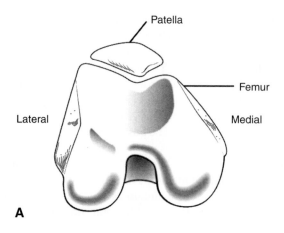

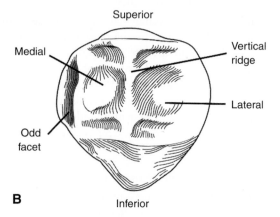

FIGURE 11-6 A, The normal position of the patella in the intercondylar groove of the distal femur. **B,** Underside of the patella with its three facets and vertical ridge. (Reprinted with permission from Belyea BC. Orthoses for the knee: The patellofemoral joint. In Nawoczenski DA, Epler ME [eds], *Orthotics in Functional Rehabilitation of the Lower Limb*. Philadelphia: Saunders, 1997. pp. 32-33.)

normally between 114 and 120 degrees; however, it can vary significantly from person to person.[16] Wiberg[17] divides the patellofemoral joint into six types based on the size and shape of facets (Table 11-1). The depth of the patellar trochlea and the facet pattern are important in patellar stability.

Dynamic stability of the patellofemoral joint is derived primarily from activity of the quadriceps femoris as well as from the tensile properties of the patellar ligament (Figure 11-7). The four components of the quadriceps muscle act together

TABLE 11-1   *Classification of Patellar Types, Listed from Most to Least Stable*[17]

Patellar Type	Description
I	Equal medial and lateral facets, both slightly concave
II	Small medial facet, both facets slightly concave
II/III	Small, flat medial facet
III	Small, slightly convex medial facet
IV	Very small, steeply sloped medial facet, with medial ridge
V (Jagerhut)	No medial facet, no central ridge

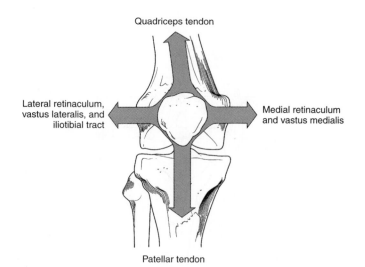

FIGURE 11-7 A schematic diagram of structures that act on the patella. (Reprinted with permission from Neumann DA. *Kinesiology of the Musculoskeletal System: Foundations for Rehabilitation*, 2nd ed. St. Louis: Mosby Elsevier, 2010.)

to pull the patella obliquely upward along the shaft of the femur, whereas the patellar ligament anchors it almost straight downward along the anatomical axis of the lower leg. The tibial tubercle is typically located at least 6 degrees lateral to the mechanical axis of the femur.

Because the structure of the patellofemoral articulation and the muscular/ligamentous forces that act on the patella are complex, patellar dynamics involve much more than simple cephalocaudal repositioning as the knee is flexed or extended. Van Kampen and Huiskes[15] describe the three-dimensional motions of the patella as flexion rotation, medial rotation, wavering tilt, and lateral shift. All of these patellar movements (except flexion) are influenced by the rotation of the tibia and the dynamic stabilization of the muscles that act on the patella.

BIOMECHANICS OF KNEE MOTION

Although it is beyond the scope of this book chapter to comprehensively cover the biomechanics of knee motion, it is important to have a basic foundation of knee biomechanics to understand the use of knee orthoses as an intervention for knee pathology. Evaluating and managing injuries of the knee requires an in-depth understanding of the biomechanical characteristics of the knee joint. The *kinematics of the knee* describe its motion in terms of the type and location and the magnitude and direction of the motion.[18] The *kinetics of the knee* describe the forces that act on the knee, causing movement.[18] Kinetic forces are classified as either external forces that work on the body (e.g., gravity) or as internal, body-generated forces (e.g., friction, tensile strength of soft tissue structures, muscle contraction).

Motion in the tibiofemoral joint can be best understood by separating the motion into its physiological and accessory components. Physiological motion can be controlled consciously, most often through voluntary contraction of muscle. Osteokinematic (bone movement) and arthrokinematic (joint surface motion) are examples of physiological motion. Accessory motion occurs without conscious control and cannot be reproduced voluntarily. Joint play, which is elicited by passive movement during examination of a joint, is an example of an accessory motion. The magnitude and type of accessory motion possible are determined by the characteristics of a particular articulation and the properties of the tissues that surround it. The arthrokinematics of the tibiofemoral joint will vary depending upon whether the lower-extremity is in a weight-bearing or loaded position. For example, with tibial-femoral extension the tibia moves anteriorly relative to the femur and with femoral on tibia extension the femoral condyles slide from anterior to posterior, while rolling anteriorly.[8]

One of the important accessory component motions of the tibiofemoral joint is its *screw home* or locking mechanism. In the final degrees of knee extension, the tibia continues to rotate around the large articular surface of the medial femoral condyle. This motion cannot be prevented or changed by volitional effort; it is entirely the result of the configuration of the articular surfaces. When the knee is flexed to or beyond 90 degrees, however, conscious activation of muscles can produce physiological (osteokinematic) external (lateral) or internal (medial) rotation of the tibia on the femur.

Three osteokinematic motions are possible at the tibiofemoral joint. Knee flexion/extension occurs in the sagittal plane around an axis in the frontal plane (x-axis). Internal/external rotation of the tibia on the femur (or vice versa) occurs in the transverse plane around a longitudinal axis (y-axis). Abduction and adduction occur in the frontal plane around a horizontal axis (z axis). The arthrokinematic movements of the tibiofemoral joint are rolling, gliding, and sliding (Figure 11-8). It is important to note that the roll-glide ratio is not constant during tibiofemoral joint motion: Approximately 1:2 in early flexion, the roll-glide ratio becomes almost 1:4 in

late flexion.[19] Rolling and gliding occur primarily on the posterior portion of the femoral condyles. In the first 15 to 20 degrees of flexion, a true rolling motion of the femoral condyles occurs in concert with the tibial plateau. As the magnitude of flexion increases, the femur begins to glide posteriorly on the tibia. Gliding becomes more significant as flexion increases.[11]

From a kinematic standpoint, the ACLs and PCLs operate as a true gear mechanism controlling the roll-glide motion of the tibiofemoral joint. With rupture of either or both of the cruciate ligaments, the gear mechanism becomes ineffective, and the arthrokinematic motion is altered. In an ACL-deficient knee, the femur is able to roll beyond the posterior half of the tibial plateau, increasing the likelihood of damage or tear of the posterior horn of the medial or lateral meniscus.

Because the knee has characteristics of a hinge joint and an arthrodial joint, two types of motion (translatory and rotatory) can occur in each plane of motion (sagittal, frontal/coronal, transverse). For this reason, knee motion is described as having six degrees of freedom. The three translatory motions of the knee include anteroposterior translation of 5 to 10 mm, mediolateral translation of 1 to 2 mm, and compression-distraction motion of 2 to 5 mm. The three rotatory motions occur in flexion/extension, varus/valgus, and internal (medial)/external (lateral) rotation.[7,19] Hinge design of an orthosis will be discussed further in this chapter to help control these motions. Single, dual, or multiple hinged orthoses that do not conform with the A/P translation (or roll back) and the rotation of the joint, will exert adverse mechanical effects.[20]

Orthoses for the Knee

As discussed previously, there are a few different categories of orthoses for the knee. A sample of the many types of knee orthoses that are commercially available to health professionals is listed in Table 11-2. The clinician should be aware that the

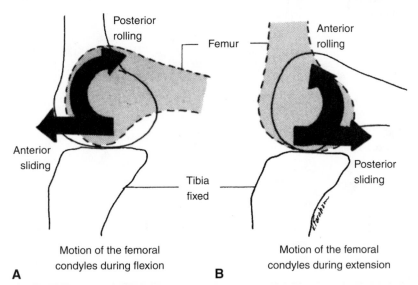

FIGURE 11-8 Diagram of femoral motion on a fixed tibia. **A,** As the knee flexes, the femoral condyles roll posteriorly *(curved arrow)* while gliding/sliding forward *(straight arrow)*. **B,** As the knee extends, the condyles roll forward *(curved arrow)* while gliding posteriorly *(straight arrow)*. (From Hartigan E, Lewek M, Snyder-Mackler L. The knee. In Levangie PK, Norkin CC [eds], *Joint Structure and Function: A Comprehensive Analysis*, 5th ed. Philadelphia: Davis, 2011. p. 355.)

TABLE 11-2   *A Few Examples of Knee Orthoses by Manufacturer and Category*

Manufacturer	Rehabilitative Knee Orthoses	Functional ACL/PCL	Functional Osteoarthritis	Prophylactic	Patellofemoral
Bauerfeind USA Kennesaw, Ga. (800) 423-3405 www.bauerfeindusa.com		Softech Genu Secutech Genu	Softtech OA		Genutrain P3
Bledsoe by Medical Technology Grand Prairie, Texas (888) 253-3763 www.bledsoebrace.com	Extender Plus Leverlock Revolution 3	Ultimate Dynamic U²CI Kneecage Forcelite	Thruster RLF Aligner ESE		20.50 Patella-femoral
Brace International Atlanta, Ga. (800) 545-1161 www.braceint.com					FLUK Infrapatellar Strap
Cropper Medical, Inc./Bio Skin Ashland, Ore. (800) 541-2455 www.bioskin.com	Gladiator Sport			Standard Knee Skin	Q Lok Patella Stabilizer Q Baby
dj Orthopedics, Inc. Vista, Calif. (800) 336-6569 www.djortho.com	IROM Telescoping IROM Bilateral with Shells	Defiance III Armor Legend 4titude	OA Defiance OA Full Force OA Assist	Protective-Knee Guard Playmaker	TruPull Wraparound H-Buttress
Generation II USA, Inc./Ossur Bothell, Wash. (800) 462-7252 www.gen2.com		Generation II 3DX Matrix Extreme Select GII Trainers	Unloader Select Unloader Adj Unloader Spirit Unloader Bi-Com		Patellar Stabilizer PS1
Innovation Sports, Inc. Irvine, Calif. (800) 222-4284 www.isports.com	Sentry Knee MD Quicklock Option	CTi Edge C180 XCI Aspire CTI²	CTI²OA		Powerflex Donut Stabilizer Lateral J Stabiliz
McDavid Sports/Medical Products Woodridge, Ill. (800) 237-8254 www.mcdavidusa.com				428R McDavid Level 3 Knee Brace with Polycentric Hinges	419R McDavid Level 2 Knee Support
Pro Orthopedic Devices, Inc Tuscon, Ariz. (800) 523-5611 www.proorthopedic.com	PRO 190 Hinged Stabilizing Knee Brace				PRO 105 Spiral Knee Support Sleeve Patellar Strap PRO 135
Townsend Design Bakersfield, Calif. (800) 700-2722 www.townsenddesign.com	ROM-SS EZ-Pads	Premier Series Rebel Series Sports Series	RelieverOne		

ACL, Anterior cruciate ligament; PCL, posterior cruciate ligament.

brace names tend to change. Some are designed to immobilize the knee after surgical repair of damaged or ruptured ligaments or menisci during the acute phases of healing, whereas other knee orthoses are used to improve biomechanical efficiency at the knee joint and/or prevent injury. *Rehabilitative orthoses* are designed to protect the knee and allow progressive increase in active range of motion during rehabilitation. *FKOs* provide additional protection as rehabilitation is completed and a patient returns to normal activities. *Prophylactic knee orthoses*, attempt to prevent injury (or at least lessen the extent of injury) in athletes who are at risk of injury during competition. A *patellofemoral knee bracing* allows for improved tracking of the patella during knee motions, whereas *unloader knee braces* dissipate increased varus and valgus forces across the tibiofemoral joint. The complexity of the knee joint (with its polycentric axis of rotation for flexion/extension, asymmetry of the lateral and medial compartments, and the arrangement of its muscular and ligamentous attachments) creates a challenge when trying to design a knee orthosis that is able to support, protect, and stabilize the knee in a multiplanar fashion with the same efficiency as its own physiological motion.

Rehabilitation Knee Orthoses

Orthoses used in the postoperative and early rehabilitation of patients who have had surgical repair of damaged cartilage, ligaments, or bone are designed to control knee motion carefully to minimize excessive loading on healing tissues (Figures 11-9 and 11-10).[3] Although many rehabilitation knee orthoses are on the market, an effective orthosis has several important characteristics. The orthosis must be adjustable to accommodate changes in limb girth due to edema or atrophy. It must remain in the desired position on the limb during functional activities in stance and in sitting. It must be comfortable, easy to don and doff, durable, and economical. Most physicians require an adjustable knee unit so that active range of motion can be increased incrementally as the tissue heals and the patient's condition improves. The ability to move in carefully controlled ranges of motion is thought to improve ligamentous strength and to minimize the risk of scar formation in the intracondylar notch that is associated with flexion contracture.[19]

Functional Knee Orthoses

Use of knee orthoses as functional braces parallels the development of the discipline of sports medicine since the early 1970s.[21] In the years before 1970, orthoses that were designed for patients with neuromuscular dysfunction were adapted to meet the needs of injured athletes with a functionally unstable knee. Typically, the adapted orthosis was cumbersome and significantly impaired the quality of the athlete's performance. To assist professional athletes in quickly and safely returning to competition, the sports medicine community explored alternative orthotic interventions to manage an unstable knee. The development of FKOs as alternatives to surgery (which often sidelined athletes for considerable periods of time) was especially welcomed.[22]

One of the first FKOs, the Lenox Hill Derotation knee brace, was developed by Nicholas and Castiglia of Lenox Hill Hospital

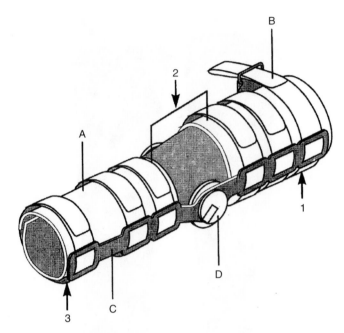

FIGURE 11-9 The components of most commercially available rehabilitation knee orthoses include open cell foam interface that encase the calf and thigh (**A**) and nonelastic adjustable Velcro strap for closures (**B**); lightweight metal, composite, or plastic sidebars (**C**); and single-axis or polycentric hinge that can be locked or adjusted to allow or restrict motion (**D**) within the therapeutically desired range of motion. The force systems of these orthoses apply a pair of anteriorly directed forces at the proximal posterior thigh (1) and distal posterior calf (3), against a posteriorly directed force (2) applied over or on either side of the patella. Varus and valgus stressors are resisted by the sidebars. (Reprinted with permission from Trautman P. Lower limb orthoses. In Redford JB, Basmajian JV, Trautman P [eds], *Orthotics: Clinical Practice and Rehabilitation Technology*. New York: Churchill Livingstone, 1995. pp. 195:230)

in the early 1970s to protect the chronically unstable knees of football quarterback Joe Namath.[23] The Lenox Hill orthosis was the primary design that was commercially available until the late 1970s. The original orthosis had medial and lateral uprights, a single-axis knee joint with a medial fulcrum pad, a broad elastic thigh and calf cuff/strap to hold the orthosis in place, and a set of derotation straps to control movement of the tibia on the femur. The intent was to control mediolateral instability, rotational instability, and multiple ligament impairment.[24] Subsequent versions of the Lenox Hill orthosis are available in standard, lightweight, and ultra-lightweight versions, with a dial-lock option to adjust available range of motion and with protective undersleeves and oversleeves (Figure 11-11).

The original design has evolved considerably: More than three dozen functional braces are manufactured in today's sports medicine market (see Table 11-2 for examples). Most are based on a lightweight rigid suprastructure made from carbon composite or titanium alloy. Many use adjustable elasticized or Velcro strapping to apply a four-point stabilizing force and hold the orthosis in position on the limb. Some have polycentric knee units; others allow variable flexion control or assisted extension. The basic design and components of most commercially available FKOs are shown in Figure 11-12.

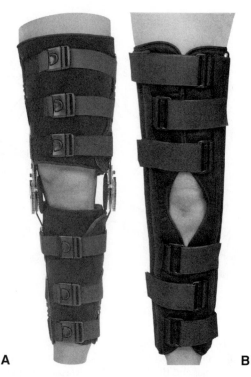

A   **B**

FIGURE 11-10 A, Townsend full shell padded knee brace typically used following knee surgery. **B,** The premium sized knee immobilizer from Ossür 2. (**A,** Reprinted with permission from Townsend Design, Bakersfield, CA. **B,** Reprinted with permission from Ossür Americas, Foothills Ranch, CA.)

According to a survey of orthopedic surgeons performed by Decoster and Vailas,[25] 87% of surgeons brace their patients who have had ACL reconstruction. In addition, DeCoster and Vailas found that typically the surgeons are more likely to prescribe "off the shelf" braces for patients with ACL deficiency compared to those patients with ACL reconstruction.[25]

Unfortunately, systematic critical evaluation of the efficacy of FKOs has not kept pace with the development of new designs; there is a paucity of clinical and laboratory research defining the indications for, roles of, or outcomes of use for these functional braces.[22]

Functional Knee Orthoses and Performance
Current available literature can be characterized by two major approaches to comparing braced and unbraced performances: (1) maximal effort tests, wherein subjects performed at maximal intensity and the criterion measure was an overall performance measure such as distance hopped or the time to run a specified distance; (2) matched effort tests, wherein subjects perform at submaximal intensity and the criterion measures tend to be specific variables such as muscle activation patterns determined via electromyography (EMG) or ground reaction forces determined via force plate.[26] Nemeth and colleagues[27] studied six expert downhill skiers who had sustained ACL injuries. Surface electrodes were used with an eight-channel telemetric EMG system to

collect recordings from the vastus medialis, biceps femoris, semimembranosus, semitendinosus, and gastrocnemius medialis muscles from both legs. Without a brace, the EMG activity level of all muscles increased during knee flexion. With a brace, the EMG activity increased in midphase during the upward push for the weight transfer and the peak activity occurred closer to knee flexion in midphase. The authors suggest the brace caused an increase in afferent input from proprioceptors, resulting in an adaptation of motor control patterns secondarily modifying EMG activity and timing.[27] Research has also shown that the use of functional knee bracing seems to protect the ACL from sagittal plane shearing in non–weight-bearing and weight-bearing, and internal torques in non–weight-bearing. However, the study also found that the braced knee did not have any decrease in strain in external torques or valgus-varus stressors in weight-bearing and non–weight-bearing when compared with the unbraced knee.[28]

Additionally, Sterett and colleagues[29] found that following ACL reconstruction, those skiers who did not use a functional brace during skiing had a higher rate of reinjury.

A number of researchers have investigated the impact of functional braces on performance and endurance in noninjured and previously injured athletes. Stephens[30] found little impact on speed of running in noninjured collegiate basketball players during straight line running tasks (end line to foul line, full court) when comparing performance in two functional braces with nonbraced speed. Although these results are positive, the in-brace time and types of activity used for the study were significantly different than those of an active, full length basketball game.

Highgenboten and colleagues[31] found a 3% to 6% increase in metabolic cost during steady-state treadmill running when functional braces were worn. Subjects also had higher ratings of perceived exertion when exercising with the brace. These effects were attributed to the weight of the brace. In addition, research by Wojtys and colleagues[32] showed that most braces appear to slow hamstring muscle reaction times at voluntary levels. The evidence from these maximal effort and matched effort performance tests suggest no advantage to use of FKOs.

Most functional knee braces weigh close to 1 pound. Despite the use of lightweight materials that are resilient to various forces, it is possible that long in-brace times can lead to fatigue or to injuries to other areas of the body that compensate for the added weight of the orthosis. This may explain the increase in injuries of the foot and ankle reported by Grace and colleagues[33] in athletes who wore braces. Styf and colleagues[34] studied changes in intramuscular pressures within the anterior compartment of the leg at rest, during exercise, and after exercise, comparing three orthoses. Intramuscular pressures at rest and muscle relaxation pressure during exercise were higher when subjects wore each of the orthoses. To evaluate whether distal strapping was responsible for this increase in pressure, distal straps were removed and subjects retested; intramuscular

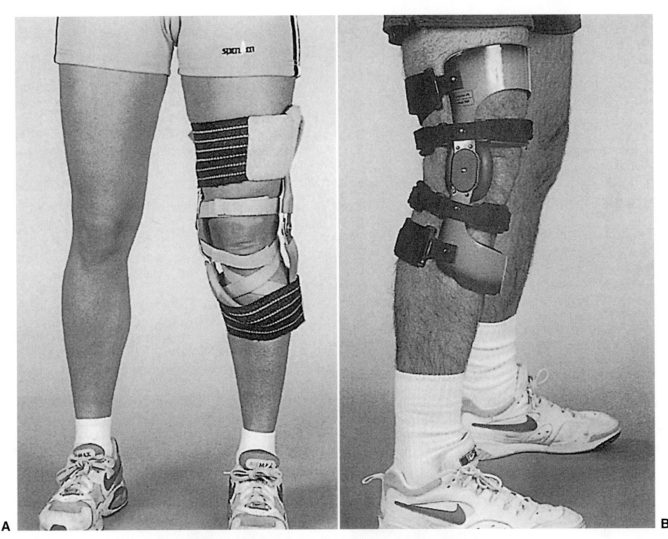

FIGURE 11-11 Comparison of the original (**A**) and current (**B**) Lenox Hill Hill Rerotation Orthosis. (From Nawoczenski DA, Epler ME [eds], *Orthotics in Functional Rehabilitation of the Lower Limb*. Philadelphia: Saunders, 1997.)

pressure and muscle relaxation pressure returned to levels that were similar to nonbraced levels. This study demonstrates the subtle yet potentially important impact of orthoses on muscle function that may contribute to injury; external compression elevates the intramuscular pressure beneath the thigh and leg straps. Local muscle blood flow is impaired by the increased intramuscular pressure, which leads to decreased oxygen tension and impaired muscle function.[35] This could possibly be the reason for premature leg muscle fatigue that has been reported in other experimental studies on individuals using knee braces.[34,36,37]

In their randomized, multicenter trial, McDevitt and colleagues[38] compared patients who wore an off-the-shelf knee brace daily for 6 months and for high-level activities thereafter with a group who did not wear any brace after 3 weeks postoperatively. The authors found that there were no significant differences between groups in multiple outcome measures, which included knee range of motion, knee stability, and function.[38]

Prophylactic Knee Orthoses

In the 1990s, considerable debate took place concerning the potential benefits or effectiveness of orthoses that were designed to prevent knee injuries or to minimize the severity of injury for athletes involved in high-risk injury activities.[33,39-41] The objective of wearing a prophylactic knee orthosis (PKO) is to provide protection to the soft tissue restraints of the knee. Most commonly, these braces have been worn by athletes who are exposed to lateral impacts.

Lateral impacts can result in MCL and cruciate ligament injuries.[42] Prophylactic orthoses are designed to protect the integrity of medial knee structures. Most prophylactic designs have a hinged lateral frame, held in place by a set of thigh and calf cuffs or straps. The hinge may be single axis, dual axis, or polycentric; many designs have also incorporated a hyperextension stop for further protection of the athlete's knee against forceful hyperextension injury (Figure 11-13). Some designs use a plastic shell with medial and lateral uprights and polycentric hinges.[43]

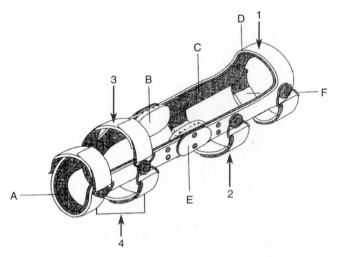

FIGURE 11-12 Components of most contemporary functional knee orthoses include the calf section/cuff with its closure (**A**); medial or lateral condylar pads, or both (**B**); medial and lateral uprights (**C**); the thigh section/cuff with its closure (**D**); an adjustable knee hinge (**E**); and the thigh strap (**F**). The stabilizing forces that are typically applied by the orthosis include (1) a posterior force over the anterior proximal thigh (1), an anterior force on the distal posterior femur (2), a posterior force at the proximal anterior tibia (3), and an anterior force at the midshaft of the posterior tibia (4). (Reprinted with permission from Trautman P. Lower limb orthoses. In Redford JB, Basmajian JV, Trautman P [eds], *Orthotics: Clinical Practice and Rehabilitation Technology*. New York: Churchill Livingstone, 1995. p. 31.)

Recommendations for the Patient with a Prophylactic Knee Orthosis

PKOs are available off-the-shelf or can be custom molded for the individual athlete. Clinical practice and research have not yet resolved the debate about the efficacy of prophylactic orthoses. Questions remain about the relationship between the biomechanical characteristics of the orthoses and the anatomical knee, the response of the orthosis to valgus loading, the impact of the orthosis on the continuum of locomotion (walking to running), and the ability of the orthosis to prevent injuries during activity as intended by its design.

Biomechanical Performance of Prophylactic Knee Orthoses

Many of the studies that have investigated the biomechanical performance of prophylactic braces have used either cadaver knees or mechanical surrogate models of the knee. Most have concluded that protection of the MCL has been inconsistent and only borderline at best.[40,44-48] Many health care providers are concerned about how the orthosis might preload the MCL before normal physiologic loading.[44,46,47] Our understanding of the interaction between the orthosis and the tissues of the knee is based on the properties of human tissue and of brace materials under static and dynamic loading conditions.

Manufacturers report high resistance of the braces to laterally directed impact loading; however, the research design and methodology on which these claims are based can be debated.

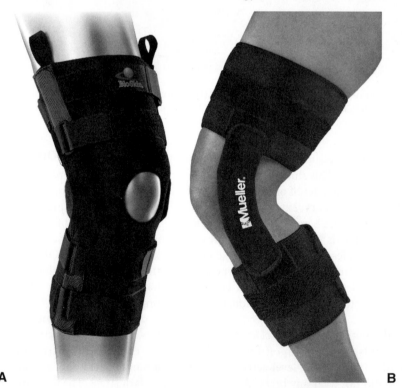

A   **B**

FIGURE 11-13 Examples of a prophylactic knee orthosis, designed to reduce risk of knee injury for athletes during practice and competition situations. **A,** BioSkin's Gladiator Sport used for knee ligament protection. **B,** Pro Level Mueller Hinge 2100 for protection of the MCL. (A, Reprinted with permission from Cropper Medical, Inc/Bioskin, Ashland, OR; B, Reprinted with permission from Mueller Sports Medicine, Inc., Prairie du Sac, WI.)

CASE EXAMPLE 1

High School Football Player

C. K., a 16-year-old high school quarterback, and his father come into your outpatient physical therapy clinic for a consultation regarding the potential benefits of wearing a knee brace during football games and practices. C. K. is a highly recruited quarterback on his high school football team. He has no history of injury that prevents him from playing or practicing football. He and his Dad are aware that football players are susceptible to knee ligament injuries due to the nature of the game. C. K.'s father is concerned that his son's ability to play college football would be compromised if he injured his knee. He wants to know whether wearing a prophylactic knee brace (PKO) would reduce the likelihood that C. K. would sustain a severe knee injury.

Questions to Consider
- Given C. K.'s history and current presentation, what additional tests and measures would provide helpful information to use in your evaluation process?
- What is your movement dysfunction-related diagnosis for C. K.?

- What is the rehabilitation prognosis for C.K.? What are his goals for intervention? What are your rehabilitation goals? How long to do you think it will take to achieve any goals that you and C. K. agree upon?
- What is the current evidence in the clinical research literature about the efficacy of PKO to reduce incidence and severity of knee injury in college football players?
- What impact does wearing a PKO have on athletic performance? What are the risks associated with wearing a PKO during athletic competition?
- Based on C. K.'s goals and expectations, your understanding of the risk for injury for football players, and evidence available in the clinical research literature, what recommendations would you make for intervention at this point in time? Is the evidence convincing enough that you would recommend that this high school athlete should begin to wear a PKO?
- What PKO designs might be most appropriate for this college-bound football player?
- How will you assess whether C. K.'s goals have been met?
- What type of follow-up would you recommend for C. K.?

In some cases, the braces are actually less rigid and resistant to derangement during loading than is the anatomic knee itself. The ability of a knee orthosis prepositioned in flexion to protect against major ligament damage is uncertain.[41] Joint line clearance during brace deformation is an additional concern. Theoretically, the prophylactic brace is designed to transmit valgus loads on the knee over the greatest possible area to dissipate the forces away from susceptible ligaments effectively.[41,46,47] The orthotic hinge forms a bridge over the joint line; its sites of attachment are best placed as far as possible on the proximal femur and distal tibia. Clearance between the hinge and the joint themselves must be adequate. Contact between the hinge and the joint creates a three-point bending system centered at the joint, inadvertently preloading the MCL.[46,47]

Evidence of Efficacy of Prophylactic Knee Orthoses
There have been many studies directed at determining the effectiveness of PKOs in preventing knee ligament injuries in football players.[33,49–52] In 1987, Teitz and colleagues[52] reported on data collected in 1984 and 1985 regarding football players from Division I NCAA schools. Players who wore PKOs had more injuries to the knee than players who did not wear these braces. This study, however, did not control for players' history of prior knee injury.[52] In 1986, Hewson and colleagues[49] reported findings on University of Arizona football players from a study that spanned 8 years. The injury records of four academic years in which players wore PKOs were compared with the preceding 4 years in which players did not use PKOs. It was mandatory for the players who were at the greatest risk for injury, that is, linebackers, defensive linemen, and tight

ends to wear PKOs in the years when brace wear was being monitored in this study. The results of this research indicated that, when comparing groups of braced players to unbraced players, there were no reductions in the number, rate, or type of knee injuries that players sustained.[49]

A 3-year study of NCAA Division I college football players in the Big Ten Conference by Albright and colleagues[53] revealed slightly different results. These researchers identified some trends that players who wore PKOs experienced lower rates of MCL injuries when compared with their unbraced peers. These trends were evident only when influential factors such as playing position, skill level of the player, and session (game or practice) in which the injury was sustained were considered in the analysis. Starting players and those who were substitutes in line positions, linebackers, and tight end positions had lower injury rates in practices and games. Backs, receivers, and kickers exhibited trends indicating higher injury rates in games when using a PKO.[53]

The implications that the benefits of PKO use may be related to player position is also suggested in a study by Sitler and colleagues.[51] Participants in this study included young men in an eight-man intramural tackle football program at West Point between 1986 and 1987. Variables such as the athletic shoe, playing surface, knee injury history, type of brace, and injury assessment and documentation were all controlled. Subjects wearing PKOs while on defense had significantly fewer knee injuries than their nonbraced counterparts. There were no significant differences for these parameters noted when players were on offense.[51]

Researchers and athletic trainers have concerns about the risk of injury to other areas of the limb when these orthoses are worn during competition. In a two-season prospective study of potentially protective benefits of prophylactic bracing in a sample of 580 high school football players, Grace and colleagues[33] found a dramatic increase in the number of injuries of the ankle and foot among athletes who wore the braces. In contrast, Sitler and colleagues[51] found no significant difference in the frequency of ankle injuries between a knee brace group and a control group of military cadets. Additionally, the severity of MCL and ACL knee injury was not reduced with the use of unilateral-biaxial prophylactic knee braces.[51]

It is difficult to make an unequivocal statement regarding the need for high school and college athletes to wear a PKO. The research examining this issue is confusing because data collection cannot take into account yearly variations in coaching techniques or completely control the data collection methods employed by all of the schools participating in the studies. Furthermore, there is no standardization in injury diagnosis between these studies. This makes it difficult to compare results of the studies to each other.[42] Many of the studies have methodological problems and limited sample size, making interpretation of their findings challenging.[54-58] Despite the inconsistency of research methods and findings, however, France and Paulos[42] conclude that there is sufficient evidence to indicate that bracing can be beneficial in reducing the number of MCL injuries sustained from direct lateral blows to the knee, especially when the knee is near full extension. They recommend that a PKO be carefully fit, so that the hinge maintains its position at the lateral joint line during activity, that the brace provides enough clearance from the joint line during impact, and that the materials used in the brace construction are sufficient to control the amount of impact delivered to the knee.[42] The literature does not provide enough information about the protection that these braces offer to the other soft tissue structures of the knee.

A study of high school football players by Deppen and Landfried[59] found no significant reduction in knee injuries in those football players wearing prophylactic knee braces compared with unbraced football players.

An additional concern regarding the use of prophylactic knee bracing is whether it diminishes athletic performance. Greene and colleagues[60] found that in football players prophylactic knee bracing did not significantly reduce 40-yard dash speed or agility during four-cone drills.[60] Sforzo and colleagues[61] found that the use of prophylactic bracing in college football players did not decrease performance, whereas, in female lacrosse players, prophylactic bracing negatively impacted athletic performance. In healthy college aged subjects, Borsa and colleagues[62] found that during the use of prophylactic bracing, subjects had decreased peak torque and torque acceleration energy during isokinetic testing, as well as slower sprint speed time.[62] Liggett and colleagues[63] found that gait pattern was not significantly altered when a prophylactic knee brace was used during running in healthy males and females.[63] In

"Technical Report: Knee Brace Use in the Young Athlete," the American Academy of Pediatrics stated that there was "insufficient evidence to recommend prophylactic knee bracing in the young athlete."[64]

In a descriptive epidemiological study, Sanders and colleagues[65] found that incidence of ligamentous knee injury decreased with prophylactic knee bracing in off-road motorcyclists compared with motorcyclists who did not wear a brace.

If prophylactic braces are intended to prevent or reduce the severity of injury, clinicians and brace manufacturers must work to be responsible for critical evaluation of these devices to define better define their appropriate use and outcomes. Clinicians must hold vendors accountable for their products, requesting well-designed and clearly reported quantitative studies to support the narrative accounts in marketing brochures about design criteria. Lastly, the clinician should have a discussion with the patient that focuses on the patient's goals and how using a brace may help the patient achieve those goals.

INFORMED CLINICAL DECISION MAKING

Because of the large number of FKOs currently marketed, it is very challenging and often frustrating for clinicians and surgeons to evaluate the information published in marketing literature when research support is not always available. As a clinician it may be challenging to remain well informed because orthotic designs are constantly being modified and improved. Making a sound decision about which design can best meet the stability and activity needs of a given individual can be a daunting task and must not be based on which sales representative most recently shared information or which orthosis is currently the most popular choice. Clinicians should keep apprised of all bracing that is commercially available. Although patients may seek a functional orthosis to protect their knee or to improve their performance, many do not have the knowledge or resources to understand the specifics and idiosyncrasies of each brace. To make the best informed decision, the clinician must consider the patient's specific injury and pattern of instability, the present and anticipated strength and bulk of their muscles around the injured knee, and the activities and likely mechanism of being reinjured in the patient's preferred activities. Decisions about orthotic options must be deliberately made, with discussion involving the patient, physical therapist or athletic trainer, orthotist, brace manufacturer, and physician. Quick decisions about an FKO, made without carefully evaluating the match between the patient's needs and the orthotic design, lead to frustration and dissatisfaction for all involved.

In evaluating information presented about knee orthoses published in the literature, health professionals must look closely at research design and methodology and evaluate the clinical relevance of the conclusions drawn from study results. Important questions to ask include the following:

1. What type of brace is being studied?
2. What patient demographic is being used to evaluate the efficacy of a knee orthosis?

3. Does the study evaluate the orthosis under static conditions or during dynamic use?
4. Does the study used cadaveric models or physiologically active joints in the evaluation of orthotic performance?
5. Did the study test reconstructed ACL knees in the use of knee orthosis?
6. What outcome measures were used to determine positive outcomes?

Many of the most frequently cited studies evaluate brace performance under static conditions, specifically the ability of particular orthoses to prevent anterior excursion of the tibia on the femur as measured by standard clinical tests for ligamentous instability (e.g., Lachman's, pivot shift, or Losee's tests). Some studies have used electronic and mechanical instrumentation to evaluate orthotic performance more precisely under static and controlled dynamic conditions. Although many studies demonstrate the efficacy of knee orthoses in prevention of excessive anterior excursion under static conditions, to generalize these static results to dynamic activity for patients with ACL-deficient knees is audacious. Because an orthosis can provide a degree of stability for the knee under static conditions does not guarantee that it can also stabilize the knee during high demand, multiplanar activity. The low load levels applied to knee ligaments during static or cadaver model testing do not accurately reflect load levels during functional and athletic activities. Decisions to choose a particular orthosis based on this type of research alone are not well informed.

The selection of a functional brace today is even more challenging as third-party payers have dictated to the consumer where and from what vendor they can get their brace, either in a custom-made or off-the-shelf model. This limits the choice and type of brace used and puts the patient in a one-brace-for-all scenario.

Another dilemma that clinicians face is the aggressive rehabilitation protocols for ACL reconstruction that are currently being used show close to normal range and strength by the third to sixth month. The decision to have the patient advance through the rehabilitation protocols and perform activities such as jumping, hopping, turning, or twisting is a complex decision that is based on many factors. These factors include strength of the ACL graft, graft fixation, and known biological factors that affect healing. A knee joint that is stabilized by a strong isometric graft, has healthy tissue healing capability, and goes through a controlled rehabilitation program should not need a functional brace. The most important part of the patient's return to activity/work is the physical rehabilitation and/or surgery.

HINGE DESIGN

Hinge options for knee orthoses range from simple single-axis (unicentric) designs to complex four-bar polycentric designs. Most commercially available off-the-shelf FKOs have hinges in one of three categories: (1) the single-axis hinge, (2) the posterior offset hinge, or (3) the polycentric or genucentric hinge.

All single-axis/unicentric hinges act as a simple hinge; a unicentric hinge becomes incongruent with the anatomic joint axis as the instantaneous axis of rotation of the knee changes with movement through the range of motion. Posterior offset designs attempt to improve the match between orthotic and anatomical axis of motion by approximating the location of the sagittal radius of curvature of the posterior femoral condyles as it articulates with the tibia in flexion.[66] Polycentric designs attempt to replicate the instantaneous axis of rotation of the anatomical knee joint, using two geared surfaces that mechanically constrain motion into a defined path.[67] Theoretically, polycentric or genucentric hinges are better able than unicentric hinge designs to match the rolling and gliding of the tibiofemoral joint as the knee flexes and extends. This closer match to physiological motion is meant to reduce pistoning, discomfort, and slippage of the orthosis on the limb during activity.

When considering which hinge design to select, consider that the soft tissue of the knee between the orthosis and the bone compromises the impact of any hinge on the kinematics of the knee. The most important characteristic of the hinge is its ability to transfer load during activity. Poorly designed or constructed hinges, or those made of weak or pliable materials, cannot effectively accomplish this task, and abnormal translations and rotations will not be well controlled. The work of Lew and colleagues[67] demonstrated greater variation in the pistoning constraint forces in a particular joint design than across designs when three orthoses were compared during specific activities.

Regalbuto and colleagues[68] evaluated the performance of four hinge designs fit into a custom-fit knee orthosis in three healthy subjects. Subjects wore the orthosis while performing a squat, an 8-inch step-up, a stand-to-sit activity, and an open chain knee extension exercise. The researchers found that accurate hinge placement was a more important influence on function and comfort than hinge kinematics. Differences in kinematics among the four designs were masked by the compliance of the soft tissues between the brace cuffs and the bones of the knee.

FUNCTIONAL ORTHOSES FOR ANTERIOR CRUCIATE LIGAMENT INSUFFICIENCY

Physical therapists are often involved in conservative and in postsurgical rehabilitation for patients with ACL insufficiency. For more than 30 years, FKOs have been used to prevent forward subluxation of the tibia on the femur for patients with ACL insufficiency. A variety of designs have evolved to be used for partial ACL tears or for complete ACL rupture (Figure 11-14).

Biomechanical Performance of Functional Knee Orthoses for Anterior Cruciate Ligament Insufficiency

For patients with an ACL tear and/or deficiencies, one of the primary goals of bracing is to control the excessive anterior drawer movement of the tibia. A number of research studies have attempted to evaluate whether these orthoses

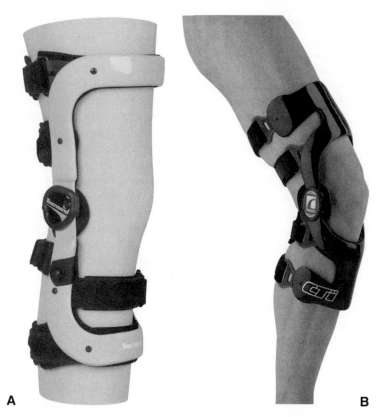

A   **B**

FIGURE 11-14 Examples of commercially available, custom-fit functional knee orthoses. **A,** The Townsend Design Premier Series is marketed as both a custom functional knee brace and prophylactic brace. **B,** CTi. (**A,** Reprinted with permission from Townsend Design, Bakersfield, CA. **B,** Reprinted with permission from Ossür Americas, Foothills Ranch, CA.)

are effective in controlling tibial movement. One strategy is to use cadaver models to evaluate the efficacy of functional knee orthoses for support of the ACL.[69,70] The major drawback of this type of study, however, is the difference between living and preserved tissue. Because active muscle contraction and normal soft tissue compliance contribute to strain on the ACL, the lack of active musculature and compliance changes in soft tissue around the knee limit the application of cadaver study findings. Similarly, the magnitude and sequence of muscle contraction alter the stiffness between the brace and the soft tissue of the leg. It is not possible to reproduce this dynamic relationship in cadaveric studies.

Another strategy is to compare forward excursion of the tibia on the femur using clinical tests of knee instability performed on a subject with and without bracing.[21,48,71] Wojtys and colleagues[72,73] conducted two studies in which anterior tibial translation was measured while subjects were seated on an ischial support, in both braced and unbraced conditions. Patients were instructed to stay relaxed throughout a test in which the tibia was forced anteriorly. Reflexive contraction of the hamstrings, quadriceps, and gastrocnemius muscles to this initial perceived force occurred more quickly in the braced than the unbraced condition. However, these muscles reacted more slowly in the braced condition when patients were told to actively resist this movement as soon

as they perceived it. Beynnon and colleagues[74] found no significant improvement in subjects' ability to detect passive anterior tibial translation in braced conditions when subjects were tested in a seated position. Also, the use of a functional knee brace in patients with ACL deficiency has been shown to improve hamstring reflex, but not as the muscle fatigues with activity.[75]

In a randomized controlled clinical trial by Birmingham and colleagues[76] the authors compared functional knee bracing to use of a neoprene sleeve in patients following an ACL reconstruction. At the patient's 6-week postoperative visit, the patient received either a functional knee brace or a neoprene sleeve. The authors found no significant difference in quality of life (ACL-QOL) and activity, KT-1000 arthrometer findings, or hop limb symmetry. The authors concluded that use of a functional knee brace following ACL reconstruction yields no better outcomes that using a neoprene sleeve.[76] However, functional knee bracing after ACL reconstruction has been found to have positive impacts in proprioception.[77]

It is difficult to draw a clinical conclusion regarding the effects of bracing on anterior tibial translation in patients with ACL-deficient knees given the conflicting results of these studies. Although the studies seem to indicate that subjects' ability to perceive passive anterior tibial motion did not improve, one must also consider that subjects were tested in nonfunctional, non–weight-bearing conditions versus dynamic situations. Additionally, the relationship between static testing and actual physiological loading during sport activity has not been well established. Noyes and colleagues[69] have demonstrated that manual examination cannot duplicate the magnitude of force that is present during activity.

Although static and cadaver studies have been the first step in critically evaluating the efficacy of FKOs for patients with ACL insufficiency, the most informative research would be done in vivo. This is especially important because static and cadaver studies cannot replicate the real-life physiological loading that occurs in the knee during activities.[69,70,78–81]

Soma and colleagues[82] found that custom made braces did a better job at preventing anterior tibial translation than off-the-shelf functional knee braces.

The next challenge for clinical researchers is to develop methodology to evaluate FKOs worn during functional activities.

Evidence of Efficacy of Functional Knee Orthoses for Anterior Cruciate Ligament Insufficiency

In 1997, Kramer and colleagues[26] published a review of research conducted between 1982 and 1992, which summarized the evidence regarding use of FKOs on dynamic performance. Collectively, these studies did not provide overwhelming evidence to support or refute the use of FKOs by individuals with ACL-deficient knees. This review cited 16 maximal effort experimental situations in which subjects' performance in braced and unbraced conditions for one-leg hop test, figure-of-eight runs, stair climbing, sprinting, and agility was recorded. Results across the studies were mixed: FKOs either improved, hindered, or had no effect on performance.

Kramer and colleagues' review[26] also summarized the results of several matched effort tests that measured biomechanical variables. The variables assessed in these studies included ground reaction forces, range of motion, EMG, joint moment, and power. These studies were difficult to interpret whether FKO use provided wearers with advantages or disadvantages because it was not assessed how changes in the measured variables impacted overall performance. Three of the matched effort studies demonstrated that bracing subjects during testing resulted in detrimental effects on energy costs. Overall, this literature review noted that five of the included studies indicated that many of the subjects reported feeling more stable when wearing the FKO. Given the mixed results of these studies, it is difficult to make a conclusive statement about whether or not patients with ACL deficiency should expect enhanced performance when wearing FKOs.

The ability of subjects to control anterior tibial translation during functional testing was examined by Ramsey and colleagues.[83] This study demonstrated that there was negligible reduction in the anterior drawer movement of the tibia between braced and unbraced conditions when patients performed horizontal, one-legged jumps.

Another strategy is to evaluate muscle function when subjects with ACL deficiency use a functional knee orthosis. Branch and colleagues[84] found little difference in electromyographic firing patterns between in-brace and out-of-brace testing. Because muscle activity was similarly reduced under both conditions (as referenced to an ACL intact limb), the researchers suggest that FKOs do not have a significant proprioceptive influence on muscle function. A study by Wu and colleagues[85] looked at 31 subjects who had undergone a unilateral ACL reconstruction with three bracing conditions: (1) a manufactured brace, (2) a mechanical placebo brace, and (3) no brace. Using an isokinetic machine to measure specific knee joint angles and peak torques, they found that knee bracing can improve static proprioception but not muscle function. The manufactured and mechanical placebo brace groups performed better than the no brace group. The apparent improvement in proprioception with knee bracing was not due to the mechanical restraining action of the brace.[85] Other studies show similar results when measuring proprioceptive improvement on ACL reconstructed knees when doing functionally relevant tasks.[86,87]

Nemeth and colleagues[27] studied the effects of bracing and not bracing on six downhill skiers who had ACL-deficient knees during a series of downhill ski runs. Surface electrodes were placed over the muscle bellies of vastus medialis, gastrocnemius medialis, biceps femoris, and semimembranosus and semitendinosus muscles to record these muscles' activity during skiing and determine whether there were differences in the patterns of muscle firing between the braced and unbraced conditions. Statistical analysis did not reveal significant differences between subjects' muscle response in either of these conditions. However, they found that subjects with greater knee instability, compared with subjects with less knee instability, had increased levels of lateral hamstring muscle activity during knee flexion when they were braced. In theory, this muscle activation may help control excessive anterolateral shifting of the tibial plateau, thereby helping the patient feel greater lower extremity stability. Despite the lack of definitive results in this study, all subjects who wore the FKO reported feeling more safe and stable during their skiing activity.

Another study by Ramsey and colleagues[88] examined the muscle firing patterns of rectus femoris, semitendinosus, biceps femoris, and the lateral head of the gastrocnemius of four subjects with ACL-deficient knees who were braced and not braced during one-legged jumps. They also measured anterior tibial displacement during the testing activity. Interestingly, their findings indicated that the subjects who were braced demonstrated decreased levels of hamstring activity and increased levels of quadriceps activity. The braced condition resulted in small reductions of anterior displacement in two subjects, no change in one subject, and small increases in this translation for one subject.

Cook and colleagues[89] compared the ability of subjects with absent ACLs (n = 14) to perform running and cutting maneuvers with and without a commercially available orthosis. Subjects' performance with the orthosis was objectively and subjectively better. In a similar study that compared the performance of subjects with ACL deficiency in several orthoses, Marans and colleagues[90] reported improved performance in two of the six orthoses evaluated.

A number of studies have examined the metabolic cost using dynamic analysis of orthotic use to test the validity and reliability of functional knee braces on ACL-insufficient knees.[31,91] Whether the slight increase in energy requirements noted is offset by protection and improved function while wearing the orthosis is not yet understood.

The authors in these studies that examined the effects of bracing subjects with ACL-deficient knees during dynamic test conditions suggest that there may be afferent inputs from knee proprioceptors and the brace-skin-bone interface to the central nervous system. This neural input may evoke adaptive motor responses when patients wear the knee brace during functional activities. The number of subjects used in each of these studies is fewer than 10, making it difficult to draw conclusions if one is to consider each study independently. Collectively, however, the results of each of the studies are similar, which may help the physical therapist formulate an opinion about the merits of using a brace on patients with an ACL-deficient knee.

CASE EXAMPLE 2

Individual with History of ACL Tear

B. J. is a 23-year-old female alpine ski racer who is 6 months postop ACL reconstruction with a patellar tendon-bearing graft to her left knee. B. J. has worked diligently in her postoperative rehabilitation. She denies pain, but still reports limited agility and quickness.

B. J. is anxious to return to the ski slopes and resume ski racing. You have been in communication with her orthopedic surgeon who recommends that B. J. can only return to skiing if she wears a knee brace. B. J. asks you what benefits the brace will provide as she relates that she has heard conflicting information about whether or not knee braces were beneficial. B. J. wonders if a specialized knee brace will help her maintain the stability of her knee during her alpine ski races. Also, she is concerned that the extra weight of a knee brace will slow her down on the slopes. She wants advice from the physical therapist about the merits of obtaining such a brace.

The therapist wanted to find evidence to support whether or not B. J. should invest in an FKO brace to enhance her knee stability. The clinical question that will direct review of the evidence is, "Will a brace designed for patients with ACL-deficient knees enhance the control and stability of the knee during recreational activities?"

Questions to Consider
- Given this patient's history and current presentation, what additional tests and measures would provide helpful information to use in your evaluation process?
- What is your movement dysfunction-related diagnosis for this patient?
- What is B. J.'s prognosis?
- What are your rehabilitation goals?
- How long to do you think it will take to achieve the goals that you and B. J. agree upon?
- What is the role of exercise and/or FKO in the management of a patient like B. J. following ACL reconstruction?

- What evidence is available in the clinical research literature about the efficacy of FKO to protect the integrity of the ACL following reconstruction?
- Based on B. J.'s goals and expectations, your understanding of the underlying disease process, and evidence from the clinical research literature, what recommendations would you make for intervention at this point in time?
- Is the evidence convincing enough, given the level of impairment that B. J. demonstrates and her prognosis, that you would recommend she purchase an FKO to wear during recreational activities?
- Would you recommend an off-the-shelf or custom-made FKO?
- Of the various FKO designs available, which might be most appropriate for B. J. following ACL reconstruction and accelerated rehabilitation?
- How will you assess whether B. J.'s rehabilitation goals have been met?
- What type of follow-up would you recommend for this patient?

Recommendations for the Patient Following Anterior Cruciate Ligament Reconstruction

After reviewing the evidence, the physical therapist discusses what she has discovered with B. J., that the research to support or refute the use of an FKO is equivocal. There is evidence to suggest that some patients feel more stable when they wear a brace, but it is unknown whether patients' feelings of enhanced stability are due to biomechanical or neuromuscular changes that are the result of FKO wear. Specific to skiers, there is evidence that the use of an FKO may help reduce the risk for reinjury.[29] The therapist recommends that B. J. rehabilitate her knee through participation in a dynamic, sport-specific exercise program before she considers returning to Alpine ski racing.

The Role of Exercise in ACL Rehabilitation

There is literature to support the premise that hamstrings and gastrocnemius muscles assist in stabilizing ACL-deficient knees as well as evidence to support that patients with ACL-deficient knees benefit from closed kinetic chain exercise programs and perturbation training.[92-96] If the patient perceives the need for an FKO after participating in a rehabilitation program, the therapist can direct the patient to braces that are available while cautioning that the patient must continue with a home strengthening program.

ORTHOSES FOR OSTEOARTHRITIS

Narrowing of the medial or lateral compartment of the knee is a common source of discomfort and pain for many adults. OA is a condition in which the collagen fibers of the articular cartilage are compromised. The breakdown of the articular cartilage in the medial or lateral compartment will result in the uneven distribution of the load forces.[97] There are currently five general methods of management for OA:

1. Pharmaceuticals
2. Surgery: unicompartmental or total knee arthroplasty (TKA)
3. Foot orthoses
4. Injections
5. Use of valgus or varus knee orthoses

Valgus/varus knee bracing evolved in the early 1990s with the theory that by unloading the medial or lateral compartment, pain could be altered enough to ward off surgery and prolong the function of an osteoarthritic knee.

Most individuals with OA of the knee demonstrate functional losses and report pain when the knee is loaded during the stance phase of gait, beginning at heel strike and ending with toe-off. Biomechanical analysis on healthy subjects reveals that loading in the knee is 62% on the medial side and 38% on the lateral side during stance; in those with a varus deformity associated with medial joint OA, the medial compartment loading can increase to 100% of the total compressive load on the knee joint during this phase of gait.[98] Based on this premise, the conservative and surgical strategy in treating these individuals is to reduce the load on the medial side of the joint to reduce the painful symptoms that the patient experiences.[99]

Valgus (unloading) orthoses (Figure 11-15) are designed to unload the medial knee compartment noted to have degenerative changes and provide a similar type of advantage as realignment osteotomy.[98] These orthoses unload the medial compartment of the knee through use of adjustable tension straps crossing the lateral aspect of the knee joint, lateral condylar pads, or lateral hinge systems, which are fixed to a brace shell at the calf and thigh.[98-100]

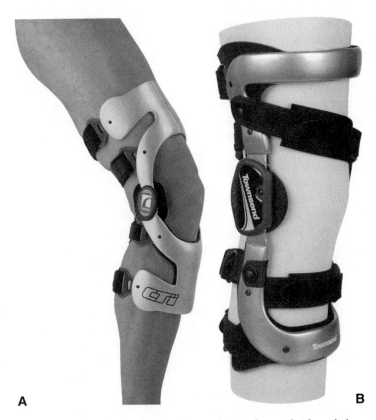

A   **B**

FIGURE 11-15 Examples of unloader knee orthoses designed to unload medial compartment of the knee for individuals with painful osteoarthritis (OA). **A,** The CTi OA brace from Ossür 2. **B,** The Single Upright Premier Series OA Knee Brace from Townsend Design. (**A** and **B,** Reprinted with permission from Ossür Americas, Foothills Ranch, CA.)

Evidence of Efficacy of Valgus/Unloading Orthoses

Research over the past 10 years has attempted to validate manufacturer's claims that valgus/varus bracing will achieve significant reductions in the amount of pain and swelling in the involved joint region. Pollo[101] looked at nine subjects (mean age 46 ± 11 years) with a varus mechanical alignment of 0 to 10 degrees. Each subject was tested during walking with and without a commercially available brace. Kinematic and kinetic data were recorded using a video-based six-camera Motion Analysis System in conjunction with two Bertec force platforms. Comparisons were made at the initial test and at the 3-month follow-up. There was a statistically significant improvement in pain and function along with a reduction in the external varus moment about the knee when wearing the commercially available brace. Other authors have found similar results with unicompartmental OA and the improved function that the valgus brace affords to the patients.[102]

A study by Katsuragawa and colleagues[102] demonstrated an increase in bone mineral density more in the lateral tibial condyle than the medial condyle due to the transfer of forces across the knee joint from the medial to the lateral side after use of a valgus orthosis. Research by Horlick and colleagues[103] demonstrated a significant reduction of pain when wearing a valgus brace, but did not find a change in functional status or in the femoral-tibial angle and joint space as viewed via radiographs.

Self and colleagues[98] examined the effects of valgus knee bracing on the varus moment at the knee during level gait on five patients who had confirmed medial compartment knee arthrosis. The varus moment causes greater loading on the medial compartment and may be responsible for the pain that patients with medial knee arthrosis experience. The researchers collected kinematic data on subjects' patterns of walking with and without their orthoses. The use of a valgus brace reduced the net varus moment on the medial compartment of the knee during the time when this moment was typically at its maximum load.[98] Lindenfeld and colleagues[99] examined the pain intensity and function scores for subjects with confirmed medial compartment knee arthrosis and persistent pain during ambulation. They hoped to determine whether valgus knee bracing altered the loads at the knee joint. Most patients who wore the prescribed brace had excellent clinical responses in terms of increased function and decreased pain, and demonstrated medial compartment unloading during radiographic testing.[99]

In patients with medial compartment knee OA, Birmingham and colleagues[104] found proprioception was improved in patients during use of a custom-fit brace. However, patients did not show a significant increase in postural control.

Finally, Hewett and colleagues[100] examined the effects of valgus bracing on a group of 19 adults with chronic medial knee joint pain, which limited their ability to participate in sports or perform activities of daily living (ADLs). Study participants were assessed after 9 weeks and again after about 1 year of orthotic wear to determine whether there were changes in their symptoms and function. Fifteen of 18 subjects reevaluated after 9 weeks reported reduction in their pain symptoms and/or an increase in walking tolerance. Thirteen patients continued to wear the brace for an average of a year. Ten of these patients felt an improvement in pain or function after using the brace. The most dramatic improvements were related to the amount of time participants were able to walk before onset of pain. Wearing the orthosis did not have much impact on returning participants to sports activities. Despite the improvements in symptoms and function for many patients, gait analysis did not reveal any changes in loading at the varus moment or any gait adaptations during brace wear.[100]

Furthermore, Nadaud and colleagues[105] performed an in vivo study examining the effectiveness of five commercial types of functional knee braces across five subjects. They found variability among the average amount of medial condylar separation among braces but found consistent off-loading of the knee upon heel-strike during gait and decreased ability to off-load at midstance.[105]

These studies, reviewed independently, include relatively small numbers of subjects. However, the conclusions in all of the studies regarding patients who wore valgus braces to control the detrimental effects of medial tibiofemoral arthrosis were similar. If pain associated with medial joint compartment arthritis is related to varus loading of the knee joint, it appears that valgus bracing can be effective in controlling some of the painful symptoms that are associated with this pathology.

The impact of valgus bracing on function and gait kinematics is not as clear. Despite the conflicting evidence regarding the influence that these braces have on gait kinematics and joint loading, there does seem to be evidence to support the notion that patients may benefit from valgus brace wear to diminish pain and increase function if these individuals do not want to consider surgery as an immediate option.

There is clear evidence that weakness of the quadriceps muscle is related to osteoarthritic conditions at the knee joint.[106,107] Ramsey and colleagues[108] found that, in subjects with medial compartment OA that decreased muscle, co-contraction of the vastus lateralis and lateral hamstrings resulted in decreased pain while using an unloader brace.[108] In a review of research related to guidelines for management of OA in the knee, Hochberg and colleagues[109] cite the need for patients to participate in quadriceps strengthening and range of motion exercises as well as aerobic conditioning exercises. In their review of the literature, Raja and Dewan[110] cited the lack of homogeneity of studies analyzing the use of knee bracing for OA, which did not allow for a conclusive statement supporting the use of knee braces. However, the authors do mention that use of knee braces and foot orthoses may prove to be less costly than other interventions.[110]

Divine and Hewett[111] suggest that clinicians should prescribe a knee brace on a trial basis in order to provide lower extremity biomechanical changes to decrease pain.

Patient with Osteoarthritis of the Knee

R. P. is a 55-year-old man who has completed 8 weeks of physical therapy (PT) with the goal of managing his right knee pain. An orthopedic surgeon referred R. P. for PT with a diagnosis of degenerative joint disease. Radiographs of R. P.'s right knee showed medial compartment tibiofemoral OA. R. P. has a 1-year history of increasing knee pain, concentrated around the medial joint line. The symptoms had worsened to the point where he felt compromised in his ADLs. R. P.'s past medical history is significant for a right partial medial meniscectomy 4 years before the onset of his knee pain.

Functionally, R. P. reported that he could not stand for more than 10 minutes or walk more than 30 minutes. His goals were to walk 60 minutes on a level surface for exercise and stand for 45 minutes. R. P. came to the PT clinic three times per week; his program emphasized quadriceps strengthening and exercises to maintain his knee range of motion. At the conclusion of 4 weeks of therapy, R. P. felt that there had been little change in his function. The referring physician recommended surgery because R. P.'s symptoms had not changed. R. P., however, did not want to consider surgery, based on the length and intensity of postoperative rehabilitation. He asked if there were any other interventions that might be considered to manage his knee pain.

Questions to Consider
- Given R. P.'s history and current presentation, what additional tests and measures would provide helpful information to use in your evaluation process?
- What is your movement dysfunction-related diagnosis for this patient?
- What is R. P.'s prognosis?
- What are physical therapy goals for R. P.?
- How long to do you think it will take to achieve the goals that you and R. P. agree upon?

- Based on R. P.'s goals and expectations, as well as your understanding of the underlying disease process, what recommendations would you make for intervention at this point in time? What evidence from the clinical research literature supports your recommendations? Why have you chosen and/or prioritized these possible interventions?
- How will you assess whether the patients and rehabilitation goals have been met?
- What type of follow-up would you recommend for this patient?

Recommendations for a Patient with Osteoarthritis of the Knee
After reviewing the evidence, and in light of the R. P.'s goals for intervention, the physical therapist recommends that wearing a valgus brace may diminish RP's knee pain and improve his functional activities, such as standing and walking. R. P. and the physical therapist consult with an orthotist to select the most appropriate orthosis. The physical therapist and orthotist caution R. P., but there is little evidence to suggest how long the potentially positive effects of this brace wear will last. The physical therapist encourages R. P. to continue exercising on a regular basis because there is clear evidence that weakness of the quadriceps muscle is related to osteoarthritic conditions at the knee joint. The physical therapist and R. P. agree on a home exercise program that includes range of motion, aerobic, and quadriceps resistive exercise, and they discuss appropriate intensity. The physical therapist helps R. P. understand that brace wear and exercise should not induce increased pain or swelling or loss of function, and instructs him to return to his physician, , or orthotist for follow-up.

ORTHOSES FOR PATELLOFEMORAL DYSFUNCTION

Just as evidence to support prophylactic and functional orthoses for tibiofemoral joint instability is inadequate, research support for the efficacy of patellofemoral taping and bracing is lacking. Nevertheless, orthotic management of patellofemoral dysfunction has become widespread in athletic and in nonathletic practice environments. The need for well-designed clinical research studies is pressing.

Physical therapy interventions for patients with patellofemoral stress syndrome (PFSS) are most often directed at optimizing patellofemoral mechanics, while reducing symptoms. Interventions may include pain relief modalities such as iontophoresis and phonophoresis, patellofemoral taping, soft tissue stretching and mobilization to enhance medial patella gliding, and extensibility of the soft tissue along the lateral aspect of the patella. An exercise program, guided by the

patient's tolerance, typically focuses on restoring appropriate tissue length and suppleness, as well as strengthening exercises (especially eccentric) for the quadriceps muscle group.

Patellofemoral orthoses (Figure 11-16) are often used as adjuncts to exercise to do the following[112]:

1. Provide pain relief and improve function for patients with patellofemoral pain syndrome
2. Prevent or control patellar subluxation or dislocation in patients with patellar tracking problems
3. Provide pain relief and support tissue healing for patients with irritation of the quadriceps or patellar tendon (e.g., patellar tendinopathy or Osgood-Schlatter disease)
4. Manage patients with chondromalacia and other symptomatic degenerative articular changes of the patellofemoral joint

There are a variety of knee orthoses directed at controlling the pain associated with PFSS. Typically these braces consist of an elasticized or neoprene sleeve worn over the knee

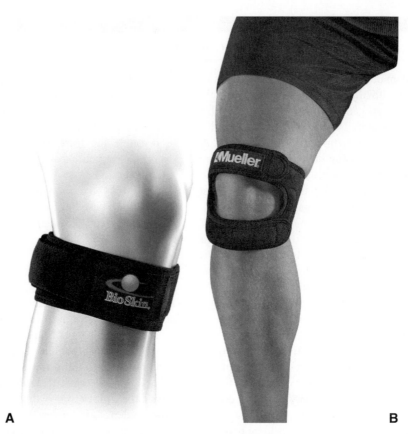

A   **B**

FIGURE 11-16 Examples of orthoses used for patellofemoral stress syndrome and/or patellar tracking problems. **A,** The Q Baby Patella Tendon infrapatellar strap from BioSkin. **B,** The Mueller #6479 Max Knee Strap. (**A,** Reprinted with permission, Cropper Medical, Inc/Bioskin, Ashland, OR. **B,** Reprinted with permission, Mueller Sports Medicine, Prairie du Sac, WI.)

(see Figures 11-2 and 11-16). Most have a circular opening to accommodate the patella and a semicircular crescent-shaped buttress that is sewn in place or held by Velcro closures and reinforcing straps. The purpose of the buttress and straps is to stabilize the position of the patella as it slides in the intracondylar groove during knee motion.[14] The goal of the PFSS orthosis is to control the undesirable, excessive lateral movement of the patella that is thought to be the underlying cause of PFSS. Some of these braces have a hinge system that, theoretically, resists knee extension, thereby reducing the potential for the unfavorable coupling effect of knee extension and excessive lateral patella excursion.[42] Other braces allow the buttress to be positioned in a number of positions around the patella, depending on the type of patella malalignment the patient demonstrates.[4] Another design uses a curved vinyl-covered strap worn snugly at the patellar tendon to support and elevate the patella during activity for more efficient tracking.[113] Normalization of tracking can, theoretically, minimize abnormal compressive forces on the articular surfaces, reduce the likelihood of further degenerative changes, and provide relief of symptoms.[114]

Biomechanics of Patellofemoral Orthoses

The mechanism for pain in those who suffer PFSS is unclear. Various theories propose that pain can be caused from patellar maltracking, tightness of the surrounding soft tissues, and/or less than optimal firing of various aspects of the quadriceps.[115]

Based on these assumptions, several studies have examined the effect of patellofemoral orthoses on the biomechanic function of the patellofemoral joint. Powers and colleagues[115] studied 10 female subjects with 12 symptomatic patellae, all of whom had a kinematic procedure done with magnetic resonance imaging (MRI), which documented lateral subluxation in their knees. The subjects performed resisted knee extension during an MRI, which recorded patella movement in braced and unbraced conditions. The patellofemoral orthosis used in this study had no significant effect on patella tracking (i.e., patellar tilt or medial/lateral displacement) from 45 to 0 degrees of knee flexion. The research did show a subtle patellar position change in the sulcus angle of the patella such that the patella moved to a more shallow portion of the trochlear groove when the knees were braced.[114]

Timm[116] used a Protonics orthosis, a brace that can be set to offer resistance to the knee flexor and extensor muscle groups while subjects perform functional activities, such as walking. There was a reduction in patellofemoral pain and improvement in patellofemoral congruence for patients who wore the brace as much as possible for 4 weeks.[116] A systematic review by D'hondt and colleagues[117] concluded in 2003 that the strength of the scientific evidence to support the use of patellofemoral orthoses is limited. The authors stated that one must take clinicians' clinical expertise and patient preferences into account when prescribing a knee orthosis.

Sleeve type braces and wrap braces have been shown to make positive changes in patellofemoral contact area.[118,119]

Evidence of Efficacy of Patellofemoral Orthoses

There have been a number of studies that have examined the effectiveness of these braces. It has been difficult to make comparisons of the research because different braces have been used and the measured outcomes also vary within these studies.

In a longitudinal study of 25 patients with unilateral retropatellar pain syndrome, Reikeras[120] found patellofemoral bracing to be minimally effective for symptom relief and for return to functional activities. In contrast, comprehensive conservative management of chondromalacia and of patellofemoral pain staged for acute symptom management, exercises to build flexibility and strength, maintenance exercise for eccentric control and muscular endurance, and return to activity using patellofemoral bracing were effective for 77% to 82% of patients.[121,122] A preliminary report by Crocker and Stauber demonstrated that use of a patellar stabilizing brace enabled four of five subjects to generate normal strength curves and increased power during isokinetic testing.[123] Subjects in this study also experienced improved performance in functional and sport activities when wearing the patellofemoral brace. In a larger study, 59 of 62 patients with diagnoses of patellar subluxation, patellofemoral arthritis, or Osgood-Schlatter disease were able to perform activities that typically provoked symptoms (pivoting, running, stair climbing, and long-distance walking) when wearing a patellofemoral brace.[14]

Powers and colleagues found that the use of a patellofemoral knee orthoses improved patellofemoral joint contact area and decreased pain in women with PFSS.[119] In a cadaveric study, Bohnsack and colleagues[124] found that the use of a patellar brace decreased patellofemoral contact area and decreased pressure of infrapatellar tissue. Additionally, Selfe and colleagues[125] found that the use of a patellofemoral brace could reduce coronal plane alterations and torsional angles.

Although some of these results are encouraging, the use of a patellofemoral brace as the primary intervention for patients with patellofemoral pain is not well supported. Conservative management strategies with established efficacy include activity modification, limited use of nonsteroidal antiinflammatory medications, and strengthening and flexibility exercises. Further clinical research to evaluate carefully the added benefit of patellofemoral bracing in the conservative management of patellofemoral dysfunction is necessary.

The literature regarding the appropriate rehabilitation protocol for management of PFSS is not consistent. A systematic review by Crossley and colleagues,[126] which examined the efficacy of a number of nonpharmacological and nonsurgical physical interventions for PFSS, illustrates this notion. The recommendation made by the authors based on the evidence from studies included in this review, is that stretching exercises, patient education, and quadriceps strengthening, including eccentric exercises, should be included in a physical therapy program. However, the evidence to support these protocols is inconclusive.[126]

A study by Finestone and colleagues[127] demonstrated that a group of Army recruits having patellofemoral pain had diminished symptoms with use of a simple elastic sleeve or an elastic sleeve with a silicone patella ring compared with symptoms in a control group that did not have any brace. However, 80% of the recruits who did not receive a brace were found to be asymptomatic at a 2-month follow-up visit.[127] In a study by Greenwald and colleagues,[128] subjects who wore a brace with a neoprene undersleeve and plastic exoskeleton with an extension stop reported that use of this brace significantly reduced the frequency and severity of their pain. BenGal and colleagues[129] demonstrated that there may be some evidence to support the use of a knee brace to prevent anterior knee pain.

Strengthening of the joints proximal and distal to the patellofemoral joint have been shown to result in decreased pain, function, and biomechanics with PFPS.[130]

CASE EXAMPLE 4

Patient with Patellofemoral Stress Syndrome

B. G. is a 25-year-old woman referred for PT with a diagnosis of left PFSS. She reports that 4 months ago, she began training for a marathon, and that she has experienced a diffuse ache around her anterior left patella for the last 2 months. She had increased her mileage gradually to the point that she was jogging 3 to 7 miles, four times per week. After 1 month of participation in the program, B. G. was experiencing left knee pain after completing her jog. This pain resolved within about 1 hour after stopping the activity. B.G.continued to jog, but noticed that her pain got progressively worse over the next 2 months. Currently, B. G. reports that she experiences pain in her left knee if she sits with her knee flexed for more than 45 minutes,

when ascending and descending stairs, and when she runs more than 1 mile.

Examination reveals that B. G. has pain on palpation of the posterolateral aspect of the left patella. She also has a positive Ely's test, a measurement of rectus femoris tightness.[131] On visual inspection, the patella orientation was consistent in demonstrating some malalignments. At 20 degrees of knee flexion, B. G.'s patella was sitting 10 mm closer to the lateral femoral epicondyle than the medial femoral epicondyle. When B. G. is positioned in supine with her knee extended, the medial border of the patella is higher than the lateral border. These patterns of patella alignment may contribute to the symptoms of PFSS.[132]

Continued

Questions to Consider

- Given this patient's history and current presentation, what additional tests and measures would be helpful information in your evaluation process?
- What is your movement dysfunction-related diagnosis for this patient?
- What might the prognosis be for this patient? What are the patient's goals for intervention? What are your rehabilitation goals? How long to do you think it will take to achieve the goals that you and the patient agree upon?
- Based on the patient's goals and expectations, as well as your understanding of the underlying disease process, what recommendations would you make for intervention at this point in time?
- What evidence from the clinical research literature supports your recommendations? Why have you chosen and/or prioritized these possible interventions?
- How will you assess whether the patients and rehabilitation goals have been met?
- What type of follow-up would you recommend for this patient?

Recommendations for a Patient with Patellofemoral Stress Syndrome

B. G. states that her pain decreased after her course of therapy. She had greater sitting tolerance, can ascend and descend stairs with no pain, and has resumed running. However, she runs 3 miles 4 days a week. She experienced mild discomfort at the end of her run, but this resolved after 30 minutes. B. G.'s goal was to increase her jogging distance to that of her original exercise program; however, she was concerned that her symptoms would recur. She asked the therapist whether wearing a knee orthosis during exercise would be beneficial. The therapist recommended a patellofemoral brace with a lateral buttress for long-distance running. This orthosis would help minimize B. G.'s excessive lateral patella tracking and, hopefully, reduce her pain. The therapist also strongly recommended that B. G. continue with her exercise program for soft tissue work, strengthening her hip abductors, external rotators, and quadriceps muscle, even as her running time and distance increases.

SUMMARY

This chapter reviews the normal structure and function of the tibiofemoral and patellofemoral joints, with special focus on arthrokinematics and osteokinematics of the knee joint. The different categories of knee orthoses for the knee complex are rehabilitation orthoses, functional orthoses, prophylactic orthoses, unloader orthoses, and patellofemoral orthoses. A review of the research literature offers some support to the use of knee orthoses. However, there appears to be a gap between what many of the braces are designed to do and evidence of their efficacy. This chapter identifies research strategies that are most frequently used in the study of knee orthoses and discusses problems with research design, methods, and generalizability to patients and athletes involved in dynamic activities. Similar problems exist when the role of patellofemoral orthoses in sports medicine and rehabilitation are considered. It is important for clinicians to realize that although there is a lack of clear consensus supporting the use of knee orthoses, that knee orthoses should be a consideration as an intervention for a patient who presents with knee pain. Despite the lack of consensus amongst evidence-based data, the subjective reports of patients can always give the most important information about whether a knee orthosis may be beneficial.

This chapter is intended to give health care professionals the ability to better evaluate the intent and design of knee orthoses and to ask for clinically applicable evidence of efficacy from brace designers and manufacturers. This chapter is also intended to encourage clinicians to contribute to the understanding of knee orthoses in rehabilitation and long-term management of patients with ligamentous instability by participating in clinical research.

REFERENCES

1. Cawley PW. *Is Knee Bracing Really Necessary? A Review of Current Research on Brace Function, the Natural History of Graft Remodeling, and Physiologic Implications.* Carlsbad, CA: Smith & Nephew Donjoy Biomechanics Research Laboratory; 1989.
2. Trautman P. Lower limb orthoses. In: Redford JB, Basmajian JV, Trautman P, eds. *Orthotics: Clinical Practice and Rehabilitation Technology.* New York: Churchill Livingstone; 1995:13–54.
3. Drez D, DeHaven K, D'Ambrosia R. *Knee Braces Seminar Report.* Chicago: American Academy of Orthopaedic Surgeons; 1984.
4. Paluska SA, McKeag DB. Knee braces: current evidence and clinical recommendations for their use. *Am Fam Physician.* 2000;61(2):411–418, 423–424.
5. Chew KT, Lew HL, Date E, et al. Current evidence and clinical applications of therapeutic knee braces. *Am J Phys Med Rehabil.* 2007;86(8):678–686.
6. Nordin M, Frankel VH. Biomechanics of the knee. In: Nordin M, Frankel VH, eds. *Basic Biomechanics of the Musculoskeletal System.* 3rd ed. Philadelphia: Lippincott Williams & Wilkins; 2001.
7. Levangie PK, Norkin CC. The knee complex. In: *Joint Structure and Function: A Comprehensive Analysis.* 3rd ed. Philadelphia: FA Davis; 2001.
8. Neumann DA. Knee. In: Neumann DA, ed. *Kinesiology of the Musculoskeletal System: Foundations for Rehabilitation.* 2nd ed. St. Louis: Mosby Elsevier; 2010.
9. Antich TJ. Orthoses for the knee: the tibiofemoral joint. In: Nawoczenski DA, Epler ME, eds. *Orthotics in Functional Rehabilitation of the Lower Limb.* Philadelphia: Saunders; 1997:57–76.
10. Terry GC, Hughston JC, Norwood LA. Anatomy of the iliopatellar band and iliotibial tract. *Am J Sports Med.* 1986;14(1):39–45.
11. Greenfield BH. Functional anatomy of the knee. In: Greenfield BH, ed. *Rehabilitation of the Knee: A Problem Solving Approach.* Philadelphia: Davis; 1993:1–42.

12. Cox AJ. Biomechanics of the patello-femoral joint. *Clin Biomech (Bristol, Avon)* 1990;5:123–130.

13. Grabiner MD, Koh TJ, Draganich LF. Neuromechanics of the patellofemoral joint. *Med Sci Sports Exerc.* 1994;26(1):10–21.

14. Palumbo PM. Dynamic patellar brace: a new orthosis in the management of patellofemoral disorders. *Am J Sports Med.* 1981;9(1):45–49.

15. Van Kampen A, Huiskes R. The three-dimensional tracking pattern of the human patella. *J Orthop Res.* 1990;8(3):372–382.

16. Larson RL, Cabaud HE, Slocum DB, et al. The patellar compression syndrome: surgical treatment by lateral retinacular release. *Clin Orthop.* 1978;34:158–167.

17. Wiberg G. Roentgenographic and anatomic studies on the femoropatellar joint: with special references to chondromalacia patellae. *Acta Orthop Scand.* 1941;12:319–409.

18. Ward SR. Biomechanical applications to joint structure and functio n. In: PK Levangie, CC Norkin, eds. *Joint Structure and Function: A Comprehensive Analysis.* 5th ed. Philadephia: FA Davis; 2011.

19. Muller W. *The Knee: Form, Function, and Ligament Reconstruction.* Berlin: Springer-Verlag; 1985.

20. Regalbuto MA, Rovic JS, Walker PS. The forces in a knee brace as a function of hinge design and placement. *Am J Sports Med.* 1989;17:535–543.

21. Bassett GS, Fleming BW. The Lenox Hill brace in anterolateral rotatory instability. *Am J Sports Med.* 1983;11(5):345–348.

22. Branch TP, Hunter RE. Functional analysis of anterior cruciate ligament braces. *Clin Sports Med.* 1990;9(4):771–797.

23. Nicholas JA. Bracing the anterior cruciate ligament deficient knee using the Lenox Hill derotation brace. *Clin Orthop.* 1983;172:137–142.

24. Beets CL, Clippinger FW, Hazard PR, et al. Orthoses and the dynamic knee: a basic overview. *Orthot Prosthet.* 1985;39(2):33–39.

25. DeCoster LC, Vailas JC. Functional anterior cruciate ligament bracing: a survey of current brace prescription patterns. *Orthopedics.* 2003;26(7):701–706.

26. Kramer JF, Dubowitz T, Fowler P, et al. Functional knee braces and dynamic performance: a review. *Clin J Sports Med.* 1997;7:32–39.

27. Nemeth G, Lamontagne M, Tho KS, et al. Electromyographic activity in expert downhill skiers using functional knee braces after anterior cruciate ligament injuries. *Am J Sports Med.* 1997;25(5):635–641.

28. Fleming BC, Renstrom PA, Beynnon BD, et al. The influence of functional knee bracing on the anterior cruciate ligament strain biomechanics in weightbearing and nonweightbearing knees. *Am J Sports Med.* 2000;28(6):815–824.

29. Sterett WI, Briggs KK, Farley T, et al. Effect of functional bracing in skiers with anterior cruciate ligament reconstruction: a prospective cohort study. *Am J Sports Med.* 2006;34(10):1581–1585.

30. Stephens DL. The effects of functional knee braces on speed in collegiate basketball players. *JOSPT.* 1995;22(6):259–262.

31. Highgenboten CL, Jackson A, Meske N. The effects of knee brace wear on perceptual and metabolic variables during horizontal treadmill running. *Am J Sports Med.* 1991;19(6):639–643.

32. Wojtys EM, Kothari SU, Huston LJ. Anterior cruciate ligament functional brace use in sports. *Am J Sports Med.* 1996;24(4):539–546.

33. Grace TG, Skipper BJ, Newberry JC, et al. Prophylactic knee braces and injury to the lower extremity. *J Bone Joint Surg.* 1988;70A(3):422–427.

34. Styf JR, Nakhostine M, Gershuni DH. Functional knee braces increase intramuscular pressures in the anterior compartment of the leg. *Am J Sports Med.* 1992;20(1):46–49.

35. Styf J. The effects of functional knee bracing on muscle function and performance. *Sports Med.* 1999;(2):77–81.

36. Sforzo GA, Chen NM, Gold CA, et al. The effect of prophylactic knee bracing on performance. *Med Sci Sports Exerc.* 1989;1:254–257.

37. Styf JR, Lundin O, Gershuni DH. Effects of a functional knee brace on leg muscle function. *Am J Sports Med.* 1994;22:830–834.

38. McDevitt ER, Taylor DC, Miller MD, et al. Functional bracing after anterior cruciate ligament reconstruction: a prospective, randomized, multicenter study. *Am J Sports Med.* 2004;32(8):1887–1892.

39. Black KP, Raasch WG. Knee braces in sports. In: Nicholas JA, Hershman EB, eds. *The Lower Extremity and Spine in Sports Medicine.* 2nd ed. St. Louis: Mosby; 1995:987–998.

40. Erickson AN, Yasuda K, Beynnon B. An in vitro dynamic evaluation of prophylactic knee braces during lateral impact loading. *Am J Sports Med.* 1993;21:26–35.

41. Garrick JG, Requa RK. Prophylactic knee bracing. *Am J Sports Med.* 1987;15(5):471–476.

42. France PE, Paulos LE. Knee bracing. *J Am Acad Orthop Surg.* 1994;2(5):281–287.

43. Edelstein JE, Bruckner J. *Orthotics: A Comprehensive Clinical Approach.* Thorofare, NJ: Slack Inc; 2002:59–71.

44. Baker BE, VanHanswyk E, Bogosian SP, et al. The effect of knee braces on lateral impact loading of the knee. *Am J Sports Med.* 1989;17(2):182–186.

45. Baker BE, VanHanswyk E, Bogosian SP. A biomechanical study of the static stabilizing effect of knee braces on medial stability. *Am J Sports Med.* 1987;15:566–570.

46. France EP, Paulos LE, Jayaraman G, et al. The biomechanics of lateral knee bracing. Part II: Impact response of the braced knee. *Am J Sports Med.* 1987;15(5):430–438.

47. Paulos LE, France EP, Rosenberg TD, et al. The biomechanics of lateral knee bracing. Part I: Response of the valgus restraints to loading. *Am J Sports Med.* 1987;15(5):419–429.

48. Paulos LE, Cawley PW, France EP. Impact biomechanics of lateral knee bracing. The anterior cruciate ligament. *Am J Sports Med.* 1991;19(4):337–342.

49. Hewson GF, Mendini RA, Wang JB. Prophylactic knee bracing in college football. *Am J Sports Med.* 1986;14(4):262–266.

50. Rovere GD, Haupt HA, Yates CS. Prophylactic knee bracing in college football. *Am J Sports Med.* 1987;15(2):111–116.

51. Sitler M, Ryan J, Hopkinson W, et al. The efficacy of a prophylactic knee brace to reduce injuries in football. A prospective, randomized study at West Point. *Am J Sports Med.* 1990;18(3):310–315.

52. Teitz CC, Hermanson BK, Kronmal RA, et al. Evaluation of the use of braces to prevent injury to the knee in collegiate football players. *J Bone Joint Surg.* 1987;69A(1):2–9.

53. Albright JP, Powell JW, Smith W, et al. Medial collateral ligament knee sprains in college football. *Am J Sports Med.* 1994;22(1):12–18.

54. Borsa PA, Lephart SM, Fu FH. Muscular and functional performance characteristics of individuals wearing prophylactic knee braces. *J Athletic Training.* 1993;28(4):336–342.

55. Liggett CL, Tandy RD, Young JC. The effects of prophylactic knee bracing on running gait. *J Athletic Training.* 1995;30(2):159–161.

56. Osternig LR, Robertson RN. Effects of prophylactic bracing on lower extremity joint position and muscle activation during running. *Am J Sports Med.* 1993;21(5):733–737.

57. Van Horn DA, Makinnion JL, Witt PL. Comparison of the effects of the Anderson knee stabler and McDavid knee guard on the kinematics of the lower extremity during gait. *JOSPT.* 1988;9(7):254–260.

58. Veldhuizen JW, Koene FM, Oostvogel HJ. The effects of a supportive knee brace on leg performance in healthy subjects. *Int J Sports Med.* 1991;12(6):577–580.

59. Deppen RJ, Landfried MJ. Efficacy of prophylactic knee bracing in high school football players. *JOSPT.* 1994;20(5):243–246.

60. Greene DL, Hamson KR, Bay RC, et al. Effects of protective knee bracing on speed and agility. *Am J Sports Med.* 2000;28(4):453–459.

61. Sforzo GA, Chen NM, Gold CA, et al. The effect of prophylactic knee bracing on performance. *Med Sci Sports Exerc.* 1989;21(3):254–257.

62. Borsa PA, Lephart SM, Fu FH. Muscular and functional performance characteristics of individuals wearing prophylactic knee braces. *J Athletic Train.* 1993;28(4):336–344.

63. Liggett CL, Tandy RD, Young JC. The effects of prophylactic knee bracing on running gait. *J Athletic Train.* 1995;30(2):159–161.

64. Martin TJ, Committee on Sports Medicine and Fitness. American Academy of Pediatrics. Technical Report: knee brace use in the young athlete. *Pediatrics.* 2001;108(2):503–507.

65. Sanders MS, Cates RA, Baker MD, et al. Knee injuries and the use of prophylactic knee bracing in off-road motorcycling: results of a large-scale epidemiological study. *Am J Sports Med.* 2011;39(7):1395–1400.

66. Gardner HF, Clippinger FW. A method for location of prosthetic and orthotic knee joints. *Artif Limbs.* 1979;13:31–35.

67. Lew WD, Patrnchak CM, Lewis JL, et al. A comparison of pistoning forces in orthotic knee joints. *Orthot Prosthet.* 1984;36(2):85–95.

68. Regalbuto MA, Rovick JS, Walker PS. The forces in a knee brace as a function of hinge design and placement. *Am J Sports Med.* 1989;17(4):535–542.

69. Noyes FR, Grood ES, Butler DL, et al. Clinical laxity tests and functional stability of the knee: biomechanical concepts. *Clin Orthop.* 1980;146:84–89.

70. Wojtys EM, Loubert PV, Samson SY, et al. Use of a knee-brace for control of tibial translation and rotation. *J Bone Joint Surg.* 1990;72A(9):1323–1329.

71. Colville MR, Lee CL, Ciullo JV. The Lenox Hill brace. An evaluation of effectiveness in treating knee instability. *Am J Sports Med.* 1986;14(4):257–261.

72. Wojtys E, Kothari W, Huston L. Anterior cruciate ligament functional brace use in sports. *Am J Sports Med.* 1996;24(2):539–546.

73. Wojtys E, Huston L. "Custom-Fit" versus "Off-the-Shelf" ACL functional braces. *Am J Knee Surg.* 2001;14(3):157–162.

74. Beynnon B, Ryder S, Konradsen L, et al. The effect of anterior cruciate ligament trauma and bracing on knee proprioception. *Am J Sports Med.* 1999;27(2):150–155.

75. Lam RY, Ng GY, Chien EP. Does wearing a functional knee brace affect hamstring reflex time in subjects with anterior cruciate ligament deficiency during muscle fatigue? *Arch Phys Med Rehabil.* 2002;83:1009–1012.

76. Birmingham TB, Bryant DM, Griffin JR, et al. A randomized controlled trial comparing the effectiveness of functional knee brace and neoprene sleeve use after anterior cruciate ligament reconstruction. *Am J Sports Med.* 2008;36(4):648–655.

77. Birmingham TB, Kramer JF, Kirkley A, et al. Knee bracing after ACL reconstruction: effects on postural control and proprioception. *Med Sci Sports Exerc.* 2001;33(8):1253–1258.

78. Beck C, Drez D, Young J, et al. Instrumented testing of functional knee braces. *Am J Sports Med.* 1986;14(4):253–256.

79. Beynnon BD, Pope MH, Wertheimer CM, et al. The effect of functional knee-braces on strain on the anterior cruciate ligament in vivo. *J Bone Joint Surg.* 1992;74A(9):1298–1312.

80. Jonsson H, Kärrholm J. Brace effects on the unstable knee in 21 cases. A roentgen stereophotogrammetric comparison of three designs. *Acta Orthop Scand.* 1990;61(4):313–318.

81. Mishra DK, Daniel DM, Stone ML. The use of functional knee braces in the control of pathologic anterior knee laxity. *Clin Orthop.* 1989;241:213–220.

82. Soma CA, Cawley PW, Liu S, et al. Custom-fit versus premanufactured braces. *Orthopedics.* 2004;27(3):307–310.

83. Ramsey D, Lamontagne M, Wretenberg P, et al. Assessment of functional knee bracing: an in vivo three-dimensional kinematic analysis of the anterior cruciate deficient knee. *Clin Biomech (Bristol, Avon).* 2001;16:61–70.

84. Branch TP, Hunter RE, Donath M. Dynamic EMG analysis of anterior cruciate deficient legs with and without bracing during cutting. *Am J Sports Med.* 1989;17(1):35–41.

85. Wu GK, Ng GY, Mak AF. Effects of knee bracing on the sensorimotor function of subjects with anterior cruciate ligament reconstruction. *Am J Sports Med.* 2001;29(5):641–645.

86. Moller E, Forssblad M, Hanson L, et al. Bracing versus nonbracing in rehabilitation after anterior cruciate ligament reconstruction: a randomized prospective study with 2-year follow-up. *Knee Surg Sports Traumatol Arthrosc.* 2001;9(2):102–108.

87. Wu GK, Ng GY, Mak AF. Effects of knee bracing on the functional performance of patients with anterior cruciate ligament reconstruction. *Arch Phys Med Rehabil.* 2001;82(2):282–285.

88. Ramsey D, Wretenberg P, Lamontagne M, et al. Electromyographic and biomechanic analysis of anterior cruciate ligament deficiency and functional knee bracing. *Clin Biomech (Bristol, Avon).* 2003;18:28–34.

89. Cook FF, Tibone JE, Redfern FC. A dynamic analysis of a functional brace for anterior cruciate ligament insufficiency. *Am J Sports Med.* 1989;17(4):519–524.

90. Marans HJ, Jackson RW, Piccinin J, et al. Functional testing of braces for anterior cruciate ligament–deficient knees. *Can J Surg.* 1991;34(2):167–172.

91. Zetterlund AE, Serfass RC, Hunter RE. The effect of wearing the complete Lenox Hill derotation brace on energy expenditure during horizontal treadmill running at 161 meters per minute. *Am J Sports Med.* 1986;14(1):73–76.

92. Yanagawa T, Shelburne K, Serpas F, et al. Effect of hamstrings muscle action on stability of anterior cruciate ligament-deficient knee in isokinetic extension exercise. *Clin Biomech (Bristol, Avon).* 2002;17(9–10):705–712.

93. Giove TP, Miller 3rd SJ, Kent BE, et al. Higher levels of sports participation in patients whose hamstring strength was equal to or greater than quadriceps. *J Bone Joint Surg.* 1983;65A(2):184–192.

94. Lass P, Kaalund S, LeFevre S, et al. Muscle coordination following rupture of anterior cruciate ligament. Electromyographic studies of 14 patients. *Acta Orthop Scand.* 1991;62(1):9–14.

95. Kirst J, Gillquist J. Sagittal plane knee translation and electromyographic activity during closed and open kinetic chain exercise in anterior cruciate ligament-deficient patients and control subjects. *Am J Sports Med.* 2001;29(1):72–82.

96. Chmieleski TL, Rudolph KS, Snyder-Mackler L. Development of dynamic knee stability after acute anterior cruciate ligament injury. *J Electromyogr Kinesiol.* 2002;12(4):267–274.

97. Loomer R, Horlick S. Valgus knee bracing for medial gonarthrosis. *Clin J Sport Med.* 1993;3:251–255.

98. Self B, Greenwald RM, Pflaster D. A biomechanical analysis of a medial unloading brace for osteoarthritis in the knee. *Arthritis Care Res.* 2000;14(4):191–197.

99. Lindenfeld T, Hewett T, Andriacchi TP. Joint loading with valgus bracing in patients with varus gonarthrosis. *Clin Orthop Relat Res.* 1997;344:290–297.

100. Hewett TE, Noyes FR, Barber-Westin SD, et al. Decrease in knee joint pain and increase in function in patients with medial compartment arthrosis: a prospective analysis of valgus bracing. *Orthopedics.* 1998;21(2):131–138.

101. Pollo FE, Otis JC, Wickiewicz TL, et al. Biomechanical analysis of valgus bracing for the osteoarthritic knee. Presentation at the first North American clinical gait lab conference, Portland, Oregon; 1994.

102. Katsuragawa Y, Fukui N, Nakamura K. Change of bone density with valgus knee bracing. *Int Orthop.* 1999;23(3):164–167.

103. Horlick SG, Loomer RL. Valgus knee bracing for medial gonarthrosis. *Clin J Sports Med.* 1993;3(4):251–255.

104. Birmingham TB, Kramer JF, Kirkley A, et al. Knee bracing for medial compartment osteoarthritis: effects on proprioception and postural control. *Rheumatology (Oxford).* 2001;40(3):285–289.

105. Nadaud MC, Komistek RD, Mahfouz MR, et al. In vivo three-dimensional determination of the effectiveness of the osteoarthritic knee brace: a multiple brace analysis. *J Bone Joint Surg Am.* 2005;87:114–119.

106. Slemenda C, Brandt KD, Heilman DK, et al. Quadriceps weakness a primary risk factor for knee pain. *Ann Intern Med.* 1997;127(2):97–104.

107. Hurley MV. The role of muscle weakness in pathogenesis of osteoarthritis. *Rheum Dis North Am.* 1999;25(2):283–298.

108. Ramsey DK, Briem K, Axe MJ, et al. A mechanical theory for the effectiveness of bracing for medial compartment osteoarthritis of the knee. *J Bone Joint Surg Am.* 2007;89:2398–2407.

109. Hochberg MC, Altman RD, Brandt KD, et al. Guidelines for the medical management of osteoarthritis. *Arthritis Rheum.* 1995;38(11):1541–1546.

110. Raja K, Dewan N. Efficacy of knee braces and foot orthoses in conservative management of knee osteoarthritis: a systematic review. *Am J Phys Med Rehabil.* 2011;90:247–262.

111. Divine JG, Hewett TE. Valgus bracing for degenerative knee osteoarthritis: relieving pain, improving gait, and increasing activity. *Phys Sports Med.* 2005;33(2):40–46.

112. Belyea BC. Orthoses for the knee: the patellofemoral joint. In: Nawoczenski DA, Eppler ME, eds. *Orthotics in Functional Rehabilitation of the Lower Limb.* Philadelphia: Saunders; 1997:31–56.

113. Levine J, Splain S. Use of the infrapatellar strap in the treatment of patellofemoral pain. *Clin Orthop.* 1979;139:179–181.

114. Levine J. A new brace for chondromalacia patella and kindred conditions. *Am J Sports Med.* 1978;6(3):137–140.

115. Powers CM, Shellock FG, Beering TV, et al. Effect of bracing on patellar kinematics in patients with patellofemoral joint pain. *Med Sci Sports Exerc.* 1999;31(12):1714–1720.

116. Timm K. Randomized controlled trial of Protonics on patellar pain, position, and function. *Med Sci Sports Exerc.* 1998;30(5):665–670.

117. D'hondt NE, Struijs PA, Kerkhoffs GMJ, et al. Orthotic devices for treating patellofemoral pain syndrome (Cochrane Review). In: *The Cochrane Library.* Issue 2, 2003.

118. Wilson NA, Mazahery BT, Koh JL, et al. Effect of bracing on dynamic patellofemoral contact mechanics. *J Rehabil Res Dev.* 2010;47(6):531–542.

119. Powers CM, Ward SR, Chan LD, et al. The effect of bracing on patella alignment and patellofemoral contact area. *Med Sci Sports Exerc.* 2004;36(7):1226–1232.

120. Reikeras O. Brace with a lateral pad for patellar pain: 2 year follow-up of 25 patients. *Acta Orthop Scand.* 1990;61:319–320.

121. DeHaven KE, Lolan WA, Mayer PJ. Chondromalacia patellae in athletes: clinical presentation and conservative management. *Am J Sports Med.* 1979;7(1):5–11.

122. Malek M, Mangine R. Patellofemoral pain syndromes: a comprehensive and conservative approach. *J Orthop Sports Phys Ther.* 1981;2(3):108–116.

123. Crocker B, Stauber WT. Objective analysis of quadriceps force during bracing of the patella: a preliminary study. *Aust J Sci Med Sport.* 1989;21:25–28.

124. Bohnsack M, Halcour A, Klagen P, et al. The influence of patellar bracing on patellar and knee load-distribution and kinematics: an experimental cadaver study. *Knee Surg Sports Traumatol Arthrosc.* 2008;16:135–141.

125. Selfe J, Richards J, Thewlis D, et al. The biomechanics of step descent under different treatment modalities used in patellofemoral pain. *Gait Posture.* 2008;27:258–263.

126. Crossley K, Bennell K, Green S, et al. A systematic review of physical interventions for patellofemoral pain syndrome. *Clin J Sport Med.* 2001;11(2):103–110.

127. Finestone A, Radin EL, Lev B, et al. Treatment of overuse patellofemoral pain. Prospective randomized controlled clinical trial in a military setting. *Clin Orthop Relat Res.* 1993;293:208–210.

128. Greenwald AE, Bagley AM, France P, et al. A biomechanical and clinical evaluation of a patellofemoral knee brace. *Clin Orthop Relat Res.* 1996;324:187–195.

129. BenGal S, Lowe J, Mann G, et al. The role of the knee brace in the prevention of anterior knee pain syndrome. *Am J Sports Med.* 1997;25(1):118–122.

130. Earl JE, Hoch AZ. A proximal strengthening program improves pain, function, and biomechanics in women with patellofemoral pain syndrome. *Am J Sports Med.* 2011;39(1):154–163.

131. Magee DJ. Hip. In: *Orthopedic Physical Assessment.* New York: Saunders; 2002: 632.

132. McConnell J. Management of patellofemoral problems. *Man Ther.* 2000;1(2):60–66.

ADDITIONAL RESOURCES

Bellamy MM. Controversy faces braces. *Sportcare Fitness.* 1988; Sept/Oct:17–24.

Burns GS, Hull ML, Patterson HA. Strain in the anteromedial bundle of the anterior cruciate ligament under combination loading. *Orthop Res.* 1992;10:167–176.

Cawley PW. Postoperative knee bracing. *Clin Sports Med.* 1990;9(4):763–770.

Cawley PW, France EP, Paulos LE. The current state of functional knee bracing research. A review of the literature. *Am J Sports Med.* 1991;19(3):226–233.

France EP, Cawley PW, Paulos LE. Choosing functional knee braces. *Clin Sports Med.* 1990;9(4):743–750.

Fuss FK. Anatomy of the cruciate ligaments and their function in extension and flexion of the human knee joint. *Am J Anat.* 1989;184(2):165–176.

Gray HG. *Gray's Anatomy.* Philadelphia: Running Press; 1974: 274–276.

Henry JH. The patellofemoral joint. In: Nicholas JA, Hershman EB, eds. *The Lower Extremity and Spine in Sports Medicine.* 2nd ed.Philadelphia: Mosby; 1995:940–970.

Hofmann AA, Wyatt RWB, Bourne MH, et al. Knee stability in orthotic knee braces. *Am J Sports Med.* 1984;12(5):371–374.

Houston ME, Goemans PH. Leg muscle performance of athletes with and without knee support braces. *Arch Phys Med Rehabil.* 1982;63(9):431–432.

Liu SH, Daluiski A, Kabo JM. The effects of thigh soft-tissue stiffness on the control of anterior tibial displacement by functional knee orthoses. *J Rehabil Res Dev.* 1995;32(2):135–140.

Seebacher JR, Inglis AE, Marshal JL. The structure of the posterolateral aspect of the knee. *J Bone Joint Surg.* 1982;64(4):536.

Sell KE. On the field again: knee bracing options. *Adv Rehabil.* 1996:March:51–53.

Silbey MB, Fu FH. Knee injuries. In: Fu FH, Stone DA, eds. *Sports Injuries. Mechanisms, Prevention, Treatment.* Baltimore: Williams & Wilkins; 1994:949–976.

Terry GC. The anatomy of the extensor mechanism. *Clin Sports Med.* 1989;8(2):163–177.

Warren LF, Marshall JL. The supportive structures and layers on the medial side of the knee. An anatomical analysis. *J Bone Joint Surg* 1979;61(1):56.

12

Orthoses in Orthopedic Care and Trauma

MICHELLE M. LUSARDI, WILLIAM J. BARRINGER, MELVIN L. STILLS, JOSHUA L. CARTER,
AND MARK CHARLSON

LEARNING OBJECTIVES

On completion of this chapter, the reader will be able to:

1. Describe the most common musculoskeletal injuries that occur at various points in the life span.
2. Describe orthotic intervention for congenital and growth-related musculoskeletal impairments.
3. Classify fracture of bone by type and severity and describe the interventions most often used by orthopedists and orthopedic surgeons on the basis of fracture type.
4. Delineate the roles of health care team members in the rehabilitation and orthotic management of individuals with congenital and acquired musculoskeletal impairment.

Orthoses play a significant role in orthopedic and rehabilitative care of individuals with many different types of musculoskeletal pathologies and impairments. Dysfunction of the musculoskeletal system can be the result of congenital or developmental disorders or can be acquired as a result of overuse injury, systemic disease, infection, neoplasm, or trauma at any point in the life span. This chapter focuses on the use of orthoses to manage congenital and developmental musculoskeletal problems in children and fractures of long bones of the lower extremity.

The understanding of how orthoses are helpful in the care of those with musculoskeletal impairments is founded on knowledge of the development and physiology of musculoskeletal tissues (bone, cartilage, ligaments, menisci, muscles, and their tendons or aponeuroses); the kinesiological relationships among these tissues; and an understanding of how these tissues remodel in response to physical stressors (forces).[1,2] This chapter begins with an overview of the anatomy of bone, its growth and remodeling, and the principles behind the rehabilitation (examination and intervention) of persons with disorders of bone. Then the authors look specifically at disorders of the hip joint and orthotic/orthopedic strategies for limb fractures.

BONE STRUCTURE AND FUNCTION

In anatomy classes and texts, students learn that the mature adult human skeleton is composed of 206 bones (Figure 12-1), ranging from the long bones of the extremities, the blocklike vertebrae of the spine, the encasing protective ribs and skull, and the multiarticulating carpals and tarsals of the wrist and ankles that enable positioning of the hands and feet for functional activities.[3,4] Bony prominences formed during development from the force of muscle contraction at tendinous origins and insertions are identified.[1] Students scrutinize articular surfaces to understand how joints move, consider the hyaline cartilage that protects the joint from repeated loading and shear during activity, and learn to examine the ligaments that maintain alignment for normal joint function. From a skeletal model or examination of bone specimens in anatomy laboratory, it is not intuitively apparent that living bone is a dynamic and metabolically active tissue serving multiple purposes and physiological roles.[5] These include storage and homeostasis of calcium, phosphate, magnesium, sodium, and carbonate (via ongoing osteoblastic and osteoclastic activity in conjunction with kidney function); production of erythrocytes, granular leukocytes, and platelets in the marrow; physical growth and development (by responsiveness to the pituitary's hormones at the epiphyseal plate); provision of a protective and functional frame for the organs of the thorax and abdomen (how would people breathe without ribs?); and body weight support when the body is either at rest or in motion during functional activities.[6]

Bone is a dense, regular, connective tissue derived from embryonic mesoderm. It contains a combination of specialized cells (osteoblasts, osteocytes, osteoclasts) embedded in a matrix of minerals (70%), protein (22%), and water (8%). The many bones of the human body can be described as long or short tubular bone (e.g., the femur, tibia, metatarsals, phalanges), flat bone (e.g., the pelvis or skull), irregular bone (e.g., the tarsals and carpals), sesamoid bone embedded within tendons (e.g., patella), or accessory bones (e.g., ossicles of the middle ear). Alternatively, they can be classified as primarily cortical (dense) or cancellous (trabecular) bone on the basis of the density and arrangement of their components. Long bones are subdivided into regions, each of which has its own blood supply (Figure 12-2). The diaphysis (shaft) is supplied by one or more nutrient arteries that penetrate the layers of the bony cortex, dividing into central longitudinal arteries within the marrow cavity. The flared metaphyses serve as an area of transition from cortical to cancellous bone and are supplied by separate metaphysical arterioles. The epiphyses are metabolically active areas of cancellous bone with supportive trabeculae, with an extensive capillary network derived from

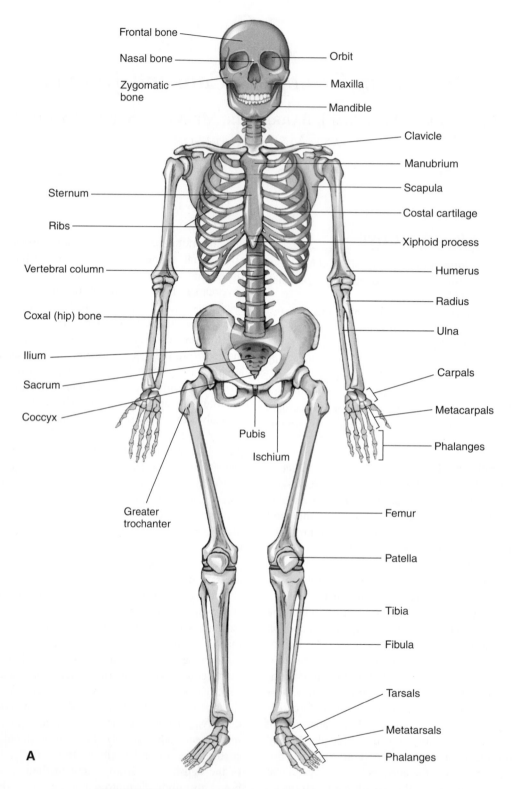

Frontal bone

Nasal bone

Zygomatic bone

Orbit

Maxilla

Mandible

Clavicle

Manubrium

Scapula

Sternum

Ribs

Costal cartilage

Xiphoid process

Vertebral column

Humerus

Radius

Ulna

Coxal (hip) bone

Ilium

Sacrum

Coccyx

Carpals

Metacarpals

Phalanges

Pubis

Ischium

Greater trochanter

Femur

Patella

Tibia

Fibula

Tarsals

Metatarsals

Phalanges

A

FIGURE 12-1 The bones of the human skeleton. **A,** Anterior view.

epiphyseal arteries. The epiphysis is actively remodeled over the life span in response to weight bearing and muscle contraction during activity.[7] In childhood and adolescence, before skeletal maturation, the bony metaphyses and epiphyses are connected by cartilaginous epiphyseal (growth) plate, which calcifies and fuses throughout various periods of development.

The periosteum is a layer of less dense, vascularized connective tissue that overlies and protects the external surface of all bone and houses osteoblastic cells necessary for bone deposition and growth. The periosteum is replaced by articular (hyaline) cartilage within the joint capsule. The endosteum, a thin connective tissue lining of the marrow cavity of long

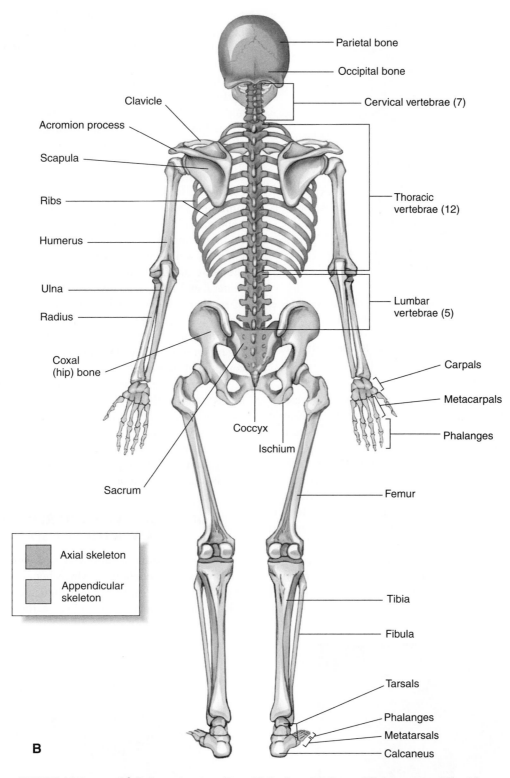

FIGURE 12-1—cont'd B, Posterior view. (From Thibodeau GA, Patton KT. *Anatomy and Physiology.* 5th ed. St. Louis: Mosby, 2003.)

bones and the internal spaces of cancellous bone of the marrow space, also houses osteoblasts. Both linings are active as part of osteogenesis during growth and fracture healing.

Cortical bone is the most highly mineralized type of bone found in the shafts (diaphyses) of the long bones of the body and serves as the outer protective layer of the metaphysis and epiphysis of tubular bone, as well as the external layers of flat, irregular, and sesamoid bones. Most of the bones in the human skeleton (80% to 85%) are primarily cortical with cancellous/trabecular bone in the metaphyseal and epiphyseal region. Cross section of a long tubular bone reveals three layers of cortical bone: the inner or endosteal region next to

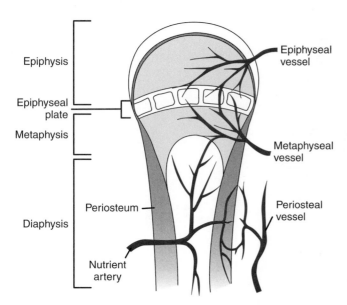

FIGURE 12-2 Diagram of the regions (epiphysis, epiphyseal plate, metaphysis, and diaphysis) of a long bone and their arterial vascular supply. (Modified from Lundon K. *Orthopedic Rehabilitation Science, Principles for Clinical Management of Bone.* Boston: Butterworth Heinemann, 2000.)

the marrow cavity, the metabolic intracortical or haversian region with its haversian canals surrounded by concentric layered rings (osteons) and Volkmann's canals containing a perpendicularly arranged anastomosing capillary network, and the dense outer periosteal region (Figure 12-3).

Cancellous (trabecular) bone with its honeycomb or spongy appearance is much more metabolically active and much less mineralized than cortical bone. Cancellous bone is composed of branching bony spicules (trabeculae) arranged in interconnecting lamellae to form a framework for weight bearing (Figure 12-4A). In the vertebral bodies, for example, trabeculae are arranged in an interconnecting horizontal and vertical network oriented perpendicular to the lines of weight-bearing stress into a boxlike shape (see Figure 12-4B).

In contrast, trabeculae in the proximal femur form an arch-like structure to support weight-bearing forces between the hip joint and femoral shaft (see Figure 12-4C). In living bone, cavities between trabeculae are filled with bone marrow.

Three types of cells are embedded within the various compartments of bone. *Osteoblasts*, bone building cells, synthesize and secrete the organic matrix of bone (osteoid) that mineralizes as bone matures. They are located under periosteum and endosteum and are active in times of bone growth and repair. *Osteocytes* are matured and inactive osteoblasts that have become embedded within bone matrix. Osteocytes remain connected to active osteoblasts via long dendritic processes running through the canaliculi (small channels) within the bone matrix. Both osteoblasts and osteocytes are responsive to circulating growth hormones, growth factors, and cytokines, as well as mechanical stressors and fluid flow within the bone itself.[8,9] Osteocytes are thought to be involved in mineral exchange, detection of strain and fatigue, and control of mechanically induced remodeling.[10] *Osteoclasts*, derived from precursor cells in bone marrow, are macrophage-like cells that can move throughout bone to resorb bone by releasing minerals from the matrix and removing damaged organic components of bone.[11,12]

The epiphyses of long bones, the vertebrae, and large flat bones house nociceptors and mechanoreceptors and a network of afferent sensory neurons that contribute to exteroceptive (primarily pain) pathways.[13] The periosteum has a particularly rich neural network with branches that continue along with penetrating nutrient arteries into the haversian canals into the diaphysis.

BONE GROWTH AND REMODELING OVER THE LIFE SPAN

During childhood and adolescence, growth occurs through the process of modeling, in which bones increase in length and diameter and are reshaped until the epiphyseal plates calcify and skeletal maturity is achieved (typically in

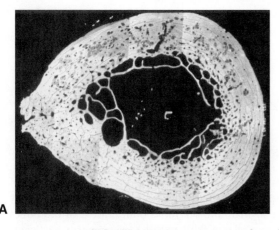

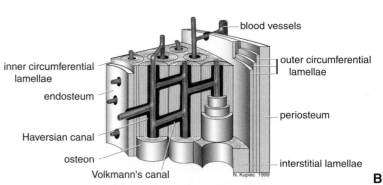

FIGURE 12-3 A, A cross section through the diaphysis of a long bone, with the external periosteal layer, the middle haversian/intracortical layer, the inner endosteal layer, and the marrow cavity. **B,** Diagram of a cross section through the diaphysis of a long bone. (From Lundon K. *Orthopedic Rehabilitation Science: Principles for Clinical Management of Bone.* Boston: Butterworth-Heinemann, 2000.)

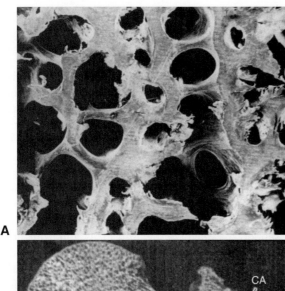

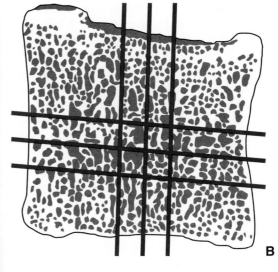

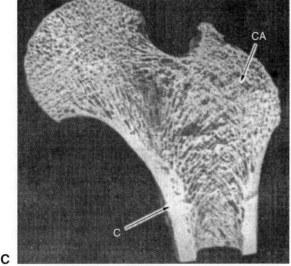

FIGURE 12-4 A, Scanning electron microscope view of cancellous/trabecular bone. **B,** The trabecular pattern in a healthy lumbar vertebra demonstrates bone tissue's response to vertical and horizontal forces during upright activity. **C,** The relationship of form and function is demonstrated by the arched bridgelike trabecular pattern in this cross section of the proximal femur. (From Lundon K. *Orthopedic Rehabilitation Science: Principles for Clinical Management of Bone.* Boston: Butterworth Heinemann, 2000.)

mid-adolescence for females and early adulthood for males).[14] In adulthood, bone health is maintained by the ongoing process of remodeling, in which there is a balance and coupling between osteoblastic deposition of new bone substance and osteoclastic resorption of existing bone.[15] This ongoing process of turnover means that the internal architecture of living bone is actively restructured and replaced at a rate of approximately 5% per year in cortical bone and up to 20% per year in cancellous bone.[5] The rate of bone formation, resorption, and turnover is influenced by both systemic hormones and other substances (e.g., parathyroid hormone, calcitonin, vitamin D from the kidney, growth hormone, adrenocorticosteroids, estrogen, progesterone, androgens); local cell-derived growth factors; and availability of essential nutrients (calcium, fluoride, vitamin A, vitamin D, and vitamin E).[16-18] These substances, along with blood or urinary levels of certain enzymes active during turnover and metabolites of bone resorption, are monitored as biomarkers to track progression of bone diseases associated with high rates of bone resorption (e.g., Paget's disease, osteoporosis, hyperparathyroidism) and to determine efficacy of medical-pharmaceutical interventions for these diseases.[19-21]

In the prenatal period and in infancy, the flat bones of the skull develop as the fetal mesenchyme that forms as the periosteum begins to ossify (intramembranous ossification). Most long bones, as well as the vertebrae and pelvis, develop from a cartilaginous framework or template. In this process of endochondral bone formation, cartilage cells mature and eventually ossify.[7] During childhood and adolescence, bones grow in both length and diameter and are dynamically modeled toward their mature configurations.[22] During puberty, accumulation of bone mass accelerates; by the end of puberty, as much as 90% of mature bone mass is established.[23] For young children with abnormal skeletal development, orthoses attempt to capitalize on the dynamic modeling process, applying external forces to influence bone shape and length.[24] For approximately 15 years following puberty, after closure of the epiphyseal plates of the long bones, bone mass continues to increase—a process described as *consolidation*.[22] Gender differences in peak bone mass have been well documented: Average peak bone mass in women is approximately 20% less than that of men. Early in the midlife period, both men and women enter a period of gradual endochondral bone loss that appears to be genetically determined; the rate of bone loss is also influenced by hormonal status, nutrition, smoking and alcohol use, and activity level.[25-28] It is estimated that males will lose between 15% and 40% of cancellous bone mass and 5% to 15% of cortical bone mass over their lifetime. In women, menopause accelerates the rate of bone loss; there may be up to a 50% decrease from peak cancellous bone mass and 30% decrease in cortical bone mass over their lifetimes.[29] Significant loss of bone mass is associated with increasing vulnerability to fracture, especially among postmenopausal women.

ORTHOSES IN THE MANAGEMENT OF HIP DYSFUNCTION

Hip orthoses are important in the management of hip disorders in infants and children, as well as in the postsurgical care of children and adults. An understanding of the designs of and indications for various hip orthoses is essential for physicians and rehabilitation professionals working with individuals who have orthopedic problems of the pelvis, hip joint, or proximal femur. For children with developmental dysplasia of the hip (DDH) or Legg-Calvé-Perthes disease (LCPD), hip orthoses are the primary intervention for prevention of future deformity and disability. Hip orthoses are essential elements of postoperative care and rehabilitation programs for children with musculoskeletal and neuromuscular conditions who have had surgical intervention for bony deformity or soft tissue contracture. Hip orthoses can also be major postoperative interventions for adults who have had repair of a traumatic injury or a complex total hip arthroplasty. The efficacy of orthotic intervention is influenced by patient and caregiver adherence: The key to successful use of these orthoses is clear, and open communication exists among the physician, therapist, orthotist, and family concerning the primary goals of the orthosis, its proper application and wearing schedule, and the possible difficulties that may be encountered. Positive health care outcomes and happy patients and families are contingent on the ability of the health care team to communicate.

When are Hip Orthosis Indicated?

Most nontraumatic hip joint dysfunction or pathology occurs either in childhood or in late adult life and is frequently related to one or more of the four following factors:

1. Inadequate or ineffective development of the acetabulum and head of the femur in infancy
2. Avascular necrosis of the femoral head associated with inadequate blood supply during childhood
3. Loss of cartilage and abnormal bone deposition associated with osteoarthritis
4. Loss of bone strength and density in osteoporosis

Orthotic intervention is an important component in the orthopedic management of many of these conditions. Most often, hip orthoses are used to protect or position the hip joint by limiting motion within a desirable range of flexion/extension and abduction/adduction. It is important to note that hip orthoses alone are not effective in controlling internal/external rotation of the hip joint. If precise rotational control is desired, a hip-knee-ankle-foot orthosis (HKAFO) must be used.

Hip Structure and Function

The hip (coxofemoral) joint is a synovial joint formed by the concave socketlike acetabulum of the pelvis and the rounded ball-like head of the femur (Figure 12-5). Because of the unique bony structure of the hip joint, movement is possible in all three planes of motion: flexion/extension in the sagittal plane, abduction/adduction in the frontal plane, and internal/external rotation in the transverse plane. Most functional activities blend movement of the femur on the pelvis (or of the pelvis on the femur) across all three planes of motion.

The hip joint has two important functions. First, it must support the weight of the head, arms, and trunk during functional activities (e.g., erect sitting and standing, walking, running, stair climbing, transitional movements in activities of daily living). Second, it must effectively transmit forces from the pelvis to the lower extremities during quiet standing, gait, and other closed chain activities.[30]

The acetabulum is formed at the convergence of the pubis, ischium, and ilium. Its primary orientation is in the vertical, facing laterally, but it also has a slight inferior inclination and an anteverted, or anterior-facing tilt. Developmentally, the depth of the acetabulum is dynamically shaped by motion of the head of the femur during leg movement and weight bearing. The acetabulum is not fully ossified until late adolescence or early young adulthood. The articular surface of the acetabulum is a horseshoe-shaped, hyaline cartilage–covered area around its anterior, superior, and posterior edges. A space along the inferior edge, called the acetabular notch, is nonarticular, has no cartilage covering, and is spanned by the transverse acetabular ligament. The acetabular labrum is a fibrocartilaginous ring that encircles the exterior perimeter of the acetabulum, increasing joint depth and concavity. The center of the acetabulum, the acetabular fossa, contains fibroelastic fat and the ligamentum teres, and is covered by synovial membrane.

The femoral components of the hip joint include the femoral head, the femoral neck, and the greater and lesser trochanters. The spherical articular surface of the femoral head is covered with hyaline cartilage. Because the femoral head is larger and somewhat differently shaped than the acetabulum, some portion of its articular surface is exposed in any position of the hip joint. The femur and acetabulum are most congruent when positioned in a combination of flexion, abduction, and external rotation. The proximal femur, composed primarily of trabecular bone, is designed to withstand significant loading while also permitting movement through large excursions of range of motion. The orientation of the femoral head and neck in the frontal plane, with respect to the shaft of the femur, is described as its angle of inclination (Figure 12-6).

In infancy the angle of inclination may be as much as 150 degrees but decreases during normal development to approximately 125 degrees in mid-adulthood and to 120 degrees in later life.[31] The orientation of the proximal femur to the shaft and condyles in the transverse plane, called the *angle of anteversion*, is also a key determinant of hip joint

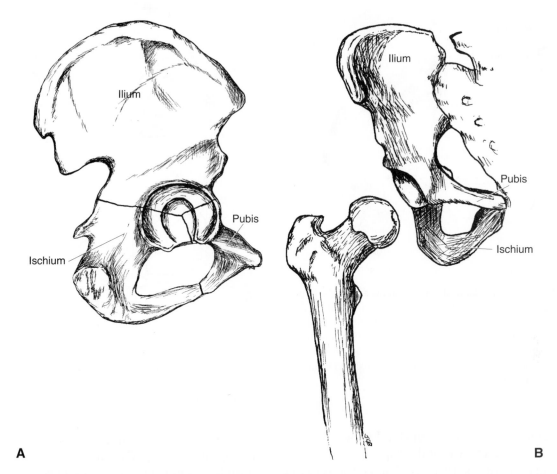

FIGURE 12-5 Anatomy of the hip joint. **A,** The articular surface of the socketlike acetabulum, a horseshoe-shaped area covered by hyaline cartilage, is extended by the acetabular labrum. **B,** The proximal femur is angled to seat the femoral head optimally within the acetabulum, to support the upper body and to transmit loading forces to or from the lower extremity.

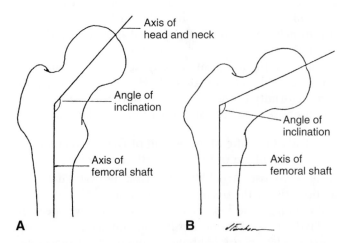

FIGURE 12-6 A, Normal angle of inclination between the neck and shaft of the femur is 125 degrees in adults. A pathological increase in the angle of inclination is called *coxa valga,* and a pathological decrease in the angle of inclination **(B)** is called *coxa vara.* (From The hip complex. In Norkin CC, Levangie PK [eds], *Joint Structure and Function: A Comprehensive Analysis*, 2nd ed. Philadelphia: FA Davis, 1992. p. 305.)

function (Figure 12-7). Anteversion may be as much as 40 degrees at birth, decreasing during normal development to approximately 15 degrees in adulthood.[31] These two angulations determine how well the femoral head is seated within the acetabulum and, in effect, the biomechanical stability of the hip joint. The functional stability of the hip joint is supported by a strong fibrous joint capsule and by the iliofemoral, ischiofemoral, and pubofemoral ligaments. Fibers of the capsule and ligaments are somewhat obliquely oriented, becoming most taut when the hip is in an extended position.

Infants and Children with Developmental Dysplasia of the Hip

DDH is the current terminology for a condition previously called *congenital dislocation of the hip.* This new term includes a variety of congenital hip pathologies including dysplasia, subluxation, and dislocation. This terminology is preferred because it includes those infants with normal physical examination at birth who are later found to have a subluxed or dislocated hip, in addition to those who are immediately identified as having hip pathologies.[32-34]

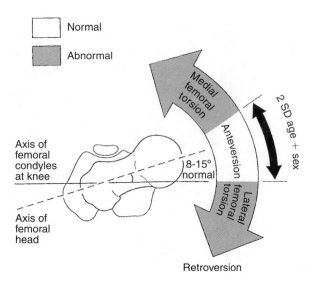

FIGURE 12-7 Normal relationship between the axis of the femoral neck and the axis of the femoral condyles (viewed as if looking down the center of the femoral shaft) is between 8 and 15 degrees. Excessive anteversion leads to medial (internal) femoral torsion. Insufficient angulation, retroversion, is associated with lateral (external) femoral torsion. (From Staheli LT.Medical Femoral Torsion. *Orthop Clin North Am.* 1980;11:40.)

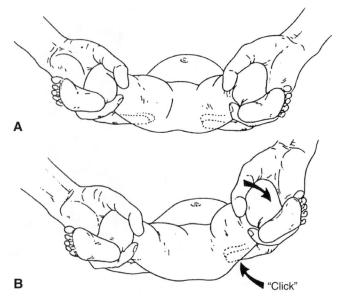

FIGURE 12-8 Test position for developmental dysplasia of the hip in the newborn. **A,** The hip is moved into flexion, adduction, and internal rotation. **B,** A "click" when upward pressure is applied at the greater trochanter suggests that the dislocation has been reduced. (From Magee DJ. *Orthopedic Physical Assessment.* 3rd ed. Philadelphia: Saunders, 1997. p. 477.)

Incidence and Etiology of Developmental Dysplasia of the Hip

Instability of the hip due to DDH occurs in 11.7 of every 1000 live births, with most of these classified as hip subluxation (9.2/1000), followed by true dislocation (1.3/1000) and dislocatable hips (1.2/1000).[33,35] Hip dislocation is more common in girls (70%) than in boys and among white than among black newborns. Approximately 20% of all hip dislocations are associated with breech presentation, although the incidence of breech presentation in the normal population is approximately 4%.[36] A familial tendency is also found: DDH is much more likely to occur when an older sibling has had congenital subluxation or dislocation. The risk of dysplasia increases with any type of intrauterine malpositioning leading to extreme flexion and adduction at the hip. This occurs more commonly during first pregnancies if and when tightness of maternal abdominal or uterine musculature is present, when the infant is quite large, or when insufficient amniotic fluid restricts intrauterine motion.[32,37] A higher incidence of DDH is also found among newborns with other musculoskeletal abnormalities including torticollis, metatarsus varus, clubfoot, or other unusual syndromes.

At birth the acetabulum is quite shallow, covering less than half of the femoral head. In addition, the joint capsule is loose and elastic. These two factors make the neonate hip relatively unstable and susceptible to subluxation and dislocation. Normal development of the hip joint in the first year of life is a function of the stresses and strains placed on the femoral head and acetabulum during movement. In the presence of subluxation or dislocation, modeling of the acetabulum and femoral head is compromised.

The most common clinical sign of DDH is limitation in hip abduction.[38] On clinical examination, a "click" (Ortolani sign) felt when upward pressure is applied at the level of the greater trochanter on the newborn or infant's flexed and abducted hip (Figure 12-8) indicates that a dislocated hip has been manually reduced.[39] The goal of orthotic management in developmental dysplasia is to achieve optimal seating of the femoral head within the acetabulum while permitting the kicking movements that assist shaping of the acetabulum and femoral head for stability of the hip joint.[40,41] This is best achieved if the child is routinely positioned in flexion and abduction at the hip. If DDH is recognized early and appropriate intervention is initiated, the hip joint is likely to develop normally. If unrecognized and untreated, DDH often leads to significant deformity of the hip as the child grows, resulting in compromised mobility and other functional limitations.

Early Orthotic Management of Developmental Dysplasia of the Hip: Birth to 6 Months

In 1958 Professor Arnold Pavlik of Czechoslovakia described an orthosis for the treatment of dysplasia, subluxation, and dislocation of the hip.[42,43] The orthosis he developed, the Pavlik harness, relies on hip flexion and abduction to stabilize the hip at risk. Although a multitude of braces and orthoses have been used historically in the treatment of hip instability, including hip spica casts, the Frejka pillow, the Craig splint, the Ilfeld splint, and the von Rosen splint, the Pavik harness, has become widely accepted as a mainstay for the initial treatment for the unstable hip in neonates from birth to 6 months of age.

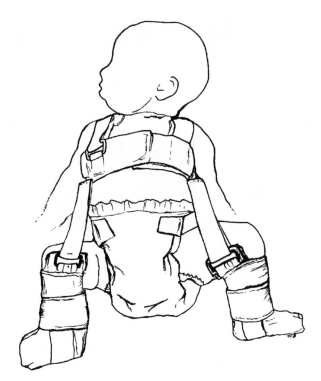

FIGURE 12-9 A Pavlik harness positions the infant's lower extremities in hip flexion and abduction in an effort to position the femoral head optimally within the acetabulum, assisting normal bony development of the hip joint. The anterior leg straps allow hip flexion but limit hip extension; the posterior flaps allow abduction but limit adduction.

At first glance, the Pavlik harness seems a confusing collection of webbing, hook-and-loop material, padding, and straps. In reality, this dynamic orthosis (Figure 12-9) has three major components:

1. A shoulder and chest harness that provides a proximal anchor for the device
2. A pair of booties and stirrups used as the distal attachment
3. Anterior and posterior leg straps between chest harness and booties used to position the hip joint optimally

The anterior strap allows flexion but limits extension, whereas the posterior strap allows abduction but limits adduction. The child is free to move into flexion and abduction, the motions that are most likely to assist functional shaping of the acetabulum in the months after birth.[42–44] To be effective, however, the fit of the harness must be accurately adjusted for the growing infant and the orthosis must be properly applied. The family caregiver must be involved in an intensive education program when the newborn is being fit with the Pavlik harness. Nurses, physical and occupational therapists, pediatricians, and orthopedic residents who work with newborns also need to understand the function and fit of this important orthosis. The guidelines for properly fitting a Pavlik harness include the following key points[40,45]:

1. The shoulder straps cross in the back to prevent the orthosis from sliding off the infant's shoulders.
2. The chest strap is fit around the thorax at the infant's nipple line.

3. The proximal calf strap on the bootie is fit just distal to the knee joint.
4. The anterior leg straps are attached to the chest strap at the anterior axillary line.
5. The posterior leg straps are attached to the chest strap just over the infant's scapulae.

In a correctly fit orthosis, the lower extremity is positioned in 100 to 120 degrees of hip flexion, as indicated by the physician's evaluation and recommendation. The limbs are also positioned in 30 to 40 degrees of hip abduction. The distance between the infant's thighs (when the hips are moved passively into adduction) should be no more than 8 to 10 cm. In a well-fit orthosis, extension and adduction are limited, whereas flexion and abduction are freely permitted: The infant is able to kick actively within this restricted range while wearing the orthosis. This position and movement encourage elongation of adductor contractures, which in turn assists in the reduction of the hip and enhances acetabular development. Three common problems indicate that the fit of the harness requires adjustment[40,46]:

1. If the leg straps are adjusted too tightly, the infant cannot kick actively.
2. If the anterior straps are positioned too far medially on the chest strap, the limb is positioned in excessive adduction rather than the desired abduction.
3. If the calf strap is positioned too far distally on the lower leg, it does not position the limb in the desired amount of hip flexion.

Optimal outcomes in infants with DDH are associated with early aggressive intervention of the unstable hip using the Pavlik harness.[47,48] Families and health care professionals must seek proper orthopedic care to avoid misdiagnosis and mistreatment. One of the most common misdiagnoses is mistaking dislocation for subluxation and implementing a triple- or double-diapering strategy for intervention. Although this strategy does position the infant's hip in some degree of flexion and abduction, bulky diapers alone are insufficient for reducing dislocation.

Initially, most infants wear the Pavlik harness 24 hours a day. The parents can be permitted to remove the harness for bathing, at the discretion of the orthopedist. Importantly, especially early in treatment, the fit and function of the orthosis must be reevaluated frequently to ensure proper position in the orthosis. The many straps of the Pavlik harness can be confusing to the most caring of families. The proper donning and doffing sequence should be thoroughly explained and demonstrated to the family. Additional strategies to enhance optimal reduction of the hip such as prone sleeping should be encouraged.

Families must be instructed in proper skin care and in bathing the newborn or infant wearing the orthosis. Initially, they may be advised to use diapers, but not any type of shirt, under the orthosis. The importance of keeping regularly scheduled recheck appointments for effective monitoring of hip position and refitting of the orthosis as the infant grows cannot be overstressed to the parents or caregivers.[48–50] Missed appointments often result in less than optimal positioning of the femoral head with respect to the acetabulum, a less than satisfactory outcome of early intervention, and the necessity of more invasive treatment procedures as the child grows.

As a general rule, the length of treatment in the harness is equal to the child's age when a stable hip reduction is achieved plus an additional three months. Thus if a stable reduction is achieved at 4 months of age, the total treatment time would be 7 months. Over time, when hip development is progressing as desired, the wearing schedule can be decreased to night and naptime wear. This often welcomed change in wearing time can begin as early as 3 months of age if x-ray, ultrasound, and physical examination demonstrate the desired bone development. When the orthopedist determines that the hip is normal according to radiographs and ultrasound and is satisfied with the clinical examination, the orthosis can be discontinued. If development of the hip is slow or the infant undergoes rapid growth, it may be advisable to continue the treatment with another type of hip abduction orthosis designed for older and larger babies, to maintain the position of flexion and abduction for a longer period of time.

Management of Developmental Dysplasia of the Hip: 6 Months and Beyond

For older infants and toddlers (6 to 18 months) whose DDH was unrecognized or inadequately managed early in infancy, intervention is often much more aggressive and may include an abduction brace, traction, open or closed reduction, and hip spica casting.[33,51] For infants who are growing quickly or whose bone development has been slow, an alternative to the Pavlik harness is necessary. After the age of 6 months, especially as the infant begins to pull into standing in preparation for walking, the Pavlik harness can no longer provide the desired positioning for reduction. Often, the infant is simply too large to fit into the harness. By this time, families who have been compliant with harness application and wearing have grown to dislike it and are ready for other forms of intervention.

A custom-fit prefabricated thermoplastic hip abduction orthosis is often the next step in orthotic management of DDH. This orthosis consists of a plastic frame with waist section and thigh cuffs, waterproof foam liner, and hook-and-loop material closures. The static version is fixed at 90 degrees of hip flexion and 120 degrees of hip abduction (Figure 12-10). An adjustable joint can be incorporated into the abduction bar; however, hip flexion is maintained at 90 degrees. This orthosis appears to be static, but the child is able to move within the thigh sections while the safe zone for continued management of hip position is maintained.

Many families view the hip abduction orthosis as an improvement over the Pavlik harness: The caregivers and the infant are free from cumbersome straps, the orthosis is easily removed and reapplied for diaper changing and hygiene, and the orthosis itself is waterproof and easier to keep clean. Parents and caregivers can hold the infant without struggling with straps, and the baby is able to sit comfortably for feeding and play.

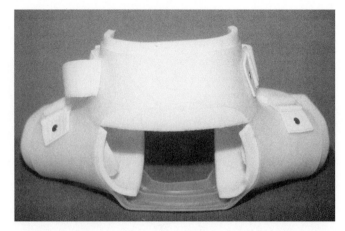

FIGURE 12-10 A posterior view of a static hip abduction orthosis, which positions the infant in 90 degrees of hip flexion and 120 degrees of abduction.

Because most hip abduction orthoses are prefabricated, the knowledge and skills of an orthotist are necessary to ensure a proper custom fit for each child. To determine what the necessary modifications are, the orthotist evaluates three areas:

1. The length of the thigh cuffs. Thigh cuffs are trimmed proximal to the popliteal fossae. Cuffs that are too long can lead to neurovascular compromise if the child prefers to sleep in a supine position, as the risk of compression of the legs against the distal edge of the cuffs is present.
2. The width of the anterior opening of the waist component. Although the plastic is flexible, the opening may need to be enlarged for heavy or large-framed infants.
3. The foam padding of the thigh and waist components. All edges must be smooth to avoid skin irritation or breakdown, and the circumference of the padding should fit without undue tightness.

Modifications may require reheating or trimming of the plastic or foam padding. Usually this fitting takes place in the orthotist's office or the clinic setting, where the necessary tools are readily available. Once the fit is evaluated and modified as appropriate for the individual child, the parents or caregivers are instructed in proper donning/doffing and orthotic care.

The static hip abduction orthosis is used in either of two ways. First, the orthosis may be a continuation of the course of treatment established by the Pavlik harness, as determined by the orthopedist's evaluation of the child's hip. As a continuation of treatment, the orthosis can be worn day and night; most often, however, it is reserved for nighttime use while the child is sleeping.[38,40,51] The use of the orthosis at night is believed to assist development of acetabular growth cartilage. If the orthosis is worn consistently for several months and evidence of effective reduction and reshaping of the joint is present, it is less likely that more aggressive forms of treatment will be necessary as the child grows.

The second application for the hip abduction orthosis is for follow-up management for children with DDH who require an orthopedic intervention such as traction, surgical reduction, or casting. In this case the orthosis provides external stability to the hip during the postoperative weeks and months, while the baby regains range of motion and continues to grow and progress through the stages of motor development. This extra stability reduces parental and physician concern about dislocation and other undesired outcomes of the orthopedic procedure.

The static hip abduction orthosis has obvious advantages over plaster or synthetic hip spica casts including greater ease in diaper hygiene and bathing and is often welcomed by families as a positive next step in treatment. Fitting requires the knowledge and skills of an orthotist familiar with proper fitting techniques and who can manage potentially irritable babies just freed from a confining hip spica cast.

Goals of Orthotic Intervention for Children with Developmental Dysplasia of the Hip

To be effective, orthotic intervention for DDH must have a set of clearly described treatment objectives against which success can be measured. The components necessary for effective orthotic interventions for children with DDH include the following:

1. Clearly presented verbal, psychomotor, and written instructions for the child's family or caregivers, with an additional goal of minimizing stress in an already stressful situation.
2. Effective communication among members of the health care team about the appropriate use and potential pitfalls of the orthosis. This often includes education about the orthosis provided by the orthotist and careful monitoring of family compliance and coping by all members of the team (orthotists, orthopedists, pediatricians, therapists, nurses, and other health professionals who may be involved in the case).
3. Safe and effective hip reduction to minimize the necessity of more aggressive casting or surgery. This requires proper orthotic fit and adjustment, as well as consistency in wearing schedules.

The ultimate goal is to facilitate normal development of the hip joint, providing the child with a pain-free, stable, functional hip that will last throughout his or her lifetime.

Complications of Orthotic Management of Developmental Dysplasia of the Hip

In most cases the Pavlik harness, perhaps followed by abduction splint use as the child grows, is a successful intervention for DDH. A small percentage of infants with DDH managed by the Pavlik harness (<8%) develop complications, the most serious of which is avascular necrosis of the femoral head, which may be caused by overtightening the posterior straps to force a position of abduction.[33,49-54] Children who have complications differ from those without complications in a number of ways. They tend to have larger acetabular angles (>35 degrees) and less total coverage of the femoral head within the acetabulum (<20%) on radiography or ultrasound, have an irreducible dislocation at initiation of orthotic intervention, have delayed diagnosis and intervention (older than 3 months of age), and have not demonstrated a prior ossific nucleus on radiograph or ultrasound.[49,50,52,55]

Orthotic Management of Legg-Calvé-Perthes Disease

LCPD is a hip pathology that affects otherwise healthy school-aged children. Although the clinical signs and symptoms of LCPD, as they differ from tuberculosis involving the hip, were first described by Arthur T. Legg in 1910,[56] the etiology of this condition is not clearly understood and its treatment and orthopedic management continue to be controversial. The hallmark of LCPD is a flattening of the femoral head, thought to be a result of an avascular necrosis insult. Left untreated, LCPD leads to permanent deformity and eventual osteoarthritis in the adult hip. The disease is four times as common in boys between the ages of 4 and 8 years old as in girls, although outcomes in girls tend to be less satisfactory.[57-59] LCPD generally involves only one hip; only approximately 12% of cases are bilateral. It is rare within the black population. Several options for orthotic management of LCPD have evolved. All are designed to help maintain a spherical femoral head and normal acetabulum.

Etiology of Legg-Calvé-Perthes Disease

The etiology of LCPD remains controversial more than 100 years after it was first described. Most researchers believe that LCPD is a result of some event or condition that compromises blood flow to the femoral head and leads to avascular necrosis. The exact mechanism that triggers this compromise is unknown. Some theories focus on an acute trauma that damages the vascular system of the femoral head, whereas others suggest that repeated episodes of a transient synovitis may compromise blood flow.[58,60,61] Another theory suggests an abnormality of thrombolysis in children who develop LCPD.[62] A genetic predisposition to delayed bone age that exposes vessels to high rates of compression as they pass through cartilage to the bony head has also been suggested.[60] Although the exact etiology of LCPD remains a mystery, it is certainly linked to episodes of avascular necrosis in the femoral head. The goal of intervention in children with LCPD is to assist revascularization of the femoral head and to restore normal anatomical shape and alignment of the hip joint.

Evaluation and Intervention for Legg-Calvé-Perthes Disease

LCPD should be suspected in children with one or more of the following signs or symptoms[63,64]:

1. A noticeable limp, often with a positive Trendelenburg sign
2. Pain in the hip, groin, knee, or a combination of these locations
3. Loss of range of motion of the hip joint

When these symptoms are present, radiographic, ultrasound, or magnetic resonance imaging studies of the hip are used to discriminate between LCPD (Figure 12-11) and other hip disorders (e.g., slipped capital femoral epiphysis, fracture, rheumatic disease, infection).[65] These studies are used by the orthopedist to determine severity and progression of the disease, considering stage of disease, shape of femoral head,

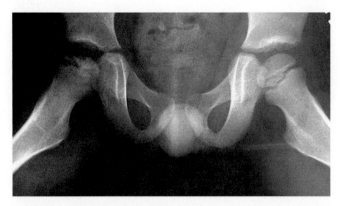

FIGURE 12-11 A radiograph of a child with Legg-Calvé-Perthes disease comparing the shape and density of the head of the femur and of the capital epiphysis on the normal (right side of image) and affected (left side of image) right hip.

degree of congruence with the acetabulum, and length and angle of the femoral neck.[66,67] A variety of classification systems have been developed to rate severity of involvements. The Catterall system describes four groups on the basis of the location of involvement and identifies four "head at risk" signs for the orthopedist or radiologist to focus on in interpreting radiographs.[68] Studies of the interrater and concurrent reliability of the Catterall systems have not all been positive.[69-71] The Salter-Thompson system rates severity of involvement on the basis of the location and extent of subchondral fracture that may be observed early in the disease process.[72,73] The Herring system examines the condition of the lateral pillar of the femoral head on radiographs.[65,71,74] Refer to texts on orthopedic conditions in pediatrics for further information about classification.[60,61]

LCPD is a self-limiting process that often resolves in 1 to 3 years. The disease progresses through three stages:
1. Necrotic stage: avascular necrosis
2. Fragmentation stage: resorption of damaged bone
3. Healing/reparative stage: revascularization, reossification, and bony remodeling

Factors that influence the eventual outcome of the disease include age at onset, severity of damage to the femoral head and epiphysis, and quality of congruency of the acetabulum and femoral head.[58-61]

Because the disease process is self-limiting, the optimal intervention strategy is controversial. The three most commonly used avenues of treatment for LCPD are observation, surgical intervention, and conservative orthotic management. Decisions about treatment are often guided by age of the child, extent of femoral head deformity, and severity of incongruency between the femoral head and acetabulum.[60,61,75] More recent data suggest that patients younger than 6 years of age at the time of disease onset are best managed nonsurgically, whereas the treatment for patients older than 8 years may involve surgery and is less well defined.[76]

For children with minimal bony deformity, observation and exercise may be the most appropriate intervention.[77] Because the child is likely to continue to limp until sufficient revascularization and remodeling have occurred

(which may require several years), parents may be uneasy, preferring instead a more aggressive intervention. Parents are reassured when close clinical follow-up is performed, with periodic reexamination by x-ray evaluation to monitor progression of the disease process.

Surgical intervention is based on the principle of containment, optimally positioning the femoral head within the acetabulum. Proximal femoral derotation osteotomy is used to decompress and center the femoral head within the acetabulum for more functional weight bearing in an extended position.[78,79] A pelvic osteotomy, which repositions the acetabulum over the femoral head, is sometimes necessary when a significantly enlarged or subluxed femoral head cannot be effectively repositioned by femoral derotation osteotomy.[80,81] Shelf arthroplasty to reshape the acetabulum to better accept the femoral head has also been used as an intervention.[82,83] The outcome of surgery is likely to be most positive for children who have full hip range of motion preoperatively. Parents must understand the goals and risks of the surgical procedure and must be actively involved in postoperative rehabilitation efforts.

The goal of conservative orthotic management of LCPD is similar to that of surgical intervention: to contain the femoral head within the acetabulum during the active stages of the disease process so that optimal remodeling can occur.[41,84] Much debate has taken place concerning whether surgery or orthotic intervention is most efficacious. If both are viable methods of treatment, the end result should be the same: a well-shaped femoral head and pain-free hip. Comparing the efficacy of surgical versus orthotic management of LCPD is challenging because of relatively low incidence as well as differences in study design and definition of control for variables such as age of onset, duration of the disease, gender, and inadequate interobserver reliability of classification systems.[84,85] Although two reports published in 1992 question the efficacy of orthotic treatment,[86,87] other studies advocate orthotic treatment even in severe cases of the disease. Because studies have reported success, as well as lack of success for all three types of intervention (noncontainment/observation, surgery, and the use of orthoses), the most appropriate management of LCPD has not been clearly determined.

Orthotic Management in Legg-Calvé-Perthes Disease

Currently the most commonly used orthosis in the nonoperative management of LCPD is the Atlanta/Scottish-Rite hip abduction orthosis (Figure 12-12). The design of this orthosis allows the child to walk and be involved in other functional activities while containing the femoral head in the acetabulum with abduction of the hips.[88-90] The Atlanta/Scottish-Rite orthosis has three components: a pelvic band, a pair of single-axis hip joints, and a pair of thigh cuffs. An abduction bar may also be included, interconnecting the thigh cuffs with a ball-and-socket joint as an interface. This orthosis holds each hip in approximately 45 degrees of hip abduction, permits flexion and extension of the hip, and can be worn over clothing. While in the orthosis the hips are abducted and flexed but the patient has no limitation in knee range of

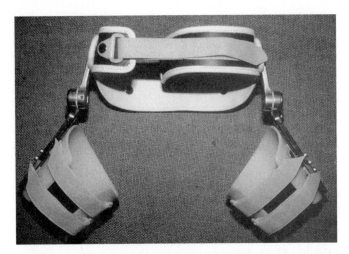

FIGURE 12-12 The Atlanta/Scottish-Rite hip abduction orthosis (anterior view), used in the conservative management of Legg-Calvé-Perthes disease. This orthosis has three components: the pelvic band, the free-motion hip joints, and the thigh cuffs. An abduction bar can be placed between the thigh cuffs to provide extra stability in the desired position of 45 degrees of hip abduction.

motion and therefore can sit or walk without difficulty. The orthosis is not designed to control internal rotation of the hip. This type of orthosis is most effective if the child who is wearing it has close to normal range of motion at the hip joint. Limitations in range of motion cause the child to stand asymmetrically in the orthosis, which effectively reduces the amount of abduction and containment of the femoral head.

Historically (in the 1960s and 1970s), a number of other orthoses were developed on the basis of the principles of containment of the femoral head. The Toronto orthosis (Figure 12-13A) and the Newington orthosis (see Figure 12-13B) hold both limbs in 45 degrees of abduction with internal rotation, but unlike the Atlanta/Scottish Rite orthosis, require the use of crutches for safe mobility.[91,92] Both of these orthoses

are cumbersome to wear and significantly affect the ease of daily function. Because the efficacy of the Atlanta Scottish-Rite orthosis is as high as or higher than the efficacy of the Toronto and Newington orthoses, the latter two orthoses are not commonly used in current management of children with LCPD.[41,93] In addition, orthoses like an "A-frame" may be used after several weeks of Petrie casting, another nonsurgical treatment option enforcing hip abduction.[76]

If the disease process progresses and the hip begins to lose additional range of motion, the orthotist may be the first to recognize this problem. The parents may bring the child to the clinic for an orthotic adjustment because the thigh cuffs have become uncomfortable. If loss of additional range of motion is noticed by parents or by therapists who are working with the child, an immediate referral to the orthotic clinic or physician is necessary. The Atlanta/Scottish-Rite orthosis is not designed to increase range of motion; its primary function is to hold the hips in abduction comfortably. Using the orthosis to restore range of motion defeats the purpose of the orthotic design and compromises treatment principles.

Communication among the orthopedist, orthotist, therapist, and family is essential. Parents must understand that this is a demanding form of treatment. Typically, the orthosis is worn continually for 12 to 18 months. Once radiographic evidence of femoral head reossification is seen, time in the orthosis is gradually reduced.

Absolute compliance with the wearing schedule is necessary for maximum effectiveness: A well-designed and well-fit orthosis can only work if it is being used. The first few days and weeks in the orthosis are often stressful for the parent and the child. With the hips held in an abducted position, routine tasks including walking may require assistance until the child learns effective adaptive strategies. Physical therapists may work with the child on crutch-walking techniques on level surfaces, stairs, inclines, and uneven surfaces. They may

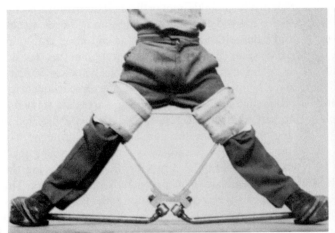

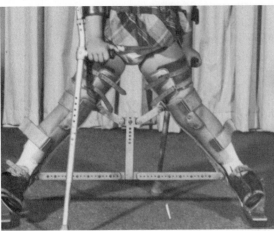

A B

FIGURE 12-13 Earlier designs for hip abduction knee-ankle-foot orthoses used to manage Legg-Calvé-Perthes disease. The Toronto hip-knee-ankle foot orthosis (**A**) and Newington orthoses (**B**) were more cumbersome to don and to function with than the Atlanta/Scottish-Rite hip abduction orthoses. (From Goldberg B, Hsu JH [eds], *Atlas of Orthotics and Assistive Devices.* 3rd ed. St. Louis: Mosby, 1997.)

make suggestions for adaptation of the home and school environments so that sitting and transitions from flooring, chairs, and standing quickly become manageable. If family education and support efforts are effective and enable parents and children to weather this difficult initial stage in orthotic management well, the likelihood of compliance in the remaining months of intervention is significantly enhanced.

Pediatric Postoperative Care

Numerous musculoskeletal and neuromuscular conditions, in addition to LCPD and developmental dysplasia, may necessitate surgical intervention for children with hip and lower extremity dysfunction or deformity. Orthoses that control hip and leg position are often used in the weeks and months after surgery as an alternative to traditional plaster casts or as a follow-up strategy once casts are removed. Although a cast may be applied in the operating room for immediate postoperative care, orthoses are often fit soon afterward and effectively shorten the time that a child spends in a cast. Hip orthoses are used when immobilization and support will be required for a long period of time, when complications arise, or when a child's special needs demand their use.

One of the major benefits of an orthosis (as compared with a plaster cast) is in regard to hygiene, especially for children who have not yet developed consistent bladder and bowel control. Additional benefits of postoperative hip orthoses include the following:

1. Being much lighter than traditional casts, hip orthoses reduce the burden of care for parents and caregivers who must lift or carry the child.
2. Hip orthoses can be removed for inspection of surgical wounds and for bathing and skin care.
3. Hip orthoses can be removed for physical therapy, range of motion, mobilization, strengthening, or other appropriate interventions.
4. Thermoplastic orthoses are waterproof; therefore, residues of perspiration or urine can be easily cleaned and sanitized with warm soap and water.
5. A well-fit orthosis is less likely to cause skin irritation or breakdown and, unlike a cast, can often be adjusted if areas of impingement develop.
6. The position and amount of abduction can be easily adjusted.
7. A hip orthosis can be custom designed for a patient with complicated needs, especially those who have had multiple surgical procedures.

Postoperative Hip Orthoses

Two basic designs are available for children's postoperative orthoses. The first is composed of thigh cuffs that fit between the knee and hip joint, an abduction bar, and hook-and-loop material closures (Figure 12-14). This orthosis can be fabricated from measurements taken before surgery and fit with no delay as soon as the cast is removed. It can also be fit in lieu of a cast if the surgical procedure was minor or when static positioning of the hip is required. This type of orthosis is commonly used after adductor release or varus osteotomy

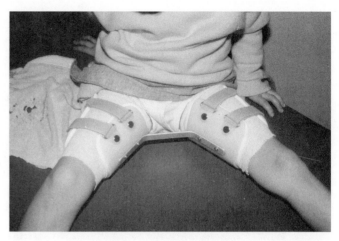

FIGURE 12-14 A postoperative hip abduction orthosis has two components: a pair of thigh cuffs held in position by an abduction bar.

with adductor release or for the management of a septic hip. A postoperative hip orthosis is most often used for extended periods of nighttime-only wear but in some circumstances can also be worn during the day.[94] In many clinics this orthosis is used after hip procedures in children with cerebral palsy.

Parents and caregivers find the postoperative hip orthosis a welcome relief from a cast. Despite its simple appearance, families should be given special instructions about how the orthosis is worn and cared for. It can be worn over clothing or pajamas or next to the skin if necessary. It should not cause skin irritation or discomfort on either side of the hip joint. If the patient experiences any hip joint pain, the orthotist should consult with the orthopedist to determine if the angle of abduction can be safely adjusted. Overzealous attempts to abduct the hip can cause pain and reduce compliance. Occasionally, this orthosis may be difficult to keep in place even though it has been properly fit. A simple suspension belt can be added to ensure optimal positioning.

The second option for postoperative care is a modification of a knee-ankle-foot orthosis. This orthosis is composed of two thermoplastic knee-ankle-foot orthoses without knee joints but with an abduction bar and hook-and-loop material closures (Figure 12-15). Fabrication of this type of orthosis requires that plaster impressions be taken: Simple length and circumferential measurements are not adequate to ensure proper fit. Ideally, these impressions are taken at the first postoperative cast change. The orthosis is then fabricated, and fitting occurs during the next clinic appointment. Taking the impressions before surgery is not advisable. Postoperatively, each joint will be at a new angle, compromising the fit of the orthosis based on preoperative impressions. This type of orthosis is recommended for patients who have had bony procedures around the hip, as well as extensive soft tissue procedures such as hamstring or heel cord release, which require protection in the early stages of healing. In our clinic, this orthosis is most often used for children with cerebral palsy or myelomeningocele. In some circumstances, when more precise control of the hip joint is desirable, the orthosis can be extended upward to include the pelvis.

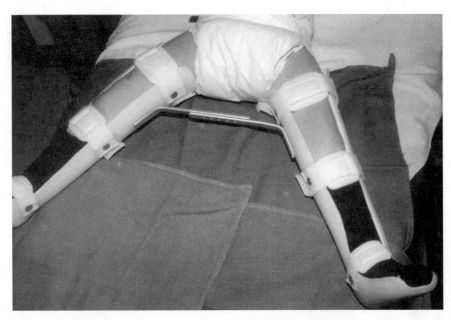

FIGURE 12-15 For postoperative management of children after extensive bony and soft tissue surgery, knee-ankle-foot orthoses with the addition of an abduction bar are often used subsequent to cast removal. Rotation of the hip is well controlled by the intimate fit of the orthosis including the ankle-foot complex. When precise control of the hip is necessary, the postoperative hip abduction orthosis encompasses the pelvis as well.

Because of the intimate fit of this orthosis, parents and caregivers must be given careful education concerning proper fit and cleaning. Especially important is a careful inspection of the posterior aspect of the calcaneus: This area is vulnerable to skin breakdown from prolonged pressure and may be overlooked during skin checks that focus on the healing surgical wounds. Because the foam lining and thermoplastic material do not breathe, perspiration cannot effectively evaporate. The orthosis should be removed periodically for cleaning to minimize the risk of skin maceration or infection from microorganisms that thrive in warm moist environments.

The postoperative orthosis has proven useful in the overall orthopedic management of children with musculoskeletal or neuromuscular diseases. The orthosis is an effective substitute for heavy casts, especially when skin irritation and incontinence are concerns. The postoperative hip orthosis helps to ensure healing in the optimal joint position and reduces the likelihood of recurrence of the deformity that prompted surgical intervention.

Management of the Adult Hip

Orthotic intervention for the hip in the adult population is limited, focusing on two groups of patients. Hip orthoses are most commonly used as postsurgical and postcast care of adult patients who have sustained a complex hip or proximal femoral fracture from a traumatic event such as a motor vehicle accident, industrial accident, or fall. In some circumstances a hip orthosis can be used for older adults after a total hip procedure, revision of a total hip, or fracture associated with total hip arthroplasty.[95,96] Although injury that affects the hip can occur at any point in the life span, most adults with trauma-related fractures who are managed with hip orthoses are young and middle aged, and many of those who are undergoing a new or revised total joint arthroplasty are 65 years or older. As the number of older adults increases in the U.S. population, so will the number of hip fractures. One estimate suggests that as many as 512,000 hip fractures will occur in the United States by the year 2040.[97]

In both of these circumstances, stabilization of the orthopedic injury and rehabilitation planning are important issues. Patients with this type of injury of the hip often require extensive physical therapy programs. Clinicians must understand age-related pathophysiological changes that affect the healing musculoskeletal system, the impact and detrimental effects of prolonged bed rest, and the optimal point at which an orthosis should be integrated into the overall treatment plan.

Total Hip Arthroplasty

Although a hip orthosis is usually not indicated in most simple, elective total hip arthroplasties, in some circumstances this orthosis can assist healing and rehabilitation. Hip orthoses can be used for patients with significant osteoporosis in whom femoral fracture occurs during total joint surgery or for those who require emergency total joint replacement as a result of trauma. Hip orthoses are also used for patients who are undergoing revision of a total hip replacement as a consequence of recurrent dislocation or of aseptic loosening of the femoral component. If control of rotation is desired, an HKAFO can be prescribed to provide additional support and protection to healing structures.

Most HKAFOs have a pelvic band and belt and an adjustable hip joint that can be locked or can allow free motion or limit motion within a specific range (Figure 12-16). An adjustable anterior panel can be added to the thigh section if a fracture

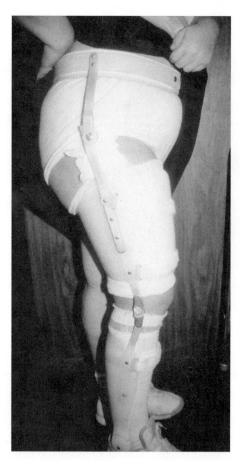

FIGURE 12-16 Lateral view of a hip-knee-ankle-foot orthosis, prescribed for postoperative management after a complex total hip arthroplasty. Note the pelvic band, free hip joint, supportive thigh cuff, and free knee joint. The ankle-foot orthosis component is necessary for effective control of rotary forces through the femur and hip joint.

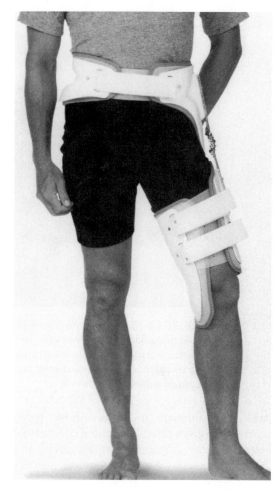

FIGURE 12-17 A postoperative hip abduction orthosis has three components. The proximal component is a padded pelvic band with a lateral extension and anterior closure that fits snugly around the upper pelvis. The distal component is a thigh cuff with a medial extension across the medial knee joint. These two pieces are connected by uprights and an adjustable hip joint, angled toward hip abduction and adjusted to limit hip flexion or extension. (From Orthomerica Newport. JPO 1995;7[1]:advertisement on front cover.)

has occurred during the surgical procedure and requires additional protection. The knee joint can also be locked, free motion, or adjustable for specific ranges of motion, depending on the patient's need. The ankle-foot orthosis component is necessary to provide maximum control of unwanted rotation of the hip.

Typically, HKAFOs are custom fabricated on the basis of an impression of the patient's limb. This increases the likelihood of an optimal fit and allows customization of the orthosis to meet the specific needs of the patient. If this approach is not amenable to certain health care environments, prefabricated custom-fit HKAFOs and hip orthoses are available as alternatives to custom-molded orthoses.[96] These orthoses are fabricated from components that are then custom fit on the basis of the patient's limb measurements. Most postoperative hip orthoses are designed to limit flexion and adduction of the hip joint (Figure 12-17). They try to prevent dislocation by supporting the optimal position of the hip joint within a safe range of motion and by providing a kinesthetic reminder when patients attempt to move beyond these ranges.[96] Many of the prefabricated hip orthoses that are commercially available are unable to provide maximum control of rotation because they do not encompass the foot. Careful evaluation

of the patient is required to determine which alternative is most appropriate. In both cases the orthosis is worn whenever the patient is out of bed and, in some instances, while the patient is in bed as well. The orthosis is usually worn for at least 8 weeks after total hip revision.

Because lower extremity orthoses add weight to a lower extremity that is already compromised, orthotists must be sensitive to the selection of lightweight materials and components. This is especially true for older patients, who may have limited endurance because of cardiac or respiratory disease. Although the initial orthosis may restrict joint motion to provide external stability to a vulnerable hip joint, the orthotic hip, knee, and ankle joints can be adjusted to meet the patient's needs as the rehabilitation program progresses. Hip orthoses and HKAFOs may be important adjuncts for rehabilitation in the following ways:

1. A well-fit hip orthosis provides protection against dislocation in patients who are predisposed to this problem.

2. Hip orthoses protect and support healing fracture sites, often allowing earlier mobility and gait training than would otherwise be possible.
3. Early and safe weight bearing for older patients with dislocation or fracture reduces the risk of secondary complications associated with prolonged bed rest or immobility.
4. The orthotic hip, knee, and ankle joints can be adjusted to restrict or permit motion to match the patient's specific needs at initial fitting and as the treatment program progresses.

Following surgical intervention after fracture or total joint arthroplasty, the focus of the rehabilitation program shifts to mobility training, strengthening, flexibility, and endurance. The decision to recommend a hip orthosis is individual, influenced by the severity of the musculoskeletal problem, the patient's particular circumstances, and the experience and preferences of the health professionals involved in postoperative care. Few definitive guidelines or documentation are available concerning the efficacy of hip orthoses in the postoperative management of hip fracture or arthroplasty. An orthosis is best used to augment the goals of rehabilitation including the return to preoperative ambulatory status, safe and protected weight bearing during activities of daily living, facilitation of union of the fracture site, and ultimately return to presurgical social and self-care independence.

Posttrauma Care

The other group of individuals who may benefit from hip orthoses are those who have experienced traumatic fractures of the femur, hip, or pelvis as a result of motor vehicle accidents, industrial accidents, or falls from great heights. Most of these patients are fit with their orthosis after stabilization of the fracture with internal fixation. The HKAFO is similar in design to the orthosis described for older patients after hip fracture or arthroplasty. Depending on the need for external support and stability, the hip joint can be locked to prevent flexion and extension or may allow motion within a limited range. For some patients, it may be necessary to incorporate a lumbosacral spinal orthosis to achieve the desired control of pelvic and hip motion. The ankle-foot orthosis component provides control of hip rotation in the transverse plane.

When complete immobilization is warranted after orthopedic trauma of the lower spine, pelvis, and hip, a custom-molded thermoplastic version of a hip spica cast can be fabricated (Figure 12-18). This hip orthosis has anterior and posterior components, extending from the mid- to lower thoracic trunk to just above the femoral condyles of the fractured extremity and to the groin of the intact extremity. This design provides maximum stability and can be used in lieu of or after casting. The position of the lower extremity within the orthosis is determined by the type and extent of the surgical repair. When the patient is lying in the supine position, the anterior component can be removed for skin inspection and personal care. Similarly, the posterior component can be removed when the patient is prone. This is an advantage for patients with open wounds or difficulty with continence and is especially appreciated if immobilization will be required for an extended period.

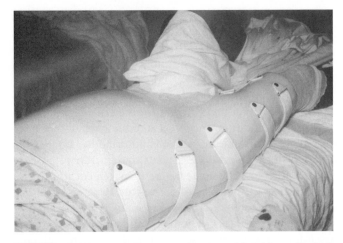

FIGURE 12-18 A postoperative custom-molded hip orthosis is sometimes used instead of a plaster hip spica cast when complete immobilization of the hip joint is required.

Many patients who are recovering from musculoskeletal trauma involving the pelvis and hip joint require physical therapy for gait and mobility training after surgery and an intensive rehabilitation program to regain preinjury muscle strength, range of motion, and functional status. The orthopedic surgeon and therapists, as well as the patient and family, must clearly understand the advantages provided and the mobility limitations imposed by postsurgical hip orthoses. An optimal orthosis can assist rehabilitation if fabricated with lightweight but durable components that can be adjusted as the patient progresses, while meeting the individual patient's need for stability or supported mobility of the hip. An appropriate hip orthosis also enhances early mobility and protected weight bearing, reducing the risk of loss of function related to bed rest and deconditioning.

FRACTURE MANAGEMENT

A fracture occurs when there is disruption in the continuity of bone.[98] Fractures are common consequences of trauma from falls, sports, work-related injuries, motor vehicle accidents, or violence.[99-101] Many disorders and diseases (e.g., osteopenia, malnutrition, paralysis, osteoporosis, medications (e.g., corticosteroids), as well as primary or metastatic malignancies of bone, increase vulnerability to fracture.[102,103] Habitual activity level over the life span, health habits (e.g., smoking), and gender and age (e.g., bone density and menopausal status) influence bone density and, subsequently, the risk of fracture during daily activity.[104-107] Orthopedic intervention for fractures is dictated by the severity of the fracture, as well as etiology. Simple fractures, those with minimal fragmentation or displacement, are often managed with closed reduction followed by initial management in a plaster or fiberglass splint to provide stabilization while allowing for swelling, and then a period of immobilization in a plaster or fiberglass cast or a custom-fit, prefabricated fracture orthosis until bony union is achieved.[108] More complex fractures, those with multiple fragments or significant displacement, often require open (surgical) reduction with internal fixation (with plates, screws, or wires) (ORIF), prosthetic replacement (arthroplasty), or stabilization in an external rigging or fixator until there has been sufficient bony healing.[109]

The care provided to individuals recovering from a fracture is founded on understanding the mechanism of injury, fracture classification, and process of bone repair and healing.[110,111] The orthopedic surgeon and orthotist choose from a variety of casts, cast braces, splints, and fracture orthoses to provide the most effective fracture management strategy for each patient on the basis of the fracture type and location, degree of reduction, skin condition, mobility needs, and likelihood of compliance. Geographical and personal preferences regarding design, device selection, and treatment influence the choice of fracture management strategy, as do the training and experience of the health professionals involved. Few strategies for immobilization can provide 100% rigid fixation. Absolute immobilization is only possible with direct skeletal attachment. A variety of factors influence the quality of fit and function of any cast, cast brace, splint, or fracture orthosis. Each device has the potential to contribute to a successful result but only if used appropriately, with absolute attention to detail by each of the treatment team members.

Mechanisms of Fracture Healing

Three distinct stages of physiological fracture healing occur: inflammation, repair, and remodeling.[111] Fracture damages bone, its periosteum, nutrient vessels, marrow, and often surrounding soft tissue and muscle. Disruption of vascular supply leads to ischemia and necrosis of bone cells and other injured tissues. These damaged tissues release inflammatory mediators into intracellular space, triggering an inflammatory response: A shift in plasma from capillary to intracellular space leads to significant edema. Migration of polymorphonuclear leukocytes, macrophages, and lymphocytes to the injured area is the first step in clearing necrosis. A hematoma forms; in a simple nondisplaced fracture on the shaft of a long bone, this hematoma provides the initial reconnection of edges of the fracture (Figure 12-19A). In more complex fractures, the process of reducing the fracture to align bony fragments further irritates tissues, augmenting the inflammatory response that is the first necessary step in fracture healing. This initial inflammatory response to fracture can last 5 or more days, depending on the severity of injury and extent of tissue disruption.

The next stage of healing is the repair stage, a period of cell migration, proliferation, and granulation. The combination of chemotactic factors and bone matrix proteins released by damaged bone and during inflammation triggers the initiation of bony repair. The hematoma organizes into a fibrin "scaffold," and cells within the hematoma begin to release growth factors and other proteins that trigger cell migration and proliferation of osteoblasts from the periosteum and endosteum, as well as synthesis of a fracture callus matrix for bony repair (see Figure 12-19B and C).[112] Initially the pH of the area around the fracture is acidic, and the fracture callus is primarily cartilaginous. As the repair stage progresses, the pH becomes more alkaline, creating an environment that enhances activity of the alkaline phosphatase enzyme, and subsequently mineralization of the cartilage of the fracture callus into woven bone tissue (see Figure 12-19D). The deposition of new cartilage within the callus is accompanied by both endochondral and intramembranous ossification. Clinical union of the fracture during the repair stage can last up to 3 months postinjury (hence the need for long periods of immobilization).

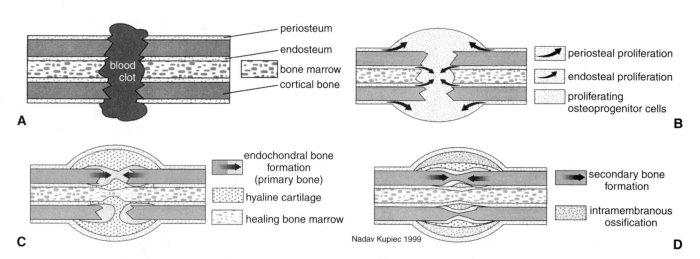

FIGURE 12-19 Healing and repair of a long bone fracture. **A,** Disruption of blood vessels in the bone, marrow, periosteum, and surrounding tissue at the time of injury results in extravasation of blood at the fracture site and the formation of hematoma. **B,** Initiation and development of the fracture callus. **C,** Note the simultaneous occurrence of chondrogenesis, endochondral ossification, and intramembranous bone formation in different regions of the fracture site. **D,** Union of a long bone fracture. (From Lundon K. *Orthopedic Rehabilitation Science: Principles for Clinical Management of Bone.* Boston: Butterworth-Heinemann, 2000.)

The final stage of healing is the remodeling stage, during which the new bone woven within the callus is reshaped into the more mature lamellae of long bone and excess callus resorbed. During this phase osteoclasts are active to reshape trabeculae and lamellae along the lines of weight-bearing forces. The process of maturation of the callus into a fully repaired bone can last a year or more, especially in complex fractures, whether managed by casting or ORIF. Factors that influence the duration of the remodeling stage include age, severity of injury, nutritional status, concurrent chronic illness, and medication use (especially corticosteroids).[113]

Fracture Classifications

Fractures are classified as either open or closed injuries on the basis of the presence of an open communication between the fracture and the outside world through a disruption of the soft tissues and skin.[114] In a closed fracture, the soft tissue envelope of muscles and skin around the bone fracture site is completely intact. Although muscle around the fracture site may be significantly damaged, the intact skin provides a barrier that prevents bacterial invasion of the injured muscle or bone. When an open or compound fracture occurs, the soft tissue envelope has been violated: The wound leaves muscle and fractured bone open to the environment and susceptible to infection. In many cases bone may actually protrude through the skin. Open injuries are orthopedic emergencies; patients are taken urgently to the operating room for debridement of the wound and fracture. Severely damaged or contaminated tissue is removed, and the wound is carefully cleaned in an effort to avoid infection and provide optimal circumstances for healing.[109] The fracture is then stabilized with a cast or surgical implant.

Gustilo and Anderson[114] have developed a classification system applied interoperatively that rates the severity of open or compound fractures. The least severe is a type I injury, in which a small wound with minimal soft tissue damage (1 cm) communicates with the fracture. The wound in a type II fracture is generally between 1 and 12 cm, and significant soft tissue injury may be present underneath the laceration or wound. In a more severe, type III injury, the wound diameter is often greater than 12 cm, there is considerable periosteal stripping, and barely enough muscle or skin is present to cover the injured or fractured bone adequately. Type III open fractures are subdivided into another three categories—A, B, and C—on the basis of whether the soft tissue can cover the bone and whether neurological or vascular involvement is present in association with the open fracture. It should be noted that more important than the size of the skin defect is the damage to soft tissues and periosteum in determining type. Therefore a 1-cm open hole in a crushed and comminuted fracture may well be classified as a type III.

The particular location and pattern of fracture determine whether the fracture is stable and can be effectively managed with a cast or brace, or unstable, requiring surgical intervention. A fracture with concurrent joint dislocation

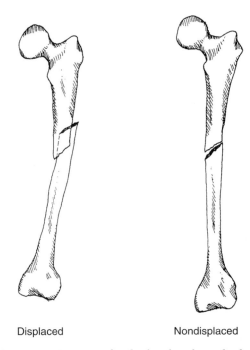

Displaced   **Nondisplaced**

FIGURE 12-20 Diagram of a displaced and nondisplaced fracture of the diaphysis of the femur. (From Gustilo RB. *The Fracture Classification Manual.* St. Louis: Mosby, 1991.)

creates an extremely unstable condition, requiring surgical management of the fracture/dislocation and a long period of rehabilitation.

Fractures (whether closed or open) are described as displaced or nondisplaced on the basis of the degree of malalignment or overlap that is observed on a radiograph (Figure 12-20). They are described as complete or incomplete, depending on whether the bone has fully transected. In children, a greenstick fracture is an incomplete oblique or spiral fracture that extends only partially through bone. Exact location of the fracture is also important: Fractures of the diaphysis or metaphysis of a long cortical bone are extraarticular (Figure 12-21), while those involving the epiphysis within the joint capsule are intraarticular. Intraarticular fractures, especially when displaced, have a high likelihood of causing posttraumatic arthritis, and often require surgical reconstruction of the joint surface.

Extraarticular fractures can be transverse (mostly perpendicular to the axis of the bone), oblique (diagonal to the axis of the bone), or spiral (typically a result of torsional forces), depending on the direction of force contributing to the injury and the resulting alteration in bone configuration. When one or more substantive fragments are seen on the radiograph, the fracture is segmental; if there are multiple small fragments, the fracture is comminuted. In high-impact, complex fractures there is often enough destruction of bone that there will be loss of bone length or substance. Fractures of the metaphysis are determined to be nondisplaced or displaced, simple, compressed, or comminuted (Figure 12-22). Before and during puberty (during times of rapid bone growth), there can be displacement of the proximal or distal epiphysis

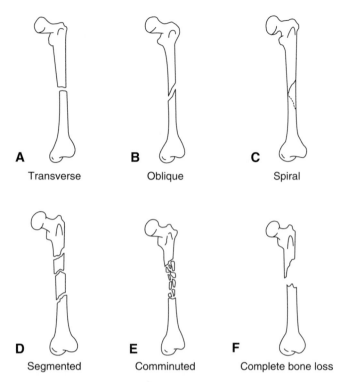

A Transverse   **B** Oblique   **C** Spiral

D Segmented   **E** Comminuted   **F** Complete bone loss

FIGURE 12-21 Examples of types of long bone fractures, illustrated in the diaphysis of the femur: A transverse fracture **(A)** is primarily perpendicular to the long axis of the bone, while an oblique fracture **(B)** diagonally transects the bone. A spiral fracture **(C)** is the result of a rotary force during injury. Segmental fractures **(D)** have one or more noncontinuous segments, while a comminuted fracture **(E)** has multiple small fragments. In cases of significant trauma, there may actually be loss of bone substance **(F)**. (Modified from Gustilo RB. *The Fracture Classification Manual*. St. Louis: Mosby, 1991.)

from the metaphysis through the cartilaginous epiphyseal plate (Figure 12-23); the proximal (subcapital) epiphysis of the femur is particularly vulnerable.

Intraarticular fractures are classified as linear, comminuted, impacted, or having a percent of bone loss (Figure 12-24); complex intraarticular fractures involve both proximal and distal components of the joint (Figure 12-25) and typically require ORIF.

In the proximal femur, fractures of the metaphysis are described as intertrochanteric fractures (extracapsular, linear or oblique, through or between the trochanters) or femoral neck fractures (intracapsular across the neck of the femur) or comminuted (with multiple fragments of neck and or trochanters) (Figure 12-26). These fractures fall into the category of hip fractures, and typically require ORIF or replacement with a femoral prosthesis (hemiarthroplasty) or even a total hip arthroplasty (Figure 12-27). Fractures of the acetabulum are the result of either a longitudinal force through the femur into the pelvis or an upward oblique lateral force through the greater trochanter; if the hip happens to be adducted at the time of injury, this may lead to posterior dislocation (Figure 12-28).

Fractures of the pelvis are classified as stable or unstable on the basis of the extent of damage that disrupts the circumferential integrity of the pelvis (Figure 12-29). Persons with unstable fractures of the pelvis are at risk for life-threatening hemorrhage, as well as residual genitourinary or neurological complications, given the vessels, nerves, muscles, and organs that are housed within the pelvis.[115]

Fractures of irregularly shaped bones such as the tarsals and vertebrae tend to fall into three categories. Stress

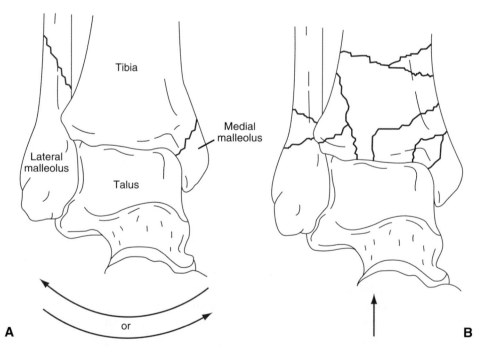

Tibia

Medial malleolus

Lateral malleolus

Talus

A   or   **B**

FIGURE 12-22 A, Extraarticular metaphyseal fracture of the malleoli of the tibia and fibula is often the result of rotational injuries. **B,** Intraarticular fractures of the ankle mortis (also called plafond or pylon fractures) result from high-energy compressive injury. (Modified from Clark CR, Bonfiglio M [eds], *Orthopaedics: Essentials of Diagnosis and Treatment*. Philadelphia: Churchill Livingstone, 1994.)

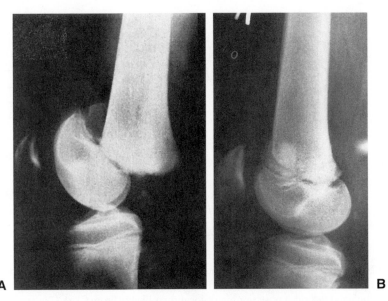

FIGURE 12-23 Lateral view of an avulsed distal femoral condyle **(A)** before and **(B)** following closed reduction. (From Clark CR, Bonfiglio M [eds], *Orthopaedics: Essentials of Diagnosis and Treatment.* Philadelphia: Churchill Livingstone, 1994.)

fractures result from repetitive loading of the bone, are often nondisplaced, and can disrupt either the inner scaffolding of the cancellous bone or the outer shell of cortical bone. Simple stress fractures typically heal well with immobilization; more complex stress fractures may require surgical stabilization. Pathological fractures occur when there is underlying disease (e.g., osteoporosis, Charcot's osteopathy, neoplasm) that compromises bone density or metabolism. In pathological fractures the trabeculae are overwhelmed by the magnitude of force exerted through the bone, and the bone

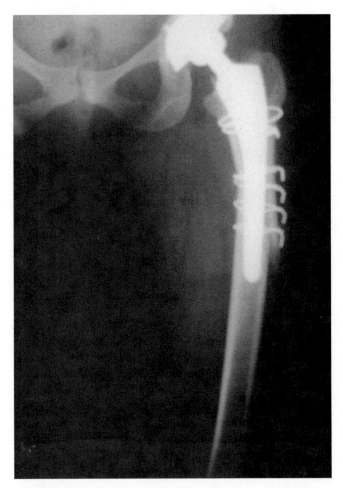

FIGURE 12-25 A radiograph of a repaired complex fracture of the proximal femur, with prosthetic total hip replacement and open reduction internal fixation with circumferentially wrapped wires to stabilize a spiral fracture of the proximal femoral diaphysis.

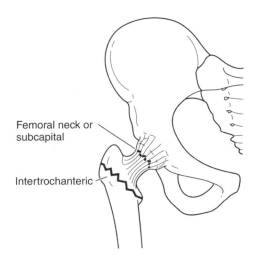

Femoral neck or subcapital

Intertrochanteric

FIGURE 12-24 Femoral neck fractures are intracapsular and traverse the blood supply to the femoral head. Intertrochanteric fractures spare the blood supply but are a greater risk for failure of fixation. (From Clark CR, Bonfiglio M [eds], *Orthopaedics: Essentials of Diagnosis and Treatment.* Philadelphia: Churchill Livingstone, 1994.)

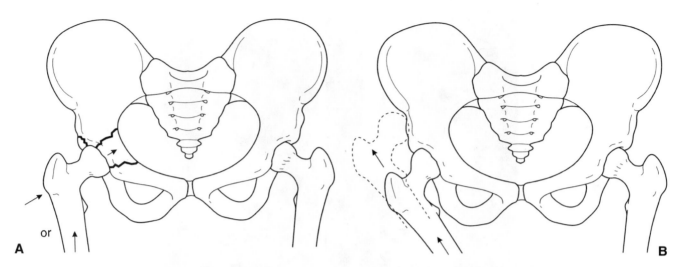

FIGURE 12-26 A, Acetabular fractures occur from a lateral blow over the greater trochanter or a proximally directed force transmitted up the length of the femur. **B,** If the limb is injured with the hip in adduction and flexion, a posterior hip dislocation is likely. (From Clark CR, Bonfiglio M [eds], *Orthopaedics: Essentials of Diagnosis and Treatment.* Philadelphia: Churchill Livingstone, 1994.)

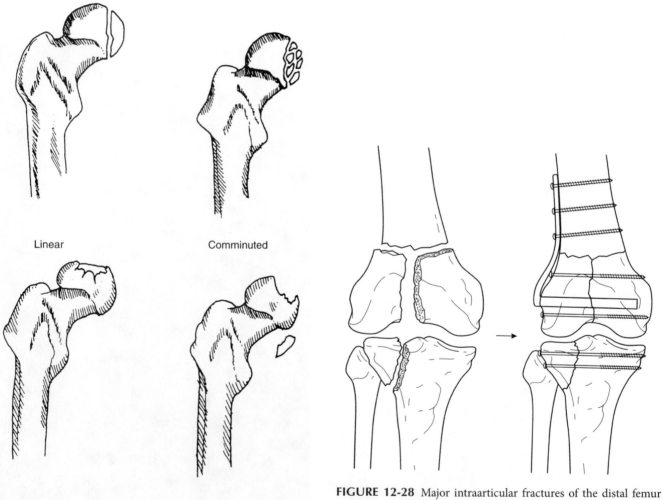

Linear

Comminuted

Impacted

Articular bone loss

FIGURE 12-27 Examples of types of intraarticular fractures, using the head of the femur as an example. (From Gustilo RB. *The Fracture Classification Manual.* St. Louis: Mosby, 1991.)

FIGURE 12-28 Major intraarticular fractures of the distal femur and proximal tibia are typically managed by surgical open reduction internal fixation using a combination of bone screws or nail and an external plate. (From Clark CR, Bonfiglio M [eds], *Orthopaedics: Essentials of Diagnosis and Treatment.* Philadelphia: Churchill Livingstone, 1994.)

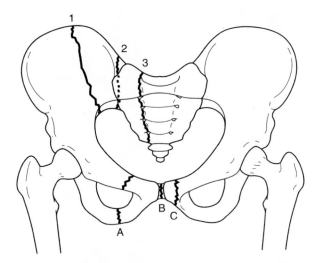

FIGURE 12-29 Unstable pelvic fractures occur when pubic rami fractures (**A**), symphysis disruption (**B**), or pubic body fractures (**C**) are accompanied by fractures through the iliac wing (1), sacroiliac joint (2), or sacrum (3). (From Clark CR, Bonfiglio M [eds], *Orthopaedics: Essentials of Diagnosis and Treatment.* Philadelphia: Churchill Livingstone, 1994.)

is compressed or fractured into fragments. Management of pathological fractures can be challenging, as bone healing is often compromised by the underlying disease process. Traumatic fractures are often comminuted; depending on severity, they may be managed by immobilization in a cast or orthosis, ORIF, or placement of an external fixation apparatus (Figure 12-30).

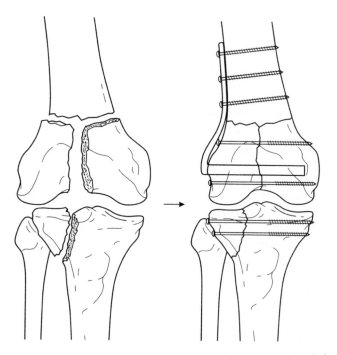

FIGURE 12-30 Open fractures of the tibial shaft often require skeletal stabilization with external fixation, as well as soft tissue repair. (From Clark CR, Bonfiglio M [eds], *Orthopaedics: Essentials of Diagnosis and Treatment.* Philadelphia: Churchill Livingstone, 1994.)

Casts and Splints

The primary goal of fracture management is to restore musculoskeletal limb function of the injured extremity with optimal anatomical alignment, functional muscle strength, sensory function, and pain-free joint range of motion. The most common methods used for immobilization of closed fractures include casts, splints, fracture orthoses, or a hybrid cast-orthosis.[108,116] Immobilization may also be used after ORIF of open fractures.

In choosing the appropriate immobilization strategy for an individual's fracture, the orthopedist considers several issues. The first is the stability of the fracture site and how well a device will be able to maintain fracture reduction and achieve the desired anatomical result. The condition of the skin and soft tissue is also an important consideration, especially if wounds are present that must be accessed for proper care. Limb volume must be evaluated, especially if edema is present or anticipated: How will limb size change over time in the device? Length of immobilization time varies as well: Is the device designed for a short-term problem, or will protection of the limb be necessary for an extended period? Will the device need to be removed for hygiene or wound care? Can the limb be unprotected while sleeping or when not ambulating? Availability (time to application) may also influence decision making. Casts and cast braces can be applied quickly. Custom orthoses need additional fabrication and fitting time; an alternative means of protection is often required while the device is being fabricated.

The individual's ability to comply consistently and reliably with weight-bearing restrictions and other aspects of fracture management must also be considered. Factors such as cognitive ability, emotional status, motivation, and physical ability, as well as the availability of assistance and environmental demands, influence the decision to provide additional external support. An unstable fracture managed by ORIF may not require additional support for those with sufficient strength and balance who have a clear understanding of the healing process. If the individual with a fracture cannot understand the need to protect the involved limb from excessive loading or is physically unable to do so, additional external support is essential. If compliance is questionable, the device of choice is usually a nonremovable cast or cast brace.

To effectively stabilize a fracture, the joints above and below the fracture site must be immobilized. The period of immobilization varies with fracture severity and location; in most cases the cast remains in place from 6 to 8 weeks or until a radiograph indicates that bone healing has progressed sufficiently for safe weight bearing and function. The time for immobilization is often less for children, due to their rapid healing response. Although immobilization is essential for effective bone healing, it also has significant consequences on other tissues: while in a cast, patients are likely to develop significant joint stiffness (contracture), as well as disuse atrophy and weakness of the muscles of the immobilized limb. Once the cast is removed, rehabilitation professionals are called on to help the patient regain preinjury muscle performance, flexibility, and range of motion.

A cast is a rigid, externally applied device that provides circumferential support to an injured body part.[108] Casts immobilize a body segment to maintain optimal skeletal alignment (Figures 12-31 and 12-32). Once a cast has been applied, a radiograph can be used to assess the effectiveness of skeletal alignment. The cast may need to be modified, wedged, or replaced to improve alignment.[117]

A splint is a temporary supportive device, usually fabricated from rigid materials, held in position on the fractured extremity with bandages or straps. Splints can be used for temporary immobilization before casting or surgical stabilization. They can be used to maintain fracture reduction while waiting for swelling to diminish or fracture blisters to clear or to provide comfort. The most commonly used splints include

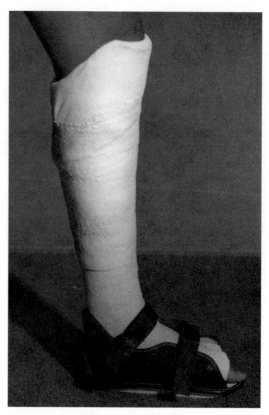

FIGURE 12-32 A medial view of a patellar tendon–bearing short leg cast. The proximal anterior area of the cast has been molded by pressing inward at the level of the patellar tendon, while the proximal posterior of the cast has been molded over the calf and then trimmed to allow knee flexion. (From Moore TJ. Functional bracing of lower extremity fractures. In Goldberg B, Hsu JD [eds], *Atlas of Orthoses and Assistive Devices*. St. Louis: Mosby; 1997.)

sugar tong splints (a long, U-shaped, padded plaster forearm splint named for its similarity to the tool used to pick up sugar cubes), short or long leg splints, thumb spica splints, ulnar or radial gutter splints, and coaptation splints.[117]

Casting and Splinting Materials

Before the 1800s, fracture casts were made from linen bandages soaked in beaten egg whites and lime. The modern era in fracture care began with the discovery of plaster of Paris (calcium sulfate), first used in the Turkish Empire as reported by Eaton in 1798.[118] Plaster of Paris was used in Europe in the early nineteenth century, and a Flemish surgeon (Mathijsen) is credited with combining the use of plaster of Paris and cloth bandages to form casts for the treatment of fractures in 1852.[117-119]

Plaster of Paris is created when heat is used to dehydrate gypsum. When water is added to plaster of Paris powder, the dehydration process is reversed, and crystals of gypsum are formed again. The new crystals interlock in a chemical exothermic (heat-producing) process.[120] The setting process is complete when heat is no longer being produced, although the cast remains wet to the touch until the excess water used in the process evaporates. Maximum cast strength is not reached until the plaster is completely dry. Drying time varies

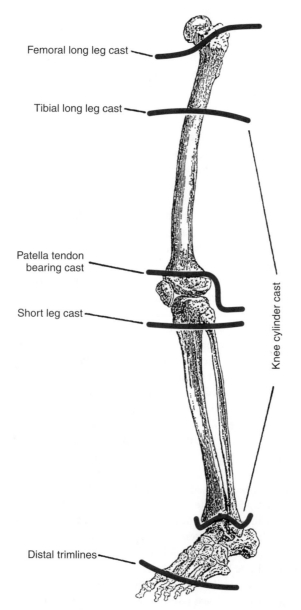

Femoral long leg cast

Tibial long leg cast

Patella tendon bearing cast

Short leg cast

Knee cylinder cast

Distal trimlines

FIGURE 12-31 Proximal and distal trimlines used in standard lower extremity casts. Typically, the joints above and below the fracture site are immobilized. Trimlines can be extended to provide better control and stabilization.

with the thickness of the cast, ambient humidity, and the type of plaster used. In most instances maximum cast strength is reached in approximately 24 hours.

Various types of plaster of Paris with different working characteristics are available. Manufacturers may add accelerators to the material that shorten the setting time: The limb has to be held still for less time while the plaster sets. Although this may be advantageous when a cast is applied to the limb of an anxious child or when an unstable fracture is cast, it also means that less working time is available to manipulate the extremity and optimally shape the cast. Setting time can be prolonged slightly if cold water is used. If warm or hot water is used to reduce setting time, care must be taken to protect the limb from injury from the higher heat that can be generated during the setting process.[117] Cast temperatures as high as 68.5°C have been reached with water temperatures of 40°C; burns can occur if cast temperature is maintained at 44°C for 6 hours or more.[121,122] To minimize any potential for burns in cast or splint application, room temperature tepid water (24°C) is recommended. If higher water temperatures have been used, the newly casted limb must not be placed on a pillow or other type of support that is likely to retain or reflect heat. Cast burns can also occur when insufficient padding has been placed between the plaster of Paris and the surface of the skin. Cast burns are avoidable if simple procedures are followed.

Cast strength is determined by three factors: the type of casting material used, the thickness of the cast, and the effectiveness of lamination among the layers of the cast material. The cloth mesh material that serves as the carrier for the plaster of Paris provides little strength for the cast. A plaster cast must be kept absolutely dry to prevent it from becoming soft and ineffective in immobilization.

The difficulties associated with the use of plaster of Paris have led to the development of newer and improved casting materials. Polyurethane-impregnated casting tapes have gained widespread popularity because of their superior strength, light weight, shorter setting time, cleaner application, and low exothermic reaction. Polyurethane casts are also radiolucent, permitting x-ray evaluation of fracture site healing while the limb remains encased in the cast.

Polyurethane is a plastic material that can be impregnated into a fabric substrate. Although the polyurethane bonds the layers of substrate together, it is actually the substrate that determines the strength of the cast. A variety of substrate materials are available. The weave determines how elastic the material will be during cast application and how strong the cast will be when set. Cotton, polyester, fiberglass, polypropylene, and blends of these materials and others are used in synthetic casting tapes.[120,121,123,124]

Immersing the synthetic casting tape in room temperature water for 10 seconds begins a heat-producing exothermic reaction and causes the material to harden (polymerize). Setting is complete for most synthetic casting materials in 5 to 10 minutes. Because of this short setting time, the rolls of bandage material cannot be opened until they are ready to be applied as a cast. The application process requires skill and must move quickly to ensure adequate molding time. Unlike plaster of Paris, the plastic bandage does not need to be massaged to ensure proper lamination between the layers of material. Also unlike plaster of Paris, which can easily be washed from the hands or clothing, polyurethane is not easily removed: Adequate protective padding must be placed around the patient's limb, and protective gloves worn to safeguard the applicator's hands. Polyurethane resin in its natural state is tacky. An additive may be incorporated into the casting tape to reduce its tackiness. In some cases the manufacturer provides special gloves with an antitacky additive to further minimize the tack.[120] The exothermic polymerization of polyurethane resin produces much less heat (44.9°C in 40°C water) than that of setting plaster of Paris. In addition, heat is quickly dissipated so that burns are much less likely to occur when synthetic materials are used. To further minimize the risk of burns, immersion of cast tape in room temperature water (24°C) is recommended.[117,121,125]

Cast Application

Stockinet is the first layer of a cast, applied over the skin, before any padding is added. The most common stockinet material is cotton. Synthetic materials such as polyester or polypropylene or Gore-Tex can be chosen in place of cotton because they do not retain water like cotton materials do. Stockinet also helps to position dressings over wounds and provides extra circumferential control of soft tissue within the cast. Stockinet is folded over the proximal and distal edges to finish the cast (and prevent inadvertent removal of cast padding by a nonresponsible individual or a child).

Next, a layer of cast padding is added over the stockinet. A variety of materials are available to pad casts. Sheet cotton comes in various forms and is used to provide a barrier between the rigid walls of the cast and surface of the skin. Some cast materials have been elasticized for easier application and conformation, and others require more technique to ensure that they uniformly conform to the body part being casted.

Although synthetic cast tapes are not affected by water, cast padding or stockinet does retain water. The risk of skin maceration and breakdown is present if the inside of a cast remains damp for long periods of time. Some manufacturers market cast padding that reportedly permits exposure to water; however, manufacturer recommendations must be followed carefully.

The thickness of cast padding varies; ⅛ to ¼ inch is sufficient for most individuals. The goal is to protect bony prominences and soft tissue from the rigid walls of the cast while effectively immobilizing the fracture site. Soft tissue usually does well with a fairly thin, uniform two- or three-layer wrap. Extra padding is added to smooth and protect the irregular surfaces around bony prominences. Excessive padding reduces the ability of the cast to provide adequate immobilization. A well-molded cast that accurately follows the anatomical contours of the extremity requires less padding. Cast padding also provides a barrier so that the cast can be removed more easily when it needs to be changed or is no longer necessary.

Lower Extremity Casts

The short leg cast is used in the management of fractures involving the distal tibia or fibula, or both; the ankle joint; or the rear foot or midfoot. The foot is positioned in a functional neutral ankle position (90 degrees) or in slight dorsiflexion. This positioning prevents a plantarflexion contracture from developing by the time of cast removal. The foot can also be casted in a plantarflexed position to accommodate repair of an Achilles tendon rupture. The proximal trimline falls at the level of the tibial tubercle; the distal trimline usually encloses the metatarsal heads. The area around the fibular head is protected by adding extra cast padding to minimize the risk of compression of the peroneal nerve. A cast shoe should be used to protect the bottom of the cast if weight bearing is to be permitted.

For persons with midshaft fractures of the tibia, a patellar tendon–bearing cast (PTB) may be applied. This design incorporates a patellar tendon bar, which directs some of the limb loading force to the external shell of the cast, thus protecting the full length of the tibia against bending moments (see Figure 12-32). This type of cast is not effective, however, in reducing axial loading of the tibia or hind foot. The PTB is most often used when extra stability is desired for individuals who will be allowed some degree of weight-bearing activity. The cast is applied with the ankle maintained in neutral or slightly dorsiflexed position, to minimize potential hyperextension moment at the knee in stance. Trimlines are similar to those used for a PTB transtibial prosthetic socket: at the midpatella (or sometimes suprapatella) anteriorly but trimmed and slightly flared posteriorly to permit knee flexion of at least 90 degrees. Proximally, the cast is well molded to the tibia in the area of the medial flare and around the patella.[126,127] Care must be taken to ensure that no pressure is placed on the peroneal nerve.

A knee cylinder cast is often applied when there have been fractures of the patella or surgical repair of the knee joint when the knee must be immobilized in full extension. To ensure the necessary stability for the knee joint, the proximal trimline encompasses the lower two thirds of the thigh and the distal trimline the entire tibial segment to just above the malleoli. The cast can be applied using either plaster of Paris or synthetic casting tape. To limit the risk of pistoning when the person wearing the cast is standing or walking, the cast is carefully molded to fit the contours of the medial femoral condyle.

For closed fractures of the upper tibia, knee joint, or lower femur, a long leg cast provides the necessary stability for healing. Depending on the site of fracture and its relative stability, the limb is immobilized in nearly full extension or in a bent knee position.[127] A straight knee cast is usually applied with a slight (5-degree) knee flexion angle to enhance patient comfort. Bent knee casts are usually chosen when non-weight bearing must be ensured during ambulation or to aid in controlling rotation of the tibia. With the relatively mobile arrangement of soft tissue that surrounds the femur, it is challenging to provide adequate immobilization, especially for persons who are particularly muscular or overweight. For this reason, control of rotational forces through the femur within a long leg cast is questionable. If the cast is being used to stabilize the tibia, the proximal trimline is at the junction of the middle and proximal third of the femur. If the cast is being used to stabilize the distal femur, the proximal trimline is at the level of the greater trochanter. Distally, the cast immobilizes the ankle and extends to a point just beyond the metatarsal heads. The fibular head should be well padded within the cast to minimize the risk of entrapment of the peroneal nerve.

A hip spica cast, which encases the hip and pelvis in addition to the lower extremity, is necessary for effective control of fractures of the proximal femur and of the hip joint[128] (Figure 12-33). The hip spica is the primary method of treatment of femoral fractures in children under five years of age and is used in adults when a prefabricated hip orthosis is not appropriate. Several variations of the hip spica are available. In a single hip spica, the plaster or synthetic cast material is anchored around the entire pelvis and lower trunk but immobilizes only the hip and knee of the involved side, allowing fairly unrestricted hip motion of the opposite limb. In a 1½ hip spica, the cast encases the entire lower extremity on the affected side, as well as the lower trunk, pelvis, and thigh on the uninvolved side. Usually the knee on the affected side is completely immobilized; however, an articulated knee joint can be incorporated if specific circumstances so dictate. In most instances the hip joint of the affected limb is immobilized in 30 degrees of flexion and 30 degrees of abduction, and the perineal edges are trimmed back to allow for personal care and hygiene. The knee is usually positioned in 30 degrees of flexion. The proximal cast encases the lower to middle trunk (to the level of the costal margin or nipple line), depending on the amount of spinal immobilization required.

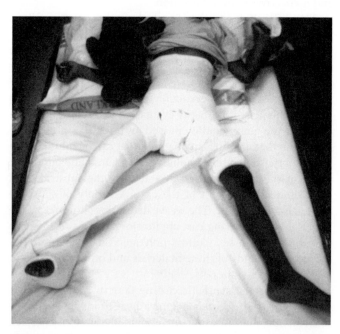

FIGURE 12-33 This child has been placed in a 1½ hip spica cast to stabilize a fracture of the proximal femur. Note the opening for personal hygiene and the additional diagonal support bar incorporated between the short and long sections of the cast.

The 1½ hip spica cast is often reinforced by the incorporation of a lightweight diagonal bar between the short and long extremity segments. Ambulation is possible but often quite challenging, requiring significant upper body strength to manage the adapted crutch-walking gait that the cast position makes necessary.

Cast Removal

A cast cutter or saw with a vibrating disk is used to cut the cast during cast removal. Modern cast cutter blades reciprocate back and forth approximately ⅛ inch in either direction. The vibrating blade easily cuts rigid materials such as metal, wood, plaster, or synthetic cast materials but does not cut through materials that are elastic or mobile. If used properly, a cast cutter does not cut skin. Incorrect or inappropriate use of a cast cutter can seriously cut or burn a patient. To reduce the risk of injury, the blade should not directly contact the patient's skin. Friction between the blade and cast significantly heats the blade, creating a potential for burns. A sharp new blade has less potential for burning the patient than does a blade that has become dull or worn out. The noise of the cast cutter can be quite frightening to children or other particularly anxious patients. A careful explanation and a demonstration of the cast cutter's action are the first steps in the process of cast removal.

To remove a cast safely, the cutter is used in a repetitive in-out motion, to progressively open the cast, instead of sliding the blade through the cast. This strategy reduces the risk of a cut or burn on the patient's skin.[129] Safety strips may be incorporated into the cast at the time of application to allow for a safe path for the saw blade to penetrate through without damaging skin. These strips are especially important when friable liners like Gore-tex are used under the cast. Safe technique involves the operator's thumb serving as a fulcrum on the cast as downward pressure is applied through the wrist. The thumb also controls the depth of the blade. Care is taken to avoid positioning the cast cutter in areas where skin is vulnerable: over a bony prominence or where significant edema or fragile healing skin is present. As the blade breaks through the inner wall of the cast, the sensation of reduced resistance to downward pressure, as well as a change in sound, occurs. Once an area of cast has been cut, the blade is repositioned farther along the cast and the process is repeated until the cast can be pried open completely. Bandage scissors are used to cut through padding and stockinet, and the limb is then extracted from the open cast. For infants and young children with small limbs, an alternative strategy can be used: A plaster of Paris cast can be removed by soaking in water. This method works particularly well when a corrective clubfoot cast is removed from an infant's limb.

Hybrid Cast Braces

Hybrid cast braces were first developed as a method of management of proximal tibial and distal femoral fractures near the knee just after World War I but then fell out of use until the mid-1960 s[130–132] (Figure 12-34). In some centers the cast brace is the method of choice for the management of nondisplaced tibial plateau fractures. The cast brace is often used for additional support of fractures near the knee or of the femur that have been stabilized via ORIF surgery for external fixation (Figure 12-35). This method is also used to control motion after knee ligament injury or reconstruction.

Cast braces incorporate orthotic components (e.g., hinge joints, range of motion locks) into a plaster or synthetic cast in an effort to provide additional stability to a healing limb.[133–141] The cast brace can be applied using either plaster of Paris or synthetic cast materials. Depending on the nature of the fracture and its stability, the orthotic knee joints incorporated into the cast brace may be chosen to provide limited, controlled, or free-knee range of motion. Because the anatomical center rotation of the knee moves in an arc centered over the femoral condyles, it is essential that the mechanical joints be carefully aligned with the anatomical knee joint to reduce the abnormal stress that occurs across the joint and fracture site.[142,143]

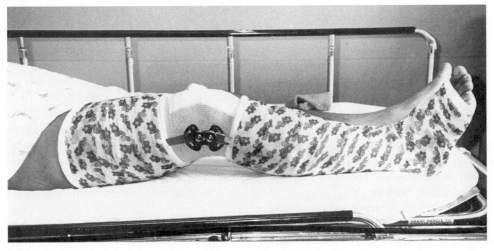

FIGURE 12-34 A tibial cast brace with polycentric adjustable range of motion hinges. The patient has undergone an open reduction internal fixation surgery after fracture of the tibial plateau. Note that synthetic cast tape is available in a wide variety of colors and patterns.

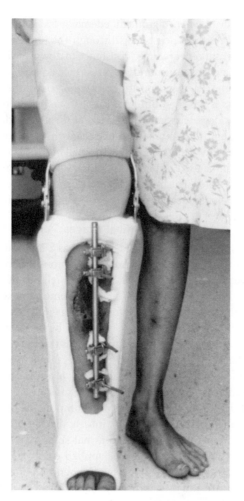

FIGURE 12-35 This cast brace provides medial/lateral stability for a comminuted grade 3 open tibial fracture. The length of the tibia is being maintained by an external fixation device. The patient also sustained a closed femoral fracture, which has been supported by an intramedullary rod fixation. Because the proximal portion of the cast must not terminate near a fracture line, the femoral portion of the cast has been extended up to the level of the trochanter to avoid stress on the femoral fixation.

Many orthotists and orthopedic surgeons choose a polycentric orthotic knee joint because its motion more closely follows anatomical motion and reduces the torque-related stress that results from a single-axis mechanical joint. Palpating the condyles on a patient who has had recent trauma about the knee is difficult; the midpatella is a somewhat less precise alternative landmark for alignment. A properly placed polycentric metal joint will be proximal to the joint line and slightly posterior to the midline. Orthotic knee joints are positioned close to but not quite contacting skin. This is especially important medially, where contact between the knees during functional activity is likely.

Medial and lateral uprights are incorporated into the cast above and below the orthotic knee joint to provide protection against unwanted varus and valgus stress and help control anteroposterior displacement of the tibia or femur.

The distal tibial cast holds the ankle in a neutral position and extends distally to encompass the metatarsal heads.

The proximal trimline of the tibial cast is typically at the tibial tubercle, and the distal trimline of the femoral cast is an equal distance from the midpatella. Posteriorly, both tibial and femoral casts are trimmed to permit at least 90 degrees of knee flexion. If warranted, a slight varus or valgus stress can be applied at the time of cast brace application, or a varus/valgus strap can be added to aid in unloading a knee compartment. For persons with fractures of the upper tibia and knee, the proximal component encases the lower two thirds of the femur. If fracture of the femur has occurred, the proximal component extends upward to the level of the greater trochanter. To be effective, careful molding of the proximal portion of the cast around the trochanter and medial wall is required. For fractures of the mid to upper femur, an orthotic hip joint and pelvic band must be added to ensure alignment and stability.

Fracture Orthoses

A custom-fabricated or custom-fit fracture orthosis is designed to maintain a body part in an optimal anatomical position, limit joint motion, and unload weight-bearing forces.[144-147] The major advantage of a fracture orthosis, as compared with a cast brace, is that the orthosis can be removed for wound or skin care. Fracture orthoses are fabricated from high-temperature thermoplastic materials. They are designed to provide total contact, circumferential control of a fracture while allowing the individual with a healing fracture to have functional mobility. Fracture stability is enhanced in two ways: by hydrostatic pressure forces created as the rigid walls of the orthosis compress soft tissue and muscles in the extremity and by the lever arm created by extension of the orthosis above and below the fracture site. Fracture orthoses do not entirely unload the lower extremity during weight bearing. If complete unloading or reduced loading is required to protect the fracture site, an appropriate assistive device (crutches or a walker) and a single limb gait pattern must be used.[139]

Two types of fracture orthoses are available: (1) those that are custom fabricated from a mold of the patient's limb and (2) prefabricated orthoses that are custom fit to match the patient's needs. Because of the wide variation in anatomical characteristics among individuals, it is not always possible to use a prefabricated orthosis. Likewise, because of anatomical similarities in the human skeleton, it is not always necessary to create a custom-fabricated device. In certain instances an orthosis must be precisely fit to provide the desired stabilization of the fracture; in other cases the orthosis must be heavily padded so that a precise fit is less important. The orthotic prescription must clearly designate the motions to be permitted and controlled, the corrective forces to be applied, and a precise diagnosis and description of the fracture.

Types of Fracture Orthoses

Fracture orthoses are named by the joints they encompass and the motion that they are designed to control. An ankle-foot orthosis (AFO) with an anterior shell is used to control ankle and distal tibia motion (Figure 12-36). It encases

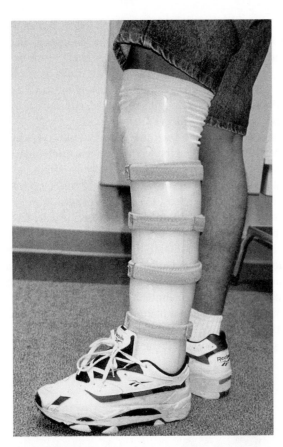

FIGURE 12-36 Ankle-foot fracture orthosis with a patellar tendon–bearing design incorporated to protect the tibia for bending moments during weight bearing. This patient was originally managed with an external fixation device, which had to be removed secondary to pin loosening before union of the fracture was solid. Note that the shoe has been modified with a cushion heel and rocker sole to compensate for a fixed ankle position and to improve forward progression during the stance phase of gait.

the injured limb completely, limiting motion of the foot or ankle for patients with distal tibial or fibular fractures. The AFO fracture orthosis has two advantages: It can be removed for wound care and hygiene, and it can be worn with standard lace-up shoes if weight bearing is permitted. The application of a cushion heel and rocker sole may be necessary on the shoe to compensate for limited heel, ankle, and toe rocker motion during gait. Because total contact is essential, this thermoplastic orthosis is vacuum molded over a positive impression of the patient's limb. The anterior shell may be lined with soft-density foam to accommodate bony deformity or insufficient soft tissue. Perforated thermoplastic material is often used for the anterior section as a means of ventilation for patient comfort. The proximal anterior trimline is at the tibial tubercle. Adequate clearance must be provided for the head of the fibula and the peroneal nerve. The distal posterior section usually extends to just beyond the metatarsal heads on the plantar surface, whereas the anterior section is trimmed just proximally. A stocking or thin sock is worn to protect the skin and for comfort. The anterior section is held in place with a series of hook-and-loop material straps. Shoes must be worn if weight bearing is permitted.

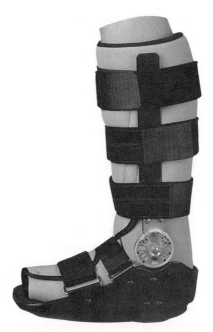

FIGURE 12-37 An example of a commercially available short leg walker with a rocker bottom sole that can be used for individuals with Achilles tendon repair, stable healing fractures of the distal tibia/fibula, ankle, or foot, or with severe ankle sprain. This particular walker has an orthotic ankle joint that can be preset to limit or allow motion at the ankle joint. (Courtesy of DJ Orthopedics, Vista, CA.)

A number of prefabricated short leg walkers are also commercially available; these devices are designed to substitute for a short leg cast and are intended to be removable by the patient. They are heavily padded and, if properly fit, provide excellent immobilization of the distal tibia, ankle, rear foot, and forefoot (Figure 12-37). The various designs are similar, but manufacturers' instructions should be followed to maximize their effectiveness. The short leg walker's advantage is that it can be removed for wound and skin care. Its disadvantage may be slightly less effective immobilization. The ankle is positioned at a neutral (90-degree) angle. Some designs have an adjustable orthotic ankle joint that permits a controlled, limited range of motion, to assist forward progression during walking. The components of a short leg walker include a rigid foot piece that is attached to a pair of metal or thermoplastic uprights and a proximal cuff that helps to suspend a foam liner. Short leg walkers are manufactured in various styles and sizes. To ensure proper fit, the manufacturer's recommendations must be followed carefully.

The PTB fracture orthosis is the removable version of the PTB cast, providing significant protection from bending and rotatory torque for the tibia during weight-bearing activities. This thermoplastic orthosis is most often vacuum molded over a positive mold of the patient's limb for optimal total contact fit. Ankle position within the orthosis is often in slight dorsiflexion, once again to minimize hyperextension moment at the knee during the stance phase of gait. Trimlines are similar to those of an AFO with anterior shell, with the proximal trimline extending somewhat more proximally to the proximal pole of the patella anteriorly, medially, and laterally. The posterior trimline should permit free knee flexion beyond

90 degrees. Hook-and-loop material straps are used to secure the anterior and posterior sections together. The anterior and the posterior sections can be hinged at the proximal edge for improved anteroposterior control.

The purpose of the knee-ankle-foot fracture orthosis is to provide long-term protection for fractures of the distal to middle femur or for fractures about the knee (Figure 12-38). This orthosis is often used as an alternative to a hybrid cast brace for persons who have had ORIF for fractures of the proximal tibia, knee, or distal femur. The orthosis is removable for wound care and personal hygiene and when protection is not required. Depending on the location of the fracture, the orthosis can be designed to limit range of motion or to permit full motion of the knee. Drop locks can be used to stabilize the knee in full extension during ambulation. The design of the orthosis also protects the knee from excessive mediolateral and anteroposterior shear stress during ambulation. If maximum stability is necessary, a solid-ankle design can be incorporated; if mobility of the ankle is desired, an articulated ankle joint with an appropriate motion stop mechanism can be used. The orthosis requires total contact within the femoral and tibial components. Proximal trimlines follow the anatomical contours of the proximal femur to the greater trochanter to provide femoral protection. To stabilize the knee or proximal tibia, encasement of the lower two thirds of the femur is sufficient. The orthosis alone cannot effectively unload the femur, tibia, or foot: If axial unloading is desired, appropriate assistive devices (crutches or walker) must be used.

For individuals with proximal femoral fractures, a hip joint and pelvic band are often incorporated into a total contact knee-ankle-foot orthosis in an effort to control motion and rotational forces through the femur (Figure 12-39). Depending on the patient's specific needs, hip flexion/extension motion can be restricted or free; abduction/adduction is usually restricted. The placement of the orthotic hip joint is approximately 1 cm anterior and 1 cm proximal to the tip of the greater trochanter in most adults. Knee and ankle motion can be free or limited, given the location and stability of the fracture. A variety of single-axis or polycentric orthotic hip joints can be incorporated. A pelvic belt is used to maintain the orthotic hip joint in proper functional position. The belt should fit midway between the crest of the ilium and the greater trochanter.

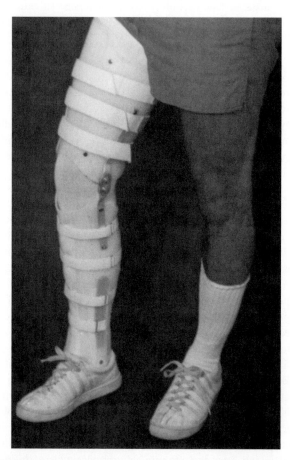

FIGURE 12-38 A prefabricated functional fracture orthosis must be adjusted regularly to ensure snug compression of soft tissues so that stability and alignment across the fracture will be maintained. (From Moore TJ: Functional bracing of lower extremity fractures. In Goldberg B, Hsu JD [eds], *Atlas of Orthoses and Assistive Devices.* St. Louis: Mosby, 1997.)

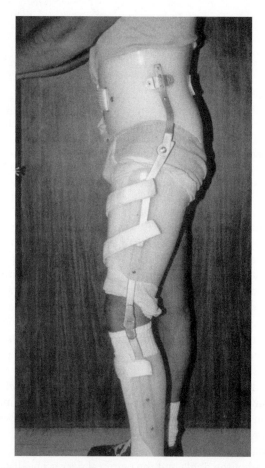

FIGURE 12-39 A lumbar sacral orthosis with an orthotic hip joint has been added to this knee-ankle-foot orthosis to provide better control of hip abduction/adduction and rotation while a proximal femoral fracture heals. The lateral uprights limit angulation through the healing femur during ambulation. Weight-bearing status is determined by the physician on the basis of the severity of the fracture and stability of the reduction.

External Fixation Devices

External fixation devices have evolved primarily to care for initial management of complex open or severely comminuted, unstable fractures that are most often the result of high-energy injury or multiple trauma (see Figures 12-30 and 12-35).[148-152] In particular, external fixation is used for severe metaphyseal fractures, severe intraarticular fractures, when there has been nonunion, in cases of substantial bone loss with allograft, and for fractures in osteoporotic bone.[150,153] They are particularly useful when fracture disrupts pelvic stability.[154-156]

Pins are placed into bone on either side of the fracture and then clamped onto lightweight rods in an external frame. The external frame can be a single rod, a set of articulated rods that cross the joint axis, circumferential, or a combination of these options.[157-161] The goal is to provide optimal skeletal alignment while providing visual access to healing skin and muscle. The external fixator permits active range of motion of the joint above and below the fracture. It is removed when soft tissues have adequately healed and radiographs demonstrate healing of the fracture. Casts or orthoses can be used to provide immobilization after fixator removal to support and protect the fracture until healing is complete.

Postfracture Management and Potential Complications

The postfracture issues and complications that are of concern to the managing physician and rehabilitation team include vascular injury, compartment syndrome, appropriate weight-bearing status, loss of reduction, delayed or nonunion, infection, implant failure (for ORIF), compression neuropathy, and skin breakdown. Each patient who presents to the emergency department with a fracture must be assessed for potential vascular injury and risk of developing compartment syndrome by careful physical examination. Whether a splint, cast, surgical ORIF, or placement of external fixators has been used to stabilize the fracture, the condition of the extremity must be monitored carefully by the physician, rehabilitation professional, patient, and family caregivers.

Fractures or dislocations around joints may have a concomitant arterial injury that can bruise or completely disrupt an artery, compromising or completely interrupting blood flow beyond the site of fracture.[162-164] This creates a grave situation: The physician has a window of less than 6 to 8 hours in which to restore blood supply and nutrition to the distal muscle and bone before significant tissue death occurs. The longer the period of ischemia, the greater the likelihood of delayed healing, infection, and necrosis.

Compartment syndrome evolves when bleeding or inflammation exceeds the expansive capacity of semirigid muscle or soft tissue anatomical spaces (compartments) of the fractured limb.[165-167] Once interstitial pressure exceeds a critical level, blood vessels and muscle are compressed and oxygen supply to the muscles is significantly compromised. Irreversible muscle or nerve damage occurs if compartment syndrome continues for longer than 6 to 8 hours. Presenting signs and symptoms include extreme pain and significant swelling of the extremity with taut skin. Passive motion of the fingers or toes causes excruciating pain. Compartment syndrome is considered a medical emergency: The treating physician must be notified immediately so that a fasciotomy can be performed to relieve excessive compartment pressures. All health professionals who are involved in the treatment of extremity trauma should be aware of the signs and symptoms of compartment syndrome. If unrecognized and untreated, compartment syndrome has devastating results.

One of the most important considerations for lower extremity fractures is weight-bearing status. A patient's weight-bearing status (full weight bearing, weight bearing as tolerated, partial weight bearing, toe-touch weight bearing, or non–weight bearing) is determined by the physician on the basis of the stability of the fracture and the immobilization method used. Once a patient is stable after an operation or a cast has been applied and is properly set, rehabilitation professionals work with the patient and family on mobility and gait training. The rehabilitation professional selects the appropriate assistive device for a patient's weight-bearing status, given the patient's physical and cognitive status and the characteristics of his or her usual living environment. Communicating quickly to the referring physician any signs of developing complications or difficulty with compliance that might put the fracture site at risk is important.

Loss of reduction of the fracture is a serious complication and can occur whether a splint, cast, ORIF, or external fixator has been used to realign and stabilize the limb.[158,167-169] A progressive angular deformity or abnormal position of the limb suggests loss of reduction and must be quickly reported to the managing physician. Even if reduction appears to be appropriate, inadequate immobilization within a splint or cast can lead to delayed union, nonunion (nonhealing), or malunion (healing in an abnormal position).

Any patient who has sustained an open fracture is at risk of developing infection of skin, deep tissue and muscle, or even bone. Both intravenous and local antibiotics are administered in the emergency department and operating room to minimize likelihood of infection from contamination sustained at the time of injury.[170,171] Infections may also be iatrogenic.[171,172] An infection is a serious complication that requires aggressive antibiotic treatment or debridement, or both. If an infection occurs after ORIF, the implanted hardware may have to be removed and an external fixation device applied. For individuals with external fixation, the pins provide a tract for infectious organisms directly into bone.[173] Appropriate wound and pin care is essential to minimize the risk of infection.[174] Osteomyelitis, or infection of bone, is a serious situation that can result in deformity; joint destruction; and, in some circumstances, amputation.[174-177]

Patients who have undergone ORIF are at risk of implant failure if repeated loading causes fatigue and ultimately exceeds the strength of the implant material and design.[178-180] Loosening or breakage of implanted screws, plates, or other devices also indicates excessive motion of the fracture site and increases the risk of delayed healing or nonunion. The patient's ability to function within weight-bearing limits established by the physician must be carefully assessed and monitored to reduce the risk of implant failure.

Complications also occur in patients whose fractures are managed by casting. The patient's neurovascular function is documented before cast application and carefully monitored while the cast is in place. In the distal lower extremity, the peroneal nerve is susceptible to prolonged pressure (compression-induced peroneal palsy) as it wraps around the head of the fibula.[108,181,182]

Complaints of edge pressure or toes being squeezed can be solved with cast modifications; however, excessive pressure and discomfort inside the cast often require removal and reapplication of a new cast.[183] On initial application, a cast is designed to have a snug but not tight fit. Signs of distal vascular compromise such as delayed capillary refill on compression of the nail bed suggest that the cast may be excessively tight.[108,183] It is not uncommon for cast fit to loosen over time as a result of several factors: Initial edema resolves, compressive forces modify soft tissue composition, disuse atrophy occurs, and cast padding compresses over time. Fit must be carefully monitored over time: A loose cast provides less control of the skeleton, and fracture reduction may be lost. Pistoning of a loose cast on the extremity is likely to lead to skin breakdown and shear over bony prominences.

Casts applied postoperatively while the patient is anesthetized are usually univalved (split down the front) to accommodate postoperative swelling.[109] Excessive swelling is accompanied by significant pain. Limb elevation is the first defense against excessive swelling and pain; however, the cast can be opened further or bivalved to relieve extreme pressure.[3] The risk of compartment syndrome must always be considered: If the patient experiences significant pain on passive motion of the fingers or toes, the physician must be contacted immediately. Failure to recognize and appropriately treat a compartment syndrome results in muscle necrosis and possible loss of the limb.[165]

Occasionally, a window can be cut into a cast to inspect a wound or relieve a pressure area. If the limb is edematous, it is likely that soft tissue will begin to protrude through the window, resulting in additional skin irritation and breakdown. For this reason, any piece of cast that is removed to make a window must be reapplied and secured to the cast after modifications have been made.[183]

Patients with foot pain try to reposition the foot within the cast to make it more comfortable. Inappropriate plantar flexion of the foot within the cast creates excessive pressure on the posterior heel and dorsum of the foot. Discomfort can be reduced if the patient is able to push the relaxed foot gently downward while pulling the cast upward, as if pulling on a boot. If this fails to relieve pressure, the cast must be removed and reapplied.[183]

Foreign objects introduced into a cast are the most common cause of discomfort and pressure. In an attempt to relieve itching of dry skin, patients are sometimes tempted to insert coat hangers, rulers, sticks, pens, and similar objects into the cast to scratch the itchy areas. This strategy often leads to displacement of cast padding, creating lumps and bumps where smooth surface contact is essential. Objects can break off or become trapped within the cast as well. The best way to relieve itching is by tapping on the cast or blowing cool air into it.

Another common complication is skin maceration, which is the result of prolonged exposure to water or a moist environment within the cast. Although, ideally, a cast is kept completely dry, many become wet at some point after application. Plaster casts that become wet lose significant stability and must be replaced. Synthetic casts can be towel dried as much as possible and then further dried using a cool setting on a blower or hairdryer.

SUMMARY

In this chapter the reader has discovered that orthoses play an important role in the management of traumatic (e.g., fracture) and developmental (e.g., DDH, LCPD) musculoskeletal conditions. Each member of the interdisciplinary rehabilitation team has a contribution to make to the care of individuals with pathologies of the musculoskeletal system, as well as shared responsibility to monitor for changes in function and potential complications. Although many prefabricated orthoses are available, knowledge of appropriate fit, design, and dynamics of the orthoses is essential so that the device will most closely match the intention of intervention. Precise communication about the goals of the orthosis (e.g., to fully immobilize the limb or to allow joint motion within a restricted range), wearing schedule (e.g., all the time or during particular activities), and weight-bearing status while using the orthosis has a major impact on efficacy of the orthotic intervention. All team members participate in patient and family education about the orthosis and its purpose, maintenance and cleaning, signs that indicate problems, and strategies to put in place should problems arise.

REFERENCES

1. Levangie PK. Biomechanical applications to joint structure and function. In: Levangie PK, Norkin CC, eds. *Joint Structure and Function: A Comprehensive Analysis.* 4th ed. Philadelphia: FA Davis; 2005:3–68.
2. Mueller MJ, Maluf KS. Tissue adaptation to physical stress: a proposed "physical stress theory" to guide physical therapist practice, education, and research. *Phys Ther.* 2002;82(4):383–403.
3. Williams PL, ed. *Gray's Anatomy.* 38th ed. New York: Churchill Livingstone; 1995.
4. Netter FH, Hansen JT. *Atlas of Human Anatomy.* 3rd ed. Teterboro, NJ: ICON Learning Systems; 2002.
5. Lundon K. Anatomy and biology of bone tissue. In: *Orthopedic Rehabilitation Science: Principles for Clinical Management of Bone.* Boston: Butterworth-Heinemann; 2000:5–23.
6. Curwin S. Joint structure and function. In: Levangie PK, Norkin CC, eds. *Joint Structure and Function: A Comprehensive Analysis.* 4th ed. Philadelphia: FA Davis; 2005:69–111.
7. Lundon K. Changes in bone across the lifespan. In: *Orthopedic Rehabilitation Science: Principles for Clinical Management of Bone.* Boston: Butterworth-Heinemann; 2000:33–47.
8. Bidwell JP, Alvarez M, Feister H, et al. Nuclear matrix proteins and osteoblast gene expression. *J Bone Miner Res.* 1998;13(2):155–167.

9. Rodan GA. Control of bone formation and resorption: biological and clinical perspective. *J Cell Biochem.* 1998; 30–31(suppl):55–61.

10. Lanyon LE. Osteocytes, strain detection, bone modeling and remodeling. *Calcif Tissue Int.* 1993;53(suppl 1):S102–S107.

11. Suda T, Nakamura I, Eijirio J, et al. Regulation of osteoclastic function. *J Bone Miner Res.* 1997;12(6):869–879.

12. Blair HC. How the osteoclast degrades bone. *BioEssays.* 1998;20(10):837–846.

13. Payne R. Mechanisms and management of bone pain. *Cancer.* 1997;80(suppl 8):1608–1613.

14. Stevens DA, Williams GR. Hormone regulation of chondrocyte differentiation and endochondral bone formation. *Mol Cell Endocrinol.* 1999;151(1–2):195–204.

15. Mundy GR. Bone resorption and turnover in health and disease. *Bone.* 1987;8(suppl 1):S9–S16.

16. Watkins BA. Regulatory effects of polyunsaturates on bone modeling and cartilage function. *World Rev Nutr Diet.* 1998;83:38–51.

17. Rosen GJ. Insulin-like growth factors I and calcium balance: evolving concepts of an evolutionary process. *Endocrinology.* 2003;144(11):4679–4681.

18. Lundon K. Physiology and biochemistry of bone tissue. In: *Orthopedic Rehabilitation Science: Principles for Clinical Management of Bone.* Boston: Butterworth-Heinemann; 2000:25–32.

19. Jilka RL. Cytokines, bone remodeling, and estrogen deficiency; a 1998 update. *Bone.* 1998;23(2):75–81.

20. Christenson RH. Biochemical markers of bone metabolism; an overview. *Clin Biochem.* 1997;30(8):573–593.

21. Seibel MJ, Baylink DJ, Farley JR, et al. Basic science and clinical utility of biochemical markers of bone turnover—a Congress report. *Exp Clin Endocrinol Diabetes.* 1997;105(3):125–133.

22. Riggs B, Melton L. Involutional osteoporosis. *N Engl J Med.* 1986;314(26):1676–1686.

23. Sabateir JP, Guaydiersouquieres G, Laroche D, et al. Bone mineral acquisition during adolescence and early adulthood: a study of 574 healthy females 10–24 years of age. *Osteoporosis Int.* 1996;6(2):141–148.

24. Crawford AH, Ayyangar R, Durrett GL. Congenital and acquired disorders. In: Goldberg B, Hsu JH, eds. *Atlas of Orthoses and Assistive Devices.* 3rd ed. St. Louis: Mosby; 1997:479–500.

25. Shipman AJ, Guy GW, Smith I, et al. Vertebral bone mineral density, content and area in 8789 normal women aged 33–73 who have never had hormone replacement therapy. *Osteoporosis Int.* 1999;9(5):420–426.

26. Stevens DA, Williams GR. Hormonal regulation of chondrocyte differentiation and endochondral bone formation. *Mol Cell Endocrinol.* 1999;151(1–2):195–204.

27. Torgerson DJ, Campbell MK, Reid DM. Lifestyle, environmental, and medical factors influencing peak bone mass in women. *Br J Rheumatol.* 1995;34(7):620–624.

28. Mazess RB, Barden HS. Bone density in pre-menopausal women: effects of age, dietary intake, physical activity, smoking, and birth control pills. *Am J Clin Nutr.* 1991;53(1):132–142.

29. WHO Scientific Group on Prevention and Management of Osteoporosis. Prevention and management of osteoporosis. *World Health Organ Tech Rep Ser.* 2003;921:1–164.

30. Levangie PK. The hip complex. In: Levangie PK, Norkin CC, eds. *Joint Structure and Function: A Comprehensive Analysis.* 4th ed. Philadelphia: FA Davis; 2005:355–392.

31. Steinberg ME, ed. *The Hip and Its Disorders.* Philadelphia: Saunders; 1991.

32. Guille JT, Pizzutillo PD, MacEvew GD. Development dysplasia of the hip from birth to six months. *J Am Acad Orthop Surg.* 2000;8(4):232–242.

33. Vitale MG, Skaggs DL. Developmental dysplasia of the hip from six months to four years of age. *J Am Acad Orthop Surg.* 2001;9(6):401–411.

34. Ilfeld FW, Westin GW, Makin M. Missed or developmental dislocation of the hip. *Clin Orthop.* 1986;Feb(203):276–281.

35. Mubarik SJ, Leach JL, Wenger DR. Management of congenital dislocation of the hip in the infant. *Contemp Orthop.* 1987;15:29–44.

36. Shapiro F. Developmental dysplasia of the hip. In: Shapiro F, ed. *Pediatric Orthopedic Deformities: Basic Science, Diagnosis and Treatment.* San Diego: Academic Press; 2002:153–271.

37. Hesinger RN. Congenital dislocation of the hip; treatment in infancy to walking age. *Orthop Clin North Am.* 1987;18(4):597–616.

38. Leach J. Orthopedic conditions. In: Campbell SK, Vander Linden DW, Palisano RT, eds. *Physical Therapy for Children.* 2nd ed. Philadelphia: Saunders; 2000:398–428.

39. Lotito FM, Rabbaglietti G, Notarantonio M. The ultrasonographic image of the infant hip affected by developmental dysplasia with a positive Ortolani's sign. *Pediatr Radiol.* 2002;32(6):418–422.

40. Walker JM. Musculoskeletal development: a review. *Phys Ther.* 1991;71(12):878–889.

41. Riester JA, Eilert RE. Hip disorders. In: Goldberg B, Hsu JD, eds. *Atlas of Orthotic and Assistive Devices.* St Louis: Mosby; 1997:509–526.

42. Pavlik A. The functional method of treatment using a harness with stirrups as the primary method of conservative therapy for infants with congenital dislocation of the hip. *Clin Orthop.* 1992;Aug(281):4–10.

43. Mubarak SJ. Pavlik: the man and his method. *J Pediatr Orthop.* 2003;23(3):342–346.

44. Song KM, Lapinsky A. Determination of hip position in the Pavlik harness. *J Pediatr Orthop.* 2000;20(3):317–319.

45. Wenger DR, Rang M. Developmental dysplasia of the hip. In: Wenger DR, Rang M, eds. *The Art and Practice of Children's Orthopaedics.* New York: Raven; 1993:272–280.

46. Mubarak S, Garfin S, Vance R, et al. Pitfalls in the use of the Pavlik harness for treatment of congenital dysplasia, subluxation, and dislocation of the hip. *J Bone Joint Surg.* 1981;63A(8):1239–1247.

47. Kim HW, Weinstein SL. Intervening early in developmental hip dysplasia: early recognition avoids serious consequences later. *J Musculoskel Med.* 1998;15(2):70–72, 77–81.

48. Harding MG, Harke HT, Bowen JR, et al. Management of dislocated hips with Pavlik harness treatment and ultrasound monitoring. *J Pediatr Orthop.* 1997;17(2):189–198.

49. Inoue T, Naito M, Nomiyama H. Treatment of developmental dysplasia of the hip with the Pavlik harness: factors for predicting unsuccessful reduction. *J Pediatr Orthop B.* 2001;10(3):186–191.

50. Leman JA, Emans JB, Millis MB, et al. Early failure of Pavlik harness treatment for developmental hip dysplasia: clinical and ultrasound predictors. *J Pediatr Orthop.* 2001;21(3):348–353.

51. Hedequist D, Kasser J, Emans J. Use of an abduction brace for developmental dysplasia of the hip after failure of the Pavlik harness. *J Pediatr Orthop.* 2003;23(2):175–177.

52. Segal LS, Boal DK, Borthwick L, et al. Avasucular necrosis after treatment of DDH: the protective influence of the ossific nucleus. *J Pediatr Orthop*. 1999;19(2):177–184.

53. Suzuki S, Kashiwagi N, Kasahara Y, et al. Avascular necrosis and the Pavlik harness: the incidence of avascular necrosis in three types of congenital dislocation of the hip as classified by ultrasound. *J Bone Joint Surg Br*. 1996;78(4):631–635.

54. Carey TP, Guidera KG, Ogden JA. Manifestations of ischemic necrosis complicating developmental dysplasia. *Clin Orthop*. 1992;Aug(281):11–17.

55. Luhman SJ, Schoenecker PL, Anderson AM, et al. The prognostic importance of the ossific nucleus in the treatment of congenital dysplasia of the hip. *J Bone Joint Surg Am*. 1998; 80(12):1719–1727.

56. Legg AT. An obscure affection of the hip joint. *Boston Med Surg J*. 1910;162–202.

57. Canale ST. Osteochondroses. In: Canale ST, Beatty JH, eds. *Operative Pediatric Orthopedics*. St. Louis: Mosby–Year Book; 1991:743–776.

58. Stulberg SD, Cooperman DR, Wallensten R. The natural history of Legg-Calvé-Perthes disease. *J Bone Joint Surg Am*. 63(7):1095–1108.

59. Guille JT, Lipton GE, Szöke G, et al. Legg-Calvé-Perthes disease in girls: a comparison of results with those seen in boys. *J Bone Joint Surg*. 1998;80A(9):1256–1263.

60. Herring JA, Tachdjian MO. *Tachdjian's Pediatric Orthopaedics*. 3rd ed. Philadelphia: Saunders; 2002.

61. Guile JT, Bowen JR. Legg-Calvé-Perthes disease. In: Dee R, ed. *Principles of Orthopaedic Practice*. 2nd ed. New York: McGraw-Hill; 1997:723–734.

62. Balasa VV, Gruppo RA, Glueck CJ, et al. Legg-Calvé-Perthes disease and thrombophilia. *J Bone Joint Surg Am*. 2004; 86(12):2642–2647.

63. Hamer AJ. Pain in the hip and knee. *BMJ*. 2004;328(7447): 1067–1069.

64. Gerberg LF, Micheli LJ. Nontraumatic hip pain in active children. *Phys Sports Med*. 1996;24(1):69–74.

65. Eich GF, Supertis-Furga A, Umbricht FS, et al. The painful hip: evaluation of criteria for clinical decision making. *Eur J Pediatr*. 1999;158(11):923–928.

66. Herring JA, Kim HT, Browne R. Legg-Calvé-Perthes disease part 1: classification of radiographs with use of the modified lateral pillar and Stulberg classifications. *J Bone Joint Surg Am*. 2004;86(10):2103–2121.

67. Yazici M, Aydingoz U, Aksoy MC, et al. Bipositional MR imaging for the evaluation of femoral head sphericity and containment in Legg-Calvé-Perthes disease. *Clin Imaging*. 2002;26(5):342–346.

68. Catterall A. Natural history, classification, and x-ray signs in Legg-Calvé-Perthes disease. *Acta Orthop Belg*. 1980; 46(4):346–351.

69. Christensen F, Soballe K, Ejsted R, et al. The Catterall classification of Perthes disease: an assessment of reliability. *J Bone Joint Surg Br*. 1986;68(4):614–615.

70. Hardcastle PH, Ross R, Hamalalnen M, et al. Catterall grouping of Perthes disease: an assessment of observer error and prognosis using the Catterall classification. *J Bone Joint Surg Br*. 1980;62(4):428–431.

71. Ritterbusch JF, Shantharam SS, Gellnas C. Comparison of lateral pillar classification and Catterall classification of Legg-Calvé-Perthes disease. *J Pediatr Orthop*. 1990;13(2):200–202.

72. Salter RB, Thompson GH. Legg-Calvé-Perthes disease: the prognostic significance of the subchondral fracture and a two group classification of the femoral head involvement. *J Bone Joint Surg Am*. 1984;66(4):479–489.

73. Sponseller PD, Desai SS, Mills MB. Abnormalities of proximal femoral growth after severe Perthes disease. *J Bone Joint Surg Br*. 1989;71(4):479–489.

74. Podeszwa DA, Stanitski CL, Stanitski DF, et al. The effect of pediatric orthopedic experience on interobserver and intrabserver reliability of the Herring lateral pillar classification of Perthes disease. *J Pediatric Orthop*. 2000;20(5):562–565.

75. Herring JA, Kim HT, Browne R. Legg-Calvé-Perthes disease part II: Prospective multi-center study on the effect of treatment outcome. *J Bone Joint Surg*. 2004;86(10):2121–2134.

76. Kim HKW. Legg-Calve-Perthes disease. *J Am Acad Orthop Surg*. 2010;Nov(18):676–686.

77. MacEwen GD. Conservative treatment of Legg-Calvé-Perthes disease conditions. In: Fitzgerald FH, ed. *The Hip: Proceedings of the 13th Open Scientific Meeting of the Hip Society*. St. Louis: Mosby; 1985:17–23.

78. Wenger DR, Ward WT, Herring JA. Current concepts review: Legg-Calvé-Perthes disease. *J Bone Joint Surg*. 1991;73(5): 778–788.

79. Poussa M, Yrjonen T, Holkka V, et al. Prognosis after conservative and operative management of Perthes disease. *Clin Orthop*. 1993;Dec(297):549–553.

80. Noonan KJ, Price CT, Kupiszewski SJ, et al. Results of femoral varus osteotomy in children older than 9 years of age with Perthes disease. *J Pediatr Orthop*. 2001;21(2):198–204.

81. Paterson DC, Leitch JM, Foster BK. Results of innominate osteotomy in the treatment of Legg-Calvé-Perthes disease. *Clin Orthop*. 1991;May(266):93–103.

82. Kruse RW, Gulle JT, Bowen JR. Shelf arthroplasty in patients who have Legg-Calvé-Perthes disease: a long term study of results. *J Bone Joint Surg Am*. 1991;73(9):1338–1347.

83. Willett K, Hudson I, Catterall A. Lateral shelf acetabuloplasty: an operation for older children with Perthes disease. *J Pediatr Orthop*. 1992;12(5):563–568.

84. Grzegorzeski A, Bowen JR, Guille JT, et al. Treatment of the collapsed femoral head by containment in Legg-Calvé-Perthes disease. *J Pediatr Orthop*. 2003;23(1):15–19.

85. Herring JA. Current concepts review. The treatment of Legg-Calvé-Perthes disease; a critical review of the literature. *J Bone Joint Surg*. 1994;76A(3):448–458.

86. Martinez AG, Weinstein SL, Deat FR. The weight bearing abduction brace for the treatment of Legg-Perthes disease. *J Bone Joint Surg*. 1992;74A(1):12–21.

87. Meehan TL, Angel D, Nelson JM. The Scottish-Rite abduction orthosis for the treatment of Legg-Perthes disease. A radiographic analysis. *J Bone Joint Surg*. 1992;74A(1):2–12.

88. Purvis JM, Dimon JH, Meehan PL, et al. Preliminary experience with the Scottish Rite hospital abduction orthosis for Legg-Perthes disease. *Clin Orthop*. 1980;July-Aug(150):49–53.

89. Meehan PL, Angel D, Nelson JM. The Scottish Rite abduction orthosis for the treatment of Legg-Perthes disease: a radiographic analysis. *J Bone Joint Surg Am*. 1992;74(1):2–12.

90. Martinez AG, Weinstein SL, Dietz FR. The weight bearing abduction brace for the treatment of Legg-Perthes disease. *J Bone Joint Surg Am*. 1992;74(1):12–21.

91. Bobechko WP, McLaurin EA, Motloch WM. Toronto orthosis for Legg-Perthes disease. *Artif Limbs*. 1968;12(2):36–41.

92. Curtis HD, Gunther SF, Gossling HR, et al. Treatment for Legg-Perthes disease with the Newington ambulation abduction brace. *J Bone Joint Surg.* 1974;56(6):1135–1146.

93. Edelstein JE, Brukner J. *Orthotics: A Comprehensive Clinical Approach.* Thorofare, NJ: Slack; 2002.

94. Drennan JC. *Orthopaedic Management of Neuromuscular Disorders.* Philadelphia: Lippincott; 1983.

95. Walker WC, Keyser-Marcus LA, Cifu DX, et al. Inpatient inter-disciplinary rehabilitation after total hip arthroplasty surgery: a comparison of revision and primary total hip arthroplasty. *Arch Phys Med Rehabil.* 2001;82(1):123–133.

96. Lima D, Magnus R, Paproshy WG. Team management of hip revision patients using a post-op hip orthosis. *J Prosthet Orthot.* 1994;6(1):20–24.

97. Cummings SR, Rubin SM, Black D. The future of hip fractures in the United States: numbers, costs, and potential effects of post-menopausal estrogen. *Clin Orthop.* 1991;March(252):163–166.

98. Schultz RJ. *The Language of Fractures.* 2nd ed. Baltimore: Williams & Wilkins; 1990.

99. Islam SS, Biswas RS, Nambiar AM, et al. Incidence and risk of work-related fracture injuries; experience of a state-managed worker's compensation system. *J Occup Environ Med.* 2001;43(2):140–146.

100. Tiderius CJ, Landin L, Duppe H. Decreasing incidence of frac-tures in children. *Acta Orthop Scand.* 1999;70(6):622–626.

101. Estrada LS, Alonso JE, McGwin G, et al. Restraint use and lower extremity fracture in frontal motor vehicle collisions. *J Trauma.* 2004;57(2):323–328.

102. Edwards BJ, Bunta AD, Madison LD, et al. An osteoporosis and fracture intervention program increases the diagnosis and treatment for osteoporosis for patients with minimal trauma fractures. *Jt Comm J Qual Patient Saf.* 2005;31(5):267–274.

103. Jacofsky DF, Haidukewych GJ. Management of pathologi-cal fractures of the proximal femur: state of the art. *J Orthop Trauma.* 2004;18(7):459–460.

104. Ringsberg KA, Gardsell P, Johnell O, et al. The impact of long-term moderate physical activity on functional performance, bone mineral density, and fracture incidence in elderly women. *Gerontology.* 2001;47(1):15–20.

105. Boden BP, Osbahr DC, Jimenez C. Low risk stress fractures. *Am J Sports Med.* 2001;29(1):100–111.

106. Vanderschueren D, Boonen S, Bouillon R. Action of andro-gens versus estrogens in male skeletal homeostasis. *Bone.* 1998;23(5):391–394.

107. Seeman E. Advances in the study of osteoporosis in men. In: Meunier PH, ed. *Osteoporosis: Diagnosis and Management.* London: Dunitz; 1998:211–232.

108. Charnley J. *The Closed Treatment of Common Fractures.* 4th ed. London: Cambridge University Press; 2002.

109. Cole AS, McNally MA. The management of open fractures. In: Bulstrode CJ, Buchwalker J, Carr A, et al., eds. *Oxford Textbook of Orthopedics and Trauma.* New York: Oxford University Press; 2002:1636–1651.

110. DeCoster TA. Fracture classification. In: Bulstrode CJ, Buchwalker J, Carr A, et al., eds. *Oxford Textbook of Orthopedics and Trauma.* New York: Oxford University Press; 2002:1575–1580.

111. Lundon K. Injury, regeneration, and repair in bone. In: *Orthopedic Rehabilitation Science: Principles for Clinical Management of Bone.* Boston: Butterworth-Heinemann; 2000:93–113.

112. Reddi AH. Initiation of fracture repair by bone morphogenetic proteins. *Clin Orthop.* 1998;Oct(355 suppl):S66–S72.

113. Hayda RA, Brighton CT, Esterhai JL. Pathophysiology of delayed healing. *Clin Orthop.* 1998;Oct(355 suppl):S31–S40.

114. Gustilo RB, Anderson JT. Prevention of infection in the treat-ment of one thousand and twenty-five open fractures of long bones. *J Bone Joint Surg.* 1976;58(4):453–458.

115. Rose DD, Rowven DW. Perioperative considerations in major orthopedic trauma: pelvic and long bone fractures. *Am Assoc Nurse Anesth J.* 2002;70(2):131–137.

116. Gugenheim JJ. External fixation in orthopedics. *JAMA.* 2004;291(17):2122–2134.

117. Harkess JW, Ramsey WC, Harkess JW. Principles of fracture and dislocations. In: Rockwood CA, Green DP, Bucholz RW, eds. *Rockwood and Green's Fractures in Adults.* Vol 1, 3rd ed. Philadelphia: Lippincott Williams & Wilkins; 1991:1–180.

118. Bick EM. *Source Book of Orthopaedics.* New York: Hafner; 1968.

119. Wytch R, Mitchell C, Ratchie IK, et al. New splinting material. *Prosthet Orthot Int.* 1987;11(1):42–45.

120. Richard RE. Polymers in fracture immobilization. In: Salamore JC, ed. *The Polymeric Materials Encyclopedia.* Boca Raton, FL: CRC Press; 1996.

121. Lavalette RN, Pope M. Dickstein H. Setting temperatures of plaster casts. *J Bone Joint Surg.* 1982;64(6):907–911.

122. Wytch R, Mitchell CB, Wardlaw D, et al. Mechanical assess-ment of polyurethane impregnated fiberglass bandage for splinting. *Prosthet Orthot Int.* 1987;11(3):128–134.

123. Wytch R, Ashcroft GP, Ledingham WM, et al. Modern splint-ing bandages. *J Bone Joint Surg.* 1991;73(1):88–91.

124. Wytch R, Ross N, Wardlaw D. Glass fiber versus non-glass fiber splinting bandages. *Injury.* 1992;23(2):101–106.

125. Pope M, Callahan G, Leveled R. Setting temperature of syn-thetic casts. *J Bone Joint Surg.* 1985;67A(2):262–264.

126. Mooney V. Cast bracing. *Clin Orthop.* 1974;(102):159–166.

127. Brown PW. The early weight-bearing treatment of tibial shaft fractures. *Clin Orthop.* 1974;(105):167–178.

128. Beatty JH. Congenital anomalies of the hip and pelvis. In: Crenshaw AH, ed. *Campbell's Operative Orthopaedics.* St. Louis: Mosby; 1987:2721–2722.

129. Hilt NE, Cogburn SB. Cast and splint therapy. In: Hilt NE, Cogburn SB, eds. *Manual of Orthopaedics.* St. Louis: Mosby; 1980:459–516.

130. Pellegrini VD, Evarts CM. Complications. In: Rockwood CA, Green DP, Bucholz RW, eds. *Rockwood and Green's Fractures in Adults,* Vol 1. 3rd ed. Philadelphia: Lippincott Williams & Wilkins; 1991:390–393.

131. Connolly JF, Dahne E, Lafollette B. Closed reduction and early cast-brace ambulation in the treatment of femoral fractures. Part 2. *J Bone Joint Surg.* 1973;55A(8):1581–1599.

132. Moll JH. The cast brace walking treatment of open and closed femoral fractures. *South Med J.* 1973;66(3):345–352.

133. Lenin BE, Mooney V, Ashy ME. Cast-bracing for fractures of the femur. *J Bone Joint Surg.* 1977;59S(7):917–923.

134. Maggot B, Gad DA. Cast bracing for fractures of the femoral shaft. *J Bone Joint Surg.* 1981;63B(1):12–23.

135. Stills M, Christiansen K, Bucholz RW, et al. Cast bracing bicon-dylar tibial plateau fractures after combined internal and exter-nal fixation. *J Prosthet Orthot.* 1991;3(3):106–113.

136. DeCoster TA, Nepola JU, El-khoura GY. Cast brace treatment of proximal tibia fractures. *Clin Orthop.* 1988;231:196–204.

137. Sutcliffe JR, Wilson-Storey D, Mackinlay GA. Children's femo-ral fractures: the Edinburgh experience. *J R Coll Surg Edinb.* 1995;40(6):411–415.

138. Segal D, Mallik AR, Wetzler MJ, et al. Early weight bearing of lateral tibial plateau fractures. *Clin Orthop Relat Res.* 1993;Sept(294):232–237

139. Tang SF, Au TL, Wong AM, et al. Modified fracture brace for tibial fracture with varus angulation: a case report. *Prosthet Orthot Int.* 1995;Aug(2):115–119.

140. Hardy AE. The treatment of femoral fractures by cast-brace application and early ambulation. *J Bone Joint Surg.* 1983;65(1):56–65.

141. Hohl M, Johnson EE, Wiss DA. Fractures of the knee. In: In: Rockwood CA, Green DP, Bucholz RW, eds. *Rockwood and Green's Fractures in Adults*, Vol 2. Philadelphia: Lippincott Williams & Wilkins; 1991:1725–1761.

142. Kapandji IA. *The Knee. The Physiology of the Joints.* 25th ed. New York: Churchill Livingstone; 1991.

143. Snyder-Macker L, Lewek M. The knee. In: Levangie PK, Norkin CC, eds. *Joint Structure and Function—A Comprehensive Analysis.* 4th ed. Philadelphia: FA Davis; 2005:393–436.

144. Moore TJ. Functional bracing of lower extremity fractures. In: Goldberg B, Hsu JD, eds. *Atlas of Orthoses and Assistive Devices.* 3rd ed. St. Louis: Mosby; 1997:401–408.

145. Goss J. Developments in orthotic deweighting technology. *Phys Med Rehabil Clin North Am.* 2000;11(3):497–508.

146. Pritham Beatty JH. Congenital anomalies of the hip and pelvis. In: Crenshaw AH, ed. *Campbell's Operative Orthopaedics.* St. Louis: Mosby; 1987:2721–2722.

147. Stills ML. Vacuum-formed orthosis for fractures of the tibia. *Orthot Prosthet.* 1976;30(2):43–55.

148. Sarmiento A. On the behavior of closed tibial fractures. *J Orthop Trauma.* 2000;14(3):199–205.

149. Chapman MW. Open fractures. In: Rockwood CA, Green DP, Bucholz RW, eds. *Rockwood and Green's Fractures in Adults.* Vol 1. 3rd ed. Philadelphia: Lippincott Williams & Wilkins; 1991:223–264.

150. Pacheo RJ, Saleh M. The role of external fixators in trauma. *Trauma.* 2004;6:143–160.

151. Weigel DP, Marsh JL. High energy fractures of the tibial plateau: knee function after longer follow-up. *J Bone Joint Surg Am.* 2002;84(9):1541–1551.

152. Babar IU. External fixation in close comminuted femoral shaft fractures in adults. *J Coll Physicians Surg Pak.* 2004;14(9):553–555.

153. Haidukewych GJ. Temporary external fixation for the management of complex intra- and periarticular fractures of the lower extremity. *J Orthop Trauma.* 2002;16(9):678–685.

154. Chui FY, Chuang TY, Lo WH. Treatment of unstable pelvic fractures: use of a transiliac sacral rod for posterior lesions and anterior lesions. *J Trauma.* 2004;57(1):141–145.

155. Ponsen KJ, van Dijke GA, Joosse P, et al. External fixators for pelvic fractures. *Acta Orthop Scand.* 2003;74(2):165–171.

156. Yang AP, Iannacone WM. External fixation for pelvic ring disruptions. *Orthop Clin North Am.* 1997;28(3):331–344.

157. Hayek TE. External fixators in the treatment of fractures in children. *J Ped Orthopaed B.* 2004;13(2):103–109.

158. Garcia-Cimbrelo E. Circular external fixators in tibial non-unions. *Clin Orthopaed Relat Res.* 2004;1(419):65–70.

159. Gordon JE. A comparison of monolateral and circular external fixation of diaphysial tibial fractures in children. *J Pediatr Orthopaed.* 2003;12(5):338–345.

160. Krieg JC. Proximal tibial fractures: current treatment, results, and problems. *Injury.* 2003;34(suppl 1):A2–A10.

161. Robberts CS, Dodds JC, Perry K, et al. Hybrid external fixation of the proximal tibia: strategies to improve frame stability. *J Orthop Trauma.* 2003;17(6):415–420.

162. Stannard JP, Sheils TM, Lopez-Ben RR, et al. Vascular injuries in knee dislocations: the role of physical examination in determining the need for arteriography. *J Bone Joint Surg Am.* 2004;86(5):910–915.

163. Rozycki GS, Tremblay LN, Feliciano DV, et al. Blunt vascular trauma in the extremity: diagnosis, management, and outcome. *J Trauma Inj Infect Crit Care.* 2003;55(5):814–824.

164. Lin C, Wei F, Levin LS, et al. The functional outcome of lower-extremity fractures with vascular injury. *J Trauma Inj Infec Crit Care.* 1997;43(3):480–485.

165. Olson SA, Rhorer AS. Orthopaedic trauma for the general orthopaedist: avoiding problems and pitfalls in treatment. *Clin Orthop Relat Res.* 2005;April(433):30–37.

166. Altizer L. Compartment syndrome. *Orthop Nurs.* 2004;23(6):391–396.

167. Leyes M, Torres R, Guillén P. Complications of open reduction and internal fixation of ankle fractures. *Foot Ankle Clin.* 2003;8(1):131–147.

168. Im GI, Shin YW, Song YJ. Potentially unstable intertrochanteric fractures. *J Orthop Trauma.* 2005;19(1):5–9.

169. Narayanan UG, Hyman JE, Wainwright AM, et al. Complications of elastic stable intramedullary nail fixation of pediatric femoral fractures, and how to avoid them. *J Pediatr Orthop.* 2004;24(4):363–369.

170. Zalavras CG, Patzakis MJ. Open fractures: evaluation and management. *J Am Acad Orthop Surg.* 2003;11(3):212–219.

171. Benirschke SK, Kramer KA. Wound healing complications in closed and open calcaneal fractures. *J Orthop Trauma.* 2004;18(1):1–6.

172. Khatod M, Botte MJ, Hoyt DB, et al. Outcomes in open tibia fractures: relationship between delay in treatment and infection. *J Trauma Inj Infect Crit Care.* 2003;55(5):949–954.

173. Weitz-Marshall AD, Bosse MJ. Timing of closure of open fractures. *J Am Acad Orthop Surg.* 2002;10(6):379–384.

174. Parameswaran AD, Roberts CS, Seligson D, et al. Pin tract infection with contemporary external fixation: how much of a problem? *J Orthop Trauma.* 2003;17(7):503–509.

175. Temple J, Santy J. Pin site care for preventing infections associated with external bone fixators and pins. *Cochrane Database Syst Rev.* 2004;CD004551.

176. Thordarson DB, Ahlmann E, Shepherd LE, et al. Sepsis and osteomyelitis about the ankle joint. *Foot Ankle Clin.* 2000;5(4):913–928.

177. Holtom PD, Smith AM. Introduction to adult posttraumatic osteomyelitis of the tibia. *Clin Orthop Relat Res.* 1999;Mar(360):6–13.

178. Bedi A, Toan Le T. Subtrochanteric femur fractures. *Orthop Clin North Am.* 2004;35(4):473–483.

179. Bhandari M, Audige L, Ellis T, et al. Operative treatment of extra-articular proximal tibial fractures. *J Orthop Trauma.* 2003;17(8):591–595.

180. Sadowski C, Lübbeke A, Saudan M, et al. Treatment of reverse oblique and transverse intertrochanteric fractures with use of an intramedullary nail or a 95 degrees screw-plate: a prospective, randomized study. *J Bone Joint Surg Am.* 2002;84(3):372–381.

181. Russell TA, Taylor JC, LaVelle DG. Fractures of the tibia. In: Rockwood CA, Green DP, Bucholz RW, eds. *Rockwood and Green's Fractures in Adults*, Vol 2. 3rd ed. Philadelphia: Lippincott Williams & Wilkins; 1991:1915–1982.

182. Weiss AP, Schenck RC, Sponseller PD, et al. Peroneal nerve palsy after early cast application for femoral fractures in children. *J Pediatr Orthop.* 1992;12(1):25–28.

183. Morgan S, Upton J. *Plaster casting: patient problems and nursing care.* Boston: Butterworth-Heinemann; 1990.

13

Orthoses for Spinal Dysfunction

Jeff Coppage and S. Elizabeth Ames

LEARNING OBJECTIVES

On completion of this chapter, the reader will be able to:

1. Identify the nomenclature for spinal orthoses.
2. Describe the basic structural and functional anatomy of the spine and its alignment.
3. Discuss the three-column concept of spine stability as it pertains to spine trauma.
4. Identify the types of injury and pathology for which spinal orthoses are used.
5. List the different types and functional use of spinal orthoses.
6. Describe the potential complications associated with the use of spinal orthoses and methods of prevention.
7. Evaluate different areas of the spine as being amenable to bracing.
8. Discuss indications and contraindications for using spinal orthoses.
9. Describe basic pathophysiology of scoliosis and its implications.
10. Identify common braces used in the treatment of scoliosis.
11. Discuss the prescription process for a spinal orthoses.
12. Value the importance of a multidisciplinary team approach in treating disorders of the spine.

External orthoses are used to manage a variety of spinal conditions. The general purpose of a brace is to limit the motion of a spinal region, decreasing the amount of load applied to the region treated. Orthoses are most frequently used when there is concern that loading the spine may result in deformity (i.e., treating an unstable fracture), when the spine is compromised in a way that requires additional support for healing (i.e., postsurgical management or osteoporosis), when the patient is experiencing low back pain that can be relieved by either limiting motion or increasing abdominal support, or when there is existing spinal deformity such as scoliosis. Another major function of a spinal orthosis is to serve as a psychological reminder to restrict trunk or neck motion, or at least to encourage the patient to move cautiously.[1]

For spinal conditions, an orthosis is defined as an external device applied to the body to restrict motion in a particular body segment or spinal region. The American Academy of Orthopaedic Surgeons standardized the nomenclature used for describing orthoses in spinal management in 1973 and divided them broadly into five categories (Table 13-1)[2]:

- Sacroiliac
- Lumbosacral
- Thoracolumbosacral
- Cervical thoracic
- Cervical

Orthoses may also be classified by their rigidity (i.e., rigid, semirigid, or flexible) or by a combination of their materials and whether they are prefabricated or custom fit. Historically, orthoses have been named according to their inventor or city of invention. This chapter provides an overview of spinal anatomy and biomechanics as they apply to orthotic use, highlights tips to ensure optimal fit and avoid complications, and discusses each of the three major spinal regions that are amenable to orthotic management and the orthoses used in each region as well as the various types of pathology for which brace treatment is used. This chapter describes common spinal orthoses, grouped by region (cervical, thoracic, and lumbosacral) and describes the clinical conditions that are most often assisted by the use of spinal orthoses.

Managing a patient who may benefit from a spinal orthosis requires an interdisciplinary team approach. Direct communication between the patient, physician, orthotist, nurse, physical therapist, and other rehabilitation personnel is necessary to ensure that the health care professionals, the patient, and caregivers all understand the rationale, limitations, and expected outcomes when prescribing and using an orthosis. In the use of spinal orthoses there are specific instructions that accompany orthotic management to avoid complications and promote optimal care. Rehabilitation professionals are responsible for designing therapeutic interventions that optimize function while carefully observing precautions and treatment goals of patient management for persons with spinal orthoses. Understanding the design of and rationale for the orthosis being used is critical to the overall success of the program.

ANATOMY AND BIOMECHANICS

The spine consists of seven cervical vertebrae, 12 thoracic vertebrae, five lumbar vertebrae, five sacral vertebrae, and three to four coccygeal segments. Load sharing intervertebral

TABLE 13-1 *Nomenclature for Spinal Orthoses*

Acronym	Name
RIGID THERMOPLASTIC OR METAL ORTHOSES, OR BOTH	
SIO	Sacroiliac orthosis
LSO	Lumbosacral orthosis
TLSO	Thoracolumbosacral orthosis
CTLSO	Cervicothoracolumbosacral orthosis
CTO	Cervicothoracic orthosis
CO	Cervical orthosis
SOFT GARMENTS AND SUPPORTS	
SI belt	Sacroiliac belt
LS corset	Lumbosacral corset
DL corset	Dorsolumbar corset
Soft collar	Nonreinforced cervical collars made from foam or any low modulus material

discs are interposed between adjacent vertebrae in the cervical, thoracic, and lumbar segments; in the sacral and coccygeal regions, the segments are fused. Two adjacent vertebrae and the intervertebral disc define the functional spinal unit (FSU). Multiple FSUs are combined in a superstructure capable of lateral bending, flexing, extending, and axial rotation. Different levels of the spine vary in their contribution to overall spine range of motion. In the cervical spine, the majority of motion in the sagittal plane (flexion-extension) occurs through Occ-C2, C4-5, and C5-6 (Figure 13-1).[3] The majority of axial rotation occurs at the level of C1-C2 and is made possible by the unique anatomy of the atlantoaxial articulations. Lateral bending of the cervical spine is more evenly distributed with the upper subaxial cervical spine contributing only slightly more than other regions. Sagittal motion in the thoracic spine increases in a cranial to caudal direction. The upper segments provide approximately 4 degrees at each level and the lower segments provide approximately 6 degrees and increase to approximately 12 degrees per level at the thoracolumbar junction.[3] Axial rotation is greatest in the upper thoracic spine and gradually decreases caudally. Segmental

contribution to lateral bending is fairly well distributed over the length of the thoracic spine. The lumbar spine contributes more flexion-extension (Figure 13-2) but significantly less axial rotation. These regional differences in motion are related to anatomical differences, primarily articular process orientation, between the thoracic and lumbar vertebrae. The ligamentous structures of the spinal column play an important role in spine kinematics by augmenting overall spinal stability while maintaining flexibility.

The normal spine is essentially vertical in the coronal plane but exhibits four curves in the sagittal plane. The terms *kyphosis* and *lordosis* are used to describe sagittal curves. Kyphosis refers to a curve in the sagittal plane with a posterior convexity (forward bend). The thoracic and sacral portions of the spine demonstrate kyphosis. The normal amount of thoracic kyphosis ranges from 20 to 50 degrees.[4] The term *lordosis* describes a curve in the sagittal plane with an anterior convexity (posterior bend). The cervical and lumbar portions of the spine demonstrate lordosis. The mean lordosis in the cervical spine is 35 to 40 degrees.[5,6] The normal range of lordosis in the lumbar spine is from 20 to 60 degrees.[4] Although multiple curves are present, an overall sagittal balance is maintained (Figure 13-3). The sagittal balance of the spine can be assessed using a plumb-line, or gravity-line, technique. In a normal balanced spine, a plumb-line from the center of the C7 should fall ±2 cm from the sacral promontory in the sagittal plane (see Figure 13-3).[7] These curves, as well as appropriate coronal and sagittal balance, allow for increased flexibility and shock-absorbing capacity while maintaining necessary stiffness and stability.[3]

The major load on the spine under normal physiological conditions is axial. Axial loading causes compression of the vertebral column and its individual FSUs. The natural kyphotic and lordotic curves of the spine increase in magnitude and components of individual FSUs (vertebrae and intervertebral discs) deform slightly in response to compression.[3] Soft tissue (ligaments and musculature) as well as bony architecture serve limit the degree to which the gross architecture of the

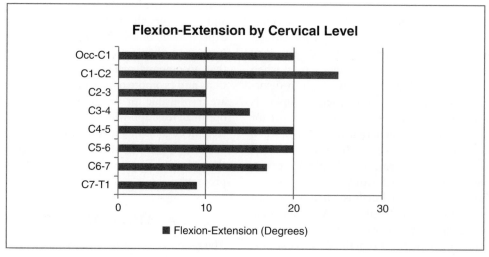

FIGURE 13-1 Flexion-Extension by cervical level. (Adapted from White AA, Panjabi MM. *Clinical Biomechanics of the Spine*, 2nd ed. Philadelphia: JB Lippincott, 1990.)

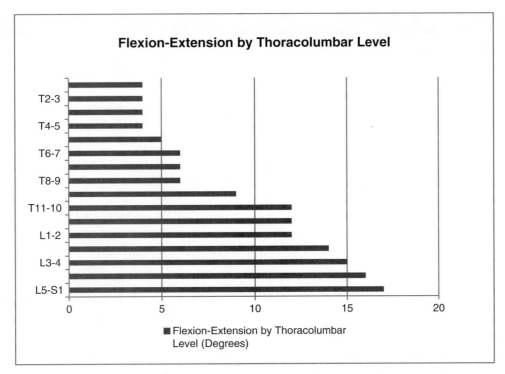

Flexion-Extension by Thoracolumbar Level

FIGURE 13-2 Flexion-extension by thoracolumbar level. (Adapted from White AA, Panjabi MM. *Clinical Biomechanics of the Spine*, 2nd ed. Philadelphia: JB Lippincott, 1990.)

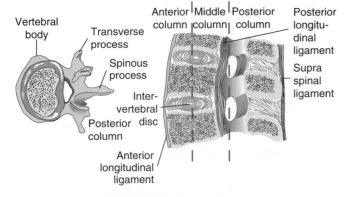

FIGURE 13-3 Three columns.

spine can be deformed and the properties intrinsic to the vertebrae and intervertebral discs counter the effects of compressive forces. The spine must resist tension and shear forces in addition to axial loads. The properties of the spine conform to Wolff's law, which states that form follows function. Studies of the spine reveal that the spine as a whole can resist higher compressive loads than tension or shear.[3] Furthermore, segments of the spine that experience greater compressive loads in vivo have been found to be capable of withstanding higher loads before failure. Biomechanical studies demonstrate that the ability of the spine to withstand forces increase in a cephalocaudal direction such that the lumbar spine, which must withstand the sum weight of the body above it, has the greatest compressive strength.[8,9] The vertebral body (anterior column and anterior aspect of the middle column) provide the majority of this resistance to compression, which translates into increased overall stability in fractures in which the vertebral body is intact and a greater likelihood that bracing may not be necessary. This structure-function relationship is vital to understanding the rationale behind bracing and other treatments of back pain, spinal deformity, or spine injury.

THE THREE-COLUMN CONCEPT

An understanding of spine injury and stability is vital to understanding the role that bracing and various orthoses play. The concept of the three-column spine was initially described by Denis[10] in 1984 and is widely used as a means to help define spinal stability. Denis used the three-column model as a basis for his classification of traumatic spine injuries. The three columns are the anterior, middle, and posterior columns (Figure 13-3). The anterior column consists of the anterior aspect of the vertebral body, anterior annulus fibrosis, and anterior longitudinal ligament. The middle column includes the posterior longitudinal ligament, posterior annulus fibrosis, and posterior aspect of the vertebral body. The posterior column consists of the posterior vertebral arch as well as the supraspinous and interspinous ligaments, facet joints, and ligamentum flavum. Debate exists as to whether injury to the posterior column or the middle column is the main factor that destabilizes thoracolumbar spine fractures[3,11-15]; a combination of both, however, results in a highly unstable spine. Compression fractures and burst fractures are the most common clinical entities where orthoses are considered. Denis defined these types of fractures using the three-column concept (Box 13-1).

Compression fractures are defined as failure and wedging of the anterior column and occur with axial forces combined

---

BOX 13-1   *Classification System for Traumatic Fractures of the Thoracolumbar Spine*

COMPRESSION FRACTURES (DENIS TYPE 1)
Mechanism of Injury: Spinal Flexion with Compression

Subtype	I-A	Anterior fracture only
	I-B	Anterior fracture with lateral components

BURST FRACTURES (DENIS TYPE II)
Mechanism of Injury: Spinal Compression with Flexion

Subtype	II-A	Fracture of both end plates or retropulsion, or both, of the posterior wall as a free fragment
	II-B	Fracture of the superior end plate, occasional retropulsion of inferior wall as a free fragment
	II-C	Fracture of the inferior end plate
	II-D	Burst fracture with rotational injury
	II-E	Burst fracture with lateral flexion injury

SEAT BELT INJURIES (DENIS TYPE III)
Mechanism of Injury: Spinal Flexion with Distraction

Subtype	III-A	(Chance fracture) single segment, posterior or middle column opening
	III-B	(Slice fracture) single segment, posterior and middle column opening through soft and bony tissue
	III-C	Two segments, posterior and middle column opening through soft and bony tissue
	III-D	Two segments, posterior and middle column opening through soft tissue only

FRACTURE DISLOCATIONS (DENIS TYPE IV)
Mechanism of Injury: Translation, Flexion, Rotation, with Shear

Subtype	IV-A	Flexion and rotation injury with disruption through bone or intervertebral disc, or both
	IV-B	Due to shear (anterior-posterior or posterior-anterior) with fracture and dislocation of facet joints
	IV-C	Ligamentous injury to posterior and middle column, with failure (marked instability) of the anterior column
	IV-D	Oblique shear forces resulting in significant instability of involved segment (bone or disc)

---

with spine flexion about an axis located in the middle column. The middle column remains intact, which provides stability and prevents retropulsion of bony fragments into the spinal canal. Some degree of partial failure of the posterior ligamentous structures may be present due to the tension forces present during the initial forced flexion. Depending on the degree of anterior column failure, some compression fractures may undergo progressive collapse and lead to increasing posttraumatic kyphosis.[16] Compression fractures with greater than 50% of vertebral body height loss are more likely to have instability due to associated posterior ligamentous involvement, which may result in progressive injury and kyphotic deformity due to the compressive forces conveyed by an upright posture.[3,16]

Burst fractures generally involve failure of the anterior and middle columns due to axial loading with or without additional moments, depending on the fracture pattern.[17] Although these fractures are defined as two-column involvement, Holdsworth[13] described an associated greenstick fracture of the lamina (posterior column). These injuries are referred to as *three-column burst fractures.* Involvement of the middle column is significant because it may lead to retropulsion of bony fragments in the spinal canal and lead to spinal cord injury. Controversy exists regarding which burst fractures are "stable" and are amenable to bracing, and which require surgery. A recent randomized trial of hyperextension casting followed by brace management compared with operative management demonstrated that patients treated operatively experienced improved functionality more rapidly than those immobilized, but long-term outcomes in terms of deformity, chronic pain, and neurological status were equivalent.[18]

FIT AND FUNCTION OF THE SPINAL ORTHOSIS

All spinal orthoses have several common effects on the spinal region they treat. Their primary action is to reduce gross spinal motion, and the degree to which they accomplish this depends on both their materials and their design. Secondary effects include the stabilization of individual FSUs, reducing the range of motion of one vertebra relative to another. Spinal orthoses also apply closed chain forces designed to counter a deforming force, such as providing hyperextension to a fracture that is vulnerable in flexion. Finally, they reduce loads on the spine itself by preventing specific actions, such as preventing bending and twisting to reduce stress on surgical implants. Each region of the spine has specific needs based on its predominant motions, loads, anatomic features, and physical condition.

The shape of a spinal orthotic, much like the natural shape of the spine, has an intimate relationship with the desired function. Braces often help restore or exaggerate natural spine structure. When thoracolumbar body casts were more commonplace in clinical practice, the casts were applied with the patient positioned supine on a casting table with a belt under their lumbar spine such that they were casted in a position of hyperextension.[19] This hyperextension (hyperlordosis) has been used in many types of braces (i.e., Jewett and CASH) because it removes or decreases the amount of flexion, which reduces compressive force on the fractured vertebral body and limits distraction of the posterior elements. Hyperextension braces achieve the intended positioning by using a three-point mold. A three-point mold refers to three points of applied force: one posteriorly and two anteriorly, with one located cephalad to the level of the posterior force and one caudal.[3] An analogy to this concept is if one was trying to break a pencil using two hands with his or her thumbs in the center and fingers located at either end. The bending that results is the intended effect of the three-point mold. The desired result is prevention of the progressive kyphotic deformity that is associated with significant compression and burst fractures. Another example of three-point molding is seen in corrective braces used for scoliosis, except that the forces are directed in a coronal plane instead of a sagittal plane. It is imperative to ensure that the contour and fit of the brace promotes adequate alignment of the spine and avoids potential complications associated with forces applied to the body for long periods of time.

An orthosis must have intimate contact with bony prominences to be effective.[20] The biomechanical principles of bracing the spine itself can be understood in these terms; in reality, however, using an orthosis to treat a human condition is subject to other variables. Compliance and the psychological effects of bracing can be significant issues including developing a psychological dependence on the orthosis.[21-26] The financial burden can be significant, with costs ranging from $32 to greater than $5000.[1] Physical issues also apply, particularly in an increasingly obese population. The ability of a brace to apply appropriate forces, either stabilizing or corrective, depends on its ability to act on the structures of the spine. This in turn depends on the soft tissue envelope in the contact areas around the spine. Too little or excessive pressures transmitted through soft tissues can result in significant physical complications including skin breakdown, loss of reduction or spinal alignment, pain due to the brace, weakening of the immobilized muscles, and soft tissue contractures.[26-32] The prescription and use of a spinal orthotic should always be prescribed with an appropriate monitoring system and rehabilitation program. Orthoses must be modified periodically, and a comfortable and appropriate fit is critical to preventing skin problems and ensuring compliance.

Compliance with brace wear is a significant clinical issue, particularly because the orthosis is specifically designed to restrict motion, which is neither an accommodating nor pleasant approach to therapy. Studies in adolescent patients with scoliosis wearing "smart braces" that can track wear time indicate compliance rates of 9% to 30%; similar studies have not been done for orthoses used for other conditions. In the current health care environment most patients with significant spinal conditions recover at home rather than in rehabilitation facilities. Orthosis designs that increase the difficulty of donning or doffing decrease the patient's ability to use the brace effectively if they are not supervised and assisted daily. The only orthoses that ensure compliance are fiberglass casts, which are very rarely used in current times.

Regional Orthoses

Cervical

The cervical spine is the most intuitively easy structure to consider bracing, in that the bony occiput, mandible, sternum, and clavicles provide appropriate supporting structures. Unfortunately this advantage is offset by the limited surface area available for contact and the fact that the mandibles and clavicles are often in motion during normal activities. The complexity of the cervical soft tissues—vessels, airway, esophagus—is a disadvantage, in that significant forces cannot be applied directly to the spine without significant visceral effects. Orthoses for the cervical spine can be limited to the subaxial spine itself—a cylinder that fits around the neck with a trimline at the occiput, mandible, and sternoclavicular structures—or may extend proximally and distally (halo vest) or distally onto the thoracic cage for additional control (cervicothoracic orthosis [CTO]).

Cylindrical cervical braces limit a variable degree of motion depending on the design and primarily provide proprioceptive feedback as a reminder to limit the range of motion of the neck. Available choices are many and this list is not exhaustive; commonly used choices include the soft collar, the Stifneck (Laerdal, Armonk, NY), the Philadelphia (Philadelphia Cervical Collar, Thorofare, NJ), and the Miami J (Össer, Foothill Ranch, CA) (Figure 13-4).

Soft collars tend to be the most comfortable of the available cervical collars but provide little stability to the cervical spine. The collar is a soft foam rubber covered with stockinet or other gentle fabric with a Velcro-type fastener. These collars have been shown to provide up to 10% restriction to cervical motion in all planes.[33-35] Conversely, Miller et al[36] analyzed differences in functional cervical spine motion between no collar, a soft collar, and a rigid collar while performing 15 different activities of daily living* (ADLs). The authors found that there was no significant difference in limitation of sagittal range of motion between the soft and rigid collars during 13 of the 15 ADLs tested (significant differences were noted while reversing a car and sitting down in a chair). No significant differences were noted during lateral bending, and the difference in rotational movement restriction was only significant while reversing a car. The soft cervical orthosis is used primarily as a comfortable reminder to the patient to limit exaggerated neck movements and may be useful in cases of minor whiplash, cervical spondylosis, or as a postoperative adjunct with a stable spine.[3] Soft collars are inappropriate for an unstable cervical spine.

A great deal more support is required in patients with injuries that compromise spinal stability. This prompted the

---

*ADLs tested include standing to sitting, backing up a car, putting on socks, tying shoelaces, reading a magazine in lap, cutting food with knife and fork and bringing food to mouth, rising from a sitting position, washing hands in a standing position, shaving facial hair (men)/applying makeup (women), washing hair in shower, picking up object from floor (bending technique), picking up object from floor (squatting technique), walking, walking up stairs, walking down stairs.

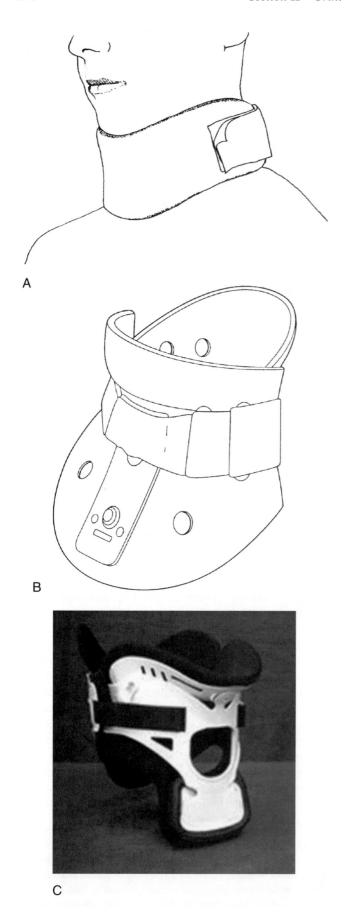

A

B

C

FIGURE 13-4 A, Soft collar. **B,** Philadelphia collar. **C,** Miami J collar.

development of the reinforced cervical collar, which is a commercially produced, prefabricated orthosis that combines some of the soft materials found in soft collars with a semirigid, contoured plastic external frame. Many different types of reinforced collars are available, such as the Philadelphia, Aspen (Aspen Medical Products, Irvine, CA), Miami J, NecLoc (Össur, Foothill Ranch, CA), and Stifneck. Most reinforced collars have anterior and posterior shells with inner padding and trim that close around the neck and fasten with Velcro-type fasteners. The collars are contoured such that they abut the sternum, clavicles, trapezius, and upper thoracic spine inferiorly and the mandible and occiput superiorly, which provides some degree of end-point control. Most have openings anteriorly to accommodate respiratory and ventilator equipment.

Although there are many similarities between the different cervical collars, studies have found significant differences in the degree to which different collars restrict cervical spine motion. The ability for a cervical collar to provide cervical stability is very important in that approximately 3% to 25% of spinal cord injuries occur after the initial spine injury.[37] Multiple studies have evaluated the various reinforced collars for their ability to promote cervical stability as well as avoid complications. Askins and Eismont[37] studied five common reinforced cervical collars by using anteroposterior and lateral radiographs to assess cervical spine motion in normal, healthy volunteers. They found the NecLoc to be statistically superior with respect to limitation of cervical motion in all planes, followed by the Miami J collar, when compared the Philadelphia and Aspen collars. Kaufman and colleagues[38] found the NecLoc to provide superior restriction of motion versus the Philadelphia collar and a soft collar. Ducker[39] found the NecLoc and Miami J collars to be statistically superior to the Stifneck, Philadelphia, and soft collars.

The treating physician must consider fit and skin protection when selecting a reinforced cervical collar in addition to selecting a collar that is capable of providing adequate stability. Fisher[29] studied the importance of proper fit of a cervical orthosis and found that an inappropriately fitted collar was equivalent to not wearing any collar at all. Bell and colleagues[32] analyzed the effects that ill-fitted Miami J collars have on the degree of cervical motion restriction. They found that in flexion-extension, the braces that were too large and too small allowed increased motion but only extension in the too large brace produced a statistically significant increase in allowed motion. Both the too small and too large braces allowed significantly more motion in left and right axial rotation. The too large and too small braces allowed significantly more lateral bending motion to the right but only the too small brace allowed a significant increase in left lateral bending. Plaisier and colleagues[28] evaluated common cervical collars and the pressures they exerted on craniofacial tissues with respect to capillary closing pressure. The pressure at the collar-skin interface was measured using an electropneumatic sensor placed between the collar and skin. This measurement was compared with a value of 32 mm Hg, which represents capillary closing pressure as defined by Berne and colleagues.[40] They found significant differences between collars in the amount of pressure exerted on the tissues. The Stifneck collar produced pressures in excess of capillary closing pressure at most collar-tissue interfaces, whereas the Miami J collar exerted pressures well below the capillary closing pressure.

Braces that need to immobilize the occipitocervical spine require fixation to the skull and significant rotational control. The most commonly used example is the halo vest (Figure 13-5). Facial fracture fixation with traction applied through a skull ring was developed by Frank Bloom, MD, during World War II to treat pilots with facial fractures and severe burns. The device was then adapted by Vernon Nickel, MD, and first reported in 1959.[8] Primary features include a ring anchored to the skull with skeletal pins and connected to a body jacket by four vertical uprights. Changes in material design and advances in plastic technology have allowed significant modifications to the halo vest—molded thermoplastic jackets, radiolucent rings and uprights, shaped rings open posteriorly for patient comfort while supine, and multidirectional adjustments in the connecting mechanisms—but the principles of fixation have remained the same. Six to eight transcranial pins provide secure proximal fixation (end point control), and full contact support around the thorax and torso provide the distal fixation.

The ring of the halo is positioned 1 cm above the eyebrows and the tip of the ears, with care taken to keep the ring well clear of the skin surface. Four pins are inserted into the outer table of the skull with 6 to 8 lb/in of torque.[41] The anterior pins are placed at the equator (widest point) of the skull above the lateral one third of the eyebrow to avoid the frontal sinus, supraorbital and supratrochlear nerves, and temporalis muscle. Posteriorly, pins are placed 1 to 2 cm posterior to the ear diagonally opposite the anterior pins. This provides secure fixation to allow for manipulation in both flexion/extension and in translation.

The halo vest itself was originally a plaster cast fit over the torso with a trimline at or slightly above the inferior costal margin of the last rib.[42] Advances in materials allow for bivalved thermoplastic shells that can be released with the patient supine to allow for hygiene, and some designs are fleece lined. A four-pad halo vest that completely avoids the shoulder girdle has been proposed to avoid scapular movements transferring loads to the neck.[43,44] Two anterior and two posterior rods link the vest to the ring through a series of connectors. Modern connectors allow translation in multiple planes with the ability to lock them into position once reduction has been achieved.

Complications can occur with halo vest use, including pressure sores, loss of reduction (particularly in injuries involving the posterior elements), and pin infection and loosening.[45–49] A higher rate of complications occurs in older patients. In a review of 53 patients with a mean age of 79.9 years, Horn and colleagues[50] recorded 31 complications in 22 patients. Serious complications included respiratory distress and dysphagia, and the cause of death in 6 of 8 patients who died within the treatment period was thought to have some relationship to the halo treatment. Modern day halo vests should always have a wrench attached to the front of the halo vest for quick removal in case of a cardiac emergency.

Studies comparing the halo to other types of cervical bracing with respect to the ability to limit motion have had variable findings. Johnson et al[51] found that the halo allowed only 4% of normal sagittal motion, 1% of normal rotation, and 4% of lateral bending in normal subjects. A cadaveric study of simulated odontoid fractures demonstrated the halo was superior in all planes versus a Miami J collar, a Minerva brace, and a soft collar.[34] In vivo studies comparing subjects in various positions and activities demonstrated a maximum reduction of sagittal motion of only 30%.[52] A study of injured patients by Benzel et al[53] demonstrated paradoxically increased movement at the injured levels in the halo versus a Minerva brace, which they attributed to the pull of the neck muscles with attempted flexion or extension against the rigidly fixed head. Ivancic and Telles[54] studied neck motion in a normal versus loosely applied halo vest in the supine and prone positions using a cadaveric cervical spine between an anthropometric dummy and surrogate head. Results showed significantly increased motion in the loose vest with respect to the normal vest. The authors conclude that such increased motion may play a role in delayed unions and nonunions of cervical spine fractures.

The halo vest is useful in providing reduction and provisional stabilization of injuries or conditions causing instability at

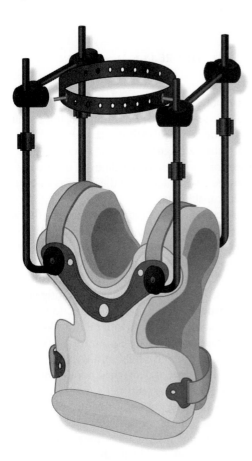

FIGURE 13-5 Halo vest.

the occipitocervical junction, and can be used to provide additional support after these patients have surgery. It is best used for reducing angular and translational deformities in cervical spinal fractures at the proximal and distal regions of the spine; in the midportion, studies have shown that a halo actually increases the forces on the injured vertebrae.[53] It is commonly used for complex combined C1 and C2 fracture patterns where internal stabilization is not possible without extension to the occiput, which results in severe loss of motion for the patient.[55,56] It is used to provide additional stability after complex surgical reconstructions or noninstrumented fusion or wiring constructs after surgery at C1-2, and may be used to supplement instrumented fusions in situations with poor bone quality or significant instability, such as in osteoporosis or rheumatoid arthritis patients.[57] The halo is no longer used as frequently in subaxial (i.e., C3-C7) trauma due to the advances in spinal instrumentation. It is still considered the treatment of choice for some types of fractures of the axis (hangman's fractures) and in some flexion-compression injuries.[58,59] A fracture of the odontoid process at C2 is a common injury among older patients and historically has often been treated with a halo vest.[60-62] Currently the optimal treatment for these patients is a topic of debate, with some authors reporting that simple collar immobilization provides equivalent results.[63-69] Significantly higher mortality has been reported in older patients treated with a halo compared with those treated with a cervical collar.[61,70] Daentzer and colleagues[71] performed a retrospective study of 29 patients divided into two groups based on age less than or greater than 65 and found that while clinical and radiographic results were equivalent between the two groups, the interval to healing and rate of complications were higher in the older than 65 age group.

Rehabilitation of the patient with a halo is challenging. The fixed head position results in a different ability to use visual cues, and the weight of the vest and position of the head combine to change the patient's center of mass. Ambulatory patients in halo vests may exhibit a forward-flexion posture to accommodate this; a cane or walker may be required while the halo is in place. Likewise, there is a readjustment period after the halo is removed that may require postural reeducation as part of the rehabilitation strategy.

Cervicothoracic and Thoracic

CTO can be divided into two categories: those that use the thoracic spine to support treatment of a subaxial cervical spine or upper thoracic spine problem, and those that support treatment at the upper cervical spine. Examples in the first category include thoracic extensions added to a cylindrical cervical orthosis (i.e., Extended Miami J), or an orthosis that utilizes pads on the chin and occiput to connect to the trunk by four stiff uprights or circumferential supports (i.e., Minerva). The Minerva brace (Figure 13-6) is the most effective method for immobilizing C1-2, and has been shown to limit flexion-extension by approximately 79%, axial rotation by 88%, and lateral bending by 51%.[72] The cervicothoracic area is a particularly challenging area to immobilize in that it is a transitional area between the very mobile and lordotic cervical spine and the kyphotic thoracic spine. Little

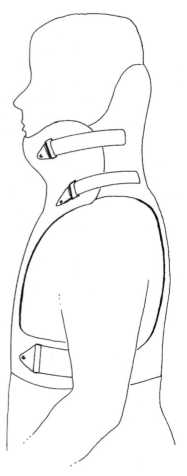

FIGURE 13-6 Minerva brace.

data exist in the literature regarding immobilization of the upper thoracic spine; for those conditions not requiring surgery, an extended cervical orthosis can be used.[1] The Minerva brace, SOMI brace (Figure 13-7), or a custom-molded CTO can be used for conditions extending as far caudally as T5. In general, increasing the length of the orthosis down the trunk enhances its capabilities.[51]

The most common condition that affects the thoracic spine is the vertebral compression fracture (VCF). Approximately 700,000 vertebral compression fractures occur each year, and it is estimated that 25% of American women will experience at least one VCF in their lifetime.[73] Most patients will have a benign course, but up to 30% are significantly symptomatic and seek treatment for pain that limits function either short or long term.[74] A study of patients with multiple VCFs found significant decreases in trunk extension torque, spinal motion, functional reach, mobility skills, and walking distance compared with the normal age-matched population.[75] The treatment of VCF is aimed at pain relief, rather than at fracture treatment as with other types of fracture management. The main objective is to improve quality of life and decrease pain.

Treatment of painful fractures may necessitate a short period of bed rest followed by gradual mobilization. Bracing with an orthosis may be beneficial for the first 6 to 8 weeks until the acute pain resolves. Unfortunately bracing is often

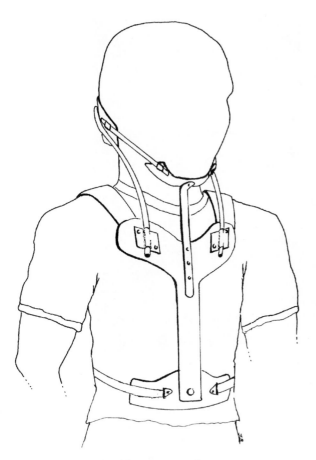

FIGURE 13-7 SOMI brace.

poorly tolerated. The efficacy of bracing VCF has not been established.[76] For osteoporotic women in general, one study demonstrated that wearing a TL orthosis that emphasized postural control for 6 months resulted in improvements in back extensor strength, abdominal flexor strength, decreased kyphosis, decrease in pain, increase in well-being, and decrease in limitations.[77] One study suggested efficacy for this orthosis in patients with VCF and demonstrated potentially better tolerance than other braces.[78] Further study is required to outline optimal general management strategies for using spinal orthoses in this population.[79] Typically a symptomatic patient requesting bracing is trialed in an extended cervical orthosis, a hyperextension TL brace (CASH or Jewett, see later), or a CTO depending on the level involved.[53] If the orthosis is not helpful it is discarded.

Thoracolumbar

The thoracolumbar region is the most common region of the spine affected by traumatic fracture, and the most likely region of the spine to benefit from orthotic support for the surgically treated spine. The integrity of the vertebral body is of primary importance to resisting compressive forces and axial loads, and this region is a transitional zone that should be neutral in alignment. Fractures involving the anterior body greatly decrease the spine's ability to withstand compressive load and tend to collapse into kyphosis, particularly if the posterior elements are also involved (i.e., a burst

fracture). This results in displacement of the patient's sagittal balance, spinal deformity, pain, and in the worst cases, neurological deficit. Fractures of this area may be treated with orthoses or surgically, and there is some consensus in the literature for surgical management when the vertebral body is severely comminuted, the patient has a neurological deficit, or the initial fracture alignment is unacceptable.[76,80] Advances in spinal instrumentation and techniques such as interbody support have improved the surgeon's ability to counteract kyphosis, but at the thoracolumbar junction this requires a combined thoracolumbar surgical approach through the thoracic and abdominal cavities, which carries significant morbidity. Surgeons often choose to use posterior spinal instrumentation alone in these cases. Posterior instrumentation is least effective in resisting kyphosis, so orthoses that reduce kyphotic forces on the thoracolumbar spine may be used to supplement internal fixation techniques.

When orthoses are used for thoracolumbar fracture management, the same principles apply. Optimal management includes a strategy to resist anterior flexion and therefore the development of a kyphotic deformity. They are best used for fractures from T10 to L2, although some types of orthoses can be adjusted to control up to T8. Several thoracolumbar hyperextension orthoses are designed to unload the anterior column.[1] The most common types are the Jewett brace (Figure 13-8A) and the cruciform anterior spinal hyperextension brace (CASH) (see Figure 13-8B). Both of these braces are available in prefabricated styles from various manufacturers. The Jewett orthosis has an aluminum frame anteriorly that is stabilized on the pubis, sternum, and lateral midline of the trunk against a posterior pad. The frame is open and is particularly suitable for patients with coexisting abdominal trauma or obesity. Trunk flexion is limited by a single three-point pressure system with posteriorly directed forces at the sternum and pubis opposing an anteriorly directed force applied by the posterior pad. Therefore it is contraindicated in patients with sternal fractures or an inability to tolerate direct pressure from the posterior pad. The goal of the Jewett is to prevent flexion while still allowing active hyperextension. The CASH brace uses the same three-point system. It has an adjustable-length anterior cross with sternal and pelvic pads at the end of the vertical bar, and lateral pads on the horizontal bar. It also uses an anteriorly directed force provided by a posterior belt. Both the Jewett and the CASH are options for those patients who cannot tolerate the constriction of a molded thermoplast thoracolumbosacral orthosis (TLSO) but are contraindicated in patients with injuries including significant three-column instability such as the thoracolumbar burst fracture.

The TLSO is the recommended treatment for significant fractures at the thoracolumbar junction being treated conservatively. TLSOs can be used to manage fractures from T6 to L4. Molded TLSOs provide total contact designed to restrict range of motion in all planes. In one study, a custom-molded thermoplastic TLSO showed 94% restriction in lateral bending and 69% restriction of flexion-extension in the lumbar spine.[81] In the thoracic spine, there was 49%

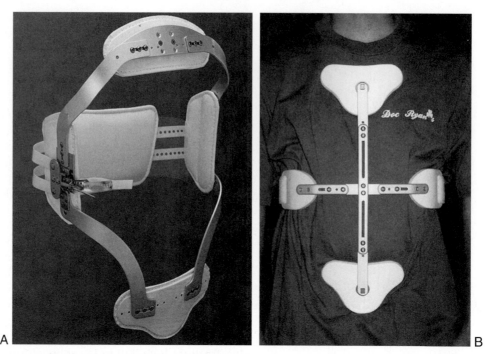

A

B

FIGURE 13-8 A, Jewett brace. **B,** CASH brace.

restriction of flexion-extension and 38% restriction of lateral bending. The thoracic spine normally also allows rotation, and a reduction of 60% in total rotation was also shown. The superior trimlines of the TLSO are at the sternal notch and have an anterior-inferior trimline at the groin; they are carefully shaped to envelop the pelvis, arching slightly laterally anteriorly to accommodate the thigh while sitting and trimmed low at the sacrococcygeal junction posteriorly. The superior-posterior trimline falls just below the spine of the scapula. The custom molds are made of a ventilated thermoplastic, which may be lined with closed cell foam to increase comfort. They can be bivalved with side closures to facilitate donning and doffing, and are generally worn over a light T-shirt for comfort and hygiene. Straps over the shoulders may increase the rigidity, particularly if a semiflexible or prefabricated model is chosen. TLSOs are also available in prefabricated models, although for maximum control of motion, a custom mold is preferred. There is some controversy as to whether the made-to-measure or prefabricated orthoses fit and function as well as the custom-fabricated ones.

Lumbosacral

Immobilization of the lumbosacral spine presents a unique set of challenges. It is a transition zone between the highly mobile, lordotic, lumbar spine and the rigid sacropelvic structures; it has the largest absolute range of flexion-extension motion, and it bears the most load of any of the spinal regions. A rigid LSO, which is simply a shorter version of the TLSO braces described earlier, is appropriate for bracing fractures at L2, L3, and L4, but the FSU at L4-5 and L5-S1 require special treatment. Fidler and Plasmans[82] found that a unilateral thigh extension is necessary to effectively immo-

bilize L4-5 and L5-S1. A thigh extension is generally a cuff attached by two longitudinal struts that have hinges, allowing a variable degree of flexion at the hip to facilitate toileting and sitting; generally, it is set at allowing 20 to 30 degrees of flexion at a maximum. The mean percentage of motion allowed in the brace was 32% at L4-5 and 70% at L5-S1 in a brace without the extension; adding the extension resulted in an additional 15% to 30% reduction of motion.[83,84] At best, restriction at the L5-S1 level still allows 40% of normal range. For this reason fractures at these levels are best treated with surgery (using an orthosis for postoperative support if necessary) if the treating physician desires to mobilize that patient during the healing period.

LSOs have commonly been used in the postoperative period up until the last few years. Advances in spinal instrumentation with the advent of pedicle screws and interbody techniques now allow many patients to go without bracing postoperatively. Pedicle screws connect the anterior load bearing portion of the spine with a posterior construct by crossing the middle column (Figure 13-9) and provide better limitation of motion and load sharing than previous hook/rod constructs. Interbody techniques place a block of bone between the vertebral bodies, either through placement by an intraabdominal approach or with hybrid approaches accessing the disc space from the posterior part of the spine. The placement of bone in the middle and anterior columns facilitates healing because of increased surface area and favorable biomechanical conditions allowing the bone graft to experience compression forces. A recent randomized trial that assessed the benefit of wearing a lumbar corset for 8 weeks after lumbar fusion did not find a significant advantage or disadvantage with respect to healing rates or patient comfort.[85]

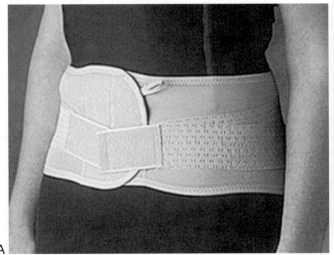
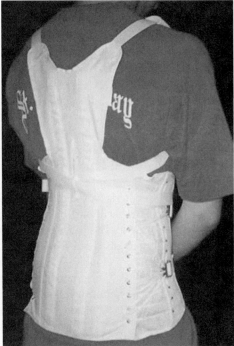

A
B

FIGURE 13-9 A, Lumbar corset. **B,** Chairback orthosis.

Today, postoperative bracing is reserved for patients who feel more comfortable with support (a lumbar corset) or those with poor bone quality or technical issues leading to concerns about healing or the stabilization provided by the instrumentation.

Patients with acute low back pain may find the additional support and postural reminder of a lumbar corset helpful for pain reduction. Lumbar corsets are generally semirigid or flexible braces (see Figure 13-9A). Their function is to reduce gross trunk motion and increase intracavitary pressure in the abdomen by transmitting a three-point pressure system to the lumbar spine. They are designed to support the trunk in a neutral sagittal alignment and provide a kinesthetic reminder to limit motion. The lumbar corset has little resistance to gross body motion during sitting and standing.[86] Typically, the anterior borders of the lumbosacral corset are superior to the symphysis pubis and inferior to the xiphoid process. The posterior borders extend between the sacrococcygeal junction of the pelvis and the inferior angle of the scapulae; some may incorporate shoulder straps. The Chairback Orthosis (see Figure 13-9B) is an LS corset with both a thoracic and a pelvic band connected by two paraspinal bars for optimized sagittal control. A pair of lateral bars can also be added for improved coronal control (the Knight orthosis).

The literature on the effectiveness of the corset is conflicting. In 2001, a systematic review of randomized and nonrandomized controlled trials demonstrated no evidence that spinal orthoses are effective in the prevention or management of low back pain.[87] An orthosis should be used in conjunction with a rehabilitation program focused on core strengthening and stabilization in these patients.

Spinal orthoses have been found to have a deconditioning effect on the paraspinal muscles and trunk stabilizers. Electromyographic studies have found conflicting results, with some demonstrating a significant reduction in muscle activity in the brace and others finding either unchanged or increased activity.[83,88] An exercise regimen should be maintained when the clinical situation allows, and the orthosis should be discontinued as soon as possible.

SCOLIOSIS

Scoliosis is a general term that refers to a three-dimensional spinal deformity characterized by coronal displacement of vertebral bodies away from the axis of gravity combined with abnormal vertebral rotation. There are many types of scoliosis as well as many etiologies. In current times, the only type of scoliosis that is typically and frequently managed with spinal orthoses is the idiopathic curve. Adolescent idiopathic scoliosis (AIS) refers to a curvature and rotational deformity of the spine that develops with growth. It can occur in the upper thoracic, thoracic, thoracolumbar, or lumbar spine or some combination of these. There is often a primary curve (the curve with abnormal growth) and a compensatory curve, which is a second region of the spine curving in the opposite direction to the primary curve to keep the head centered over the pelvis. The age of the child, growth remaining, and curve pattern all have implications for prognosis.

Prevalence and Natural History

Idiopathic scoliosis has been studied and documented for many years and maintains a consistent prevalence of approximately 1% to 2% of school-age children.[89-91] Ninety percent of children have adolescent onset curves, although this figure may be falsely elevated because younger children are not routinely evaluated.[92] The prevalence of curves that do not require treatment (<20 degrees) is 20 to 30 per 1000, the prevalence of moderate curves amenable to bracing (20 to 30 degrees) is 3 to 5 per 1000, and the prevalence of large curves likely to go on to surgical management is 2 to 3 per 1000 people.[91] The prevalence of curves is greater in females, particularly with respect to curves over 20 degrees (6.4 F:1 M).[93] The single right thoracic curve is the most prevalent pattern.[94] The most important determinants of the likelihood of progression are those that reflect skeletal maturity: age, menarchal status, and the presence of mature growth centers on radiographs of the pelvis (Risser sign) or hand. The likelihood of progression determines the need for treatment; those at highest risk are those with a younger age at diagnosis, a curve that appears before the onset of menstruation, a double curve pattern, and a curve that is documented to change more than 5 degrees on serial radiographs taken at 6-month intervals. Curve magnitude and rotation are both correlated with increased progression rates.[95] This is the basis for the recommendation that curves greater than 50 degrees in a growing child be treated surgically.

Biomechanics

Curves progress when buckling loads change during growth, along with other hormonal and developmental factors. A straight, flexible column fixed at the base and free at the other end subjected to axial forces will buckle, which in the spine results in a combination of curvature and rotation. The loads at which these processes occur are related to length and rigidity of the spine. The adolescent growth spurt results in a significant increase in spinal length and may result in increased flexibility as well, which contributes to the drastic increases in curve progression commonly observed during adolescent years. As the curve progresses, a feed-forward cycle is created. With curve progression, the spine is subjected to increasingly abnormal force vectors and deviates further from the normal anatomic alignment at which it is best equipped to resist such loading. Braces used for scoliosis are designed to interrupt this feed-forward cycle.

There are three primary mechanisms by which an orthosis exerts forces on a developing spine: end point control, curve correction, and transverse loading.[96] End point control is the ability of the orthosis to constrain the spine. An example of end-point control is the neck ring at the proximal end of the Milwaukee brace, which can control the position of the upper thoracic spine relative to the pelvis. Curve correction has the greatest effect because it stiffens the spine and reduces the curve, which in turn decreases the load on the spine and slows the rate of deformation. Transverse loading at the apex is the primary mode of correction within modern orthoses, but begins to lose efficacy as the curves get larger.[97] It is important to note that brace treatment often does not significantly correct the curve that exists but rather prevents it from increasing in size during growth. Some degree of curve correction should be achieved within the brace (ideally 50%

or more) because the curve will regress back to its initial magnitude once the brace is removed. [98,99] The overall concept is to halt curve progression.

Evaluation

The first step in evaluating a child with a spinal curvature is a thorough orthopedic history including age, growth patterns, family history of spinal problems, the age the curve was discovered, and any treatment that has been used to date. The primary goal of an orthosis in treating a scoliotic deformity is to control remaining spinal growth so that the spine reaches maturity with an acceptable curvature. There is no role for using an orthosis to prevent scoliosis and the ability of an orthosis to make a curvature ultimately smaller is limited.[100-102] Scoliosis progresses as the spine grows, so an adolescent at the end of spinal growth has very little risk of progression, and there is no role for bracing a curve that has already reached a size where surgery is indicated.[103] Therefore it is critical to identify children with scoliosis at the early stages. A national screening program has been adopted in many countries for this purpose.

Physical examination and radiographs are used to measure the size, flexibility, and effects of each spinal curvature. The Scoliosis Research Society has adopted a set of terms and definitions to describe scoliosis as well as to describe the multitude of spinal conditions that can lead to scoliosis. Curves can be described either by etiology of the structural changes (Box 13-2) or by the spinal level of the anatomical apex of the curve. In a cervical scoliosis, the apex of the curve is at or between the vertebral body of C1 and C6. In a cervicothoracic curve, the apex is at C7, C8, or T1. A thoracic curve has an apex at or between T2 and T11. A thoracolumbar curve reaches its apex at the T12 or L1 vertebral body. A lumbar curve occurs at L2, L3, or L4, whereas a lumbosacral curve reaches its apex at L5 or S1. Numerous descriptive terms are also used in the diagnosis, evaluation, and management of scoliosis (Table 13-2). These standards and definitions are used throughout this chapter.

Scoliosis can also be described by etiology. A child or adolescent who develops scoliosis after relatively typical growth and development is diagnosed as having idiopathic scoliosis. An individual who develops scoliosis as a secondary complication of nervous system or muscle disease is described as having neuromuscular scoliosis. Clinical examination includes an assessment of the patient's posture, noting any asymmetry in trunk alignment, shoulder height, scapular prominence, and pelvic rotation. Special attention is paid to the degree of thoracic kyphosis and lumbar lordosis, and any tendency toward trunk shift to the right or left (spinal decompensation) (Figure 13-10). The Adams forward bending test assesses the rotation of each curve by the degree of prominence over the apices, and the patient can be flexed laterally while bent forward to assess the degree of curve flexibility (Figure 13-11). Complete neurological, skin, and cardiac examinations are then performed.

The timing of orthotic treatment is an important determinant of efficacy. Principles have remained the same regardless of the orthosis used. First, treatment should

---

BOX 13-2 *Classification System for Idiopathic and Neuromuscular Structural Scoliosis*

IDIOPATHIC
Infantile (0-3 years)
Resolving
Progressive

Juvenile (3-10 years)

Adolescent (older than 10 years) Neuropathic

NEUROMUSCULAR
Upper motor neuron
   Cerebral palsy
   Spinocerebellar degeneration
   Friedreich's ataxia
   Charcot-Marie-Tooth disease
   Roussy-Lévy disease
   Syringomyelia
   Spinal cord tumor
   Spinal cord trauma
   Other

Lower motor neuron
   Poliomyelitis
   Other viral myelitides
   Trauma
   Spinal muscular atrophy
   Werdnig-Hoffmann disease
   Kugelberg-Welander disease
   Myelomeningocele (paralytic)
   Dysautonomia (Riley-Day syndrome)

Other
Myopathic
Arthrogryposis
Muscular dystrophy
   Duchenne's (pseudohypertrophy)
   Limb-girdle
   Fiber-type disproportion
Congenital hypotonia
Myotonic dystrophica
Other

TABLE 13-2 *Glossary and Definitions of Terms in Scoliosis*

Term	Definition
Adolescent scoliosis	Spinal curvature presenting at or about the onset of puberty and before maturity
Adult scoliosis	Spinal curvature that develops after skeletal maturity
Angle of thoracic	The angle between the horizontal plane and inclination plane across the posterior rib cage at the greatest prominence of a rib hump, assessed with the trunk flexed 90 degrees at the hips
Apical vertebra	The most rotated vertebra in a curve; the most deviated vertebra from the vertical axis of the patient
Body alignment	1. Alignment of the midpoint of the occiput over the sacrum in the same vertical plane as the shoulders over the hips 2. In radiography, when the sum of the angular deviations of the spine in one direction is equal to that in the opposite direction (also described as balance or compensation)
Café au lait spots	Light-brown, irregular areas of skin pigmentation; if they are sufficient in number and have smooth margins, they suggest neurofibromatosis
Cobb angle or method	On radiograph, the uppermost and lowermost vertebrae in the curve are identified; a perpendicular line (curve measurement) is drawn from the transverse axes of these vertebrae, and the angle formed at their intersection (Cobb angle) measures the severity of the curve; if vertebral end plates are poorly visualized, a line through the bottom or top of the pedicles can be used
Compensatory curve	A curve, which can be structural, above or below the major curve that tends to maintain normal body alignment
Congenital scoliosis	Scoliosis due to congenitally anomalous vertebral development
Double major scoliosis	Scoliosis with two structural curves
Double thoracic curves	Two structural curves within the thoracic spine
End vertebra	1. Uppermost vertebra of a curve, the superior surface of which tilts maximally toward the concavity of the curve 2. The most caudal vertebra, the inferior surface of which tilts maximally toward the concavity of the curve
Fractional curve	Compensatory curve that is incomplete because it returns to the erect; its only horizontal vertebra is its caudad or cephalad one
Full curve	Curve in which the only horizontal vertebra is at the apex

(Continued)

TABLE 13-2   *Glossary and Definitions of Terms in Scoliosis—cont'd*

Term	Definition
Gibbus	Sharply angular kyphos
Hyperkyphosis	Sagittal alignment of the thoracic spine in which more than the normal amount of kyphosis is present (a kyphos)
Hypokyphosis	Sagittal alignment of the thoracic spine in which less than the normal amount of kyphosis is present but not so severe as to be lordotic
Hysterical scoliosis	Nonstructural deformity of the spine that develops as a manifestation of a conversion reaction
Idiopathic scoliosis	Structural spinal curvature for which no cause is established
Iliac epiphysis or apophysis	Epiphysis along the wing of an ilium
Inclinometer	Instrument used to measure the angle of thoracic inclination or rib hump
Infantile scoliosis	Spinal curvature that develops during the first 3 years of life
Juvenile scoliosis	Spinal curvature that develops between the skeletal age of 3 years and the onset of puberty (10 years)
Kyphos	Change in alignment of a segment of the spine in the sagittal plane that increases the posterior convex angulation; an abnormally increased kyphosis
Kyphoscoliosis	Spine with scoliosis and a true hyperkyphosis; a rotatory deformity with only apparent kyphosis should not be described by this term
Kyphosing scoliosis	Scoliosis with marked rotation such that lateral bending of the rotated spine mimics kyphosis
Lordoscoliosis	Scoliosis associated with an abnormal anterior angulation in the sagittal plane
Major curve	Term used to designate the largest structural curve
Minor curve	Term used to refer to the smallest curve, which is always more flexible than the major curve
Nonstructural curve	Curve that has no structural component and that corrects or overcorrects on recumbent side-bending radiographs
Pelvic obliquity	Deviation of the pelvis from the horizontal in the frontal plane; fixed pelvic obliquities can be attributable to contractures either above or below the pelvis
Primary curve	First or earliest of several curves to appear, if identifiable
Risser sign	Rating system used to indicate skeletal maturity, based on degree of ossification of the iliac epiphysis
Rotational prominence	In the forward-bending position, the thoracic prominence on one side is usually due to vertebral rotation, causing rib prominence; in the lumbar spine, the prominence is usually due to rotation of the lumbar vertebrae
Skeletal age (bone age)	Age obtained by comparing an anteroposterior radiograph of the left hand and wrist with the standards of Greulich and Pyle's atlas
Structural curve	Segment of the spine with a lateral curvature that lacks normal flexibility; radiographically, it is identified by the complete lack of a curve on a supine film or by the failure to demonstrate complete segmental mobility on supine side-bending films
Vertebral end plates	Superior and inferior plates of cortical bone of the vertebral body adjacent to the intervertebral disc
Vertebral growth plate	Cartilaginous surface covering the top and bottom of a vertebral body, which is responsible for linear growth of the vertebra
Vertebral ring apophyses	Most reliable index of vertebral immaturity, seen best in lateral radiographs or in the lumbar region in side-bending anteroposterior views

be initiated before skeletal maturity when there is growth remaining because bracing is only effective in a growing child; curves less than 20 degrees are generally observed, but once a curve is greater than 20 degrees and/or demonstrates significant progression bracing is initiated. Second, the brace should be worn full time, which was defined by Blount[104] as 23 hours per day and recently confirmed by metaanalysis of available studies.[105] Third, the brace should be worn until skeletal maturity. Lastly, there should be a weaning period accompanied by a rehabilitation program to rebuild muscle strength once skeletal maturity is reached.

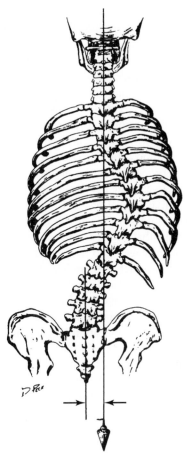

FIGURE 13-10 Trunk shift.

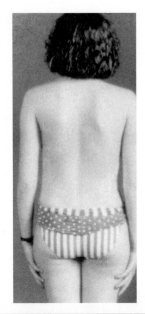

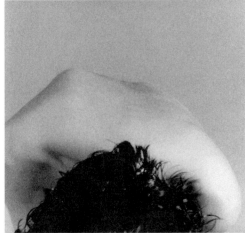

FIGURE 13-11 Adams forward bend test.

Types of Braces

Milwaukee Brace

In 1944 the Milwaukee brace was developed by Blount and Schmidt. The Milwaukee brace, a cervicothoracolumbosacral orthosis (CTLSO), was initially employed as a postoperative modality but soon found a more important role. Since 1954 it has been used in the nonoperative treatment of idiopathic scoliosis.[106] The brace consists of a pelvic section, which helps reduce lumbar lordosis, and an attached "superstructure." The superstructure consists of three metal uprights that are attached to a neck ring superiorly. It provides an end point of control to make the spine structurally more rigid, better aligned, and provide a means of attachment for the spinal pads (Figure 13-12). This style is considered a full-time brace and should be worn 23 hours each day. The initial design incorporated distraction; however, this has since been modified due to problems with malocclusion of the jaw. Subsequent to the Milwaukee brace, various low-profile TLSOs have been introduced. Most of these spinal orthoses are named for the city in which they were developed (e.g., Boston brace, Miami orthosis, Wilmington brace, Lyon brace). These spinal orthoses share one characteristic: All control the alignment of the thoracolumbosacral spine but have no superstructure. The Milwaukee brace is mentioned here primarily for historical significance. It remains the most

effective brace for upper thoracic curves but requires a dedicated patient and family for compliance.

Boston Thoracolumbosacral Orthosis

In 1972, Hall created a more low-profile, modular TLSO known as the *Boston brace* in response to patient concerns about the bulkiness and neck ring of the Milwaukee brace.[107] Watts and Hall[108] reported on the Boston brace in 1977. The Boston is a rigid underarm TLSO that has become the most prevalent form of orthosis used, with various modifications. The original Boston brace consisted of multiple modules that were fabricated in different sizes and could be combined to provide a custom-fitted brace that did not require as much time or expertise on the part of the orthotist.[107] Several studies have demonstrated equivalent results with the use of the Boston brace or its related products compared with the Milwaukee brace, with the possible exception of use for high thoracic curves.[98,99,109-111] Boston braces are popular due to their low-profile and partially open design, which is comfortable and well-tolerated.

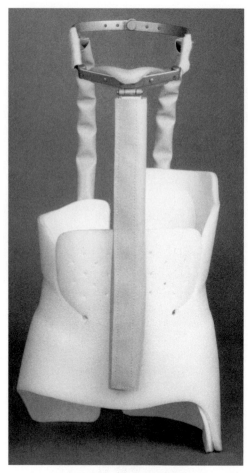

FIGURE 13-12 Milwaukee brace.

Charleston Nighttime Brace

The Charleston Nighttime brace was created in 1979 by Reed and Hooper.[107] This orthosis is manufactured so that curve is maximally corrected while the patient sleeps; the correction is so significant that an upright position is not comfortable.[112] Price and colleagues[112] reported on the prevention of progression of curvature in 66% of patients with curves less than 49 degrees and significant growth remaining. One comparative study between the Boston and the Charleston orthoses showed the Boston orthosis to be more effective in all curve patterns but the Charleston orthosis to have equal efficacy in 25- to 35-degree single thoracolumbar or lumbar curves.[113] The theoretical advantages to the Charleston orthosis in terms of body image and socialization issues are intuitive, but have not been shown in rigorous studies; likewise, compliance problems are similar to those of other braces.

SpineCor

Traditionally, corrective spinal orthoses used in the treatment of adolescent and juvenile scoliosis have been rigid or semirigid devices. Rigid orthoses have been shown to be effective for some patients with adolescent idiopathic scoliosis (AIS) but are associated with drawbacks related to cosmesis and physical discomfort, which create a barrier to adequate patient compliance. In the early 1990s, Coillard and Rivard developed the SpineCor

brace. The SpineCor brace is a dynamic bracing system that uses nonrigid, harness-like bands to apply corrective forces to the patient's torso. The components of the brace include a pelvic base, two thigh bands, two crotch bands, a cotton bolero, and four corrective elastic bands that may be arranged in a number of different configurations, depending on the specific deformity being treated. The pelvic base is a belt that includes three pieces of soft thermoplastic material. Fitting patients with the brace is done in a systematic fashion using supplementary computer software and a training course is offered to providers for education on proper fitting technique.

Coillard and Rivard, the developers of the SpineCor brace, published the initial clinical results in 2003.[114] They reported on the treatment results of 195 patients between 6 and 14 years of age with idiopathic scoliosis curves between 15 and 50 degrees and Risser stages 0 to 3. Success in their study was defined as either a correction or stabilization of ± 5 degrees or more. Failure was defined as worsening of the curve by more than 5 degrees. The authors found that, at 2 years of follow-up, there was an overall correction of greater than 5 degrees in 55% of patients, curve stabilization in 38%, and worsening by greater than 5 degrees in 7% of patients. This equates to 93% success at 2 years. At 4 years of follow-up, the probability of success was 0.88 to 0.92. Coillard and Rivard published results of the same prospective cohort again in 2007 using the Scoliosis Research Society scoliosis research inclusion criteria.[115] One-hundred-seventy patients were included in the study. The authors reported that successful treatment was achieved in 59.4% of patients at the time of brace discontinuation with 22.9% requiring fusion during the treatment period and 1.2% of patients with curves exceeding 45 degrees at maturity. These initial results reported by the developers of the SpineCor brace were promising; however, further study by independent investigators have yielded some conflicting results.

Weiss and Weiss[116] published the results of a small study which compared treatment with a SpineCor brace with TLSO bracing. The authors compared 12 SpineCor patients with 15 TLSO patients and found that the SpineCor patients, with a starting Cobb angle of 21 degrees, progressed an average of 10 degrees after 21 months of treatment versus 0.2 degrees in the TLSO patients who had a starting Cobb angle of 33 degrees. Wong and colleagues[117] compared 22 SpineCor patients with 21 TLSO patients and demonstrated that only 68% of SpineCor patients maintained curve progression of less than or equal to 5 degrees compared with 95% of TLSO patients. Gammon and colleagues[118] compared 35 patients treated with a TLSO with 32 patients treated with the SpineCor brace and found no significant differences between the two outcomes with respect to progression of less than or equal to 5 degrees (60% in TLSO and 53% in SpineCor) or success in avoiding curve progression past 45 degrees (80% in TLSO and 72% in SpineCor).

An important aspect of any brace is the degree of physical comfort and cosmetic considerations. As is true with the literature regarding the efficacy of the SpineCor brace versus TLSO bracing, the literature addressing the impact of the SpineCor brace on comfort and cosmesis is scant. In their 2008 study comparing the SpineCor brace with TLSO bracing, Wong and colleagues[117] administered a questionnaire at 3, 9, and 18 months of treatment to gain information about patient acceptance of her brace. The only significant differences noted were problems with toileting (greater in the SpineCor group) and donning/doffing the orthosis (greater in the TLSO group).

ORTHOTIC PRESCRIPTION

An orthosis should initially improve the magnitude of the curve.[119] An orthosis that provides some correction theoretically decreases the load on the developing vertebrae, increasing the likelihood of long-term control of the deformity.[120] Over time the orthosis should be capable of preventing curve progression for long periods, frequently until the patient reaches skeletal maturity. Finally, an orthosis should be designed to be well tolerated and allow normal social and physical development; even then, compliance with brace wear is a significant issue for adolescents.[121-124] The effectiveness of an orthosis has been shown to be directly related to time spent in the brace, so the patient's willingness to wear the brace is of utmost importance.[105,113,125-127] "Smart braces" that measure compliance have demonstrated that even the most apparently compliant patient spends much less time in the brace than actually prescribed.[122,124,128-131]

The prescribing physician should specify the particular requirements for the orthosis based on the deformity, the goals of treatment, and his or her assessment of the likelihood for compliance. The exact type of brace, generally CTLSO or TLSO, with specifications of thoracic pad placement, lumbar pad placement, need for axillary slings, anterior gussets, trochanteric extensions, kyphosis pads, and the like depends on the type of deformity being treated. Each pad requires a specified location, medial-lateral orientation, and placement instructions. The choice between a CTLSO and TLSO is dictated by the location of the curve, with high thoracic curves most effectively treated by the former. A TLSO has a much lower profile and is therefore more socially acceptable. The orthosis may be prefabricated and adjusted to fit, or custom molded for patients who require additional adaptability.

The time in the orthosis is slowly increased over several weeks and then assessed both physically and radiographically by the prescribing physician. Specific pressure point relief and corrective pad adjustments may be required periodically because these patients are in a period of rapid spinal growth. For the youngest patients, multiple braces may be required before growth concludes.

Complications

Complications with scoliosis orthoses are generally mild from a physical standpoint. Compression of abdominal viscera can result in increased intragastric pressure, leading to gastroesophageal reflux and, potentially, esophagitis.[132] Mild to moderate decreases in kidney function and lung volumes have been described, but neither has been found to have significant long-term consequences.[133,134] Brace treatment in adolescence has been found to produce psychological disturbances that are measurable into adult life.[135,136] Finally, the successful use of bracing requires a supportive, constructive family and a similar relationship between the physician and the adolescent.

Future Directions

The key to scoliosis treatment is to identify which children are likely to develop curve progression, avoiding treating those with curves that will remain in the 25- to 35-degree range through their growth and therefore not require any intervention. Epidemiological studies and skeletal maturity indicators have traditionally been used for this purpose and continue to be refined.[89,103,137-139] Recently, genes that control the growth of scoliotic curves have been identified.[140-143] With this new information in combination with traditional methods, it may become possible to predict which children will develop significant curves with a high degree of certainty. Surgical treatments that harness asymmetrical growth in the spine are also becoming available.[144-152] This combination of techniques may allow intervention before bracing becomes necessary.

SUMMARY

Spinal orthoses are used to treat patients with a variety of spinal disorders ranging from low back pain to complex spine trauma and deformity. Selection of the appropriate orthosis for a specific patient is based on many factors such as the indication for bracing and its severity, the age and body habitus of the patient, the willingness and ability to commit to a potentially long and difficult treatment course, and weighing the risks and benefits of orthotic treatment against other treatment modalities. These challenging treatment decisions are best managed by a multidisciplinary team comprised of the treating physician, the orthotist, the physical and occupational therapists, and the patient and his or her personal support network. Frequent follow-up and close communication between all members of the treatment team is essential to ensure thorough patient and family education, to ensure adequate fit of the orthosis, to evaluate for treatment efficacy, to monitor for complications, and to provide psychosocial support to the patient. Adequately addressing all of the issues surrounding orthotic treatment of spinal disease requires a thorough understanding of the natural history of the pathology being treated, the indications for bracing and use of specific braces, the mechanism of action of the orthosis, potential outcomes of the treatment, and potential complications and methods to minimize them. Comparative studies, long-term outcome analysis, and biomechanical studies have helped promote understanding of and appropriate and effective use of spinal orthoses. Despite the large body of knowledge about these topics, there are still many unknowns surrounding spinal orthoses and their role in treating disorders of the spine. This chapter provides a brief overview of basic functional anatomy of the spine, the fundamentals of spine trauma and scoliosis, the various types of braces and their mechanisms of action and indications, and the potential complications. The ability to use spinal orthoses safely and effectively requires a comprehensive understanding of these topics.

REFERENCES

1. Agabegi SS, Asghar FA, Herkowitz HN. Spinal orthoses. *J Am Acad Orthop Surg.* 2010;18(11):657–667.
2. American Association of Orthopaedic Surgeons. *Atlas of Orthotics.* St. Louis: CV Mosby; 1975.
3. White AA, Panjabi MM. *Clinical Biomechanics of the Spine.* 2nd ed. Philadelphia: JB Lippincott; 1990.
4. Bernhardt M, Bridwell KH. Segmental analysis of the sagittal plane alignment of the normal thoracic and lumbar spines and thoracolumbar junction. *Spine (Phila).* 1989;14(7):717–721.
5. Harrison DD, Harrison DE, Janik TJ, et al. Modeling of the sagittal cervical spine as a method to discriminate hypolordosis: results of elliptical and circular modeling in 72 asymptomatic subjects, 52 acute neck pain subjects, and 70 chronic neck pain subjects. *Spine (Phila).* 2004;29(22):2485–2492.
6. Hardacker JW, Shuford RF, Capicotto PN, et al. Radiographic standing cervical segmental alignment in adult volunteers without neck symptoms. *Spine (Phila).* 1997;22(13):1472–1480.
7. Knight RQ, Jackson R, Stanley E, et al. *Scoliosis Research Society: White paper on sagittal Balance.* Available at www.srs. org; September 2002.
8. Perry J, Nickel VL. Total cervical spine fusion for neck paralysis. *J Bone Joint Surg Am.* 1957;39:111–139.
9. Bell GH, Dunbar O, Beck JS, et al. Variation in strength of vertebrae with age and their relation to osteoporosis. *Calcif Tissue Res.* 1967;1(75).
10. Hsu J, Michael J, Fisk J. *AAOS Atlas of Orthoses and Assistive Devices.* 4th ed. Philadelphia: Mosby-Elselvier; 2008.
11. Whitesides Jr TE. Traumatic kyphosis of the thoracolumbar spine. *Clin Orthop Relat Res.* 1977;128:78–92.
12. Lindahl S, Willen J, Nordwall A, et al. The crush-cleavage fracture. A "new" thoracolumbar unstable fracture. *Spine (Phila)* 1983;8(6):559–569.
13. Holdsworth F. Fractures, dislocations, and fracture-dislocations of the spine. *J Bone Joint Surg Am.* 1970; 52(8):1534–1551.
14. James KS, Wenger KH, Schlegel JD, et al. Biomechanical evaluation of the stability of thoracolumbar burst fractures. *Spine (Phila).* 1994;19(15):1731–1740.
15. Panjabi MM, Oxland TR, Kifune M, et al. Validity of the three-column theory of thoracolumbar fractures. A biomechanic investigation. *Spine.* 1995;20(10):1122–1127.
16. Ferguson RL, Allen Jr. BL. An algorithm for the treatment of unstable thoracolumbar fractures. *Orthop Clin North Am.* 1986;17(1):105–112.
17. Denis F. Spinal instability as defined by the three-column spine concept in acute spinal trauma. *Clin Orthop Relat Res.* 1984;189:65–76.
18. Wood KB, Bohn D, Mehbod A. Anterior versus posterior treatment of stable thoracolumbar burst fractures without neurologic deficit: a prospective, randomized study. *J Spinal Disord Tech.* 2005;18(suppl):S15–S23.
19. Weninger P, Schultz A, Hertz H. Conservative management of thoracolumbar and lumbar spine compression and burst fractures: functional and radiographic outcomes in 136 cases treated by closed reduction and casting. *Arch Orthop Trauma Surg.* 2009;129(2):207–219.
20. Lumsden 2nd RM, Morris JM. An in vivo study of axial rotation and immoblization at the lumbosacral joint. *J Bone Joint Surg Am.* 1968;50(8):1591–1602.
21. Weiss HR, Werkmann M, Stephan C. Brace related stress in scoliosis patients—comparison of different concepts of bracing. *Scoliosis.* 2007;2:10.
22. Sapountzi-Krepia DS, Valavanis J, Panteleakis GP, et al. Perceptions of body image, happiness and satisfaction in adolescents wearing a Boston brace for scoliosis treatment. *J Adv Nurs.* 2001;35(5):683–690.
23. Misterska E, Glowacki M, Harasymczuk J. Brace and deformity-related stress level in females with adolescent idiopathic scoliosis based on the Bad Sobernheim Stress Questionnaires. *Med Sci Monit* 2011;17(2):CR83–CR90.
24. MacLean Jr WE, Green NE, Pierre CB, et al. Stress and coping with scoliosis: psychological effects on adolescents and their families. *J Pediatr Orthop.* 1989;9(3):257–261.
25. Andersen MO, Andersen GR, Thomsen K, et al. Early weaning might reduce the psychological strain of Boston bracing: a study of 136 patients with adolescent idiopathic scoliosis at 3.5 years after termination of brace treatment. *J Pediatr Orthop B.* 2002;11(2):96–99.
26. Sypert GW. External spinal orthotics. *Neurosurgery.* 1987; 20(4):642–649.
27. Powers J, Daniels D, McGuire C, et al. The incidence of skin breakdown associated with use of cervical collars. *J Trauma Nurs.* 2006;13(4):198–200.
28. Plaisier B, Gabram SG, Schwartz RJ, et al. Prospective evaluation of craniofacial pressure in four different cervical orthoses. *J Trauma.* 1994;37(5):714–720.
29. Fisher S. Proper fitting of the cervical orthosis. *Arch Phys Med Rehabil.* 1978;59(11):505–507.
30. Webber-Jones JE, Thomas CA, Bordeaux Jr. RE. The management and prevention of rigid cervical collar complications. *Orthop Nurs.* 2002;21(4):19–27.
31. van den Hout JA, van Rhijn LW, van den Munckhof RJ, et al. Interface corrective force measurements in Boston brace treatment. *Eur Spine J.* 2002;11(4):332–335.
32. Bell KM, Frazier EC, Shively CM, et al. Assessing range of motion to evaluate the adverse effects of ill-fitting cervical orthoses. *Spine J.* 2009;9(3):225–231.
33. Hartman JT, Palumbo F, Hill BJ. Cineradiography of the braced normal cervical spine. A comparative study of five commonly used cervical orthoses. *Clin Orthop Relat Res.* 1975;109:97–102.
34. Richter D, Latta LL, Milne EL, et al. The stabilizing effects of different orthoses in the intact and unstable upper cervical spine: a cadaver study. *J Trauma.* 2001;50(5):848–854.
35. Podolsky S, Baraff LJ, Simon RR, et al. Efficacy of cervical spine immobilization methods. *J Trauma.* 1983;23(6):461–465.
36. Miller CP, Bible JE, Jegede KA, et al. Soft and rigid collars provide similar restriction in cervical range of motion during fifteen activities of daily living. *Spine (Phila).* 2010;35(13):1271–1278.
37. Askins V, Eismont FJ. Efficacy of five cervical orthoses in restricting cervical motion. A comparison study. *Spine (Phila).* 1997;22(11):1193–1198.
38. Kaufman W, Lunsford TR, Lunsford BR, et al. Comparison of three prefabricated cervical collars. *Orthot Prosthet.* 1986;39:21–28.
39. Ducker T. Restriction of cervical spine motion by cervical collars. Scientific exhibit presented at the 58th annual meeting of the American Association of Neurologic Surgeons. In 58th annual meeting of the American Association of Neurologic Surgeons. Nashville, Tenn; 1990.
40. Berne RM, Levy MN, eds. *Physiology.* St Louis: CV Mosby; 1983.
41. Bono CM. The halo fixator. *J Am Acad Orthop Surg.* 2007; 15(12):728–737.

42. Wang GJ, Moskal JT, Albert T, et al. The effect of halo-vest length on stability of the cervical spine. A study in normal subjects. *J Bone Joint Surg Am*. 1988;70(3):357–360.

43. Krag MH, Beynnon BD. A new halo-vest: rationale, design, and biomechanical comparison to current halo-vest designs. *Spine (Phila)*. 1988;13:228–235.

44. Fukui Y, Krag MH, Huston D, et al. Halovest 3-D dynamic loads: full crossover comparison of 3 vest types. *Spine (Phila)*. 2002;27:241–249.

45. Garfin SR, Botte MJ, Waters RL, et al. Complications in the use of the halo fixation device. *J Bone Joint Surg Am*. 1986;68(3):320–325.

46. Koch RA, Nickel VL. The halo vest: an evaluation of motion and forces across the neck. *Spine (Phila)*. 1978;3(2):103–107.

47. Nickel VL, Perry J, Garrett A, et al. The halo. A spinal skeletal traction fixation device. *J Bone Joint Surg Am*. 1968;50(7):1400–1409.

48. Whitehill R, Richman JA, Glaser JA. Failure of immobilization of the cervical spine by the halo vest. A report of five cases. *J Bone Joint Surg Am* 1986;68(3):326–332.

49. Botte MJ, Garfin SR, Byrne TP, et al. The halo skeletal fixator. Principles of application and maintenance. *Clin Orthop Relat Res*. 1989;239:12–18.

50. Horn EM, Theodore N, Feiz-Erfan I, et al. Complications of halo fixation in the elderly. *J Neurosurg Spine*. 2006;5(1):46–49.

51. Johnson RM, Hart DL, Simmons EF, et al. Cervical orthoses. A study comparing their effectiveness in restricting cervical motion in normal subjects. *J Bone Joint Surg Am*. 1977;59(3):332–339.

52. Lind B, Sihlbom H, Nordwall A. Forces and motions across the neck in patients treated with halo-vest. *Spine (Phila)*. 1988;13(2):162–167.

53. Benzel EC, Hadden TA, Saulsbery CM. A comparison of the Minerva and halo jackets for stabilization of the cervical spine. *J Neurosurg*. 1989;70(3):411–414.

54. Ivancic PC, Telles CJ. Neck motion due to the halo-vest in prone and supine positions. *Spine (Phila)*. 2010;35(10):E400–E406.

55. Longo UG, Denaro L, Campi S, et al. Upper cervical spine injuries: indications and limits of the conservative management in Halo vest. A systematic review of efficacy and safety. *Injury*. 2010;41(11):1127–1135.

56. Kakarla UK, Chang SW, Theodore N, et al. Atlas fractures. *Neurosurgery*. 2010;66(3 suppl):60–67.

57. Dickman CA, Sonntag VK. Surgical management of atlanto-axial nonunions. *J Neurosurg*. 1995;83(2):248–253.

58. Vaccaro AR, Madigan L, Bauerle WB, et al. Early halo immobilization of displaced traumatic spondylolisthesis of the axis. *Spine (Phila)*. 2002;27(20):2229–2233.

59. Fisher CG, Dvorak MF, Leith J, et al. Comparison of outcomes for unstable lower cervical flexion teardrop fractures managed with halo thoracic vest versus anterior corpectomy and plating. *Spine (Phila)*. 2002;27(2):160–166.

60. Elgafy H, Dvorak MF, Vaccaro AR, et al. Treatment of displaced type II odontoid fractures in elderly patients. *Am J Orthop*. 2009;38(8):410–416.

61. Tashjian RZ, Majercik S, Biffl WL, et al. Halo-vest immobilization increases early morbidity and mortality in elderly odontoid fractures. *J Trauma*. 2006;60(1):199–203.

62. Pryputniewicz DM, Hadley MN. Axis fractures. *Neurosurgery*. 2010;66(3 suppl):68–82.

63. Seybold EA, Bayley JC. Functional outcome of surgically and conservatively managed dens fractures. *Spine (Phila)*. 1998;23(17):1837–1846.

64. Lennarson PJ, Mostafavi H, Traynelis, et al. Management of type II dens fractures: a case-control study. *Spine (Phila)*. 2000;25(10):1234–1237.

65. Ryan MD, Taylor TK. Odontoid fractures in the elderly. *J Spinal Disord*. 1993;6(5):397–401.

66. Greene KA, Dickman CA, Marciano FF, et al. Acute axis fractures. Analysis of management and outcome in 340 consecutive cases. *Spine (Phila)*. 1997;22(16):1843–1852.

67. Polin RS, Szabo T, Bogaev CA, et al. Nonoperative management of types II and III odontoid fractures: the Philadelphia collar versus the halo vest. *Neurosurgery*. 1996;38(3):450–457.

68. Apuzzo ML, Heiden JS, Weiss MH, et al. Acute fractures of the odontoid process. An analysis of 45 cases. *J Neurosurg*. 1978;48(1):85–91.

69. Glaser JA, Whitehill R, Stamp WG, et al. Complications associated with the halo-vest. A review of 245 cases. *J Neurosurg*. 1986;65(6):762–769.

70. Majercik S, Tashjian RZ, Biffl WL, et al. Halo vest immobilization in the elderly: a death sentence? *J Trauma*. 2005;59(2):350–358.

71. Daentzer D, Florkemeier T. Conservative treatment of upper cervical spine injuries with the halo vest: an appropriate option for all patients independent of their age? *J Neurosurg Spine*. 2009;10(6):543–550.

72. Sharpe KP, Rao S, Ziogas A. Evaluation of the effectiveness of the Minerva cervicothoracic orthosis. *Spine (Phila)*. 1995;20(13):1475–1479.

73. Melton 3rd LJ. Epidemiology of spinal osteoporosis. *Spine (Phila)*. 1997;22(24 suppl):2S–11S.

74. Wasnich RD. Vertebral fracture epidemiology. *Bone*. 1996;18(3 suppl):179S–183S.

75. Lyles KW, Gold DT, Shipp KM, et al. Association of osteoporotic vertebral compression fractures with impaired functional status. *Am J Med*. 1993;94(6):595–601.

76. Kim DH, Vaccaro AR. Osteoporotic compression fractures of the spine; current options and considerations for treatment. *Spine J*. 2006;6(5):479–487.

77. Pfeifer M, Begerow B, Minne HW. Effects of a new spinal orthosis on posture, trunk strength, and quality of life in women with postmenopausal osteoporosis: a randomized trial. *Am J Phys Med Rehabil*. 2004;83(3):177–186.

78. Kaplan RS, Sinaki M. Posture Training Support: preliminary report on a series of patients with diminished symptomatic complications of osteoporosis. *Mayo Clin Proc*. 1993;68(12):1171–1176.

79. Lane JM, Johnson CE, Khan SN, et al. Minimally invasive options for the treatment of osteoporotic vertebral compression fractures. *Orthop Clin North Am*. 2002;33(2):431–438.

80. Shen M, Kim Y. Osteoporotic vertebral compression fractures: a review of current surgical management techniques. *Am J Orthop*. 2007;36(5):241–248.

81. Buchalter D, Kahanovitz N, Viola K, et al. Three-dimensional spinal motion measurements. Part 2: A noninvasive assessment of lumbar brace immobilization of the spine. *J Spinal Disord*. 1988;1(4):284–286.

82. Fidler MW, Plasmans CM. The effect of four types of support on the segmental mobility of the lumbosacral spine. *J Bone Joint Surg Am*. 1983;65(7):943–947.

83. Nachemson A. Orthotic treatment for injuries and diseases of the spinal column. *Phys Med Rehabil.* 1987;1:11–24.

84. Vander Kooi D, Abad G, Basford JR, et al. Lumbar spine stabilization with a thoracolumbosacral orthosis: evaluation with video fluoroscopy. *Spine (Phila).* 2004;29(1):100–104.

85. Yee AJ, Yoo JU, Marsolais EB, et al. Use of a postoperative lumbar corset after lumbar spinal arthrodesis for degenerative conditions of the spine. A prospective randomized trial. *J Bone Joint Surg Am.* 2008;90(10):2062–2068.

86. Lantz SA, Schultz AB. Lumbar spine orthosis wearing. I. Restriction of gross body motions. *Spine (Phila).* 1986; 11(8):834–837.

87. Jellema P, van Tulder MW, van Poppel MN, et al. Lumbar supports for prevention and treatment of low back pain: a systematic review within the framework of the Cochrane Back Review Group. *Spine (Phila).* 2001;26(4):377–386.

88. Cholewicki J, Reeves NP, Everding VQ, et al. Lumbosacral orthoses reduce trunk muscle activity in a postural control task. *J Biomech.* 2007;40(8):1731–1736.

89. Kane WJ. Scoliosis prevalence: a call for a statement of terms. *Clin Orthop Relat Res.* 1977;126:43–46.

90. Lonstein JE, Bjorklund S, Wanninger MH, et al. Voluntary school screening for scoliosis in Minnesota. *J Bone Joint Surg Am.* 1982;64(4):481–488.

91. Willner S, Uden A. A prospective prevalence study of scoliosis in Southern Sweden. *Acta Orthop Scand.* 1982; 53(2):233–237.

92. Riseborough EJ, Wynne-Davies R. A genetic survey of idiopathic scoliosis in Boston, Massachusetts. *J Bone Joint Surg Am.* 1973;55(5):974–982.

93. Weinstein SL, Ponseti IV. Curve progression in idiopathic scoliosis. *J Bone Joint Surg Am.* 1983;65(4):447–455.

94. Duval-Beaupere G, Lamireau T. Scoliosis at less than 30 degrees. Properties of the evolutivity (risk of progression). *Spine (Phila).* 1985;10(5):421–424.

95. Kehl DK, Morrissy RT. Brace treatment in adolescent idiopathic scoliosis. An update on concepts and technique. *Clin Orthop Relat Res.* 1988;229:34–43.

96. Patwardhan AG, Bunch WH, Meade KP, et al. A biomechanical analog of curve progression and orthotic stabilization in idiopathic scoliosis. *J Biomech.* 1986;19(2):103–117.

97. Bunch WH, Patwardhan A, eds. Biomechanics of Orthoses. In: *Scoliosis: Making Clinical Decisions.* St. Louis: Mosby; 1989.

98. Emans JB, Kaelin A, Banel P, et al. The Boston bracing system for idiopathic scoliosis. Follow-up results in 295 patients. *Spine (Phila).* 1986;11(8):792–801.

99. Willers U, Normelli H, Aaro S, et al. Long-term results of Boston brace treatment on vertebral rotation in idiopathic scoliosis. *Spine (Phila).* 1993;18(4):432–435.

100. Hassan I, Bjerkreim I. Progression in idiopathic scoliosis after conservative treatment. *Acta Orthop Scand.* 1983;54(1):88–90.

101. Kahanovitz N, Levine DB, Lardone J. The part-time Milwaukee brace treatment of juvenile idiopathic scoliosis. Long-term follow-up. *Clin Orthop Relat Res* 1982;(167):145–151.

102. Mellencamp DD, Blount WP, Anderson AJ. Milwaukee brace treatment of idiopathic scoliosis: late results. *Clin Orthop Relat Res.* 1977;126:47–57.

103. Lonstein JE, Carlson JM. The prediction of curve progression in untreated idiopathic scoliosis during growth. *J Bone Joint Surg Am.* 1984;66(7):1061–1071.

104. Blount WP, Schmidt AC. The Milwaukee brace in the treatment of scoliosis. *J Bone Joint Surg Am.* 1957;47:693.

105. Rowe DE, Bernstein SM, Riddick MF, et al. A meta-analysis of the efficacy of non-operative treatments for idiopathic scoliosis. *J Bone Joint Surg Am.* 1997;79(5):664–674.

106. Blount WP, Schmidt AC, Keever ED, et al. The Milwaukee brace in the operative treatment of scoliosis. *J Bone Joint Surg Am.* 1958;40A(3):511–525.

107. Fayssoux RS, Cho RH, Herman MJ. A history of bracing for idiopathic scoliosis in North America. *Clin Orthop Relat Res.* 2010;468(3):654–664.

108. Watts HG, Hall JE, Stanish W. The Boston brace system for the treatment of low thoracic and lumbar scoliosis by the use of a girdle without superstructure. *Clin Orthop Relat Res.* 1977;126:87–92.

109. Bassett GS, Bunnell WP, MacEwen GD. Treatment of idiopathic scoliosis with the Wilmington brace. Results in patients with a twenty to thirty-nine-degree curve. *J Bone Joint Surg Am.* 1986;68(4):602–605.

110. Hanks GA, Zimmer B, Nogi J. TLSO treatment of idiopathic scoliosis. An analysis of the Wilmington jacket. *Spine (Phila).* 1988;13(6):626–629.

111. Olafsson Y, Saraste H, Sodelund V, et al. Boston brace in the treatment of idiopathic scoliosis. *J Pediatr Orthop.* 1995;15(4):524–527.

112. Price CT, Scott DS, Reed FR, et al. Nighttime bracing of adolescent idiopathic scoliosis with the Charleston bending brace. *J Prosthet Orthop.* 1987;17:703–707.

113. Katz DE, Richards BS, Browne RH, et al. A comparison between the Boston brace and the Charleston bending brace in adolescent idiopathic scoliosis. *Spine (Phila).* 1997;22(12):1302–1312.

114. Coillard C, Leroux MA, Zabjek KF, et al. SpineCor–a non-rigid brace for the treatment of idiopathic scoliosis: post-treatment results. *Eur Spine J.* 2003;12(2):141–148.

115. Coillard C, Vachon V, Circo AB, et al. Effectiveness of the SpineCor brace based on the new standardized criteria proposed by the scoliosis research society for adolescent idiopathic scoliosis. *J Pediatr Orthop.* 2007;27(4):375–379.

116. Weiss HR, Weiss GM. Brace treatment during pubertal growth spurt in girls with idiopathic scoliosis (IS): a prospective trial comparing two different concepts. *Pediatr Rehabil.* 2005;8(3):199–206.

117. Wong MS, Cheng JC, Lam TP, et al. The effect of rigid versus flexible spinal orthosis on the clinical efficacy and acceptance of the patients with adolescent idiopathic scoliosis. *Spine (Phila).* 2008;33(12):1360–1365.

118. Gammon SR, Mehlman CT, Chan W, et al. A comparison of thoracolumbosacral orthoses and SpineCor treatment of adolescent idiopathic scoliosis patients using the Scoliosis Research Society standardized criteria. *J Pediatr Orthop.* 2010;30(6):531–538.

119. Uden A, Willner S, Pettersson H. Initial correction with the Boston Thoracic Brace. *Acta Orthop Scand.* 1982; 53(6):907–911.

120. Bunch WH, Patwardhan AG, Vanderby R, et al. Stability of scoliotic spines. *Orthop Trans.* 1983;8(1):145.

121. Morton A, Riddle R, Buchanan R, et al. Accuracy in the prediction and estimation of adherence to bracewear before and during treatment of adolescent idiopathic scoliosis. *J Pediatr Orthop.* 2008;28(3):336–341.

122. Nicholson GP, Ferguson-Pell MW, Smith K, et al. Quantitative measurement of spinal brace use and compliance in the treatment of adolescent idiopathic scoliosis. *Stud Health Technol Inform.* 2002;91:372–377.

123. Takemitsu M, Bowen JR, Rahman T, et al. Compliance monitoring of brace treatment for patients with idiopathic scoliosis. *Spine (Phila)*. 2004;29(18):2070–2074.

124. Nicholson GP, Ferguson-Pell MW, Smith K, et al. The objective measurement of spinal orthosis use for the treatment of adolescent idiopathic scoliosis. *Spine (Phila)*. 2003;28(19):2243–2251.

125. Katz DE, Durrani AA. Factors that influence outcome in bracing large curves in patients with adolescent idiopathic scoliosis. *Spine (Phila)*. 2001;26(21):2354–2361.

126. Howard A, Wright JG, Hedden D. A comparative study of TLSO, Charleston, and Milwaukee braces for idiopathic scoliosis. *Spine (Phila)*. 1998;23(22):2404–2411.

127. Lou E, Hill D, Raso J, et al. Prediction of brace treatment outcomes by monitoring brace usage. *Stud Health Technol Inform*. 2006;123:239–244.

128. Vandal S, Rivard CH, Bradet R. Measuring the compliance behavior of adolescents wearing orthopedic braces. *Issues Compr Pediatr Nurs*. 1999;22(2–3):59–73.

129. Lou E, Raso JV, Hill DL, et al. The daily force pattern of spinal orthoses in subjects with adolescent idiopathic scoliosis. *Prosthet Orthot Int*. 2002;26(1):58–63.

130. Lou E, Raso JV, Hill DL, et al. Correlation between quantity and quality of orthosis wear and treatment outcomes in adolescent idiopathic scoliosis. *Prosthet Orthot Int*. 2004;28(1):49–54.

131. DiRaimondo CV, Green NE. Brace-wear compliance in patients with adolescent idiopathic scoliosis. *J Pediatr Orthop*. 1988;8(2):143–146.

132. Kling Jr TF, Drennan JC, Gryboski JD. Esophagitis complicating scoliosis management with the Boston thoracolumbosacral orthosis. *Clin Orthop Relat Res*. 1981;159:208–210.

133. Aaro S, Berg U. The immediate effect of Boston brace on renal function in patients with idiopathic scoliosis. *Clin Orthop Relat Res*. 1982;170:243–247.

134. Sevastikoglou JA, Linderholm H, Lindgren U. Effect of the Milwaukee brace on vital and ventilatory capacity of scoliotic patients. *Acta Orthop Scand*. 1976;47(5):540–545.

135. Apter A, Morein G, Munitz H, et al. The psychologic sequelae of the Milwaukee brace in adolescent girls. *Clin Orthop Relat Res*. 1978;1131:156–159.

136. Nachemson A, Cochran TP, Fallstrom K, et al. Somatic, social and psychologic effects on treatment for idiopathic scoliosis. *Orthop Trans*. 1983;7:508.

137. Sanders JO, Browne RH, McConnell SJ, et al. Maturity assessment and curve progression in girls with idiopathic scoliosis. *J Bone Joint Surg Am*. 2007;89(1):64–73.

138. Bruszewski J, Kamza Z. Incidence of scoliosis based on an analysis of serial radiography. *Chir Narzadow Ruchu Ortop Pol*. 1957;22(2):115–116.

139. Rogala EJ, Drummond DS, Gurr J. Scoliosis: incidence and natural history. A prospective epidemiological study. *J Bone Joint Surg Am*. 1978;60(2):173–176.

140. Ogilvie JW, Braun J, Argyle V, et al. The search for idiopathic scoliosis genes. *Spine (Phila)*. 2006;31(6):679–681.

141. Cheng JC, Tang NL, Yeung HY, et al. Genetic association of complex traits: using idiopathic scoliosis as an example. *Clin Orthop Relat Res*. 2007;462:38–44.

142. Miller NH. Genetics of familial idiopathic scoliosis. *Clin Orthop Relat Res*. 2007;462:6–10.

143. Ward K, Ogilvie J, Argyle V, et al. Polygenic inheritance of adolescent idiopathic scoliosis: a study of extended families in Utah. *Am J Med Genet A*. 2010;152A(5):1178–1188.

144. Braun JT, Akyuz E, Udall H, et al. Three-dimensional analysis of 2 fusionless scoliosis treatments: a flexible ligament tether versus a rigid-shape memory alloy staple. *Spine (Phila)*. 2006;31(3):262–268.

145. Braun JT, Hines JL, Akyuz E, et al. Relative versus absolute modulation of growth in the fusionless treatment of experimental scoliosis. *Spine (Phila)*. 2006;31(16):1776–1782.

146. Braun JT, Hoffman M, Akyuz E, et al. Mechanical modulation of vertebral growth in the fusionless treatment of progressive scoliosis in an experimental model. *Spine (Phila)*. 2006;31(12):1314–1320.

147. Puttlitz CM, Masaru F, Barkley A, et al. A biomechanical assessment of thoracic spine stapling. *Spine (Phila)*. 2007;32(7):766–771.

148. Lavelle WF, Samdani AF, Cahill PJ, et al. Clinical outcomes of nitinol staples for preventing curve progression in idiopathic scoliosis. *J Pediatr Orthop*. 2011;31(1 suppl):S107–S113.

149. Betz RR, Ranade A, Samdani AF, et al. Vertebral body stapling: a fusionless treatment option for a growing child with moderate idiopathic scoliosis. *Spine (Phila)*. 2010;35(2):169–176.

150. Guille JT, D'Andrea LP, Betz RR. Fusionless treatment of scoliosis. *Orthop Clin North Am*. 2007;38(4):541–545.

151. Newton PO, Farnsworth CL, Faro FD, et al. Spinal growth modulation with an anterolateral flexible tether in an immature bovine model: disc health and motion preservation. *Spine (Phila)*. 2008;33(7):724–733.

152. Newton PO, Upasani VV, Farnsworth CL, et al. Spinal growth modulation with use of a tether in an immature porcine model. *J Bone Joint Surg Am*. 2008;90(12):2695–2706.

14

Orthoses in the Management of Hand Dysfunction

Noelle M. Austin and MaryLynn Jacobs

LEARNING OBJECTIVES

On completion of this chapter, the reader will be able to:

1. Define immobilization, mobilization, and restriction orthoses and give examples of orthoses in each category.
2. Explain the differences among static, dynamic, serial static, and static progressive orthoses and discuss which may be appropriate at each of the three wound healing stages.
3. Identify the three arches of the hand along with creases and discuss their significance.
4. Identify a 90-degree angle of pull and explain its importance in the application of force.
5. Describe the various handling and physical characteristics of thermoplastic materials and discuss how they affect orthotic fabrication.
6. Explain the importance of patient education related to proper orthosis wear, care, and precautions.

He who works with his hands is a laborer,
He who works with his hands and his mind is a craftsman,
He who works with his mind and his heart is an artist.
Unknown

The hand is the body's tool to interact with the surrounding environment. A hand afflicted with disease or injury greatly impairs the ability to function, even if normal functioning proximal joints and muscles are present. The therapist's ability to provide clinical intervention can positively affect the use of the hand and therefore overall function. One tool at a therapist's disposal is orthotic intervention. The appropriate use of orthoses during specific phases of tissue healing, depending on the diagnosis, can be an effective adjunct to traditional therapy techniques for restoring use of the limb. Treatment decisions must be based on an integration of knowledge and clinical experience along with information specific to the individual patient, including diagnosis, general medical status, and the physician's prescription. Clinicians need to understand the principles associated with orthotic design and fabrication.

This chapter focuses on orthotic fabrication for the hand and upper extremity and includes discussion of nomenclature, materials, mechanical and anatomical principles, and case studies to provide examples of orthotic intervention with an emphasis on critical thinking.

NOMENCLATURE

In the medical literature, the terms *splint, brace, support,* and *orthosis* have similar definitions.[1,2] This is often confusing to physicians, therapists, students, insurance companies, and even those who fabricate these devices. Are splints made by a therapist? Is an orthosis made by an orthotist? In 1989, the American Society of Hand Therapists (ASHT) put together a task force to address issues such as proper nomenclature and redefinition of orthoses in an attempt to enhance and clarify communication among all disciplines.[1] The task force developed a Splint Classification System (SCS) and addressed the similarity in definitions of the words *splint, brace, support,* and *orthosis* (Figure 14-1). The task force's review confirmed that these words were so similar in nature that they were used interchangeably in the hand therapy literature. Another key issue that challenged the task force was how to define orthoses to provide universal comprehension and approval. Currently, there is a shift in nomenclature from the word 'splint' to 'orthosis' in order to follow Center for Medicare and Medicaid Services (CMS) guidelines for billing and reimbursement purposes. Therefore, the word orthosis will be utilized throughout this chapter and should be adopted in clinical and billing documentation as well.[3]

Traditionally, orthoses have generally been described according to their form (e.g., thumb spica splint, wrist cock-up splint, ulnar gutter splint).[4] This form-based nomenclature, however, can often lead to confusion and misunderstanding regarding the actual orthosis requested. The SCS painstakingly describes most universally used orthoses according to their specific function (e.g., thumb immobilization splint, wrist/hand extension mobilization splint). This functional-based description of orthoses gives clinicians a clear concept of what the orthosis must look like and what its function should be. The specific categories described by the SCS are outlined in Figure 14-1.

Articular and Nonarticular Orthoses

Orthoses are classified into two broad categories: articular and nonarticular. Articular orthoses, the most common

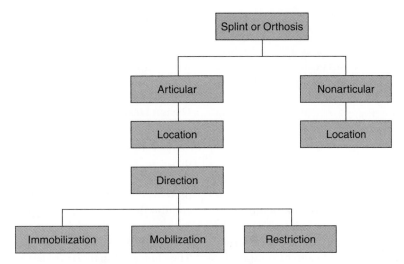

FIGURE 14-1 The American Society of Hand Therapists Splint Classification System.

type of fabricated orthosis, are those that cross a joint or series of joints. Examples of articular orthoses include a wrist immobilization orthosis, proximal interphalangeal (PIP) joint extension mobilization orthosis, and elbow flexion restriction orthosis. The word *articular* is implied in the orthosis description and is not necessary in the title of the orthosis.

Nonarticular orthoses do not cross a joint; instead, they stabilize the body segment to which they are applied. The ASHT recommends that clinicians include the term *nonarticular* before an orthosis description; an orthosis used to stabilize the humerus would be called a *nonarticular humerus orthosis*, and an orthosis designed to soley stabilize a metacarpal would be called a *nonarticular metacarpal orthosis*. Without this designation, the orthosis fabricator may not know whether to include or exclude proximal or distal joints in the orthotic design.

Location

Location refers to the specific body part or joint levels acted on by the orthosis. The primary joint is the target joint. The secondary joints are included for protection, stabilization, or comfort. When several primary joints are involved (e.g., crush injury to the hand), the description of the orthosis can be simplified by grouping all the joints together, such as *hand orthosis* or *digit orthosis*.

Direction

Direction refers to the primary direction of the force applied when the orthosis is worn. This includes flexion, extension, radial or ulnar deviation, supination, pronation, abduction, and adduction. Information regarding direction is essential because it tells the clinician the desired joint positioning. Direction notation is also critical when fabricating a mobilization orthosis; accurate application of the direction of force is essential to achieve the goal of joint or soft tissue mobility.

Purpose of Orthosis

The purpose or intent of the orthosis is the single most important aspect documented in the description. The purpose of the orthosis can be to (1) immobilize a structure, (2) mobilize a tissue, or (3) restrict an aspect of joint motion.

Immobilization

The purpose of an immobilization orthosis is simply to place a structure in its anatomical or most comfortable resting position. Immobilization orthoses are perhaps the most common and simple form, although it can be used for complex injuries. Immobilization orthoses immobilize the joints they cross.

Mobilization

Mobilization refers to moving or stretching specific soft tissues or joints to create change. The benefits of using mobilization orthoses as a treatment modality have been well documented in the literature.[5-8] The effectiveness of mobilization does not rely on stretching tissue but rather on the facilitation of cell growth. The target tissue lengthens when the living cells of the contracted tissues are stimulated (by the application of force) to grow. This stimulation occurs when steady tension is applied through the orthosis over a specific period of time. The living cells recognize the tension applied and permit the older collagen cells to be actively absorbed and replaced with new collagen cells oriented in the direction of tension.[9-16] Tissue growth has been clearly demonstrated in certain cultures in which elongating certain body parts, such as earlobes and lips, is popular. In these cultures, dowels are used to serially increase the diameter of the intended structure, slowly allowing expansion and accommodation of the new tension and diameter. Another common example includes the use of braces and retainers in the dental field. There are three choices of orthotic design to mobilize tissue, including serial static, static progressive, and dynamic orthoses.

Restriction

Restriction orthoses restrict or block an aspect of joint motion. These are generally simple orthoses applied in such a way that they limit motion. Therapists can construct static orthoses, dynamic orthoses, and forms of taping to become types of restrictive orthoses because they can be made to restrict some portion of joint motion while allowing full motion in the opposite direction.

Examples

Figure 14-2 demonstrates the critical impact that the words *immobilization, mobilization,* and *restriction* can have when describing an orthosis. Within the PIP immobilization orthosis (see Figure 14-2A), the PIP joint is immobilized in a comfortable resting position to allow the involved structures to heal, commonly used for a PIP ligament sprain. The PIP flexion mobilization orthosis stretches the PIP joint into flexion to address a PIP extension contracture (using a static

progressive approach) (see Figure 14-2B). The PIP joint is restricted from full extension but allowed to flex fully within the boundaries of the PIP extension restriction orthosis, which is commonly used for swan neck deformities when the PIP joint pulls into hyperextension (see Figure 14-2C).

Design Descriptors

Design descriptors are used to increase clarity of the specific orthosis request and provide detail in notes or for correspondence to physicians or reimbursement sources. The design descriptors are non-SCS nomenclature but are commonly used by the hand therapy and surgery community.[17] The most commonly used descriptors are summarized in Box 14-1.

Choices of Orthotic Designs

The choices of orthotic design include familiar terminology: static, serial static, dynamic, and static progressive orthoses. An orthotic design should be chosen to achieve the goals of immobilization, mobilization, or restriction of a specific tissue.

Static Orthoses

Static orthoses have a rigid base, immobilizing the joints they traverse (Figure 14-3). A static orthosis provides stabilization, protection, and support to a body segment such as the elbow, wrist, or finger. Static orthoses are perhaps the most common orthoses made. They can be used as an adjunct to treatment, an exercise device, by blocking a distal or proximal joint to increase glide of another joint or improve tendon excursion.

Serial Static Orthoses

Serial static orthoses or casts are applied with the joints, soft tissue, or musculotendinous units they cross in a lengthened position (near maximum) and are worn for extended periods

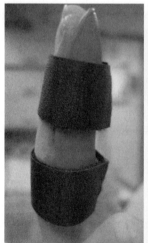
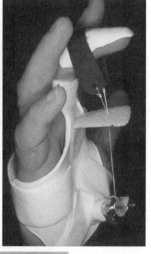

A

B

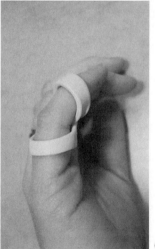

C

FIGURE 14-2 Three different proximal interphalangeal (PIP) joint orthoses. **A,** PIP immobilization orthosis. **B,** PIP flexion mobilization orthosis. **C,** PIP extension restriction orthosis.

BOX 14-1 *Orthosis Design Descriptors*

Digit-based: Originates from the digit, allowing metacarpophalangeal joint motion

Hand-based: Originates from the hand, allowing wrist motion

Thumb-based: Originates from the thenar eminence or thumb, incorporating one or more joints of the thumb

Forearm-based: Originates from the forearm, allowing full elbow motion

Circumferential: Encompasses the entire circumference of the involved body part or limbsegment

Gutter: Includes only the radial or the ulnar portion of the limb

Radial: Incorporates the radial aspect of the limb

Ulnar: Incorporates the ulnar aspect of the limb

Dorsal: Traverses the dorsal (posterior) aspect of the hand or forearm

Volar: Traverses the volar (palmar, anterior) aspect of the hand or forearm

Anterior: Traverses the anterior aspect of the body part

Posterior: Traverses the posterior aspect of the body part

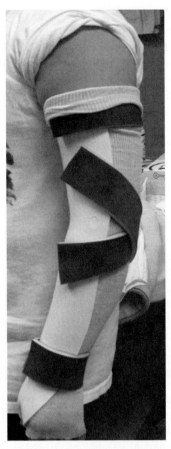

FIGURE 14-3 This anterior elbow mobilization orthosis, including the wrist, is used to prevent forearm rotation.

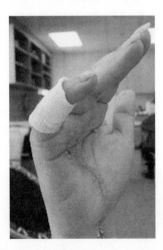

FIGURE 14-4 This proximal interphalangeal extension mobilization orthosis is designed to address a flexion contracture using a serial static approach.

of time (Figure 14-4). Tissue held in this end-range position should react and accommodate by stretching into the desired direction of correction. Serial static orthoses are often removed during therapy and exercise sessions so that the clinician and patient can work on the involved structures with modalities such as heat, ultrasound, joint mobilization, and range

of motion (ROM). The orthosis or cast is then remolded to maintain the gains made during the exercise session. This design may provide greater patient compliance and ensures that the tissue is being continually stressed without the risk of the tissue rebounding (reverting back to original shortened state) upon removal of the orthosis. Some therapists use an approach with serial static orthoses when the orthosis is worn continuously for a few days and then removed in therapy. In other cases, using these orthoses at night only can help maintain the gains made throughout the day with exercise and stretching. Nonremovable serial static orthoses may also be a better choice for patients who are young, who have cognitive or behavioral issues, or who have fluctuating tone and spasticity.

Dynamic Orthoses
Dynamic orthoses use an elastic-type force to mobilize specific tissues to achieve increases in ROM (Figure 14-5). Most dynamic orthoses have a base that permits the attachment of various outriggers and components. The mobilizing forces applied through a dynamic orthosis are elastic (stretchy) in nature, such as rubber bands, springs, or wrapped elastic cord. The dynamic force applied continues as long as the elastic component can contract, even when the tissue reaches the end of its elastic boundary.[18]

Static Progressive Orthoses
Static progressive orthoses achieve tissue mobilization by applying low-load force to the tissue's end range in one direction over a long period of time (Figure 14-6).[5] The goal is that the tissue will eventually accommodate to this position. The fabrication of a static progressive orthosis is similar to a dynamic orthosis, but the force applied is static or nonelastic. The mobilization force can be generated through static line, nonelastic strapping materials, hinges, turnbuckles, and vari-

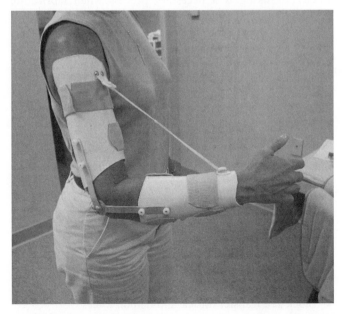

FIGURE 14-5 This elbow flexion mobilization orthosis uses a rubber band to apply a dynamic force.

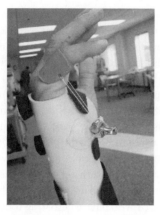

FIGURE 14-6 This metacarpophalangeal flexion mobilization orthosis uses a static line and component to apply a static progressive force.

ous types of inelastic tape. When the joint position is achieved and the tension on the static progressive component is set, the orthosis will not continue to stress the tissue beyond its elastic limit.[18] Force can be altered by the patient or therapist through progressive adjustments. Some patients may tolerate static progressive orthoses better than dynamic. One reason may be that the joint position is constant while the tissue accommodates gently and gradually to the tension, without the influences of gravity and motion.[18,19]

Objectives for Orthotic Intervention

The key objective for orthotic fabrication may not always be straightforward. The objectives for orthotic intervention may be multiple, as in a wrist and hand immobilization orthosis (resting hand orthosis) used on a patient with rheumatoid arthritis. The orthosis may be constructed to immobilize inflamed arthritic joints, yet place the metacarpophalangeal (MP) joints serially in a gently extended and radially deviated position to minimize ulnar drift and periarticular deformity. Critical thinking is a necessary process when fabricating orthoses; multiple injuries, wound status, age, and lifestyle are a few of the key factors that must be taken into consideration. More skilled clinicians can appreciate that there can be several purposes for one orthosis; therefore creative problem solving must be used when fabricating orthotic devices for the more involved, complex injury.

Immobilization Orthoses

Orthoses designed to hold or immobilize a joint or limb segment can be used to do the following[17]:

- Provide symptom relief
- Protect and position edematous structures
- Aid in maximizing functional use
- Maintain tissue length
- Protect healing structures and surgical procedures
- Provide support and protection for soft tissue healing
- Maintain and protect reduction of fracture
- Improve and preserve joint alignment
- Block and transfer muscle and tendon forces
- Influence a spastic muscle
- Prevent possible contracture development

Mobilization Orthoses

Orthoses designed to change or mobilize tissues or structures are used to do the following[17]:

- Remodel long-standing, dense, mature scar
- Elongate soft tissue contractures, adhesions, and musculotendinous tightness
- Increase passive joint ROM
- Realign or maintain joint and ligament profile
- Substitute for weak or absent motion
- Maintain reduction of an intraarticular fracture with preservation of joint mobility
- Provide resistance for exercise

Restriction Orthoses

Orthoses designed to restrict or limit motion may be used to do the following[17]:

- Limit motion after nerve injury or repair
- Limit motion after tendon injury or repair
- Limit motion after bone or ligament injury or repair
- Provide and improve joint stability and alignment
- Assist in functional use of the hand

ANATOMY-RELATED PRINCIPLES

Therapists treating the upper extremity need to have a thorough understanding of the complex anatomical features of the hand and arm to manage patients with dysfunction effectively. Disturbance of the delicate relationship between the bones, muscles, nerves, and other soft tissue structures, either by disease or trauma, can result in disruption of normal function. Knowledge of normal anatomical features and how pathological conditions affect them is important for therapists to make appropriate clinical decisions regarding treatment interventions.[11,20–22]

Arches of the Hand

The configuration of the bones in the hand, along with the tension of the muscles and ligaments in this region, contribute to the creation of an arch system composed of the proximal transverse, distal transverse, and longitudinal arches (Figure 14-7).[23,24] This arch system is vital for positioning

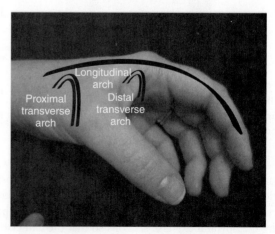

FIGURE 14-7 The fixed proximal transverse arch, the flexible distal transverse arch, and the mobile longitudinal arch of the hand.

the hand to allow for normal function related to grasp and prehension.[24,25] Incorporating these arches within an orthosis is essential to allow maximal function and comfort. Including the arches also prevents orthosis migration on the extremity.

The fixed proximal transverse arch is created by the configuration of the distal row of the carpal bones and the taut volar carpal ligament. This region is also referred to as the carpal tunnel, through which the long flexors and median nerve pass en route to the hand.[26] This fixed structure provides mechanical advantage to the flexors, maximizing grasp function.

The mobile distal transverse arch is located at the level of the metacarpal heads. This arch is adaptive by the mobile ulnar fourth and fifth carpometacarpal (CMC) joints and highly mobile thumb trapeziometacarpal joint.[27] This increased mobility of the peripheral digits allows for optimal grasping abilities.

The longitudinal arch spans the length from the metacarpal to the distal phalanx. A disruption of this arch occurs in patients who have sustained an ulnar nerve injury with resulting loss of intrinsic muscle function. In this situation, the hand takes on an intrinsic minus position with the MP joints hyperextended and the PIP and distal interphalangeal joints flexed (clawlike deformity).[23]

Palmar Creases

The regular arrangement of creases is easily visible on the volar surface of the hand (Figure 14-8). The thick palmar skin is fixed

to the underlying structures by fibrous connections that aid in formation of these creases.[27] Therapists need to appreciate the location of these creases and how they correlate with the underlying anatomy. Commonly, these creases are used by therapists as an anatomical guide when creating orthosis patterns. For example, the distal palmar crease and proximal palmar crease must be fully cleared when fabricating a wrist immobilization orthosis to allow for unrestricted ROM at the MP joints. However, care must be taken not to clear too much because the mechanical advantage of the orthosis can be adversely altered.[17]

Metacarpal Length and Mobility

Dual obliquity is a concept relating to the anatomy of the metacarpals.[23,25] Because of the differing lengths of the metacarpals (radial side of hand longer than ulnar), when an object is held in the hand, an oblique angle is formed compared with the distal ends of the radius and ulna (Figure 14-9A). In addition, the object is angled in accordance with the distal transverse arch and increasing mobility of the ulnar metacarpals (see Figure 14-9B). This dual obliquity should be incorporated into the orthosis to provide a comfortable and functional orthosis that resists migration because of the incorporation of the arches.

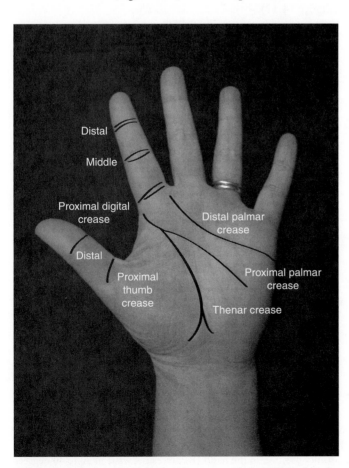

FIGURE 14-8 Creases of the hand can provide helpful landmarks during the orthotic fabrication process.

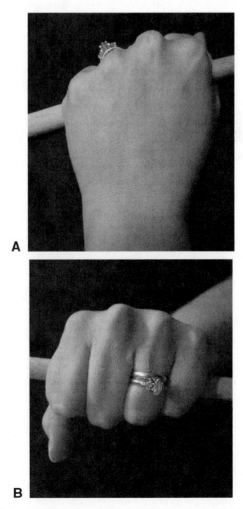

FIGURE 14-9 The dual obliquity of the hand, from the dorsal (**A**) and transverse (**B**) perspectives.

Positioning the Hand

When deciding how to position the hand within an orthosis, many factors must be considered, including the patient's diagnosis, healing time frame, and intervention goals. Being mindful of proper positioning within an orthosis initially can help prevent future joint and soft tissue contractures. The two most common positions described in the literature include the position of function and the position of rest.[17,28] See Figure 14-10 for the general joint angles described for each position.

The antideformity position considers the unique anatomical characteristics of the MP and PIP. The length of the collateral ligaments at the MP joint varies according to the position of the MP joint (Figure 14-11).[29] The collateral ligaments are slack with MP joint extension, whereas tension in the collateral ligaments increases with greater amounts of MP joint flexion. Placing the joints in flexion within an orthosis helps prevent MP joint extension contractures (limited flexion). If the joints were placed in extension with resulting MP contractures, the disruption of the longitudinal arch would greatly impair grasping abilities.

Similarly at the PIP joint level, the volar plate is placed on tension with PIP joint extension, whereas flexion at the PIP joint places the volar plate at risk for shortening (see Figure 14-11A and B).[29] Shortening of the volar plate could result in debilitating PIP joint flexion contractures, which can significantly affect the ability to grasp and especially release objects. Therefore careful positioning of the PIP joint in extension (as long as not contraindicated per the diagnosis) is crucial to maintain the length of the volar plate.

Tissue Precautions

In the upper extremity, a number of areas exist where bony protuberances or superficial nerves are highly susceptible to compression from orthoses (Box 14-2).[30] If these areas are not accounted for in the fabrication process, the orthosis will likely be uncomfortable for the patient and therefore possibly not worn. Special consideration must be given to the patient with impaired sensation (those with peripheral nerve injury, neuropathy, nerve root compression, or central nervous system disorders). Those with limited or absent sensation do not have the normal ability to feel or detect areas of excess pressure; instead, they must rely on visual inspection to determine integrity of skin and soft tissue.

Because superficial bony prominences have minimal soft tissue coverage, they are vulnerable to compression. Excessive external pressure can place the tissue at risk for irritation and eventual breakdown (necrosis). Older adults may be at most risk because they commonly have minimal subcutaneous fat combined with extremely fragile skin, making the bony areas more apparent. Patients may report pain, redness, and irritation over the bone area. To prevent such occurrences, these at-risk areas on the orthosis can either be padded with foam/gel or flared away during the molding process (Figure 14-12).[17]

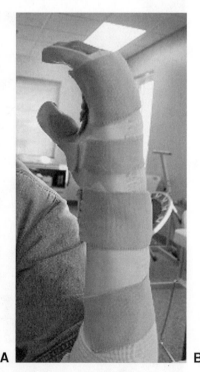

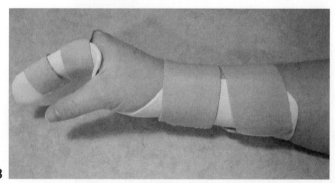

FIGURE 14-10 The functional position of the hand (**A**) places the wrist in 20 to 30 degrees of extension, the metacarpophalangeal (MP) joints in 35 to 45 degrees of flexion, the proximal interphalangeal (PIP) joints in 45 degrees of flexion, the distal interphalangeal joints in a relaxed flexed position, and the thumb in palmar abduction. The antideformity position of the hand (**B**) places the wrist in 30 to 40 degrees of extension, the MP joints in 60 to 90 degrees of flexion, the PIP and distal interphalangeal joints in extension, and the thumb in palmar abduction.

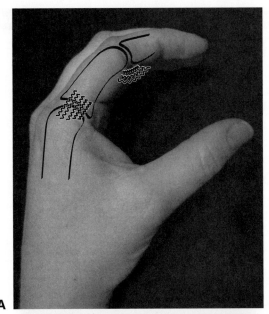

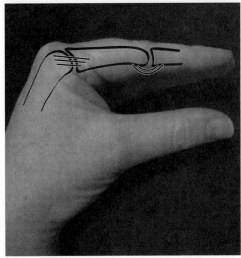

FIGURE 14-11 Soft tissue length changes associated with joint positioning. **A,** Placing the metacarpophalangeal (MP) joint in extension will cause the MP collateral ligaments and the proximal interphalangeal (PIP) volar plate to become "slack" and at risk of becoming shortened. **B,** Placing the MP joint in flexion elongates both the MP collateral ligaments and the volar plate of the PIP joint to minimize risk of shortening (contractures) of these structures.

Therapists must also appreciate peripheral nerve anatomy and how orthoses and strapping may place undue pressure over these regions where nerves become relatively superficial, potentially leading to nerve compression.[31] Patients may report pain, redness, paresthesias (tingling), and numbness in that nerve's distribution. Timely modification of the orthosis is necessary to prevent long-term nerve irritation. Orthotic fabrication over gel or the use of wider straps to disperse the pressure better are two techniques that may be useful to address this issue.[17]

Also of note is the potential for compression of vascular structures when an orthosis is worn or an elasticized product is applied.[32] Symptoms of vascular compromise include throbbing, color changes, temperature changes, and pain

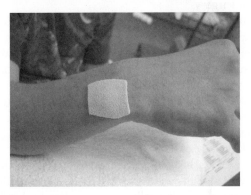

FIGURE 14-12 Padding bony prominences, such as the ulnar styloid, before molding of the orthosis can decrease the risk of high-pressure areas and potential for skin irritation or breakdown.

should immediately be dealt with. Reporting these symptoms is especially important if any surgical reconstruction of vascular structures was performed. Wide straps and slings to distribute pressure maximally along with the appropriate use of elasticized wraps can aid in preventing this problem.[24] Most important, educating the patient regarding these potential signs and symptoms of bony and neurovascular compromise is key to preventing any long-term problems caused by orthotic application.

TISSUE HEALING

The phases of specific tissue healing (e.g., bone, nerve, tendon, ligament) aid in directing appropriate orthosis selection, fabrication, and wearing schedule.[33,34] Appreciation of what role an orthosis can play during each phase is a critical step in the critical thinking process (i.e., knowing when to rest tissue versus mobilize tissue). Clinicians must recognize that although the stages of tissue healing are described as chronological, overlap in their incidence can occur. For example, in a patient who has suffered a traumatic snow blower injury and sustained soft tissue, bone, tendon, and nerve damage, depending on the severity of each of these injuries, healing rates of each specific tissue may be different even though it is the same hand. As the healing stages overlap, so may the time frames for using specific orthosis designs.

Stages of Tissue Healing

Therapists must understand how each specific injury affects the surrounding tissues. For example, immobilization orthoses may be indicated throughout the length of the healing process but are most commonly used during the inflammatory stage. The three main phases of tissue healing are the inflammatory, proliferative (fibroplasia), and remodeling (maturation) phases (Figure 14-13).

During the inflammatory phase, an influx of white blood cells occurs to cleanse the area (edema).[35,36] Clinically the tissue feels soft, boggy, and easy to mobilize. This stage typically lasts for 1 week or less. Rest is normally more important than exercise during the inflammatory stage, so immobilization orthoses are appropriate in the days immediately after tissue injury or surgery.[24]

During the proliferative phase, collagen is laid down and the wound gains strength. The clinician begins to see and feel more tissue resistance (scar adherence), although the tissue is still soft and "movable" with tension. This phase lasts from 1 to 6 weeks. Mobilization orthoses that gently stretch tissue can be effective during this time frame. They provide gentle stress that can facilitate tissue growth, resulting in tissue lengthening.[1,13]

The last phase of tissue healing is referred to as the remodeling phase. During this stage the collagen is organized as it remodels along lines of stress. The tensile strength of the tissue is enhanced. Clinically, the tissues involved feel dense, hard, and inelastic. Tissues may actually shorten because of a decrease in elasticity; therefore stretching is a valuable tool to address unwanted contractures. Superficial scars also begin to soften during this stage. This stage begins as early as 6 weeks and can last up to 12 to 24 months. Serial static and static

> **BOX 14-3** *Factor That Influence Tissue Healing*
>
> **COMMON FACTORS**
> - Age
> - Nutritional status
> - Tobacco use
> - Diabetes
> - Edema
> - Infection
> - Rheumatoid arthritis
>
> **LESS COMMON FACTORS**
> - Alcohol use
> - Sickle cell disease
> - Steroids
> - Radiation therapy
> - Peripheral vascular disease
> - Raynaud's disease
> - Systemic lupus erythematosus

progressive approaches (or a combination of the two with day and night orthoses) to mobilize tissue during this phase are most appropriate.[5]

Factors That Influence Tissue Healing

Tissue healing is influenced by several factors. For example, tissue that is deprived of oxygen requires a longer healing time and influences the orthosis wearing time. Therapists must thoroughly discuss medical history and lifestyle habits with the patient to determine any factors that may delay or impair tissue healing. Tobacco (nicotine), for example, diminishes the body's ability to heal, decreasing blood flow and nutrition to the tissue.[37] Excessive alcohol intake can impair the immune system, leading to malnourishment and liver damage.[38] There are various factors that influence the rate of tissue healing (Box 14-3).[17]

MECHANICAL PRINCIPLES

Before fabricating an orthosis, therapists need to know basic mechanical principles and be able to integrate this information into the orthotic design and construction process.[17,24,33,39,40] This section briefly reviews the most common principles to consider. Careful attention to the following principles will improve the fabrication, function, and fit of an orthosis.

Levers

Levers are rigid structures through which a force can be applied to produce rotational motion about a fixed axis.[17] A lever system is composed of a fulcrum, or fixed axis, and two arms: the effort arm and resistance arm. The effort arm, also referred to as the force arm, is the segment of the lever between the fulcrum and the effort force that is attempting to stabilize or mobilize a structure. In orthotic design, the fulcrum corresponds with the anatomical axis of the target joint, the effort arm is the segment of the orthosis that applies the effort force, and the resistance arm is the segment of the limb that resists the effort force. Ideally, the effort and resistance forces work in concert to create opposing torques

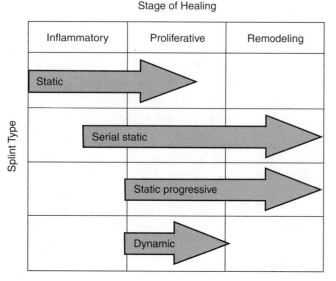

FIGURE 14-13 An algorithm for the uses of various types of orthoses according to the stages of healing.

about the fulcrum. However, cases occur in which the axis of rotation (fulcrum) has been interrupted from disease or injury (e.g., fracture, rheumatoid arthritis).

Most orthoses are categorized as first-class levers in which the fulcrum is between the effort and resistance arms (Figure 14-14). Common examples of first-class lever systems are a seesaw, a pair of scissors, or a pair of pliers. The goal when designing an orthosis is to create the most efficient work. The length of the resistance arm greatly influences the mechanical advantage of the force applied. The effort arm of the orthosis can also influence mechanical advantage by how carefully it is molded about the body part.

Both the effort and resistance arms should be vigilantly formed, incorporating arches, clearing for creases, and allowing adequate surface area for maximal distribution of pressure. As forces actively influence a joint, a balance-counterbalance effect must occur. If the opposing force (effort arm) is not distributed well to counterbalance the distal forces (resistance arm), the orthosis may not sit flush with the body part. This may create high-pressure areas, shear stress, and an unproductive application of force. Clinicians can generate "mechanical advantages" through careful application of orthotic principles and meticulous attention to detail while molding. Clinically, orthoses tend to be most comfortable when well molded, incorporating adequate length and depth. Short, narrow, and shallow orthoses can cause increases in localized pressure and overall discomfort.

Stress

Stress can occur in various forms. The most common types that relate directly to application of orthoses are compression, shear, tension, bending, and torsion.[17] Compressive stress (also referred to as pressure) is defined as force per unit area. In the process of creating and planning an orthosis design, therapists must understand the various forms of stress that can be produced by the external forces of an orthosis.

For example, compression can be minimized by increasing the surface area (designing the orthosis base wider and longer) over which the force can be maximally distributed. Optimizing the conformity of materials to the shape of the body part can minimize compressive stress.

A number of factors can result in areas of high pressure. Narrow strap width, especially in conjunction with "shallow" orthoses, can produce high compressive stress on the soft tissue. Orthosis borders should lie flush with the skin surface that the strap traverses. The strap should not bridge the two borders of the orthosis; it should come in contact with the skin.

The slings used in mobilization orthoses are another possible source of compression stress that should be considered, especially if edema or neurovascular issues are evident in the patient's limb. Compression to the lateral, dorsal, or volar aspects of the digit can be avoided by using several techniques. The orthosis line can be attached to each side of a sling (two pieces of line), then joined after they pass through the pulley. This design prevents the circumferential compression created when one line is threaded through both ends of the sling. Alternatively, a custom-fabricated thermoplastic "pan" can be placed under the sling as a support. The digital pan disperses the compressive forces applied through the sling by lifting the borders away from the skin and increasing the area of force application (see Figure 14-2B).

Shear stress results from a parallel force applied to the surface and produces a tendency for an object to either deform or slide along the surface.[17] When fabricating mobilization orthoses, the mobilizing force, which is attached to the proximal orthosis base, usually traverses the length of the orthosis and terminates distally at the body segment. If the proximal portion (base) of the orthosis is not adequately secured to the limb with appropriate strapping, there will be an undesirable migration or dragging and shearing of the proximal base over the skin when the mobilization force is distally applied (Figure 14-15). Being mindful of incorporating the arches of the hand as well

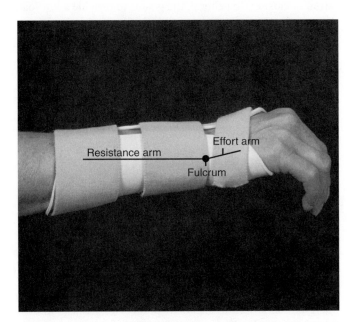

FIGURE 14-14 The fulcrum of a orthosis is placed at the axis of joint motion. The resistance arm is applied by the proximal segment of the orthosis; the effort arm is applied by the distal segment of the orthosis.

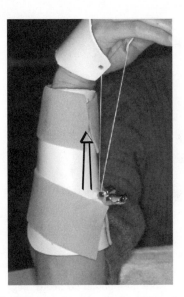

FIGURE 14-15 When tension is applied to this wrist flexion mobilization orthosis, shear stress is created as the proximal orthosis migrates distally on the forearm.

and obtaining a well-contoured orthosis during the molding process aid in preventing this migration. In some cases, a nonskid material such Dycem (Dycem Technologies Limited, Bristol, England) or foam tape to line the orthosis can also help keep the orthosis stable on the extremity.

Angle of Force Application

The angle of force application is critical to the proper design and fabrication of mobilization orthoses. Ideally, the force should be applied 90 degrees to the body segment being mobilized (Figure 14-16), which maximizes the therapeutic effect of the force being applied.[17,24] With a pure 90-degree orientation to the part being mobilized, there are virtually no forces disseminated in other directions (compression or distraction). However, if the angle is other than 90 degrees, a portion of the force is dissipated elsewhere, thereby diminishing the therapeutic effect and causing potentially harmful compression or shear stress.

Clinically, the use of custom-made or prefabricated line guides or pulleys can be helpful to achieve a 90-degree angle of application. The therapist must view the orthosis from all angles to ensure that the line of application is directed centrally over the segment and oriented properly in all planes. To improve flexion of the digits with a mobilization orthosis, the anatomical configuration of the hand necessitates the

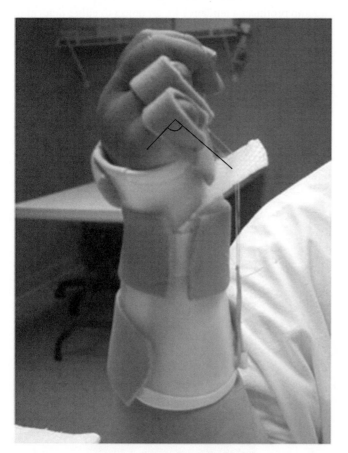

FIGURE 14-16 Note the optimal 90-degree angle formed by the proximal phalanx and the monofilament line in this metacarpophalangeal flexion mobilization orthosis.

line of force application to converge toward the scaphoid. If this orientation is not incorporated into the design of the orthosis, excessive stress is placed on the digit joints, causing discomfort and potential harm. Occasionally, a force applied in either a radial or ulnar direction is indicated, as with postoperative MP joint arthroplasties or sagittal band repairs. Except for special circumstances such as these, the line of application should be centrally located over the longitudinal axis of the bone being mobilized.

Force Application

When using elastic force to mobilize stiff structures, therapists must consider the therapeutic objectives.[41-43] Is the goal mobilization of a mature, dense joint contracture, or is it stabilization of the MP joints in extension after MP joint arthroplasty? Both situations may require an elastic force; however, both the amount of force and the materials used to achieve these goals can vary considerably.[44] The amount of force necessary to mobilize various tissues depends on such factors as individual tolerance, diagnosis, stage of tissue healing, chronicity of problem, severity of contracture, density of contracture (end feel), age, smoking, alcohol use, and other health-related issues. Ranges of 100 to 300 g have been suggested for mobilization of the small joints of the hand, whereas higher parameters (350+ g) may be more effective for larger structures.[1,24] This 300 g of force is based on what is tolerated per unit of surface area of the skin, not the tolerance of the contracted tissue to tension. In most cases, skin tolerance becomes the limiting factor in determining appropriate tension, not the risk of injury to the specific targeted tissue. The therapist can almost always rely on the tissue's response to the tension to help determine the effectiveness of the mobilizing forces. Signs of too much stress include edema, skin blanching, vascular changes, and pain. The amount of time the force is applied is another factor to consider with mobilization orthoses.[45] In general, the goal is to provide a low load stress to the tissue over a long period of time.

MATERIAL AND EQUIPMENT

Numerous companies market and distribute supplies for orthotic fabrication (Box 14-4), which include many types of thermoplastic material, strapping, component systems, and equipment. The best way to become educated regarding what is on the market is by spending time reviewing the catalogs/websites and contacting local sales representatives to request samples. In addition, attending orthotic fabrication workshops and hand therapy conferences can be a helpful means to gain knowledge and practice skills that can be used in the clinical setting.

Thermoplastic Materials

Low-temperature thermoplastics are the most commonly used material by therapists to fabricating custom orthoses. The material is sold in sheets or precut designs also known as orthosis banks. The material is softened in warm water before application to the body part. Once on the body part, the material cools and hardens into shape. Therapists can select from a wide range of thermoplastic material, making the choice of which to use for a specific patient confusing for novice practitioners. The orthosis fabricator must have a sound understanding of the differences to be able to make an informed decision, taking into account the purpose of the orthosis and the specifics of a particular patient's diagnosis. In addition to considering the patient's needs, other factors therapists must consider include level of orthotic fabrcation experience, availability of materials, and any cost constraints.

Few studies have examined the characteristics of thermoplastic materials in an attempt to categorize their differences.[46-48] However, a knowledge of handling and physical characteristics and the different categories of thermoplastic materials can help therapists make informed selections.

Handling Characteristics

Handling characteristics refer to the way a material behaves during the molding process. The three most important characteristics of orthosis materials that must be considered are conformability and resistance to stretch, memory, and bonding characteristics.

Conformability and Resistance to Stretch

The ability for a material to conform to a body part is related to its level of resistance to stretch (Figure 14-17).[49,50] A helpful system for organizing thermoplastic materials is to group them into categories according to their degree of resistance to stretch (Table 14-1).[49,50] Materials with minimal resistance to stretch are highly conforming and may not be the best choice for novice orthosis fabricators. The less hands-on the better during the fabrication process because this material tends to contour well without much assistance. Gravity-assisted positioning during the molding process is essential. These materials may be appropriate for the patient who has a high level of pain and would not tolerate hands-on molding or for those orthoses for which achieving an intimate fit is crucial to maximize comfort. Smaller orthoses such as finger or hand-based can be made with these highly conforming materials.

Materials with maximal resistance to stretch are minimally conforming and demand more hands-on work from the orthosis fabricator to obtain a desireable fit. Therapists with nominal orthotic fabrication experience may do better with these materials because they tolerate more aggressive handling. These materials are appropriate for use when fabricating larger orthoses such as for the elbow or in situations in which fabrication against gravity is not an option (e.g., in patients who are either wheelchair or bed bound). Because this material does not contour as precisely, it may be the best choice when fabrication over wound dressings when the dimensions are altered with each dressing change.

Memory

Memory refers to a material's ability to revert to its original shape once heated, ranging from 0% to 100% memory.[49,50] Materials with this property are good choices for orthoses that need to be frequently remolded, such as when fabricating a serial static orthosis that needs to be reheated and reformed to the body part as ROM increases. Caution must be used when removing the orthosis from the body part after molding to be sure the material is completely cool, or the material may shrink and the fit achieved within the orthosis lost. Also, spot heating is not advised with this material because of the possibility of altering adjacent regions.

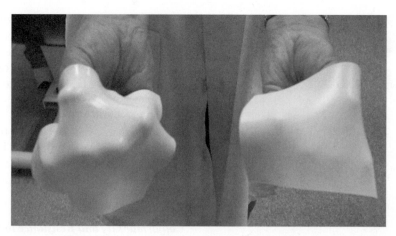

FIGURE 14-17 The drape, or contouring of the material, placed over the hand on the left indicates a low resistance to stretch, whereas the less moldable material on the right is more resistant to stretch.

TABLE 14-1   *Characteristics of Thermoplastic Materials*

| Company Name | Stretch Resistance | | |
	Minimum	Moderate	Maximal
AliMed	Polyform	Orthoplast II	Ezeform
	Multiform	Polyflex II	Orthoplast
	Multiform Clear		
DeRoyal	LMB Drape	LMB Blend	LMB Royal
		LMB Flex	
North Coast Medical	NCM Clinic	Encore	Omega Max
		NCM Preferred	Solaris
		NCM Vanilla	Omega Plus
		NCM Spectrum	NCM Classic
		Prism	Orthoplast
Orfit Industries	Orfit Drape	Orfit Natural	Bluelight
	Orfilight	Colors	Orfit Ease
	Orfit Classic Soft		Orfit Classic
	Soft Fit		Orfit Ortho
	Orfit Soft		
Patterson Medical	Polyform	Polyflex II	Ezeform
	Aquaplast ProDrape	Kay-Splint II	Aquaplast Resilient
		Aquaplast	Synergy
		Watercolors	San Splint
		ProPlast	Orthoplast
		Tailorsplint	
		Kay-Splint III	
		Orthoplast II	
WFR Corporation	Reveals XS	Reveals	Reveals LS
		Reveals Colors	

Bonding

Bonding is the ability of a material to adhere to itself when heated fully.[49,50] The presence of a protective coating prevents this occurrence. The coating can allow two pieces of material to be popped apart after the orthosis is formed, which can be particularly helpful when applying a circumferential design such as around the thumb (Figure 14-18). The coating must be removed with solvent or disrupted by scratching the surface to allow for adherence, which is commonly required for attaching mobilization components. The coating may make the orthosis easier to clean. Without a coating, the material may stick to a wound dressing, the patient's body hair, or itself. When using material without a coating, apply a barrier between the two pieces such as a wet paper towel or hand lotion to prevent adherence.

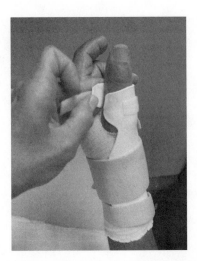

FIGURE 14-18 The presence of coating on this material allows the circumferential segment around the thumb to be pulled apart after cooling to form a "trap door" on this wrist and thumb mobilization orthosis.

Physical Characteristics

Physical characteristics are evident on visual inspection. The most relevant include the material's thickness, the presence of perforations, and the color of the material.[17]

Thickness

Low temperature thermoplastics are available in a variety of thicknesses, including ⅟₁₆, ³⁄₃₂, and ⅛ inches.[49,50] The appropriate thickness for an orthosis depends on the body part, diagnosis, and required rigidity of the orthosis. For example, an elbow immobilization orthosis for a patient who sustained a fracture and underwent surgical fixation would best be made from a thick ⅛-inch material for a more rigid support. On the contrary, a hand-based thumb orthosis for an elderly patient with arthritis might be better served with a thinner ⅟₁₆-inch orthosis to achieve a light, unbulky support. The goal should be to provide the least bulky, lightest weight orthosis possible that still performs its intended function. Thinner materials are generally quicker to heat and harden faster than their thicker counterparts.

Perforations

Thermoplastic materials with perforations allow for air exchange and produce a lighter-weight orthosis compared with those made with solid materials.[49,50] Materials with a high density of perforations create an orthosis that is flexible (less rigid), which may not be appropriate for specific diagnoses. Caution must be used to ensure that the edges of the orthosis, cut-through perforations, are smoothed to prevent irritation to the patient's skin.

Colors

A wide array of colors is available, making the fabrication process even more creative.[48,49] Choices in thermopalstic material and strap colors can improve compliance with orthosis wear in children. Providing orthosis straps in a color other than white can be helpful for patients to prevent loss within bed linens. Be sure to ask for requests from patients to make them feel they have contributed in the construction of the orthosis and hopefully improve their acceptance for wear.

Categories of Orthosis Materials

Thermoplastic materials can be categorized according to their chemical composition.[46-48] This composition determines the way the material behaves during the fabrication process and affects how the finished orthosis functions. Thermoplastic materials may be made of plastics (e.g., Polyform [Patterson Medical, Bolingbrook, Ill.] or Multiform [AliMed, Dedham, Mass.]), rubber or rubberlike materials (e.g., Ezeform [Patterson] or Orthoplast [AliMed]), combination plastic and rubberlike materials (e.g., Tailorsplint, PolyFlex II [Patterson], or Encore [North Coast Medical, Morgan Hill, Calif.), and elastic materials (e.g., Aquaplast [Patterson] or Reveal [WFR Corporation, Wyckoff, N.J.]).

Plastic materials typically have a low resistance to stretch, allowing a highly contoured finished orthosis. Rubber or rubberlike materials are highly resistant to stretch but offer more control during the fabrication process. Combination plastic and rubberlike materials offer the best of both worlds in terms of conformability and control during the molding process. Elastic materials possess memory and may be suitable for the beginner orthosis fabricator who wishes to have the ability to remold the orthosis if necessary.

Orthoses may also be fabricated from alternative materials.[17,49,50] These materials include lined materials (e.g., Rolyan AirThru [Patterson], Silon-LTS [Patterson], or Multiform Soft [Alimed]), mesh-type materials (e.g., X-Lite [Patterson]), casting materials (e.g., plaster of Paris or QuickCast [Patterson]), and soft materials (e.g., neoprene or Kinesio Tape [Patterson]).

Strapping

Many different strapping systems are offered through distributors.[49,50] The choice of appropriate strapping depends on the patient diagnosis, orthosis design and availability in the same way that the choice of the appropriate thermoplastic material does. Strapping is essential to secure the orthosis to the body part properly. If the strapping is not adequate, the orthosis will likely be uncomfortable or ineffective in achieving its desired goals. Generally, adhesive hook-and-loop material (e.g., Velcro; Velcro USA, Manchester, N.H.) is applied to the orthosis base, and strapping material secures the segment within the orthosis. The most commonly used strapping mechanisms consist of traditional loop, foam, neoprene, or elasticized straps. In small areas where adhesive hook may continually pull off, rivets may be used to permanently secure the loop material onto the thermoplastic (Figure 14-19).

Other adjuncts to strapping include D-rings that offer the ability to easily adjust the tension on the straps or circumferential wrapping (with an elasticized bandage) for those patients with significant edema. Straps should be wide and conforming to distribute the pressure maximally, but not so wide that they inhibit ROM of adjacent joints.[17,24] The patient should be educated in how to apply the straps snugly enough to secure the orthosis in place without compromising the neurovascular system.

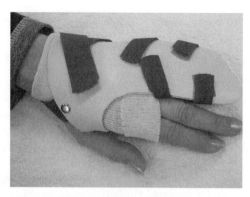

FIGURE 14-19 A rivet can be applied to permanenetly secure strapping to the orthosis by forming holes in the thermoplastic material and the strap with a hole punch; pliers are used to set the rivet in place.

Padding and Lining

Padding and lining products are available in a wide variety of thicknesses, textures, and materials.[49,50] Therapists may use padding in specific regions during the orthotic fabrication process to accommodate bony prominences or superficial nerves. Ideally, this padding should be applied to the target area before molding the orthosis so that the device can contour to its proportions. Attaching the padding after the orthosis is made can potentially cause a shift in pressure distribution and lead to problematic areas of high stress. Foam padding can also be adhered to straps at strategic places to improve joint position and prevent migration within the orthosis.

Lining an orthosis with an adhesive product may be indicated in rare cases, such as when the patient has very fragile skin. Application of these adhesive liners should be used sparingly because of hygienic concerns; they are not easily cleaned or removed. As an alternative, disposable liners on the body part can be a way to improve comfort within an orthosis by placing a barrier between the skin and the plastic (see Figure 14-19). Cotton or elasticized stockinettes are the most commonly used products.

Components

Component systems are an important element of mobilization orthoses.[49,50] Rehabilitation catalogs help therapists keep abreast of what is available. In general, outrigger systems are designed to help provide optimal force application to a body part. Ideally these devices should be highly adjustable to allow the therapist to maintain the crucial 90-degree angle of force application. If the commercial systems are not accessible, therapists can fabricate homemade ones with wire and scrap pieces of thermoplastic material. Four basic elements of an outrigger system are used in a digit mobilization orthosis: the proximal attachment device, mobilization force, pulley system, and finger slings (Figure 14-20).

The proximal attachment device provides the means to secure the mobilization force to the orthosis. The mobilization force, whether it be static line (static progressive approach) or elastic (dynamic approach), traverses through a pulley system to maintain the 90-degree angle of force application. Distally,

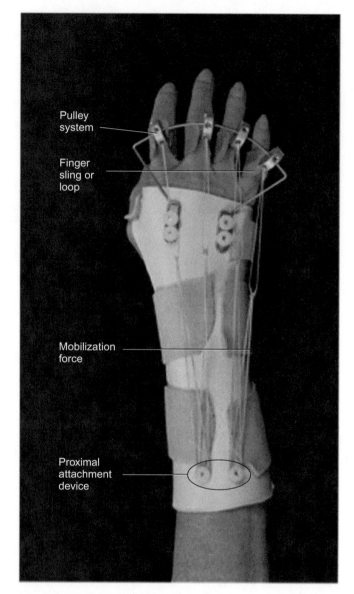

FIGURE 14-20 Elements of this forearm-based metacarpophalangeal joint extension mobilization orthosis include a proximal attachment device, a mobilization force through a pulley system, and finger slings.

the force is imparted to the body part, in this example the finger, by a sling or loop.

Mobilization orthoses can be challenging to fabricate for a new therapist. Learning through practicing and obtaining feedback from more experienced colleagues are important ways to improve fabrication skills. Patients must consistently receive follow-up in the clinic to assess and modify the orthosis to achieve a positive outcome; the orthoses need frequent adjustments as the tissue responds to the stress.

Equipment

Quality tools in the clinic can help make the orthotic fabrication process easier for the therapist. Sharp scissors designated for thermoplastic use only are essential; if the scissors are used for all products, most notably adhesive products, the blades can retain the residue and make cutting the thermoplastic difficult.

Scissors with a nonstick coating are now available and are quite effective when cutting adhesive-backed products. Dull scissors do not provide a clean cut, which can lead to frustration and unsightly orthoses. Other tools helpful to keep on hand include a hole punch and blunt nose pliers for rivet application, a hand drill for creating a hole or series of perforations, and a heat gun to make minor adjustments.

OVERVIEW OF ORTHOTIC FABRICATION PROCESS

A comprehensive prescription from the referring physician is essential for appropriate orthotic application and therapeutic intervention. In addition to the patient's name, the prescription must contain the following information:

- Diagnosis, including surgical procedures if applicable
- Date of injury and surgery
- Any precautions that must be followed
- Orthosis goals, including purpose, joint positions, and wearing schedule

Radiographs and the patient's surgical report can assist the therapist in gaining a clear understanding of the tissue involvement. As always, good communication with the physician is key in terms of gathering and sharing information regarding a patient's status.

After obtaining all the essential information regarding the patient's diagnosis and the physician's orders, the therapist should perform a comprehensive examination. This begins with a patient interview for gathering subjective information and continues with a review of systems and a detailed physical examination.[9,22] The therapist uses the results of the history and examination to form a clinical judgment and movement dysfunction diagnosis, including a list of problems. From these problems the therapist determines the prognosis for improvement of function, goals and formulates an appropriate plan of care.

To prepare a comprehensive therapeutic plan of care, therapists must use critical thinking skills to integrate all their knowledge with the information obtained from the physician and patient. The therapist has many modalities that can be used to treat the patient, only one of which is orthotic fabrication. Not all patients are appropriate for orthoses; determining if and when orthoses may be appropriate is the challenge of the therapist. Some patients may require orthoses initially and others may need one later in their rehabilitation. An individualized approach is necessary to address a patient's unique needs.[51]

If orthoses are deemed appropriate, the patient must be thoroughly educated regarding its use. This education must always include a written handout outlining the specifics of wear, care, and precautions. The key points to stress include the following:

- Purpose of orthosis, specific to the patient's diagnosis
- Key indicators of problems that might occur and information about what to do if they occur
- Any functional limitations that might result from wearing the orthosis and suggestions of how to compensate for such limitations
- Wearing schedule
- Information about washing or cleaning the orthosis
- Information or diagrams about how to properly don and doff the orthosis (if applicable)
- Precautions related to the patient's diagnosis and indicators of tissue tolerance (signs and symptoms of neurovascular compromise or bony irritation)
- Avoidance of heat to prevent loss of orthosis shape
- Contact information (the therapist's name and clinic phone number) with encouragement to call if any questions or problems should arise

---

CASE EXAMPLE 1

Patient with Osteoarthritis of the Carpometacarpal Joint

M. F. presents to the hand surgeon with progressive onset of thumb pain. Symptoms of aching and tenderness are exacerbated by activities such as turning keys, opening jars, holding a book, and writing. Deformity from joint subluxation at the first carpometacarpal (trapeziometacarpal) joint and osteoarthritis (OA) are evident (Figure 14-21). The patient also has a positive grind test—the manual application of longitudinal compression force of the first metacarpal into the trapezium. (This test is positive for carpometacarpal OA when pain and crepitation are present.) M. F. receives a steroid injection into the joint space to decrease local inflammation and a prescription for therapy.

Questions to Consider
- Given this patient's current presentation, what additional tests and measures might be important in the evaluation process?

- What is your movement dysfunction–related diagnosis for this patient?
- What do you think the prognosis will be for this patient? What are the patient's goals for intervention? What are your rehabilitation goals? How long do you think it will take to achieve the goals that you and the patient agree on?
- On the basis of the patient's goals and expectations as well as your understanding of the underlying disease process, what recommendations would you make for intervention at this point in time? What evidence from the clinical research literature supports your recommendations? What have you chosen or prioritized from these possible interventions?
- What type of follow-up would you recommend? How might the goals and interventions change as the patient progresses through the stages of tissue healing? How would you assess the outcomes of your interventions?

Continued

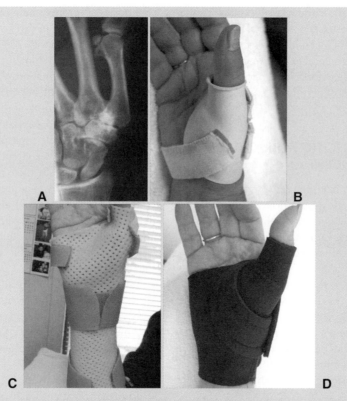

FIGURE 14-21 A, A radiograph indicating osteoarthritis at the carpometacarpal (CMC) joint of the thumb. **B,** A custom thumb orthosis designed to reduce stress on the CMC joint during activities of daily living (ADLs). **C,** After ligament reconstruction and arthroplasty, a forearm-based wrist and thumb immobilization orthosis is used during the proliferative stage of healing. **D,** When adequate healing and fixation have occurred, the patient transitions into a neoprene orthosis to support the thumb during ADLs.

Recommendations for a Patient with OA of the Carpometacarpal Joint

A custom thumb orthosis is fabricated from a lightweight thermoplastic material (thickness: ¹⁄₁₆ inch) (see Figure 14-21B). M. F. is instructed to use this during the day to decrease stress on the joint during activities of daily living (ADLs). She is also educated in activity modification and joint protection principles. Some of the strategies include avoiding forceful, repetitive, and sustained pinching along with using pens and kitchen utensils with larger handles.

Despite these interventions, M. F. continues to have symptoms and returns to the physician to discuss her treatment options. M. F. undergoes a ligament reconstruction with tendon interposition arthroplasty, which includes a trapezium excision with a slip of the flexor carpi radialis interposed between the scaphoid and the first metacarpal.[24] For the initial 3-week postoperative period, during the initial inflammatory stage of healing when resting the tissue is important, a cast is used to immobilize the region. As healing progresses into the proliferative stage at 3 weeks, the patient is placed in a removable forearm-based wrist/thumb immobilization orthosis that is removed for periodic range of motion exercises (see Figure 14-21C).

At approximately 6 weeks after surgery, as the healing continues to progress, the patient uses a prefabricated neoprene thumb orthosis to aid in the transition from the rigid thermoplastic orthosis (see Figure 14-21D). The neoprene material offers a restrictive support combining warmth and gentle support for use during ADLs. At 12 weeks, all orthoses are discontinued and M. F. returns to normal activities without pain.

CASE EXAMPLE 2

Patient with a Wrist Fracture

V. A. presents to the hand surgeon's office after a fall onto an outstretched hand. The radiograph reveals a comminuted wrist fracture requiring surgical fixation. The surgeon performs an open reduction internal fixation with a plate and screws (Figure 14-22). At 5 days after surgery, the patient is referred to therapy for a protective orthosis and an early ROM program.

Questions to Consider
- Given this patient's current presentation, what additional tests and measures might be important in the evaluation process?
- What is your movement dysfunction–related diagnosis for this patient?

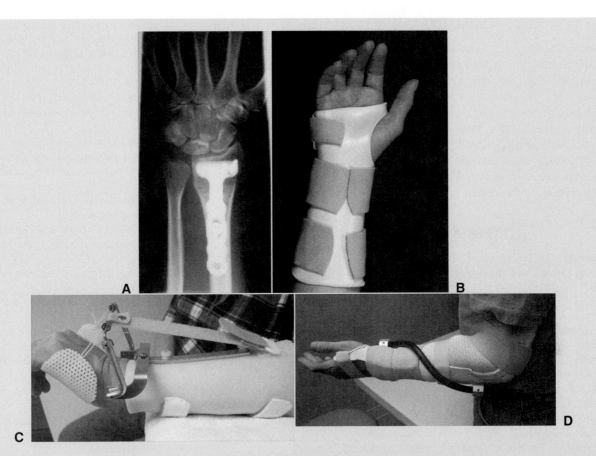

FIGURE 14-22 A, A radiograph of open reduction and internal fixation of a comminuted wrist fracture. **B,** A forearm-based wrist immobilization orthosis used during the initial stages of healing. When adequate healing had occurred, a wrist extension mobilization orthosis (**C**) and a forearm supination mobilization orthosis (**D**) are fabricated to help increase functional range of motion.

- What do you think the prognosis will be for this patient? What are the patient's goals for intervention? What are your rehabilitation goals? How long do you think it will take to achieve the goals that you and the patient agree on?
- On the basis of the patient's goals and expectations, as well as your understanding of the underlying disease process, what recommendations would you make for intervention at this point in time? What "evidence" from the clinical research literature supports your recommendations? What have you chosen or prioritized from these possible interventions?
- What type of follow-up would you recommend? How do you anticipate your intervention will need to be modified as the patient progresses through the phases of tissue healing? How would you assess the outcomes of your interventions?

Recommendations for a Patient with Open Reduction and Internal Fixation of Wrist Fracture

A forearm-based wrist immobilization orthosis is fabricated with a ⅛-inch material to obtain a rigid support to be used during the proliferative stage of healing (see Figure 14-22B). The patient is instructed to remove the orthosis six times a day for gentle range of motion of the wrist and digits. As expected, all wrist motions are significantly limited. He is encouraged to move the digits frequently while in the orthosis between exercise sessions and incorporate the hand in light ADLs.

At 4 weeks after surgery, because the radiograph revealed adequate healing along with the stable fixation provided by the plate and screws, the wrist orthosis is discontinued (except for stressful activities) and therapy progresses with the addition of gentle passive range of motion. All movements of the wrist improve except wrist extension and forearm supination, which are significantly restricted passively. At 6 weeks, these limitations continue to be problematic and the physician recommends the addition of a wrist extension mobilization orthosis (see Figure 14-22C) and a forearm supination mobilization orthosis (see Figure 14-22D).

The wrist extension mobilization orthosis is fabricated with a standard hook-and-loop material to provide the mobilization force by a static progressive approach. This method is chosen because of the high degree of wrist stiffness. The supination mobilization orthosis is fabricated with a tubing mechanism to provide the stretching force. The patient is instructed to wear each device four times a day for 30 minutes, increasing the passive stretch on the tissue as tolerated. The previously used wrist immobilization orthosis continues to be used at night as a serial static device, by remolding to position the wrist at maximal extension to maintain all the gains made throughout the day.

After 4 weeks of use, V. A. begins to plateau at 55 degrees of wrist extension and 70 degrees of supination, which is functional and, because of the severity of the injury, quite acceptable.

SUMMARY

Orthotic fabrication is a commonly used intervention for clinicians treating the upper extremity. Gaining an appreciation for how different orthoses can be created for specific purposes aids in obtaining maximal patient outcome. This chapter reviews many aspects of orthotic fabrication, including nomenclature, tissue healing, and anatomical and mechanical principles, and provides an overview of the various products on the market. Through comprehensive study and practice, fabrication of orthoses can be another tool used successfully in the clinic.

REFERENCES

1. American Society of Hand Therapists. *Splint Classification System*. Garner, NC: The American Society of Hand Therapists; 1992.

2. Fess EE. A history of splinting: to understand the present, view the past. *J Hand Ther*. 2002;15(2):97–132.

3. Coverdell J. An editorial note on nomenclature: Orthosis versus splint. *J Hand Ther*. 2012;25:3–4.

4. Tenney CG, Lisak JM. *Atlas of Hand Splinting*. Boston: Little, Brown; 1986.

5. Schultz-Johnson K. Static progressive splinting. *J Hand Ther*. 2002;15(2):163–178.

6. Raphael J, Skirven T. Contractures and splinting. In: *Atlas of Hand Clinics*, Vol 6(1). Philadelphia: Saunders; 2001.

7. Glasgow C, Tooth LR, Fleming J. Mobilizing the stiff hand: combining theory and evidence to improve clinical outcomes. *J Hand Ther*. 2010;23(4):392–401.

8. Lucado AM, Li Z, Russell GB, et al. Changes in impairment and function after static progressive splinting for stiffness after distal radius fracture. *J Hand Ther*. 2008;21(4):319–325.

9. Bell-Krotoski JA. Plaster cylinder casting for contractures of the interphalangeal joints. In: Mackin EJ, Callahan AD, Osterman AL, et al., eds. *Rehabilitation of the Hand and Upper Extremity*. 5th ed. St. Louis: Mosby; 2002:1839–1845.

10. Bell-Krotoski JA, Figarola F. Biomechanics of soft tissue growth and remodeling with plaster casting. *J Hand Ther*. 1995;8(2):131–137.

11. Brand P, Hollister A. *Clinical Mechanics of the Hand*. 3rd ed. St. Louis: Mosby Year Book; 1999.

12. Colditz JC. Therapist's management of the stiff hand. In: Skirven TM, Osterman AL, Fedorczyk JM, et al., eds. *Rehabilitation of the Hand and Upper Extremity*. 6th ed. St. Louis: Mosby; 2011:894–921.

13. Flowers KR, LaStayo P. Effect of total end range time on improving passive range of motion. *J Hand Ther*. 1994;7(3):150–157.

14. Gyovai JE, Wright Howell J. Validation of spring forces applied in dynamic outrigger splinting. *J Hand Ther*. 1992;5(1):8–15.

15. Prosser R. Splinting in the management of proximal interphalangeal joint flexion contracture. *J Hand Ther*. 1996;9(4):378–386.

16. Bell Krotoski JA. Tissue remodeling and contracture correction using serial plaster casting and orthotic positioning. In: Skirven TM, Osterman AL, Fedorczyk JM, et al., eds. *Rehabilitation of the Hand and Upper Extremity*. 6th ed. St. Louis: Mosby; 2011:1599–1609.

17. Jacobs M, Austin NM. *Splinting the Hand and Upper Extremity: Principles and Process*. Baltimore: Lippincott Williams & Wilkins; 2003.

18. Schultz-Johnson KS. Splinting: a problem solving approach. In: Stanley BG, Tribuzi SM, eds. *Concepts in Hand Rehabilitation*. Philadelphia: FA Davis; 1992:238–271.

19. Schultz-Johnson KS. Splinting the wrist: mobilization and protection. *J Hand Ther*. 1996;9(2):165–175.

20. Skirven TM, Osterman AL, Fedorczyk JM, et al., eds. *Rehabilitation of the Hand and Upper Extremity*. 6th ed. St. Louis: Mosby; 2011.

21. Wolf SW, Hotchkiss RN, Pederson WC, et al. *Green's Operative Hand Surgery*. 6th ed. New York: Churchill Livingstone; 2010.

22. Stanley BG, Tribuzi SM, eds. *Concepts in Hand Rehabilitation*. Philadelphia: FA Davis; 1992.

23. Tubiana R, Thomine JM, Mackin E. *Examination of the Hand and Wrist*. 2nd ed. St. Louis: Mosby; 1996.

24. Fess EE, Gettle KS, Philips C, et al. *Hand and Upper Extremity Splinting: Principles and Methods*. 3rd ed. St. Louis: Mosby Year Book; 2005.

25. Kiel J. *Basic Hand Splinting: A Pattern Designing Approach*. Boston: Little, Brown; 1983.

26. Rotman MB, Donovan JP. Practical anatomy of the carpal tunnel. *Hand Clin*. 2002;18(2):219–230.

27. Pratt NE. Anatomy and kinesiology of the hand. In: Skirven TM, Osterman AL, Fedorczyk JM, et al., eds. *Rehabilitation of the Hand and Upper Extremity*. 6th ed. St. Louis: Mosby; 2011:3–17.

28. Coppard BM, Lohman H. *Introduction to Splinting: A Clinical Reasoning & Problem-Solving Approach*. 3rd ed. St. Louis: Mosby; 2008.

29. Austin N. The wrist and hand complex. In: Levangie PK, Norkin CC, eds. *Joint Structure and Function: A Comprehensive Analysis*. 5th ed. Philadelphia: FA Davis; 2011.

30. Fess EE. Splints: mechanics versus convention. *J Hand Ther*. 1995;8(2):124–130.

31. Cannon NM, Foltz RW, Koepfer J, et al. *Manual of Hand Splinting*. New York: Churchill Livingstone; 1985.

32. Bell-Krotoski JA, Breger-Stanton DE. Biomechanics and evaluation of the hand. In: Mackin EJ, Callahan AD, Osterman AL, et al., eds. *Rehabilitation of the Hand and Upper Extremity*. 5th ed. St. Louis: Mosby; 2002:240–262.

33. Van Lede P, van Veldhoven G. *Therapeutic Hand Splints: A Rational Approach*. Antwerp, Belgium: Provan; 1998.

34. Fess EE, McCollum M. The influence of splinting on healing tissue. *J Hand Ther*. 1998;11(2):157–161.

35. Strickland JW. Biologic basis for hand and upper extremity splinting. In: Fess EE, Gettle KS, Philips C, et al., eds. *Hand and Upper Extremity Splinting: Principles and Methods*. 3rd ed. St. Louis: Mosby Year Book; 2005:87–103.

36. Smith KL, Dean SJ. Tissue repair of the epidermis and dermis. *J Hand Ther*. 1998;11(2):95–104.

37. Smith J, Feske N. Cutaneous manifestations and consequences of smoking. *J Am Acad Dermatol*. 1996;34(5 pt 1):717–726.

38. Rund C. Postoperative care of skin graft, donor sites, and myocutaneous flaps. In: Krasner D, Kane D, eds. *Chronic Wound Care: A Clinical Source Book for Healthcare Professionals*. 2nd ed. Wayne, NJ: Health Management Publication; 1997.

39. Wilton JC. *Hand Splinting: Principles of Design and Fabrication*. Philadelphia: Saunders; 1997.

40. McKee P, Morgan L. *Orthotics in Rehabilitation*. Philadelphia: FA Davis; 1998.

41. Bell Krotoski JA, Breger-Stanton D. The forces of dynamic orthotic positioning: ten questions to ask before applying a dynamic orthosis to the hand. In: Skirven TM, Osterman AL, Fedorczyk JM, et al., eds. *Rehabilitation of the Hand and Upper Extremity*. 6th ed. St. Louis: Mosby; 2011:1581–1587.

42. Flowers KR. A proposed decision hierarchy for splinting the stiff joint, with an emphasis on force application parameters. *J Hand Ther.* 2002;15(2):158–162.

43. McClure PW, Blackburn LG, Dusold C. The use of splints in the treatment of joint stiffness: biological rationale and an algorithm for making clinical decisions. *Phys Ther.* 1994;74(12):1101–1107.

44. Mildenberger LA, Amadio PC, An KN. Dynamic splinting: a systematic approach to the selection of elastic traction. *Arch Phys Med.* 1986;67(4):241–244.

45. Glasgow C, Wilton J, Tooth L. Optimal daily total end range time for contracture: resolution in hand splinting. *J Hand Ther.* 2003;16(3):207–218.

46. Lee DB. Objective and subjective observations of low-temperature thermoplastic materials. *J Hand Ther.* 1995;8(2):138–143.

47. Breger Lee DE, Buford WL. Properties of thermoplastic splinting materials. *J Hand Ther.* 1992;5(3):202–211.

48. Breger Lee DE, Buford WL. Update in splinting materials and methods. *Hand Clin.* 1991;7(1):569–585.

49. *Patterson Medical Hand Rehab Catalog.* Bolingbrook, IL 2011.

50. North Coast Medical Inc. *Hand Therapy Catalog.* San Jose, CA; 2007–2008.

51. McKee PR, Rivard A. Biopsychosocial approach to orthotic intervention. *J Hand Ther.* 2010;1–8.

15

Splinting, Orthoses, and Prostheses in the Management of Burns

R. Scott Ward

LEARNING OBJECTIVES

On completion of this chapter, the reader will be able to:

1. Identify the elements of burn injury that contribute to decision making regarding splints, orthotics, and prosthetics.
2. Describe how wound care may affect the use and application of splints, orthotics, and prosthetics.
3. Discuss components of rehabilitation interventions that may incorporate or affect the use of splints, orthotics, and prosthetics.
4. Describe the use of splints and orthotics in the care of patients with burn injuries.
5. Describe the use of prosthetics for patients with amputations associated with burn injuries.

Rehabilitation of a patient with burns involves programs that focus on restoring functions compromised by the burn injury.[1] Treatment strategies used by therapists address five important goals:

1. Improve or promote wound healing by reducing wound infection
2. Prevent or reduce deformity
3. Increase mobility and strength to achieve maximal function
4. Reduce effects of hypertrophic scarring
5. Educate the patient about recuperation

The rehabilitation plan for patients with burns centers on wound care, positioning, range-of-motion (ROM) exercises, splinting, strengthening exercises, endurance and functional exercises, gait training, and scar control. Burn care emphasizes the need for a comprehensive team approach to achieve maximal clinical results.[1,2]

BURN INJURY

Each year in the United States, 450,000 to 500,000 individuals sustain and seek medical care for burn injuries and an estimated 3500 of these injuries result in death.[3] Estimates are that burn injuries result in approximately 45,000 hospitalizations per year.[3] The American Burn Association has outlined criteria for determining the severity of burn injury, which include cause of the injury, burn depth, total body surface area (TBSA) burned, location of the burn, and patient age.[4,5] A burn injury of any given size is more severe for patients who are very young or very old. The deeper the injury, the more serious the burn. Involvement of the face, eyes, ears, perineum, hands, and feet make the injury more critical. Associated trauma, smoke inhalation injury, and poor preinjury health status are factors that increase severity of the injury.[6] An appropriate understanding of the nature of burn injury and the location and depth of the burn wound is important in understanding and anticipating the possible problems a patient may face during rehabilitation.

Causes of Burns

Types of burn injury include flame, scald, flash (radiant heat explosions), contact, chemical, electrical, and other (e.g., irradiation, radioactivity) burns.[7] Scald and flame injuries are common causes of burn injury. Preschool-aged children are at the highest risk for suffering scald injuries.[8-10] Flame burns are generally the leading cause of burn injury in other age groups.[8,11] Chemical and electrical burns present differently than other burn injuries. Burns resulting from chemical agents require identification of the causative agent so that proper neutralization of the chemical can take place. Assessment of the depth of chemical burns is difficult at first, but these wounds are predictably deep.[12] An electrical injury may have areas of significant surface burn; however, these areas are often the result of associated flash burns. Small, deep wounds where the current enters or exits the body are more typical.[13] The major complication with rehabilitative consequence of electrical injury is musculoskeletal necrosis, which frequently results in the need for amputation.[14,15]

Burn Depth

Thomsen[16] has studied Indian writings dating back to approximately 600 BC that describe four levels or degrees of burn depth and declare that deep burns heal slowly and with scarring.[16] There are two methods to describe burn depth: by degree (first, second, or third degree) or thickness (superficial, partial thickness, and full thickness).[17] The thickness terminology is more commonly used in clinical practice. A superficial injury corresponds to a first-degree injury, a partial thickness to a second-degree injury, and a full thickness to a third-degree injury (Figure 15-1).

Clinical characteristics associated with the injury thickness are helpful in identification of the depth of burn.[17]

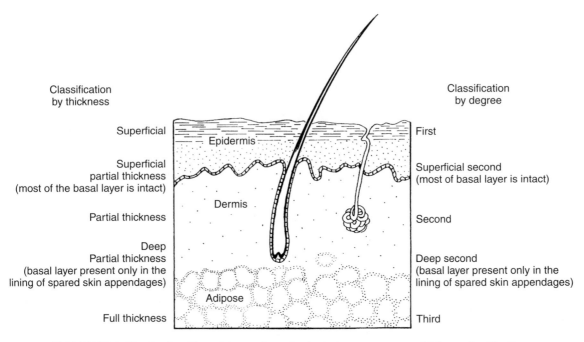

FIGURE 15-1 The depths of burn injury, referencing both the contemporary thickness classification with the more traditional degree terminology. (From Ward RS. The rehabilitation of burn patients. *CRC Crit Rev Phys Med Rehabil* 1991;2[3]:121-138.)

Superficial (first degree) injuries involve only the epidermis. They are often painful, erythematous, and mildly edematous. Superficial burn injuries usually heal in 3 to 7 days and they rarely result in scarring. Superficial partial-thickness burns (superficial second degree) compromise the epidermis and upper dermis. These burns are very painful, very red, and often have blisters or weeping wounds. Superficial partial-thickness burns usually heal in 14 to 21 days and rarely develop scar. In deep partial-thickness burns (deep second degree), deeper layers of the dermis are damaged. The wound may or may not be painful, it may be cherry red or pale, and the skin is still pliable. Deep partial-thickness burns require more than 21 days to heal spontaneously and will scar. In full-thickness burns (third degree) all layers of the skin are destroyed. The wound generally has a tan or brown appearance and exhibits a leathery texture. Full-thickness wounds are painless and need several weeks to heal without surgical intervention. Deep partial-thickness burns are often managed by skin grafting; full-thickness injuries require skin grafting. A deeper burn generally correlates with an increased severity of injury.

Surgical Management of Burns

Small burn wounds may be excised and primarily closed; however, most burn wounds require excision of the burn followed by coverage of the site with a skin graft.[18] Excision of the burn wound is ordinarily performed tangentially; that is, thin layers of the burn are removed until viable tissue is reached.[19] Autografts (split-thickness grafts) are harvested from undamaged areas of the body for coverage of the excised wound.[19] Skin grafts placed on tangentially excised wounds demonstrate good long-term functional results.[20] Full-thickness skin grafts can also be used. Interestingly, split-thickness grafts scar more than full-thickness grafts.[20]

Progress has been made in the use of skin substitutes and cultured skin for the coverage of the excised burn.[21-23] Areas treated in this fashion tend to be fragile and susceptible to breakdown.[24] Wounds treated with cultured epithelium do not aggressively scar; however, little information is available about the rehabilitative ramifications of this treatment approach.[25]

Burn Size

Burn wound size is reported as a percentage of the TBSA that is injured. Lund and Browder[26] describe a method for estimating percent TBSA. Variations in body part ratios during development and diversified proportions of individual anatomical parts are considered in the estimation (Figure 15-2). The "rule of nines" is another technique for estimating surface area by dividing the body into 11 different areas equal to 9% each; the genitalia make up the remaining 1% of the total 100% estimate.[27] A burn injury increases in severity as the percentage of TBSA burn increases. Large burns usually require longer convalescence, which in turn increases the rehabilitative needs of the patient.

Location of the Burn

Burns of the face, perineum, hands, and feet create special problems.[6] Burns of the face are distressing because there may be cosmetic disfigurement, visual impairment, or compromised nutrition (intake of food). Injuries of the face are often accompanied by inhalation injuries. Hands and feet

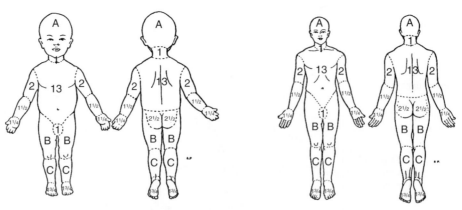

Relative Percentages of Areas Affected by Growth

Area	Age	0	1	5		Area	Age	10	15	Adult
A = 1/2 of head		9 1/2	8 1/2	6 1/2		A = 1/2 of head		5 1/2	4 1/2	3 1/2
B = 1/2 of one thigh		2 3/4	3 1/4	4		B = 1/2 of one thigh		4 1/4	4 1/2	4 3/4
C = 1/2 of one leg		2 1/2	2 1/2	2 3/4		C = 1/2 of one leg		3	3 1/4	3 1/2

FIGURE 15-2 The original Lund and Browder chart outlines the accepted method for determining the TBSA of a burn injury. (From Lund CC, Browder NC. The estimation of areas of burns. *Surg Gynecol Obstet* 1944;79:352-358.)

have broad functional importance that can be substantially compromised after burn injury. Severity of injury is significantly magnified as the total surface area of the hand or foot encompassed by the burn increases. Any burn that crosses a joint increases the risk for functional compromise and creates challenges in rehabilitation.

WOUND CARE

The time it takes to heal a burn wound is directly related to depth of the injury. The more superficial a wound, the faster it heals. Surgical intervention, such as skin grafting, is often used to reduce healing time for deep wounds. Wound infection can significantly delay healing and lead to increased scar formation.[28]

Topical Agents and Wound Dressing

The outermost layer of epidermis (stratum corneum) in intact skin is too dry to support microbial growth and serves as an effective barrier to microbial penetration. As a result, skin infections seldom occur unless the skin is opened.[29] Because this protective barrier is compromised or destroyed in burn injury, the risk for infection is greatly increased. Personal protective equipment, particularly gloves, gowns, and masks, must be worn when caring for patients with burn wounds.[30] Topical agents may be applied to these open wounds after each cleansing and debridement to prevent or manage infections. Topical agents are particularly important for ischemic wounds in which systemic delivery of natural substrates to fight infection is compromised.[29,31] A well-applied dressing minimizes discomfort and allows mobility.

Mild lotions help relieve dryness and itching in maturing healed wounds.[29] The use of moisturizers helps prevent healed wounds from cracking or splitting. Because alcohol is a desiccant to the skin and exacerbates dryness, lotions that

contain alcohol should be avoided. Fragrance-free moisturizers are recommended; most hypersensitivity reactions are triggered by perfumes. Moisturizers can also be beneficial when applying a splint, orthotic, or prosthetic device to a patient with healed burns or scar because they help protect the skin from desiccation and shear.

Rehabilitative personnel often take an active role in the wound care of a patient with burns. Involvement in wound care provides a better understanding of the reasons for discomfort. Familiarity with wound care procedures is often necessary for outpatient therapy sessions.[32,33] Adjustments in the treatment plan are often necessary as the wound heals and tolerance of certain rehabilitative procedures changes. Consideration of the effects of pressure, shear, and friction on a healing wound or newly healed, fragile skin is especially important when splints, orthotics, prosthetics, or other external devices are being used.

PSYCHOLOGY OF BURN INJURY

An acute burn injury creates emotional distress. Treatment of the burns is often traumatic as well; stress and anxiety continue during the period of recovery. The psychological consequences of burn trauma in the adult include depression, posttraumatic stress disorder, despair, fear, anxiety, and survivor's guilt.[34-37] Children often feel guilt and manifest loss of interest in play, unpredictable sadness, avoidance, and regression.[38-40]

Psychological adaptation in early phases after burn injury includes denial (often manifest by a feeling of calmness), and concern about prognosis, pain, personal issues, and dependence on medical staff (depression).[39,41] Individuals who become actively involved in the process of rehabilitation and self-care often are more encouraged and optimistic about the future.[38,41]

Rehabilitation professionals can facilitate psychological function and recovery of patients with burns in several ways. Encouraging independence by allowing individuals as much control over medical procedures as possible helps them focus on recovery and empowers them to a certain degree.[41,42] Patients feel more comfortable with caregivers if they have the opportunity to get to know one another outside painful treatment settings.[38,42] Support and understanding demonstrate a caring attitude. Tactful but honest answers to questions about prognosis, cosmesis, and functional outcome help establish trust.[38] Ongoing education about the recovery process helps the patient develop realistic expectations about recovery.

REHABILITATION INTERVENTION

Early surgical intervention, availability of nutritional support, and pharmaceutical advances have improved survival after burn injury and the American Burn Association has reported a survival rate of 94.8% from 2000 to 2009.[3] As a result of improvement in care, treatment, and survival of burned patients, more physical therapists will become responsible for treating these patients for a significant portion of their rehabilitation in settings other than a hospital burn center (e.g., outpatient clinics, community hospitals).

This improvement, in turn, has increased the emphasis on and need for rehabilitation of patients with burns. Physical therapists and occupational therapists are important members of the burn care team.

After examination and evaluation, the team establishes goals and designs and implements an appropriate plan of care. Important rehabilitation goals for patients with burns might include the following as put forward in *The Guide to Physical Therapist Practice*: (1) wound and soft tissue healing is enhanced; (2) risk of infection and complications is reduced; (3) risk of secondary impairments is reduced; (4) maximal ROM is achieved; (5) preinjury level of cardiovascular endurance is restored; (6) good to normal strength is achieved; (7) independent ambulation is achieved; (8) independent function in activities of daily living (ADLs) is increased; (9) scar formation is minimized; (10) patient, family, and caregivers understanding of expectations and goals and outcomes is increased; (11) aerobic capacity is increased; and (12) self-management of symptoms is improved.[43]

Burn rehabilitation interventions emphasize patient independence through achievement of maximal functional recovery.[44]

Wound Healing and Scar Formation

Unhealed burn wounds can create challenges during rehabilitation. Most problems in burn rehabilitation are caused by the ceaseless contraction and hypertrophy of immature burn scars.[45] Scar contracture can lead to visible cosmetic deformity of involved body parts, particularly of the face and hands. Functional limitations are common when the scar crosses a joint. The contraction of scar has been classically associated with a type of fibroblast called myofibroblasts, which have contractile properties.[46–48]

Burn wound healing encompasses three phases: the inflammatory phase, the proliferative phase, and the maturation, or remodeling, phase.[49] The inflammatory phase is characterized by the formation of new blood vessels, an initial defense against infection, and migration of fibroblast and epithelial cells into the injured area. Treatment focuses on proper wound care to encourage vascular regrowth and retard contamination of the site. The proliferative phase is marked by continued revascularization, rebuilding, and strengthening of the wound site as a result of vigorous synthesis of collagen by fibroblasts, and reepithelialization.[50] Treatment is directed toward promoting epithelialization and encouraging proper alignment of newly deposited collagen fibers. During the maturation phase, the wound site is further strengthened by protracted deposition of collagen fibers by active fibroblasts. Treatment during maturation stresses lengthening the scar, reconditioning the patient, and returning the patient to preburn functional levels. Activity and rehabilitation interventions aimed at opposing wound and scar tightness and education about the process of recovery are critical in all phases of healing.

While fibroblasts deposit collagen during the proliferative phase, macrophages and endothelial cells release enzymes that degrade collagen. The severity of scar formation is determined by the balance between collagen synthesis and lysis: the more that collagen deposition exceeds its breakdown, the more likely a significant scar will form.[51,52] A hypertrophic scar is raised above the normal surface of skin (Figure 15-3).[53-55] A keloid occurs when the scar extends beyond the initial boundaries of the wound.[53-55]

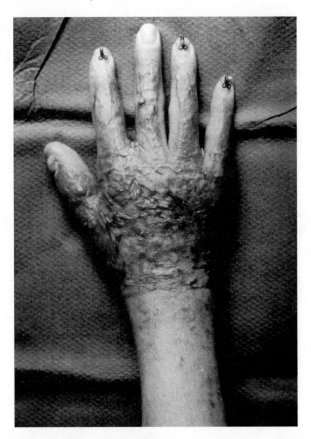

FIGURE 15-3 The dorsum of this patient's hand exhibits hypertrophic scarring. (From Ward RS. Pressure therapy for the control of hypertrophic scar formation after burn injury: a history and review. *J Burn Care Rehabil* 1991;12[3]:257-262.)

An immature scar is raised, red, leathery, and stiff. As the scar matures, it becomes pale, relatively soft and flattened, and more yielding.[56-58] The process of scar maturation requires 6 to 18 months after wound closure; scars actively contract during maturation.[56,57,59] Contraction is most vigorous in the early months of maturation but continues throughout this period of remodeling.

Superficial and partial-thickness burns usually do not scar; full-thickness burns almost always do. Full-thickness wounds closed by a skin graft scar significantly less than a similar wound allowed to heal spontaneously. Very dark-skinned or very fair-skinned individuals and those with familial history of susceptibility to scarring are more likely to form hypertrophic scar.[60-63] The larger the burn, the greater the likelihood of scar formation.[62-64] A contracture occurs when a portion or distortion of the shortening scar becomes fixed or semifixed.[65] The axilla, elbow, hand knee, face, and neck are common and most problematic sites of scar contracture formation.[61,63,65] One of the most important goals of burn rehabilitation is to prevent, counteract, and minimize the adverse effects of scar contraction.[65]

Operative Scar Management

Surgery is used to correct scar contractures that have created specific functional deficits or deformities.[66] Surgical techniques used to release scar contracture include split-thickness or full-thickness skin grafts, skin flaps, Z-plasties, and tissue expansion.[66,67] Most surgeries are deferred until at least 6 months after the burn or until the scar is sufficiently mature.[66,67] Although surgery alleviates contracture-related problems, it also creates a new wound with its own subsequent scar maturation process. Rehabilitation is necessary after a majority of reconstructive surgeries to again avert the affects of contraction.

Nonoperative Scar Management

The nonoperative control of hypertrophic scarring most commonly involves pressure therapy and the application of silicone gel sheeting. The use of continuous pressure for the treatment of burn scars was described in 1971.[68] Pressure has also been shown to relieve other aggravating discomforts of the healing burn wound, such as itching and blistering.[69-72] ROM is not significantly impeded with pressure garments despite the restriction felt by patients (particularly initially) when fit with pressure garments.[73]

Pressure therapy is indicated when healing requires more than 14 days or if skin grafting has been performed. There are several strategies to assess burn scar condition. The Vancouver Scar Scale developed by Sullivan and colleagues describes severity of the scar by rating pigmentation, vascularity, pliability, and height of the scar tissue (Box 15-1).[74]

Early pressure therapy is used to control edema in a wound even if there is no ensuing scar formation. Some of the most common elastic materials used on newly healing, still fragile wounds include elastic bandages, Coban self-adherent wrap (3M Medical, St. Paul, Minn.), or elasticized cotton tubular bandages such as Tubigrip (SePro Healthcare, Inc., Montgomeryville, Pa.).[75-77] These materials are useful while the patient is waiting for the arrival of custom-fit, antiburn scar supports.[75-77]

Individuals with scars are commonly fitted with custom-fit pressure garments for the duration of the maturation phase of healing. Custom-fit, antiburn scar supports are available from manufacturers such as Bio-Concepts (Phoenix, Ariz.), Barton-Carey Medical Products (Perrysburg, Ohio), Gottfried Medical (Toledo, Ohio), and Medical Z (San Antonio, Texas). Although the measuring procedure varies by manufacturer, most require measurements approximately every 1 to 1.5 inches along each extremity, with special guidelines for the torso, face, and hands. Burn scar supports can be fabricated to fit almost any body part, including the face, torso, upper extremity, hand, and lower extremity. Some burn centers fabricate rigid or semirigid face masks (essentially orthotics) in an attempt to gain a better match with facial contours.[78]

Pressure garments and devices are worn through the entire process of scar maturation, to be discontinued only when the scar has completely matured.[1] Fit of pressure garments is

---

BOX 15-1	*Vancouver Scar Scale Ratings for Assessing Burn Scar*

PIGMENTATION
 0 = Normal (scar color closely resembles that of the rest of the body)
 1 = Hypopigmentation
 2 = Hyperpigmentation

PLIABILITY
 0 = Normal
 1 = Supple (flexible with minimum resistance)
 2 = Yielding (gives way to pressure)
 3 = Firm (inflexible, not easily moved, resistant to manual pressure)
 4 = Banding (ropelike tissue that blanches with extension on the scar)
 5 = Contracture (permanent shortening of scar, producing deformity or distortion)

VASCULARITY
 0 = Normal (scar color closely resembles that of the rest of the body)
 1 = Pink
 2 = Red
 3 = Purple

HEIGHT
 0 = Normal (flat)
 1 = Raised less than 2 mm
 2 = Raised less than 5 mm
 3 = Raised more than 5 mm

Modified from Sullivan T, Smith J, Kernoda J, et al. Rating the burn scar. *J Burn Care Rehabil* 1990;11(3):256-260.

regularly reassessed to ensure the desired therapeutic effect. Regular follow-up provides an opportunity for the patient to discuss other ongoing rehabilitative problems associated with the burn.

Silicone gel sheets or pads can be put right on a maturing scar. Silicone gel sheeting is generally applied over small areas or on scar where it is otherwise difficult to provide sufficient pressure. The mechanism of action for the effect of silicone gel on scar is not known.[79,80]

BURN REHABILITATION INTERVENTIONS

Many different types of rehabilitation interventions are appropriate in the care of patients with burns. Although many interventions are briefly described in the following section, the emphasis is on the use of splints, orthoses, and prosthetic devices.

Therapeutic Exercise

Exercise helps minimize outcomes of burn injury and burn scar formation by improving mobility and function.[81] As important and effective as exercise is in burn rehabilitation, some individuals may be reluctant to exercise (and some therapists may be reluctant to encourage them) because of the anticipation of increased pain or anxiety about damaging newly healing tissue. Exercise programs for patients with burns are principally directed at the prevention of burn scar contractures and the side effects of inactivity and disuse. Additional consequences of immobilization in these patients can include progressive contracture of the joint capsule and pericapsular structures, atrophy and contracture of muscle, deleterious effects on articular cartilage, and possible decrease in bone strength. Exercise is a significant health promotion and disability prevention component in the rehabilitation of patients with burns.

Assessment of location and depth of burn injury identifies those areas most at risk of burn scar contracture. This assessment also guides design of an exercise program to improve mobility, strength, and functional status. Past and present medical conditions influence rehabilitative expectations; a previous orthopedic injury may have already reduced ROM of a particular joint whereas a concomitant inhalation injury may limit exercise tolerance.

Active Exercise

After a burn, exercise may be difficult because of edema, pain (particularly over areas of partial-thickness burns), the loss of skin elasticity in the burned tissue, and wound contraction.[44,82] Early on, edema is a major contributor to stiffness of joints; active exercise is valuable in reducing the edema.[32,83] Positioning and compressive wraps or devices are used for edema control in addition to exercise. Pain tolerance varies widely among individuals. The therapist is challenged to help the patient understand the importance of activity despite the pain involved. Many individuals have relief of their pain and stiffness after exercise periods, which may encourage them to participate in the subsequent therapy sessions. Persons who

understand the advantages of exercise may be asked to confer with, and encourage, newly injured individuals or those having difficulty with their exercises.

General stiffness from the loss of skin elasticity and wound contracture is a short-term problem but often persists during the process of scar maturation, especially for those who form a hypertrophic scar. Exercise targeting those areas most vulnerable to scar formation identified in the initial evaluation must begin as early as possible after admission.[44,84] Early presentation of an exercise routine aids edema control, relieves stiffness, and prevents loss of strength and ROM. The early introduction of active exercise reinforces the importance of exercise to the individual, who will incorporate daily exercise as a important contributor to overall recovery. Because of the wide scope of benefits derived from active exercises, they are the preferred form of ROM exercises for patients with burns. A survey of physical and occupational therapists, 96% reported instituting active ROM exercises within 24 hours of acute burn center admission.[85]

Patients are also encouraged to perform independent activities of daily living.[44,83] Self-reliance is important after burn injury, and independence can increase the patient's self-confidence.[44,83] It is likely that the more patients can do, particularly in directing their exercise programs, the more compliant they will become.[84] Independence in an exercise program is therefore an important goal for those recovering from burn injury.

The primary goals of active exercise for patients with acute burns are opposition of tissue contraction and strengthening. For an individual with a burn crossing the antecubital fossa and weakness of the biceps brachii, exercise is focused on preservation of elbow-extension ROM and functional strength of the muscle. If a patient with a burn encompassing the lower leg and ankle also has weakness and atrophy of the triceps surae, appropriate strengthening exercises may be performed, but certainly not at the sacrifice of active ankle ROM.

Conditioning exercises can be incorporated to improve the cardiovascular status of the patient.[86] Occupation-specific training programs may be a part of the long-term rehabilitation plan as patients plan to return to their jobs. This type of activity may be directed at one or a few specific functions or may incorporate a traditional work-hardening program.

Gait Training

The functional nature of ambulation makes it an important exercise for burned lower extremities.[87] Ambulation assists with edema control, ROM, and strengthening in all lower extremity joints. Ambulation also helps with the function of other physiological systems such as the cardiovascular, gastrointestinal, and renal systems. Individuals with lower extremity burns exhibit gait deviations related to compromised joint function, such as incomplete hip and knee flexion in initial swing and incomplete knee extension in terminal swing. Initial contact may be made with the entire foot (foot flat) instead of the heel, and loading response may be compromised by lack of plantar flexion ROM or an unwillingness to perform the controlled knee flexion necessary for shock absorption. Excessive knee flexion in midstance, poor or absent heel-off and weight shift in terminal stance, and inadequate knee flexion in preswing are often present.[33] Differences in individual gait deviations in gait phases are generally based on variations in the location, size, and depth of the burn injury and levels of pain. Any gait deviation caused by the burn may accentuate the need for vigilant gait training of a patient with burns who also has a lower extremity prosthesis. Exercise is an important adjunct to gait training because it can address specific movement limitations of the lower limbs.

Passive Exercise and Stretching

Passive exercise is included in therapy regimens when patients are unable to move on their own or cannot actively complete normal ROM. Passive ROM and slow, gentle stretching exercises that elongate healing soft tissues are used to preserve and improve joint ROM.[88] Eighty-four percent of physical and occupational therapists reported initiating passive ROM stretching exercises within the first 24 hours after burn center admission.[85] Blanching of the scar indicates an appropriate amount of stretch. Although the scar should be stretched to the point of tolerance, joint movement should not be forced because of possible tissue damage and the potential for heterotopic ossification.[89-91]

Positioning or splints are used after a stretching session to maintain the achieved ROM. Suitable stretching positions must also consider scars that cross multiple joints and therefore affect a broad kinematic chain.

Most of the exercise equipment typically found in rehabilitation settings is appropriate for patients with burns. The therapist must decide when certain equipment will be most beneficial and incorporate the use of this resource into the plan of care. The use of latex rubber tubing for strengthening and overhead reciprocal pulleys for increasing ROM are a few examples of simple equipment that have been described in the literature.[92-94] Bicycle ergometers for either the upper or lower extremities assist with motion, provide resistance, and allow for some cardiovascular workout.

Physical Agents

Because of the variety of treatment goals important for burn rehabilitation, many different types of modalities may be used for appropriate intervention. Hydrotherapy, functional electrical stimulation (neuromuscular electrical stimulation), transcutaneous electrical nerve stimulation, ultrasound, continuous passive motion (CPM), and paraffin are physical agents that have been reported to be used in burn care. Hydrotherapy is most often used for wound care but may also be used for dressing removal and exercise.[95] If hydrotherapy is chosen as a thermal modality, precautions similar to those used for any open wound care are necessary to reduce the chance of cross-contamination.

Functional electrical stimulation has been successfully used to treat hands that have responded poorly to typical treatment.[96] Burn pain has been altered by transcutaneous electrical stimulation in some cases.[97] Ultrasound has been used to treat pain and ROM impairments in patients with burns; however, the efficacy of ultrasound in either decreasing

pain or improving motion is still a matter of some debate.[98-100] Successful use of CPM has been specifically reported for hand burns and lower extremity burns at the knee.[101] The gentle heat provided by paraffin, as well as the potential skin softening from the mineral oil in the paraffin, may be reasons for the use of this modality in burn care.[102]

Healing skin and recently healed skin are often very sensitive. Scar tissue has varying levels of sensory deficit.[103,104] Accordingly, heat, cold, coupling agents, and electrode adhesives may lead to skin breakdown. Caution must be exercised when applying any modality; thorough pretreatment and posttreatment inspection of the site is warranted.

Positioning

Positioning is an important component of any burn rehabilitation program. Positioning is used for acute burn and postsurgical edema control and to prevent or treat scar contractures.[105] The initial burn therapy evaluation identifies sites at risk for contracture formation; appropriate counteractive positions become part of the therapy plan. Contracture prevention is more successful when a program of positioning and activity is instituted as soon after burn as possible.[44,63]

Postexercise positioning extends the effects of activity; positioning is also fundamental for individuals who cannot move or exercise. Manufactured positioning devices, such as arm boards that attach to the side of the bed, are available to assist in proper positioning of extremities. Positioning need not be expensive or require intricate equipment. Avoiding the use of a pillow behind the head is a simple way of decreasing neck flexion and facilitating a neutral alignment of the head and neck. A pillow or several folded blankets placed under the arms can effectively elevate the burned limb while keeping the elbows extended and supporting the hands. At least some horizontal flexion of the shoulders is indicated to minimize prolonged stretch of the brachial plexus.[106,107] A washcloth, towel, or gauze roll placed in the palm helps hold the hand in a functional position. Pillows, high-top tennis shoes, towels, blankets, and foot boards help position the foot with a neutral ankle.[44] Positions of choice for a patient with burns are shown in Box 15-2 (see next page).

SPLINTS AND ORTHOSES

Hippocrates described burn scars as "tetanus," and Wilhelm Fabry illustrated a splint to treat a hand for hyperextension scar contractures.[16] In the early to mid-1900s, patients with burns were placed in splints immediately on admission to the hospital in an effort to prevent contraction; splints were removed for brief periods to permit wound care. Most burns were not covered by skin graft until at least 5 weeks after injury. The advent of surgical excision and grafting in the mid-1900s decreased the time required for a burn to heal. As a result, prophylactic splinting became a less common procedure, and in the late 1970s and early 1980s active exercise became the primary treatment method used by physical therapists working with burn patients.[44] The use of splints has, however, become a critical adjunct to active exercise and positioning of individuals with burns. The term *splint* is used in burn care more often than *orthosis*, even though the terms and the devices they represent are nearly synonymous.

Splints may have a multiplicity of purposes.[108] Splinting is often used to protect fragile wounds or newly grafted burn wounds. Splints are also used to position joints to maintain achieved ROM or as dynamic devices to apply gentle prolonged stretch to increase ROM. Splints cannot replace active exercise; contractures will form even in desirable positions if a patient is constantly splinted in a particular position. Static splints are designed to maintain a position of choice by immobilizing the joint.[109,110] Dynamic splints are designed to exercise or mobilize a joint.[110-113] A splint may also enhance the pressure applied to a scar by a pressure support. If unusual pain (other than from gentle tissue elongation or stretch), sensory impairment, or wound maceration occurs at the site of the splint, it must be removed and the fit adjusted.[114]

A splint should be fabricated with a proper, secure fit to minimize friction injuries or skin breakdown at pressure points. Pressure points over bony prominences are particularly vulnerable in this regard. Large, broad surface contact areas better distribute forces and reduce the likelihood of pressure-related tissue injury. The splint is worn only when it will not impede the functional activities or requisite exercises of the patient; splints are often donned during rest periods and at night when the patient is sleeping. The corners and edges of the splint are rounded and sometimes padded to avoid shear stresses. The design of the splint may also need to be adapted for orthopedic hardware such as surgical pins or for intravenous line sites. The splint design should, whenever possible, allow for ease of application and removal to enhance compliance among staff and family members who otherwise might struggle while maneuvering the splint.

Careful consideration should be given as to the rationale for the application of a splint in any clinical case.[115]

Material used in fabricating splints include thermoplastics, plaster, and elastomer compounds. Thermoplastics resource companies include Orthoplast (Johnson and Johnson, New Brunswick, NJ), Orfit (Orfit Industries, Jericho, NY), Supracor (Supracor Inc., San Jose, Calif.), and Hexalite (Reebok International, Canton, Mass.), among others. Hexalite and plaster are most often used to make temporary splints. Thermoplastic material, which can be remolded to adjust fit, make it an ideal splinting material for patients with burns. The amount of material to be used is determined by measuring the area to be splinted and the design of the splint. The splint is then molded to the individual. When the splinting material is set, or hardened, the splint should be inspected for correct fit to avoid pressure- and shear-related problems. Splints are often padded with gauze or any of the numerous cushion or foam materials available. For areas where fragile skin is problematic, foam is a soft alternative splinting material; however, it does not provide the same resistance to force that more rigid materials do. The advantages and disadvantages, as well as indications and contraindications of therapist-fabricated splinting and burn care, are summarized in Box 15-3. Although a number of appropriate splint designs for each anatomical site are possible, some are chosen more commonly than others and the choices are based on clinical indications and are not generally evidence based.[115]

Neck

The possible consequences of anterior neck burns include flexion contracture, facial disfiguration, loss of cosmetic contours of the neck, and difficulty with mastication.[114,116] A molded neck conformer splint helps prevent neck flexion contracture and provides compression on the forming scar. A rectangular piece of low-temperature thermoplastic splinting material is cut to span the distance from ear to ear along the jaw line and from below the lower lip to the sternoclavicular notch. After heating, the splint is molded directly on the patient's neck. Padding is added to protect vulnerable areas, and a hook-and-loop material strap is attached over the back of the neck to secure the splint.[114] Because this type of splint is occlusive and covers many bony prominences, the splint must be frequently removed to inspect the skin for any areas of irritation or breakdown.

For wounds that do not involve much of the chin, soft cervical collars have also been successful in providing positioning, pressure, and contour.[114,116] Although soft collars are more comfortable to wear, they do not extend over the chin for increased moment arm resistance. Commercially available Philadelphia collars may be an alternative. Watusi splints can also be designed to assist with conforming neck scarring and maintaining neck position.[117]

Axilla and Shoulder

Burns involving the axilla and shoulder may lead to adduction contracture and webbing of the axillary folds. This type of deformity contributes to difficulty in reaching and overhead use of the arm, components of many functional activities. A custom-fit conforming splint is often used to inhibit development of such contracture and webbing. Conforming splints for axillary burns support the entire arm, from the wrist through the axilla, and extend down the trunk to at least waist level.[118] The splint wraps around the trunk from umbilicus to spine, one third of the circumference of the chest, at the axilla around both folds, and one half of the circumference of the arm at the brachium, elbow, and wrist.[114,119,120] The splint is molded directly to the patient (flaring at the iliac crest may be necessary) and appropriate padding is applied. Hook-and-loop material strapping or other wraps around the trunk, shoulder, arm, and wrist secure the splint. A more traditional airplane splint may also be used to counteract the problems at the shoulder (Figure 15-4). Clavicle straps or soft foam may also be used to help conform the axillae.

Elbow and Forearm

The most common deformities caused by burns involving the elbow and forearm are elbow flexion and pronation contractures. The elbow joint is most often fit with a conformer splint designed as either an anterior or posterior gutter or trough (Figure 15-5).[114,116,119] The splint is fit to the arm from the proximal third of the brachium to the distal third of the forearm. Partial circumference measurements are taken at the proximal and distal sites and the elbow. The splint is molded directly on the patient, with padding added. The splint should be flared or "bubbled" at the bony prominences of the elbow. The splint is held in place by hook-and-loop material straps

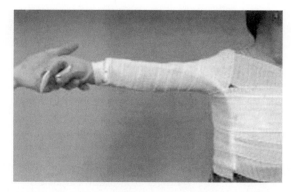

FIGURE 15-4 An example of a thermoplastic airplane splint designed to reduce the likelihood of development of an axillary contracture during burn healing. (Courtesy Shriners Hospitals for Children, Cincinnati Burn Hospital, Cincinnati, Ohio.)

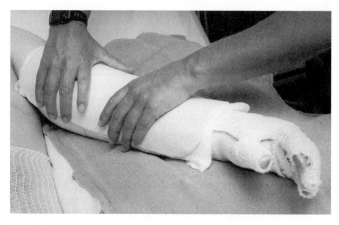

FIGURE 15-5 A thermoplastic anterior elbow gutter splint being custom fit for a patient with burns of the antecubital fossa.

or by circular gauze or elastic wrapping. Commercially available three-point extension or air splints may also be used.

Wrist and Hand

Burns of the wrist may lead to contractures in extension or flexion or ulnar or radial deviation, depending on the location of the burn. The prevention of flexion or extension contractures of the hand and fingers is important, as is maintenance of the web space of the thumb. Many different designs of wrists and hand splints exist; the best option for a particular individual is based on the anticontracture position of the joint or joint complex that is involved.

The most common splint used at the wrist and the hand is the Antideformity Splint.[114,116,119,121,123] This splint is designed to position the wrist and hand in the functional position. A modification of this splint, the pan splint, positions all finger joints in extension (Figure 15-6). Splints that conform to the thumb, thumb web space, and the index finger can help preserve the thumb web space.[114,116,119] Dorsal- or palmar-resting extension splints, used when the wrist has been burned but the hand is not damaged, may be custom molded or are commercially available. Finger gutter or trough splints are used to treat individual fingers, on the basis of the same principles used in elbow conformer splints.

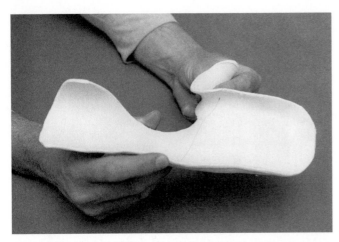

FIGURE 15-6 A thermoplastic pan splint that been molded to support the wrist in a functional position, with fingers in full extension.

Another easily fabricated splint that is useful to minimize formation of either flexion or extension contractures when multiple joints of the fingers have been burned is the sandwich splint.[116,122] Foam padding is attached to two pieces of splinting material that have been cut large enough to cover the hand. The burned hand is "sandwiched" between these two padded supports, which are held in place with a circumferential wrap (Figure 15-7).[124]

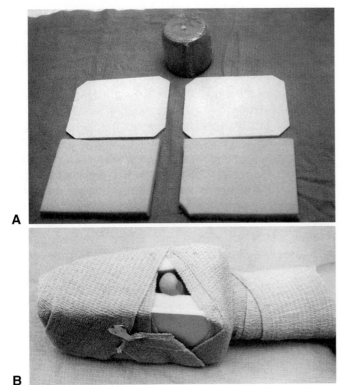

FIGURE 15-7 A, Materials used for a sandwich splint include thermoplastic splinting material, foam, and a compression wrap. **B,** A sandwich splint applied to the hand with burns. (From Ward RS, Schnebly WA, Kravitz M, et al. Have you tried the sandwich splint? A method of preventing hand deformities in children. *J Burn Care Rehabil* 1989;10[1]:83-85.)

Trunk and Pelvis

Patients with burns involving the anterior trunk are at risk for developing kyphosis. Clavicular straps in a figure-of-eight design have been used to position the shoulders in retraction and counteract the flexion forces in healing upper trunk burns.[114,116] Commercially available corsets or thoracolumbar spinal orthotics may be prescribed to help maintain posture for individuals with burns of the mid and lower trunk if it is being compromised by scar contracture.

For burns of the pelvis, groin, and hip, the problem is the likelihood of hip flexion and adduction contractures. Hip abduction splints reinforced with a spreader bar or an anterior hip spica splint may be necessary for some patients.[116]

Lower Extremity

At the knee, flexion contracture is an important concern. Splinting of the knee is similar to that of the elbow, adjusted to fit the longer segments of the lower extremity.[114,116,119,125] Although knee conformer splints are most often chosen for patients with burns involving the knee, three-point extension splints or air splints have also been used to reduce risk of flexion contracture as the burn scar matures.

Because of the complexity of structure and arthrokinematics, burns of the ankles and feet often present challenges for splinting similar to those of the wrist and hand. The location of the burn dictates whether the patient is at risk for contracture in either a plantar flexion or dorsiflexion direction (or both). Posterior foot drop splints, or anterior or posterior ankle conformers, are the most commonly fabricated ankle splints.[114,116,119] The distance from toes to calf is measured, and limb half-circumferences determine the width of the splint. After the desired splint pattern is cut from thermoplastic material, the splint is molded directly on the patient. Necessary padding is applied and the splint is flared at the malleoli and often on the posterior heel. Successful treatment of burns to the dorsum of feet can be difficult.

Another important consideration is the extrapolation of splint designs for other anatomical areas to a seemingly unrelated location. In 2001, Guild[126] reported an application of the designs from various splints for dorsal hand burns to a splint for the treatment of burns of the dorsal foot. The splint has a base and a dorsal thermoplastic piece that fits over the toes and is secured with a hook-and-loop material strap. This splint is intended to minimize or prevent contractures of the dorsal foot during scar maturation. "Bunny boots" and other commercial foot drop splints can also be used for positioning ankles that have been burned.[114] Molded leather shoes can be useful in positioning both the ankles and toes of involved feet.[116] High-top gym shoes provide a less expensive but similar option for foot splinting.[38,116] Toe conformer splints can be fabricated for the dorsal surface of the foot to prevent toe extension contracture.

Face and Mouth

Burns of the face can affect the eyes and eyelids, the contours of the face, and the soft tissue around the mouth.[127-130] Contracture of the mouth (microstomia) is particularly

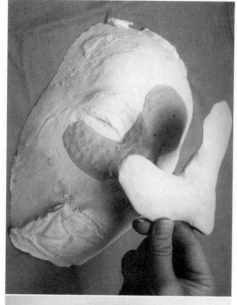

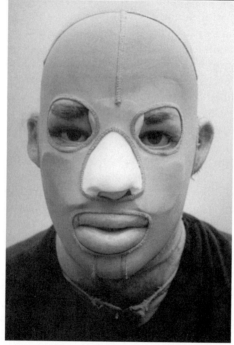

FIGURE 15-8 **A,** This elastomer mold of the patient's nose and cheeks will be reinforced with rigid thermoplastic material. **B,** When worn under a compression garment, the insert will deliver pressure more effectively to areas of the face than the compression garment alone. Splint inserts may help minimize ectropion (eversion) of the lower eyelids. Both would be worn during the maturation phase of healing to prevent excessive contracture and hypertrophic scarring. (From Ward RS. The rehabilitation of burn patients. *CRC Crit Rev Phys Med Rehabil* 1991;2[3]:121-138.)

troublesome because it interferes with feeding (and subsequently nutrition), speaking, and dental care.[131] Splints designed to support the functional contours of specific areas of the face are often fabricated (Figure 15-8). This type of splint helps decrease scar hypertrophy and minimize or prevent ectropion (eversion) deformity of the lower eyelids and the lips.

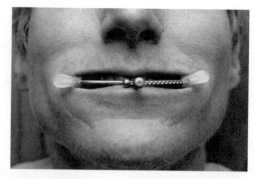

FIGURE 15-9 A microstomia prevention appliance is used to preserve the oral opening.

Microstomia prevention splints, designed to apply pressure or stretch to commissures and fibrotic oral muscles, are commercially available or may be custom made (Figure 15-9).[132-134] This type of splint or appliance is worn at all times when the patient is not eating or receiving oral care or is speaking.[134] In cases in which contracture affects the actual opening of the mouth, cone-shaped splints of thermoplastic material can be used to increase the opening of the mouth progressively. The cone is placed between the teeth after the mouth is opened. As the mouth is able to open wider, the narrower portions of the cone are cut off and the patient progresses to a wider part of the splint to widen the opening of the mouth.

Additional Considerations

Simple materials such as tongue depressors secured with gauze wrapping at various joints have been described as "splints."[135] Elastic wraps have also been used to increase ROM much like dynamic splints.[136,137] These methods may be useful as temporary devices but are not effective substitutes for more stable splinting materials.[136]

For patients with existing contractures, a serial splinting protocol is often used to assist in stretching the deformity. Plaster casts, thermoplastic materials, and Dynasplints (Dynasplint Systems Inc., Severna Park, Md.) have been successfully used in this manner.[138,139] Individually fabricated dynamic splints are also helpful for individuals with contracture after burns.

Any splint worn over an open wound may be a transfer agent for microorganisms from the burn.[140] In fact, organisms can be cultured from splint surfaces 50% of the time.[141] Effective strategies for cleaning burn splints are imperative. Simple washing and drying of the splint is not always effective in eliminating all organisms. The use of quaternary ammonia (1 oz per gallon of water) has been found to be 100% effective as a cleaning agent and is the recommended splint-cleaning strategy.[141]

Occasionally, special rehabilitative complications arise after burn injury, especially in patients who have sustained deep thermal wounds or an electrical injury. The most commonly encountered complications are exposed tendons and peripheral neuropathy with motor or sensory deficit. Splints can be useful in protecting or supporting these areas. Exposed tendons must be kept moist with an ointment-based gauze or biological dressing. The limb is splinted in a position where the tendon is slack, and exercise is avoided.[88] Idiopathic neuropathy occurs most often in patients with 20% or more TBSA burn involvement.[1] Secondary neuropathies may be caused by overelongation or compression of a peripheral nerve; such problems can be prevented by careful systematic monitoring of a patient's position, tightness of dressings, and the fit of splints and may be more common following deeper burn injury.[88,142,143] Splints may also be fit to overcome a temporary or long-term neurological deficit such as a drop foot.

CASE EXAMPLE 1

A Patient with Burns of Both Upper Extremities

M. J. is a 17-year-old girl who was injured in a house fire 3 weeks ago and sustained 11% TBSA burns to her face and both upper extremities. Facial burns were partial thickness in depth and spontaneously healed within 2 weeks. The burn injuries affecting both arms from midbrachium down each forearm and the dorsum of each hand were full thickness and required skin grafting for wound closure. Skin grafting procedures were completed during the first 2 weeks of hospitalization in a series of three surgeries.

Questions to Consider
- What tests and measures would be most appropriate to document and track changes in M. J.'s ROM, strength, endurance, and functional status? How might they need to be modified or adapted because of the severity of her burns?
- How will the medical care of her healing partial-thickness facial burns and her full-thickness, grafted upper extremity burns be similar or different in terms of pain control, likelihood of scarring, and wound care? What factors might influence maturation of burn scars in this young woman?
- At this point in time, what are the primary rehabilitation goals for this young woman? How do rehabilitation goals change over the stages of wound healing (inflammatory, proliferative, and maturation)?
- What joints are most at risk for developing contracture in the early phases of healing? What positions would be optimal to reduce risk of contracture development? What type of orthosis might you recommend at this time? What other interventions would be important to consider as she progresses through the stages of wound healing?
- What passive and active exercise strategies might you recommend to enhance ROM, flexibility of healing tissues, strength, and endurance?
- What education and supportive strategies might be necessary?
- How long would you expect M. J. to be involved in rehabilitation activities? How will you assess whether your interventions are accomplishing the rehabilitation goals?

Interventions and Outcomes
When M. J. is not immobilized after surgery, she is involved in a treatment program that includes upper extremity mobility exercises and strengthening exercises and an aerobic conditioning exercise program. Early ROM is generally mildly limited because of edema and wound contraction. After the skin-grafting procedures, ROM at all affected joints is improving, with the exception of declines in left elbow extension and left hand metacarpophalangeal flexion (digits 2 through 5). An anterior elbow-conforming splint is fabricated for the left arm and a functional position splint with approximately 40 degrees of metacarpophalangeal flexion is made for the left hand. Both splints are made of thermoplastic material and secured with hook-and-loop material strapping. These splints are applied during rest periods, naps, and during the night to prevent further loss of ROM. When awake, M. J. participates in therapy sessions and a home program of passive stretching and active exercise of all the affected joints, with emphasis on the troublesome left elbow and hand. Use of the splints is discontinued after 2 weeks because the ROM has improved to normal.

AMPUTATION AND PROSTHESES IN BURN REHABILITATION

Electrical burn injuries are more likely to lead to amputation than any other types of burns. Significant damage occurs as electrical current passes through nerve tissue, vascular tissue, and other deep structures. The current can cause destruction of cells, coagulation of tissues, thrombosis of blood vessels, neuropathies, and tissue necrosis. Other types of burn injuries and frostbite injuries may necessitate amputation if the wound is very deep or has associated tissue trauma. Some amputations, however, can be the consequence of an unrelenting infection.

Patients with burns who require limb amputation may have complications that delay prosthetic fitting and training as a result of multiple wound or scar sites, skin grafting on the residual limb, repeated surgical procedures (not necessarily associated with the residual limb), and burn-induced catabolic atrophy. Individuals with burns are also susceptible to the same postoperative complications faced by any patient with a new amputation: edema, phantom pain, and formation of neuroma or bone spur. Patients with amputation as a result of electrical injury may be susceptible to the formation of bone spurs.[144] Otherwise, heterotopic bone formation does not appear to be more prevalent in a burn population. Edema after burn injury is generally a short-term problem and seldom creates long-term delays in prosthetic training. There are no reports that suggest individuals with burns with amputations are more likely to develop phantom limb pain than other patients with amputation.[145]

Any of these complications may intensify discomfort or the amount of work and time required for prosthetic training, which can be reasons for limited use or rejection of the prosthesis. Despite these concerns, patients with burn-related amputations are successfully rehabilitated with standard protocols.[146-148]

Skin Condition

For individuals with skin graft sites on the residual limb, fragility of skin (its tolerance of pressure and shear forces) is an important concern. Blisters or small open wounds may appear where a skin graft or a fragile scar breaks down as a result of forces on the residual limb during gait. Wearing of the prosthesis is often discontinued until the new wound is adequately healed. Wounds or skin grafts on areas associated with the prosthesis use, such as the shoulder or scapula under an upper extremity prosthetic harness, may demonstrate these same initial problems with wound breakdown. Even though the presence of a skin graft or fragile scar may delay or prolong prosthetic training, most patients with burn-related amputation are eventually successful in using their prostheses on skin-grafted limbs.[146-150] New "antishear" prosthetic socket suspension and lining materials may be especially helpful for individuals with burn-related amputation.

Contracture

The typical postamputation contracture in patients with burns is a result of muscle and soft tissue shortening related to a decreased moment arm of the affected extremity. When there is a maturing burn scar or graft site over the joint of the residual limb, the risk of contracture significantly increases (Figure 15-10). Such contractures may form more rapidly with the additional shortening force of the contracting scar tissue (Figure 15-11). The prevention of joint contracture after amputation requires vigilant positioning and stretching, which may be augmented by knee extension splints for individuals with transtibial amputation.

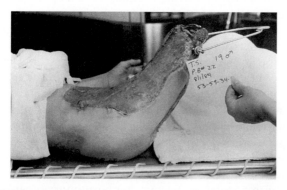

FIGURE 15-10 This patient with burn-related transfemoral amputation has increased risk of flexion contracture caused by scarring of the graft sites over the anterior surface of the hip. (From Ward RS, Hayes-Lundy C, Schnebly WS, et al. Rehabilitation of burn patients with concomitant limb amputation: case reports. *Burns* 1990;16[5]:390-392.)

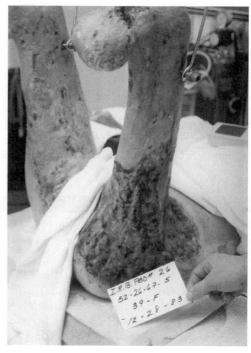

FIGURE 15-11 This patient has sustained bilateral transtibial amputation as a result of severe burn injury. She is at risk of significant knee flexion contracture because of the positioning required for her burn care and the inevitable contraction and scarring of her extensive graft sites. The areas of skin graft in her distal residual limbs may not initially tolerate the pressure and shear forces associated with prosthetic use, leading to delays in prosthetic fit and training.

Delayed Fitting

For patients with large TBSA burns, repeated surgical skin-grafting procedures are often necessary to cover the burn wound adequately. Repeated surgical procedures often delay prosthetic fitting and training. Individuals may be placed on postoperative bed rest for up to 7 days to ensure initial healing of the grafted area. To protect the new graft site and promote healing, the limb may be temporarily positioned in a less than optimal position for prosthetic use. Continued monitoring by the therapist, along with conscientious wrapping of the residual limb, can help overcome some of the problems caused by successive surgeries.

Stabilization of Body Weight

It is common for patients with burns to lose weight because of hypermetabolism. A large burn can nearly double the body's metabolic requirements. Although individuals with significant burns receive nutritional supplementation, this often slows but does not prevent catabolic weight loss. Most individuals regain the weight lost in the catabolic process; this may require a series of revisions or refabrications of temporary sockets until weight stabilizes enough to fit a permanent prosthesis.

A Patient with Amputation After Electrical Burns

C. T. is a 32-year-old man who was injured when a metal ladder he was using to trim tree branches made contact with overhead electrical wires. He sustained 35% TBSA burns to his face, trunk, both upper extremities (including the right axilla), and his right lower leg. A right transhumeral amputation and a right transtibial amputation were required because of significant tissue damage from the electrical current. The amputations were performed on the third day after the burn; both residual limbs required several revisions of the amputation sites. Both residual limbs were successfully covered with a skin graft by the sixth day after the initial amputation.

Questions to Consider

- What tests and measures would be most appropriate to document and track changes in C. T.'s ROM, strength, endurance, and functional status? How might they need to be modified or adapted because of the severity of his burns?
- Given the cause of his burns, what are the possible issues related to wound healing, contracture formation, and preprosthetic care that will influence your clinical decision making? What are the most pressing rehabilitation goals considering both his burns and his amputations in this early period of rehabilitation? In the months ahead?
- What will pain management and wound healing be like for someone like C. T., who has undergone amputation after electrocution, compared with someone with thermal burns who has had skin grafting?
- What factors will influence C. T.'s readiness for prosthetic fitting for this transtibial limb? For his transhumeral limb? What is C. T.'s prognosis for prosthetic use at both transtibial and transhumeral levels? How might the presence of skin grafts influence the prosthetist's recommendation for socket type and suspension of the prostheses? How will maturation of the residual limb and likely changes in body weight over time influence prosthetic fit and function?
- What are the key components in your preprosthetic plan of care for C. T.'s residual limbs? How might tissue healing influence his progression through prosthetic training? What passive and active exercise strategies might you recommend to enhance ROM, flexibility of healing tissues, strength, and endurance?
- What education and supportive strategies might be necessary for this young man with serious burns and amputation?
- How long would you expect C. T. to be involved in rehabilitation activities? How will you assess whether your interventions are accomplishing the rehabilitation goals?

Interventions and Outcomes

Although C. T. was fitted with a transtibial prosthesis within 3 weeks of skin grafting, the fitting of C. T.'s initial upper extremity prosthesis must be postponed because of the time required to obtain closure of the remaining burn wounds on the right upper extremity (6 weeks). Given the extent of his burns, signal sites for a myoelectric (externally powered) prosthesis are difficult to identify; thus, C. T. is fit with a conventional body-powered transhumeral prosthesis with a hook as a terminal device. (See Chapters 30 and 31 for more information about prosthetic options and rehabilitation for individuals with upper extremity amputation.) Deep burns on both shoulders and the left trunk further delay (10 weeks) this fitting because of intolerance of the newly healed skin to the prosthetic harness.

C. T. quickly becomes functional with his transtibial prosthesis although susceptibility to pressure requires a special antishear, pressure-distributing liner. (See Chapters 23 and 26 for more information on prosthetic options and rehabilitation for patients with transtibial amputation.) During the fitting and training delays for his transhumeral prosthesis, an aggressive treatment program, including mobility exercises and strengthening exercises, is directed at the right upper extremity. The residual limb is also shaped with compression wraps and stockinet. C. T. also participates in similar mobility and strengthening exercises for other affected areas as well as an aerobic exercise program aimed at improving his endurance.

Twelve weeks after injury, C. T. is fit for and begins formal training with his prosthesis (dual-control cable system). There is one incident of skin breakdown under the harness over the left scapula. This area is dressed and padded with dense foam. There are no further incidences of skin breakdown. C. T. is discharged from physical therapy associated with the amputation 15 weeks after injury.

During his episode of care for rehabilitation and prosthetic training, C.T. endured several delays in management of his amputations as a result of the care related to other burn injuries, particularly those in strategic anatomical regions. It was important to maintain focus on preparation of the transtibial residual limb for containment within and functional use of the prosthesis and to prepare his transhumeral residual limb and opposite arms for the figure-of-eight harness and control system. Much of C.T.'s rehabilitation care concentrated on mobility ROM, and strength (especially of his upper extremities and the shoulder girdle) and endurance training.

EDUCATION

The patient with burns is the most important member of the rehabilitative burn care team. Family members and any others who will be caregivers outside the hospital must be included as early as possible to learn about the process of burn recovery and rehabilitation. Effectiveness of education is reflected by the individual's and caregiver's ability to demonstrate knowledge and understanding of the rehabilitation program.[151] Skin care, exercise programs, use of pressure supports, positioning techniques, and splint protocols are the obvious items that need to be taught to the patient.[152,153] Reinforcement, reasoning, and reassurance are key words to remember when designing an educational process.

SUMMARY

Optimal care of individuals recovering from burn injury taps the knowledge and skills of many different health care providers. Rehabilitation professionals are actively involved in many facets of postburn care, such as wound care and surgical grafting procedures; education about the burn rehabilitation process; and preventive care to minimize risk of hypertrophic scarring, contractures, deformity, and subsequent disability. Postburn rehabilitation care requires knowledge of and expertise in splint design and fabrication, exercise prescription (stretching and flexibility, strengthening, endurance), adaptive and assistive devices for gait and activities of daily living, and often prosthetic prescription and training.

REFERENCES

1. Petro JA, Salisbury RE. Rehabilitation of the burn patient. *Clin Plast Surg.* 1986;13(1):145–150.
2. Helm PA, Head MD, Pullium G, et al. Burn rehabilitation: a team approach. *Surg Clin North Am.* 1978;58(6):1263–1278.
3. American Burn Association. *Burn Incidence and Treatment in the US: 2011 Fact Sheet.* Chicago, IL: American Burn Association, 60611 Retrieved February 28, 2011, from www.ameriburn.org.
4. Ryan MR, Schoenfeld DA, Thorpe WP, et al. Objective estimates of the probability of death from burn injuries. *N Engl J Med.* 1998;338:362–366.
5. Bessey PQ, Arons RR, Dimaggio CJ, et al. The vulnerabilities of age: burns in children and older adults. *Surgery.* 2006;140:715–717.
6. Burn center referral criteria. *Guidelines for the operation of burn centers resources for optimal care of the injured patient.* Chicago, IL: Committee on Trauma, American College of Surgeons; 2006:79–86.
7. Van Rijin OJL, Bouter LM, Meertens RM. The aetiology of burns in developed countries: review of the literature. *Burns.* 1989;15(4):217–221.
8. Pruitt Jr BA, Mason Jr AD. Epidemiological, demographic and outcomes characteristics of burn injury. In: Herndon DN, ed. *Total Burn Care.* 3rd ed. Philadelphia: Saunders; 2007:20–23.
9. Dissanaike S, Rahimi M. Epidemiology of burn injuries: highlighting cultural and socio-demographic aspects. *Int Rev Psychiatry.* 2009;21:505–511.
10. Guzel A, Aksu B, Aylanc H, et al. Scalds in pediatric emergency department: a 5-year experience. *J Burn Care Res.* 2009;30:450–456.
11. Renz BM, Sherman R. The burn unit experience at Grady Memorial Hospital: 844 cases. *J Burn Care Rehabil.* 1992; 13:426–436.
12. Herbert K, Lawrence JC. Chemical burns. *Burns.* 1989; 15(6):381–384.
13. Monafo WW, Freedman BM. Electrical and lightning injury. In: Boswick JA, ed. *The Art and Science of Burn Care.* Rockville, MD: Aspen; 1987:241–253.
14. Haberal M. Electrical burns: a five years experience. *J Trauma.* 1986;26(2):103–109.
15. Cancio LC, Jimenez-Reyna JF, Barillo DJ, et al. One hundred ninety-five cases of high-voltage electric injury. *J Burn Care Rehabil.* 2005;26(4):331–340.
16. Thomsen M. It all began with Aristotle: the history of the treatment of burns. *Burns Incl Therm Inj.* 1988;(suppl):S1–S46.
17. Richard RL, Ward RS. Burns. In: O'Sullivan SB, Schmitz, ed. *Physical Rehabilitation.* Philadelphia: FA Davis; 2007:1093–1097.
18. Miller SF, et al. Surgical management of the burn patient. In: Richard RL, Staley MJ, eds. *Burn Care and Rehabilitation: Principles and Practice.* Philadelphia: FA Davis; 1994:180.
19. Mosier MJ, Gibran NS. Surgical excision of the burn wound. *Clin Plast Surg.* 2009;36(4):617–625.
20. Jones T, McDonald S, Deitch EA. Effect of graft bed on long-term functional results of extremity skin grafts. *J Burn Care Rehabil.* 1988;9(1):72–74.
21. Sheridan R. Closure of the excised burn wound: autografts, semipermanent skin substitutes, and permanent skin substitutes. *Clin Plast Surg.* 2009;36:643–651.
22. Chern PL, Baum CL, Arpey CJ. Biologic dressings: current applications and limitations in dermatologic surgery. *Dermatol Surg.* 2009;35:891–906.
23. Fohn M, Bannasch H. Artificial skin. *Methods Mol Med.* 2007;140:167–182.
24. Desai MH, Mlakar JM, McCauley RL, et al. Lack of long-term durability of cultured keratinocyte burn-wound coverage: a case report. *J Burn Care Rehabil.* 1991;12(6):540–545.
25. Stern R, McPherson M, Longaker MT. Histologic study of artificial skin used in the treatment of full-thickness thermal injury. *J Burn Care Rehabil.* 1990;11(1):7–13.
26. Lund CC, Browder NC. The estimation of areas of burns. *Surg Gynecol Obstet.* 1944;79:352–358.
27. Artz C, Saroff HS. Modern concepts in the treatment of burns. *JAMA.* 1955;159:411–417.
28. Singer AJ, McClain SA. Persistent wound infection delays epidermal wound maturation and increases scarring in thermal burns. *Wound Repair Regen.* 2002;10:372–377.
29. Ward RS, Saffle JR. Topical agents in burn and wound care. *Phys Ther.* 1995;75(6):526–538.
30. Weber J, McManus A. Infection control in burn patients. *Burns.* 2004;30:A16–A24.
31. Saffle JR, Schnebly WA. Burn wound care. In: Richard RL, Staley MJ, eds. *Burn Care and Rehabilitation: Principles and Practice.* Philadelphia: FA Davis; 1994:19–176.
32. Wright PC. Fundamentals of acute burn care and physical therapy management. *Phys Ther.* 1984;64(8):1217–1231.
33. Ward RS. The rehabilitation of burn patients. *CRC Crit Rev Phys Med Rehabil.* 1991;2(3):121–138.
34. Steiner H, Clark WR. Psychiatric complications of burned adults: a classification. *J Trauma.* 1977;17(2):134–143.
35. Williams EE, Griffiths TA. Psychological consequences of burn injury. *Burns.* 1991;17(6):478–480.
36. Smith JS, Smith KR, Rainey SL. The psychology of burn care. *J Trauma Nurs.* 2006;13(3):105–106.
37. Dyster-Aas J, Willebrand M, Wikehult B, Gerdin B, Ekselius L. Major depression and posttraumatic stress disorder symptoms following severe burn injury in relation to lifetime psychiatric morbidity. *J Trauma Inj Infect Crit Care.* 2008;64(5):1349–1356.

38. Goodstein RK. Burns: an overview of clinical consequences affecting patient, staff, and family. *Compr Psychiatry.* 1985;26(1):43–57.

39. Stoddard FJ. Body image development in the burned child. *J Am Acad Child Psychiatry.* 1982;21(5):502–507.

40. Mahaney MB. Restoration of play in a severely burned three-year-old child. *J Burn Care Rehabil.* 1990;11(1):57–63.

41. Watkins PN, Cook EL, May SR, et al. Psychological stages of adaptation following burn injury: a method for facilitating psychological recovery of burn victims. *J Burn Care Rehabil.* 1988;9(4):376–384.

42. Tollison CD, Still JM, Tollison JW. The seriously burned adult: psychologic reactions, recovery and management. *J Med Assoc Ga.* 1980;69(2):121–124.

43. American Physical Therapy Association. *Guide to Physical Therapist Practice.* 2nd ed. Alexandria, Va: American Physical Therapy Association; 2001.

44. Schnebly WA, Ward RS, Warden GD, et al. A nonsplinting approach to the care of the thermally injured patient. *J Burn Care Rehabil.* 1989;10(3):263–266.

45. Ward RS. Pressure therapy for the control of hypertrophic scar formation after burn injury: a history and review. *J Burn Care Rehabil.* 1991;12(3):257–262.

46. Li B, Wang JH. Fibroblasts and myofibroblasts in wound healing: force generation and measurement. *J Tissue Viability.* 2011;20(4):108–120.

47. Shin D, Minn KW. The effect of myofibroblast on contracture of hypertrophic scar. *Plast Reconstr Surg.* 2004;113:633–640.

48. Nedelec B, Ghahary A, Scott PG, et al. Control of wound contraction. Basic and clinical features. *Hand Clin.* 2000;16:289–302.

49. Hardy MA. The biology of scar formation. *Phys Ther.* 1989;69(12):1014–1024.

50. Steed DL. Wound-healing trajectories. *Surg Clin North Am.* 2003;83:547–555, vi–vii.

51. Ladin DA, Garner WL, Smith Jr DJ. Excessive scarring as a consequence of healing. *Wound Repair Regen.* 1995;3:6–14.

52. Armour A, Scott PG, Tredget EE. Cellular and molecular pathology of HTS: basis for treatment. *Wound Repair Regen.* 2007;15(suppl 1):S6–S17.

53. Burd A, Huang L. Hypertrophic response and keloid diathesis: two very different forms of scar. *Plast Reconstr Surg.* 2005;116:150e–157e.

54. Kose O, Waseem A. Keloids and hypertrophic scars: are they two different sides of the same coin? *Dermatol Surg.* 2008;34:336–346.

55. Slemp AE, Kirschner RE. Keloids and scars: a review of keloids and scars, their pathogenesis, risk factors, and management. *Curr Opin Pediatr.* 2006;18:396–402.

56. Hunt TK. Disorders of wound healing. *World J Surg.* 1980;4(3):289–295.

57. Clark JA, Cheng JCY, Leung KS, et al. Mechanical characterization of human postburn hypertrophic skin during pressure therapy. *J Biomech.* 1987;20(4):397–406.

58. Rudolf R. Wide spread scars, hypertrophic scars, and keloids. *Clin Plast Surg.* 1987;14(2):253–260.

59. Gangemi EN, Gregori D, Berchialla P, et al. Epidemiology and risk factors for pathologic scarring after burn wounds. *Arch Facial Plast Surg.* 2008;10(2):93–102.

60. Rockwell WB, Cohen IK, Erlich HP. Keloids and hypertrophic scars: a comprehensive review. *Plast Reconstr Surg.* 1989;84:827–837.

61. Davies D. Scars, hypertrophic scars, and keloids. *BMJ.* 1985;290(6474):1056–1058.

62. Deitch EA, Wheelahan TM, Rose MP. Hypertrophic burn scars: analysis of variables. *J Trauma.* 1983;23(10):895–898.

63. Rudolf R. Construction and the control of contraction. *World J Surg.* 1980;4(2):279–287.

64. Stern PJ, Law EJ, Benedict FE, et al. Surgical treatment of elbow contractures in postburn children. *Plast Reconstr Surg.* 1985;76(3):441–446.

65. Schneider JC, Holavanahalli R, Helm P, et al. Contractures in burn injury: defining the problem. *J Burn Care Res.* 2006;27(4):508–514.

66. Wainwright DJ. Burn reconstruction: the problems, the techniques, and the applications. *Clin Plast Surg.* 2009;36(4):687–700.

67. Kreymerman PA, Andres LA, Lucas HD, et al. Reconstruction of the burned hand. *Plast Reconstr Surg.* 2011;127(2):752–759.

68. Larson DL, Abston S, Evans EB, et al. Techniques for decreasing scar formation and contractures in the burned patient. *J Trauma.* 1971;11(10):807–823.

69. Kischer CW, Shetlar MR, Shetlar CL. Alteration of hypertrophic scars induced by mechanical pressure. *Arch Dermatol.* 1975;111(1):60–64.

70. Leung PC, Ng M. Pressure treatment for hypertrophic scars. *Burns.* 1980;6:224.

71. Ward RS. Pressure therapy for the control of hypertrophic scar formation after burn injury: a history and review. *J Burn Care Rehabil.* 1991;12(1):257–262.

72. Torring S. Our routine in pressure treatment of hypertrophic scars. *Scand J Plast Reconstr Surg.* 1984;18(1):135–137.

73. Ward RS, Hayes-Lundy C, Reddy R, et al. Influence of pressure supports on joint range of motion. *Burns.* 1992;18(1):60–62.

74. Sullivan T, Smith J, Kerrnode J, et al. Rating the burn scar. *J Burn Care Rehabil.* 1990;11(3):256–260.

75. Lowell M, Pirc P, Ward RS, et al. Effect of 3M Coban Self-Adherent Wraps on edema and function of the burned hand: a case study. *J Burn Care Rehabil.* 2003;24(4):253–258 discussion 252.

76. Ward RS, Reddy R, Brockway C, et al. Uses of Coban self-adherent wrap in management of postburn hand grafts: case reports. *J Burn Care Rehabil.* 1994;15(4):364–369.

77. Rose MP, Deitch EA. The clinical use of a tubular compression bandage, Tubigrip, for burn-scar therapy: a critical analysis. *Burns Incl Therm Inj.* 1985;12(1):58–64.

78. Powell BW, Haylock C, Clarke JA. A semi-rigid transparent face mask in the treatment of postburn hypertrophic scars. *Br J Plast Surg.* 1985;38(4):561–566.

79. O'Brien L, Pandit A. Silicon gel sheeting for preventing and treating hypertrophic and keloid scars. *Cochrane Database Syst Rev.* 2006:CD003826.

80. Berman B, Perez OA, Konda S, et al. A review of the biologic effects, clinical efficacy, and safety of silicone elastomer sheeting for hypertrophic and keloid scar treatment and management. *Dermatol Surg.* 2007;33:1291–1302; discussion 302–303.

81. Dobbs ER, Curreri PW. Burns: analysis of results of physical therapy in 681 patients. *J Trauma.* 1972;12(3):242–248.

82. Parry SW. Reconstruction of the burned hand. *Clin Plast Surg.* 1989;16(3):577–586.

83. Howell JW. Management of the acutely burned hand for the nonspecialized clinician. *Phys Ther.* 1989;12(12):1077–1089.

84. Parrot M, Ryan R, Parks DH, et al. Structured exercise circuit program for burn patients. *J Burn Care Rehabil.* 1988;9(6):666–668.

85. Whitehead C, Serghiou M. A 12-year comparison of common therapeutic interventions in the burn unit. *J Burn Care Res.* 2009;30(2):281–287.

86. de Lateur BJ, Magyar-Russell G, Bresnick MG, et al. Augmented exercise in the treatment of deconditioning from major burn injury. *Arch Phys Med Rehabil.* 2007;88(12 suppl 2):S18–S23.

87. Trees DW, Ketelsen CA, Hobbs JA. Use of a modified tilt table for preambulation strength training as an adjunct to burn rehabilitation: a case series. *J Burn Care Rehabil.* 2003;24(2):97–103.

88. Helm PA, Kevorkian CG, Lushbaugh M, et al. Burn injury: rehabilitation management in 1982. *Arch Phys Med Rehabil.* 1982;63(1):6–16.

89. Chen HC, Yang JY, Chuang SS, et al. Heterotopic ossification in burns: our experience and literature reviews. *Burns.* 2009;35(6):857–862.

90. Crawford CM, Vaeghese G, Mani M, et al. Heterotopic ossification: are range of motion exercises contraindicated? *J Burn Care Rehabil.* 1986;6(4):323–327.

91. VanLaeken N, Snelling CFT, Meek RN, et al. Heterotopic bone formation in the patient with burn injuries: a retrospective assessment of contributing factors and methods of investigation. *J Burn Care Rehabil.* 1989;10(4):331–335.

92. Tafel JA, Thacker JG, Hagemann JM, et al. Mechanical performance of exertubing for isotonic hand exercise. *J Burn Care Rehabil.* 1987;8(4):333–335.

93. Johnson CL. Physical therapists as scar modifiers. *Phys Ther.* 1984;64(9):1381–1387.

94. Richard RL, Miller SF, Finley RK, et al. Home exercise kit for the shoulder. *J Burn Care Rehabil.* 1987;8(2):144–145.

95. Carrougher GJ. Burn wound assessment and topical treatment. In: Carrougher GJ, ed. *Burn Care and Therapy.* St. Louis: Mosby; 1998:142.

96. Apfel LM, Wachtel TL, Frank DH, et al. Functional electrical stimulation in intrinsic/extrinsic imbalanced burned hands. *J Burn Care Rehabil.* 1987;8(2):97–102.

97. Lewis SM, Clelland JA, Knowles CJ, et al. Effects of auricular acupuncture-like transcutaneous nerve stimulation on pain levels following wound care in patients with burns: a pilot study. *J Burn Care Rehabil.* 1990;11(4):322–329.

98. Bierman W. Ultrasound in the treatment of scars. *Arch Phys Med Rehabil.* 1954;35:209–214.

99. Baryza MJ. Ultrasound in the treatment of postburn skin graft contracture: a single case study. *Phys Ther.* 1996;76:S54.

100. Ward RS, Hayes-Lundy C, Reddy R, et al. Evaluation of therapeutic ultrasound to improve response to physical therapy and lessen scar contracture after burn injury. *J Burn Care Rehabil.* 1994;15(1):74–79.

101. Covey MH, Dutcher K, Marvin JA, et al. Efficacy of continuous passive motion (CPM) devices with hand burns. *J Burn Care Rehabil.* 1988;9(4):397–400.

102. Head M, Helm P. Paraffin and sustained stretching in treatment of burn contracture. *Burns.* 1977;4(2):136–139.

103. Ward RS, Saffle JR, Schnebly WA, et al. Sensory loss over grafted areas in patients with burns. *J Burn Care Rehabil.* 1989;10(6):536–538.

104. Ward RS, Tuckett RP. Quantitative threshold changes in cutaneous sensation of patients with burns. *J Burn Care Rehabil.* 1991;12(6):569–575.

105. Serghiou M, Cowan A, Whitehead C. Rehabilitation after a burn injury. *Clin Plast Surg.* 2009;36:675–686.

106. Cooper S, Paul EO. An effective method of positioning the burn patient. *J Burn Care Rehabil.* 1988;9(3):288–289.

107. Heeter PK, Brown R. Arm hammock for elevation of the thermally injured upper extremity. *J Burn Care Rehabil.* 1986;7(2):144–147.

108. Richard R, Ward RS. Splinting strategies and controversies. *J Burn Care Rehabil.* 2005;26:392–396.

109. Waymack JP, Fidler J, Warden GD. Surgical correction of burn scar contractures of the foot in children. *Burns.* 1988;4(2):156–160.

110. Duncan RM. Basic principles of splinting the hand. *Phys Ther.* 1989;69(12):1104–1116.

111. Richard RL. Use of Dynasplint to correct elbow flexion burn contracture: a case report. *J Burn Care Rehabil.* 1986;7:151.

112. Richard RL, et al. Dynamic versus static splints: a prospective case for sustained stress. *J Burn Care Rehabil.* 1995;16:284.

113. Richard R, Miller S, Staley M, Johnson RM. Multimodal versus progressive treatment techniques to correct burn scar contractures. *J Burn Care Rehabil.* 2000;21:506.

114. Malick MH, Carr JA. *Manual on Management of the Burn Patient.* Pittsburgh: Harnarville Rehabilitation Center; 1982: 32–62.

115. Richard R, Ward RS. Splinting strategies and controversies. *J Burn Care Rehabil.* 2005;26(5):392–396.

116. Daugherty MB, Carr-Collins JA. Splinting techniques for the burn patient. In: Richard RL, Staley MJ, eds. *Burn Care and Rehabilitation Principles and Practice.* Philadelphia: FA Davis; 1994:242–317.

117. Mathew Jose R, Varghese S, Nandakumar UR. Modified Watusi splint: a simple and economical device. *Br J Plast Surg.* 2002;55(3):270.

118. Manigandan C, Gupta AK, Venugopal K, et al. The wrist in axillary burns—a forgotten focus of concern. *Burns.* 2003; 29(5):497–498.

119. Walters C. *Splinting the Burn Patient.* Laurel, MD: RAMSCO; 1987: 9–97.

120. Manigandan C, Gupta AK, Venugopal K, et al. A multi-purpose, self-adjustable aeroplane splint for the splinting of axillary burns. *Burns.* 2003;29(3):276–279.

121. Kwan MW, Ha KW. Splinting programme for patients with burnt hand. *Hand Surg.* 2002;7(2):231–241.

122. Van Straten O, Sagi A. "Supersplint": a new dynamic combination splint for the burned hand. *J Burn Care Rehabil.* 2000;2:71–73.

123. Tilley W, McMahon S, Shukalak B. Rehabilitation of the burned upper extremity. *Hand Clin.* 2000;16(2):303–318.

124. Ward RS, Schnebly WA, Kravitz M, et al. Have you tried the sandwich splint? A method of preventing hand deformities in children. *J Burn Care Rehabil.* 1989;10(1):83–85.

125. Yildirim S, Avci G, Akan M, et al. Anterolateral thigh flap in the treatment of postburn flexion contractures of the knee. *Plast Reconstr Surg.* 2003;19(4):225–233.

126. Guild S. A new splinting approach for dorsal foot burns. *J Burn Care Rehabil.* 2001;22:454–456.

127. Kung TA, Gosain AK. Pediatric facial burns. *J Craniofac Surg.* 2008;19(4):951–959.

128. Dougherty ME, Warden GD. A thirty-year review of oral appliances used to manage microstomia, 1972 to 2002. *J Burn Care Rehabil.* 2003;24(6):418–431, discussion 410.

129. Lehman CJ. Splints and accessories following burn reconstruction. *Clin Plast Surg.* 1992;19(3):721–731.

130. Taylor LB, Walker J. A review of selected microstomia prevention appliances. *Pediatr Dent.* 1997;19(6):413–418.

131. Moore DJ. The role of the maxillofacial prosthetist in support of the burn patient. *J Prosthet Dent.* 1970;24(1):68–76.

132. Wust KJ. A modified dynamic mouth splint for burn patients. *J Burn Care Res.* 2006;27(1):86–92.

133. Heinle JA, Kealey GP, Cram AE, et al. The microstomia prevention appliance: 14 years of clinical experience. *J Burn Care Rehabil.* 1988;9(1):90–91.

134. Sela M, Tubiana L. A mouth splint for severe burns of the head and neck. *J Prosthet Dent.* 1989;62(6):679–681.

135. Kaufman T, Newman RA, Weinberg A, et al. The kerlix tongue depressor splint for skin-grafted areas in burned children. *J Burn Care Rehabil.* 1989;10(5):462–463.

136. Wilder RP, Doctor A, Paley RJ, et al. Evaluation of cohesive and elastic bandages for joint immobilization. *J Burn Care Rehabil.* 1989;10(3):258–262.

137. Richard RL, Miller SF, Finley Jr RK, et al. Comparison of the effect of passive exercise vs static wrapping on finger range of motion of the hand. *J Burn Care Rehabil.* 1987;8(6):576–578.

138. Richard RL. Use of the Dynasplint to correct elbow flexion burn contracture: a case report. *J Burn Care Rehabil.* 1986;7(2):151–152.

139. Bennett GB, Helm P, Purdue GF, et al. Serial casting: a method for treating burn contractures. *J Burn Care Rehabil.* 1989;10(6):543–545.

140. Faoagali JL, Grant D, Pegg S. Are thermolabile splints a source of nosocomial infection? *J Hosp Infect.* 1994;26(1):51–55.

141. Wright MP, Taddonio TE, Prasad JK, et al. The microbiology and cleaning of thermoplastic splints in burn care. *J Burn Care Rehabil.* 1989;10(1):79–83.

142. Lee MY, Liu G, Kowlowitz V, et al. Causative factors affecting peripheral neuropathy in burn patients. *Burns.* 2009;35(3):412–416.

143. Helm PA. Peripheral neurological problems in acute burn patients. *Burns.* 1977;3(2):123–125.

144. Helm PA, Walker SC. New bone formation at amputation sites in electrically burn-injured patients. *Arch Phys Med Rehabil.* 1987;68(5 part 1):284–286.

145. Thomas CR, Brazeal BA, Rosenberg L, et al. Phantom limb pain in pediatric burn survivors. *Burns.* 2003;29(2):139–142.

146. Ward RS, Hayes-Lundy C, Schnebly WS, et al. Rehabilitation of burn patients with concomitant limb amputation: case reports. *Burns.* 1990;16(5):390–392.

147. Ward RS, Hayes-Lundy C, Schnebly WS, et al. Prosthetic use in patients with burns and associated limb amputation. *J Burn Care Rehabil.* 1990;11(4):361–364.

148. Meier RH. Amputations and prosthetic fitting. In: Fisher SA, Helm PA, eds. *Comprehensive Rehabilitation of Burns.* Baltimore: Williams & Wilkins; 1984:267–310.

149. Rosenfelder R. The below-knee amputee with skin grafts. *Phys Ther.* 1970;50(9):1338–1346.

150. Wood MR, Hunter GA, Millstein SG. The value of stump split skin grafting following amputation for trauma in adult upper and lower limb amputees. *Prosthet Orthot Int.* 1987;11(2):71–74.

151. Wallace LM, Lees J. A psychological follow-up study of adult patients discharged from a British burn Unit. *Burns.* 1988;14(1):39–45.

152. Kaplan SH. Patient education techniques used at burn centers. *Am J Occup Ther.* 1985;39(10):655–658.

153. Neville C, Walker S, Brown B, et al. Discharge planning for burn patients. *J Burn Care Rehabil.* 1988;9(4):414–418.

16

Adaptive Seating in the Management of Neuromuscular and Musculoskeletal Impairment

Barbara Crane

LEARNING OBJECTIVES

On completion of this chapter, the reader will be able to do the following:

1. Describe the population of individuals who use wheelchairs and adaptive seating.
2. Identify the elements of a basic wheelchair and seating evaluation.
3. List potential outcomes for adaptive seating and mobility intervention.
4. Summarize biomechanical principles related to adaptive seating and wheeled mobility.
5. Rank the major types of wheelchair technologies in order from lowest technical sophistication to highest technical sophistication.
6. Explain various factors related to development of pressure ulcers for wheelchair users with a spinal cord injury.
7. Specify which of the current technologies for postural control in seating would be most effective in the management of severe spasticity in a patient with cerebral palsy.
8. Recommend an appropriate wheeled mobility base and adaptive seating system for a patient after a cerebrovascular accident.

Neuromuscular and musculoskeletal impairments often limit a person's functional gait potential. When this occurs, adaptive seating support and wheeled mobility interventions are essential in returning a person to a maximal level of independent function. Individuals use their wheeled mobility device for many hours each day. People who use wheeled mobility devices (wheelchairs or scooters) for some or all of their mobility often require adaptive seating support. Additionally, individuals who use wheeled mobility devices often require assistance for other activities of daily living and may require postural support and balance in a seated position. Individuals with neuromuscular impairments typically require specialized seating support to attain a maximal level of independent function, comfort, safety, and quality of life. Individuals with musculoskeletal impairment in the absence of neurological deficits may also require postural support because of the amount of time

they spend in a seated posture or, in some cases, because of the inability to either stand or walk.

Individuals who use wheelchairs and adaptive seating systems are of all age groups and races. They use their wheelchairs in many different environments and for many different reasons. Some are full-time wheelchair users because they cannot stand or walk. Others spend part of their day in the wheelchair to augment their mobility over long distances or on uneven surfaces. Some use wheelchairs for short-term conditions that resolve within weeks or months, such as lower extremity fractures or joint replacement surgeries. Others use wheelchairs long-term because of permanent disabling conditions.

There are approximately 1.7 million community-dwelling people in the United States who use wheelchairs or powered scooters to assist them with mobility.[1] Of these, approximately 1.5 million use manual wheelchairs, 155,000 use electric-powered wheelchairs, and 142,000 use electric-powered scooters.[2] In addition to these permanent users, there are likely to be several million part-time or temporary wheeled mobility device users at any given time in the United States, not including individuals residing in institutional settings. The National Medical Expenditure Survey conducted in 1987 indicated there were 2.5 million individuals residing in long-term care facilities, and of these, more than 50% use wheelchairs for mobility.[3,4] Individuals who use wheelchairs range from very young children who never attain the ability to walk to very old adults who have lost this ability because of various disabling conditions and processes.

Among all age groups, the leading condition associated with wheelchair use is cerebrovascular disease. Among individuals ages 18 to 64 years, the leading condition associated with wheelchair use is multiple sclerosis.[1] Other conditions commonly associated with wheelchair use include osteoarthritis and rheumatoid arthritis, congenital absence or amputation of lower extremities, tetraplegia and paraplegia, cardiopulmonary diseases and disorders (e.g., emphysema) that limit endurance, cerebral palsy, diabetes, and orthopedic impairment of the lower extremities.[1]

Individuals who use adaptive seating and wheeled mobility live in many different environments. Many live in the community independently or with assistance or support. Others live in long-term care settings or in assisted-living environments. Individuals use wheelchairs at home, school, work, and outdoors. People rely on their wheeled mobility devices to allow them to work, learn, play, care for themselves, and meet their personal goals. Therefore the assessment for and recommendation of a wheeled mobility device and seating support system is an important responsibility, which is typically undertaken by a team of trained individuals.

WHAT IS A WHEELCHAIR?

A wheelchair, or wheeled mobility device, is a complex piece of assistive technology. In addition to providing a means for mobility, this device provides the foundation for all other function, that is, activities of daily living such as bathing and dressing, work activities, and recreation. To do this, several interrelated components of the wheeled mobility device must work together to meet the needs of the individual user. The three major components of a wheelchair are the seating system (the postural support component), the wheelchair frame (the supporting structure), and the propelling structure (Figure 16-1).[5] All three components provide different functions but must form an integrated unit for efficient and safe wheeled mobility. Successful integration is critical to the function of the wheelchair user.

Seating System

The seating system, or adaptive seating component, of the wheeled mobility device is primarily responsible for support and positioning of the wheelchair user or wheelchair rider.

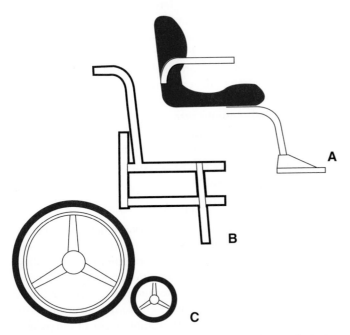

FIGURE 16-1 The three components of a wheelchair include the postural support (**A**), the supporting structure (**B**), and the propelling structure (**C**).

This component can be thought of as an orthotic intervention in wheeled mobility prescription.

Adaptive seating is used to promote postural support and positioning so that the user may function optimally.[6] To do this, it must accomplish the following five goals:

1. Provide effective postural support and positioning for the pelvis, trunk, lower body, and sometimes extremities and head
2. Provide optimal soft-tissue loading by pressure redistribution to minimize the risk of pressure ulcer development
3. Provide optimal comfort so that the seating system may be tolerated for long periods
4. Facilitate distal extremity function by providing a stable base of support for the user
5. Permit optimal access to the mobility interface component (e.g., the wheel rims of a manual chair or the power controller of a powered wheelchair) of the wheelchair

Although all these goals are critical to the optimal function of any wheeled mobility device, goals must be prioritized on the basis of personal needs of each user. For example, a wheeled mobility device user with a spinal cord injury who has good overall posture but lacks sensory function requires greater emphasis on pressure management goals than on postural support.

The seating system is often divided into several components, each with responsibility for supporting different body segments. Table 16-1 summarizes the indications for each type of seating component.

Support Frame and Mobility Components

The support frame is integrated with the seating component and is closely linked with the propelling structure. The main purpose of the support frame is to provide a smooth integration or connection of the seating support system and the mobility component of the wheeled mobility device. Many styles of frames are available; some provide specialty purposes, such as tilt, recline, or standing frames, but the majority are configured to allow attachment of adaptive seating systems and facilitate access to the mobility structures of the device by the user.

The mobility base, or propelling structure, of the wheelchair is composed of the drive wheels, caster wheels, tires, and some type of user interface component. Goals for the mobility base focus on the facilitation of mobility within the user's environment and can include the following:

1. Independent mobility in all environments encountered by the individual
2. Safe access to mobility and the prevention of injuries, such as overuse or secondary injuries
3. Maximum efficiency in mobility
4. Facilitation of overall function within the person's environment

In Cook and Hussey's Human Activity Assistive Technology model, wheeled mobility devices and seating systems are defined as "extrinsic enablers."[5] These devices facilitate or allow the user to perform many functions. A seating support system is referred to as a "general-purpose extrinsic enabler"[5]

TABLE 16-1   *Postural Support Components and Indications for Use*

Postural Support Component	Indications for Use
Seat cushion	Wheelchair use for any amount of time (see Table 16-6 for detailed descriptions of types of seat cushions)
Solid seat support	Wheelchair use for any amount of time, particularly a folding wheelchair with sling seat upholstery
Solid back support	Wheelchair use of 4 hours or more per day Impaired sitting balance or trunk control Scoliosis or any need for lateral and posterior spinal support
Lateral thoracic supports	Impaired sitting balance or trunk control Flexible or fixed spinal scoliosis Need for additional lateral support for safe or efficient activities of daily living (e.g., driving)
Lateral pelvic supports	Impaired pelvic and lower trunk control Flexible or fixed scoliosis Medial knee supports Lower extremity adduction while sitting Hypertonicity (spasticity) of lower extremities Windswept deformities of lower extremities
Knee blocks	Impaired anterior stability of pelvis in wheelchair If the patient slides out of wheelchair on a regular basis Severe extensor spasticity in lower extremities
Head support	Impaired head control from weakness or abnormal muscle tone
Anterior pelvic support	Anterior/posterior instability of pelvis while sitting (e.g., falling into posterior pelvic tilt or excessive anterior tilt, sliding out of chair)
Anterior trunk support	Anterior trunk instability If additional support is needed for safe and efficient functional activities (e.g., wheelchair propulsion, mobility over rough terrain, driving activities, or transportation needs)

because it facilitates many different functions for the user, such as self-care, recreation, or mobility. The wheeled mobility device is a "specific purpose extrinsic enabler," meaning it specifically allows users to be mobile within their environment.

SEATING AND MOBILITY ASSESSMENT

Seating and mobility assessment is a highly complex process involving multiple component evaluations and tests.[7] Seating and mobility assessments have many similarities to physical therapy and occupational therapy assessments but are more specific to the seating and wheeled mobility needs of the patient. The major difference in the outcome between more traditional therapy assessment and seating and mobility assessment is the intervention. The intervention plan in a seating and mobility assessment involves recommending a particular wheeled mobility device and adaptive seating system. As with any therapeutic intervention, the first step is an examination of the patient.[8] This examination allows the therapist to collect all appropriate information to evaluate the patient's needs and determine the most appropriate intervention plan.

Members of the Assessment Team

Specially trained clinicians, organized in a team structure, are usually responsible for performing seating and mobility assessments (Figure 16-2). This team may consist of physical or occupational therapists with specialized training in

wheelchair seating and mobility, physicians, rehabilitation technology suppliers, orthotists, and other health care professionals. The rehabilitation technology supplier is the team member who is ultimately responsible for providing the equipment to the patient. The rehabilitation technology supplier participates in the assessment process, compiles an equipment quotation and cost estimate, orders the equipment from the manufacturer, submits the justification and billing information to the equipment funding source(s), and then assembles the components in preparation for delivery of the wheeled mobility system. When an individual with seating or mobility problem is referred to the team, a multistep process of assessment, prescription, and training begins (Figure 16-3). The team must carefully document its findings and recommendations.

History

As with most therapeutic examinations, a detailed history is an essential component of a seating and mobility assessment. This history typically includes information related to diagnosis, nature of the disabling condition, related health problems, current and past assistive technology use, description of the home environment and other environments in which the equipment will be used, transportation needs of the patient, and funding source information for the equipment. All these elements are critical to the selection of an appropriate seating and wheeled mobility device.

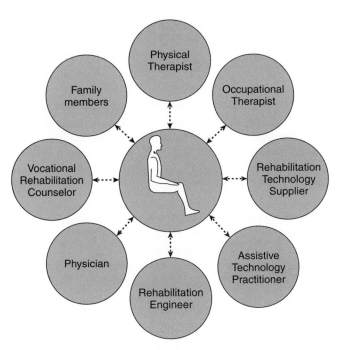

FIGURE 16-2 The interdisciplinary seating and mobility assessment team is most successful if it is consumer focused.

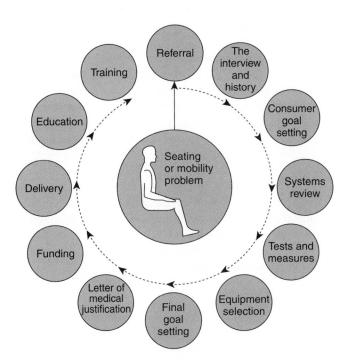

FIGURE 16-3 When a patient is referred to the team, the first steps in the process involve collecting relevant information and examination, including specific tests and measures. The team uses this information to select appropriate components on the basis of prognosis and the patient's functional needs. Once ordered and delivered, the team works with the patient on mobility, safety, and maintenance issues.

The diagnosis of the patient is a critical component of the history—particularly diagnoses related to why years requires a wheeled mobility device. If a patient has a gait disability, the cause of the disability must be described both to evaluate the most effective intervention and to justify the need for the

equipment to the funding source. Important questions to ask include the following:

1. When was the onset of the disability?
2. Was it sudden or slow?
3. Is the disability progressive or nonprogressive?

In addition to the major diagnosis, information about associated health problems is also important. Related health problems may include breathing problems, cardiovascular or circulatory problems, seizure disorders, bowel and bladder continence problems, nutrition and digestion, medications the individual takes, surgeries in the past or planned surgeries, orthopedic concerns such as subluxation or dislocation of the hip or shoulder, osteoporosis, other orthotic interventions (including any leg or foot orthoses or trunk orthoses), skin condition problems or concerns, sensation, pain problems, visual deficits, hearing deficits, and cognitive and behavioral problems.[9] Diagnostic information and related health concerns have a direct impact on the selection of appropriate equipment.

The history must also include elements related to the patient's equipment use and the environmental demands. Gathering information about current and past assistive technology use is important. Knowing what the individual has tried and the outcomes of these interventions helps avoid the repetition of mistakes. Also, knowledge of previously used assistive technology is important for interfacing any new devices with already existing devices, such as alternative communication systems. Also, knowledge of the mode of transportation (e.g., car, adapted van, public transportation, school-provided transportation) is critical because equipment must be chosen to meet these transportation needs. The demands of the patient's home environment or other environments in which the equipment will be used must be understood, including school or workplace environment and recreational activities.[7] Last, but certainly not least, the funding source or sources for the equipment must be discerned. Different funding sources have different requirements for evidence documented in support of patient needs and benefits of selected devices and for medical necessity to justify reimbursement for the equipment.

Systems Review

Once this detailed history is gathered, the therapist may move on to a systems review.[8] A systems review includes a limited examination of the major systems affecting the selection of the assistive device (Table 16-2), including the cardiovascular and pulmonary system, the integumentary system, the musculoskeletal system, the neuromuscular system, and the communication and cognitive abilities of the individual.[8] During the systems review, additional questions may arise related to the history of the patient, particularly related to past equipment use; these questions should be incorporated into the remainder of the examination and the responses integrated with the history already recorded.

If an individual is already using a wheeled mobility device, the systems review must include an assessment of the patient's use of the current equipment. The make and model

TABLE 16-2   *Components of the Systems Review for Seating and Wheelchair Assessment*

Systems	Issues to Assess

Musculoskeletal	Range of motion
	Strength of all muscles
	Postural asymmetry
	   Pelvic obliquity
	   Pelvic rotation
	   Pelvic tilt (anterior/posterior)
	   Scoliosis
	   Excessive kyphosis
	   Lordosis
	Flexibility of any noted asymmetries

Integumentary	History of skin breakdown Surgeries performed Skin inspection to identify current problems Performance of active pressure reliefs Condition of pressure management equipment Success/failure of technologies in the past
Neurological	Motor control Abnormal muscle tone Abnormal primitive reflexes
Cardiovascular	Heart rate Blood pressure (at rest and with activity) Edema
Pulmonary	Respiratory rate Shortness of breath (dyspnea) Blood oxygenation (pulse oximetry) Change in pulmonary status with activity Change in pulmonary status with position

Communication	Verbal and nonverbal
	Use of alternative or augmentative systems
	Effectiveness of communication
	   With family or familiar individuals
	   With unknown or unfamiliar individuals

Cognitive status	Type of cognitive impairments present Developmental delay Progressive dementia Overall mental health and judgment Ability to learn Understanding of wheeled mobility function

of any devices currently used should be recorded, along with the sizes of all items and their present condition. In addition to the condition of the equipment, the patient's posture and function while using this equipment should be noted. Determining why the person needs an assessment for new equipment is extremely important. Questions to ask include the following:

- Did the patient outgrow the equipment or did the equipment exceed its expected lifespan?
- Did the patient's needs change because of a change in medical condition or functional status?

Specific details of how the current equipment is used and whether such use is appropriate and effective help with setting goals and determining the most effective equipment intervention for the future.

The reason for the seating and wheeled mobility assessment often translates into the justification for the recommended equipment, so this information is critical to ascertain during the examination. If the patient has not used any device in the past, why is one needed now? What change has triggered the referral for an evaluation? During this review, the specific, patient-centered, functional goals related to wheeled mobility device use also should be determined. These goals are incorporated into the intervention after all the data are collected and the evaluation is made.

Cardiovascular and pulmonary assessment, including blood pressure, heart rate, pulse oximetry, respiratory rate, and edema, are also important. Skin condition must be assessed, particularly overall seating contact areas. Gross musculoskeletal status should be assessed and the patient's height and weight recorded. General assessments of function and movement ability in the current wheeled mobility system and the patient's communication skills and abilities and cognition should also be performed.

Tests and Measures Used in Seating and Mobility Assessment

The systems review helps determine which areas require a more comprehensive assessment in the form of specific tests and measures, including seated and supine mat evaluation, seating simulation, equipment simulation, and pressure mapping (Table 16-3). If a patient has a cardiovascular condition, such as postural hypotension, then more extensive testing of different seated positions and interventions along with detailed tracking of changes in blood pressure are necessary during the mat evaluation and the seating simulation. Many tests and measures are used during the seating and wheeled mobility examination process. Some are necessary for all patients requiring adaptive seating, and some are used only in particular instances. Tests and measures for adaptive seating and mobility intervention can be classified according to postural and technical or instrumentation requirements, such as mat table or seat simulator.

Mat Evaluation

Many of the tests and measures used are incorporated into the mat evaluation, which consists of an evaluation with the patient in both seated and supine postures.[7] During a seated mat evaluation, the therapist measures or determines a person's unsupported seated posture, postural asymmetries, sitting balance, joint flexibility (particularly of the spine and pelvis) and functional abilities in terms of transfers and seated function, such as reaching ability. A supine mat evaluation is essential for measuring specific joint range of motion, strength, coordination, and abnormal muscle tone and reflexes. Particular attention must be paid to true hip joint mobility, orthopedic deformities such as pelvic asymmetries, hip joint subluxations or dislocations, and flexibility of spinal postures.[7] The supine mat evaluation is critical in determining the flexibility of postural deformities because of

TABLE 16-3 *Tests and Measures Used in Seating and Wheelchair Assessment*

Component of Evaluation	Measures or Task Analysis

Seated mat evaluation	Unsupported seated posture
	Sitting balance
	Postural flexibility
	Functional abilities
	   Transfers
	   Reaching
	   Activities of daily living
	     simulation

Supine mat evaluation	Seating angles
	   Thigh-to-trunk angle
	   True hip flexion range of motion
	   Thigh-to-lower leg angle
	   Hamstring tightness
	   Lower leg-to-foot angle
	Pelvic flexibility
	Abnormal muscle tone
	Mobility skills and abilities
	Supine to/from sitting transition

Mat (hand) simulation	Position of supports required Amount of force required Ability to reduce flexible asymmetries

Seated simulation testing	Desired seating dimensions
	Desired seating angles
	   Seat tilt or orientation
	   Seat to back angle support
	   Need for biangular back support
	Other simulated supports and
	   effects
	   Lateral pelvic supports
	   Lateral trunk supports
	   Arm supports
	   Leg and foot supports
	   Head support

Equipment simulation	What equipment was used
	Results of mobility assessment in
	   mock-up
	Consumer comfort
	Ability to meet goals with simulated
	   system
	Photos to include with justification
	   documents

Pressure mapping	Note cushions used during testing
	Results of cushions tested
	   Pressure distribution patterns
	Consumer education
	   Importance of proper seat
	     cushion use
	   Optimal pressure relief methods

Other	Custom molding simulation Pulse oximetry Circulatory testing Functional wheelchair propulsion testing

the change in the effects of the gravitational pull on the body. If a postural deformity is present during the sitting assessment and then disappears during the supine mat evaluation, that deformity is "flexible" in nature and may be correctible in the adaptive seating system. If, on the other hand, the postural asymmetry is present in both seated and supine postures, in spite of any attempt at repositioning, then this asymmetry is described as a "fixed" posture.

SIMULATION TECHNIQUES AND EQUIPMENT

The other tests and measures of a seating and mobility assessment are performed by using simulation techniques or equipment. Three primary simulation techniques are used: hand simulation, simulation with a commercial seated simulator, and simulation with commercial seating and mobility products similar to those likely to be selected.[9,10]

Hand simulation is often performed with the patient seated on the mat. During this simulation the therapist uses his or her hands to simulate or mimic forces applied by various components of an adaptive seating system. In this manner, the therapist can determine if external supports are capable of providing the desired effect on the patient's posture and how much force is required or what is the optimal application point on the body.[7]

After hand simulation, a seating simulator may be used to verify the manual data. A seating simulator is a highly adjustable wheelchair frame with many interchangeable components.[10] This device is first preset to provide the desired supports; then the patient sits in it so the therapist can determine if the settings actually produce the desired postural or functional outcomes.

The third simulation method involves assembling actual commercial products into a system similar to that being recommended to assess its effect. This may be done if a commercial simulator is not available as an additional component after performing the other types of simulation. This final simulation provides evidence of the effectiveness of actual products in meeting the desired goals of the seating and mobility assessment and may be an excellent way of providing the funding source with information regarding why specific equipment is being recommended.

Other tests and measures used for seating and mobility assessment include pressure mapping (Figure 16-4),[11] custom contour seat simulation, pulse oximetry during simulation, specific circulatory assessments during simulation, and functional wheelchair propulsion testing.[12] These specific measures may not be used in all seating and mobility assessments but can be mixed and matched according to the needs of the patient. All these tests and measures provide the therapist with necessary information required for evaluation and determination of final equipment selections.

Plan of Care and Equipment Prescription

The evaluation of all this information will lead to a diagnosis related to the patient's level of function and a plan to address specific adaptive seating and wheeled mobility device needs that have been identified (Table 16-4). The clinician

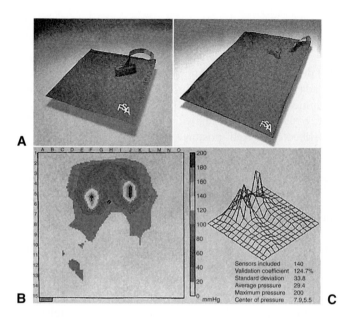

FIGURE 16-4 An example of a pressure measurement system. The pressure-sensitive mat that the patient sits on is connected to a computer (**A**). The computer generates a two-dimensional (**B**) or three-dimensional (**C**) display of seating pressures. (From Cook AM, Hussey SM [eds]. *Assistive Technologies: Principles and Practice, vol 1*, 2nd ed. St. Louis: Mosby, 2002. p. 196.)

TABLE 16-4   *Components Included in Final Recommendations*

Category	Details
Wheelchair propulsion ability	Distance Speed Safety In recommended wheelchair In less expensive options

Final equipment selection	Mobility base
	    Access method
	    Postural support components

Goals of the seating system	Based on consumer's stated goals Objective Measurable Related to recommended equipment
Wheelchair and seating fitting and delivery needs	Is preliminary fitting required? How many visits will be necessary? Estimated time to delivery

Training and education plans	When will the training begin?
	Who will carry out the training?
	    Referral for additional training?
	Written materials to be provided
	    Product manuals
	    Care and maintenance instructions
	    Safety recommendations and concerns
	    Guidelines for proper and effective use

Plan for follow-up care	When will follow-up occur?
	    Scheduled visits or as needed?
	    Frequency of reevaluation?

and patient also set specific goals for use of the equipment within various environments. The actual intervention process in seating and wheeled mobility is often called the equipment recommendation or equipment prescription. During this process a specific mobility base is selected and adaptive seating equipment is specified.

Other major components of adaptive seating and mobility intervention involve coordination, communication, and documentation. The physical or occupational therapist typically has the primary responsibility of coordinating the seating team and assuring that all team members are working together to assist in the attainment of the patient's goals. Communication with all team members is essential during this process. All team members must be made aware of the results of the examination and the ultimate goals involved. Each team member may have some responsibilities in this process; the rehabilitation technology supplier, for example, has a primary responsibility to provide specific manufacturer's specifications for the equipment needed. These specifications will then be used to prepare the letter of medical justification. In addition to all the typical documentation of the history and physical assessment, the therapist also has a primary responsibility, in the case of adaptive seating intervention, to prepare the letter of medical justification. The letter is critical because it is the primary means of communication with all funding sources involved to obtain necessary funding for the seating and wheeled mobility system.

Documentation: The Letter of Medical Justification

The intention of the letter of medical justification is to provide the funding source with a clear picture of the patient with a disability and the equipment being recommended, with a focus on why the specific equipment being prescribed is required. This letter must contain several elements. The introductory paragraph should describe the person with a disability. This description includes the diagnoses, onset dates, prognosis, and a summary of the history and the systems review.

Next, detailed information is provided about the specific tests and measures used during the examination and outcomes of the evaluation. These include, but are not limited to, the individual's functional status, strength, range of motion, orthopedic deformities, motor coordination, abnormal tone or reflex findings, and the results of the equipment simulation. This information can be organized and reported on a standardized form or in a narrative style.

Specific measurable, functional goals for the adaptive seating and wheeled mobility system should be clearly stated. All the specifications of the selected equipment must be included, and the reason for each item must be effectively justified as to why the person requires this specific piece of equipment (Box 16-1). The funding source sometimes also requires a description of other possible lower cost options and an explanation of why these options are not effective for the patient. Finally, a summary of the patient information and contact information for the primary therapist and the prescribing physician should be provided so that the funding source may contact these individuals if any questions arise during the review process.

BOX 16-1   *Examples of Adaptive Seating and Wheeled Mobility Interventions and Goals*

EXAMPLE 1

Reason for referral:	Frequent falls in the home
Evaluation finding:	Only able to ambulate for 20 feet and unsteady; high risk of falling
Goals:	Safe and independent mobility for functional distances, at least 200 feet for indoor environments
Equipment feature:	Manual, power assist, or power wheeled mobility device
Justification:	Patient able to safely and independently propel the selected wheeled mobility device for functional distances in his or her environment

EXAMPLE 2

Reason for referral:	Having problems sitting upright in wheelchair; falls to the left and has difficulty propelling chair
Evaluation findings:	Impaired sitting balance noted during mat evaluation, poor trunk muscle strength resulting in poor trunk control, no ability to react to sitting balance challenges
Goals:	Able to maintain upright sitting posture and perform all functional activities without falling, such as wheelchair propulsion, activities of daily living
Equipment feature:	Solid seat cushion and back support, possible lateral trunk supports, seat tilt posterior or open seat to back angle if simulation shows increased stability in these postures without compromising function
Justification:	Patient able to sit upright with adequate support for pelvis and spine to allow maximal function of upper body for activities of daily living or other functional activities (e.g., access to propulsion)

EXAMPLE 3

Reason for referral:	Impaired endurance; fatigues easily and cannot go into community
Evaluation findings:	Unable to tolerate wheelchair propulsion farther than 100 feet and becomes quite short of breath with indoor manual propulsion, even in lightweight wheelchair
Goals:	Ability to tolerate mobility for functional distances in all desired environments, in home and community
Equipment feature:	Powered wheelchair or powered scooter
Justification:	Patient independent for all mobility with selected device for functional distances for the patient's home environment

EXAMPLE 4

Reason for referral:	Pressure ulcer under the left ischial tuberosity
Evaluative findings:	Stage 2 pressure ulcer under left ischial tuberosity observed during mat evaluation skin inspection; pelvic obliquity noted in sitting, disappears in supine (flexible)
Goals:	Improve pressure distribution and correct pelvic obliquity to minimize pressure under left ischial tuberosity; provide equipment and training for active pressure relief while seated in wheelchair
Equipment features:	Skin protection and positioning seat cushion that redistributes pressure, minimizing pressure under the ischial tuberosities, and supports pelvis in a neutral position; may also require increased trunk support, possibly lateral supports for correcting pelvic obliquity posture
Justification:	Equipment will provide safe seating for up to 4-hour intervals without worsening of pressure ulcer and will facilitate healing of current ulcer over time; seating will correct pelvic obliquity and minimize weight bearing under left ischial tuberosity, to be verified with pressure mapping

EXAMPLE 5

Reason for referral:	Right shoulder pain and weakness; difficulty with transfers and manual wheelchair propulsion
Evaluative findings:	Right shoulder rotator cuff tear with resulting pain and muscle weakness
Goals:	Maximize functional abilities while minimizing pain and decreasing stress on right shoulder
Equipment features:	Powered wheelchair with access method that minimizes stress on right shoulder; sliding board and training for transfers that minimize stress on right shoulder
Justification:	Patient will function independently with minimal pain in right upper extremity and will be independent for all mobility and transfer activities

Meticulous preparation of the letter of medical justification may mean the difference between efficient funding of the seating and mobility system and a long, drawn-out review process that may delay the delivery of equipment by several months.

When the Seating and Mobility System Is Delivered

After approval by the funding source and after the adaptive seating equipment is ordered and obtained, the rehabilitation technology supplier notifies the therapist that the seating and mobility system is ready for delivery. The patient then returns to the seating clinic and the adaptive seating and mobility device is delivered and adjusted to ensure proper fit and efficient function. Delivery of the wheelchair or seating system is a critical element in the intervention process and directly affects the outcomes related to use of the equipment.

Delivery of equipment typically occurs several months after the examination and prescription process. The therapist is responsible for ensuring that the status and needs of the patient have not changed since the initial seating and mobility assessment. If the needs have changed, then recommended modifications to the equipment must be specified at this time. The equipment must then be verified to ensure it meets all the recommended specifications. Finally, the equipment must be adjusted for proper fit and the patient must be trained in its safe use, adjustment, maintenance, and care.

The patient should have the opportunity to function in and use the equipment during the initial delivery to ensure that the goals set during the examination can be effectively attained. This may require a period of training and further rehabilitation intervention as an outpatient or in the patient's living environment. In addition, the patient and caregivers are instructed in routine maintenance and cleaning of the equipment, by verbal instruction, demonstration, and in written format, such as review of the owner's manuals provided by the equipment manufacturers. The patient and caregivers also need to learn when they should return to the clinic for adjustment or modification of the equipment.

Assessment of Seating and Mobility Outcomes

The final critical component of an adaptive seating evaluation is reexamination, or followup and follow-along. Adaptive seating equipment needs are fluid over time. Fixed orthopedic deformities may change or progress, and functional abilities often change. Equipment needs must be reevaluated when the patient's needs are no longer met by the equipment. This may happen as equipment ages and falls into disrepair, or as the patient's functional or physical status changes over time. Most adaptive seating equipment has a usable life span of 3 to 5 years. If a person is particularly active or if the equipment is used in harsh and demanding environments, the equipment may have a shorter functional life span. Periodic reexamination of equipment and patient needs is essential to maintain optimal function. Although planning reexamination appointments is important, the patient needs to understand when and why contacting the therapist and requesting a reexamination between

scheduled visits might be necessary. The patient is the most knowledgeable person regarding the adequacy of the equipment and whether goals are being met.

BIOMECHANICAL PRINCIPLES IN SEATING AND MOBILITY

Adaptive seating for persons who use wheelchairs involves the strategic application of forces to provide postural support and stability for optimal function. All applications of forces in this context are governed by the laws of physics and described in the field of biomechanics, the study of body position and movement.[5] All adaptive seating components exert forces or torques on the body that ultimately affect changes in posture and static or dynamic equilibrium. Improperly applied forces or improper fit of components can lead to a variety of seating and mobility problems. Table 16-5 summarizes the most commonly encountered problems.

Propulsion of a wheeled mobility device, particularly manual propulsion, depends on the forces and torques applied by the user. These forces must be understood because of their possible long-term effects on the body; wheelchair users are at risk of repetitive motion and overuse injuries.[13] Understanding basic biomechanical principles and how they affect the design of adaptive seating and wheeled mobility is critical to the strategic application of forces to maximize function and minimize risk of injury for the wheeled mobility device user.

No single strategy, or even a small set of strategies, works for every wheelchair user. Each wheelchair user is unique, with a unique set of problems and goals, and each therefore requires an individualized approach to adaptive seating.[14] Many biomechanical and ergonomic principles govern the application of forces in adaptive seating, but all center on basic principles, as outlined by Engstrom.[14] These principles include the following:

1. Providing a stable base of support for the pelvis
2. Providing adequate pressure distribution
3. Allowing an individual to move into an active position (e.g., to lean forward)
4. Allowing variations in positions
5. Providing support for the back
6. Allowing free movement of the feet and legs if possible
7. Providing the user with a feeling of safety, security, and comfort

Providing adaptive seating that meets all these requirements is often quite challenging.

Stability of the Pelvis

A basic challenge inherent in seated posture is achieving pelvic stability. Although the base of support is larger and the body's center of gravity is lower when sitting than standing,[15] the pelvis is actually more unstable when seated. In standing, ligamentous tension and balanced muscle activity contribute to stability of the pelvis. When sitting, many of the ligaments become slack, and the flexed hip position alters the line of pull and efficiency of muscles around the hip. If, in addition,

TABLE 16-5 *Potential Problems Resulting from Improper Biomechanics in Support or Propulsion*

Support or Access Problem	Possible Resultant Biomechanical Problem	Potential Equipment Solutions
Seat too long	Posterior pelvic tilt Sliding out of wheelchair	Shorten seat or provide additional back support (effectively shortening seat)
Seat too short	Pressure ulcer, lack of support under femurs Sliding out of seat	Increase seat depth of wheelchair or add longer seat cushion with solid support underneath
Seat too wide	Lateral shift of pelvis in chair Pelvic obliquity Trunk scoliosis Feeling of instability	Narrow wheelchair seat or add lateral pelvic supports to properly center pelvis in wheelchair
Seat too narrow	Pressure ulcers over greater trochanters Difficulty transferring in and out of wheelchair	Widen wheelchair seat
Back too wide	Flexible scoliosis Lateral trunk leaning Pelvic obliquity Feeling of instability	Narrower back support Lateral thoracic supports Lateral pelvic supports
Back too narrow	Lack of movement needed for function Skin breakdown on lateral trunk Discomfort caused by inability to move	Widen wheelchair back support
Back too low	Upper trunk instability; limited function Excessive thoracic kyphosis Posterior pelvic tilt	Higher back support Solid back support (if current back is sling)
Back too high	Falling forward in wheelchair Inability to propel wheelchair optimally	Lower back height Narrower upper back support to allow increased scapular excursion
Rear wheels too far back	Shoulder pain; impingement Inability to optimally propel wheelchair	Move rear wheels forward
Rear wheels too far forward	Wheelchair tipping backwards; user unable to control	Move rear wheels back on frame

the patient who is sitting demonstrates a lack of flexibility (shortening or tightness) in the hamstring muscles, the pelvis rotates posteriorly and the spine adopts a more flexed posture than in standing (Figure 16-5).[15] This flexed posture has been implicated in muscle fatigue and abnormally high disk pressures, both of which contribute to discomfort and pain in prolonged sitting.

Forces exerted in an adaptive seating system must overcome these natural tendencies as well as any postural asymmetries caused by abnormally high muscle tone or other disability-related impairments. To do this, forces to the body must be applied as strategically as possible by considering both the lever arm and the surface area through which the force will be applied.

When a torque is applied to control or influence the position of a body part, the force necessary is inversely related to the lever arm, the distance from the axis of rotation of the body part, and the point of application of the force. As the distance away from the point of rotation increases, the force required to achieved the desired outcome decreases.[5] This principle is very important for adaptive seating, because in dealing with application of forces on the surface of the body, decreasing the force necessary is critical to a person being able to tolerate that

force. One way to accomplish this is to apply the force as far from the part to be controlled as reasonably possible.

Pressure is directly related to the force applied but inversely related to the area over which the force is distributed. This means that, if high forces are necessary to achieve the desired outcome, providing a larger area of contact will decrease the pressure exerted on the body.[5] Applying forces over as large an area as possible is critical to avoiding pressure-related skin ulcers as well as increasing comfort and tolerance for the wheelchair user.

Understanding and applying these two biomechanical principles assists the clinician in designing adaptive seating systems that accomplish the goals of postural support and positioning for function while being comfortable and well tolerated by the patient.

One of the main forces that adaptive seating systems must balance is the force of gravity (Figure 16-6). Gravity is a constant force exerted on the body that must be counteracted for an individual to remain in an upright-seated posture. The adaptive seating components must provide enough external support so that, combined with the internal muscular forces generated by the wheelchair user, an individual can sit in a desired position for long periods of time and perform all

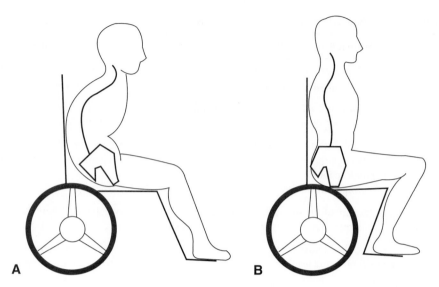

FIGURE 16-5 **A,** In the presence of hamstring tightness, if knees are relatively extended, the pelvis falls into a position of posterior rotation, with a decrease in lumbar lordosis, an increase in thoracic kyphosis, and cervical lordosis. **B,** One strategy to achieve optimal alignment of pelvis and spine in the presence of hamstring tightness is to reduce seat depth and position slightly under the seat.

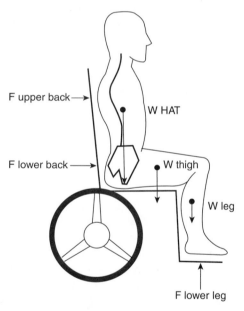

FIGURE 16-6 Each body segment has its own center of mass (W HAT, W thigh, W leg). These downward forces must be counterbalanced by opposing forces from support surfaces (seat, upper back, sacral, foot). *W,* weight = gravity acting on center of mass; *F,* opposition forces.

desired functional activities. This can be quite challenging, depending on the ability of the wheelchair user to generate muscular forces that work in opposition to the force of gravity. Body positions should allow gravity to facilitate desired postures or functions if an individual has severe weakness or muscle fatigue. This is often a main reason for using tilt or recline seating systems. These systems allow the person's body to be reoriented in space, allowing the force of gravity to facilitate desired postures or functions rather than requiring the user to generate muscular forces to counteract the force of gravity at all times.

Propulsion

Biomechanical principles are also extremely important in the propulsion of manual wheelchairs.[13] Manual wheelchair users have many problems associated with shoulder and wrist pain and injuries.[16] Understanding wheelchair propulsion biomechanics and the importance of wheelchair configuration and wheelchair propulsion training is critical to minimizing or preventing these overuse injuries. The weight of the wheelchair user should be distributed rearward (with the seat moved back in relation to the rear wheels) to decrease rolling resistance and make the wheelchair easier to propel.[17] This will also make the wheelchair easier to tip backward, so the skill of the user in controlling this tipping must be carefully considered.

The seat surface should be low enough to allow a 100- to 120-degree bend in the elbow when the user's hand is placed at the top of the wheel rim (Figure 16-7). This position tends to minimize impact on the shoulders and maximize efficiency in propulsion.[17,18]

Individuals who self-propel manual wheelchairs must master and consistently use proper propulsion techniques.[19] Long, smooth strokes limit excessive forces on upper extremity joints and soft tissue and decrease the rate of loading on the push rims. In contrast, short, choppy pushes are associated with higher energy expenditure and the development of repetitive use syndromes. Allowing the hands to drop below the rims during the "recovery," or nonpropulsion part of the stroke, aids in smooth motion and protects the shoulders from injury.[17]

SEATING CLASSIFICATION AND MATERIALS

Many new wheeled mobility and adaptive seating technologies have been developed over the last 20 years.[7] Technological development has helped meet the challenges involved in two major wheelchair seating objectives: postural support and pressure management. Individuals with neuromuscular

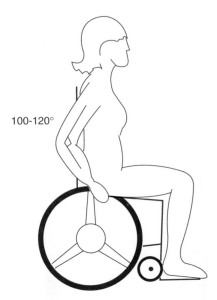

FIGURE 16-7 For maximum biomechanical efficiency in manual wheelchair propulsion, the elbow should be flexed between 100 and 120 degrees when the hand is resting on top of the push rim.

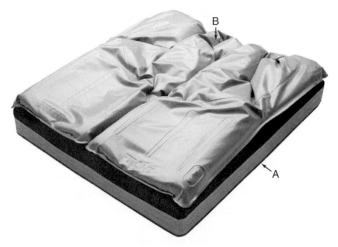

FIGURE 16-8 The J2 cushion is an example of a passive seat cushion with two objectives. Its firm, contoured foam base provides postural support (**A**), and its fluid-filled bladder provides increased contact area so that weight-bearing pressures are reduced (**B**). (Courtesy Sunrise Medical, Longmont, CO.)

impairments leading to wheelchair use for significant portions of their day require critical support for maintaining optimal postures that maximize function and minimize fatigue and discomfort while still attending to pressure buildup issues that might cause local tissue damage.

Seating support surfaces, often referred to as "wheelchair cushions," are actually far more complex. Seating components can be classified in many different ways, such as by their shape and contour or their component materials. Garber[20] divides wheelchair seating into two basic categories based on purpose: seating for positioning and seating for pressure

management. Many patients require seating that optimizes both positioning and pressure management. Although this classification helps us understand the basic functional division in seating products, it is too simplistic for most seating devices. Many seating support surfaces are designed to address both positioning and pressure management needs, especially for individuals with neuromuscular impairments (Figure 16-8). Those who use a wheelchair on a part-time basis generally do not rely on external support for positioning and may sit on a "general use" foam cushion to enhance comfort. Table 16-6 summarizes the advantages and disadvantages of wheelchair cushions on the basis of purpose.

TABLE 16-6   *Wheelchair Seat Cushions: Advantages and Disadvantages*

Primary Purpose of Seat Cushion	Features of Seat Cushions	Typical Client Problems Addressed
General use (comfort)	Composed of foam, flexible material, air, fluid, gel, or a combination of materials	General wheelchair use: fewer than 4 hours per day May be for temporary or intermittent use Individual has protective sensation Individual has good posture and sitting balance
Pressure management	Composed of two or more materials that may include foam, flexible material, air, fluid, gel Deeper contour when loaded than general use cushion Design must enhance pressure redistribution	Wheelchair use greater than 4 hours per day Individual with limited sensation Individual with limited ability to shift or reposition his or her body Individual at high risk for skin breakdown
Postural support and positioning	Composed of same materials as skin protection; includes additional postural supports that may include preischial bar (antithrust seat), lateral pelvic support, medial thigh support, lateral thigh supports	Wheelchair use greater than 4 hours per day User with abnormal muscle tone User with flexible postural asymmetries User with poor sitting balance or pelvic/lower extremity control in sitting
Pressure management, postural support, and positioning	Combination of properties found in both skin protection and postural support cushion above	User who sits more than 4 hours per day User has impaired sensation or high risk for skin breakdown User has postural support needs as listed above

Passive and Active Seating Systems

Seating surfaces can also be described or classified as active or passive devices.[21] Most support surfaces discussed in this chapter are passive in nature; they react to pressure exerted by the body but do not actively exert or change any forces. Recently, however, active cushion technologies have led to the development of various pressure management devices. These cushions have an active (mechanical) mechanism, such as a battery-powered pump system, that actually causes the cushion to change in some way to systematically alter pressure distribution. Although active cushions may be highly effective at pressure management for certain individuals, they are quite expensive and rely on a pumping system and a battery pack that make them heavier than typical seat cushions. They also are subject to malfunction and require more maintenance to be effective.

Noncontoured and Contoured Seating Systems

Regardless of the specific purpose of the cushion, seating surfaces can be classified according to their shape or amount of contour.[22] The most basic surfaces are planar or noncontoured. These surfaces are most easily manufactured. They are also most readily modified to allow for growth or other changes in the patient's needs. The drawback for noncontoured seating surfaces is their inability to accommodate the many body surfaces that are not flat in nature; the result is a less-than-optimal surface area for contact with the body, creating areas of relatively high pressure under bony prominences and soft tissues that contact the seating surface. To increase the amount of contact area and better distribute pressures, increasing the surface's contour is typically necessary to match the shape of the body more closely.[22]

Two levels of contoured surfaces exist: precontoured (generically contoured) seating surfaces and custom-contoured seating surfaces. Precontoured seating surfaces are designed around generic molds intended to match the body's shapes more precisely than planar components. Many are available in a number of sizes. Precontoured surfaces are available as seat components designed to match the shape of the pelvis better and as trunk support components to match alignment of the spinal column better (Figure 16-9). The effectiveness of these surfaces for either postural support or pressure management depends on the precision of fit. The clinician determines precision of fit at the time of the initial assessment and prescription.

Custom-contoured surfaces are constructed directly from the shape of the patient. Many technologies are available to assist measurement for custom seating surfaces, including hand-shaping foam, computer-assisted design/computer-assisted manufacturing systems, and "foam-in-place" technologies, among others.[23] All these systems have the same general purpose: to record the shape of a person's body as precisely as possible to manufacture a support surface that precisely matches the contours of the person.

Material

Another method of classifying seat cushions or other postural supports is according to the component materials included in the support device. A variety of materials are being used

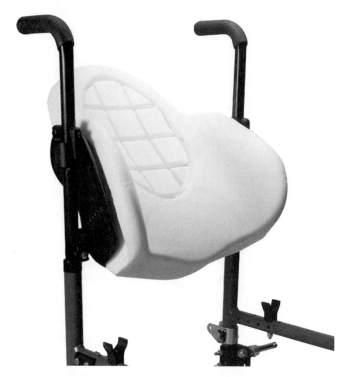

FIGURE 16-9 The Jay Care Back is an example of a precontoured back support. The back can be tilted as necessary, and the cross-hatched foam distributes pressures away from spinous processes for patients with pronounced thoracic kyphosis. (Courtesy Sunrise Medical, Longmont, CO.)

to create postural support devices. The most commonly used materials include various foams, air, gel materials, water-based materials, or a combination of these. The properties and characteristics (including advantages and disadvantages) of the each material must be carefully considered to select the seating system that will best meet a patient's seating needs and minimize the major risk factors for the development of pressure ulcers, such as pressure over bony prominences, shear and friction forces, temperature, and moisture.[24]

Foams are the most common component material used in making support surfaces. Two major categories of foam are available: elastic (available as either a closed-cell or open-cell material) and viscoelastic. Both types have advantages that make them well suited for use in postural supports as well as disadvantages that must be considered. Elastic foams deform in proportion to the applied load, which helps them reduce peak pressure over bony prominences.[24] They do not, however, provide good envelopment characteristics and they tend to insulate heat and keep it near the body. Viscoelastic foams are temperature sensitive, meaning they become softer and more compliant at higher temperatures.[24] This characteristic helps them provide even better pressure distribution than elastic foams, but it depends on the heating effect of being positioned near the body.

Fluid-filled cushions are often composed of materials such as air, water, or viscous fluids contained in one or more containers, either large or small.[24] Most of these products provide greater immersion into the cushion, thus distributing pressure over larger areas of the body and reducing pressures at bony prominences (see Figure 16-8). The type of material used in the cushion influences both skin temperature and the moisture buildup where the body makes contact with the support surface.[25] Understanding the different kinds of material helps the clinician select an appropriate seat cushion for pressure management and support or positioning in wheelchair seating.

Covering material is important to the function of postural support devices, especially seat cushions and back cushions. Regardless of the materials comprising the support itself, the covering material alters the performance characteristics of the support.[25] For example, an inflexible covering material prevents a cushion from providing optimal envelopment for the user. Also, if a covering material with a high coefficient of friction encloses a material selected for its low coefficient of friction, the advantage of the selected cushion material is lost. Covering material also needs to be resilient, easy to clean, in some cases moisture repellent, and aesthetically pleasing to the user.

ACCESSING THE MOBILITY UNIT

For wheelchair users to be independent in mobility in their environment, they must be able to perform some movement that can be translated into wheel movement of the mobility base. This movement is called the *access method for wheeled mobility*.[5] The access method can be entirely manual, entirely powered, or manual with power assistance. The access method for a manually propelled chair is different from that needed for an electrically powered chair. Table 16-7 summarizes the advantages, disadvantages, and indicators for the various wheeled technologies. The best access method and frame characteristics are those that allow wheelchair users to obtain the most efficient mobility from their access method (Figure 16-10).

Whether ordering a manual or powered wheelchair, the team must also carefully consider the need for back support, support of extremities, and type of locking mechanism that is most appropriate for each patient's needs. Table 16-8 provides an overview of the advantages and disadvantages of various limb support and locking mechanisms.

MANUAL WHEELCHAIRS

Manual wheelchairs typically have one large pair of wheels, most often at the rear, that cause the wheelchair to move when pushed. These are sometimes called the drive wheels. The diameter of these wheels is typically between 20 and 26 inches. The wheels are most often equipped with push rims that are slightly smaller in diameter, attached to the outside of the wheel itself. The push rims, rather than the wheel, are the access point for most manual wheelchair users. By pushing the wheel rims, the user has control over both the speed and direction of the wheelchair depending on how the user pushes each of the wheels.

The axle position of these drive wheels is critical for optimal wheel rim access for the user, as well as for maximal efficiency in manual propulsion. Standard wheelchairs do not have adjustable axle attachment points and are therefore quite difficult to optimize for efficient mobility. Many ultralightweight and maximally adjustable wheelchairs do have adjustability of this axle location, allowing for adjustment of the wheelchair to the user's needs (Figure 16-11).

Although the majority (90%) of manual wheelchair users propel in a traditional push rim propulsion method with both upper extremities,[26] this is not the only method for wheelchair propulsion and may not be the best in light of problems such as repetitive strain injuries. Some wheelchair users have only one functional upper extremity or one upper extremity and one lower extremity, often on the same side of the body (such as individuals with hemiplegia). Still others have severely weakened upper extremities but somewhat stronger lower extremities. For individuals with these different skills, alternative access for manual wheelchairs exists.[26]

Wheelchair users with only one strong upper extremity may use a one arm drive or lever drive system on their wheelchairs. These systems connect the axles of both drive wheels (either with a dual push rim or a lever system) so that the user can control both wheels and have effective directional control from one side of the chair. Wheelchair users with one functional arm and leg often propel their wheelchairs by pushing on one wheel rim and using their functional lower extremity on the ground to assist in directional control and to increase their speed or power of propulsion. Likewise, wheelchair users with stronger lower extremities and weaker upper extremities often "foot propel" their wheelchairs by using both lower extremities on the ground, bypassing the typical wheel rim input and controlling the movement of the chair by interfacing with the ground and indirectly causing the wheels of the chair to react to these forces.

Regardless of the method used for manual wheelchair propulsion, maximal efficiency is critical to functional mobility.[13] Upper extremity musculature is poorly suited to providing the body with ambulation, and without efficiency obtained through the technology, manual propulsion may be highly stressful and fatiguing for the wheelchair user. The environments in which most wheelchair users must function are much better suited to bipedal mobility, making it even more difficult for wheeled mobility to be an adequate substitute when an individual loses the ability to walk.

Many risks are associated with the use of a manual wheelchair. Some of these risks are manageable through other therapeutic interventions (e.g., training) or technological modifications. Others are more serious and must be carefully considered when a manual mobility system is prescribed for a user. Short-term risks include the potential for injury for a new user who is not fully able to control the balance of a wheelchair. This may lead to tipping a wheelchair over (most often falling backwards) when maneuvering up or down ramps or curbs. Other common injuries include trauma involving fingers and hands inadvertently caught in the wheel spokes or wheel lock mechanisms, injuries to lower extremities that are

TABLE 16-7   *Advantages, Disadvantages and Possible Applications of Various Wheeled Mobility Technologies*

Wheeled Mobility Device	Advantages	Disadvantages	Possible Application
Semiadjustable manual wheelchair (lightweight)	Simple to use Folds for transportation Lighter weight than standard wheelchair Partial adjustability Easier to propel Durable Will accommodate custom seating	Not custom fit Lack of axle adjustability may limit manual propulsion by user Still may be too heavy for many users	Intermittent or temporary use Possible use for in-home applications if environment tolerates
Fully adjustable manual wheelchair with a folding frame (ultra-lightweight)	Very light frame Maximal adjustability, especially of rear axle position Custom fit to user Accommodates custom seating Accommodates to uneven ground by flexing Folds side to side for easy transportation	Many adjustable or removable parts More complex design, requires more maintenance Some propulsion energy lost in flex of frame	Full-time wheelchair user with permanent disability User wants to transport in trunk of vehicle Environment includes travel over uneven surfaces
Fully adjustable manual wheelchair with a rigid frame (ultra-lightweight)	Very light frame Maximal adjustability, especially of rear axle position Custom fit to user Fewer removable or adjustable parts than folding frame Accommodates custom seating	Does not accommodate to uneven terrain as easily as folding frame May be more difficult to transport in trunk of car (less compact when folded)	Full-time wheelchair user with permanent disability User wants most efficient system for propulsion Used mainly indoors or on even terrains
Power assist manual wheelchair	Light frame Maneuvers like manual wheelchair Minimizes stress on shoulders	Heavier than nonpower assist More difficult to disassemble for transport	Lightweight manual wheelchair user with limited endurance or shoulder limitations Manual wheelchair user with long-distance ambulation needs or difficulty managing outdoor terrain independently

Type	Advantages	Disadvantages	Indications
Tilt-in-space frame wheelchair	Allows rotation in space for pressure management or other benefits Available for both manual and powered wheelchairs	Frame often heavier and bulkier Usually does not fold for transportation If on manual wheelchair, typically has small rear wheels, requiring an attendant to propel	Wheelchair user requires rotation in space for pressure management or other medical reason, such as respiratory disease
Reclining frame wheelchair	Allows for change in seat-to-back angle, often to full supine position Available for both manual and powered wheelchairs	Frame often heavier and bulkier Rear wheels set further back to provide larger base of support when in recline position Difficult to propel if used with manual wheelchair	Used when a need for change in seat to back angle is required Used for pressure management May be used for self-care in wheelchair May be used when supine bed transfers are required Often used when building sitting tolerance during initial rehabilitation
Powered scooter	Allows simple-to-learn powered mobility Good outdoor access Swivel seat for ease of transfers Baskets and other accessories for function, such as shopping	Only one access method Large turning radius; difficult to use in many homes Does not accommodate custom seating; few seating support options	Used with individuals who have limited endurance Often used for primarily outdoor mobility purposes
Powered wheelchair	Full access to powered mobility for both indoor and outdoor use Multiple access methods possible Accommodates custom seating supports Accommodates power seating options, such as tilt or recline	Heavy Requires van for transportation Less maneuverable than manual wheelchair Requires more initial training for optimal safety and function	Individuals who cannot propel manual wheelchair effectively Used for indoor and outdoor mobility for long distances May be used in work or school applications for part-time manual wheelchair users

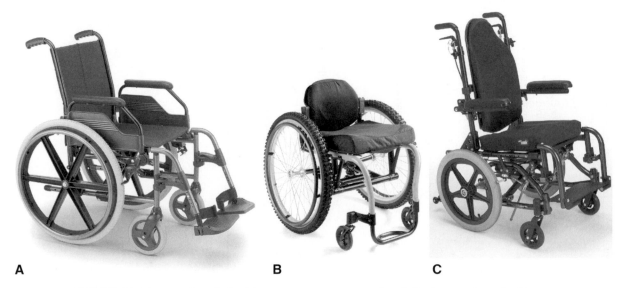

A   **B**   **C**

FIGURE 16-10 Examples of wheelchair support structure and mobility base options. **A,** A standard lightweight, semiadjustable wheelchair with arm support and swing-away leg rests. **B,** An ultralightweight wheelchair with rigid frame, precontoured seat and back support, and shock-absorbing mechanism. **C,** A pediatric wheelchair with reclining back and precontoured seating system. (Courtesy Sunrise Medical, Longmont, CO.)

TABLE 16-8   *Advantages and Disadvantages of Various Wheelchair Components*

Wheelchair Component	Options	Advantages	Disadvantages
Leg and foot supports	Swing-away foot rests	Lightweight	Add to weight of wheelchair (vs. platform)
		Support for lower extremities	Require maintenance
		Removable for transfers	Require management by wheelchair user
	Flip-up foot platform	Lightweight	Very little adjustability
		Few moving parts	Both lower extremities supported at same angle
		Very stable	Unable to accommodate moderate or severe ankle contractures
		Often allows increased knee flexion angle; more comfortable and compact for user	Not removable; may interfere with transfers for some users
	Manual elevating leg rests	Allows multiple leg positions	Heavier than standard leg supports
		May prevent some dependent edema (true edema management also requires recline or tilt to elevate the legs above the heart level)	Many moving and adjustable parts; higher maintenance needs
		May increase lower extremity comfort	More strength and dexterity needed to manage
Arm supports	Flip-back arm rests	Stable arm support	Multiple moving parts
		Typically lightweight	Require maintenance to work properly
		Easy to manage	May not be adjustable enough for all individuals
	Tubular swing-away arm rest	Extremely lightweight	May not feel stable to user
		Easy for wheelchair user to manage	May not tolerate extreme or repeated stresses
		Requires very little hand dexterity and strength	Attachment hardware requires maintenance
	Detachable, adjustable-height arm rest	Support upper extremities in multiple positions	Heavier
		Removable for transfers	More moving parts; higher maintenance requirement
			May be difficult for users to manager; especially to replace parts on the wheelchair
	Desk-length arm rest	Allow wheelchair user to approach tables, sinks, desks for improved function	May not provide adequate support during transfers
		Lighter in weight than full-length arm supports	Do not provide full arm support
	Full-length arm rest	Provide full arm support	Heavier than desk-length arm
		Provide improved support during transfers	Do not allow close approach to tables, sinks, or desks

TABLE 16-8   *Advantages and Disadvantages of Various Wheelchair Components—cont'd*

Wheelchair Component	Options	Advantages	Disadvantages
Wheel locks	Pull-to lock	Allow closer access for transfers to surfaces Move away from wheels so hands do not hit with propulsion	May be more difficult to lock
	Push-to lock	Lock easily and securely	May interfere with propulsion May interfere with transfers
	Under-seat or scissor locks	Complete clearance for hands during propulsion No interference in transfers	Significantly better balance and coordination required for locking and unlocking More difficult to adjust

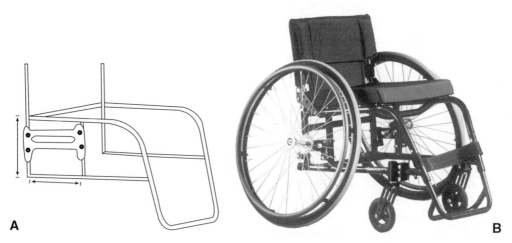

FIGURE 16-11 In maximally adjustable wheelchair frames, wheel position can be tailored to meet the user's specific needs by adjusting the location of the wheel axis in an anteroposterior slide and vertical position on the frame. **A,** A rigid frame in which the wheel bracket can be positioned as needed on the frame. **B,** An actual chair. (Courtesy Sunrise Medical, Longmont, CO.)

not properly supported, and injuries to limbs that fall off their supports during propulsion. Most of these risks can be minimized by adequate training and safety mechanisms added to a wheelchair during the initial training period. The most common of these strategies is the use of rear antitip tubes until a new wheelchair user gains enough strength and postural control to master the "wheelie" maneuver and managing steep inclines or steps.

Other risks associated with manual wheelchair propulsion are less-well understood and are the focus of much current research. These risks include long-term risks of manual wheelchair user for repetitive use strain injuries, leading to impairment in function or pain in the shoulders and upper extremities.[16] The two main areas of focus are the shoulders (e.g., rotator cuff tears) and wrists (e.g., carpal tunnel syndrome).[27] These risks may be much larger than previously thought, particularly for individuals who have depended on wheeled mobility use over long periods. Because of the increased longevity of persons with different types of disabilities who have relied on manual wheeled mobility for 20 years or more, these injuries are becoming much more prevalent and may be extremely detrimental to continued independent function.

WHEN IS A POWERED CHAIR APPROPRIATE?

The choice of manual or powered mobility is straightforward for many wheelchair users. For example, an individual with tetraplegia who has little movement in the upper extremities benefits most from powered mobility. Likewise, persons with minimal trunk and upper body impairment are obvious manual wheelchair candidates. The problem arises when individuals have skills and abilities that are not so clearly indicative of a particular variety of mobility, or when the environmental demands placed on the individual really require use of powered mobility in spite of the individual's basic ability to propel a manual mobility device.

One of the most important decisions for any wheelchair user is that of manual versus powered mobility. Both types of mobility have advantages and disadvantages, and overall function is greatly affected by this basic selection. Conditions and impairments that often indicate need for powered mobility include the following:

1. Severe upper extremity or upper trunk weakness leading to an inability to propel any type of manual wheelchair
2. Ataxic or uncoordinated movement of the upper extremities

3. Endurance limitations, whether from muscular or cardiopulmonary impairment
4. Progressive conditions that will likely lead to loss of upper extremity strength or poor endurance (particularly a rapidly progressing condition)
5. Orthopedic problems in the upper extremity joints (e.g., arthritis or preexisting rotator cuff or carpal tunnel impairments)
6. Environments that require long-distance travel on a regular basis or travel over rough terrain

Once a determination has been made that powered mobility is necessary, one of the next decisions is the access method for control of the device. If the powered mobility device is a powered scooter, this decision is uncomplicated; a tiller mechanism is the most efficient and effective choice. If, however, the device under consideration is a powered wheelchair (Figure 16-12), the access methods available are far more complex. Powered wheelchair access methods include standard joysticks, switch arrays, sip and puff input devices, and head-controlled devices, among others. These options make it more likely that an effective control system can be designed for powered wheelchair users with various and significant impairments and functional limitations. The decision making process, however, is more complex for clinicians who must evaluate and assist in the selection of an access method.

The best method of powered wheelchair access allows the wheelchair user optimal control and function in the environment over the long term. Sometimes the simplest method to learn may not ultimately be the best for the user over the long-term. Some input methods, such as head control systems, require a longer training period, but the ultimate function of the user may be superior to a simpler joystick system. A thorough evaluation with multiple episodes of training may be required before an ultimate access method is selected. To

select appropriate power access options and effectively train a wheelchair user in the proper use of these devices, clinicians must be aware of the different types of equipment and how each works to stop and start, turn or change direction, lock and unlock, and alter velocity of movement. Ideally, clinicians also must know how to adjust the control mechanism to allow the user to be most energy efficient and effective. These skills may take many years of training to develop, most often when the clinician functions as a specialist who works with individuals with highly complex access needs on a regular basis.

TRAINING STRATEGIES

Regardless of the type of wheelchair selected or the access method chosen, intensive training of the person using the wheelchair is necessary. Training takes place across settings and over time. Wheelchair skills are typically introduced during inpatient rehabilitation but training usually continues either in home care or outpatient settings until the new user gains independence with advanced skills. Initial training may actually be accomplished with loaner or temporary equipment used to assess options and designs that will allow optimal mobility before a wheelchair prescription is finalized. Additional training is typically necessary once the permanent wheelchair and associated equipment have been delivered.

Functional manual wheelchair users are well trained in the safe use of equipment, are able to effectively manage obstacles in the home environment and community (work and leisure settings), are able to perform or direct basic maintenance of the equipment (including cleaning procedures and maintaining moving parts), and know when and whom to contact if something out of the ordinary occurs with the wheelchair.

Power wheelchair users often require more extensive periods of training than manual chair users to achieve optimal mobility and function. This training must include management of indoor terrain and obstacles such as turning in tight spaces, managing door frames and transitions between flooring surfaces, and negotiating other indoor obstacles such as elevators. Training should also include outdoor terrain and obstacles, such as ramps, curbs, side slopes, grassy surfaces, gravel surfaces, and safe operation on crowded sidewalks or when crossing streets. If a powered seating system is prescribed, the user must be educated regarding the proper and safe use of this powered seating system, including how often to use it, under what conditions it should (and should not) be used, and whom to contact if the powered seating system is not functioning properly.

Although the assessment and prescription for a wheelchair usually takes place in a specialty clinic, functional training after delivery of the equipment is typically provided by outpatient or home care therapy services. A therapist who has questions about a particular piece of equipment that a patient is learning to use should contact the seating clinician and work on a training protocol that will be most effective.

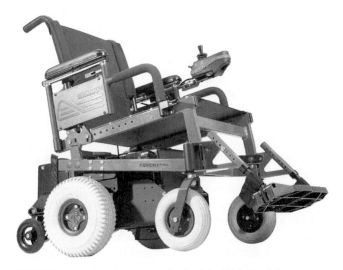

FIGURE 16-12 In this powered wheelchair, the mobility component includes the wheelbase as well as the joystick (or alternative access method) used to control the movement of the chair. Note that anterior–posterior wheelbase dimension is longer to accommodate the weight of the batteries and motors of the chair. (Courtesy Sunrise Medical, Longmont, CO.)

SEATING SYSTEMS FOR PRESSURE MANAGEMENT

Selection of the wheeled mobility device itself is only part of the equation when working with individuals who use wheelchairs for much or all of their mobility. The seating system or postural support system is as important as the wheeled mobility base and access method. The seating system is critical to integrating the person and the wheeled mobility system, and several major issues must be considered in its selection.

A major issue for many wheelchairs users is pressure management. Any person who sits for more than 4 hours per day is at increased risk for pressure-related damage to the skin.[28] This risk is exacerbated by many factors, including impaired sensation, increased heat or moisture buildup near the skin, inadequate nutrition or hydration status, and atrophy of muscle tissue leading to decreased soft-tissue protection for bony prominences.[29]

The major problem associated with pressure sustained over long durations is skin breakdown. This problem has been the focus of a great deal of research for more than 30 years and is better understood than it used to be, but still mysterious. The individual and interactive effects of pressure, friction, and shear are the current focus of research regarding skin breakdown, its causes, and ways to prevent it. Skin breakdown is an extremely costly and debilitating problem for many wheelchair users.[30,31] Treatment for skin breakdown often involves costly surgical interventions and prolonged hospital and rehabilitation stays. Skin breakdown may also be responsible for ultimately reducing the life expectancy for individuals with disabilities who use wheelchairs for mobility.[30]

Active and Passive Strategies

Many technologies have been developed to provide pressure management. Recognizing that low pressure exerted over long periods can be as dangerous for skin as high pressures exerted over short periods, pressure management technologies provide options either to distribute pressure over as wide a surface area as possible or to change position so that the forces exerted on weight-bearing surfaces vary over time. Most rely on good user training and use of the systems for optimal function and outcome; no pressure management system can entirely prevent skin breakdown if used improperly or inconsistently.

Technologies can be grouped into three general categories on the basis of whether they use an active, rotational, or passive strategy to provide pressure relief. Active technologies, such as active or dynamic seat cushions, are designed to relieve areas of high pressure periodically. Dynamic seat cushions are often divided into a series of alternating chambers. A motor pumps air or fluid through chambers to change the configuration of the support surface gently and continuously (much like an alternating-pressure mattress used in hospital beds for patients who are unable to change position). Rotational seating systems include those with a powered tilt or recline mechanism, a manual tilt or recline system, or a standing system (Figure 16-13). Passive technologies for pressure management focus on increasing seating surface area, usually by increasing envelopment or compliance of the seating surface or by shifting pressure from traditionally high-risk areas, such as ischial tuberosities, to lower-risk areas, such as distal femurs. Some passive technologies completely offload areas such as the ischial tuberosities, and others simply aim to reduce pressure in these areas by using more compliant materials in certain zones of the cushion (see Figure 16-8).

Some supports can cause skin "hammocking," or stretching the skin and soft tissues across bony surfaces such as the coccyx, when unloading other regions such as the ischial tuberosities. This effect can cause skin breakdown even in the absence of direct external tissue loading.

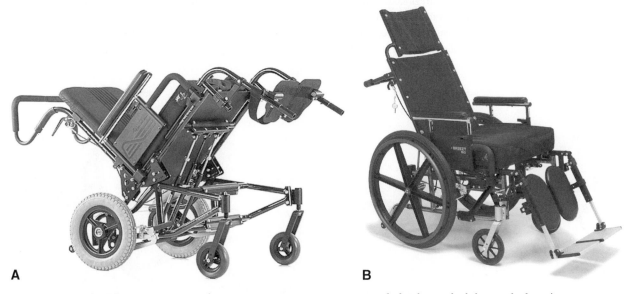

A   **B**

FIGURE 16-13 Rotational pressure management strategies include tilt, in which hip angle doesn't change (**A**), and reclining (**B**), in which hip angle (extension) is opened (increased). Rotational pressure management systems are available for both manual and powered wheelchairs. (Courtesy Sunrise Medical, Longmont, CO.)

Size and Setup

In addition to the technological development of products for pressure management, clinicians have learned a great deal about seating intervention to manage pressure as effectively as possible. Proper size and setup of wheelchairs is often critical in appropriately managing pressure.[21] The strategic use of contoured surfaces, different types of materials and coverings, and a well-planned mobility system and any active seating choices, such as tilting or reclining seating systems (also known as *rotational systems*) must be integrated in a holistic approach to protect wheelchair users from skin breakdown.[28]

Training

In addition to choices of technologies, proper training and education of wheelchair users is essential to the effective application of this technology. Most of the technologies developed rely on proper use, either through correct positioning on the wheelchair and proper maintenance and adjustment, or schedules by the user. Sometimes an apparent failure of a particular technology has more to do with how it was used or in what combinations different technologies were used than the actual failure of the technology itself.

Seating for Function and Comfort

Although pressure management in seating often dominates research and technological development, maximal function and optimal comfort are equally important.[7] Wheelchair users who are not able to function optimally or become uncomfortable when seated will probably not reach their full potential. Individuals who have discomfort when seated also have satisfaction problems with their equipment, which may cause equipment abandonment.[32] To function optimally individuals must be comfortable and secure in their seating systems.

The priorities of a seating system depend on the problems and goals identified during the assessment process. If a patient has a lack of sensation and a history of skin breakdown problems, then seating for pressure management will most likely be the highest priority. However, if the problems identified focus on a lack of optimal function or feelings of discomfort when using the equipment, then goals for enhanced function and comfort may be more critical. For some patients all three issues are priorities, and equipment must be carefully selected that will balance all needs and allow the individual to meet all goals of seating.

The determination of these priorities is often quite challenging. For a health care team, the primary medical concern might be pressure management or improving comfort, but the user may be focused on a particular functional goal that the user believes is more critical than pressure management. Occasionally, equipment selection will be difficult because some needs may have to be compromised to meet other needs optimally. An air–fluid cushion, for example, may provide the maximal pressure management desired by the team but might feel unstable to the wheelchair user, disrupting comfort, function, or both.

When compromises must be made, a conflict can occur between the health care or seating team and the wheelchair user. The best way to resolve conflicts is to find a technology intervention that meets all the stated needs. If this is not possible, then the wheelchair user must be properly educated regarding the risks and benefits of the equipment selected and ultimately make an informed choice. Health professionals should remember that the user is the only one who can decide what is best for the user's circumstances. Forcing choices on an individual often has very negative consequences in terms of equipment abandonment or improper use and can also negatively affect the individual's satisfaction with the process and equipment provided. The best solution is one that meets all the needs to the greatest extent possible and that yields optimal consumer satisfaction.

SUMMARY

The science associated with adaptive seating and mobility for persons with disabilities is still in its infancy. Significant research in this field only began in the 1960s, and serious growth of this research has only been happening for the last 10 to 20 years.[33] Recent work has focused on the development of wheeled mobility that allows individuals to participate in a variety of leisure and competitive sport activities (Figure 16-14). In spite of this, several important research findings related to wheelchair

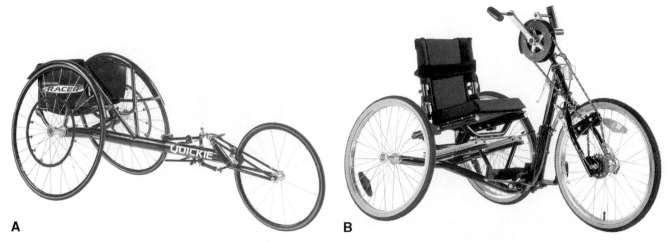

A   **B**

FIGURE 16-14 Examples of wheelchairs designed for wheelchair racing (**A**) and upper-extremity–powered bicycling (**B**). (Courtesy Sunrise Medical, Longmont, CO.)

seating and mobility are now beginning to be applied to the practice of wheelchair mobility seating.

A great deal of research has contributed to and resulted from the development of international and national seating and wheelchair standards. The Rehabilitation Engineering and Assistive Technology Society of North America has been actively working toward the development of wheelchair seating standards since 1979.[34] These standards are intended to provide objective information to consumers about the safety and performance of wheelchairs.[34] In addition, wheelchair standards have facilitated improvements in quality and performance of wheeled mobility equipment.[35] Standards development also has provided a platform for research into characteristics of wheelchairs that are most beneficial to consumers and allowed the justification of higher-quality products based on ultimate cost effectiveness.[36-39] Wheelchair seating standards regarding the strength, efficacy, and safety of postural support devices are currently under development to provide many of these same benefits to the development and research related to adaptive seating products.

In addition to the research being performed in the standards arena, a great deal of interest and research in evidence-based practice exist for wheelchair seating and mobility. Although many seating clinicians prefer to practice with an evidence-based model, little research exists to support the efficacy of either the intervention process used or the equipment prescribed.[40,41] Several researchers are developing and validating outcomes measures to facilitate development of evidence-based practice in this field.[6,12,42-45] Once appropriate seating and wheeled mobility outcomes measures are developed, applying these outcomes in clinical and research settings and building the evidence so desperately needed in this field will be possible. Few randomized, controlled clinical trials assessing efficacy of seating and mobility intervention have been performed.[46,47] Such studies have primarily focused on preventing pressure ulcers as an outcome of seat cushion intervention. More research regarding the many other possible outcomes of wheelchair seating and mobility intervention is still needed.

CASE EXAMPLE 1

Patient with a C5/C6 Complete Spinal Cord Injury

J. J. is a 24-year-old man who sustained an injury to his spine at the C5 vertebral level in a motor vehicle accident 8 weeks ago. He has total loss of motor function on his right side below the level of the C5 nerve root and on his left side below the C6 nerve root level. He was referred to the clinic for an evaluation for his first wheelchair after his in-patient rehabilitation.

J. J.'s sensation is severely impaired below the level of his shoulders, although he has some ability to feel in localized areas of his body. At the time of his visit to the seating clinic, he was using a cervical orthosis for stabilization

of his surgically repaired cervical spinal column. He has undergone surgery consisting of a spinal fusion from C4 through T1 vertebrae. J. J. will be returning home to live with his wife and 2-year-old child. He is an architect and works in an office approximately 20 miles from his home. His job responsibilities include visiting construction sites involved in his design projects.

During his rehabilitation, J. J. has been propelling a fully adjustable manual wheelchair with specialty wheelchair propulsion gloves and plastic-coated wheel rims. He is able to propel his wheelchair on indoor surfaces for 300 feet at a time but still has problems with fatigue and neck pain. He requires assistance for outdoor surfaces and for propelling up or down ramps. J. J. lives in a home with 3 steps to enter, but his neighbors are building him a ramp that will be ready by the time he returns home. He has wall-to-wall carpeting throughout his home with the exception of the kitchen and bathroom floors.

J. J.'s stated goals include the following:
- Being as independent as possible in his home and workplace
- Being able to transport his wheelchair in a car
- Returning to work as soon as possible
- Helping care for his 2-year-old son and his home
- Improving his endurance and reducing his level of neck pain so that he can sit up and function for a full day
- Maintaining skin integrity

Questions to Consider
- Given his history and stated goals, what should the systems review include?
- What specific tests and measures will likely be used in the examination?
- How might his current functional status and his prognosis for recovery or accommodation of impairments and associated functional limitations influence the assessment of his needs?

Evaluation and Prognosis
J. J. has no active movement in his legs or trunk. He has good strength in elbow flexion on the left side, fair strength in elbow flexion on the right side, good strength in both of his shoulders, but no evidence of triceps activity on either side. His range of motion is normal with the exception of his neck range, which cannot be tested because of the cervical orthosis. His conscious sensation is spotty, and he has no sensation in his buttock region. He requires assistance for all transfers and other mobility and for activities of daily living, such as bathing and dressing. J. J. has a healed pressure sore in the region of his coccyx; it developed during his acute hospitalization but is now healed, and he is able to sit for 6 to 8 hours per day. He has been using an ultra-lightweight, folding-frame, manual wheelchair and a foam and gel seat cushion.

Continued

- What will the team's priorities be for J. J.'s seating and mobility system? How are these priorities similar or different from J. J.'s priorities? What compromises might be necessary?
- What options might be considered for J. J. in terms of seating system (noncontoured, contoured, or custom)? Support frame (lightweight, heavy duty)? Mobility component (manual or powered chair)?
- What recommendations should be made for managing pressure in J. J.'s seating system (active, rotational, reclined, or passive)? Why?

Recommendations

General recommendations for J. J. include a manual wheelchair with a power assist add-on component to allow him more independent mobility and access to all his environments while minimizing stress on his shoulders and neck and accomplishing his goal of transportability by car. Seating will consist of a gel and foam seat cushion contoured to match the shape of his buttocks and manage pressure distribution as evenly as possible. J. J. requires a solid back support with generic contour and angle adjustability to allow appropriate upright posture to maximize his function and balance and minimize future development of spinal deformities. Plastic-coated wheel rims and specialty gloves will maximize his wheel/rim interface, allowing him optimal propulsion as well.

CASE EXAMPLE 2

Patient with Cerebral Palsy

S. W. is a 35-year-old woman with spastic quadriplegia attributable to cerebral palsy. She has been using a fully adjustable manual wheelchair for most of her life with good success. Her current wheelchair is 10 years old and she reports that it is falling apart (her rehabilitation technology supplier confirms the extensive repair history of this wheelchair). She came to the seating clinic for an assessment for a replacement wheelchair and seating system.

S. W. has no functional movement in her lower extremities and has severe extensor tone in both legs. She has impaired motor control in her arms but is able to propel her manual wheelchair with some difficulty. She transports her wheelchair in her car with some assistance from others for disassembling the seating and folding the wheelchair for stowing. The muscle tone in her trunk and arms fluctuates, but she has significant intermittent extensor tone.

S. W. works independently in an office as an administrative assistant. Her home is wheelchair accessible and her office setting does not require long-distance propulsion. When she shops or goes to the mall, her friends assist her with her mobility or she borrows a powered scooter from the grocery store.

S.W.'s goals include the following:
- Maintaining or improving her current level of mobility
- Improving her perception of postural stability in her wheelchair
- Being able to transport her wheelchair in her car with no more difficulty than she currently has
- Having a wheelchair that is easy to manage and maintain (fewer moving parts to break)

Questions to Consider
- Given her history and her stated goals, what should the systems review include?
- What specific tests and measures would likely be used in the examination?
- How might her current functional status and the chronic nature of her neuromuscular condition (coupled with the aging process), with its associated impairments and functional limitations, influence the assessment of her needs?

Evaluation and Prognosis

S. W. has severely impaired strength in her legs and trunk, poor unsupported sitting balance, severe extensor spasticity in both legs, hip flexion limited to a 100-degree pelvis-to-thigh angle, moderate weakness in her arms with poor motor control, and fluctuating muscle tone. S. W. also has a severe scoliosis and a pelvic rotation and pelvic obliquity. With moderate trunk support she is able to use her arms functionally and feels secure.

Questions to Consider
- What will the team's priorities be for S. W.'s seating and mobility system? How are the team's priorities similar to or different than S. W.'s priorities? What compromises might be necessary?
- What options might be considered for S. W. in terms of seating system (noncontoured, contoured, or custom)? Support frame (lightweight, heavy duty)? Mobility component (manual or powered chair)?
- What recommendations should be made for managing pressure in S. W.'s seating system (active, rotational, or passive)? Why?

Recommendations

General recommendations for S. W. may include a new custom manual wheelchair with a folding titanium frame with a fixed-axle position specified to her particular needs, a custom-contoured seat and back cushion to support and position her, spring-loaded foot rests with elevating leg rests for her lower extremities, a push-button pelvic belt with special loops so that she can fasten and secure it around her hips, and a hook-and-loop material chest belt to stabilize her upper body. The combination of custom-contoured seating and anterior support devices that she can tighten herself will improve her feeling of stability and the overall fit of the wheelchair seating. This wheelchair will be more durable with fewer moving parts and will meet her mobility needs.

A Patient with Cerebrovascular Accident

M. L. is an 80-year-old woman who has been referred for an assessment for wheeled mobility because of a recent decline in her ability to walk. M. L. had a stroke 10 years ago that impaired the strength on the left side of her body. Although she regained the ability to walk and can do so with a quad cane, she has begun to fall more frequently and currently is severely limited by her mobility impairment. She can walk only a distance of 10 feet and must have assistance from another person to do so safely. Because of this limitation, she spends most of her time sitting in a recliner chair in her living room and is becoming quite depressed. She has always been an active woman and would like to be able to participate in activities outside her home as well as move around inside her home by herself.

Questions to Consider

- Given her history and her stated goals, what should the systems review include?
- What specific tests and measures should be used in the examination?
- How might her current functional status and the chronic nature of her neuromuscular condition (coupled with the aging process), with its associated impairments and functional limitations, influence the assessment of her needs?
- What will the team's priorities be for M. L.'s seating and mobility system? How are the team's priorities similar or different from M. L.'s priorities? What compromises might be necessary?
- What options should be considered for M. L. in terms of seating system (noncontoured, contoured, or custom)? Support frame (lightweight, heavy duty)? Mobility component (manual or powered chair)?
- What recommendations should be made for managing pressure in M. L.'s seating system (active, rotational, reclined, or passive)? Why?

Recommendations

M. L. was evaluated in the seating and mobility clinic. The team arranged for her to borrow a semiadjustable, lightweight manual wheelchair and a powered wheelchair for a week so that she could assess which might best meet her needs. She was only able to propel the manual wheelchair on smooth indoor surfaces and could not move the chair up an incline without great difficulty. She was fully independent in operating the powered wheelchair but was discouraged by its large size.

The rehabilitation technology supplier obtained a smaller powered wheelchair considered transportable and that more closely resembles a manual wheelchair in overall size and shape. M. L. evaluated this wheelchair in her home environment and was pleased with her increased independence and access to all areas of her home and immediate outdoor environment. For seating, M. L. was prescribed a generically contoured foam seat cushion and a solid, adjustable back support. With this equipment, her posture was improved and she felt comfortable and secure.

REFERENCES

1. Kaye HS, Kang T, LaPlante MP. *Mobility Device Use in the United States*. Washington, DC: U.S. Department of Education, National Institute on Disability and Rehabilitation; 2000.
2. Jones ML, Sanford JA. People with mobility impairments in the United States today and in 2010. *Assist Technol.* 1996;8(1):43–53.
3. Schoenman JA. Description of the US working age disabled populations living in institutions and in the community. *Disabil Rehabil.* 1995;17(5):231–238.
4. Simmons SF, Schnelle JF, MacRae PG, et al. Wheelchairs as mobility restraints: predictors of wheelchair activity in nonambulatory nursing home residents. *J Am Geriatr Soc.* 1995;43(4):384–388.
5. Cook AM, Hussey SM. Seating systems as extrinsic enablers for assistive technologies. In: Cook AM, Hussey SM, eds. *Assistive Technologies: Principles and Practice*, vol 1, 2nd ed. St. Louis: Mosby; 2002:165–211.
6. Pedersen JP, Lange ML, Griebel C. Seating intervention and postural control. In: Olson DA, DeRuyter F, eds. *Clinician's Guide to Assistive Technology*. St. Louis: Mosby; 2002:209–236.
7. Minkel JL. Seating and mobility considerations for people with spinal cord injury. *Phys Ther.* 2000;80(7):701–709.
8. American Physical Therapy Association. Guide to Physical Therapist Practice. *Phys Ther.* 2001;81(1):21–138.
9. Zollars JA, Knezevich J. *Special seating: an illustrated guide*. Minneapolis, MN: Otto Bock Orthopedic Industry; 1996.
10. Trefler E. Then and now. *Team Rehab Report.* 1999;10(2):32–36.
11. Ferguson-Pell M, Cardi MD. Prototype development and comparative evaluation of wheelchair pressure mapping system. *Assist Technol.* 1993;5(2):78–91.
12. Kirby RL, Swuste J, Dupuis DJ, et al. The Wheelchair Skills Test: a pilot study of a new outcome measure. *Arch Phys Med Rehabil.* 2002;83(1):10–18.
13. McLaurin CA, Brubaker CE. Biomechanics and the wheelchair. *Prosthet Orthot Int.* 1991;15(1):24–37.
14. Engstrom B. *Seating and Mobility for the Physically Challenged, Risks and Possibilities When Using Wheelchairs*, vol 1. 2nd ed. Sweden: Posturalis Books; 2002.
15. Zacharkow D. *Posture: Sitting, Standing, Chair Design and Exercise*. Springfield, IL: Charles C. Thomas; 1988.
16. Curtis KA, Drysdale GA, Lama D, et al. Shoulder pain in wheelchair users with tetraplegia and paraplegia. *Arch Phys Med Rehabil.* 1999;80(4):453–457.
17. Koontz AM, Boninger ML. Proper propulsion. *Rehab Manag.* 2003;16(6):18–22.
18. van der Woude LH, Veeger DJ, Rosendal RH, et al. Seat height in hand rim wheelchair propulsion. *J Rehabil Res Dev.* 1989;26(4):31–50.
19. van der Woude LH, Veeger HE, Rozendal RH. Propulsion technique in hand rim wheelchair ambulation. *J Med Eng Technol.* 1989;13(1–2):136–141.
20. Garber SL. Wheelchair cushions: a historical review. *Am J Occup Ther.* 1985;39(7):453–459.

21. Ham R, Aldersea P, Porter D. *Wheelchair Users and Postural Seating: A Clinical Approach*, vol 1. New York: Churchill Livingstone; 1998.

22. Hobson DA. Seating and mobility for the severely disabled: Technology overview and classification. In: Leslie J, ed. *Rehabilitation Engineering*. Boca Raton, FL: CRC Press; 1988:201–218.

23. St-Georges M, Valiquette C, Drouin G. Computer-aided design in wheelchair seating. *J Rehabil Res Dev*. 1989;26(4):23–30.

24. Brienza DM, Geyer MJ. Understanding support surface technologies. *Adv Skin Wound Care*. 2000;13(5):237–244.

25. Stewart SFC, Palmieri V, Cochran GVB. Wheelchair cushion effect on skin temperature, heat flux, and relative humidity. *Arch Phys Med Rehabil*. 1980;61(5):229–233.

26. van der Woude LH, Dallmeijer AJ, Janssen TWJ, et al. Alternative modes of manual wheelchair ambulation: an overview. *Am J Phys Med Rehabil*. 2001;80(10):765–777.

27. Boninger ML, Cooper RA, Roberson RN, et al. Wrist biomechanics during two speeds of wheelchair propulsion: an analysis using a local coordinate system. *Arch Phys Med Rehabil*. 1997;78(4):364–372.

28. Bergman-Evans B, Cuddigan J, Bergstrom N. Clinical practice guidelines: prediction and prevention of pressure ulcers. *J Gerontol Nurs*. 1994;20(9):19–26.

29. Bergstrom N, Braden BJ, Laguzza A, et al. The Braden Scale for predicting pressure sore risk. *Nurs Res*. 1987;36(4):205–210.

30. Allman RM. Pressure ulcer prevalence, incidence, risk factors, and impact. *Clin Geriatr Med*. 1997;13(3):421–436.

31. Cuddigan J, Berlowitz DR, Ayello AE. Pressure ulcers in America: prevalence, incidence, and implications for the future. *Adv Skin Wound Care*. 2001;14(4):208–215.

32. Weiss-Lambrou R. Satisfaction and comfort. In: Scherer MJ, ed. *Assistive Technology: Matching Device and Consumer for Successful Rehabilitation*. Washington, DC: American Psychological Association; 2002:77–94.

33. McLaurin CA. Current directions in wheelchair research. *J Rehabil Res Dev* 1990;(Suppl 2):88–99.

34. Axelson P, Minkel J, Chesney DA. *Guide to Wheelchair Selection: How to Use the ANSI/RESNA Standards to Buy a Wheelchair*. Washington, DC: Paralyzed Veterans of America; 1994.

35. Hartridge M, Seeger BR. International wheelchair standards: a study of costs and benefits. *Assist Technol*. 1990;2(4):117–123.

36. Cooper RA, Boninger ML, Rentschler A. Evaluation of selected ultralight manual wheelchairs using ANSI/RESNA standards. *Arch Phys Med Rehabil*. 1999;80(4):462–467.

37. Cooper RA, DiGiovine CP, Rentschler A, et al. Fatigue-life of two manual wheelchair cross-brace designs. *Arch Phys Med Rehabil*. 1999;80(9):1078–1081.

38. Cooper RA, Gonzalez J, Lawrence B, et al. Performance of selected lightweight wheelchairs on ANSI/RESNA tests. *Arch Phys Med Rehabil*. 1997;78(10):1138–1144.

39. Cooper RA, Robertson RN, Lawrence B, et al. Life-cycle analysis of depot versus rehabilitation manual wheelchairs. *J Rehabil Res Dev*. 1996;33(1):45–55.

40. Rader JD, Jones D, Miller L. The importance of individualized wheelchair seating for frail older adults. *J Gerontol Nurs*. 2000;26(11):24–32 46–47.

41. Scherer MJ. Outcomes of assistive technology use on quality of life. *Disabil Rehabil*. 1996;18(9):439–448.

42. Aissaoui R, Boucher C, Bourbonnais D, et al. Effect of seat cushion on dynamic stability in sitting during a reaching task in wheelchair users with paraplegia. *Arch Phys Med Rehabil*. 2001;82(2):274–281.

43. Demers L, Wessels R, Weiss-Lambrou R, et al. Key dimensions of client satisfaction with assistive technology: a cross-validation of a Canadian measure in The Netherlands. *J Rehabil Med*. 2001;33(4):187–191.

44. Hobson D, Crane B. State of the science white paper on wheelchair seat comfort. *Wheelchair Seating: A State of the Science Conference on Seating Issues for Persons with Disabilities*. Orlando, FL: Rehabilitation Engineering Center on Wheeled Mobility and the School of Health and Rehabilitation Sciences at the University of Pittsburgh; 2001;29–33.

45. May LA, Butt C, Minor L, et al. Measurement reliability of functional tasks for persons who self-propel a manual wheelchair. *Arch Phys Med Rehabil*. 2003;84(4):578–583.

46. Conine TA, Hershler C, Daechsel D, et al. Pressure ulcer prophylaxis in elderly patients using polyurethane foam or Jay wheelchair cushions. *Int J Rehabil Res*. 1994;17(2):123–137.

47. Geyer MJ, Brienza DM, Karg P, et al. A randomized control trial to evaluate pressure-reducing seat cushions for elderly wheelchair users. *Adv Skin Wound Care*. 2001;14(3):120–129.

III

Prostheses in Rehabilitation

17

Etiology of Amputation

CAROLINE C. NIELSEN AND MILAGROS JORGE

LEARNING OBJECTIVES

On completion of this chapter, the reader will be able to do the following:
1. Describe the epidemiology of nontraumatic, traumatic and congenital amputation.
2. Compare and contrast the major causes of amputation.
3. Describe the interrelationships of the major risk factors for dysvascular/neuropathic-related amputation.
4. Explain the differences in risk factors of amputation among various racial and ethnic groups.
5. Describe health-promotion efforts for the prevention of dysvascular disease.
6. Identify key issues considered by the rehabilitation team when caring for older adults with amputation.

Throughout the history of medicine, amputation has been a relatively frequently performed medical procedure and has often been the only available alternative for complex fractures or infections of the extremities. The earliest amputations were generally undertaken to save lives; however, their outcomes were often unsuccessful—many resulted in death from shock caused by blood loss or onset of infection and septicemia in those who survived the operation. In these early amputations, removal of the compromised limb segment as quickly as possible was essential. With the advent of antisepsis, asepsis, and anesthesia in the mid nineteenth century, physicians focused increasingly on the surgical procedure and conservation of tissue.[1] The development of modern medical treatment has provided alternatives to amputation. Today, when amputation is necessary, surgery is undertaken with consideration for the functional aspects of the residual limb. This chapter reports the epidemiology of amputation; reviews the causes for amputation; describes the expected outcomes for persons with limb pathology resulting in amputation; and discusses approaches to rehabilitation of the person with limb loss.

EPIDEMIOLOGY OF AMPUTATION

Surveillance data on persons living with limb loss is limited, because in the United States there is no national database for compiling data specific to persons with amputation. Information on persons with amputation is derived from a variety of sources including hospital discharge diagnoses information. The 1996 National Health Interview Survey has the most comprehensive data on amputation and persons living with limb loss.[2] The number of Americans living with limb loss is estimated at 1.6 million.[3] In the United States, each year, an estimated 185,000 persons lose a limb. Limb loss occurs for a variety of reasons including dysvascular diseases, trauma, cancer, and congenital anomalies (Figures 17-1 and 17-2). In 2008, Ziegler-Graham and colleagues[3] conducted an epidemiological study that estimated the prevalence of limb loss in the United States for the period 2005 to 2050. According to statistical analysis based on the figure that 1.6 million Americans were living with limb loss in 2005, it is estimated that the number of persons living with limb loss will increase to 3.6 million by the year 2050. It is anticipated that the number of persons living with amputation will more than double in the next 45 years. Increase in life span and health-related age factors will figure significantly in the increase number of persons living with limb loss (Figure 17-3).[3]

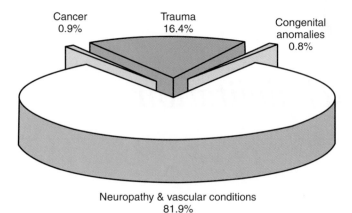

Cancer
0.9%

Trauma
16.4%

Congenital
anomalies
0.8%

Neuropathy & vascular conditions
81.9%

FIGURE 17-1 Causes of amputation by percent. The majority of amputations result from a disease process. (From Dillingham TR, Pezzin LE, Mackenzie EJ. Limb amputation and limb deficiency: epidemiology and recent trends in the United States. *South Med J.* 2002;95[8]:875-883.)

The leading cause of amputation is dysvascular disease. Predisposing factors for amputation include diabetes, hypertension, and dyslipidemia. Health conditions that affect the blood vessels such as peripheral vascular disease (PVD), peripheral arterial disease (PAD), and diabetes are the leading cause of amputation. Dysvascular disease accounts for approximately 82% of all limb loss hospital discharges.[4] Between 1988 and 1996, the estimated increase in the rate of dysvascular amputations was 27%, with the highest percentage of disease-related amputations occurring in persons 65 years of age and older.[4] Most of these were lower-extremity amputations, which are performed 11 times more frequently than upper-extremity amputations.[5] More amputations occur among men than women, and amputation rates increase steeply with age.[3,6] The health condition most frequently related to amputation is dysvascular disease including PVD and PAD complicated by neuropathy. Although PVD and neuropathy are frequently associated with type 2 diabetes,

vascular disease also occurs independently of diabetes. The increased frequency of amputation for PVD likely reflects increased growth in the older population. This increase is likely to continue with current population projections. The population in the age group 45 to 64 years is projected to increase 23.8% between 2002 and 2020, and the population at greatest risk for amputation, those 65 to 85 years and older, is expected to increase by 71%.[7] The population of individuals older than 85 years of age is projected to increase at the highest rate. Because the prevalence of dysvascular increases with age, these demographic changes will likely have a large impact on the amount of vascular reconstruction and amputation that will be performed.[3]

Diabetes and smoking are the strongest risk factors for developing PAD. Other well-known risk factors are advanced age, hypertension, and hyperlipidemia.[8] The number of Americans with diabetes with limb loss will continue to rise because of the persistent reports that diabetes is a national health problem. In 2007, approximately 1.6 million new cases of diabetes were diagnosed in people age 20 years or older. If current trends continue, one in three Americans will develop diabetes sometime in their lifetime.[9] Diabetes is the leading cause of new cases of nontraumatic lower-extremity amputations among adults (Figure 17-4).[9] The number of hospital discharges for nontraumatic lower-extremity amputation with diabetes as a listed diagnosis increased from 45,000 in 1991 to 86,000 in 1996. From 1988 to 2006, the number of hospital discharges for persons with diabetes who had amputation increased by 20%.[10,11]

The second leading cause of amputation is trauma. Traumatic amputation is most common in the young adult age group (20-29 year olds). The leading causes of trauma-related amputation are injuries involving machinery (40.1%), power tools and appliances (27.8%), firearms (8.5%), and motor vehicle crashes (8%).[4] The incidence of trauma-related major amputation continues to decrease over time. This reduction in traumatic amputation is attributable to

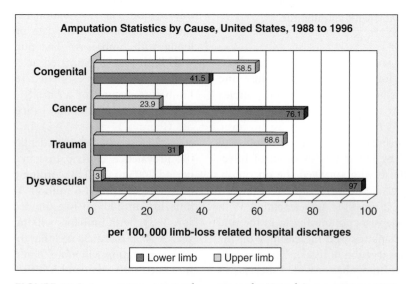

FIGURE 17-2 Amputation statistics by cause in the United States, 1988 to 1996. Causes of amputation per 100,000 as reported by the Amputee Coalition of America. (From http://www.amputee-coalition.org/fact_sheets/amp_stats_cause.html.)

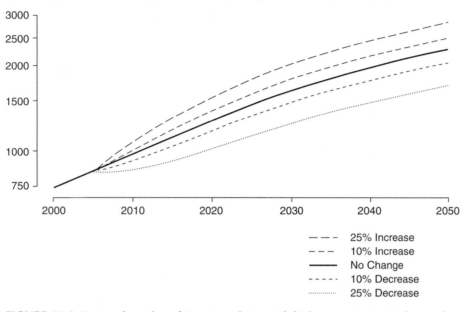

FIGURE 17-3 Projected number of Americans living with limb amputation secondary to dysvascular disease (log scale) from year 2000 to 2050. (From Ziegler-Graham K, MacKenzie EJ, Ephraim PL, et al. Estimating the prevalence of limb loss in the United States: 2005 to 2050. *Arch Phys Med Rehabil.* 2008; 89:426.)

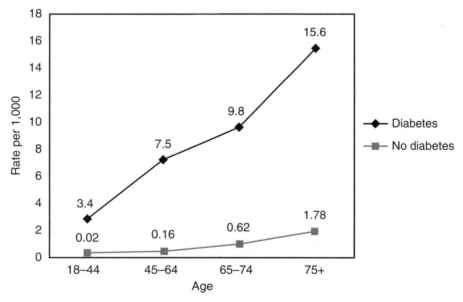

FIGURE 17-4 Hospital discharge rates for nontraumatic lower-extremity amputation for persons with diabetes as a listed diagnosis in the United States for the period 1988 to 2006. (From http://www.ahrq.gov/data/hcup/highlight1/high1fig2.htm.)

implementation of new safety regulations, the development of safer farm and industrial machinery, improved safety in work conditions, and medical advancement in techniques for salvaging traumatized limbs. Whenever there is a period of significant armed conflict, the number of veterans with traumatic amputation increases. U.S. engagement in the wars in Afghanistan and Iraq, has resulted in more

than 1000 service men and women who have sustained traumatic amputations.[12]

The third cause of limb loss is cancer related. In the data compiled by the U.S. National Center for Health Statistics, Healthcare and Utilization Project 1988–1996, limb loss as a consequence of cancer showed a marked decrease over this period, from 0.62 per 100,000 persons in 1988 to 0.35 per

100,000 persons in 1996.[4] The tumor most commonly associated with amputation is osteosarcoma, which primarily affects children and adolescents in the 11- to 20-year-old age group. Currently amputation is no longer the primary intervention for osteosarcoma, and the current rate of amputation for this disease is less than 1%.[5] With development of new surgical techniques, including bone graft and joint replacement, and advancement in chemotherapy and radiation, the incidence of amputation as a consequence of osteosarcoma has decreased significantly.

Congenital limb deficiencies, as well as the amputations used to adjust or correct them, are relatively rare, and little has changed over time in the birth prevalence of congenital limb deficiencies. Rates have been reported ranging from 3.8 per 10,000 births to 5.3 per 10,000 births.[4] This percentage has remained relatively stable and is less than 1% of all amputations.

LEVELS OF AMPUTATION

Amputation can be performed as a disarticulation of a joint or as a transection through a long bone. The level of amputation is usually named by the joint or major bone through which the amputation has been made (Table 17-1).[5] An amputation that involves the lower extremity can affect an individual's ability to stand and walk, requiring the use of prosthetics and, often, an assistive device for mobility. Amputation involving the upper extremity can affect other activities of daily living, such as feeding, grooming, dressing, and a host of activities that require manipulative skills. Because of the complex nature of skilled hand function, prosthetic substitution for upper limb amputation does not typically restore function to the same degree that lower extremity prosthetics do.

The levels of amputation surgery that are most commonly performed today involve the lower extremity below the knee (including transtibial, foot, and toe amputations), accounting for 97% of all dysvascular limb loss hospital discharges (Table 17-2). This high percentage reflects the prevalence of PVD of the lower extremities. Transfemoral amputations account for approximately 26% of all dysvascular amputations.[4]

TABLE 17-1   *Terminology Used to Describe the Site of Lower-Extremity Amputation*

Site	Terminology
Toe	Phalangeal
Forefoot	Ray resection (one or more complete metatarsal)
	Transmetatarsal (across the metatarsal shaft)
Midfoot	Partial foot (e.g., Chopart, Boyd, Pirogoff)
At the ankle	Syme
Below the knee	Transtibial (long, standard, short)
At the knee	Knee disarticulation
Above the knee	Transfemoral (long, standard, short)
At the hip	Hip disarticulation
At the pelvis	Hemipelvectomy

TABLE 17-2   *Incidence of Lower-Limb Amputation: Average Annual Number and Percent of Hospital Discharges After Lower-Extremity Amputation, 1988-1996*

Level of Amputation	Number	Percent (%)
Toe	338,288	33.11
Foot and ankle	116,302	11.38
Transtibial	287,295	28.12
Knee disarticulation	5291	0.52
Transfemoral	266,465	26.08
Hip and pelvis	6588	0.64
Bilateral amputations	1504	0.15
Total	1,021,733	100

Source: From Dillingham TR, Pezzin LE, Mackenzie EJ. Limb amputation and limb deficiency. Epidemiology and recent trends in the United States. *South Med J.* 2002;95(8):875-883.

In general, the proportion of lower-limb amputations in relation to upper-limb amputations is increasing. This most likely reflects an increase in the number of older persons with lower-extremity amputations rather than an actual decrease in the number of upper-extremity amputations.

Because dysvascular disease typically affects both lower extremities, a significant number of individuals eventually undergo amputation of both lower extremities. Approximately 50% of persons undergoing diabetes-related amputation will have contralateral amputation within 3 to 5 years.[13] Between 25% and 45% of persons with amputations have had amputations of both lower extremities, most often at the transtibial level in both limbs, or a combination of transtibial amputation of one limb and transfemoral amputation of the other.[13]

Today, the majority of transtibial and transfemoral amputations are performed with an understanding of wound healing and the functional needs and constraints of prosthetic fitting, so that rehabilitation outcomes are usually positive. Other levels of amputation, although less commonly performed procedures, continue to pose challenges for the surgeon, prosthetist, physical therapist, and patient during prosthetic fitting and rehabilitation.

CAUSES OF AMPUTATION

Currently the most likely reasons for amputation are poor wound healing associated with diabetes[4,14] and dysvascular disease,[4,15] trauma,[4,16] or cancer.[4,17] Children with congenital limb deficiencies are a special population group and may require surgical revision during or after periods of significant growth or after conversion to a more functional level for prosthetic fitting.

Diabetes and Peripheral Arterial Disease

Diabetic foot ulceration is a common complication of diabetes that often results in lower-extremity amputation. Elevated blood sugars associated with diabetes damage blood vessels and nerve fibers, and impair circulation. Nerve damage causes peripheral neuropathy, a condition of loss of sensation to the feet. The loss of protective sensation in the feet would not alert an individual to foreign substance in their shoe such as pebbles or gravel. This lack of awareness may lead to blisters or other minor injuries. Once the skin is broken, sores on the feet may not heal because of poor circulation. The Centers for Disease Control confirms that neuropathy is a major contributor to diabetic amputations.[18]

The prevalence of PAD in persons with diabetes is four times greater than in persons without diabetes.[19] Dysvascular disease is the most common contributing factor for lower-extremity amputations. In epidemiological studies, two symptoms are classic indicators of vascular insufficiency: (a) intermittent claudication and (b) loss of one or more lower-extremity pulses. Intermittent claudication is a significant cramping pain, usually in the calf, that is induced by walking or other prolonged muscle contraction and relieved by a short period of rest. In arteriosclerosis obliterans, at least one major arterial pulse (dorsal pedis artery at the ankle, popliteal artery at the knee, or femoral artery in the groin) is often absent or markedly impaired (Figure 17-5).[20] The major risk factors for development of PAD are the same as those for cardiovascular and cerebrovascular disease, most notably poorly managed hypertension, high serum cholesterol and triglyceride levels, and a history of tobacco use and smoking. Peripheral neuropathy and PAD are the major predisposing factors for lower-extremity amputation in individuals with diabetes.[21]

According to the National Hospital Discharge Survey, the number of hospital discharges that listed diagnoses of amputation and diabetes increased 27% from 1988 to 1996.[4] The prevalence of PAD among persons with diabetes, whether men or women, is significantly greater than in those without diabetes. The Framingham Heart Study[22] found a four to five times greater relative risk of intermittent claudication in persons with diabetes, even when controlling for

blood pressure, cholesterol, and smoking. The age-adjusted rate of lower-extremity amputation among persons with diabetes in the United States is approximately 28 times that of the nondiabetic population. More than 50% of the lower-limb amputations in the United States are diabetes related, although persons diagnosed with diabetes represent only 3% of the population.[23] Although major improvements have been made in noninvasive diagnosis, surgical revascularization procedures, and wound-healing techniques, between 2% and 5% of individuals with PAD and without diabetes and between 6% and 25% of those with diabetes eventually undergo an amputation.[24,25]

The three most common predisposing factors for lower extremity amputation appear to be (a) concurrent diabetes and hypertension, (b) hypertension without diabetes, and (c) diabetes without hypertension (Figure 17-6). Other predisposing factors include race, gender, history of smoking, and previous vascular surgery. The incidence of lower-extremity amputation among persons with diabetes is almost 50% higher for men than for women.[4] The most frequently cited criteria for amputation among persons with diabetes include gangrene, infection, nonhealing neuropathic ulcer, severe ischemic pain, absent or decreased pulses, local necrosis, osteomyelitis, systemic toxicity, acute embolic disease, and severe venous thrombosis.[19,21]

In individuals with diabetes, the prevalence and severity of dysvascularity increases significantly with age and the duration of diabetes, particularly in men. Initial amputation may involve a toe or foot; subsequent revision to transtibial or transfemoral levels is likely to occur with progression of the underlying disease. In individuals with diabetes, dysvascular disease increases the risk of a nonhealing neuropathic ulcer, infection, or gangrene, all of which increase the likelihood of amputation. Twenty percent to 50% of patients will have

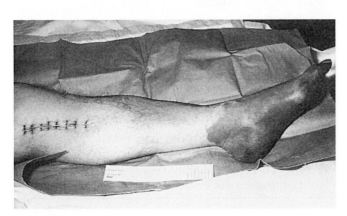

FIGURE 17-5 This patient with atherosclerosis obliterans underwent a femoral-distal popliteal bypass in an attempt to revascularize the foot. The demarcation indicating ischemia at the ankle and foot is clear. Transtibial amputation is necessary when revascularization is unsuccessful. (From Robinson KP. The dilemma: amputation or revascularization. In Murdock G, Wilson AB [eds], *Amputation: Surgical Practice and Patient Management.* Oxford, UK: Butterworth-Heinemann, 1996. p. 169.)

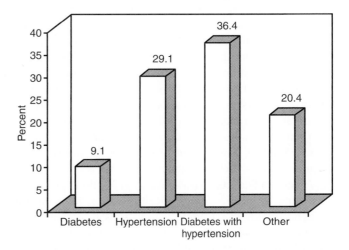

FIGURE 17-6 Lower-extremity amputations, classified by predisposing factors. Hypertension, especially in the presence of diabetes, is a powerful risk factor. "Other" includes a combination of risk factors including race, gender, cigarette smoking, and previous vascular surgery. (Based on data reported by Lee CS, Sariego J, Matsumoto T. Changing patterns in the predisposition for amputation of the lower extremities. *Am Surg.* 1992;5[8]:474-477.)

amputation of the contralateral leg in 1 to 3 years.[13,19] Patients with diabetes who are 65 years old or older account for most diabetes-related lower-extremity amputations. The estimated amputation rate in 1996 was 1.4 times higher for persons with diabetes who were 65 to 74 years old and 2.4 times higher for those 75 years of age or older, compared with those 0 to 64 years of age.[26,27]

Peripheral neuropathy is a common complication of diabetes. Neuropathy is as important and powerful as dysvascular disease as a predisposing factor for lower-extremity amputation. Peripheral neuropathy is suspected when one or more of the following clinical signs are present: deficits of sensation (loss of Achilles and patellar reflexes, decreased vibratory sensation, and loss of protective sensation), motor impairments (weakness and atrophy of the intrinsic muscles of the foot), or autonomic dysfunction (inadequate or abnormal hemodynamic mechanism, tropic changes of the skin, and distal loss of hair).[20] The resulting loss of thermal, pain, and protective sensation increases the vulnerability of the foot to acute, high-pressure and repetitive, low-pressure trauma. Patients may also experience significant numbness or painful paresthesia of the foot and lower leg. Individuals with peripheral neuropathy may not be aware of minor trauma, pressure from poorly fitting shoes along the sides and tops of their feet, or pressure from thickening plantar callus, all of which contribute to the risk of ulceration, infection, and gangrene. Motor neuropathy and associated weakness and atrophy contribute to development of bony deformity of the foot. The bony prominences and malalignments that are associated with foot deformity change weight-bearing pressure dynamics during walking, further increasing the risk of ulceration. Peripheral neuropathy is one of the most crucial precursors of foot ulceration, especially in the presence of dysvascular disease. Nonhealing or infected neuropathic ulcers precede approximately 85% of nontraumatic lower extremity amputations in individuals with diabetes.[23]

Lower-extremity amputation continues to be a major health problem for the diabetic population. For this group of patients, amputation is associated with significant morbidity, functional limitation and disability, mortality, and high health care costs. Approximately 185,000 persons undergo amputation each year in the United States.[3] The average cost for a patient per hospitalization for amputation is approximately $30,000. The cost of health care for persons with chronic diseases such as diabetes and PAD is estimated by the American Diabetes Association at $174 billion per year.[28] According to the U.S. Public Health Service, reducing the incidence of lower-extremity amputations in persons with diabetes is a key health care objective in terms of quality of life and containment of health care costs. It is estimated that the current prevalence of 1.6 million persons living with limb loss will more than double to 3.6 million by the year 2050.[3] Planned health promotion efforts will hopefully reduce the risk of diabetes and amputation, minimizing the impact of risk factors and increasing access to care by multidisciplinary health care teams.

CASE EXAMPLE 1

A Patient with Dysvascular Disease-Related Amputation

T. S., is a 67-year-old African-American man with a 10-year history of type 2 diabetes mellitus. Until 2 years ago, he smoked one pack of cigarettes daily, but he quit after coronary artery bypass grafting (×4) following acute myocardial infarction. He became insulin dependent at the time of his myocardial infarction and coronary artery bypass grafting surgery. Comorbid medical problems include hypertension, managed pharmaceutically with a β-blocker, and moderate vision loss secondary to diabetic retinopathy.

T. S. underwent complete transmetatarsal amputation of the left foot 6 months ago because of a nonhealing plantar ulcer under the second and third metatarsal heads that had progressed to osteomyelitis. Three weeks ago, intermittent claudication of the right calf became severe enough to warrant medical attention. On evaluation T. S. was noted to have a neuropathic ulcer under his first metatarsal head, probing to bone. Doppler studies were monophasic, suggesting inadequate vascular supply for healing. Arteriography indicated markedly diminished distal arterial flow to his foot but adequate arterial supply to midtibial levels. He had failed a revascularization attempt with stent placement.

After an interdisciplinary meeting involving his internist (who helps him manage his diabetes), cardiologist (who helps him manage his hypertension and heart disease), vascular surgeon (who oversaw this evaluation), physical therapist and prosthetist (who explained the process of rehabilitation), social worker (who explained services and support available to those with amputation), and family, T. S. concurred with the recommendation for an "elective" transtibial amputation. His surgery occurred 2 weeks ago, and he is impatiently waiting for his wound to heal sufficiently to begin prosthetic training.

Questions to Consider

- What possible medical and physiological factors contributed to this patient's loss of limb?
- What impact will his current health status and comorbid conditions have on his prognosis for rehabilitation, both in terms of eventual outcome and in duration of this episode of care?
- What plan of care for the preprosthetic phase of his rehabilitation would you propose?
- How is the International Classification of Functioning (ICF) disablement framework applied to T. S.?

Amputation Rates and Racial and Ethnic Populations

Evidence indicates that certain racial and ethnic groups are at increased risk for lower-extremity amputation. This increased risk appears to be linked to a higher prevalence of diabetes complicated by PAD. Minority groups with the highest incidence of diabetes and greatest risk of lower-extremity amputation are Native Americans, African-Americans, and

Hispanic Americans. Native Americans are 3.5 times more likely to have lower-extremity amputation than their non-Hispanic white counterparts.[29] African-Americans are two to four times more likely to lose a limb as a result of diabetes complications.[30] Hispanic Americans are diagnosed with diabetes at twice the rate of whites[31] and are 1.5 times more likely to have an amputation.[31,32]

Native Americans have a two to five times higher prevalence of diabetes than the overall population in the United States. This high prevalence is directly reflected in increased amputation rates. Amputation rates among Native Americans are three to four times higher than the general population. Among Pima Indians with diabetes, the rate of amputation is 3.7 times higher than the rate of other persons with diabetes.[33,34] Why these populations have a significantly higher rate of lower-extremity amputation is unclear. Potential contributors include a genetic or familial predisposition to diabetes, a higher prevalence of hypertension and smoking, or both. Health-promotion and education efforts that target this high-risk population (including programs aimed at effective management of diabetes, minimization of other risk factors, and special foot care programs for early detection of neuropathic and traumatic lesions) are effective strategies to reduce the likelihood of amputation. Further research is necessary to better understand the causes of racial differences in amputation rates and to identify and promote health initiatives that will alleviate this excess risk among minority populations.

Outcome of Dysvascular Conditions and Amputation

The morbidity and mortality risks associated with systemic diseases, such as diabetes and vascular disease, continue after amputation. As a result, death in the years immediately after amputation is not uncommon. The 3-year survival rate after initial lower-extremity amputation for persons with diabetes is only approximately 50%; the 5-year survival rate ranges in various studies from 39% to 68%.[23] Because neuropathy and PVD occur in a symmetric distribution, the risk of subsequent amputation of the contralateral lower extremity is high. Even with successful healing of the primary amputation site, amputation of part of the contralateral limb occurs in 50% of patients within 2 to 5 years.[13] The most common causes of death in persons with amputation include complications of diabetes, cardiovascular disease, and renal disease.

Evidence is growing that the incidence of lower-extremity amputation in persons with diabetes can be significantly reduced through particular kinds of preventive care. Large clinical centers have demonstrated the effect of early intervention for the diabetic population, using an interdisciplinary team approach to preventive care. Interventions to prevent neuropathy and PVD target smoking reduction programs, as well as dietary, exercise, and pharmaceutical interventions, to obtain better control of hypertension, hyperlipidemia, and hyperglycemia. Reduction of these predisposing factors is likely to further reduce the incidence of amputation, heart disease, and stroke among people with diabetes. For those with existing diabetic neuropathy or PVD, intensive foot care programs should focus on prevention of ulceration and early intervention to prevent expansion, infection, or gangrene of small lesions.[35] Foot care programs are most effective if they develop in a team setting and focus on patient education. Surgical revascularization procedures are performed to avoid amputation in persons with chronic foot ulceration. The revascularization procedures include vascular bypass, angioplasty, stent placement, and end-stage limb-salvage procedures.[19]

The decision to undergo amputation often follows a long struggle to care for an increasingly frail foot by the patient, the family, and health care providers. In this circumstance, elective amputation is often perceived by the patient and family as a positive step toward a more active and less stressful life. The interdisciplinary team approach best addresses the complex needs of the individual with diabetes, including clinical evaluation, determination of risk status, patient education, footwear selection, decision making about amputation, and rehabilitation after surgery.

Traumatic Amputation

Traumatic amputation is defined as an injury to an extremity that results in immediate separation of the limb or will result in loss of limb as a result of accident or injury.[36] Traumatic loss of a limb, the second most common cause of amputation, occurs most frequently in vehicle- or work-related accidents, as a result of violence such as gunshots or warfare, or after severe burns and electrocution (Figure 17-7). Trauma-related amputation occurs most commonly in young adult men but can happen at any age to men or women. Because the mechanism of injury in traumatic amputation is quite variable, this type of amputation is usually classified or categorized according to the severity of tissue damage. The extent of injury to the musculoskeletal system depends on three interacting factors: (a) movement of the object that causes the injury; (b) direction, magnitude, and speed of the energy vector; and (c) the particular body tissue involved.

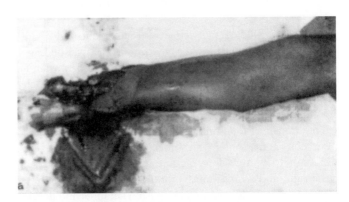

FIGURE 17-7 This patient sustained a traumatic amputation of his left foot and distal tibia when he stepped on a buried land mine. (From Coupland RM, Korver A. Injuries from antipersonnel mines: the experience of the International Committee of the Red Cross. *BMJ.* 1991;303[14]:1509. Reprinted with permission from the BMJ Publishing Group.)

In partial traumatic amputations, at least one half the diameter of the injured extremity is severed or damaged significantly. This kind of injury can incur extensive bleeding, because all of the blood vessels involved may not be vasoconstrictive. A second type of traumatic amputation occurs when the limb becomes completely detached from the body. As much as 1 L of blood may be lost before the arteries spasm and become vasoconstrictive.[37]

For optimal outcome, surgical intervention is usually necessary within the first 12 hours after the accident for revascularization or for treatment of the amputated site. One of the primary efforts of the surgical team for a person with lower extremity amputation is to preseve limb length to the extent that healing is possible.[36] Replantation is the surgical procedure to reattach a part of the body that has been amputated.[38] When replantation is considered, the window of opportunity is much narrower. The decision to replant is a difficult one and is influenced by the patient's age and overall health status, the level of extremity injury, and the condition of the amputated part. Replantation has been most successful in the distal upper extremity. The goal of upper extremity replantation is to provide a mechanism for functional grasp rather than solely for cosmetic restoration of the limb.[38] The period of recovery and rehabilitation after replantation is often significantly longer than that after amputation.

Persons with trauma-related amputation undergo extreme physiological changes, as well as psychological trauma. With the sudden loss of a body part, the patient may experience an extended period of grieving. Addressing the patient's psychological needs as well as physical needs is important for optimal outcome. An interdisciplinary team approach to rehabilitation is the most effective means of addressing the comprehensive needs of a patient who has unexpectedly lost a limb to trauma.[36–38]

CASE EXAMPLE 2

A Patient with Traumatic Amputation

C. J. was a 20-year-old female in active duty with the National Guard on a tour in Afghanistan. She sustained significant shrapnel injury to both lower extremities when a rocket-propelled grenade was aimed at the convoy in which she was riding. After emergency care on the ground, C. J.'s condition was considered critical enough to warrant immediate transport to a military hospital in Germany. Trauma surgeons at the center determined her wounds were severe enough to require midlength transtibial amputation on the right and a long transfemoral amputation on the left. Because of wound contamination from shrapnel and debris and a resulting high risk of infection, C. J.'s surgical wounds were initially left open (unsutured) while local and intravenous antimicrobials were administered. After several days of care, C. J. was returned to the operating room for revision and closure of the residual limbs. She now has

significant edema and serosanguineous drainage on the right limb with a small area of wound dehiscence in the middle of the suture line. Although the left residual limb is not as edematous, the suture line is inflamed and ecchymotic, with more than a dozen healing puncture wounds from shrapnel fragments over the anterior and lateral thigh. When medically stable, C. J. will be moved to a military rehabilitation hospital in the United States for preprosthetic care and rehabilitation.

Questions to Consider
- Given the circumstances of these traumatic amputations, how does this patient's prognosis differ from the previous patient (Case Example 1) with dysvascular-neuropathic amputation?
- How might the rehabilitation of this patient be similar to or different from the previous patient with dysvascular-neuropathic amputation, in terms of eventual outcome and duration of care?
- What plan of care would you implement to promote wound healing?

Cancer

Cancer of the bone and joint is a rare form of cancer. The U.S. National Cancer Institute Surveillance, Epidemiology and End Results data from 1988 to 2001 reported 4062 cases of bone and joint cancer. Twenty-seven percent of cases occurred in children ages 0 to 9 years. Bone cancers have three typical histological types: (a) osteosarcoma; (b) chondrosarcoma; and (c) Ewing sarcoma. The cancers arise from the growing end of long bones (osteosarcoma), cartilage (chondrosarcoma), and the axial skeleton (Ewing sarcoma).[39] The limb-presenting cancers are osteosarcoma and chondrosarcoma. Sixty-three percent of cancers were diagnosed as osteosarcoma and 54% were chondrosarcoma. Amputation because of a primary cancer generally results from osteogenic sarcoma (osteosarcoma) (Figure 17-8). This type of cancer occurs predominantly in late childhood, adolescence, or the early young adult years. The incidence is slightly higher among young males than among females. Osteosarcoma typically occurs at or near the epiphyses of long bones during times of rapid growth, especially the distal femur, proximal tibia, or proximal humerus. Most patients have a history of worsening, increasingly deep-seated pain, sometimes accompanied by localized swelling. Children with osteosarcoma are vulnerable to pathological fracture, an event that often prompts diagnosis. Since the early 1990s, the need for amputation in osteosarcoma has been greatly reduced by advances in early detection, improved imaging techniques, more effective chemotherapy regimens, and better limb resectioning and salvage procedures. Tumor resection followed by limb reconstruction frequently provides a functional extremity. Weight bearing is limited, and the limb is protected by an orthosis early in rehabilitation. Once satisfactory healing occurs, full weight bearing and near-normal activity can

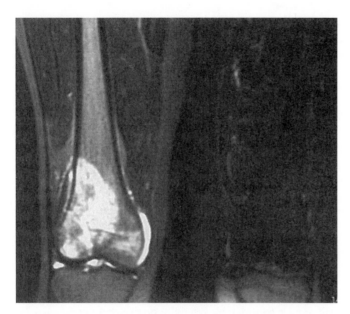

FIGURE 17-8 Magnetic resonance image of the distal femur of a patient with an osteosarcoma of the bone and marrow canal. The bright signal beyond the bone indicates invasion of surrounding soft tissue. (From Lundon K. *Orthopedic Rehabilitation Science: Principles for Clinical Management of Bone.* Boston: Butterworth-Heinemann, 2000. p. 147.)

be resumed. With new techniques, 5-year survival rates for individuals with osteosarcoma increased from approximately 20% in the 1970s to 80% in the 1990s.[40] Rhabdomyosarcoma is a rare malignant tumor occuring in the extremities that predominantly affects children. Chemotherapy and radiation therapy is often the primary medical management. On occasion amputation is performed along with chemotherapy and radiation therapy.[41,42]

CASE EXAMPLE 3

A Patient with Osteosarcoma

R. K. is a 16-year-old male high school student who sustained an unexpected fracture of the distal femur in a collision during playoffs for the state soccer title. He experienced increasing lateral knee pain for the previous 4 weeks but did not complain to his coaches and parents for fear he would have to "sit out." Examination in the emergency department reveals a swollen and tender distal femur and knee. A radiograph reveals a fracture just proximal to a radiodense lesion of the medial femoral condyle, including articular surfaces of the knee. Magnetic resonance imaging reveals that the tumor extends posteriorly, close to the neurovascular bundle in the popliteal fossa. Biopsy confirmed osteosarcoma. The orthopedic surgeon and oncologist review options for limb salvage and amputation with R. K. and his parents, recommending amputation because the location of the tumor precludes the wide clear margins at the knee required for endoprosthetic knee replacement or cadaver allograft salvage strategies. His fractured limb is

stabilized in a knee orthosis while a preoperative course of chemotherapy is undertaken and the possibility of metastasis to the lungs is evaluated by further testing. Resection of the tumor to a midlength transfemoral level of amputation will occur once the initial course of chemotherapy is completed and will be followed by a second course of chemotherapy. R. K. and his family have been encouraged by visits from a survivor of osteosarcoma who had transfemoral amputation 7 years ago and is now a competitive runner at the national and Paralympic level.

Questions to Consider
- How does the diagnosis of a serious cancer affect the rehabilitation of young people with medically necessary amputations?
- What psychological factors must be considered?
- What physiological factors must be considered?
- What are the similarities and differences in the prognosis and plan of care for this patient with cancer-related amputation, as compared with the previous patients with dysvascular-neuropathic and trauma-related etiology, in terms of eventual outcome, and duration of this episode of care?

Congenital Limb Deficiencies

The incidence of congenital limb deficiency has remained relatively stable over time, accounting for only approximately 0.8% of all limb loss-related hospital discharges. The rate in 1996 was 25.64 per 100,000 live births. A slight male preponderance in the incidence of limb reductions has been reported, as well as a slightly higher incidence of upper limb reductions among newborns with limb deficiencies.[4]

The actual incidence of congenital limb deficiencies is difficult to determine because of lack of a common definition and reporting mechanisms. Six categories of limb deficiencies have been recognized[43]:

1. Failure of formation of parts, indicating a partial or complete arrest in limb development
2. Failure of differentiation or separation of parts, when the basic structures have developed but the final form is not completed
3. Duplication of parts, such as polydactyly
4. Skeletal overgrowth, also called gigantism (not to be confused with the syndrome caused by growth hormone excess in adolescence)
5. Congenital constriction band syndrome, characterized by constriction bands, which may compromise circulation to the distal part
6. Generalized skeletal abnormalities

Upper limb deficiencies in children vary from minor abnormalities of the fingers to major limb absences. Embryological differentiation of the upper limbs occurs most rapidly at 5 to 8 weeks after gestation, often before pregnancy has been recognized or confirmed. During this period the upper limbs are particularly vulnerable to malformation. The etiology of limb

TABLE 17-3   *Classification of Longitudinal Congenital Limb Deficiencies*

Limb Segment	Upper-Extremity Bone Segment*	Lower-Extremity Bone Segment*
Proximal	Humeral	Femoral
Distal	Radial	Tibial
	Central	Central
	Carpal	Tarsal
	Metacarpal	Metatarsal
	Phalangeal	Phalangeal
Combined (indicated by the bone segments that remain)	Partial or complete	Partial or complete
	Specific carpal, ray, or phalanx remaining	Specific carpal, ray, or phalanx remaining

*May be partial or complete.
Source: Modified from May BJ. *Amputations and Prosthetics: A Case Study Approach.* Philadelphia: Davis, 1996. p. 221.

malformation is unclear. Potential contributing factors cited in the research literature include (a) exposure to chemical agents or drugs, (b) fetal position or constriction, (c) endocrine disorders, (d) exposure to radiation, (e) immune reactions, (f) occult infections and other diseases, (g) single-gene disorders, (h) chromosomal disorders, and (i) other syndromes with unknown causes.[43] For many children, an upper limb deficiency is their only anomaly. However, as many as 12% of these children have coexisting nonlimb malformations.

Limb deficiencies present at birth are classified according to an international standard based on skeletal elements (Table 17-3). These deficiencies are referred to as transverse or longitudinal. Transverse deficiencies are described by the level at which the limb terminates. In longitudinal deficiencies, a reduction or absence occurs within the long axis of the limb, but normal skeletal components are present distal to the affected bones (Figure 17-9).[43,44]

The use of prosthetics is a common intervention for children with congenital limb deficiencies. Sometimes surgery is necessary to prepare the existing limb for the most effective use of a prosthesis, especially after periods of rapid growth. The goals of prosthetic training for the child should be to enhance the function of the limb and provide a cosmetic replacement for a missing limb. Rehabilitation efforts are designed with the child's cognitive, motor, and psychological development in mind.

REHABILITATION ISSUES FOR THE PERSON WITH AN AMPUTATION

Several factors influence the success of rehabilitation after amputation. These include age, health status, cognitive status, sequence of onset of disability, concurrent disease and comorbidity, and the level of amputation.[45] With anticipated growth in the aging segments of the population, and the presence of chronic dysvascular conditions, amputation in the U.S. geriatric population will probably double from 28,000 to 58,000 per year by 2030.[3] The number of persons living with limb loss will more than double from 1.6 million in 2005 to 3.6 million in 2050. Prosthetic, physical therapy, and health care needs will increase to ensure continued independence, quality of life, and

participation in activities of daily living. Persons with limb loss will require considerable rehabilitation resources.

The physical rehabilitation process for persons with amputation occurs in different stages beginning with a postoperative acute phase where positioning, skin protection,

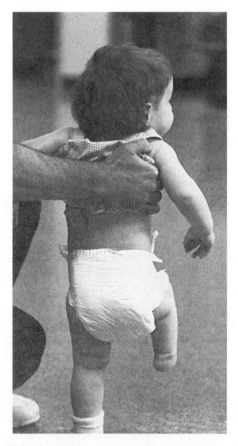

FIGURE 17-9 This child was born with a unilateral proximal focal deficiency of the right lower extremity. To facilitate prosthetic use, she has undergone an elective amputation of her foot at the ankle. Note the popliteal crease near the diaper line, indicating where her knee is located. (From Campbell SK, Vanderlinden DW, Palisano RJ [eds]. *Physical Therapy for Children*, 2nd ed. Philadelphia: Saunders, 2000. p. 380.)

sensory and proprioceptive training, joint range of motion, muscle strengthening occurs in conjunction with general conditoning activities leading to functional training for independence in mobility including transfer skills, balance exercises, wheelchair mobility, and ambulation with assistive devices that extends to the subacute phase of rehabilitation. The preprosthetic phase includes management of the residual limb including wound care, edema control, shaping, desensitization, and increasing joint and muscle flexibility. Strengthening of the trunk as well as the extremities is essential for prosthetic use. Traditionally, physical therapists have focused on the ability to perform functional activities such as walking, turning, and managing ramps and other uneven or unpredictable surfaces safely, independently, and efficiently with and without a prosthesis. Physical therapists assist physicians and prosthetists in determining an individual's readiness for prosthetic fitting and are often involved in decisions about prosthetic components. After initial fitting, physical therapists coordinate prosthetic training, consulting with prosthetists if problems with prosthetic alignment arise. Once these basic mobility activities are mastered, the therapist can serve as a consultant to assist the person with amputation in returning to preamputation employment and leisure activities. Treatment programs, predictors of outcome, and measures of success or failure are often based on these functional activities.

In one study[46] of patient progression through postamputation rehabilitation (n = 459), between 85% and 89% of persons with lower-extremity amputations mastered basic functional activities, such as moving about the bed, moving from supine into sitting position, and sitting balance, within the second postoperative week. Between 65% and 75% of persons with amputation demonstrated independence in transfers and dressing of upper and lower limbs in the third to fifth postoperative week. Although steady gains were made in the ability to doff and don the prosthesis and to walk indoors and outside during the fifth to the twelfth postoperative weeks, just one-third of people in the study achieved independence within this time frame.[46] Optimal rehabilitation outcome, achievement of the highest functional level of which the person with amputation is capable, requires ongoing contact with and support of a transdisciplinary rehabilitation team.[36]

As many as 70% of persons with a lower-extremity amputation report using their prosthesis on a full-time basis: putting it on in the early morning, wearing it all day, and taking it off in the evening.[47] Two major reasons for limited use or nonuse are generally cited: physical discomfort when walking with the prosthesis and psychological discomfort. The wide variation reported in the success of functional ambulation with a prosthesis after below-knee amputation appears to be related to age and concurrent disease.[48] Healing time, indicated by time between surgery and fitting for the first prosthesis, correlate with age but not with the cause of amputation. Age is also more important than the etiology of amputation in predicting the total length of time in rehabilitation and achievement of functional ambulation: Older adults with amputation are likely to require a longer rehabilitation period to accomplish

an ambulatory status equal to that of the younger group.[49] Although most people recovering from amputation achieve some level of upright mobility, a smaller percentage of older persons with concurrent chronic disease become functional ambulators when compared with younger persons who had amputations because of trauma or osteomyelitis.

The typical age at the time of initial lower limb amputation is between 51 and 69 years; therefore consideration must be given to the special rehabilitation needs of the older patient. The complexity of issues during rehabilitation of the older adult who is undergoing an amputation is often compounded by comorbidity, fragile social supports, and limited resources.[48] In patients with dysvascular conditions, concomitant cerebrovascular disease can have a more complicated rehabilitation process. A preamputation history of stroke or occurrence of stroke during the course of rehabilitation is not uncommon. Similarly, cardiovascular disease can limit endurance and exercise tolerance; endurance training becomes a critical component of the postamputation, preprosthetic rehabilitation program. Optimal rehabilitation care begins with consultation and patient and family education efforts before surgery. A specialized interdisciplinary team most effectively provides this presurgical and perisurgical care (Table 17-4). Team members often include a surgeon, physical therapist, certified prosthetist, occupational therapist, nurse or nurse practitioner, recreational therapist, psychologist, and social worker.[36] The patient and family members are active and essential members of the team as well. Effective communication provides the team with the necessary information to develop a tentative treatment plan from the time of amputation to discharge home.

With a specialized treatment team and the use of new lightweight and dynamic prosthetic designs, the potential for rehabilitation of the older patient has increased significantly in the past decade. At the time of surgery, special consideration is given to the optimal level of amputation. This is a particularly important concern for the older patient. The selection of the surgical level of amputation is probably one of the most important decisions to be made for the patient undergoing an amputation. A lower-limb prosthesis ideally becomes a full body-weight–bearing device. However, bony prominences, adhesions of the suture line scar, fragile skin and open areas, shearing forces at the skin/socket interface, and perspiration can complicate this function.[45] The energy cost of ambulation must be considered, especially for older patients with significant deconditioning or comorbid conditions. The higher the level of amputation and loss of joints, long bone length, and muscle insertion, the greater the impairment of normal locomotor mechanisms. This leads to increased energy costs in prosthetic control and functional ambulation and a greater likelihood of functional limitation and disability.

Preservation of the knee joint seems to be a key determinant in determining the potential for functional ambulation and successful rehabilitation outcome. Persons with transtibial amputation, who have an intact anatomical knee joint, demonstrate a more energy-efficient prosthetic gait pattern

TABLE 17-4   *Members and Roles of the Multidisciplinary Team for Rehabilitation after Amputation*

Team Member	Role
Physician	Often serves as coordinator of the team
	Assesses need for amputation, performs surgery, monitors healing of suture line
	Monitors and manages patient's overall medical care and health status
	Monitors condition of remaining extremity for patients with peripheral vascular disease (PVD), neuropathy, or diabetes
Physical therapist	Provides preoperative education about the rehabilitation process and instruction in single limb mobility
	Designs and manages a preprosthetic rehabilitation program that focuses on mobility and preparation for prosthetic training
	Evaluates patient's readiness for prosthetic fitting; can make recommendations for prosthetic fitting
	Designs and manages a prosthetic training program that focuses on functional ambulation and prosthetic management
	Monitors condition of the remaining extremity for patients with PVD, neuropathy, or diabetes
Prosthetist	Designs, fabricates, and fits the prosthesis
	Adapts the prosthesis to individuals, adjusts alignment, repairs/replaces components when necessary
	Monitors fit, function, and comfort of the prosthesis
	Monitors condition of the remaining extremity for patients with PVD, neuropathy, or diabetes
Occupational therapist	Assesses and treats patients with upper extremity amputation, monitors readiness for prosthetic fitting, recommends components
	Assists with problem solving in activities of daily living for patients with upper or lower limb amputations
	Makes recommendations for environmental modification and assistive/adaptive equipment to facilitate functional independence
Social worker	Provides financial counseling and coordination of support services
	Acts as liaison with third-party payers and community agencies
	Assists with patient's and family's social, psychological, and financial issues
Dietitian	Evaluates nutritional status and provides nutritional counseling, especially for patients with diabetes or heart disease or those who are on chemotherapy or are recovering from trauma
Nurse/nurse practitioner	Monitors patient's health and functional status during rehabilitation
	Provides ongoing patient education on comorbid and chronic health issues
	Monitors condition of remaining extremity for patients with PVD, neuropathy, or diabetes
Vocational counselor	Assesses patient's employment status and potential
	Assists with education, training, and placement

Source: Modified from May B. Assessment and treatment of individuals following lower extremity amputation. In O'Sullivan SB, Schmitz TJ (eds), *Physical Rehabilitation: Assessment and Treatment.* Philadelphia: Davis, 1994. p. 379.

and postural responses and are more likely to ambulate without additional assistive devices (walkers, crutches, or canes). They are also more likely to be full-time prosthetic wearers than are persons with transfemoral amputation. The benefits of preserving the knee, particularly among older adults, are so crucial that a transtibial amputation may be attempted even with the risk of inadequate healing; this may necessitate later revision to a higher level.[45]

The patient with a bilateral transfemoral amputation faces additional rehabilitation challenges. The significant increase in energy consumption that is required can prevent long-distance ambulation. Many older patients, as well as younger persons with bilateral transfemoral amputation, may choose wheelchair mobility as a more energy-efficient and effective means of locomotion. Ambulation potential depends on cardiac function, strength, balance, and endurance.[48]

Options for prosthetic components for the older person with an amputation have increased dramatically in the past

20 years. Selecting the most appropriate components for the individual requires the input of the complete rehabilitation team, in close communication with the patient and the family members.

REHABILITATION ENVIRONMENT

Traditionally, preprosthetic and early prosthetic programs have occurred in rehabilitation departments of acute care hospitals. In this environment, the care may or may not be specialized for the older person with an amputation. A specialized postamputation rehabilitation treatment team is best able to address the complex needs of this group of patients. However, in today's health care environment, it may not be possible for older persons with an amputation to receive inpatient intensive rehabilitation until they are ready for prosthetic fitting. For patients with multiple medical complications, rehabilitation may be continued in a subacute setting or skilled nursing facility. For patients without complications and with a strong social support network, an outpatient rehabilitation program may be preferable. This plan allows them to reintegrate into home and community while maintaining support of the treatment team. The most effective care and rehabilitation for individuals undergoing an amputation require the skills and ongoing support of an integrated treatment team.[50,51]

SUMMARY

Although the rehabilitation process after amputation presents many challenges for patients, their families, and the professionals involved in their care, it also allows many opportunities for success and rewards. Understanding the risk factors for amputation and the influence of comorbid disease and age on progression of rehabilitation is important. Optimal outcome after amputation is best achieved through the interaction of a patient-centered, interdisciplinary health care team.[52] With effective physical rehabilitation and prosthetic care, most individuals with amputation can return to a level of activity and lifestyle similar to their preamputation status.

REFERENCES

1. Wilson Jr BB. The modern history of amputation surgery and artificial limbs. *Orthop Clin North Am.* 1972;3:267–285.

2. Adams P, Hendershot G, Marano M, Centers for Disease Control and Prevention/National Center for Health Statistics. Current estimates from the National Health Interview Survey, 1996. *Vital Health Stat 10.* 1999;200:1–203.

3. Ziegler-Graham K, MacKenzie EJ, Ephraim PL, et al. Estimating the prevalence of limb loss in the United States: 2005 to 2050. *Arch Phys Med Rehabil.* 2008;89:422–429.

4. Dillingham TR, Pezzin LE, Mackenzie EJ. Limb amputation and limb deficiency: epidemiology and recent trends in the United States. *South Med J.* 2002;95(8):875–883.

5. Shurr DG, Michael JW. Introduction to prosthetics and orthotics. In: *Prosthetics and Orthotics.* 2nd ed. Norwalk, CT: Appleton & Lange; 2000:1–19.

6. Group TG. Epidemiology of lower extremity amputation in centers in Europe, North America, and East Asia. The global lower extremity amputation group. *Br J Surg.* 2000;87(3):328–337.

7. US Department of Congress, Bureau of the Census. *Projection of the Total Resident Population by Five Year Age Groups, and Sex with Special Age Categories. Middle Series.* Washington, DC: US Department of Congress, Bureau of the Census; 2000.

8. Criqui MH. Peripheral arterial disease: epidemiological aspects. *Vasc Med.* 2001;6(suppl 1):3–7.

9. *Diabetes: Successes and Opportunities for Population-Based Prevention and Control at a Glance 2011.* Available at: http://www.cdc.gov/chronicdisease/resources/publications/AAG/ddt.htm. Accessed 16.02.11.

10. Clark N. Peripheral arterial disease in people with diabetes. *Diabetes Care.* 2003;26:(12):3333–3341.

11. *Number (in Thousands) of Hospital Discharges for Non-traumatic Lower Extremity Amputation with Diabetes as a Listed Diagnosis, United States, 1988-2006.* Available at: http://www.cdc.gov/diabetes/statistics/lea/fig1.htm. Accessed 18.02.11.

12. Reiber GE, McFarland LV, Hubbard S, et al. Service members and veterans with major traumatic limb loss from Vietnam War and OIF/OEF conflicts: Survey methods, participants, and summary findings. *J Rehabil Res Dev.* 2010;47(4):299–316.

13. Meltzer DD, Pels S, Payne WG, et al. Decreasing amputation rates in patients with diabetes mellitus. An outcome study. *J Am Podiatr Med Assoc.* 2002;92(8):425–428.

14. Moulik PK, Mtonga R, Gill GV. Amputation and mortality in new-onset diabetic foot ulcers stratified by etiology. *Diabetes Care.* 2003;22:382–387.

15. Wrobel JS, Mayfield JA, Reiber GE. Geographic variation of lower extremity major amputation in individuals with and without diabetes in the Medicare population. *Diabetes Care.* 2001;24:860–864.

16. Dillingham T, Pessin L, MacKenzie E. Incidence, acute care, length of stay, and discharge to rehabilitation of traumatic amputee patients: an epidemiological study. *Arch Phys Med Rehabil.* 1998;79:279–287. 17.

17. Ebskov L. Major amputation for malignant melanoma: an epidemiological study. *J Surg Oncol.* 1993;52:89–91.

18. *2011 National Diabetes Fact Sheet.* Available at: http://www.cdc.gov/diabetes/pubs/pdf/ndfs_2011.pdf. Accessed 19.02.11.

19. Van Gils CC, Wheeler LA, Mellstrom M, et al. Amputation prevention by vascular surgery and podiatry collaboration in high-risk diabetic and non-diabetic patients. *Diabetes Care.* 1999;22:678–683.

20. Bild DE, Selby JV, Sinnock P, et al. Lower extremity amputation in people with diabetes: epidemiology and prevention. *Diabetes Care.* 1989;12(1):24–31.

21. Centers for Disease Control. Hospital discharge rates for non-traumatic lower extremity amputation by diabetes status-United States, 1997. *MMWR Morb Mortal Wkly Rep.* 2001;50(43):954–958.

22. Kannel WB, McGee DL. Diabetes and glucose tolerance as risk factors for cardiovascular disease: the Framingham study. *Diabetes Care.* 1979;2(2):120–126.

23. Reiber GE, Boyko EJ, Smith DG. Lower extremity foot ulcers and amputations in diabetes. In: Harris MI, Cowie CC, Stern MP, et al., eds. *Diabetes in America.* 2nd ed. Washington, DC: U.S. Dept of Health and Human Services, DHHS Pub No. 95-1468; 1995:409–427.

24. May B. Assessment and treatment of individuals following lower extremity amputation. In: O'Sullivan SB, Schmitz TJ, eds. *Physical Rehabilitation: Assessment and Treatment.* 4th ed. Philadelphia: Davis; 2001:619–644.

25. Centers for Disease Control. Lower extremity amputations among persons with diabetes mellitus—Washington, 1988. *MMWR Morb Mortal Wkly Rep.* 1991;40(43):737–739.

26. Humphry LL, Palumbo PJ, Butters MA, et al. The contribution of non-insulin dependent diabetes to lower-extremity amputation in the community. *Arch Intern Med.* 1994;154(8):885–892.

27. Centers for Disease Control and Prevention. *Diabetes Surveillance, 1993.* Atlanta, GA: US Department of Health and Human Services; 1993.

28. *Data 2011 Diabetes Fact Sheet.* Available at: http://www.diabetes.org/diabetes-basics/diabetes-statistics/. Accessed 19.02.11

29. Centers for Disease Control. Lower extremity amputation episodes among persons with diabetes—New Mexico, 2000. *MMWR Morb Mortal Wkly Rep.* 2003;52(4):66–68.

30. Dillingham TR, Pezzin LE, Mackenzie EJ. Racial differences in the incidence of limb loss secondary to peripheral vascular disease: a population-based study. *Arch Phys Med Rehabil.* 2002;83:1252–1257.

31. Prevalence of Diabetes Among Hispanics–Selected Areas, 1998-2002. *MMWR Morb Mortal Wkly Rep.* 2004;53(40):941–944.

32. Centers for Disease Control. *CDC Reports that Hispanics Are Diagnosed with Diabetes at Twice the Rate of Whites.* Atlanta, GA: National Center for Chronic Disease Prevention and Health, Division of Media Relations; 1999.

33. *North American Indians and Alaska Natives. In Diabetes in America.* Available at: http://www.diabetes.niddk.nih.gov/DM/pubs/america /pdf/chapter34.pdf. Accessed 19.02.11.

34. Nelson RG, Ghodes DM, Everhart JE, et al. Lower extremity amputation in NIDDM: 12-year follow-up study in Pima Indians. *Diabetes Care.* 1988;11(1):8–16.

35. Canavan RJ, Unwin NC, Kelly WF, et al. Diabetes- and nondiabetes-related lower extremity amputation incidence before and after the introduction of better organized diabetes foot care. *Diabetes Care.* 2008;31:459–463.

36. Healey AJ, Tai N. Traumatic amputation—a contemporary approach. *Trauma.* 2009;11:177–187.

37. Brown LW. Traumatic amputation. *AAOHN J.* 1990;38(10):483–486.

38. Webb JB. Replantation in trauma. *Trauma.* 2005;7:1–9.

39. Lewis DR, Gloeckler LA. *Cancers of the Bone and Joint.* Available at: http://seer.cancer.gov/publications/survival/surv_bone_joint.pdf. Accessed 15.02.11.

40. LaQuaglia MP. Osteosarcoma: specific tumor management and results. *Chest Surg Clin N Am.* 1998;8(1):77–95.

41. Phillipe PG, Rogers DA, Fontanesi J, et al. Sarcomas of the flexor fossae in children: Is amputation necessary? *J Pediatr Surg.* 1992;8:964–967.

42. Sabapathy SR, Venkatramani H, Shankar SU. Rhabdomyosarcoma of the thumb: a case report with a review of the literature. *Indian J Plast Surg.* 2007;40(2):189–193.

43. Gover AM, McIvor J. Upper limb deficiencies in infants and young children. *Infants Young Child.* 1992;5(1):58–72.

44. May BJ. The child with amputation. In: *Amputations and Prosthetics: A Case Study Approach.* 2nd ed. Philadelphia: Davis; 2002:255–268.

45. Esquenazi A. Geriatric amputee rehabilitation. *Clin Geriatr Med.* 1993;9(4):731–743.

46. Ham R, de Trafford J, Van de Ven C. Patterns of recovery for lower limb amputations. *Clin Rehabil.* 1994;8(4):320–328.

47. Dillingham TR, Pezzin LE, Mackenzie EJ, et al. Use and satisfaction with prosthetic devices among persons with trauma-related amputations: a long-term outcome study. *Am J Phys Med Rehabil.* 2001;80(8):563–571.

48. Green GV, Short K, Easley M. Transtibial amputation. Prosthetic use and functional outcome. *Foot Ankle Clin.* 2001;6(2):315–327.

49. Scremin AM, Tapia JI, Vichick DA, et al. Effect of age on progression through temporary prostheses after below-knee amputation. *Am J Phys Med Rehabil.* 1993;72(6):350–354.

50. Osterman H. The process of amputation and rehabilitation. *Clin Podiatr Med Surg.* 1997;14(4):585–597.

51. Stineman MG, Kwong PL, Kurichi JE, et al. The effectiveness of inpatient rehabilitation in the acute postoperative phase of care after transtibial or transfemoral amputation: study of an integrated health care delivery system. *Arch Phys Med Rehabil.* 2008;89(10):1863–1872.

52. Fletcher DD, Andrews KL, Hallett JW, et al. Trends in rehabilitation after amputation for geriatric patients with vascular disease: implications for future health resource allocation. *Arch Phys Med Rehabil.* 2002;83(10):1389–1393.

18

Wound Care for Vulnerable Feet

EDWARD MAHONEY AND CAROLYN B. KELLY

LEARNING OBJECTIVES

At the conclusion of this chapter the reader will be able to do the following:

1. Explain the relationship between diabetes and foot ulceration.
2. Identify the interactive factors that contribute to ulceration in the high-risk foot.
3. Describe the components of an effective high-risk foot examination.
4. Explain the importance of each component of a thorough wound examination.
5. Compare and contrast the efficacy and drawbacks of the most commonly used options for reducing pressure to promote ulcer healing and prevention.
6. Determine which wounds would benefit from the addition of therapeutic modalities.
7. Develop a comprehensive treatment plan to manage vulnerable feet, including those with open wounds.

The thought of losing a limb has to be one of the most frightening things a person will ever face. For the majority of the population, the idea likely conjures up some sort of catastrophic event that can be pushed to the back of the mind as something that is unlikely to occur. Unfortunately, individuals with a high-risk foot face the very real possibility of losing a limb in the foreseeable future. A high-risk foot is one that has an underlying disease process that puts the tissues at a greater risk of breakdown. The largest group of people with high-risk feet in the United States is the diabetic population. In 2006, approximately 65,700 amputations were performed on patients with diabetes, which accounted for more than 60% of all nontraumatic amputations performed that year.[1] In the simplest designation, amputations can be divided into traumatic and nontraumatic causes. Trauma can result in extensive tissue damage and is often complicated by infection and foreign materials in the wound bed, but healing generally proceeds appropriately when these factors are corrected. Nontraumatic causes of amputations are not as straightforward. Unlike traumatic wounds, there may not be an isolated incident that can be identified as a causative factor in nontraumatic wounds. In many cases, the wound is the result of

an underlying disease, such as diabetes, or condition that will negatively affect wound healing. In these individuals, the key to effective treatment is often early intervention. This chapter is designed to assist the reader in identifying feet at risk of ulceration and implementing comprehensive examination and treatment strategies to prevent or minimize the need for amputation.

NORMAL WOUND HEALING

To fully appreciate the impact of different disease states on wound healing, it is necessary to begin with an understanding of normal wound healing. Wound healing involves a coordinated interaction of three phases: inflammation, proliferation, and remodeling. Although these stages do overlap to some degree, they are discussed individually for purposes of clarity. The body's first response to injury during the inflammatory phase is to stop the bleeding at the site of injury through a process known as hemostasis. In response to an injury, platelets, which are formed in bone marrow and are free floating in the vascular system, are attracted to the injury site. The platelets also undergo activation, which causes them to change from a round shape into a sticky form that enables them to adhere to the injured area.[2] The platelet plug may be enough to stop the bleeding in minor injuries, or it may be augmented by the coagulation cascade to form a larger clot. An in-depth discussion on the coagulation cascade is beyond the scope of this chapter. In terms of wound healing, coagulation is only one part of the role of the platelet. The second role, which is critical to wound healing, is the secretion of numerous growth factors and cytokines that set the stage for later phases of wound healing.

The first cells to arrive at the wound site in response to the coagulation cascade are granulocytes, which are a form of white blood cells. Neutrophils are the most abundant of the granulocytes and are found in the wound within 24 hours after injury. These cells are nonspecific and phagocytic, which is crucial for disposing of damaged cells in the area. Other granulocytes include phagocytic eosinophils and basophils, which release histamine. The next leukocytic cells to respond are monocytes, which become macrophages in the wounded area. Macrophages are phagocytic, but can also be thought of as growth factor factories because they play such a critical role in producing the growth factors that guide the remainder of the healing process.

Toward the latter stages of the inflammatory response, the wound is well into the proliferative phase of healing. The goal of this phase is to resurface the wound with a layer of viable epithelium. For this to occur, a well-vascularized dermal matrix is laid down in the wound bed. To accomplish this, new blood vessels are formed (neovascularization), and collagen is created by fibroblasts (fibroplasia). At the same time, new skin is being produced through the process of reepithelialization, and wound contraction is occurring, which helps to approximate the wound margins and make the resultant scar smaller. The duration of this phase is greatly influenced by the size of the wound, but is generally considered to last up to several weeks. Despite wound closure, the healing process is not yet complete as tissues continue to remodel. In fact, the remodeling phase is by far the longest and can last for more than a year from wound closure until the tissues have reached their maximum strength. Even after the wound has completely remodeled, it will not regain the same strength that uninjured tissue has, and will continue to require close monitoring and protection to prevent reulceration.

ASSESSMENT OF THE HIGH-RISK FOOT

According to the most recent data from the Centers for Disease Control, approximately 60% of all nontraumatic lower-extremity amputations were the result of diabetes in 2006.[3] With that in mind, it is of particular importance to assess the patient's diabetes status (Figure 18-1).

Following a thorough review of systems, a quick, but thorough objective examination of the foot should occur. This examination should include assessments of the vascular, sensory, motor, and autonomic systems, as well as a mobility assessment and footwear inspection.

Vascular Assessment

It could be argued that a thorough vascular assessment is the most crucial aspect of the evaluation of a high-risk foot.

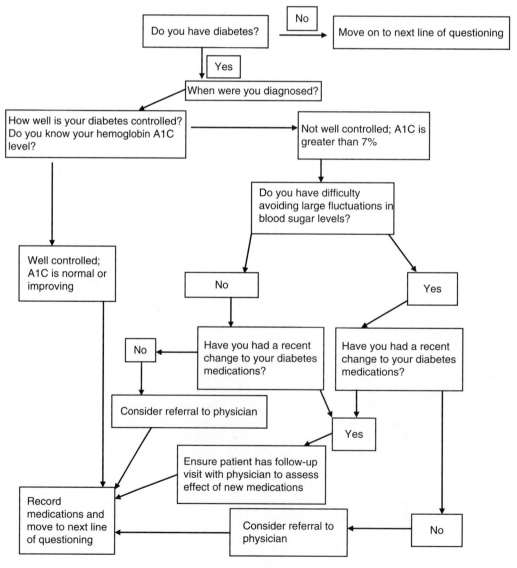

FIGURE 18-1 Flow sheet for diabetes assessment.

Not only can impaired blood flow be a causative agent for the development of ulceration, it will impact healing of ulcers regardless of the etiology. A clinical vascular examination can be performed quickly, and help the clinician decide if circulation is adequate or if further, more advanced testing is required. The examination should begin with an assessment of the pedal pulses (dorsalis pedis and posterior tibial). Pulses can be recorded as present or absent, or can be graded on a more qualitative basis (Figure 18-2):

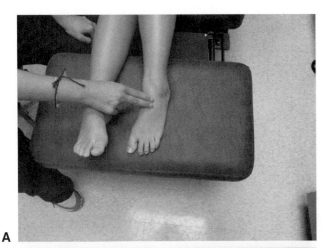

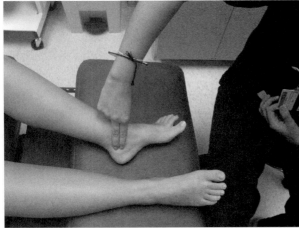

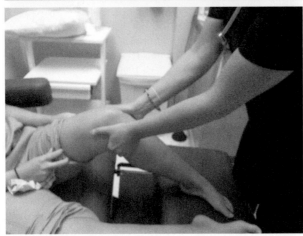

FIGURE 18-2 Palpation of pedal pulses. **A,** Dorsalis pedis pulse. **B,** Posterior tibial pulse. **C,** Popliteal pulse.

0 = Unable to palpate
1+ = Barely perceptible
2+ = Weak
3+ = Normal
4+ = Bounding pulse; possible Charcot joint or aneurysm

The assessment of pulses should not be used alone to determine the extent of arterial compromise, but should be correlated with other findings from the clinical examination. The lack of a palpable pulse (grade 0) is not sensitive for the detection of peripheral arterial disease. In a study by Collins and colleagues, more than two-thirds of limbs with diagnosed peripheral arterial disease still had palpable pulses.[4] Pulse palpation may be most useful for the comparison between the left and right limb to detect abnormalities. If there is any question as to the arterial status of a limb, an ankle-brachial index (ABI) should be performed. The ABI is a comparison of the systolic blood pressure of the pedal arteries with the brachial artery. The systolic pressure is recorded in both arms, unless contraindicated (lymphedema, dialysis port), and the higher of the two values should be used. In the foot, the dorsalis pedis and posterior tibial artery are both assessed and the highest value is used (Figure 18-3).

$$ABI = \frac{highest\ ankle\ systolic\ pressure}{highest\ brachial\ systolic\ pressure}$$

A normal ABI is 1.0, which indicates normal arterial blood flow to the foot. If an ABI value of less than 0.8 is obtained, referral to a vascular specialist is warranted for further testing. In the case of individuals with longstanding diabetes, an ABI greater than 1.2 may be obtained because of calcified vessels in the lower extremity. If this is the case, the ABI value is of no significance as it pertains to arterial flow and further testing is required. One test that can be performed is a toe pressure. By using a specially designed cuff that fits over the digit and a Doppler flowmeter, the pressure in the digital arteries, which are less affected by calcification, can be assessed (Figure 18-4). A systolic toe pressure greater than 50 mm Hg is generally considered normal; an increased risk of amputation and failure to heal is associated with pressures less than 30 mm Hg.[5]

Another noninvasive vascular assessment technique is transcutaneous oxygen pressure ($TcPO_2$). Low $TcPO_2$ measurement, a measurement of skin perfusion, is a predictor of ulceration[4] and healing.[6] In 1999, the American Diabetes Association's Consensus Development Conference on Diabetic Foot Wound Care recommended use of abnormal toe systolic pressures and $TcPO_2$ measurements to predict poor outcomes.[7] Generally, no single noninvasive test provides enough information to make decisions about vascular intervention. Analysis is usually done by a vascular specialist who interprets the results of a combination of tests.

If signs of arterial insufficiency are present and the patient has a foot wound, or if the patient has none of the typical symptoms of ischemia but has a nonhealing wound despite adequate control of infection and external pressure, referral for further vascular evaluation is warranted. Many patients

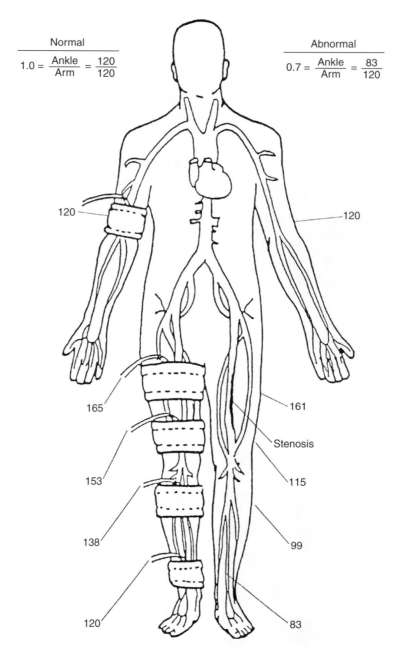

FIGURE 18-3 Segmental systolic pressures show a normal condition on the left. A 0.7 ankle-brachial index on the right indicates a reduction in flow. Also of note is the greater than 30 mm Hg drop in pressure between two successive thigh cuffs, which indicates stenosis or occlusion of the segment. (From Hoffman AF. Evaluation of arterial blood flow in the lower extremity. In Robbins J [ed], *Clinics in Podiatric Medicine, Surgery, and Peripheral Vascular Disease*. Philadelphia: Saunders, 1999. p. 42.)

have significant arterial disease but few clinical signs, such as pain or open wounds, that warrant the risks involved with an invasive vascular procedure. They should still be educated in foot care and proper shoe fit. Because better circulation may be necessary to heal an open wound than to keep unbroken skin intact, the goal for patients with arterial insufficiency is to prevent foot wounds from occurring.

Sensory Assessment

Patients in all settings, with many different diagnoses, may have impaired sensation. Diabetes is the most common reason for impaired sensation, but it is also associated with

chronic alcoholism, syphilis, Hansen's disease (formerly leprosy), spinal cord injury, and peripheral nerve injuries. Regardless of the cause, when the ability to perceive an external stimulus is diminished, it increases the risk for ulceration. In patients with diabetes, a loss of protective sensation is the leading cause of foot ulceration.[8] Simply put, if a patient cannot feel discomfort, there is no stimulus to change anything. In the case of a foot rubbing on a shoe or brace, an individual with intact sensation will stop to adjust the problem because of discomfort, whereas the person with impaired sensation may be unaware of the problem until the shoes are removed and blood is seen on the sock.

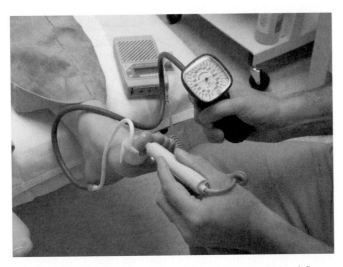

FIGURE 18-4 Toe cuff for the assessment of digital blood flow.

with enough pressure to cause it to bend. Inability to sense the monofilament is considered to be a positive test for the loss of protective sensation. Care must be taken to avoid areas with thick callus, as the test results will not be valid. Alternatively, a tuning fork can be used for vibratory testing. A study by Oyer and associates found a vibrating 128-Hz tuning fork placed on the toe was more sensitive to the onset of neuropathic changes than monofilament testing.[9] In this testing procedure, a clanging tuning fork is placed on the area to be tested and remains there until the subject can no longer feel the vibration. The tuning fork is then quickly moved to an area of known intact sensation on either the subject or examiner. If the vibration can still be felt in that site, the test is positive for a loss of vibratory sensation. Other authors have found similar results using similar methods with tuning forks of different frequencies, for example, 512 Hz, which may be more convenient as the 512 Hz tuning fork is smaller (Figure 18-6).[10]

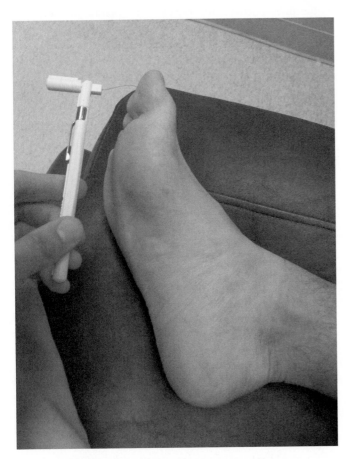

FIGURE 18-5 Semmes-Weinstein monofilament.

Protective sensation can be assessed in several different ways in the clinic, with very little special equipment needed. The two simplest methods are Semmes-Weinstein monofilaments, and tuning forks. A 5.07 monofilament, which takes 10 g of perpendicular force to bend, is the most widely used clinical tool for the assessment of protective sensation (Figure 18-5).

The patient is instructed to close his or her eyes and the monofilament is applied perpendicular to the skin surface

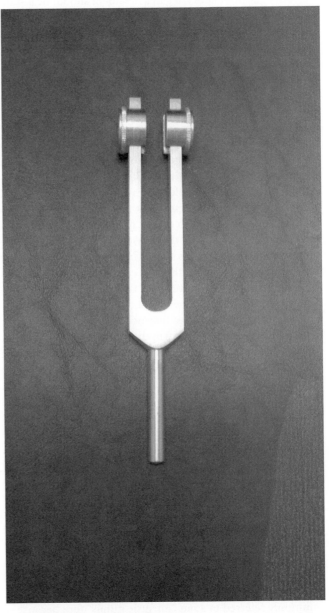

FIGURE 18-6 Tuning fork for the assessment of neuropathy.

Motor Assessment

A thorough musculoskeletal evaluation is necessary to determine a given patient's likelihood for ulceration. Deformities and abnormal biomechanics often change pressure distribution in the foot and can lead to discomfort, callus, and, ultimately, ulceration. The clinician can begin to assess for motor impairments while the patient is seated. The wear pattern on shoes, as well as the presence of calluses on the foot, can identify potential pathologies that ultimately may lead to ulcer formation. Following a visual inspection of the feet and footwear, a musculoskeletal examination that includes reflexes, strength, and range of motion should be performed. Particular attention should be paid to toe extension and dorsiflexion range of motion, as limitations in either one greatly increases weight-bearing forces through the forefoot in the latter stance phases of gait. This becomes increasingly important to assess if the patient has diabetes, as a loss of dorsiflexion has been widely documented in that population.[11,12] If a patient is ambulatory, a gait assessment should be a standard part of the high-risk foot assessment. Major deviations from the normal gait pattern can be assessed with a quick visual inspection. For example, patients with peroneal nerve injuries have difficulty with foot clearance and have a shorter loading response, which increases pressure at the forefoot. Alternatively, a patient could have increased forefoot pressure in terminal stance as a result of limited dorsiflexion range of motion. A mild limitation in motion may present as an early heel rise, while a more severe restriction can lead to excessive knee flexion for clearance during the swing phase of gait. With a static foot assessment, it may be apparent that both individuals have increased forefoot pressure, but the cause would not be known, with the result that the optimal intervention could not be selected. With careful gait analysis, the clinician can determine the cause of the pressure and choose appropriate interventions, such as a rocker bottom shoe to substitute for the midfoot rocker in the first case or an orthosis to aid in dorsiflexion in the second case. Chapter 5 provides an in-depth review of the gait assessment.

Many of the deformities that occur as a result of motor neuropathy are more subtle than the examples above. As neuropathy advances, the intrinsic muscles atrophy and become weaker, leading to muscle imbalances and changes in joint alignment.[13,14] When tissues over these joints are then loaded, they are unable to withstand the same amount of pressure and begin to break down. As extensor muscles on the dorsum of the foot overpower flexor muscles of the plantar aspect, the net result is extension at the metatarsophalangeal joint, which increases pressure at the plantar aspect of the metatarsal head (MTH). This occurs with both claw, and hammer toe deformities; the difference being that claw toes are characterized by flexion of both interphalangeal (IP) joints, whereas hammer toes have flexion at the proximal IP and extension at the distal IP joint. Care must also be taken to protect the distal tips of the toes as well as the dorsum of the IP joints, as these areas are easily injured from rubbing on shoes. Persons with diabetes who have motor neuropathy may develop a high-risk foot, commonly referred to as an "intrinsic minus" foot because of the impairment in function of the small muscles of the foot. The intrinsic minus foot presents as a pes cavus (high arch) deformity with prominent MTHs. Compounding matters is the distal migration of the metatarsal fat pad into the toe sulcus as a result of muscle imbalance. Now the metatarsal region has increased pressure because of the foot shape, as well as the loss of fat pad over the MTH that would normally increase the total surface area being loaded.[15]

Partial foot amputation is another deformity that alters plantar pressure distribution. Because the surface area to carry the force of body weight is smaller, pressure on the remaining structures increases. Studies that have looked at great toe amputation in patients with diabetes have found an increase in plantar pressure and the development of new deformities and ulcerations after amputation.[16,17] As loss of parts of the foot occurs, the mechanics of the foot change, transferring stresses to new areas with the potential for ulceration.

Plantar ulceration has been associated with lower extremity peripheral neuropathy and excessive plantar pressures.[18-21] Pressure on the soft tissues of the foot is related to three variables: the magnitude of the force applied to the foot, the amount of surface over which the force is applied, and the length of time over which the force is sustained.[22] Because much of the focus in treating and preventing foot ulcers is on reducing pressure, one must understand the relationship of pressure to these three variables. The following formula should be considered:

$$Pressure = Force/Area$$

As indicated, anything that increases the magnitude of the force applied to the foot or decreases the area over which the force is applied increases pressure and makes tissue damage more likely. Immediate injury can occur from extremely high force applied over a small area, as when a patient steps on a tack or piece of glass. Injury occurs because tremendously high pressure exceeds the tensile strength of the skin. Pressure on the foot can also become excessive when a moderate amount of force is repeatedly applied over a small surface area—when bony deformities cause small localized areas of weight bearing or when partial foot amputations decrease the patient's weight-bearing surface. The force applied to the foot (body weight) remains essentially the same, but the actual pressure on the tissues is greater because of reduction of the surface area. In patients with diabetes, factors such as limited joint mobility,[23-27] structural abnormalities,[28-30] and previous amputation[16,17] can lead to increased force or decreased surface area. All of these are associated with increased plantar pressures and ulceration.

Further complicating this picture is the time factor. In looking at tissue ischemia and resultant ulceration, Kosiak found an inverse relationship between the amount of pressure applied to tissues and length of time that the pressure was sustained.[31] Low pressures sustained over long periods of time caused tissue necrosis. This is the mechanism of tissue injury when decubitus ulceration occurs in bedridden, poorly mobile patients. Tissue necrosis also occurs along the medial or lateral borders of the feet or tops of hammer toes when patients wear shoes that are too tight. Kosiak found that as the magnitude of pressure increased, fewer hours were necessary to induce injury.

The most common cause of skin breakdown in the neuropathic foot is repeated bouts of moderate pressure during every-day walking.[32] Dr. Brand demonstrated this fact by applying repeated bouts of moderate pressure to the anesthetized foot pads of rats. Repeated bouts of moderate pressure caused inflammatory changes, and with continued repetition, this inflammation progressed to ulceration.[22] For health professionals who care for patients with diabetic foot problems, two facts from this research hold particular significance. First, when the inflammatory changes (heat and swelling) began to persist from one day to the next, breakdown of the tissue was prevented by discontinuing the repeated stress. Second, breakdown was prevented by either decreasing the amount of pressure per repetition or by reducing the number of repetitions. The findings of Brand and Kosiak suggest that the variables of force, area, and time and repetition contribute to tissue breakdown and that changing one or more of these variables must be considered in the treatment plan for patients with a high-risk foot.

Autonomic Assessment

Autonomic changes represent the third category of changes associated with polyneuropathy. With roles including the regulation of moisture and blood flow, as well as controlling hair and nail growth and overall skin integrity, the autonomic system is crucial to healthy feet. Cracks and fissures in the foot, as well as nail pathologies, can predispose people to ulceration or infection. As these are all end products of autonomic dysfunction, patients need to be educated on how to prevent them from occurring. Patients with autonomic dysfunction, most commonly from diabetes, should be educated to moisturize their feet often so as to avoid drying and cracking of the skin. Creams or non–alcohol-based lotions should be applied liberally to the feet and legs, but the areas between the toes should be avoided as the excess moisture can lead to fungal infections. Not only is moisturized skin more comfortable, it is also stronger and less likely to develop cracks and fissures, which are easy entries for infections. If nails are too thick to be trimmed safely at home with regular nail clippers, the patient should be encouraged to seek professional help for nail care.

One of the most damaging outcomes related to dysfunction of the autonomic system is diabetic neuropathic osteoarthropathy, also known as Charcot foot. This destructive process can significantly alter the bony architecture of the foot, and can lead to excessive plantar pressures[33] and subsequent ulceration if left unchecked (Figure 18-7). This process was first recognized in patients with syphilis during the nineteenth century by Jean-Martin Charcot. Although several neuropathic diseases, including syphilis and Hansen's disease, can cause a Charcot arthropathy, it is most commonly seen in persons with diabetes.[34] Charcot foot is a progressive disorder that leads to joint dislocation, fractures, and deformity of the foot.[35]

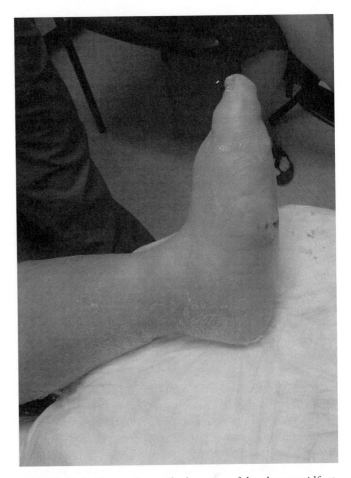

FIGURE 18-7 Charcot foot with ulceration of the plantar midfoot.

Charcot surmised that when the proper functioning of the autonomic system was impaired by disease, it led to an increase in blood flow to the bones, which then led to bone resorption. Over time, this became known as the neurovascular theory.[36] A second theory states that development of a Charcot foot is related to trauma in an insensate foot. Because of the lack of sensation, there is no perception of the trauma, and thus no adjustments to compensate for it. If the joint continues to be loaded, it will stay inflamed and eventually break down. This became the neurotraumatic theory.[36] In most experts' opinions, the cause of Charcot foot is likely to be some combination of the two theories.[35,37] A commonality of the two theories is that Charcot foot starts with an insensate foot.[36,38,39] As a result, the Charcot foot is most likely to occur in someone with sensory neuropathy, adequate blood flow, and a history of trauma, whether they were aware of it or not. Upon clinical examination, the foot is erythematous, edematous, has an elevated skin temperature, and a bounding pulse indicative of excessive blood flow.[39,40]

Charcot foot can become debilitating if not recognized early enough to arrest the development of the rocker bottom deformity that is characteristic of the disease. It is often misdiagnosed because no single diagnostic test can confirm its presence. Medical history, clinical manifestations, and radiographic findings all must be considered. Unfortunately, the clinical presentation of a red, hot, swollen foot often leads to the diagnosis of cellulitis, which is treated with antibiotics. During the time the patient is being treated with antibiotics for an infection that does not exist, they are continuing to damage the foot by walking on it. Radiographs taken in the acute phase are not sensitive to the development of neuropathic fractures and bone scans do not differentiate Charcot foot from osteomyelitis. MRI, on the other hand, is capable of identifying bone injury prior to complete fracture.[37,40] MRI may be cost-prohibitive, making the medical history and physical examination that much more important.

Charcot foot should be suspected if a patient with neuropathy presents with sudden onset of localized swelling, warmth, and erythema in the absence of an open wound. Appropriate treatment for Charcot foot should be initiated until this condition is ruled out on further testing. During acute Charcot arthropathy, joint destruction can be minimized by immobilization in a total-contact cast and avoidance of weight bearing until signs of healing become apparent (decreased temperature, decreased swelling, and improved radiographic findings). Both lack of compliance with non–weight bearing and use of orthotic devices in place of cast immobilization have shown prolonged healing times.[41,42] When cast immobilization is discontinued, the use of an orthotic device for continued protection of the joints during the initial return to weight bearing should be considered.[33,42]

The architectural changes that occur in the foot secondary to neuropathic osteoarthropathy result in high-pressure areas.[33] Because of this, following the period of immobilization and limited weight bearing, patients with a history of Charcot foot must be provided with appropriate footwear to stabilize the foot and reduce plantar pressure. Surgical intervention may be indicated for unstable or severely malaligned fractures or dislocations, which create problems with recurrent ulceration, fitting of shoes, ability to ambulate,[43,44] as well as recalcitrant ulcers.[45] Some of these procedures require months of immobilization and avoidance of weight bearing, which can be difficult for many patients with diabetes and neuropathy. Such surgery is usually advocated only if nonsurgical management fails.

Footwear Assessment

The analysis of the high-risk foot truly begins before the patient sits on the examination table. The type and appearance of the footwear they are wearing can give insight as to the cause of their pathology. Shoes that either do not fit properly or are excessively worn can cause problems including blisters, calluses, and wounds. On the other hand, shoes that someone refuses to wear are not useful as they will just sit in the closet.

Characteristics of the proper shoe for the high-risk foot include:

- Snug fit at the heel to prevent pistoning (moving up and down) of the heel
- Wide toe box to accommodate for deformities such as bunions and hallux valgus
- Deep toe box to accommodate claw/hammer toes and molded inserts
- Fashionable enough that the patient will wear the shoes

It is recommended that people shop for new shoes in the mid to late afternoon to ensure the best fit. Because foot size changes throughout the day, a shoe purchased to fit the foot early in the morning may be too small by late evening, and conversely a shoe bought at night may be too large for the foot in the morning.

Gait and Balance

Motor neuropathy causes weakness of foot and ankle musculature that may result in gait deviations that change plantar pressure patterns or contribute to instability. Gait and balance are also affected by damage to sensory nerves, which leads to an inability to sense where the foot is in space. The use of ankle-foot orthoses or shoe modifications may help restore a more normal gait, stabilize joints, or improve balance. Studies have found that patients with peripheral neuropathy secondary to diabetes have problems with gait and postural stability.[46-50] In examining a patient with a high-risk foot, physical therapists must include not only the patients' foot problems but also their overall functional status. To reduce the morbidity associated with falls, recommendations that address safety and function should be included in the treatment plan.

WOUND ASSESSMENT

Although it is clear that the most effective way to prevent amputations is to avoid getting wounds in the first place, that is not always possible. When a wound does develop, regardless of the etiology, a thorough wound assessment becomes a necessity. The comprehensive wound assessment begins with a thorough patient history, which helps the clinician not only gain a better understanding of the cause of the wound, but also forecast healing rates of the wound more accurately. Refer to the previous section on risk factor assessment for more information pertaining to patient history. It is often helpful to take the entire patient history prior to undressing the wound, as there is a tendency to focus solely on the wound once it is visible and forget about other factors that may be important.

Once the patient history is reviewed, the wound can be carefully undressed. In addition to the components already discussed for the evaluation of the high-risk foot, the assessment also includes an examination of the immediate wound and periwound area. The wound should be assessed for location, color, odor, size/depth, and drainage type and amount, and the periwound tissues should be assessed for any abnormalities (Figure 18-8).

Location

If a thorough medical history has been taken, the examiner may have a good hypothesis as to the cause of a wound before even seeing it. The objective examination can either confirm or refute this hypothesis. One of the first objective findings that should be documented is wound location. Although traumatic wounds can occur in any anatomic location, many of the common wound etiologies tend to occur most frequently in certain areas. Diabetic foot (neuropathic) ulcers are most common on the plantar aspect of the digits and MTHs, more specifically, the great toe and first MTH, but they can occur in any area of high stress.[51] Ulceration secondary to neuropathy is also common on the dorsum of the toes, as well as bony prominences, such as the lateral aspect of the first and fifth MTHs and the base of the fifth metatarsal, and anywhere a shoe or brace may be rubbing. Wounds secondary to vascular insufficiency can occur in any location that has impaired blood flow, but are most frequently found on the toes, dorsum and lateral aspects of the foot, as well as the lateral leg. In contrast, wounds of venous origin tend to be in what is often referred to as the "gaiter" area, just proximal to the medial malleolus. It should be noted that these are general guidelines, and an accurate diagnosis cannot be made based solely on location. When describing wound location, the clinician should be as precise as possible, often using bony landmarks as descriptors. This becomes increasingly important when multiple wounds are present.

Subjective exam:

Pain: Last dressing change:

Comments:

Objective exam:

Mode of arrival: Edema:

Assistive device: Sensation:

Wearing prescribed dressings/footwear?   Pulses: (L)   (R)

Wound location:

	(L)	(R)
DP		
PT		
Popliteal		
ABI		

   If other, enter location:

Wound stage:

Wound color:

Color	Pre-debridement	Post-debridement
	%	%
	%	%
	%	%

Range of motion:

Special Tests: Results:

Odor:

Size: cm^2

L: W: D:

Drainage amount:

Drainage type:

Periwound:

Nails:

FIGURE 18-8 Wound assessment flow sheet.

(Continued)

Comments:

Treatment:

Wound cleansed with

Debridement performed today?   Debridement type:

Modalities:

Dressings: Offloading:

Comments:

Assessment:

Tolerance to treatment:

Comments:

Plan:

Comments:

Follow up:

Nails:

Edema:

Sensation:

Pulses: (L)   (R)

	(L)	(R)
DP		
PT		
Popliteal		
ABI		

Range of motion:

Special Tests: Results:

FIGURE 18-8 Cont'd

Wound Color

A simple designation for wound color is to use the red-yellow-black staging system, which was first published in the United States in 1988 and had been used in Europe prior to that.[52] Red wounds are generally healthy, well vascularized, and are progressing through the normal stages of healing. The red appearance is attributed to the deposition of highly vascularized collagen, known as granulation tissue. This tissue is fragile, and may bleed with excessive force or friction. Granulation tissue that bleeds with minimal pressure or has a dusky appearance is called *friable* and should be investigated further as it is typically a sign of increased bacteria present in the wound. Yellow wounds indicate fibrinous slough or infection is present. Slough has a stringy, adherent characteristic and can be removed by a variety of methods, which are discussed later in this chapter (Preparing the Wound Bed by Eliminating the Source of Inflammation or Infection). Wounds also may have a black appearance, which signifies the presence of eschar. Eschar is often hard to the touch, but can be soft or boggy if there is a lot of fluid present.

In most cases, it is beneficial to remove the eschar because the necrotic tissue promotes the proliferation of bacteria. Several instances when this is not advised are intact eschar on heels and vascular wounds that would not be able to heal following debridement. In addition to the red-yellow-black system that is focused on the dermis, the clinician must also be aware of deeper structures that may be apparent in the wound bed. The first tissue encountered beneath the dermis is known as subcutaneous tissue, fat, or adipose. This should have a pale yellow, moist appearance when healthy, but dries out and darkens when it is nonviable. Healthy, muscle has a bright red color, and the striations are often visible in the tissue. Damaged muscle takes on a dusky gray appearance with a much-less-pliable texture. The remaining structures that will be encountered in a deep wound bed—ligaments, tendons, bone—all should be white if well vascularized. If these tissues are compromised, they will take on a dusky yellow appearance, and continue to darken as damage proceeds.

For documentation purposes, the use of percentages is helpful in describing the wound color. For example, a wound could be 80% red, with 20% firmly adhered yellow fibrin. It is also suggested that the percentage should be documented before and after treatment if there is any significant change in the wound appearance.

Odor

One of the most troubling aspects of a wound from a patient's perspective is odor. Most significant wounds will have some odor when dressings are removed. As a clinician, it is important to know whether or not the odor is caused by infection, or simply from the dressing having been in place for an extended period. Before making this determination, dressings should be removed and the wound should be rinsed with sterile water or saline. Odors that are eradicated are likely caused by drainage on the dressings. This is especially true of occlusive dressings, such as hydrocolloids. If cleansing the wound does not eliminate the odor, it is more likely caused by necrotic or infected tissue. Wounds with a strong odor often contain anaerobic and aerobic bacteria, and are referred to as *polymicrobial*[53]; anaerobic bacteria create odor by releasing compounds including putrescine and cadaverine. These odors can be extremely strong, and are often described as acrid smelling. Aerobic bacteria also are capable of producing foul odors. Because the strength of an odor is subjective, it is recommended that descriptions such as sweet, fishy, necrotic, putrid, and the like also be included in the assessment of the odor. Infection should be considered when previously odor-free wounds develop an odor, but it should also be pointed out that some infections do not produce any odor at all.

Size

Wound size should be documented on a routine basis as it is an easy way to monitor progress in wound healing. For most wounds, unless they are perfectly symmetrical, a diameter or even length and width may not give an accurate representation as to the true size of the wound. When length and width are used, the largest length is recorded, and the width is recorded perpendicular to the length. Although improvements can be seen as these numbers decrease, it is difficult to accurately calculate a total surface area for the wound or a percent area reduction because wounds are irregularly shaped. Alternative methods include photography with a transparent film over the wound, wound tracings with transparent film, and digital cameras that can calculate the surface area of the wound. All of these options enable the clinician to calculate surface area, and percent reduction in size (Figures 18-9 and 18-10).

Regardless of the method used to calculate wound size, the orientation of the wound should be standardized to ensure that subsequent measurements are assessing the same dimension. Bony landmarks can be used for this purpose, but it is most common to describe length in a cephalocaudal (head-to-toe) fashion and width perpendicular to that. Unfortunately, the largest dimensions of most wounds will not line up perfectly with axes along the cephalocaudal and perpendicular plane. For this reason many clinicians describe wound orientation using a clock face, with 12 o'clock being at the head and 6 o'clock at the feet. Using this system, a wound could be described as 6 cm in length from 10 o'clock to 4 o'clock and 3 cm in width from 1 o'clock to 7 o'clock. Undermining, tunneling, or any other abnormality in the wound can also be described using the clock face, which will help with consistency in measurement, especially if another clinician is measuring the wound.

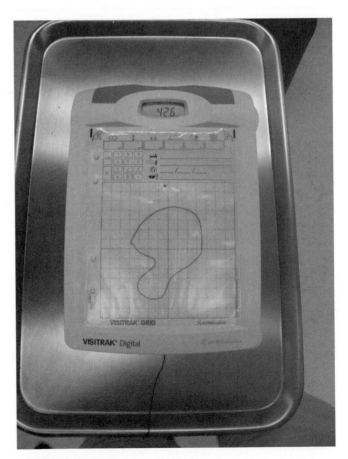

FIGURE 18-9 VISITRAK wound measurement system (Courtesy of Smith & Nephew, Hull, United Kingdom).

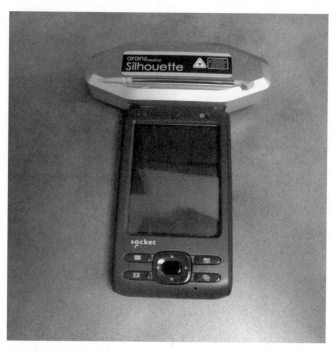

FIGURE 18-10 ARANZ Medical Silhouette wound imaging device (Courtesy of ARANZ Medical, Christchurch, New Zealand).

Depth

A thorough understanding of anatomy is necessary for an accurate staging of wounds. In turn, an accurate staging of wounds relies on being able to assess wound depth properly. Before depth can be measured, the wound must be free of nonviable tissue so the wound base can be visualized or probed. The wound can then be probed with a sterile probe held perpendicular to the skin surface. As wounds do not all have a uniform depth throughout, the deepest point should be measured and the location where the measurement was taken should be documented. After the depth measurement is obtained, wounds can be classified in several ways, depending on the etiology. Table 18-1 reviews different wound classification systems that rely on wound depth as a part of the staging criteria.

Drainage

The ideal wound will have enough moisture to prevent desiccation of the wound bed, but not so much that it causes breakdown of periwound tissues. The characteristics of wound drainage will vary depending on multiple factors, including wound location, vascular status, and presence of infection. Drainage should be classified by amount and type to accurately describe what is occurring in the wound. Assessing

TABLE 18-1   *Wound Classification Systems*

Classification System	Intended Wound Etiologies	Grades	Comments
Wagner[128]	Diabetic foot	0 = Intact skin 1 = Superficial ulcer 2 = Deep ulcer (through dermis) 3 = Infection 4 = Partial foot gangrene 5 = Full foot gangrene	
University of Texas[129]	Diabetic foot	A0 = Preulcerative or postulcerative lesion AI = Superficial wound AII = Involves tendon or capsule AIII = Involves bone or joint	Letter stage changes as follows: B = Infection C = Ischemia D = Infection and ischemia
Partial/full	All wounds	Partial = Involves epidermis and up to part of the dermis Full = Involves structures deep to the dermis	
Burns[130]	Burns	Superficial = Epidermis only Superficial partial = Superficial dermis involved Deep partial = Deep dermis involved Full thickness = Subcutaneous tissue involved Subdermal = Muscle, tendon, bone involved	Some experts do not make a distinction between full-thickness and subdermal burns, as both require surgery to heal[130]
National Pressure Ulcer Advisory Panel[131]	Pressure ulcers	I = Nonblanchable skin, or abnormal color; skin is intact II = Partial loss of dermis III = Down to, but not through fascia IV = Injury to subfascial tissues (muscle, tendon, ligament, capsule, bone) Unstageable = Wound bed cannot be visualized Suspected deep tissue injury = Purple or maroon area of discolored skin; may progress to deep, open ulceration rapidly	Do not reverse stage—a stage IV ulcer does not become a stage III ulcer, it is a healing stage IV

the amount of drainage is somewhat subjective in that it is not practical, or even possible in many cases, to weigh the amount of exudate from the wound. Instead, the clinician describes the amount of exudate along a continuum, such as the one below:

None → Scant → Minimal → Moderate → Heavy → Copious

This can be difficult to quantify, especially for the inexperienced clinician, as different dressings will absorb vastly different amounts of fluid and thus could make a heavily draining wound appear drier, or vice versa. Wounds with underlying arterial insufficiency tend to be drier because less circulation is getting to the wound bed, whereas patients with wounds that are venous in nature often experience heavy drainage because of the edema present. If the amount of exudate increases, and a reason is not clearly related to changes in treatment (i.e. surgical intervention to increase blood flow, discontinuation of compression therapy, or resting in dependent positions), then infection should be considered as a likely cause. The presence of infection causes the wound to remain in the inflammatory phase of wound healing, which results in increased drainage. Infected wounds often exhibit purulent drainage, which can be yellow, green, tan, or even creamy or cloudy. These wounds often require a combination of local and systemic agents to treat the infection. In addition to purulent drainage, drainage can also be serous (watery), sanguineous (bloody), or serosanguineous (pink or reddish, watery).

Periwound Skin

The area immediately surrounding a wound, known as the *periwound skin*, should be assessed carefully because it can give clues as to the state of the wound. Evidence of excessive pressure, excess moisture, decreased vascularity, and the presence of infection can all be found in the periwound skin with a quick visual inspection and palpation. Table 18-2 lists periwound findings and their significance.

TABLE 18-2   *Periwound Skin Assessment*

Appearance	Description	Significance
Callus	Area of hyperkeratosis, typically in response to high pressures[54,132,133]	Frequently associated with neuropathy and/or bony deformity. Indicates area susceptible to breakdown[132]
Blister	Fluid-filled area causing separation of epidermis from dermis	Shearing forces from rubbing on shoes, brace, bed, etc.; may also be caused by adhesive dressings on skin
Erythema	Redness	Indicates inflammation caused by local stress or infection; redness in immediate periwound area is normal in acute wounds, but excessive redness or redness that persists for 30 to 60 minutes after the stress is removed requires intervention; erythema associated with infection is often well demarcated; if red streaks are noted (lymphangitis), consult physician as it is a sign of spreading infection
Maceration	Changes in tissue caused by excessive moisture	Can lead to skin breakdown; may be a result of excessive sweating, heavy wound drainage, incontinence, or inappropriate dressings
Induration	Hardening of the tissue because of edema	Chronic edema impairs wound healing; induration is often associated with infection or venous disease
Hemosiderin	Brownish discoloration of the skin around a wound. Associated with deposition of hemoglobin in extravascular tissues	Often associated with venous disease
Excoriation	Wearing away of the skin	Indicates an area of trauma; often preceded by maceration and/or blistering
Presence of scars	A scar is the final result of a previous injury	May give clues to the chronicity of the problem as well as the extent of damage in the area
Temperature	Can be palpated or assessed with infrared thermometer; is typically compared with adjacent areas or to contralateral side	Nonspecific indicator of inflammation; helpful to monitor "hot spots" that may be at risk of breakdown, or for resolution of a Charcot fracture
Edema	Swelling in the tissues	Bilateral edema suggests a systemic problem; unilateral edema indicates a localized problem; can occur with infection, inflammation, venous dysfunction, and lymphedema; consider Charcot foot if insensate
Other changes	Taut, shiny, hairless, cracked skin	Taut, shiny skin with a loss of hair indicates impaired blood flow; cracked skin is associated with aging, diabetes, or vascular disease. Important to moisturize skin frequently

In addition to the factors listed in Table 18-2, the amount of soft tissue over prominent areas also can be assessed. Decreased amounts of soft-tissue bulk have been identified in persons with diabetic neuropathy in comparison to persons without diabetes used as controls.[13,54–67] With less soft tissue present, peak pressures at the prominent areas are increased, which increases the likelihood of ulceration.[12,54]

WOUND MANAGEMENT

It is truly incredible how much the field of wound management has changed over the last few decades. It can be an overwhelming endeavor for the inexperienced clinician as it seems there are constantly new modalities, dressings, and devices coming out on the market. Further complicating things is the fact that there are frequently conflicting results when one therapy is compared to another. This leaves the clinician with the difficult task of developing the best treatment plan for a given individual, without having a gold standard of treatment in many instances. Luckily, the basic tenets of wound healing have remained largely unchanged, and a practical approach remains effective. Successful wound healing interventions can be categorized into a few simple steps, which are discussed in detail. These overlapping steps are:

1. Preparing the wound bed by eliminating the source of inflammation or infection;
2. Providing an optimal wound healing environment;
3. Reducing further trauma to the wound; and, finally,
4. Keeping the wound healed once it has closed and preventing new ulcers from forming.

Preparing the Wound Bed by Eliminating the Source of Inflammation or Infection

The current model of infections that is most widely used involves the interaction between the host response and the amount of bacteria present in the wound. As outlined by this model, a patient with a healthy immune response is able to tolerate a higher bacterial load without developing signs of infection than a patient with an impaired immune response. The amount of bacteria in a wound is usually described on a continuum from sterile to a systemic infection. Sterile wounds have no bacteria, whereas systemic infections have overwhelmed the wound with bacteria and cause systemic immune responses. Intermediate stages include contaminated wounds, characterized by bacteria that is present, but not invading the tissue; colonized wounds which are still capable of healing despite invading bacteria; and critical colonization in which the bacteria are overwhelming the immune system and are creating a localized response.[58] It is in the colonized and critically colonized wounds, and in infected wounds in conjunction with systemic medications, that selective debridement, modalities, and topical dressings are most helpful in optimizing the wound environment.

A very effective means of reducing inflammation and the risk of infection is removal of the tissue that may harbor bacteria, through a process known as *debridement*. There are many ways that debridement can be performed, and all of them are within the scope of practice of the physical therapist except for surgical debridement. Because surgical debridement may involve the excision of viable and nonviable tissue to ensure that all of the necrotic or infected tissue is removed from the area, it is called *nonselective debridement*. Slightly less aggressive is sharp debridement. Sharp and surgical debridement both use sterile sharp instruments to remove tissue, but the tissue that is being debrided is limited to nonviable tissue in sharp debridement. For this reason, sharp debridement is referred to as *selective debridement*. Despite being widely accepted, or perhaps because it is so widely accepted as a standard of care, there is limited evidence on the effectiveness of sharp or surgical debridement. Debridement with sharp instruments is the quickest way to remove undesirable tissue, but is also the riskiest method, and is best employed by the experienced clinician. Risks can be minimized by using the appropriate equipment, and assessing the patient thoroughly to ensure that they do not have any of the contraindications/precautions listed in Box 18-1.

In addition to sharp and surgical debridement, mechanical, acoustic, enzymatic, larval, and autolytic forms of debridement are also viable options. Of these, all are classified as selective with the exception of mechanical debridement. Mechanical debridement can be performed using a variety of methods, including abrasion, wet-to-dry dressings, and whirlpool. All of these methods may remove nonviable tissue, but can be detrimental to healthy tissue, and if used at all, should be limited to cases in which the majority of the wound is nonviable.

Historically, whirlpools were frequently included in the treatment plan for an individual with a wound. Proposed benefits were increasing blood flow to the area because of the warm water, as well as the ability to remove dressings and necrotic tissue. The whirlpool also has many shortcomings as a wound care modality, including the risk of cross-contamination, unregulated pressures on the wound, exacerbation of dependent edema, and excessive maceration. As a result, pulsatile lavage with suction (PLWS) has largely replaced the whirlpool as the hydrotherapy of choice for wound management. There are no absolute contraindications to the use of PLWS, but care must be taken around exposed vessels, vital organs, and fistulas. Precautions must also be taken to reduce the risk of cross-contamination, including using personal protective equipment, treating in a private room, using a shield to prevent backsplash, and disposing of single-use components properly (Figure 18-11 and Table 18-3).

BOX 18-1 *Contraindications and Precautions to Sharp and Surgical Debridement*

Medically unstable patient (surgical only)[125]
Dry gangrene or lack of vascular supply to heal wound[125]
Intact, dry eschar on heel[126]
Impaired clotting mechanism or on anticoagulants[127]
Pyoderma gangrenosum[126]
Clinician without a thorough knowledge of anatomy of the area to be debrided

although PLWS seems to reduce bacterial counts in wounds, some researchers believe the effect may have less to do with mechanical debridement and more to do with the negative pressure exerted by the suction component.[63]

Acoustic, or ultrasonic, energy is the newest form of debridement to enter the wound care arena. Currently, there are several ultrasonic debridement devices on the market that are capable of performing selective debridement. These devices are classified as low frequency (kilohertz range, as opposed to megahertz with conventional ultrasound) and high-intensity ultrasound devices. Studies have demonstrated effectiveness of these devices at increasing fibrinolysis, improving blood flow to the wound, reducing bacterial counts, and anecdotally seems to be faster than sharp debridement in many cases.[64–70] Although capable of producing extremely rapid debridement and a reduction in bacteria, the use of ultrasonic debridement will likely be cost-prohibitive for clinics that do not specialize in wound healing. For that reason, an in-depth discussion of ultrasonic debridement is not included in this chapter.

The remaining forms of debridement tend to be slower, but are less harmful to healthy tissue. Larval therapy involves the use of sterile maggots, which secrete enzymes to liquefy necrotic tissue, but have no negative effect on granulation tissue. Similarly, enzymatic debridement involves the application of an enzyme to the wound surface. The enzyme works to denature the protein in the necrotic tissue on the wound bed. In the past, papain urea products were frequently used as debriding agents without the U.S. Food and Drug Administration (FDA) approval. This is no longer available as the FDA banned the manufacturing of and distribution of unapproved topical papain products in late 2008 and early 2009, respectively. As none of the papain products had FDA approval, there are currently none on the market.[71] The only enzymatic agent that is available is Santyl (Healthpoint, Fort Worth, TX), which is a collagenase, and thus breaks down unwanted collagen in the wound. The final form of debridement is autolysis, which is the most selective, but also the slowest. Autolysis, or autolytic debridement, uses moisture-retentive dressings to provide an environment that allows the body's natural enzymes to debride necrotic tissue. It is the simplest form of debridement to perform, but requires careful monitoring for infection, primarily because of the slow nature of this method. These debridement strategies should not necessarily be thought of as independent of each other. For example, sharp debridement is often done in conjunction with enzymatic or autolytic debridement. All of the forms of debridement serve to reduce the risk of infection by removing the energy source for the bacteria. There also are interventions that specifically target the bacteria, rather than the necrotic tissue.

Over the last decade or so, the number of dressings that have been developed to reduce bacteria in the wound has increased dramatically. These include a variety of dressings that contain silver, methylene blue, gentian violet, polyhexamethylene biguanide, iodine, or honey. These dressings have been shown to be superior to non–antimicrobial dressings in the reduction of bacteria, but there is insufficient evidence

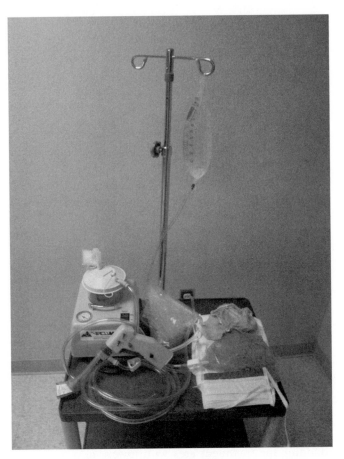

FIGURE 18-11 Pulsatile lavage with suction.

TABLE 18-3 *Pulsatile Lavage with Suction Recommendations for Infection*

Pressure	12 to 15 psi
Suction	60 to 100 mm Hg
Amount of irrigant	Dependent upon wound size
Frequency	At least daily if possible
Location	Private treatment room with closed door

Data from Albaugh K, Loehne H. Wound bed preparation/debridement. In McCulloch JM, Kloth LC (eds), *Wound Healing: Evidence-Based Management*, 4th ed. Philadelphia: Davis, 2010. pp. 155-179; and Bukowski EL, Nolan TP. Hydrotherapy: the use of water as a therapeutic agent. In Michlovitz SL, Bellew JW, Nolan TP (eds), *Modalities for Therapeutic Intervention*, 5th ed. Philadelphia: Davis, 2011. pp. 109-134.

PLWS delivers a stream of irrigant solution that can be directed at the area of interest to debride slough and reduce bacterial counts on the wound.[59,60] It appears that the effectiveness of lavage improves as the amount of irrigant used to flush out bacteria is increased.[60] With PLWS, the water pressure can be controlled, and can be delivered within the safe range of 4 to 15 psi, which is effective at removing nonviable tissue and bacteria without traumatizing healthy tissue.[61] For the purposes of reducing bacterial levels, the higher end of that range is recommended, as nearly 85% of bacteria can be removed from a wound with 15 psi.[59,62] It should be noted that to state one antimicrobial dressing is superior to another in terms of promoting wound healing.[72,73] These dressings are available in so many varieties ranging in absorptive capacity, adhesive versus nonadhesive, amorphous versus sheet form, and the like, that there is likely a good option for nearly any wound type. What is most important to remember is that none of these dressings should be used as a replacement for systemic antibiotics.

It is common to use topical antimicrobial dressings along with systemic medications, especially in the case of arterial insufficiency. For example a patient with a diabetic foot ulcer may have an infected toe, with poor vascularity. In this case, the amount of the systemic antibiotic getting to the infected area may be limited and could benefit from a topical agent to reduce the degree of surface bacteria. There are several problems with the continued use of antimicrobial dressings, namely cost and the concern over developing resistance. Because they are impregnated with antimicrobial agents, these dressings are more expensive than a comparable non–antimicrobial dressing and are not intended to be used for the duration of wound healing. Likewise, there is some concern in the wound care community that overuse of silver dressings may lead to the development of resistant strains of bacteria, similar to what happened with the widespread use of antibiotics.

In addition to antimicrobial dressings, and the interventions already discussed, two therapeutic modalities that have strong evidence supporting their use in the management of infections are electrical stimulation and ultraviolet light. Electrical stimulation is likely to be found in most physical therapy clinics because of its use in strengthening and pain reduction. The most common waveforms for electrical stimulation in wound healing are high-voltage pulsed current and low-intensity direct current (or microcurrent). Both of these currents are monophasic, meaning current will only flow in one direction. As a result of this, charged particles will be drawn toward the oppositely charged electrode, and repelled from the like-charge electrode, just as a positive pole and negative pole on a magnet will stick together and two positives will push each other apart. This concept is known as *galvanotaxis*, and is the basis for the use of electrical stimulation in tissue healing. When the goal is to treat an infection, the negative pole (cathode) should be used at the wound site, and the positive pole (anode) can be placed approximately 15 to 30 cm away. By applying cathodal stimulation to the wound, activated neutrophils are recruited which can attack the bacteria that is present.[74] The treatment electrode may be placed on the immediate periwound skin, or directly in the wound. If stimulation is applied directly to the wound, the wound must be filled with hydrogel or saline-moistened gauze. Treatment is usually continued until signs of infection are no longer present, or until progress halts, at which time polarity is reversed to jump start healing (Table 18-4).

Ultraviolet C (UVC) light is another effective modality for the treatment of infection, although it may not be readily available in many offices. The carcinogenic effects of ultraviolet A and B lights are well known, but do not seem

TABLE 18-4   *Electrical Stimulation Treatment Recommendations for Infection*

Waveform	LIDC or HVPC
Polarity	Negative
Duration	60 minutes
Frequency	Daily
Intensity	100 to 800 µA (LIDC) or 75 to 150 V (HVPC)

HVPC, high-voltage pulsed current; *LIDC*, low-intensity direct current.
Data from Kloth LC, Zhao M. Endogenous and exogenous electrical fields for wound healing. In McCulloch JM, Kloth LC (eds), *Wound Healing: Evidence-Based Management*, 4th ed. Philadelphia: Davis, 2010. pp. 450-513.

to be a problem with UVC because the light is absorbed by the epidermis, and those cells that may have been damaged are constantly sloughing off.[75] Complete eradication of bacteria has been demonstrated with UVC in vitro as well as in vivo in animals.[76,77] In humans, UVC is very effective for the treatment of colonized wounds; however, if the wound is grossly infected, or is too deep for proper application of the light, outcomes are not as impressive,[78] although positive outcomes have been demonstrated in small case series.[79] If any form of ultraviolet light is to be used, care must be taken to prevent injury to the patient and clinician by wearing protective eyewear, and covering the area surrounding the treatment area with towels, or a thick layer of petroleum jelly to prevent penetration of the ultraviolet light (Table 18-5).

Providing an Optimal Wound-Healing Environment

As mentioned previously, it is somewhat of an artificial delineation to break wound healing down into different steps because there is so much overlap. Early in the wound-healing process the primary goal may be removal of nonviable tissue, as mentioned in the previous section, but selective debridement would be of no use if concurrent steps were not taken to optimize the wound-healing environment. Once bacteria in the wound are controlled and an adequate arterial supply is assured, the focus of therapy can shift to moist wound healing. Moist wound healing includes the use of dressings, and in some cases, compression therapy to create a wound bed that is neither too wet (macerated) or too dry (desiccated) to

TABLE 18-5   *Ultraviolet C Treatment Recommendations for Infection*

Wavelength	UVC (200 to 290 nm)
Time	180 seconds
Distance from wound	1 inch
Frequency	Bacteria reduced in as little as one treatment

Data from Thai TP, Houghton PE, Keast DH. Ultraviolet light C in the treatment of chronic wounds with MRSA: a case study. *Ostomy Wound Manage.* 2002;48(11):52-60; and Kloth LC. Physical modalities in wound management: UVC, therapeutic heating, and electrical stimulation. *Ostomy Wound Manage.* 1995;41(5):18-27.

be suitable to wound healing. An analogy to a beach is commonly used to help explain this concept, in which the optimal wound environment is the wet sand, and suboptimal environments are underwater or on dry land.

To create a moist wound bed, the clinician must have a good understanding of the wound etiology, and a familiarity with the available wound care dressings. Certain wounds, such as those associated with infection, venous insufficiency, and lymphedema, tend to drain heavily and require absorbent dressings, whereas wounds without an adequate blood supply tend to be dry and often require the addition of moisture. With the appropriate use of cleansing agents, protection of the periwound skin, and selection of suitable dressings, wound healing can be positively influenced. Educating a patient about appropriate cleansing agents is particularly important if a patient will be cleansing the wound at home. The patient should be educated not to scrub the wound and to avoid the use of harsh chemicals such as bleach, iodine, hydrogen peroxide, alcohol, or surgical scrub brushes for daily cleansing, unless specifically prescribed for the management of a heavily colonized wound. Although some of these chemicals can be extremely effective at controlling bacteria, they are all cytotoxic and can impede wound healing. The general rule of thumb "if you wouldn't put it in your eye, don't put it on your wound" works well. For healthy granulating wounds, normal saline or sterile water are effective for mild cleansing and the removal of small particles of adhered dressing that may be present. Some wounds have bacteria that are adhered to the surface forming a matrix known as a biofilm. In these cases, a noncytotoxic wound surfactant is a better option.

Once the wound is clean, consideration can shift to the periwound area. This skin is vulnerable to injury from adhesive dressings or excess wound drainage, but damage can be limited or prevented with the use of a skin protectant. There are literally hundreds of dressings on the market, making it impractical, if not impossible, to keep up with all of them. By having a general understanding of each class of dressings, the clinician should be able to choose a dressing that is not only safe, but effective in the management of the wound at hand. Table 18-6 outlines the characteristics of some of the most commonly used classifications of dressings.

No single dressing is intended to treat a wound through all phases of wound healing. Nor is each patient with the same diagnosis going to respond the same. It is important to reassess the characteristics of the wound at each patient visit to ensure that the dressing being used remains the best option. Factors such as ease of use, whether or not the patient can change the dressing independently, how often it will need changing, the degree of discomfort associated with dressing changes, and cost need to be considered. For example, a hydrocolloid is easy to apply, but would not be cost-effective for a wound that needs to be changed twice per day, and a transparent film may be inexpensive and easy to use but inappropriate for an individual with poor periwound skin integrity.

Acute wounds in an otherwise healthy individual may heal without difficulty if appropriate dressings are used. In chronic wounds, or patients with impaired wound healing potential, the use of certain modalities can be used to stimulate wound healing. Electrical stimulation, pneumatic compression, negative-pressure wound therapy, ultrasound, and laser have all been shown to be effective in the management of wounds. It is beyond the scope of this chapter to go into an in-depth discussion of each of these modalities. Table 18-7 lists the proposed indications and contraindications for each modality; however, the reader is referred to other resources that will provide a more detailed analysis than space in this chapter permits.[80-82]

Reducing Further Trauma to the Wound

Regardless of the advanced wound care dressing used, wounds will not heal unless the wound can be protected from further trauma. In most cases, trauma comes in the form of weight-bearing forces. In a bed-bound individual, dynamic air mattresses and air-fluidized beds are used to disperse forces, which in turn, reduce the amount of pressure at the wound site and allow it to heal. For persons who are more active, offloading can be even more of a challenge as there is a balance that needs to be met between maintaining function and providing pressure relief to the wound. Take the case of an individual with dropfoot whose ankle foot orthosis is causing a wound on the plantar aspect of the fifth MTH. The patient needs to continue to wear the orthosis in order to walk, but if the patient does so, the wound will continue to deteriorate. The challenge for the clinician is to offload the foot so that the wound can heal as quickly as possible, enabling the patient to return to the patient's normal activities.

Many of the advances in pressure reduction strategies for the foot have come about because of diabetes. Between the years 2007 and 2011 the number of Americans with diabetes increased by more than 2 million to 25.8 million (8.3% or one of every 12 people).[1] As a result of the neuropathic and arterial changes discussed previously, many of these individuals will develop foot ulcers that will require offloading. Many of these wounds would respond well to several weeks of complete bed rest as all weight-bearing forces would be eliminated from the bottom of the foot. This is not practical for most patients, and even if it was a possibility, it is not without risk, that is, blood clots, deconditioning, and pressure ulcers. Maintaining non–weight bearing at home is also a major challenge for most patients. When a patient sustains an orthopedic fracture to the foot, pain serves as negative feedback and prevents the person from weight bearing. In the presence of neuropathy, the sensation of pain is diminished so the deterrent from putting the foot on the floor is absent. Although non–weight bearing or partial weight bearing is encouraged through the use of an assistive device, it is prudent to assume the device will not be used all the time and to protect the foot as if you intend weight bearing to occur.

Total Contact Casting

The "gold standard" for offloading the neuropathic foot has traditionally been the total contact cast (TCC) (Figure 18-12). Initially used in the management of Hansen's disease (formerly leprosy), the TCC was first brought to the United States

TABLE 18-6   *Common Wound Care Dressings*

Indication	Dressing Type	Contraindications	Comments
Absorption	Alginate	Excessively dry wounds Full-thickness burns	Secondary dressing required
	Hydrofiber	None	Secondary dressing required
	Foam	Excessively dry wounds	Adhesive and nonadhesive varieties Absorptive capacity varies between brands
Active bleeding	Alginate	Excessively dry wounds Full-thickness burns	Secondary dressing required
	Silver nitrate	Skin hypersensitivity	Effective on hypergranulation
Add moisture	Hydrogels	Moderate to heavy exudate	Gel or sheet forms
Maintain moisture	Hydrocolloids	Local or systemic infection Caution with fragile periwound skin	May increase wound odor at dressing removal
	Transparent films	Cavity wounds Tracts, tunnels, undermining Infection Excessive exudates	May decrease need for unnecessary dressing changes because wound can be visualized
Fragile skin	Silicone	None	Reduces scarring May be used to prevent an absorbent secondary dressing from adhering
Antimicrobial	Silver	Avoid use with enzymatic debriders	Most dressing classifications have a silver version
	Honey	None	Requires secondary dressing
	Polyhexamethylene biguanide	Avoid gauze-based dressing over exposed nerves, vessels, and tendons	Important to keep gauze moist to avoid adhering to wound bed
	Methylene blue/gentian violet	Full-thickness burns	Requires premoistening with sterile water or saline Requires secondary dressing
	Cadexomer iodine	Iodine sensitivity Hashimoto thyroiditis Nontoxic nodular goiter Graves disease Pregnant or lactating women	Sheet and gel forms available Requires secondary dressing
Debridement	Hydrocolloid	Local or systemic infection Caution with fragile periwound skin	May increase wound odor at dressing removal
	Transparent film	Cavity wounds Tracts, tunnels, undermining Infection Excessive exudates	No absorptive capacity
	Collagenase	Hypersensitivity to collagenase Do not use with silvers	Requires daily application Requires secondary dressing
	Gauze	Directly on healthy granulation tissue Exposed nerves, vessels, tendons	Wet-to-dry dressing is not recommended; if used, it should be restricted to necrotic wounds Effective as a secondary dressing

by Dr. Paul Brand.[83] Using the simple equation, pressure = force/area, it is evident that pressure can be reduced by reducing the amount of weight (force) going through the wound, and by increasing the total area that the patient's weight is spread over. The TCC has intimate contact with the entire plantar aspect of the foot, with the exception of the wound location. This serves to increase the weight-bearing surface area and reduce the force through the wound. Additionally, immobilization of the ankle in neutral prevents dorsiflexion

and weight transfer toward the front of the foot during the late stance phases of gait. The TCC reduces vertical and shear forces acting on the foot.[84,85]

Numerous studies report favorable results in healing diabetic foot ulcers with the use of the TCC.[51,83,84,86–88] Particularly interesting are the results of a prospective, randomized, controlled clinical trial done by Mueller and colleagues[12] that compared the effectiveness of total contact casting and reduced weight bearing with traditional treatment (debridement, daily

TABLE 18-7   *Indications and Contraindications/Precautions for Modalities Associated with Tissue Healing*

Modality	Indications Related to Tissue Healing	Contraindications/Precautions
Electrical stimulation[80,134]	Stimulates blood flow Promotes epithelialization Stimulates angiogenesis Stimulates collagen synthesis Impedes bacterial growth	Malignancy in the wound area Osteomyelitis In proximity to demand-type pacemakers or defibrillators Pregnancy Active hemorrhage Carotid bodies Eyes and gonads
Intermittent pneumatic compression[135]	Venous insufficiency Arterial insufficiency* (short duration, high-pressure pumps) Prevention of DVT Lymphedema (requires specialized pump)	Arterial compromise (ABI < 0.8) Acute infection DVT Uncompensated congestive heart failure
Negative-pressure wound therapy[136–138]	Pressure ulcers Traumatic wounds Diabetic ulcers Flaps/grafts Abdominal wounds Dehisced wounds Fasciotomy Arterial and venous ulcers	Exposed vital organs Untreated osteomyelitis or sepsis in the wound Necrotic tissue with eschar Inadequately debrided wounds Untreated coagulopathy or anticoagulant medications Malignancy in the wound Unexplored fistulas Active bleeding Exposed blood vessels
Ultrasound[81]	Accelerate inflammatory phase Stimulate capillary and blood vessel formation	Cancer Pregnancy or over reproductive tissue Circulatory impairment Epiphyseal plates in children Implants Infection Exposed neural tissue
Laser[139]	Fibroplasia Collagen synthesis Improves immune response	Cancer Over the eyes Pregnancy Over the thyroid gland

ABI, ankle-brachial index; *DVT*, deep vein thrombosis.
*Kavros SJ, Delis KT, Turner NS, et al. Improving limb salvage in critical ischemia with intermittent pneumatic compression: a controlled study with 18-month follow-up. *J Vasc Surg.* 2008;47(3):543-549.

dressing changes, the use of accommodative footwear, and instruction to avoid weight bearing through the use of assistive devices). Of 21 ulcers in the TCC group, 19 healed, compared to six of 19 in the traditional treatment group. Ulcers treated by total contact casting healed in 42 ± 29 days, whereas the traditionally treated ulcers healed in 65 ± 29 days. Five of 19 patients in the traditional treatment group required hospitalization for infection, versus no one in the TCC group.

One study showed that although some removable cast walkers were as effective as TCCs in relieving pressure from ulcer sites,[89] the TCC still healed a higher number of foot ulcers in a shorter time period.[88] The traditional TCC was made of plaster material, which required the patient to be non–weight bearing for at least 24 hours. Many clinics now do a combination of plaster and fiberglass or all fiberglass casts to allow patients to return to weight bearing more quickly.

The initial TCC also had contact with the entire foot, including the wound. Since that time, a modified approach in which the wound site is isolated has been shown to reduce pressure significantly more than the true "total contact" method.[90]

Although it has demonstrated superiority in offloading, the TCC is not appropriate for all cases. It should not be used in cases of excessive drainage, vascular insufficiency, infection, fluctuating edema, and for wounds that are deeper than they are wide. Because the condition of the foot cannot be monitored while it is enclosed in a cast, the patient must be able to recognize the warning signs indicating the need to have the cast changed. These signs include excessive swelling of the leg that causes the cast to become too tight, loosening of the cast that allows the foot and leg to move within the cast, a sudden increase in body temperature or of blood glucose level that might indicate infection, staining and drainage through

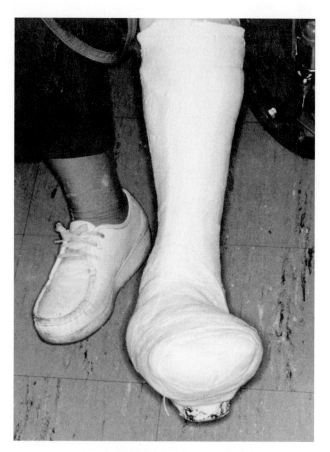

FIGURE 18-12 Total contact cast.

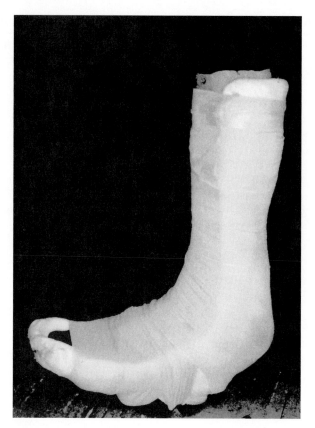

FIGURE 18-13 Posterior walking splint held in place by an elastic bandage.

the cast, excessive odor from the cast, new complaints of pain, and damage to the cast.

Posterior Walking Splints

An alternative to the TCC is the posterior walking splint (Figure 18-13). Fabrication of a walking splint is much like that of the TCC; however, with the anterior portion removed, the splint requires more reinforcement posteriorly. Elastic bandages are used to secure it to the foot and leg. The splint still allows for total contact with the plantar aspect of the foot and ankle immobilization. There are several advantages of the splint over the cast. The most obvious advantage is that it can be removed to cleanse the leg, inspect the skin, and change dressings. It is also a good alternative in most cases in which the cast is contraindicated. Another advantage is that it may reduce the cost to heal the wound since it does not need to be refabricated at each visit. Conversely, the splint is not without its disadvantages. It requires the same amount of skill and typically slightly more time to fabricate than the cast, and can be just as cumbersome. The most important clinical disadvantage is the fact that it can be removed, so there is no guarantee that the wound is being protected at all times, as it is in the cast.

Removable Cast Walkers

Despite being the "gold standard" for offloading the neuropathic foot, the TCC is not widely used because of concerns over iatrogenic complications as well as a lack of experience among clinicians. In its place, removable cast walkers have become the most widely used method to offload the foot. The removable cast walker is an orthotic device with double uprights fixed at a 90-degree angle to a rocker-soled walking platform (Figure 18-14). As with the TCC and walking splint, the fixed position of the ankle prevents propulsion at the forefoot, where the greatest pressures tend to occur. Removable cast walkers are available from various manufacturers. Because they are not custom made for each patient, care must be taken when fitting the device to ensure that it accommodates the contours of the patient's foot and ankle, particularly in the area of the uprights. A custom-molded insert can be added to most manufactured walkers. One variation of the removable cast walker, the DH Pressure Relief Walker (Ossur North America, Aliso Viejo, CA), has a removable, multidensity padded insole made up of individual plugs. This insole can be modified by removing plugs to create a relief area for the ulcer site. Studies show this walker to be more effective in reducing plantar pressures than other offloading devices.[89,91]

Instant Total Contact Cast

A major advantage of the TCC over the removable walker is the forced compliance because of the inability of the patient to remove the cast. Because the cast cannot be removed, it is assured that the wound is being offloaded 24 hours per day. Several studies show the removable cast walkers to be comparable to the TCC for pressure reduction.[91-93] However, other investigators report faster healing times with the TCC as opposed to removable cast walkers.[88,94] Under the

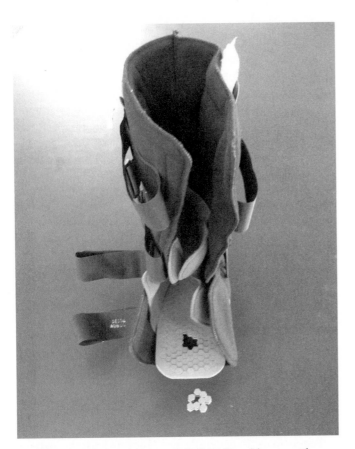

FIGURE 18-14 DH Pressure Relief Walker (shown with pegs removed) (Courtesy of Ossur North America, Aliso Viejo, CA).

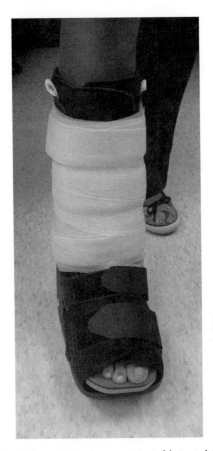

FIGURE 18-15 Instant total contact cast fabricated by applying fiberglass to a removable walker.

assumption that the seemingly conflicting data was a function of the cam walker being removed, researchers designed studies that compared TCCs and removable cast walkers to cast walkers that were made irremovable by wrapping them with a layer of fiberglass (Figure 18-15). These irremovable cast walkers were named instant total contact casts (iTCCs). Results of one study found the iTCC to be equivalent to the TCC in the proportion of wounds that healed in 12 weeks,[95] whereas the second study found healing rates with the iTCC to be comparable to healing rates of the conventional TCC in previous studies and superior to the removable cast walker.[96] Based on the available evidence, the iTCC seems like a viable option for a neuropathic wound, especially for the clinician that has not been trained in the application of, or does not have the time to apply, a TCC.

Wound-Healing Shoes

The cast, splint, and cam walker should all be considered as therapies of choice to offload neuropathic ulcerations. It is tempting to use less-restrictive devices because the devices that cover the leg seem like such an inconvenience to the patient. For most patients, putting them in devices that will be less than optimally effective is doing them a disservice. In some cases where a cast is contraindicated or the leg will not fit in a cam walker, devices that only go as high as the ankle may be useful. One of these devices is the wedge shoe, which has an elevated toe portion in relation to the heel so as to offload

the forefoot (Figure 18-16). The wedge shoe causes the body weight to shift back toward the heel, decreasing forces at the forefoot, albeit not to the same extent as the devices that transfer weight up the leg.[89] For pressure to be reduced, the area to be offloaded must be distal to the fulcrum of the shoe. To maximize pressure reduction, patients should be instructed to take short steps with the contralateral leg. This assures that they do not propel over the wedge causing contact between the distal end of the shoe and the ground. In clinical experience, this is often difficult for patients to do, and the telltale "clicking" of a patient in a wedge shoe can usually be heard as soon as

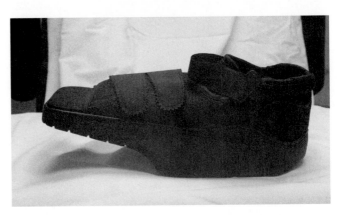

FIGURE 18-16 OrthoWedge shoe (Courtesy of Darco International, Huntington, WV).

the patient walks into the clinic. When a patient takes a large enough step to allow the front of the shoe to hit the ground, pressure at the forefoot is increased, but may still be less than if the patient was ambulating in a regular shoe because of the rigidity of the wedge shoe's sole. This rigidity serves to reduce the transfer of weight toward the forefoot that typically happens in terminal stance, but it does not isolate the at risk area in relation to the rest of the forefoot. The addition of a custom molded insert with a relief area has been shown to be effective at addressing this problem.[97]

The issue of compliance with the wedge shoe, and all shoe offloading devices, remains a question. On one side, it could be argued that wedge shoes are less cumbersome, so are more likely to be worn; and on the other side that they are easier to remove, making it more likely that the foot will be left unprotected. Another issue is that wedge shoes are difficult for patients with limited dorsiflexion, and could actually increase forefoot pressure if a patient has a limited range of motion. Walking in a wedge shoe feels very unnatural because of the functional leg-length discrepancy created. This can be difficult to manage for patients with balance issues, and can also lead to back discomfort. Finally, one last drawback to the wedge shoe is that it cannot be used to offload bilaterally because it shifts the patient's weight too far posteriorly.

An alternative shoe-type device to the wedge shoe is a shoe with modifiable insoles. An example of this device, the DH shoe by Royce Medical Co. (Ossur North America, Aliso Vejo, CA), has an insole with pegs that can quickly be removed to relieve pressure to the at-risk area (Figure 18-17). Advantages of this shoe type versus the wedge shoe include the ability to offload any part of the foot, not just the forefoot, a flat sole that is safer for those with balance issues, and the ability to offload bilateral feet simultaneously. A disadvantage to this type of shoe is that the flexible sole allows for a toe break during the gait cycle, which allows weight to transfer anteriorly.

Other Pressure-Relieving Options

There are several temporary offloading options that can be applied directly to the foot in cases in which the above options either are unavailable or undesirable. The first option is adhesive felted foam (Figure 18-18).[98,99] A custom-fit piece of ¼-inch felt-backed foam is adhered to the plantar surface of the foot. A U-shaped aperture is cut in the foam to reduce pressure around the ulcer. The margins of the aperture are positioned close to but not overlapping the wound edge, extending distally beyond the wound. The entire plantar surface of the foot must be examined to identify all vulnerable spots that need accommodation before the pad is applied. For forefoot ulcers, the pad extends proximally along the midfoot to increase the weight carriage in this area. All edges of the foam pad should be beveled to minimize chances of skin breakdown from edge pressure. When a bony deformity is particularly prominent, an additional layer of foam can be used to relieve pressure adequately from the ulcer site. A thin dressing is placed flatly over the ulcer. A healing sandal is used for ambulation. If the area is preulcerative or postulcerative, an extra-depth shoe can be worn. The felted foam should be thought of as temporary because the pressure relief provided by the foam pad decreases significantly by the fourth day.[100] Consequently, changing the pad every 3 or 4 days might be beneficial.

Felted foam is generally well accepted by the patient. Because this method allows for easier mobility than a TCC or walking splint, patients tend to walk more. This may not be desirable considering the possible effect of cumulative pressure. Despite walking more, patients using felted foam as an offloading method seem to respond well to the therapy as measured by the percentage of wounds that heal and the amount of time they take to heal.[99-103] The major benefit of the felted foam appears to constant wear time,

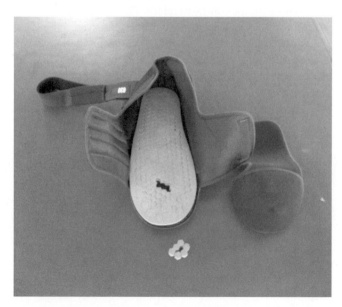

FIGURE 18-17 DH Wound Healing shoe, with pegs removed (Courtesy of Ossur North America, Aliso Viejo, CA).

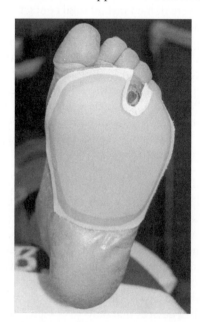

FIGURE 18-18 Felted foam pressure relief. Edges of the foam have been beveled.

without the excess bulk and seems to be a good option for patients that tend to walk barefoot, even though they are instructed not to.

A second temporary form of offloading is the football dressing. The football dressing was first proposed by Rader and Barry as a simple alternative to total contact casting for neuropathic ulcers.[104] The football dressing involves three layers of cast padding: the first is fan-folded over the toes, the second is wrapped circumferentially around the foot, and the third covers up to the lower ⅓ of the leg. A layer of gauze is then applied and covered with an elastic wrap. Although there is limited data that supports the use of the football dressing, a retrospective analysis of its use found it to have comparable effectiveness compared to the published data for the TCC and iTCC for the management of wounds across the spectrum on the University of Texas Diabetic Foot Classification System.[104] Some clinicians have had success using the football dressing in conjunction with a removable cam walker to ensure that the foot has some degree of protection even if the cam walker is removed.[105]

Prevention of Ulceration or Reulceration

The simplest and most cost-effective way to treat a wound is to avoid getting one in the first place. This is best accomplished through risk identification, patient education, fitting with appropriate footwear, and follow up for routine care. Being able to classify patients based on their risk for developing ulceration is critical for the proper management of each individual. One of the most widely used risk classifications was developed by the International Working Group on the Diabetic Foot (IWGDF) (Table 18-8). This classification system has been shown to predict foot complications (Table 18-8).[106]

In 2008, Lavery and associates published a revision of the IWGDF classification system.[107] In their new model, risk category 2 was divided into two groups labeled 2A and 2B. Group 2A included patients with sensory neuropathy and deformity, while group 2B consisted of patients with peripheral arterial occlusive disease. Group 3 was divided into those with a history of an ulcer (3A) and those with a history of amputation (3B). When they applied this new classification system to 1666 patients with diabetes, they found that there were significantly more foot complications in the "B" groups than in the "A" groups. Additionally, they found that there was little clinical difference between groups 1 and 2A, and thought those two groups could be combined. These changes

TABLE 18-8 *Diabetic Foot Risk Classification*

Risk Category	Definition
0	No neuropathy
1	With neuropathy, no deformity or peripheral vascular disease
2	With neuropathy and deformity or peripheral vascular disease
3	History of ulceration or amputation

TABLE 18-9 *Texas Foot Risk Classification*

Risk Group	Characteristics
0	No neuropathy or arterial disease
1	Neuropathy present
2	Arterial disease present
3	History of ulceration
4	History of amputation

From Lavery LA, Peters EJ, Williams JR, et al. Reevaluating the way we classify the diabetic foot: Restructuring the diabetic foot risk classification system of the International Working Group on the Diabetic Foot. *Diabetes Care.* 2008;31(1):154-156.

led to the development of the Texas Foot Risk Classification (Table 18-9).

Once a patient's risk factors have been identified, patient education can be tailored to the individual patient's needs. It is often helpful to have a small pamphlet or flier available for patients to take home that outlines what is safe and unsafe for them to do. A comprehensive educational pamphlet should include skin care, skin inspection, and footwear guidelines as shown in Box 18-2. Recommendations should be adjusted based on the patient's individual needs; for example, performing nail care at home would not be advisable for a patient with vascular compromise or who has difficulty reaching or seeing his or her feet.

Risk stratification is also important in determining the most appropriate footwear for a patient. Patients in the risk category 0 do not typically require special footwear, but should be educated on proper shoe fit. The proper shoe should match the contours of the foot, and should be comfortable at the time of purchase (no break-in period). High-risk patients should have the width and length of their feet measured every time they buy a new pair of shoes. It is also a wise investment for each clinic that deals with high risk feet to obtain a shoe-measuring device (Figure 18-19), as many problems can be avoided with proper fitting shoes. Width is measured across the widest part of the forefoot, typically across the MTHs, with the patient standing. Two measurements need to be taken for shoe length; one is the heel-to-toe length and the other is the heel-to-arch length. This extra measurement helps to ensure that the toe break in the shoe is in line with the MTHs. If the heel-to-toe and heel-to-arch lengths are the same, then that is the correct shoe size. If they are different, the patient should be fit with the larger of the two sizes. Patients should be instructed to try on new shoes in the mid to late afternoon, after they have been on their feet for most of the day. If they shop in the morning, they risk having shoes that are too tight by evening, and if they wait until evening to shop, shoes may be too large in the morning. A well-fitting shoe should have about one thumb's width between the longest toe and the end of the shoe, and the material on the dorsum of the shoe should be pinchable if the shoe is not too narrow or shallow. Patients who have a loss of sensation and no other risk factors (category 1 of original IWGDF) also do not require protective footwear, but may benefit from a soft

BOX 18-2   *Guidelines for Preventative Foot Care*

SKIN CARE

DO:
Wash feet daily. Dry them well, especially between the toes.
Apply a thin coat of moisturizer to feet daily, avoiding between the toes.
Trim toenails after washing and drying feet.
Cut toenails straight across; smooth any sharp edges with an emery board.
Have a podiatrist handle any thickened or ingrown toenails.
Thin thick corns or calluses by gently using a pumice stone or by professional care.
Check water temperature with a thermometer or elbow before bathing.
Wear socks at night if feet are cold.
Use sunscreen on the tops of feet during the summer.
Ask health care provider to check feet at each visit.

DO NOT:
Soak feet. This can dry them out and cause cracking.
Use moisturizer between toes. Moisture between the toes allows germs to grow.
Cut corns and calluses.
Use chemical agents, corn plasters, strong antiseptics, or adhesive tape on feet, because they can damage skin.
Use hot water bottles or heating pads because they can burn feet.

FOOT SELF-INSPECTION

DO:
Inspect all surfaces of the feet daily (including between the toes) for signs of injury: reddened areas, blisters, cuts, cracks, or sores.
Report any injuries to a health care provider immediately.
Feel for areas of increased temperature.
Check for tender areas on the bottom of feet.
Use a mirror if necessary to see the bottom of feet.
Have a family member, friend, or health care professional check feet if necessary.

DO NOT:
Wait to report problems to a health care provider. Early attention can often prevent small problems from becoming big ones.

FOOTWEAR

DO:
Wear shoes that fit the size and shape of feet and leave room for any necessary insoles.
Ask a health care provider to recommend the correct type of shoe.
Break in new shoes slowly, checking feet frequently for signs of irritation. Report signs of irritation to a health care provider.
Keep shoes and insoles in good repair.
Always wear socks or stockings with shoes, wearing a clean pair daily.
Before putting on shoes, check for rough areas, torn linings, or loose objects that can injure a foot.

DO NOT:
Walk barefoot (use slippers at night, special shoes or sandals for the beach).
Wear socks that are too baggy or have holes or prominent seams.
Wear socks or stockings that are constricting at the top.
Use sandals with thongs between the toes.

nonmolded insert in the shoe. It is important that they are educated on what to look for in a shoe. High heels increase forefoot pressure, shoes with narrow toes squeeze the foot, thongs can irritate between the toes, and slip on shoes do not stay in place very well. A supportive shoe allows the foot to stay in proper biomechanical alignment, while remaining relaxed. Running shoes are excellent options for this low-risk group as they reduce pressure in comparison to leather shoes.[108-110]

For higher-risk groups, specialty footwear, including custom insoles and extra-depth or molded shoes, is indicated.

Custom inserts are molded to the foot and reduce pressure at the heel and forefoot compared to flat insoles by spreading weight-bearing forces over a larger area.[111] The ideal insert strikes the perfect balance between durability and cushioning. No single material has been identified that accomplishes both tasks effectively, so most orthotics are fabricated with several different materials.[112,113] One concern with orthotic materials is that they lose their resistance to compression quickly. Some materials, such as Plastazote (Zotefoams, Inc., Hackettstown, NY) have some ability to rebound following repeated bouts of compression, but these softer materials need to be replaced

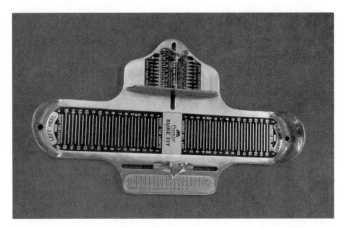

FIGURE 18-19 Brannock foot measuring device (Courtesy of The Brannock Device Co., Liverpool, NY).

frequently.[113] In one investigation, the combinations of Poron (Rogers Corporation, Rogers, CT), Plastazote #2 (Zotefoams, Inc., Hackettstown, NY), Spenco (Spenco Medical Corp., Waco, TX), and Microcel Puff Lite (Acor Orthopaedic, Inc., Cleveland, OH) were found to be the most effective.[112] Although these multidensity insoles seem to strike a balance between support and pressure relief, they are thicker than a flat insole and require the use of an extra-depth shoe. Custom-molded insoles in combination with extra-depth shoes are effective at preventing recurrent ulceration in diabetics (Figure 18-20).[114,115]

One of the most difficult times in the wound healing process is the transition from "treatment" footwear to everyday footwear. These patients comprise group 3 in the Texas Foot Risk Classification. As most people with a diabetic foot ulcer see the return to normal footwear as a goal, it is often tempting for both the patient and clinician to rush this process once the wound has completely epithelialized. At this point in the healing process, the wound may not be mature enough to handle the pressure increase from the treatment shoe to a regular shoe. As an intermediary, some of the shoe-type offloading

devices mentioned earlier in this chapter can serve as a bridge between treatment devices that immobilize the ankle and permanent footwear. Depending on the degree of deformity, individuals in these risk groups will need to be fit with custom insoles and either extra-depth or custom-molded shoes. For added pressure relief, areas surrounding the postulcerative site can be built up with firmer materials to transfer weight away from the maturing tissue. To reduce the risk of blisters caused by shear forces, any adjustments should be made to the underside of the insole so the foot remains in contact with a smooth surface.

More aggressive shoe modifications can be used for those that require pressure reduction beyond what in-shoe modifications can achieve. The most effective of these modifications is adding a rocker bottom to the outer sole of the shoe (Figure 18-21). Diabetic shoes with molded inserts and rocker bottom soles decrease pressure at the heel and forefoot, and simultaneously increase midfoot pressures, which is typically a less vulnerable area.[116] A review by Cavanagh reported mixed results pertaining to the effectiveness of rocker bottom soles, but notes several major flaws in the studies that found them to be ineffective.[117] In numerous studies, the reduced pressure associated with the rocker sole has been shown to be clinically significant as it reduced the recurrence rate compared to patients wearing their own shoes,[115,118-120] although none of these studies were randomized, controlled trials. For the rocker shoe to be effective, the sole must be rigid so that the shoe can take the place of the midfoot rocker, which would normally transfer weight anteriorly toward the toes. Another factor to consider is the placement of the axis of the rocker bottom. To maximize pressure relief at the toes, the axis of the rocker bottom needs to be shifted forward to 65% of the shoe length. For MTH pressure reduction, the most relief occurs when the axis is placed between 55% and 60% of the shoe length.[121]

Many of the strategies used for patients transitioning back to permanent footwear following an ulceration, can be applied to the Texas Foot Risk Classification group 4, or more simply, those whose status is postamputation. Pressure relief remains critical and rocker bottom shoes are effective in limiting the transfer of weight anteriorly, but there are some unique complications associated with transmetatarsal amputations.

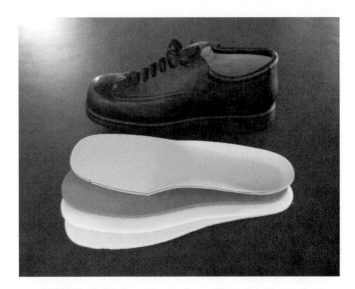

FIGURE 18-20 Extra depth shoe with removable insoles.

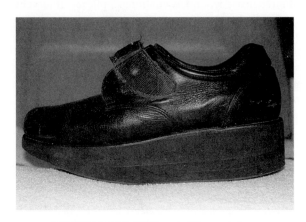

FIGURE 18-21 Rigid rocker bottom shoe.

Depending on the amputation site, the long extensors of the foot may be damaged or be put at a mechanical disadvantage relative to the intact plantar flexors which attach to the posterior heel. The result of this imbalance is an equinus deformity which increases pressure at the distal end of the foot. In a small study of 11 patients with great toe and partial metatarsal amputations, peak pressures were found to be significantly higher under the MTHs and remaining toes compared to the contralateral foot.[17] A second problem is proper shoe fit. A short shoe that is fit to the amputation, can reduce pressure on the distal foot, but also increases pressure on the contralateral foot; however, short shoes were not well received by patients because of cosmesis.[122] Appearance may seem trivial in relation to preventing the recurrence of an ulcer, but it is naïve to overlook appearance. If shoes are disliked so much that they are not worn, they serve no purpose at all. Along the same line of reasoning, patients need to be educated about the importance of not only wearing their shoes while outside, but also in the house where shoes are frequently removed.[123] If this is not feasible, some other form of offloading, such as a customized sandal may be helpful to increase compliance with offloading. Conversely, a full-length shoe is more cosmetically pleasing, but may increase shear forces as a result of the foot sliding forward in the shoe. When a full-length shoe is combined with a rigid rocker bottom and a custom-molded insert, pressures at the forefoot of both the involved and contralateral foot were reduced compared to a regular shoe with a toe filler.[122] Following a 1-month adjustment period, patients wearing this combination also had faster walking speeds and physical performance test scores compared to patients in regular footwear with a toe filler.[124] Based on these findings, the best option for those in risk category 4 is a full-length, rigid rocker bottom shoe, with a custom-molded insole.

SUMMARY

The largest group of people with high-risk feet in the United States is the population of individuals with diabetes. With an ever-increasing number of individuals diagnosed with diabetes, it is important that the clinician be able to identify risk factors so as to reduce future complications. This chapter reviewed the assessment of the high-risk foot as well as a comprehensive wound evaluation. Applicable interventions were provided and organized according to the treatment goal to assist with the development of a successful treatment plan. Finally, footwear recommendations based on risk stratification were discussed to ensure that clients are given the best chance to return to their activities without ulcer formation or recurrence.

REFERENCES

1. American Diabetes Association. *American Diabetes Association home page*. Available at: http://www.diabetes.org/diabetes-basics/diabetes-statistics. Accessed 10.08.11.
2. Pietrzak WS, Eppley BL. Platelet rich plasma: Biology and new technology. *J Craniofac Surg.* 2005;16(6):1043–1054.
3. Centers for Disease Control and Prevention. *National diabetes fact sheet: national estimates and general information on diabetes and prediabetes in the United States, 2011. from 2011 National Diabetes Fact Sheet*. Available at: http://www.cdc.gov/diabetes/pubs/pdf/ndfs_2011.pdf. Accessed 28.02.11.
4. Collins TC, Suarez-Almazor M, Peterson NJ. An absent pulse is not sensitive for the early detection of peripheral arterial disease. *Fam Med.* 2006;38(1):38–42.
5. Bonham PA. Get the LEAD out: noninvasive assessment for lower extremity arterial disease using ankle brachial index and toe brachial index measurements. *J Wound Ostomy Continence Nurs.* 2006;33(1):30–41.
6. McMahon JH, Grigg MJ. Predicting healing of lower limb ulcers. *Aust N Z J Surg.* 1995;65(3):173–176.
7. American Diabetes Association. Consensus development conference on diabetic foot wound care. *Diabetes Care.* 1999;22(8):1354–1360.
8. Steeper RA. A critical review of the aetiology of diabetic neuropathic ulcers. *J Wound Care.* 2005;14(3):101–103.
9. Oyer DS, Saxon D, Shah A. Quantitative assessment of diabetic peripheral neuropathy with use of the clanging tuning fork test. *Endocr Pract.* 2007;13(1):5–10.
10. Juma A, Mandal A. Vibration sensitivity testing with tuning fork—256 Hz or 512 Hz? *Eur J Plast Surg.* 2007;30:5–6.
11. Caselli A, Pham H, Giurini J, et al. The forefoot-to-rearfoot plantar pressure ratio is increased in severe diabetic neuropathy and can predict foot ulcerations. *Diabetes Care.* 2002;25(6):1066–1071.
12. Mueller MJ, Hastings M, Commean PK, et al. Forefoot structural predictors of plantar pressures during walking in people with diabetes and peripheral neuropathy. *J Biomech.* 2003;36(7):1009–1017.
13. Anderson H, Gjerstad MD, Jakobsen J. Atrophy of foot muscles: a measure of diabetic neuropathy. *Diabetes Care.* 2004;27(10):2382–2385.
14. van Schie C, Vermigli C, Carrington A, et al. Muscle weakness and foot deformities in diabetes: Relationship to neuropathy and foot ulceration in Caucasian diabetic men. *Diabetes Care.* 2004;27(7):1668–1673.
15. Laing P. The development and complications of diabetic foot ulcers. *Am J Surg.* 1998;176(2A suppl):11S–19S.
16. Quebedeau TL, Lavery LA, Lavery DC. The development of foot deformities and ulcers after great toe amputation in diabetes. *Diabetes Care.* 1996;19(2):165–167.
17. Lavery LA, Lavery DC, Quebedeau-Farham TL. Increased foot pressures after great toe amputation in diabetes. *Diabetes Care.* 1995;18(11):1460–1462.
18. Boulton AJ, Hardesty CA, Betts RP, et al. Dynamic foot pressures and other studies as diagnostic and management aids in diabetic neuropathy. *Diabetes Care.* 1983;6(1):26–33.
19. Veves A, Murray HJ, Young MJ, et al. The risk of foot ulceration in diabetic patients with hight foot pressure: a prospective study. *Diabetologia.* 1992;35(7):660–663.
20. Birke JA, Paout CA, Foto JG. Factors associated with ulceration and amputation in the neuropathic foot. *J Orthop Sports Phys Ther.* 2000;30(2):91–97.
21. Kastenbauer T, Sauseng S, Sokol G, et al. A prospective study of predictors for foot ulceration in type 2 diabetes. *J Am Podiatr Med Assoc.* 2001;91(7):343–350.
22. Brand PW. The diabetic foot. In: Ellenberg M, Rifkin H, eds. *Diabetes Mellitus: Theory and Practice.* 3rd ed. New Hyde Park, NY: Medical Examination; 1983:829–849.

23. Delbridge L, Perry P, Marr S, et al. Limited joint mobility in the diabetic foot: relationship to neuropathic ulceration. *Diabet Med.* 1988;5(4):333–337.

24. Mueller MJ, Diamond JE, Delitto A. Insensitivity, limited joint mobility, and plantar ulcers in patients with diabetes mellitus. *Phys Ther.* 1989;69(6):453–459.

25. Birke JA, Cornwall MW, Jackson M. Relationship between hallux limitus and ulceration of the great toe. *J Orthop Sports Phys Ther.* 1988;10(5):172–176.

26. Fernando DJS, Masson EA, Veves A, et al. Relationship of limited joint mobility to abnormal foot pressures and diabetic foot ulceration. *Diabetes Care.* 1991;14(1):8–11.

27. Birke JA, Franks BD, Foto JG. First ray joint limitation, pressure and ulceration of the first metatarsal head in diabetes mellitus. *Foot Ankle Int.* 1995;16(5):277–284.

28. Mueller MJ, Minor SD, Diamond JE, et al. Relationship of foot deformity to ulcer location in patients with diabetes mellitus. *Phys Ther.* 1990;70(6):356–362.

29. Robertson DD, Mueller MJ, Smith KE, et al. Structural changes in the forefoot of individuals with diabetes and prior plantar ulcer. *J Bone Joint Surg Am.* 2002;84A(8):1395–1404.

30. Lavery LA, Armstrong DG, Vela SA. Practical criteria for screening patients at high risk for diabetic ulceration. *Arch Intern Med.* 1998;158(2):157–162.

31. Kosiak M. Etiology and pathology of ischemic ulcers. *Arch Phys Med Rehabil.* 1959;40(2):62–69.

32. Brand PW. Repetetive stress in the development of diabetic foot ulcers. In: Levin MO, ed. *The Diabetic Foot.* 4th ed. St. Louis: Mosby; 1998:83–90.

33. Armstrong DG, Lavery LA. Elevated peak plantar pressures in patients who have Charcot arthropathy. *J Bone Joint Surg.* 1998;80A(3):365–369.

34. Banks AS, McGlamry ED. Charcot foot. *J Am Podiatr Med Assoc.* 1989;79(5):213–235.

35. Frykberg RG, Zgonis T, Armstrong DG, et al. Diabetic foot disorders: a clinical practice guideline (2006 Revision). *J Foot Ankle Surg.* 2006;45(5 suppl):S1–S66.

36. Buttke J. Stepping up foot injury diagnosis: Jones, Lisfranc, and Charcot. *Nurse Pract.* 2005;30(12):46–52.

37. Rajbhandari SM, Jenkins RC, Davies C, et al. Charcot neuroarthropathy in diabetes mellitus. *Diabetologia.* 2002;45(8):1085–1096.

38. Chantelau E, Onlyee G. Charcot foot in diabetes: farewell to the neurotrophic theory. *Horm Metab Res.* 2006;38(6):361–367.

39. Strauss E, Gonya G. Adjunct low intensity ultrasound in Charcot neuroarthropathy. *Clin Orthop Relat Res.* 1998;349:132–138.

40. Chantelau E, Richter A, Schmidt-Grigordiadis P, et al. The diabetic Charcot foot: MRI discloses bone stress injury as trigger mechanism of neuroarthropathy. *Exp Clin Endocrinol Diabetes.* 1997;114(3):118–123.

41. Boninger ML, Leonard JA. Use of bivalved ankle-foot orthosis in neuropathic foot and ankle lesions. *J Rehabil Res Dev.* 1996;33(1):16–22.

42. Morgan JM, Biehl WC, Wagner FW. Management of neuropathic arthropathy with the Charcot restraint orthotic walker. *Clin Orthop Relat Res.* 1993;296:58–63.

43. Sammarco GJ, Conti SF. Surgical treatment of neuroarthropathic foot deformity. *Foot Ankle Int.* 1998;19(2):102–109.

44. Early JS, Hansen ST. Surgical reconstruction of the diabetic foot: A salvage approach for midfoot collapse. *Foot Ankle Int.* 1996;17(6):325–330.

45. Frykberg RG, Mendeszoon E. Management of the diabetic Charcot foot. *Diabetes Metab Res Rev.* 2000;16(suppl 1):S59–S65.

46. Cavanagh PR, Derr JA, Ulbrecht JS, et al. Problems with gait and posture in neuropathic patients with insulin-dependent diabetes mellitus. *Diabet Med.* 1992;9(5):469–474.

47. Cavanagh PR, Simoneau GG, Ulbrecht JS. Ulceration, unsteadiness, and uncertainty: the biomechanical consequences of diabetes mellitus. *J Biomech.* 1993;26(suppl 1):23–40.

48. Simoneau GG, Ulbrecht JS, Derr JA, et al. Postural instability in patients with diabetic sensory neuropathy. *Diabetes Care.* 1994;17(12):1411–1421.

49. Uccioli L, Giacomini PG, Monticone G, et al. Body sway in diabetic neuropathy. *Diabetes Care.* 1995;18(3):339–344.

50. Courtemanche R, Teasdale N, Boucher P, et al. Gait problems in diabetic neuropathic patients. *Arch Phys Med Rehabil.* 1996;77(9):849–855.

51. Birke JA, Sims DS. Plantar sensory threshold in the insensitive foot. *Lepr Rev.* 1986;57(3):261.

52. Krasner D. Wound care: how to use the red-yellow-black system. *Am J Nurs.* 1995;5:44–47.

53. Bowler PG, Davies BJ, Jones SA. Microbial involvement in chronic wound malodour. *J Wound Care.* 1999;8:216–218.

54. Abouaesha F, Carine HM, Gareth D, et al. Plantar tissue thickness is related to peak plantar pressure in the high-risk diabetic foot. *Diabetes Care.* 2001;24(7):1270–1274.

55. Bus SA, Yang QX, Wang JH, et al. Intrinsic muscle atrophy and toe deformity in the diabetic neuropathic foot: A magnetic resonance imaging study. *Diabetes Care.* 2002;25(8):1444–1450.

56. Greenman RL, Khoadhiar L, Lima C, et al. Foot small muscle atrophy is present before the detection of clinical neuropathy. *Diabetes Care.* 2005;28(6):1425–1430.

57. Gooding GAW, Stess RM, Graf PM, et al. Sonography of the sole of the foot: Evidence for loss of foot pad thickness in diabetes and its relationship to ulceration of the foot. *Invest Radiol.* 1986;21(1):45–48.

58. White RJ, Cutting KF. Critical colonization—the concept under scrutiny. *Ostomy Wound Manage.* 2006;52(11):50–56.

59. Rodeheaver GT, Pettry D, Thacker JG, et al. Wound cleansing by high pressure irrigation. *Surg Gynecol Obstet.* 1975;141(3):357–362.

60. Svoboda SJ, Bice TG, Gooden HA, et al. Comparison of bulb syringe and pulsed lavage irrigation with use of a bioluminescent musculoskeletal wound model. *J Bone Joint Surg.* 2006;88:2167–2174.

61. Bergstrom N, Allman R, Alvarez O, et al. *Treatment of Pressure Ulcers. Clinical Practice Guideline. Quick Reference Guide for Clinicians.* No. 15. Publication No. 95–0652. Rockville, MD: U.S. Department of Health and Human Services, Public Health Services, Agency for Health Care Policy and Research; 1994.

62. Loehne H. Wound debridement and irrigation. In: Kloth LC, McCulloch JM, eds. *Wound Healing Alternatives in Management.* 3rd ed. Philadelphia: Davis; 2002:220.

63. Morykwas MJ, Argenta LC, Shelton-Brown EI. Vacuum-assisted closure: a new method for wound control and treatment: Animal studies and basic foundation. *Ann Plast Surg.* 1997;38(6):553–562.

64. Suchkova V, Siddiqi FN, Carstensen EL, et al. Enhancement of fibrinolysis with 40 kHz ultrasound. *Circulation.* 1998;98:1030–1035.

65. Suchkova V, Carstensen EL, Francis CW. Ultrasound enhancement of fibrinolysis at frequencies of 27 to 100 kHz. *Ultrasound Med Biol.* 2002;28:377–382.

66. Kloth LC, Niezgoda JA. Ultrasound for wound debridement and healing. In: McCulloch JM, Kloth LC, eds. *Wound Healing Evidence-Based Management.* 4th ed. Philadelphia: Davis; 2010:545–575.

67. Schoenbach SF, Song IC. Ultrasonic debridement: a new approach in the treatment of burn wounds. *Plast Reconstr Surg.* 1980;66:34–37.

68. Nichter LS, McDonald S, Gabriel K, et al. Efficacy of debridement and primary closure of contaminated wounds: a comparison of methods. *Ann Plast Surg.* 1989;23(3):224–230.

69. Connor-Kerr T, Alston G, Stovall A, et al. The effects of low-frequency ultrasound (35kHz) on methicillin-resistant *Staphylococcus aureus* (MRSA) in vitro. *Ostomy Wound Manage.* 2010;56(5):32–42.

70. Stanisic MM, Provo BJ, Larsen DL, et al. Wound debridement with 25 kHz ultrasound. *Adv Skin Wound Care.* 2005;18:484–490.

71. U.S. Food and Drug Administration. *Questions and Answers about FDA's Enforcement Action Regarding Unapproved Topical Drug Products Containing Papain.* Available at: http://www.fda.gov/Drugs/GuidanceComplianceRegulatoryInformation/EnforcementActivitiesbyFDA/SelectedEnforcementActionson UnapprovedDrugs/ucm119646.htm; 2009 Accessed 30.07.11.

72. Ovington LG. The truth about silver. *Ostomy Wound Manage.* 2004;50(9A suppl):1S–10S.

73. Ovington LG. Dressings and skin substitutes. In: McCulloch JM, Kloth LC, eds. *Wound Healing Evidence-Based Management.* 4th ed. Philadelphia: Davis; 2010:180–195.

74. Kloth LC. Electrical stimulation for wound healing: A review of evidence from in vitro studies, animal experiments, and clinical trials. *Int J Low Extrem Wounds.* 2005;4(1):23–44.

75. Sterenborg H, van der Putte SC, van der Leun JC. The dose response relationship of tumorigenesis by ultraviolet radiation of 254nm. *Photochem Photobiol Sci.* 1988;47(2):245–253.

76. Connor-Kerr TA, Sullivan PK, Keegan DS, et al. UVC reduces antibiotic-resistant bacterial numbers in living tissue. *Ostomy Wound Manage.* 1999;45(4):84.

77. Connor-Kerr TA, Sullivan PK, Gaillaird J, et al. The effects of ultraviolet radiation on antibiotic-resistant bacteria in vitro. *Ostomy Wound Manage.* 1998;44(10):50–56.

78. Thai TP, Keast DH, Campbell KE. Effects of ultraviolet light C on bacterial colonization in chronic wounds. *Ostomy Wound Manage.* 2005;51(10):32–45.

79. Thai TP, Houghton PE, Keast DH. Ultraviolet light C in the treatment of chronic wounds with MRSA: a case study. *Ostomy Wound Manage.* 2002;48(11):52–60.

80. Bellew J. Clinical electrical stimulation: Application and techniques. In: Michlovitz SL, Bellew JW, Nolan TP, eds. *Modalities for Therapeutic Intervention.* 5th ed. Philadelphia: Davis; 2011:241–277.

81. Mahoney E. Therapeutic modalities for tissue healing. In: Michlovitz SL, Bellew JW, Nolan TP, eds. *Modalities for Therapeutic Interventions.* 5th ed. Philadelphia: Davis; 2011:361–385.

82. McCulloch JM, Kloth LC, eds. *Wound Healing: Evidence-Based Management.* 4th ed. Philadelphia: Davis; 2010.

83. Coleman WC, Brand PW, Birke JA. The total contact cast: a therapy for plantar ulceration on insensitive feet. *J Am Podiatr Med Assoc.* 1984;74(11):548–552.

84. Pollard JP, LeQuesne LP, Tappin JW. Forces under the foot. *J Biomed Eng.* 1983;5(1):37–40.

85. Birke JA, Sims DS, Buford WL. Walking casts: effect on plantar foot pressures. *J Rehabil Res Dev.* 1985;22(3):18–22.

86. Helm PA, Walker SC, Pullum G. Total contact casting in diabetic patients with neuropathic ulcerations. *Arch Phys Med Rehabil.* 1984;65(11):691–693.

87. Sinacore DR, Mueller MJ, Diamond JE, et al. Diabetic neuropathic plantar ulcers treated by total contact casting. *Phys Ther.* 1987;67(10):1543–1549.

88. Armstrong DG, Nguyen HC, Lavery LA, et al. Offloading the diabetic foot wound: a randomized clinical trial. *Diabetes Care.* 2001;24(6):1019–1022.

89. Fleischli JG, Lavery LA, Vela SL, et al. Comparison of strategies for reducing pressure at the site of neuropathic ulcers. *J Am Podiatr Med Assoc.* 1997;87(10):466–472.

90. Petre M, Tokar P, Kostar D. Revisiting the total contact cast: maximizing off-loading by wound isolation. *Diabetes Care.* 2005;28(4):929–930.

91. Lavery LA, Vela SA, Lavery DC, et al. Reducing dynamic foot pressures in high-risk diabetic subjects with foot ulcerations. *Diabetes Care.* 1996;19(8):818–821.

92. Beuker BJ, van Deursen RW, Price P. Plantar pressure in off-loading devices used in diabetic ulcer treatment. *Wound Repair Regen.* 2005;13(6):537–542.

93. McGuire JB. Pressure redistribution strategies for the diabetic or at-risk foot: part II. *Adv Skin Wound Care.* 2006;19(5):270–277.

94. Mueller MJ, Diamond JE, Sinacore DR, et al. Diabetic plantar ulcers treated by total contact casting. *Phys Ther.* 1987;67:1543–1547.

95. Katz IA, Harlan A, Miranda-Palma B, et al. A randomized trial of two irremovable offloading devices in the management of plantar neuropathic diabetic foot ulcerations. *Diabetes Care.* 2005;28(3):555–559.

96. Armstrong DG, Lavery LA, Wu S, et al. Evaluation of removable and irremovable cast walkers in the healing of diabetic foot wounds: a randomized controlled trial. *Diabetes Care.* 2005;28(3):551–554.

97. Birke J, Lewis K, Penton A, et al. The effectiveness of a modified wedge shoe in reducing pressure at the area of previous great toe ulceration in individuals with diabetes mellitus. *Wounds.* 2004;16(4):109–114.

98. Birke JA, Sims DS. The insensate foot. In: Hunt G, ed. *Physical Therapy of the Foot and Ankle.* New York: Churchill; 1998:133–168.

99. Zimny S, Meyer MF, Schatz H, et al. Applied felted foam for plantar pressure relief is an efficient therapy in neuropathic diabetic foot ulcers. *Exp Clin Endocrinol Diabetes.* 2002;110(7):325–328.

100. Zimny S, Reinsch B, Schatz H, et al. Effects of felted foam on plantar pressures in the treatment of neuropathic diabetic foot ulcers. *Diabetes Care.* 2001;24(12):2153–2154.

101. Zimny S, Schatz H, Pfohl U. The effects of applied felted foam on wound healing and healing times in the therapy of neuropathic diabetic foot ulcers. *Diabet Med.* 2003;20(8):622–625.

102. Ritz G, Kushner D, Friedman S. A successful technique for the treatment of diabetic neuropathic ulcers. *J Am Podiatr Med Assoc.* 1992;82(9):479–481.

103. Birke JA, Pavich MA, Patout CA, et al. Comparison of forefoot ulcer healing using alternative off-loading methods in patients with diabetes mellitus. *Adv Skin Wound Care.* 2002;15(5):210–215.

104. Rader AJ, Barry TP. The football: an intuitive dressing for offloading neuropathic plantar forefoot ulcerations. *Int Wound J.* 2008;5(1):69–73.

105. McGuire J. Transitional off-loading: An evidence-based approach to pressure redistribution in the diabetic foot. *Adv Skin Wound Care.* 2010;23(4):175–188.

106. Peters EJ, Lavery LA. Effectiveness of the diabetic foot risk classification system of the international working group on the diabetic foot. *Diabetes Care.* 2001;24(8):1442–1447.

107. Lavery LA, Peters EJ, Williams JR, et al. Reevaluating the way we classify the diabetic foot: Restructuring the diabetic foot risk classification system of the International Working Group on the Diabetic Foot. *Diabetes Care.* 2008;31(1):154–156.

108. Perry JE, Ulbrecht JS, Derr JS, et al. The use of running shoes to reduce plantar pressure in patients who have diabetes. *J Bone Joint Surg Am.* 1995;7(12):1819–1928.

109. Lavery LA, Vela BS, Fleischli JG, et al. Reducing pressure in the neuropathic foot: a comparison of footwear. *Diabetes Care.* 1997;20(11):1706–1710.

110. Kastenbauer T, Sokol G, Auinger M. Running shoes for relief of plantar pressure in diabetic patients. *Diabet Med.* 1998;15(6):518–522.

111. Bus SA, Ulbrecht JS, Cavanagh PR. Pressure relief and load redistribution by custom-made insoles in patients with neuropathy and foot deformity. *Clin Biomech (Bristol, Avon).* 2004;19(6):629–638.

112. Foto JG, Birke JA. Evaluation of multidensity orthotic materials used in footwear for patients with diabetes. *Foot Ankle Int.* 1998;19(12):836–841.

113. Brodsky JW, Kourosh S, Stills M, et al. Objective evaluation of insert material for diabetic and athletic footwear. *Foot Ankle.* 1988;9(3):111–116.

114. Edmonds ME, Blundell MP, Morris ME, et al. Improved survival of the diabetic foot: the role of the specialized foot clinic. *Q J Med.* 1986;60(232):763–771.

115. Uccioli L, Faglia E, Monticone G, et al. Manufactured shoes in the prevention of diabetic foot ulcers. *Diabetes Care.* 1995;18(10):1376–1378.

116. Hsi WL, Chai HM, Lai JS. Comparison of pressure and time parameters in evaluating diabetic footwear. *Am J Phys Med Rehabil.* 2002;81(11):822–829.

117. Cavanagh PR. Therapeutic footwear for people with diabetes. *Diabetes Metab Res Rev.* 2004;20(suppl 1):S51–S55.

118. Chantelau E, Kushner T, Spraul M. Effect of therapeutic shoes on the diabetic foot syndrome: a two year follow up [abstract]. *Diabetes.* 1989;38:139A.

119. Chantelau E, Kushner T, Spraul M. How effective is cushioned therapeutic footwear in protecting diabetic feet? A clinical study. *Diabet Med.* 1990;7(4):355–359.

120. Busch K, Chantelau E. Effectiveness of a new brand of stock "diabetic" shoes to protect against diabetic foot ulcer relapse. A prospective cohort study. *Diabet Med.* 2003;20(8):665–669.

121. Van Schie C, Ulbrecht JS, Becker MB, et al. Design criteria for rigid rocker shoes. *Foot Ankle Int.* 2000;21(10):833–844.

122. Mueller MJ, Strube MJ, Allen BT. Therapeutic footwear can reduce plantar pressures in patients with diabetes and transmetatarsal amputation. *Diabetes Care.* 1997;20(4):637–641.

123. Armstrong DG, Abu-Rumman PL, Nixon BP, et al. Continuous activity monitoring in persons at high risk for diabetes-related lower-extremity amputation. *J Am Podiatr Med Assoc.* 2001;91(9):451–455.

124. Mueller MJ, Strube MJ. Therapeutic footwear: enhanced function in people with diabetes and transmetatarsal amputation. *Arch Phys Med Rehabil.* 1997;78(9):952–956.

125. Albaugh K, Loehne H. Wound bed preparation/debridement. In: McCulloch JM, Kloth LC, eds. *Wound Healing: Evidence-Based Management.* 4th ed. Philadelphia: Davis; 2010:155–179.

126. Kirshen C, Woo K, Ayello AE, et al. Debridement: a vital component of wound bed preparation. *Adv Skin Wound Care.* 2006;19(9):506–517.

127. Schultz GS, Sibbald R, Falanga V, et al. Wound bed preparation: A systematic approach to wound management. *Wound Repair Regen.* 2003;11(suppl 1):S1–S28.

128. Lavery LA, Armstrong DG, Harkless LB. Classification of diabetic foot wounds. *Ostomy Wound Manage.* 1997; 43(2):44–53.

129. Armstrong DG, Lavery LA, Harkless LB. Validation of a diabetic wound classification system: the contribution of depth, infection, and ischemia to risk of amputation. *Diabetes Care.* 1998;21:855–859.

130. Sittig K, Richardson K. Acute burn management. In: McCulloch JM, Kloth LC, eds. *Wound Healing: Evidence-Based Management.* 4th ed. Philadelphia: Davis; 2010:334–335.

131. National Pressure Ulcer Advisory Panel. *Updated staging system: pressure ulcer stages revised by NPUAP, 2007.* Available at: http://www.npuap.org/pr2.htm. Accessed 16.05.11.

132. Murray HJ, Young MJ, Hollis S. The association between callus formation, high pressure and neuropathy in diabetic foot ulceration. *Diabet Med.* 1996;13(11):979–982.

133. Young MJ, Cavanagh PR, Thomas G, et al. The effect of callus removal on dynamic plantar foot pressures in diabetic patients. *Diabet Med.* 1992;9(1):55–57.

134. Robinson A. Electrical stimulation to augment healing of chronic wounds. In: Robinson AJ, Snyder-Mackler L, eds. *Clinical Electrophysiology: Electrotherapy and Electrophysiologic Testing.* 3rd ed. Philadelphia: Lippincott Williams & Wilkins; 2008:275–299.

135. McCulloch JM. Compression therapy. In: McCulloch JM, Kloth LC, eds. *Wound Healing: Evidence-Based Management.* 4th ed. Philadelphia: Davis; 2010:594–601.

136. McCallon SK. Negative-pressure wound therapy. In: McCulloch JM, Kloth LC, eds. *Wound Healing: Evidence-Based Management.* Philadelphia: Davis; 2010:602–620.

137. Bollero D, Driver V, Glat P, et al. The role of negative pressure wound therapy in the spectrum of wound healing: A guidelines document. *Ostomy Wound Manage.* 2010;56(5 suppl):1–18.

138. Agency for Healthcare Research and Quality. *Negative pressure wound therapy devices: technology assessment report.* Available at: http://www.ahrq.gov/clinic/ta/negpresswtd/. Accessed 17.08.11.

139. Connor-Kerr TA. Light therapies. In: McCulloch JM, Kloth LC, eds. *Wound Healing: Evidence-Based Management.* Philadelphia: Davis; 2010:576–593.

19

Amputation Surgeries for the Lower Limb

MICHELLE M. LUSARDI AND JUDITH L. PEPE

LEARNING OBJECTIVES

On completion of this chapter, the reader will be able to do the following:

1. Compare and contrast the assessments typically used to determine the need for, and optimal level of, amputation surgery for individuals with dysvascular/neuropathic disease, trauma, neoplasm, or congenital limb deficiency.
2. Describe key perioperative concerns and issues for individuals facing lower-limb amputation (e.g., complications, hydration/nutrition, pain management, respiratory status, concurrent medical issues for each etiology of amputation).
3. Provide an overview of the most commonly used surgical approaches for each level of amputation (including myodesis, drain position, tissue manipulation, and surgical closures).
4. Apply understanding of biomechanics of surgical approaches and tissue healing to the care of new and maturing residual limbs.

WHEN IS AMPUTATION NECESSARY?

The amputation of a limb is a truly life-altering event, affecting the physical, functional, and psychological dimensions of a person's world.[1] The decision to amputate a limb is not made lightly; amputation is performed as a lifesaving measure for those affected by severe trauma,[2] infection,[3] peripheral arterial disease,[4] and certain cases of osteosarcoma.[5] Amputation can be incredibly life improving when burdensome care of a vulnerable neuropathic or painful dysvascular foot is no longer necessary.[6] Unexpected traumatic amputations, especially in younger active individuals, can contribute to significant depression in the postoperative and rehabilitation periods.[7]

Although surgical technique is one of the key determinants in the success of amputation,[8] other factors that are as important include the individual's and family's understanding and acceptance that amputation is the best option of care[9]; effective attention to and management of comorbidities during the perioperative period, as well as avoidance of postoperative complications such as pneumonia and wound infection[10,11]; and a promptly implemented rehabilitation plan

that the individual, family, surgical team, and rehabilitation team have developed and agreed on.[12]

This chapter provides an overview of the strategies used to determine if amputation is necessary for individuals with dysvascular/neuropathic disease, for those who have sustained significant trauma to their lower limbs, for those with diagnoses of bone or soft-tissue neoplasm, and for children who are growing up with congenital limb deficiency. We then describe the surgical techniques used in the most commonly performed lower-extremity amputation and discuss the rehabilitation implications for each. The goal is to help rehabilitation professionals understand what has happened to soft tissue and bone during surgery and to use this knowledge to better incorporate principles of wound healing and maturation into the preprosthetic and prosthetic care of those who have undergone amputation.

Basic Principles

The decision to amputate a limb, whether related to critical limb ischemia, infection of a neuropathic wound, trauma, or neoplasm, is based on careful consideration of prognosis for survival and for successful rehabilitation. Determination of the appropriate level of amputation is guided by two principles. The first is that there must be adequate circulation to ensure successful healing of the incision and surgical construct.[13] In addition to a physical examination (evaluation of peripheral pulses, skin color, skin condition, and skin temperature), surgeons consider the individual's ankle-brachial index,[14] results of transcutaneous oximetry,[15] and vascular studies such as magnetic resonance arteriography.[16] The second principle is to preserve as many anatomical joints as possible; having an intact anatomical knee joint typically leads to better functional outcome.[14]

At times, tension occurs between these principles. For individuals with plantar neuropathic ulcers and osteomyelitis, for example, a transmetatarsal amputation has the potential to preserve the ankle joint and permit functional gait without prosthesis and is often less difficult for individuals to accept psychologically.[17] If there is delayed or failed healing, however, the risks of complications associated with limited activity and bed rest (e.g., further deconditioning, pneumonia, deep venous thrombosis, decubitus ulcer) and repeated anesthesia if surgical revisions to more proximal levels become necessary can be significant.[18] In these instances an initial surgery at the transtibial level might improve the chances for optimal rehabilitation outcome.[19]

In individuals with traumatic crush injury to the proximal tibia but intact knee joint, an extremely short transtibial residual limb may actually be more difficult to manage prosthetically than a long transfemoral residual limb: the reduced surface area around a short residual tibia and fibula for weight bearing within the socket increases pressure on skin and soft tissue of the residual limb, reducing functional wearing time of the prosthesis despite the advantage of preservation of the anatomical knee joint.[20]

Dysvascular and Neuropathic Disease

The overall prevalence of peripheral arterial disease (PAD) in the United States, across all ethnicities, is estimated to range from approximately 2% in persons 40 to 49 years of age to 20% or higher in persons older than age 80 years.[21] Rates of PAD vary by ethnicity and gender, however; African-American men demonstrate two- to threefold greater rates than white men, whereas women demonstrate lower rates than men of their ethnicity (Table 19-1).[21,22] Likelihood of amputation increases with the number of risk factors for PAD an individual has. Risk factors include history of smoking (especially if currently smoking); untreated or poorly managed hypercholesteremia; untreated or poorly managed hypertension, obesity (body mass index >30); diabetes mellitus, kidney dysfunction (glomerular filtration rate <60 mL/min), and chronic inflammatory response (elevated high-sensitivity C-reactive protein >30 mg/L).[23] Significant morbidity and mortality is associated with PAD: It is estimated that one in four individuals with PAD undergoes some form of amputation, one in three will likely die within 5 years of diagnosis, and only one in four will survive more than 10 years after diagnosis.[24,25] Comorbid

conditions that amplify risk of death in the year following PAD-related amputation include congestive heart failure, renal failure, and liver disease, as well as postoperative systemic sepsis.[26] PAD is a significant health care issue, impacting not only on the quality of an individual's life, but also on ever-increasing health care costs.[27,28]

There are three reasons an individual might require revascularization or amputation of the lower limb because of underlying disease processes: (1) they have significant, often acute, occlusive atherosclerotic vascular disease but without neuropathy or diabetes; (2) they are without significant vascular disease but have neuropathy-related wounds that may lead to osteomyelitis; and (3) they have diabetes with a combination of vascular disease and sensory, motor, and autonomic neuropathy.[29,30] The management and prognosis for each of these groups are somewhat different. Vascular bypass surgery,[31] percutaneous endovascular stents,[32] or the use of thrombolytic intervention[33] may preserve the limbs of those with large-vessel vascular disease without neuropathy. Recent reports suggest that intramuscular injection of autologous bone marrow cells may decrease risk of amputation in persons with chronic limb ischemia who are not candidates for surgical revascularization, or when such surgeries are unsuccessful.[34,35] Persons with a combination of diabetes and vascular disease are the most likely to require amputation; advanced age and multiple comorbidities (e.g., cardiovascular and cerebrovascular disease, kidney disease, and visual impairment) provide additional challenges for healing, early mobility after amputation, and the prosthetic rehabilitation process.

Conservative management with total contact casting or felted foam may be sufficient to heal a neuropathic ulcer (when there are no indications of osteomyelitis), and accommodative orthoses and protective footwear may protect the plantar surface of the foot in those with a healing neuropathic wound.[36] Hyperbaric oxygen therapy and negative-pressure

TABLE 19-1 *Prevalence of Peripheral Arterial Disease by Age and Gender*

Gender	Ethnicity	Age Category, % (CI)				
		40-49	50-59	60-69	70-79	≥ 80
Male	NHW	1.4 (0.3-2.5)	1.9 (0.9-2.9)	5.4 (3.9-6.9)	9.2 (7.9-10.5)	22.6 (18.6-26.3)
	AA	1.2 (0.0-2.5)	5.0 (2.6-7.3)	13.2 (10.0-16.3)	24.4 (20.3-28.6)	59.0 (45.6-68.6)
	HS	0.2 (−0.4-0.8)	3.4 (1.3-5.4)	4.3 (2.1-6.5)	9.6 (6.0-13.2)	22.5 (9.4-34.5)
	AS	1.2 (−1.1-3.5)	0.9 (−0.6-2.3)	3.5 (0.7-6.4)	9.8 (8.7-11.0)	21.5 (18.8-24.0)
	AI	2.6 (1.3-4.0)	4.5 (2.9-6.1)	6.1 (3.8-8.4)	11.7 (5.5-17.8)	28.7 (24.2-32.6)*
Female	NHW	1.9 (0.7-3.2)	4.3 (2.9-5.7)	5.1 (3.7-6.4)	7.9 (6.9-9.0)	18.2 (15.2-21.2)
	AA	3.0 (1.2-4.7)	3.4 (1.7-5.1)	8.9 (6.6-11.1)	20.0 (16.8-23.2)	35.1 (27.0-43.2)
	HS	0.3 (−0.3-1.0)	0.4 (−0.2-3.0)	3.1 (1.3-4.9)	6.9 (3.7-10.2)	18.2 (7.6-28.8)
	AS	0.0 (0.0-0.0)	1.4 (−0.2-3.0)	0.7 (−0.5-2.0)	7.9 (3.4-12.4)	18.2 (3.1-33.3)*
	AI	3.2 (1.9-4.5)	3.9 (2.7-5.1)	8.6 (6.4-10.8)	14.7 (9.5-19.9)	33.8 (30.1-37.4)*

AA, African-American; *AI*, American Indian; *AS*, Asian American; *CI*, confidence interval; *HS*, Hispanic, *NHW*, non-Hispanic white; *OTH*, other.
Results are presented as prevalence estimates (95% CI).
*Imputed.
From Allison MA, Ho E, Denenberg JO, et al. Ethnic-specific prevalence of peripheral arterial disease in the United States. *Am J Prev Med.* 2007;32(4):328-333; Table 2, p. 330.

wound therapy also have been investigated as strategies to close neuropathic wounds and reduce risk of limb amputation in persons with chronic limb ischemia and diabetes.[37,38] When neuropathic or vascular foot wounds become infected or osteomyelitis is evident, conservative management can be challenging, and amputation may be necessary.[39]

Because both vascular disease and neuropathic disease are typically symmetrical in distribution, individuals in all of these groups are at risk for compromise of both lower limbs. After amputation of one limb, careful monitoring of vascular status and skin condition and appropriate conservative care of the intact limb and foot are essential. This is especially true in the postoperative–preprosthetic period when there is single-limb ambulation with assistive devices, as well as in the months and years following initial amputation.[40,41]

For all of these individuals, clinical decision making must be informed by careful assessment of (a) vascular status to determine whether revascularization or amputation is warranted, (b) cardiovascular and cardiorespiratory function to determine the most appropriate type of anesthesia to use during surgery, and (c) cognitive and psychological status to assure proper perioperative and postoperative care and patient education.

The assessment of an individual with compromised peripheral circulation begins with a careful and detailed health history and review of risk factors, continues with physical examination and routine blood work, and is followed up by additional tests or measures as needed.[42,43] Cognitive and psychological status is initially assessed by interview and as part of the neurological examination and can be followed up by more formal testing if warranted. Vascular status is initially examined using noninvasive methods such as the ankle-brachial index (ABI); values less than 0.9 suggest PAD.[44] Any suspicion of vascular compromise should be further investigated using duplex ultrasound,[45] magnetic resonance arteriography (MRA),[46] or computed tomographic arteriography (CTA). The physician's differential diagnosis process focuses on determining which component of the circulatory system is involved (arterial, venous, or lymphatic), if it is an acute problem that requires immediate medical, pharmacological or surgical intervention (e.g., vascular bypass or amputation), or a chronic problem that necessitates conservative medical management (Table 19-2).

Vascular Pain

One of the most common symptoms of chronic arterial vascular insufficiency is *intermittent claudication*.[47] This vascular-related pain has been described as a deep aching, cramping, muscle fatigue, or tightness that develops during physical activity and dissipates with rest. Although most common in the posterior compartment (gastrocnemius and soleus) of the lower leg, claudication can occur in any muscle with compromised blood supply, including the muscles of the thigh and hip. Claudication is the result of accumulation of lactic acid as a byproduct of anaerobic metabolism during muscle contraction. Several strategies are used to classify severity of PAD and of intermittent claudication. In 1954, Fontaine first defined

TABLE 19-2 *Common Peripheral Vascular Disorders*

System	Acute Conditions	Chronic Conditions
Arterial	Arterial thrombosis Embolic occlusion Vasospastic disease (Raynaud)	Atherosclerosis obliterans Thromboangiitis obliterans Buerger disease Diabetic angiopathy
Venous	Venous thromboembolism	Varicose veins Chronic venous insufficiency
Lymphatic	Lymphangiitis	Primary lymphedema (congenital) Secondary lymphedema (acquired)

four stages of PAD on the basis of the presence and severity of clinical symptoms (Table 19-3).[48] In 2007, the Trans-Atlantic Inter-Societal Consensus Task Force published a classification system (TASC II) for intermittent claudication with recommendations for appropriate intervention (endovascular angioplasty with or without stent placement, versus open surgical endarterectomy or bypass graft) based on location, length, and severity of occlusion or stenosis obtained from imaging studies.[49] Severity of PAD can be quantified using treadmill testing at a constant 2 mph speed, beginning flat and continuing with 2% increase in grade every 2 minutes, noting time to onset of claudication and time to maximum claudication. Change in the total distance that an individual is able to walk (e.g., number of city blocks or actual measured distance) before onset of symptoms is an alternative means of tracking progression of arterial vascular impairment.[50] When an individual requires opiates to manage vascular pain while at rest, or if there are arterial ulcers with dry gangrene in the toes or foot, the individual is classified as having critical limb ischemia, and is at high risk of amputation if revascularization fails or cannot be undertaken.[51]

When there is an acute or sudden occlusion of an arterial vessel (such that collateral circulation has not had sufficient time to develop), a much different pattern of pain occurs. Instead of relief with rest, pain is constant and somewhat unrelenting; it may be accompanied by feelings of tingling, numbness, or coldness as peripheral nerves of the lower limb are affected by ischemia.[34] Although a limb with chronic arterial insufficiency demonstrates dependent rubor, the skin of an acutely compromised limb may be quite pale or blanched distal to the site of occlusion (Figure 19-1). Acute occlusion is often an emergent situation, requiring pharmacological or surgical intervention to restore blood flow to the limb, and often necessitates long-term anticoagulation.

Examination: Skin and Soft Tissue

Assessment begins with visual inspection of the lower extremity and feet, concentrating on skin condition, presence or absence of hair, and nail condition.[52] Open wounds,

TABLE 19-3 *Classification of Peripheral Arterial Disease Severity (Note: Ankle-Brachial Index <0.9 in All Categories)*

	Stage				
	I: Atherosclerosis without major clinical symptoms	IIA: Atherosclerosis with claudication	IIB: Atherosclerosis with claudication	III: Atherosclerosis with resting pain; critical limb ischemia	IV: Atherosclerosis with issue damage; critical limb ischemia
Findings	Atherosclerosis without major clinical symptoms	Atherosclerosis with claudication	Atherosclerosis with claudication	Atherosclerosis with resting pain; critical limb ischemia	Atherosclerosis with issue damage; critical limb ischemia
Prognosis	No immediate threat	Marginal threat Medical or surgical intervention	Immediate threat Revascularization to salvage	Irreversible damage to nerve Revascularization to salvage Moderate risk of amputation	Revascularization may not salvage limb High risk of amputation
Vascular exam	Normal to absent pedal pulse Bruits on auscultation Arterial and venous Doppler audible (arterial not triphasic) Diminished peak flow on plethysmography	Absent pedal pulses Bruits on auscultation Inaudible arterial Doppler; audible venous Doppler Diminished peak flow on plethysmography	Absent pedal pulse Inaudible arterial Doppler, audible venous Doppler Slight elevation blood viscosity, fibrinogen, and platelet function	Toe segmental pressure <30 mm Hg Ankle segmental pressure <50 mm Hg Diminished transcutaneous oxygen pressure Arterial and venous Dopplers inaudible	All findings markedly abnormal
Pain/claudication	Distal paresthesia	Pain when walking >200 m, relieved with rest	Walking <200 m, relieved with rest	Resting pain, especially at night (or with elevation of lower limbs), relieved with dependency of limbs	Resting pain, especially at night, requiring opioids for relief
Sensory loss	Minimal; adequate protective sensation of the entire foot	Some (toes) Diminished protective sensation distally	Moderate (toes and forefoot) Diminished to absent protective sensation	Marked sensory neuropathy, anesthetic to sensory testing	Anesthetic to sensory testing
Motor deficit	None	Intrinsic muscle weakness "Claw toes" develop	Moderate weakness of toe extensors, ankle dorsiflexion	Marked weakness of foot and ankle	Marked weakness of foot and ankle
Soft tissue	Intact skin Subjectively cold extremities	Hair loss on toes and forefoot "Thin" skin	Hair loss Poor wound bed if neuropathic ulcer present, healing unlikely	Trophic changes in nails Fragile skin, foot, and lower leg Nonhealing plantar neuropathic ulcers likely	Dry gangrenous wounds in nail beds and dorsum of foot; desiccation likely High-risk infection Nonhealing plantar neuropathic ulcers likely

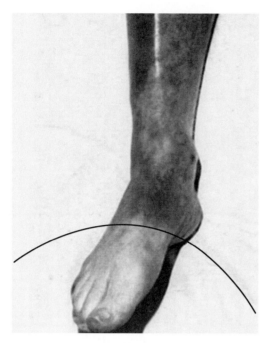

FIGURE 19-1 A chronically ischemic limb demonstrating rubor of dependency of the distal lower leg and rearfoot and significant pallor suggesting acute ischemia of the forefoot. (Courtesy Carolyn Kelly, Center for Wound Healing and Hyperbaric Medicine, Hartford Hospital, Hartford, Conn.)

callus, ecchymosis, dry necrosis and other skin lesions, as well as areas of erythema (redness), mottling, and altered pigmentation, are documented on a body chart. Circular wounds that lie under or are surrounded by callus on the plantar or weight-bearing surfaces of the foot are most likely neuropathic ulcers (Figure 19-2, *A*). Dry, blackened, or moist gangrenous wounds in the nail beds and between toes are likely signs of vascular insufficiency (Figure 19-2, *B*). Although

"healthy" traumatic wounds often display clear serosanguineous drainage, any thickened, yellowish, or foul-smelling discharge from a wound suggests soft tissue or bone infection.

Open wounds around ankles or a distal leg surrounded by areas of darkly pigmented skin are typically the result of chronic venous stasis. Progressive circumferential measurements are taken to document the presence of pitting or nonpitting edema resulting from venous or lymphatic insufficiency, localized infection, or as part of an underlying systemic disease of kidney, heart, or lung. Skin temperature is assessed subjectively (using the web space or back of the examiner's hand) or objectively using a surface thermometer. Cold areas in particular may have compromised arterial flow, while areas of increased temperature (especially if accompanied by erythema and swelling) often indicate underlying infection.[52]

In the presence of diabetic and other polyneuropathies there is often atrophy or wasting of the intrinsic muscles of the foot with apparent claw or hammer toe deformity.[53] Protective sensation (as measured by perception of Semmes-Weinstein 5.07 filament), as well as touch, pressure, vibration, and position sense, are likely to be impaired or inconsistent.[54] Additionally, impairment of the autonomic system often causes dry, tight, shining, easily cracked skin, as well as altered dynamics of blood flowing to the bones of the foot, increasing risk of Charcot arthopathy.[55,56]

Vascular Examination: Noninvasive Strategies

The least invasive and simplest strategy used to assess adequacy of vascular supply to the distal limb is palpation of distal lower-extremity pulses at the dorsalis pedis and posterior tibial arteries, popliteal pulse at the knee, and femoral pulse at the groin. Strength of pulses at each site is noted as absent (0/4), weak (1/4), normal (2/4), full (3/4), or bounding (4/4).[40] If all pulses are palpable, it is likely that there is adequate circulation to heal a neuropathic ulcer. Absent distal

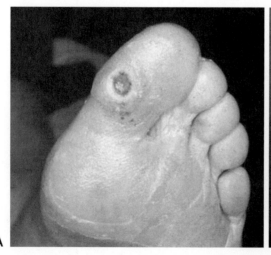 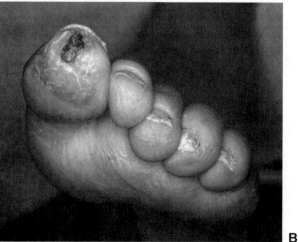

FIGURE 19-2 Comparison of neuropathic and dysvascular foot lesions: Note the typical round callus-rimmed neuropathic lesion **(A)** on the plantar surface of the hallux in an individual with diabetic neuropathy and the ischemic changes (dry gangrene) **(B)** on the tip of the hallux in an individual with peripheral arterial disease. (Courtesy Carolyn Kelly, Center for Wound Healing and Hyperbaric Medicine, Hartford Hospital, Hartford, Conn.)

pedal pulses do not, however, confirm vascular insufficiency; it is estimated that pedal pulses are nonpalpable in up to 10% of the general population.[57]

When pedal pulses are not palpable, further assessment might include positional tests of capillary and venous filling time, auscultation with Doppler ultrasound, calculation of an ABI, taking segmental blood pressure of the limb, transcutaneous oximetry (pulse oximetry), pulse-volume recordings, MRA, computed tomography (CT) angiography, or duplex scanning.[58] (Refer to Chapter 18 for a detailed description of noninvasive assessment strategies.) Table 19-4 lists reference ranges for noninvasive tests.

High-resolution B-mode imaging combined with color and power Doppler and real-time spectral analysis have made duplex scanning one of the most widely used methods of noninvasive evaluation of arterial disease.[59] Duplex scanning can accurately assess the location and degree of arterial disease from the level of the aorta to the level of the ankle. It provides accurate, objective information that supplements the physical examination. A disadvantage of this modality is the prolonged time it takes to perform an accurate examination of the entire extremity. Screening for arterial disease is done by comparing the signals from the various sites along the peripheral arterial tree and measuring the velocities at points of narrowing and comparing them with velocities in non-narrowed

areas of the arteries.[60] This velocity ratio correlates to a 50% diameter narrowing when the ratio value is greater than 2. When the velocity ratio is greater than 4, the corresponding arterial narrowing is greater than 75%. Peak velocities at sites of narrowing can also be used to estimate the degree of narrowing. The sensitivity and specificity of this test is on the order of 90% or greater.[61] Although some surgeons may rely solely on duplex scanning for preoperative peripheral arterial bypass planning, many prefer to more directly outline arterial anatomy using other imaging options.

Two additional methods that successfully outline the specific arterial anatomy are MRA and CTA (Figure 19-3).[62-65] Magnetic resonance imaging (MRI) detects radiofrequency signals given off by protons within a powerful magnet; such proton movement within body structures creates a detectable echo that can be imaged. Use of a contrast agent, such as gadolinium injected through a peripheral vein, greatly enhances the information gained from the images. MRA studies with gadolinium contrast are highly specific and 100% sensitive for identification of arterial lesions that require intervention.[66] The visualization of the distal runoff arterial tree when there are multiple levels of occlusions is much better than that seen with conventional angiography; however, the spatial resolution of MRA images is less than that available through invasive digital subtraction arteriography (DSA). Calcium

TABLE 19-4 *Reference Values for Noninvasive Examination of Peripheral Arterial Circulation*

Test/Measure	Normal Values	Abnormal Findings
Capillary refill time	Elevation of limb 20 seconds Return to dependent position Pressure on toe or nail Blanch, then refill in 1 to 2 seconds	Delayed refill or persistent blanching Rubor of dependency
Refill after occlusion	Inflation of blood pressure cuff at thigh for 5 minutes On release, flush to normal skin color at toes within 10 seconds	>10 seconds: impaired arterial perfusion
Venous refill time	Elevation of the limb 2 minutes Return to dependent position Veins on dorsum of foot refill in 10 seconds	>10 seconds: impaired arterial perfusion <10 seconds: valvular incompetence of veins
Doppler ultrasound	Triphasic on auscultation	Biphasic: mild vascular impairment Monophasic: significant impairment Absent: complete occlusion
Ankle-brachial index	0.9 to 1	<0.9 impaired arterial flow <0.5 unlikely to heal distal wound
Segmental blood pressure	<15 mm Hg drop in systolic pressure between adjacent sites (groin, thigh, just below knee, and at ankle)	>20 mm Hg decrease: possible occlusion >10 mm Hg: possible vessel calcification
Pulse volume recordings	Sharp peaks at each recorded site Similar across left and right extremities	Flattening on recording: occlusive disease
Transcutaneous oxygen pressures	>40 mm Hg suggest healing of ulcer or surgical incision is likely	<20 mm Hg predict nonhealing of ulcer or surgical incision
Duplex scanning	Low velocity ratio; constant hue and intensity of image	Velocity ratio >4 or peak velocity >400 cm/s indicates >75% stenosis

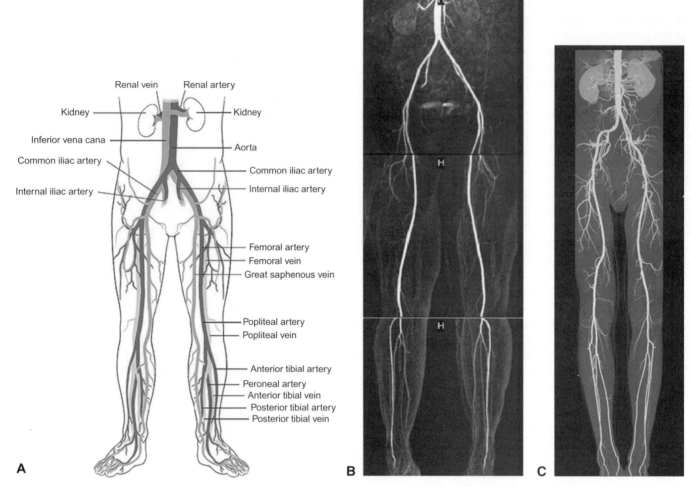

FIGURE 19-3 Examples of imaging techniques used to evaluate the arterial vascular tree in the lower extremity. **A,** Arterial and venous circulation for reference. **B,** Results of MRA in an individual with intact circulation. **C,** Results of CTA in an individual with intact circulation. (**A** courtesy of http://my.clevelandclinic.org/heart/disorders/vascular/circulationlegs.aspx; **B** reprinted with permission from Blackwell G, Wann S, Kadekar S. Clinical applications of cardiovascular magnetic resonance methods. *J Tehran Heart Cent.* 2006;1[3]:125-136; **C** courtesy of http://drugster.info/img/ail/1190_1197_2.jpg.)

within the artery, which impacts operative planning, cannot be seen in MRA. Other disadvantages include the inability to use this magnet-driven modality in patients with pacemakers, defibrillators, and intracorporeal metallic fragments that might migrate.

The advent of the helical or spiral CT scanners enabled CT technology to be applied to the diagnosis of peripheral arterial abnormalities due to the markedly reduced time required for scanning.[67] With this technology, large areas of the body can be scanned in 20 or 30 seconds. An iodinated contrast agent is given through a peripheral vein. This avoids potential complications of a direct arterial injection but does not preclude the risk of inducing renal failure. Although less-concentrated contrast agents can be used for CTA, the volumes required are larger than those for conventional angiography. Both noncontrast images and postcontrast injection images are taken. One advantage of CTA over MRA is the excellent visualization of vessel wall calcium deposits with CTA. But if there is much

calcium, these areas become indistinguishable from the areas opacified after contrast injection. CTA performed for evaluation of the arteries in the lower extremities is being increasingly used in clinical practice. However, its spatial resolution is less than that seen with DSA and small peripheral arteries are not as well visualized.

Vascular Examination: Invasive Strategies

Conventional arteriography and DSA are classified as an invasive examination strategies because both involve local surgical placement of a catheter into the femoral artery in the groin (or alternatively, the axillary, radial, or subclavian arteries, or the aorta), followed by introduction of radiopaque dye into the arterial tree and exposure to radiation.[68]

DSA computer-assisted x-ray method used to visualize vascular structures without superimposed bone and soft tissue usually seen on radiography.[65] The computer subtracts initially recorded x-ray images from those taken following ion injection of contrast medium, to isolate arteries of the limb. Contrast material (dye) is injected into the arterial tree, often at the groin into the femoral artery to assess patency of distal vessels and evaluate collateralization. This carries some risk of cholesterol embolization from atherosclerotic plaques at the site of puncture if the artery is diseases at the injection site; in addition, many of the dyes used can be nephrotoxic.[62] Despite these risks, DSA is considered the gold standard against which other less-invasive imaging methods are compared.

Because of the risks associated with invasive procedures, conventional arteriography is most typically used just prior to revascularization (bypass[69] or thrombolysis[70]) or amputation surgery to determine specific location and severity of vessel occlusion as well as the extent of collateral circulation. It may also be used in place of MRA imaging for individuals with metal implants such as pacemakers and total joint prostheses. Because contrast material used in arteriography are nephrotoxic, this procedure is not appropriate for individuals with renal dysfunction; it is also contraindicated for persons with cholesterol emboli syndrome, or allergies to substances containing iodine.[71,72]

An invasive angiography procedure can take 90 minutes or more, depending on what is being imaged and how many images are required.[73] During the procedure the area that is to be punctured is first numbed with a local anesthetic agent. If the person undergoing the procedure is particularly anxious, the physician can administer a sedative agent orally or parentally before or during the procedure. After the area is adequately anesthetized, an 18-gauge, 2.75-cm needle with a hollow, thin-walled outer cannula and a sharp, beveled, inner stylet is inserted into the artery. Once the artery has been punctured, the stylet is removed and replaced with a guide-wire that is carefully threaded farther into the vessel; this wire then guides placement of the catheter that will deliver contrast medium. Catheters as small as 1-mm outer diameter may be used (3 French), but more commonly, 4 or 5 French catheters are used with outer diameters of 1.32 mm and 1.65 mm, respectively. Once 40 to 120 mL of contrast medium has been injected, the catheter is flushed with heparinized saline to reduce the risk of clot formation. Successive still or continuous video radiographs record the progression of the dye through the limb's arterial tree (Figure 19-4). After the catheter is removed from the femoral artery, manual compression is held locally at the site for several minutes and the patients remain at bed rest for a minimum of 4 hours. To ensure healing of the puncture artery, physical activity (include rehabilitation interventions) is postponed until several hours to a day after the procedure.

Decision Making: Thrombolytic Therapy, Angioplasty, or Amputation?

Intraarterial infusion of thrombolytic agents is used to manage several situations: (a) acute thrombosis of the extremity, (b) following percutaneous angioplasty, (c) after surgical bypass procedure of an extremity, or (d) after acute thrombosis of a diseased native artery.[74–76] The most commonly used thrombolytic agents are streptokinase, urokinase, and

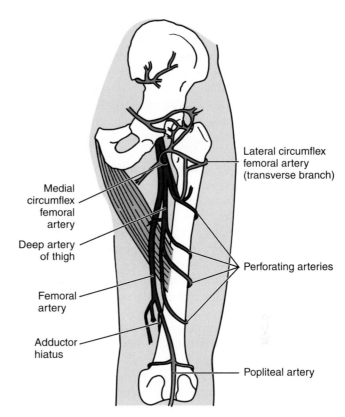

FIGURE 19-4 Diagram of arterial vessels of the pelvis and femur (posterior view) that can be visualized by MRA or by invasive arteriography.

tissue plasminogen activator.[77] Streptokinase and urokinase are non–fibrin-specific agents that convert circulating plasminogen to plasmin, which subsequently breaks down fibrin, one of the main components of clot. Tissue plasminogen activator is a fibrin-selective agent that acts locally by activating plasminogen to form plasmin, which, in turn, breaks up the fibrin in the clot. These agents are typically administered directly at the site of the clot (or as close as possible to it) via a catheter that is threaded through the arterial tree from the initial access site. Infusion may require several days; active rehabilitation begins after infusion is completed.

Intraarterial infusion of thrombolytic agents is typically followed by either systemic intravenous heparin therapy or oral warfarin therapy.[78,79] For individual's status after bypass graft, long-term warfarin therapy is used to reduce risk of graft occlusion. The heparins are a class of agents that bind to antithrombin III to effect anticoagulation. Warfarin blocks the action of the vitamin K-dependent factors in the coagulation cascade. This has implications for the patient undergoing active rehabilitation because these agents increase the risk of bleeding complications, especially with manipulation of the wound in the immediate postoperative period of about 7 to 10 days.

In the postoperative period, should an individual on anticoagulant therapy report a sudden and significant increase in pain at the bypass site or in the residual limb following amputation, the likelihood of local bleeding must be quickly evaluated.[80] Outward signs of bleeding at the operative site, such as swelling, ecchymosis, hematoma, or active bleeding, may not be readily apparent should the bleeding occur at the sub-fascial level. Sudden onset of increased pain in the wound or extremity, along with recurrence of signs of limb ischemia, may also herald occlusion of the graft or progression of disease in the native vasculature following amputation at any level. It is important to identify signs of the failing graft as early as possible because the limb could possibly be salvaged if intraarterial thrombolytic therapy, as described earlier, is initiated soon enough.

Amputation is often the best option for some individuals with dysvascular or neuropathic disease when the arterial anatomy precludes bypass or if severity of disease is such that bypass cannot salvage irreversibly ischemic and gangrenous tissue, as well as persons with complex medical conditions at high risk for intraoperative and postoperative complications. Arterial bypass or thrombolytic therapy may be adjuncts to amputation so as to allow amputation at a more distal level, as long as there is no frank infection (wet gangrene) and the person's arterial anatomy is conducive to bypass. In these cases amputation removes only nonviable portion of the limb, and the bypass or thrombolytic therapy improves the chance of healing at the more distal site.

Extensive gangrene of the foot, which is complicated by infection, is an indication for an open (guillotine) distal transtibial amputation. Time is given for the infection to be controlled by antibiotics and local wound care of the open surgical construct. The residual limb is then revised more proximally and a formal transtibial or transfemoral amputation with standard closure techniques is done.

Traumatic Injuries

Within the continental United States, traumatic amputations are the result of industrial and farming accidents, motor vehicle accidents, or injury during high-risk sport and leisure activities.[81] In areas of the world where there is current or recent armed conflict, traumatic amputations are more likely to be the result of improvised explosive devices, land mines or grenades, shrapnel, or direct gunfire.[82] Many of the injuries sustained by U.S. military personnel during the conflicts in Iraq and Afghanistan involve limb salvage or amputation.[82] In most traumatic injuries the wound is likely to be contaminated by weapon fragments and organic materials (dirt, road debris, bits of clothing, vegetation), as well as damaged bone and soft tissue. In these situations the likelihood of infection as a consequence of introduced environmental microorganism, ischemia caused by vascular damage, and tissue necrosis because of direct damage is high.[83] There may also be significant loss of blood volume and hypovolemic shock, head injury, chest or abdominal injury, and other fractures to contend with.

In emergency care the first priority is to stabilize the medical condition: maintain the airway, support respiration, and ensure adequacy of circulation to the heart and brain.[84] The mangled limb is then carefully cleaned and debrided, a "cocktail" of systemic prophylactic antibiotics (e.g., cephalosporin, gentamicin, and penicillin) is begun, and a tetanus shot is given. Next the trauma team must decide whether the limb can be salvaged or replanted.[85] The team considers many fac-

tors in making this difficult decision including severity of fracture and soft-tissue injury, likelihood of bony union, adequacy of arterial blood supply, neuromotor and sensory function of the extremity, potential for prosthetic use, recovery time, and anticipated long-term functional status and quality of life. Although there are a number of decision-making models available that attempt to quantify these dimensions when such a difficult decision is necessary (e.g., Predictive Salvage Index, Mangled Extremity Severity Score, Limb Salvage Index, Hanover Fracture Scale) most are more effective in determining need for amputation; few accurately predict the likelihood of a positive outcome of limb salvage.[86,87]

Limb Salvage

Limb salvage and replantation are associated with high health care costs because of increased likelihood of multiple hospitalizations for successive surgical procedures, complications and delayed healing, and secondary amputation if the salvage attempt failed.[88] With improving microsurgical techniques, long-term outcome (e.g., return to work, perceived health status) is fairly similar when primary amputation and successful limb salvage and reconstruction are compared; however, residual impairment, functional limitation, and disability can have a significant impact on the quality of life in both groups.[89,90] Any severe trauma to the lower extremities, whether salvage is attempted or amputation is the intervention of choice, is life altering.

In general, salvage attempts are most likely to demonstrate delayed healing or go on to secondary amputation if there has been high-energy injury, comminuted open fractures of Gustillo classification IIIC or higher, periosteal stripping, arterial injury with prolonged warm ischemia time, or complete disruption of the tibial nerve.[91] Individuals or their family health proxy must be informed of the pros and cons of limb salvage versus amputation, including risk of infection and failure, as well as intensity and time frame for rehabilitation and likelihood of returning to premorbid functional levels.[92]

If the decision is made to attempt limb salvage, the individual is taken from the emergency department to the operating room.[93] Arteriography (angiography) may be used to determine the extent of viable arterial perfusion. The next step is precise debridement of the damaged limb; surgeons must be sure that all compromised bone, muscle, and soft tissue are removed to reduce the likelihood of postoperative infection, necrosis, or later development of heterotopic ossification. It can be challenging to determine viability of cortical bone; cancellous bone is more likely to be revascularized. The biomechanical benefit of preserving as much bony length as possible must be weighed against the risk of developing osteomyelitis or delayed healing. Next, fractured fragments are stabilized with appropriate internal fixation, intramedullary rod, or external frame.

Defects in the bone may be filled with antibiotic-impregnated polymethylmethacrylate beads to further reduce the risk of infection and to preserve space for a later bone graft. The areas of the limb that were incised during surgery are stitched or stapled closed, while trauma-damaged areas may be temporarily closed with a biological dressing. The reconstructed limb is monitored closely, with sharp debridement of any nonviable tissue in the early postoperative period every 24 to 72 hours, as appropriate for the degree of wound contamination on initial injury, until a clean wound bed is obtained. Once the wound bed is consistently clean, the individual whose limb is being salvaged returns to the operating room (optimally within 1 week) for definitive closure of the surgical construct. This may be accomplished by delayed primary closure, split-thickness skin graft, local flaps, or, in some cases, vascularized pedicle graft. Subsequent to successful closure, the individual may return to the operating room for bone graft or transplantation or distraction osteogenesis to address osseous defects and limb-length discrepancy.

Amputation in Trauma Care

If limb injury is deemed too severe for salvage, a "guillotine" amputation may be performed to remove damaged tissues and restore hemostasis.[83] If there has been significant contamination of the wound, the surgical construct may be left open (without skin closure) until the trauma team is satisfied that no infection has occurred.[94] Once the individual's medical condition has stabilized and the wound is clean, revision to a definitive level of amputation can be performed. Amputation after severe injuries may require split-thickness skin graft or pedicle graft to achieve adequate skin closure. Skin pressure tolerance when wearing a prosthesis can be problematic later in the rehabilitation process when any type of grafting has been necessary.

Traumatic amputation is most likely to occur in young and midlife adults who are otherwise healthy. Once damaged tissue is removed and wound closure is achieved, circulation is often adequate for successful healing. These individuals, however, may be more likely to develop depression in the postoperative period because the injury was so sudden, and amputation so unexpected.[95] The sense of loss and alteration of body image after traumatic amputation can be more substantial than for an older adult with a diseased limb who "elected" to undergo amputation. Similarly, depression is a significant risk in those who are in the midst of limb salvage because of the likelihood of a long period of limited activity and altered appearance of the salvaged limb.

Neoplasm

Various tumors of soft tissue and bone range from slow-growing localized tumors to invasive and aggressive tumors (Box 19-1).[96] Presenting signs and symptoms may include nonpainful enlargement of the limb, persistent pain, and pathological fracture.[97] The incidence of tumors of bone and soft tissue demonstrate two age peaks: the first occurs in adolescents and young adults (especially osteosarcoma), with a second peak in mid- and late-life adults (especially metastatic).[98]

The most frequently diagnosed tumor of the skeletal system is metastatic, usually originating from a primary site in the breast, prostate, lung, or colon.[99] The most common sites of metastatic bone disease are spine and long bones of the extremities. Metastatic cells disrupt and alter the balance of osteoblastic and osteoclastic activity within bone, resulting in higher rates of

resorption and lysis of bony structure. Metastatic bone disease is most commonly manifested as a deep pain present at rest and during activity, and it carries an increasing risk of pathological fracture.[100] Metastatic bone disease is typically managed with a combination of radiation and chemotherapy as well as nonsteroidal antiinflammatory or opioid medications to relieve pain and enhance function, and administration of bisphosphonate to reduce likelihood of recurrent skeletal-related events and recurrance.[100–103] Some metastatic tumors may require an orthopedic surgical intervention such as placement of an endoprosthesis, along with orthotic intervention to preserve or restore function,

---

BOX 19-1   *Tumors of Bone and Soft Tissue*

METASTATIC TUMORS OF BONE

Primary site:	Breast
	Prostate
	Lung
	Kidney
	Melanoma
	Thyroid
Most common sites:	Rib cage
	Spine
	Pelvis
	Long bones of the extremities
	Skull
Signs and symptoms:	Pain
	Hypercalcemia
	Anemia
	Pathological fracture

PRIMARY BENIGN TUMORS OF CARTILAGE OR BONE

Osteochondroma (exostoses, bony overgrowths)
Chondroma
Chondroblastoma
Chondromyxoid fibroma
Osteoid osteoma
Osteoblastoma
Giant cell tumor

Signs and symptoms:	Nonpainful unless pathological fracture occurs

PRIMARY MALIGNANT TUMORS OF BONE, CARTILAGE, OR MARROW

Chondrosarcoma
Osteosarcoma
Ewing sarcoma
Lymphoma
Myeloma

Signs and symptoms:	Pain, with no history of injury
	Insidious asymmetry of limbs
Osteosarcoma:	Evidence of osteoblastic activity on radiograph
Chondrosarcoma:	Areas of lysis and of calcification

especially if there has been pathological fracture with neuro-muscular impairment.[104]

The incidence of primary malignant neoplasm involving bone and soft tissue is quite low when compared with tumors of other systems.[97] Because of this, the management of primary tumors of bone has evolved into a specialty practice, which means that many newly diagnosed individuals are referred to regional centers where national guidelines ensure consistency of care.[96] Although the number of amputations performed as a result of neoplasm is significantly less than those resulting from dysvascular/neuropathic disease, amputations as a consequence of neoplasm are more likely to be performed at proximal levels, including hip disarticulation. Along with trauma injury, neoplasm is the leading cause of limb loss in children and adolescents.

Decision Making: Limb-Saving Surgery or Amputation?

Until the 1990s most tumors of bone were managed by amputation with adjunctive chemotherapy or radiation.[96] Currently, localized radical resection with allograph of bone, endoprosthesis, joint replacement or rotationplasty, along with and a combination of multiagent chemotherapy, isolated limb perfusion with tumor-necrosis factors, and radiation may be used.[105-109] These strategies have significantly reduced the number of tumor-related amputations performed each year. Amputation may be necessary when there is large, multifocal, high-grade, proximally positioned sarcoma, especially if there has been pathological fracture or significant involvement of neurovascular structures and if the tumor is chemoresistant.[110-114] Amputation is also performed when there is local recurrence following previous limb salvage.[114]

Limb-sparing intervention is often staged, requiring multiple surgeries, given the comorbidities associated with concurrent chemotherapy.[115] In addition, the immunosuppression caused by chemotherapy increases risk of postoperative infection of the endoprosthesis; if such infections cannot be controlled medically, amputation of the limb is likely.[113,116] Survival rates and rehabilitation outcomes are surprisingly similar for those with primary bone or soft-tissue sarcoma managed by amputation or by limb-sparing surgery and reconstruction, although quality of life may be compromised as compared with peers without sarcoma.[117-119]

When a tumor of bone or soft tissue is suspected, initial assessment strategies may include a radiograph, bone scan, CT scan, or MRI.[120] In individuals with previous history of cancer who present with bone pain, a radiograph may reveal a "moth-eaten" area within bone, with unclear boundaries or edges (Figure 19-5), demonstrating areas of osteolysis and reactive osteoblastic activity. A whole-body bone scan may be used to determine if there are multiple metastatic sites. A CT scan may be used to assess three-dimensional structural integrity and mineral content of the bone.

An MRI determines the extent of tissue involvement in marrow, bone, and surrounding soft tissue that is especially useful in planning surgical intervention for primary malignant tumor of bone or soft tissue (Figure 19-6).[121] Laboratory tests may include blood assays, including sedimentation rate,

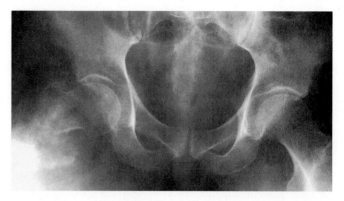

FIGURE 19-5 Radiograph of the hip joints and pelvis of an individual with a metastatic lesion of the right femoral neck and trochanter. Note the poorly defined edges of the metastatic tumor and the differences in appearance of bone when right and left femurs are compared. (From Davis AM. Bone neoplasm. In Lundon K (ed), *Orthopedic Rehabilitation Science: Principles for Clinical Management of Bone.* Boston: Butterworth-Heinemann, 2000.)

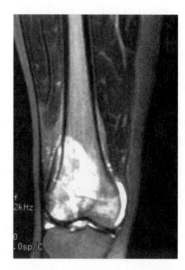

FIGURE 19-6 A magnetic resonance image of osteosarcoma of the distal femur that extends through both condyles and marrow and into surrounding soft tissue. (From Davis AM. Bone neoplasm. In Lundon K (ed), *Orthopedic Rehabilitation Science: Principles for Clinical Management of Bone.* Boston: Butterworth-Heinemann, 2000. p. 147.)

C-reactive protein levels, serum electrophoresis, alkaline and acid phosphate levels, blood calcium levels, blood sugar levels, and hemoglobin concentration.[122] For those with primary neoplastic bone disease, biopsy is used to determine cell type and contributes to pathological staging of the tumor. Depending on the tumor location, the surgeon may use an open frozen section, cannulated drill, or fine-needle aspiration to obtain a biopsy sample. For those with previous cancers of the breast, lung, bone, or colon, biopsy may not be necessary.

Once a primary tumor of bone has been typed and staged, the appropriate intervention is initiated.[123] Nonpainful localized benign tumors typically do not require surgical intervention and are followed serially to watch for tumor progression. Symptomatic benign tumors (i.e., those that are painful or interfere with function) are treated by excision with bone graft or cement to fill the resulting bony defect.[124] Localized malignant tumors are excised using limb-sparing and reconstructive strategies.[108] Those with osteosarcoma or Ewing sarcoma almost always have preoperative and postoperative chemotherapy to minimize the likelihood of recurrence, while those with chondrosarcoma may not require such intervention.[109,125]

For successful limb-saving surgery, the surgeon must first completely remove the tumor, achieving wide, clean margins in the bone above and below the lesion. A tumor in the middle of long bone that does not include epiphyses is often excised en bloc and replaced with an allograft transplantation or expandable endoprosthesis.[126] A tumor that crosses the epiphysis or extends into the joint space is also excised en bloc, and a total joint replacement performed to restore function of the limb.[127] When the tumor is large, high grade, and invasive of other soft-tissue compartments of the limb, amputation may be the most appropriate strategy.[110-114]

Following limb-sparing surgery or amputation, appropriate rehabilitation interventions may include exercise to improve strength, range of motion, and endurance; energy conservation strategies; protective weight bearing during gait training with an appropriate assistive device; prosthetic rehabilitation (for those with amputation); functional training for mobility and activities of daily living; pain management (especially for those with metastatic disease); and patient and family education.[128] The therapist's understanding of the biomechanics and tissue manipulation undertaken in the reconstructive or amputation surgery is essential for appropriate exercise prescription and activity planning. Therapists must also be aware of the impact of chemotherapy and radiation treatments on healing soft tissue and bone; on peripheral sensation; and on physiological response to exercise and activity, as well as the individual's overall health status, immune response, prognosis, and level of energy.[129,130] The most successful rehabilitation programs are individualized and adapt to any adverse effects of concurrent adjuvant oncological interventions.[131] Individuals with recent diagnosis of bone cancer often find significant support in interacting with others who have previously rehabilitated from limb-sparing or amputation surgery.[132]

Congenital Limb Deficiency

The birth of a child with a congenital limb deficiency is initially more distressing and disruptive to the new parents than to the infant.[132] The development of the child's body schema and personality is significantly influenced by the attitudes and expectations of parents and caregivers within the context of the social–cultural environment in which the child is raised.[133] The rehabilitation, prosthetic, and eventual elective surgical management of children with limb deficiency is linked to age-appropriate developmental status, with the goal of enhancing function while minimizing deformity.[134,135] The reader is referred to Chapter 29 for in-depth information on developmentally appropriate preprosthetic and prosthetic activities for mobility and skill, as well as discussion of the therapist's and prosthetist's role in counseling and educating the family and child about rehabilitation and prosthetic alternatives.

Orthopedic and surgical management of children with congenital limb deficiency focuses on enhancing appropriate growth of the residual limb, maintaining relatively equal limb length, enhancing joint function, and ensuring appropriate prosthetic fit. This may include custom-fit and fabricated orthoses or prostheses with shoe lifts; surgical and distraction procedures to lengthen bone; rotational osteotomy; simple surgical revisions to optimize shape of the residual limb; surgical correction of terminal overgrowth; and, when the deficiency is complex, conversion to a conventional level of amputation or disarticulation so as to enhance functional use of a prosthesis.[136-140] School-age children with a partial longitudinal deficiency of the femur (proximal focal femoral deficiency) may be managed with a Van Ness procedure, a rotation osteotomy that fuses a tibia that has been repositioned 180 degrees to the residual femur (if present) or pelvis so that the foot can function as a knee joint (Figure 19-7), or with an osteotomy without rotation

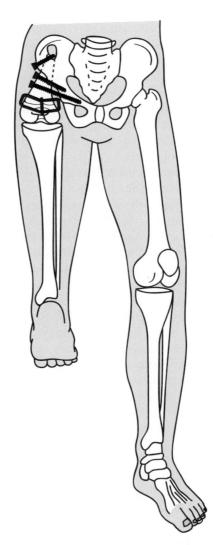

FIGURE 19-7 Diagram of the surgical resection, rotationplasty, and femoral arthrodesis (modified Van Ness procedure) used to create a functional residual limb that can be fit with a prosthesis for a child with a severe congenital proximal focal femoral deficiency. (Modified with permission, from Brown KL. Resection, rotationplasty, and femoropelvic arthrodesis in severe congenital femoral deficiency. A report of the surgical technique and three cases. *J Bone Joint Surg Am.* 2001;83-A[1]:81.)

that is subsequently followed by ankle disarticulation to achieve a weight-tolerant residual limb closely resembling traditional transfemoral residual limb.[141] Deficiencies of the fibula or tibia may be managed, depending on the severity of the defect and resulting deformity, by custom footwear and shoe lift, epiphysiodesis, ankle reconstruction or disarticulation, conversion to traditional transtibial amputation and prosthetic fitting, derotation osteotomy, and limb-lengthening procedures.[142-144]

AMPUTATIONS OF THE FOOT AND ANKLE

Amputations of one or more toes (digit, phalanx) or of part of the foot are the most frequently performed surgeries in older individuals, most often secondary to a nonhealing, often infected, neuropathic plantar ulcer. Individuals most vulnerable to development of plantar ulcers usually present with a combination of sensory impairment (loss of protective sensation); autonomic dysfunction (dry and brittle skin); foot deformity resulting from weakness of the intrinsic muscles of the foot; and impaired circulation that, although adequate to sustain an intact limb, is insufficient to allow healing to occur.[145] In these situations it is especially important to determine (before amputation) the point at which limb circulation is sufficient for successful healing of the residual foot.[146]

Physical deconditioning associated with prolonged bed rest (especially problematic in older adults) and increasing likelihood of systemic complications (in persons with cardiac and pulmonary comorbidities) associated with repeated surgical revisions of a poorly healing amputation can substantially compromise the rehabilitation process and potential for positive outcome.[147] Amputations of the foot may also be the result of severe crush injury, land mine explosion, shrapnel wounds, or similar acute trauma to the foot. The risk of wound contamination by environmental debris and microorganisms increases the likelihood of infection and may require a two-stage surgical approach.[148] Not all individuals with amputations of the toes are referred for physical therapy and prosthetic rehabilitation, unless they require instruction in non–weight-bearing or protected ambulation. Those with partial foot amputation may require adaptive footwear, shoe filler, a passive prosthesis, or accommodative foot orthoses, and may be referred to physical therapy for gait training with an appropriate assistive device.[149]

Amputations of the Toes

Phalangeal (digit) amputations are performed when there is evidence of localized dry gangrene on the toe related to vascular insufficiency, when conservative management of a neuropathic ulcer on the plantar toe surface has not been successful, or when there is infection or osteomyelitis of the phalanges.[150] Digit amputation can be performed at the distal, middle, or proximal interphalangeal joints or with removal of the metatarsal head.[151] Adequate circulation for healing of the surgical wound is a prerequisite to amputation surgery at this distal level. Depending on the age, comorbidities, and current medical condition of the individual undergoing surgery, phalangeal amputations can be performed using an ankle block, an epidural, spinal anesthesia, or general anesthesia.[152] The forefoot is thoroughly cleaned, especially between the toes, with an antiseptic solution to reduce the risk of postoperative infection. A tourniquet may be placed around the calf to be inflated to approximately 50 mm Hg above systolic blood pressure as surgery begins so as to minimize bleeding during the procedure.

For removal of digits, sagittal flaps are typically used (Figure 19-8, *A*). If there will also be resection of metatarsal head, the surgeon may opt to use a "racquet" incision. The digits are removed, either by disarticulation through the joint or transection through the shaft of the digit, using a bone cutter or oscillating saw. Transection through the phalanx is the preferred method because of the avascular nature of cartilage, which compromises wound healing. Distal nerves and tendons are cut under tension (to shorten them 5 to 10 mm) and allowed to retract into the foot. Sesamoid bones, if present, are removed, especially when the metatarsal head is resected.

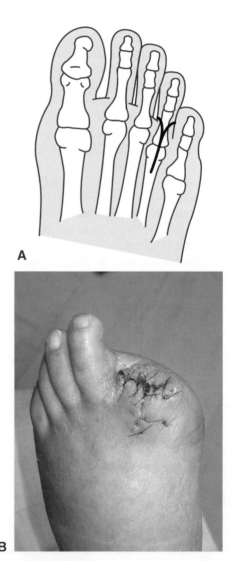

FIGURE 19-8 A, Skin incision used for amputation of the fourth toe, with disarticulation at the metatarsal-phalangeal joint. **B,** Postoperative appearance of the foot after amputation of the hallux. (Photo courtesy Michael Z. Fein, DPM, Bethel Podiatry, Bethel, Conn.)

Once the segment being amputated is removed, the tourniquet is deflated to reestablish hemostasis; the surgeon may use ligature or electrocautery to close bleeding vessels as needed. Next, the surgical site is irrigated with sterile saline or an antibiotic solution to remove any tissue debris before closure. Absorbable sutures are placed to close the internal layers of soft tissues, and then the skin is closed with either sutures (for simple digit resection) or staples (for the larger incisions used in resection of a metatarsal head) (Figure 19-8, *B*). A nonadherent dressing (e.g., Adaptic or Xeroform) is placed over the suture line, and several folded 4 × 4 gauze pads are positioned over the wound and around neighboring toes to apply slight pressure over the surgical wound. Kerlix or Ace bandages are then applied in a figure-of-eight distal toward proximal wrap, leaving remaining toes visible to monitor adequacy of circulation.

The initial dressing typically stays in place up to 5 days unless there are signs of infection (localized pain, excessive or purulent drainage, fever, loss of diabetic control).[151-153] The individual is instructed in non–weight-bearing ambulation using an appropriate assistive device (typically a walker or crutches), on level surfaces, inclines, and stairs. The individual is encouraged to keep the limb elevated as much as possible: education about avoiding prolonged dependency of the limb (i.e., elevating the limb while sitting) is essential.

If the wound heals optimally, many surgeons allow progression to protected partial weight-bearing ambulation approximately 10 days after surgery. Most do not encourage return to weight bearing as tolerated or full weight bearing until all sutures or staples have been removed, often 2 to 3 weeks postoperatively. Many individuals wear a healing sandal to protect the forefoot for several weeks or months following surgery, before returning to normal footwear. Individuals with dysvascular and neuropathic disease benefit from custom-fabricated accommodative orthosis to distribute plantar pressures and minimize the

risk of developing additional neuropathic ulcers on plantar surfaces of the remaining digits and metatarsal heads.

Metatarsal Head Resection

Metatarsal head resections are typically performed when there is a nonhealing plantar ulcer, especially if there is osteomyelitis of the metatarsal head, as long as there is evidence of adequate circulation for postamputation wound healing. The associated digit can be left in place to serve as a spacer in the shoe and to minimize the risk of subsequent foot deformity. The methods of anesthesia and preparation are similar to those used in toe amputation. Once again, a tourniquet may be placed to minimize bleeding during surgery.

A longitudinal incision is made along the dorsal shaft of the targeted metatarsal (Figure 19-9, *A*). Soft tissue structures are carefully detached from around the metatarsal head. The metatarsal is transected behind its head using an oscillating saw, and the metatarsal head is dissected from the proximal phalanx. The tourniquet is deflated to reestablish hemostasis, bleeding vessels are ligated or cauterized, and the wound is irrigated with sterile saline or antibiotic solution. Subcutaneous layers are closed with absorbable sutures, and skin closure is achieved with either staples or interrupted fine monofilament sutures (Figure 19-9, *B*). As soft tissue heals, scarring will create a pseudoarthrosis in place of the anatomical metatarsal head. A nonadherent dressing (e.g., Telfa pad) and several 4 × 4 gauze pads are placed over the dorsal incision site.

Next, the surgeon turns to the plantar surface of the foot to trim any hypertrophic callus and to debride any plantar ulcer that might be present, cleaning it and packing it with gauze soaked in saline or antibiotic solution, and covered with fluff gauze. To minimize forefoot pressure and reduce risk of recurrent or transfer ulceration once ambulation has resumed, the surgeon may also opt to simultaneously lengthen the Achilles

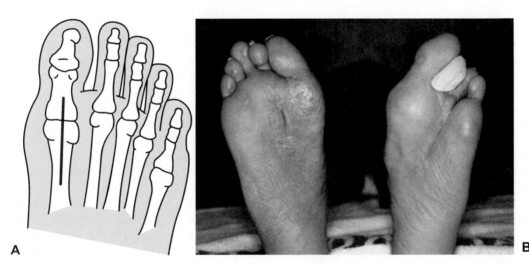

A **B**

FIGURE 19-9 A, Skin incision for excision of the first metatarsal head, when the plan is to leave the hallux intact. Soft-tissue scarring will eventually create a pseudarthrosis so that forward progression over the toe in the late stance phase of gait will not be compromised. **B,** Postoperative fully healed appearance of the feet after excision of the second metatarsal head on the right foot, and resection of the second and fourth toe and metatarsal heads on the left foot. (Courtesy Carolyn Kelly, Center for Wound Healing and Hyperbaric Medicine, Hartford Hospital, Hartford, Conn.)

tendon.[154] The foot is then wrapped, in a distal toward proximal progression, with Kerlix gauze and an Ace bandage. Because of the need to monitor and repack any plantar wounds, dressings are typically changed daily. Instruction in non–weight-bearing ambulation with the appropriate assistive device and patient education about avoiding prolonged dependency of the limb should occur as soon as feasible following surgery. Sutures or staples usually remain in place up to 2 weeks postoperatively. Adequate followup care must be provided. This usually includes an accommodative orthosis to redistribute plantar pressure to avoid the future development of a transfer neuropathic ulcer under remaining metatarsal heads.[155]

Ray Resection

Ray resections may be performed when vascular disease, neuropathic ulcer or osteomyelitis has compromised one or more "rays" of the forefoot and circulation is compromised enough to make healing unlikely at a more distal level. In this surgery, 50% or more of the metatarsal, as well as its associated digits, are removed (see Figures 19-9, *B* and 19-10). The residual metatarsal (if any) is beveled at a 30- to 45-degree angle so that there will be no sharp edge to damage tissue during the late stance phase, as body weight rolls over the distal plantar surface of the healed residual limb. If multiple rays are resected, skin graft may be required for wound closure.[156,157]

Ray resection may be the surgery of choice for problems of the fourth and fifth rays: as long as the first through third rays are intact, there is minimum compromise to forward progression in gait on the healed residual limb. When the first and second rays must be removed, however, there is significant disruption of weight bearing forces during walking and high risk of ulceration; a complete transmetatarsal amputation managed with custom footwear with a rocker bottom often has better functional outcome than leaving the third through fifth rays intact.[158]

Anesthesia and intraoperative care are similar to those described for toe amputation and metatarsal head resection. The soft dressing applied in the operating room is typically changed daily for wound inspection, especially if there has been skin graft or debridement of a plantar ulcer. As soon as feasible, the individual is instructed in non–weight-bearing mobility using a walker or crutches; non–weight-bearing status continues until sutures or staples have been removed.

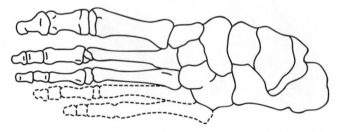

FIGURE 19-10 In this diagram of a metatarsal ray resection, the fourth and fifth rays (metatarsal and phalanges) have been removed. Surgeons can elect to transect the shaft of the metatarsal and leave the base of the metatarsals in place or to disarticulate through the tarsometatarsal joint.

The deformity that results when multiple rays have been amputated may require an accommodative orthosis or a prosthetic filler in the shoe, along with adaptive or custom footwear to protect the residual limb from high pressures resulting from altered biomechanics during forward progression and propulsion when walking.[149]

Transmetatarsal Amputation

A complete transmetatarsal amputation (TMA) is, essentially, ray resection of all five metatarsals proximal to their metatarsal heads. In this surgery, the goal is to preserve as much length of the shaft of the metatarsals and healthy plantar skin as possible so that the resulting residual limb will be long enough for an effective biomechanical lever for forward progression over the foot during gait and will have enough plantar surface such that higher shear forces and pressures exerted on the shortened forefoot during the late stance phase of gait will not compromise skin condition.[159]

It is difficult to predict whether primary healing is possible after TMA in persons with diabetes and critical limb ischemia. Rates for successful healing (primary and delayed up to 8 months) following TMA are reported as 60% to 70%; with as many as 15% requiring revision to a shorter TMA, 15% to transtibial amputation, and a 5% to 10% death rate within 6 months of surgery.[160–162] Risk factors for poor healing include concurrent kidney dysfunction, history of heaving smoking, and concurrent cardiovascular disease. Although the best predictor of healing appears to be a palpable pedal pulse, ABI, unless greater than 0.9, is not an effective indicator. Noninvasive Doppler vascular assessment may help decision making about adequacy of arterial supply for primary healing.[163]

If the surgeon determines that a TMA is necessary, the limb is carefully cleaned and draped for surgery, a tourniquet is applied to reduce distal blood flow and a guideline is marked across the dorsal foot just proximal to the metatarsal heads, continuing in a curvilinear arc along the plantar surface almost to the base of the toes (Figure 19-11). This type of incision creates a long posterior flap that will be sutured closed after bony and soft-tissue elements have been excised. An oscillating saw is used to transect each of the metatarsals, and then the toes are plantar flexed to allow careful dissection of the soft tissue that will be used as the posterior flap from the bony structures being removed. The tendons and sheaths of extrinsic muscles of the foot, as well as distal attachments of intrinsic muscles, are transected; the plantar surface of residual metatarsals are beveled or rounded (to allow rollover in gait without high distal plantar pressures); and any distal nerves are resected under slight tension and allowed to retract into the residual limb. The posterior flap is trimmed and debulked to fit it appropriately to the dorsal incisions for a smooth wound closure. Blood vessels that have been transected are tied off or cauterized, the tourniquet is released, and hemostasis is restored. Just before closure, the surgical wound is thoroughly irrigated with saline and an antibiotic solution; antibiotic beads may be used to further reduce risk of infection.[164] Meticulous attention to hemostasis should preclude the need for placement of a drain; a closed suction drain placed deep to the facial layer of closure would be the preferred choice

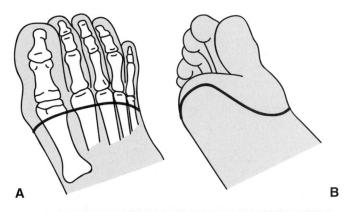

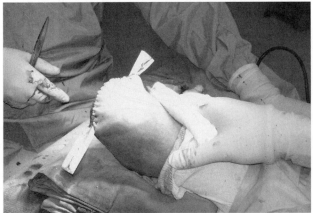

FIGURE 19-11 Dorsal (**A**) and plantar (**B**) incisions for a complete metatarsal amputation. Each metatarsal will be transected just proximal to its head to preserve as much foot length as possible, and the longer plantar flap will be drawn upward and sutured to close the wound. **C,** Postoperative appearance of the foot after transmetatarsal amputation, with surgical drain in place. (Photo courtesy Michael Z. Fein, DPM, Bethel Podiatry, Bethel, Conn.)

of drain if it is determined that one is required. The posterior flap is drawn upward to approximate edges of the wound on the dorsal surface. Deep subcutaneous fascia is sutured closed, followed by suturing and stapling of skin.

Muscle imbalance between dorsiflexors and plantar flexors increases as the length of a transmetatarsal residual limb decreases, leaving individuals with short transmetatarsal residual limb at risk of developing equinovarus deformity in an already vulnerable foot. Tendon transfers or orthopedic stabilization using screws or pins may be used to restore balance to the transmetatarsal residual limb.[165–167] Achilles lengthening may be used as a means to provide greater ankle flexibility, ultimately reducing distal plantar pressures on the TMA residual limb.[168]

Once the wound has been closed, a layer of nonadherent dressing (e.g., Adaptic or Xeroform) is placed over the suture/staple line and a bulky dressing of fluffed gauze is placed around the forefoot. Several rolls of gauze bandage are gently wrapped around the entire foot and ankle, and an Ace wrap is applied to provide gentle compression (graded distally toward proximally) and minimize postoperative swelling. Dressings are left in place 3 to 5 days unless there are indications of

infection or significant focal pain. Limited mobility and non–weight-bearing ambulation with a walker or crutches are often begun after the first dressing change, although healing is enhanced if the limb is kept elevated when in bed or in sitting in the early postoperative period. Staples and sutures are often left in place from 2 to 3 weeks postoperatively. Once the surgeon is satisfied that adequate wound closure has been achieved, the individual may be placed in a healing sandal and graded partial weight bearing during walking can begin.

Gradual progression to full weight bearing with an assistive device (walker, crutches, single cane) and independent ambulation without an assistive device is determined by skin condition of the residual limb and the individual's previous ambulatory status, postural control, and functional level. Many individuals benefit from wearing a sneaker or oxford with forefoot filler and a rocker bottom applied to the sole to dissipate higher weight-bearing forces on the distal plantar residual limb in the late stance phase; those with short residual transmetatarsal limbs may require a custom shoe that encompasses the ankle or a custom thermoplastic ankle-foot orthosis to counteract muscle imbalance leading to equinovarus position during the swing phase of gait and to ensure efficient heel strike at initial contact and appropriate forward progression in stance. Those with polyneuropathy should be cautioned not to go barefoot, even in their home environment: their ability to detect injury to the plantar (or dorsal) surface of the foot may be significantly compromised. An open wound (neuropathic or traumatic in origin) on a transmetatarsal residual limb that becomes infected or fails to heal often leads to revision to the transtibial amputation level.

Amputations and Disarticulations of the Midfoot

The two most commonly performed amputations of the midfoot are tarsometatarsal disarticulation (Lisfranc procedure) and a midtarsal disarticulation (Chopart procedure) (Figure 19-12, also see Figure 22-3). The operative approach

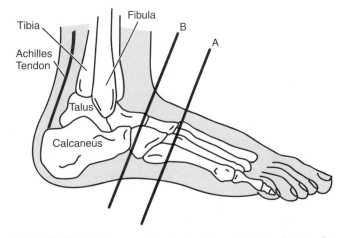

FIGURE 19-12 Diagram of the levels of amputation or disarticulation for a Lisfranc (**A**) procedure at the tarsal metatarsal joint and a Chopart procedure (**B**) at the midtarsal (talonavicular and calcaneocuboid) joints. In both surgeries, a longer plantar flap is left in place and used to close the wound.

and postoperative care for both surgeries is similar to that of a TMA. The surgical incision is made more proximally across the dorsum of the foot, and a long posterior/plantar flap is created to wrap upward toward the dorsal incision when the surgical wound is closed. In a Lisfranc procedure, the forefoot is excised from the midfoot through the tarso-metatarsal joint, usually leaving the "keystone" base of the second metatarsal in place to maintain a transverse arch of the midfoot. The midtarsal joints may be surgically fused as well to maintain the integrity of the architecture between midfoot and rearfoot.

The distal attachment of the peroneus brevis, peroneus longus, and anterior tibialis may be repositioned during surgery in an attempt to restore some level of equity (power) among muscle groups controlling dorsiflexion/plantar flexion and inversion/eversion positioning of the foot at rest and during walking. In a Chopart procedure, the disarticulation takes place in the joints between the talus and navicular bones and the calcaneus and cuboids. Both approaches may also include lengthening of the heel cord to ensure adequate dorsiflexion excursion for rollover during the stance phase of gait. A bulky dressing with an Ace wrap or a slightly dorsiflexed plaster cast is applied in the operating room.[169] Non–weight-bearing mobility with a walker or crutches begins several days after surgery, and protected weight bearing starts once adequate wound closure has been achieved and sutures or stables have been removed.

Lisfranc and Chopart surgeries may be used for individuals with significant traumatic injury or bone or soft-tissue tumor in the forefoot; they are rarely used for individuals with dysvascular or neuropathic limbs.[170] Although both approaches preserve the ability to bear weight through the calcaneus, there is even greater likelihood of development of the equinovarus deformity and prosthetic fitting can be challenging. Persons with a midfoot-level residual limbs typically require custom footwear and orthoses to protect the residual limb during functional activities and to ensure biomechanically sound, safe ambulation.[171] Those who develop significant equinovarus with pain and tissue damage during ambulation may opt return to the operating room after maturation of the residual limb, for surgical modification and subtalar arthrodesis of the residual limb, to achieve more comfortable and functional ambulation ability.[172]

Syme Amputation

The most commonly performed amputation involving the rearfoot is the Syme procedure, a surgical technique that disarticulates the talocrural, trims the malleoli to create a flat weight-bearing surface, and repositions the fat pad and soft tissue of the heel under the distal tibia and fibula. Although the Syme procedure reduces leg length because the calcaneus and talus have been removed, the well-healed distal residual limb is pressure tolerant for ambulation with a prosthesis and, if necessary, for short distances (e.g., emergencies, getting to the bathroom at night) without a prosthesis.[173] Variations of the Syme procedure retain the weight-bearing portion of the calcaneus, fusing it to the distal tibia and fibula.

When the limb has been scrubbed and prepared for surgery and a tourniquet is in place, guidelines for incision are

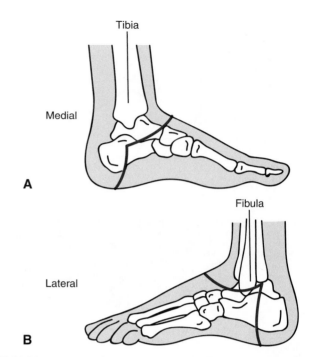

FIGURE 19-13 Medial (**A**) and lateral (**B**) views of the incision for a Syme ankle disarticulation. After the talus is removed from its mortise, the distal points of malleoli are trimmed to create a flat surface and the posterior heel pad is drawn upward to close the wound.

drawn on the anterior ankle from medial to lateral malleoli and then downward around the plantar (posterior calcaneus) surface to outline what will be the distal pad of the residual limb (Figure 19-13). After sharp incision through skin and subcutaneous tissue, toe extensor and dorsiflexor tendons are cut and the anterior capsule of the ankle is exposed. The foot is passively plantar flexed so as to access and open the joint capsule medially to laterally (with care to preserve the posterior tibialis artery going to tissue that will be the pad of the residual limb) and to disarticulate the talus. The posterior joint capsule, posterior tibialis tendon, and flexor hallucis longus tendon are transected. The periosteum of the calcaneus is carefully stripped and preserved for use in attaching the posterior flap/fat pad to the tibia later in the procedure. The Achilles tendon and plantar soft tissue are then dissected from the calcaneus, and the amputated foot completely removed. Plantar tendons and any remaining intrinsic muscle tissue are excised from the posterior flap/fat pad. The distal tips of the medial and lateral malleoli are removed using an oscillating saw, level with the articulating surface of the tibia. The flares of the malleoli are trimmed parallel to the long axis of the tibia and fibula in order to create a less bulbous residual limb.[174]

The tourniquet is deflated, and vessels are tied off or cauterized to restore hemostasis. The surgical construct is irrigated with a sterile saline antibiotic solution. Several obliquely oriented holes are drilled in the medial, lateral, and anterior edges of the tibia and fibula to be used as anchors for suturing the preserved periosteum and posterior flap/fat pad in place. A tubular drain is placed through the anterolateral skin to drain the wound as it heals, minimizing the risk of postoperative hematoma between bone and posterior flap. The flap is drawn up into position, and the preserved periosteum is sutured to bone, followed by suturing of the subcutaneous tissue and then stapling of the skin. After wound closure, a nonadherent dressing is placed over the suture line, followed by a fluffed-gauze, bulky dressing, and the limb is wrapped distally toward proximally toward the knee. Depending on surgeon preference, the limb may then be wrapped with a slightly compressive Ace bandage dressing; Unna paste, which will dry into a semirigid dressing; or plaster of Paris cast.

The drain is typically pulled and removed by postoperative day 2, leaving the dressing in place. The initial dressing change may wait until between postoperative days 5 and 7 unless there are clinical signs of infection or necrosis, to assist adherence of the fat pad to the distal surface of the tibia and fibula. Non–weight-bearing ambulation with a walker or crutches begins 2 to 3 days after surgery and continues for up to 8 weeks. This non–weight-bearing status is essential to ensure that the fat pad is not disrupted until it is firmly healed in place. Staples are typically removed after 3 weeks, and a program of gentle compression with Ace wraps or shrinker garment is initiated. Depending on the condition of the residual limb, the individual may be ready for initial prosthetic fitting by 6 to 8 weeks following amputation. Initial prosthetic training must be with careful partial weight bearing and an appropriate assistive device, with frequent inspection of the integrity and positioning of the distal pad. Progression to full weight bearing follows over the next several weeks.

The successful healing of a Syme amputation is most likely when necessitated by trauma; Persons with PAD who undergo Syme amputation often have an extremely prolonged period of healing and nearly half go on to amputation at the transtibial level.[174,175]

TRANSTIBIAL AMPUTATION

Transtibial amputation typically has positive surgical and rehabilitative outcomes, as long as there is sufficient circulation for healing of the residual limb.[176,177] In the mid-1960s the ideal transtibial surgery preserved 15 cm (approximately 6 inches) of residual tibia to allow for effective knee extension power to control the prosthesis and to minimize discomfort and skin problems in the thermosetting hard sockets that were commonly in use at that time.[178] As residual tibial length decreases toward the tibial tubercle, mechanical advantage of knee flexors exceeds that of knee extensors, making it difficult to extend the knee enough to advance a prosthesis during swing and for controlled (eccentric) knee extension for stability in the early stance phase (Figure 19-14).

Because the surface area for weight bearing within the socket decreases as the length of the residual limb decreases, limb length, the likelihood of discomfort, skin irritation, and limited use of a transtibial prosthesis increases. Conversely, in long residual limbs, the larger total surface area to distribute pressures within the socket and long lever arm potentially

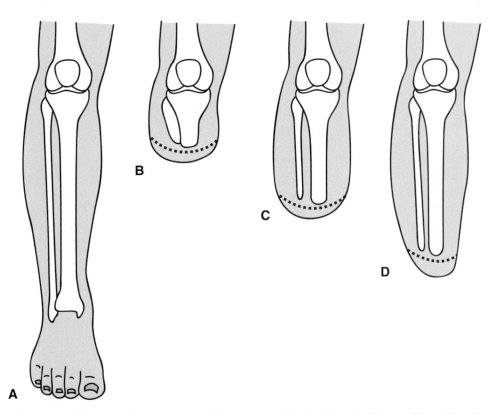

FIGURE 19-14 Anatomical diagram of the tibia and fibula (**A**) and of short (**B**), midlength, standard (**C**), and long (**D**) residual limbs after transtibial amputation. *Dotted line* represents the suture line when a posterior flap approach has been used.

enhance prosthetic control, although there is a risk of chronic skin irritation and discomfort along the sharp edge of the distal–anterior tibial crest. Recent advances in prosthetic materials and design can accommodate, to some degree, for the biomechanical and prosthetic fitting challenges of a long residual limb (i.e., with more than 66% of original tibial length) or of a short residual limb (i.e., preserving 33% or less of original tibial length). Comfort in the prosthesis, quality of gait, and energy cost of ambulation seem to be best balanced when the level of amputation preserves 40% to 50% of the tibia.[179]

The type of anesthesia chosen for transtibial amputation surgery is determined by the individual's overall health and comorbid conditions and consideration of potential adverse outcomes of each method. Options include general anesthesia, spinal anesthesia or an epidural, regional nerve blocks, and in some cases careful local anesthesia at the site of the incision and underlying tissues.[180,181] In older individuals, the likelihood of postoperative delirium and the risks associated with concurrent cardiac disease may lead the anesthesiologist to use spinal anesthesia or regional blocks. In those with multiple traumatic injuries, general anesthesia may allow for optimal physiological control during the surgery.

Depending on the condition of the skin and soft tissue, as well as the circumstances that have led to the decision to amputate, the surgeon selects from a number of surgical approaches. Until recently, the most commonly used approach is the long posterior (myofasciocutaneous) flap described by Burgess in the 1960s: This technique preserves the highly vascular gastrocnemius as well as all anterior compartment muscles beyond the residual tibia, brings the flap up and forward, and positions the suture line across the distal anterior residual limb below the cut surface of the tibia (Figure 19-15, *A*).[182]

Muscles of the anterior compartment are somewhat susceptible to necrosis which contributes to delayed healing and may require revision to a higher level. A modification of the posterior flap procedure described by Bruckner removes all of the tibialis anterior as well as the bulk of the soleus to the level of the residual tibia (see Figure 19-15, *B*), so as to reduce the likelihood of muscle tissue necrosis and increase likelihood of successful primary healing. The modified Bruckner method also removes the fibula.[183,184]

A third options, first described by Ertl in 1949 as an osteomyoplastic amputation with tibia–fibula synostosis, preserves more residual length and incorporates a bone bridge between the distal tibia and fibula for stability (Figure 19-16).[185,186] Although not frequently used in the presence of dysvascular disease, this approach has reemerged for persons with traumatic and military-related lower limb injury.[187] While there is some evidence that the Bruckner and Ertl procedures are more likely to heal successfully (i.e., without need of revision) than the traditional Burgess posterior flap, which surgical technique to use is based on surgeon preference.[188]

When a posterior flap cannot be achieved, the surgeon may create equal anterior–posterior skin flaps in which the

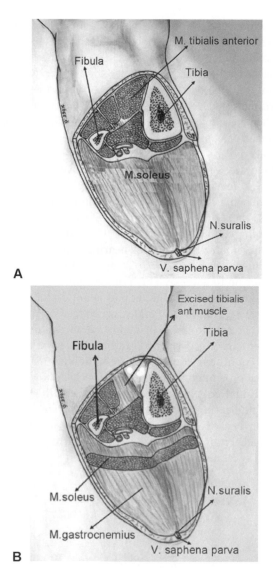

FIGURE 19-15 Comparison of the (**A**) traditional posterior flap transtibial amputation (Burgess procedure) in which all muscles in the residual limb are preserved and the amputation closed with a long posterior flap, and (**B**) the modified Burgess procedure described by Brückner, with removal of all of the tibialis anterior and of the soleus beyond the distal end of the tibia, so as to reduce likelihood of muscle tissue necrosis in the postoperative period. (Reprinted with permission from Yurttas Y, Kurklu M, Demiralp B, Atesalp A. A novel technique for transtibial amputation in chronic occlusive arterial disease: modified Burgess procedure. *Prosthet Orthot Int.* 2009;33[1]:25–32.)

incision runs in a U shape medially to laterally across the bottom of the residual limb, or equal medial-lateral flaps, in which the incision runs in a U anteriorly to posteriorly across the bottom of the residual limb (Figure 19-17). The surgeon may even use a long medial or long lateral flap that positions the incision on the distal opposite side of the limb.[189] In all approaches the surgeon seeks to retain enough soft tissue so that there is little or no tension across the closed incision, but not so much that there will be redundant skin and tissue that might challenge prosthetic fitting.

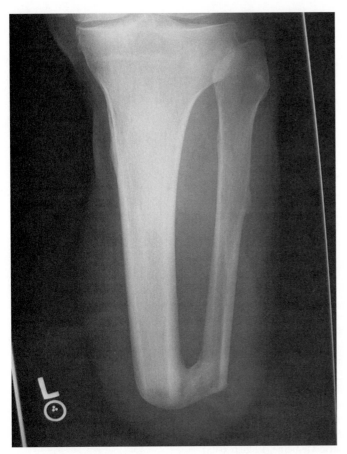

FIGURE 19-16 Radiograph of a healed bone bridge (tibia–fibula synostosis) several months following a transtibial amputation using the Ertl approach. (Reprinted with permission from Dionne CP, Ertl WJ, Day JD. Rehabilitation for those with transtibial osteomyoplastic amputation. *J Prosthet Orthot*: 2009;21[1]:64-70.)

Modified Burgess Posterior Flap Surgery

The limb is cleansed, prepped, and draped for surgery, and a tourniquet is applied at mid-thigh level.[190] A guideline for tibial length and for anterior incision sweeping into a distally curved posterior flap is drawn on the leg. The anterior incision is made through skin and then soft tissue to the periosteum of the tibia, and subcutaneous blood vessels are clamped. Next, muscles in the anterior compartment are incised so that the anterior tibial artery, vein, and deep peroneal nerve can be identified, clamped, transected, and ligated.[194] Soft tissue is carefully removed from around the fibula approximately 2 cm (¾ inch) shorter than the residual tibia. An oscillating saw or double-action bone cutter is used to transect the fibula. The surgeon then bevels the anterior tibia at an approximate 45-degree angle with an oscillating saw and repositions the saw to complete the transection in the transverse plane, controlling the wedge to be removed with a clamp. The skin and subcutaneous incision are now continued along what will become the posterior flap.[191,192]

The transected lower tibia and fibula are pulled up and forward to allow access to structures in the posterior compartment and carefully beveled following the line of the posterior incision to create the posterior flap. Once the amputated limb has been removed, the posterior tibial and peroneal arteries and veins are clamped. Major nerves are elongated with gentle traction, resected at the most accessible proximal point, and allowed to retract into the residual limb.[193] The soleus muscle is then dissected from the medial and lateral heads of the gastrocnemius and removed to debulk the posterior flap for optimal wound closure. The blood vessels of the posterior and lateral compartments are clamped, transected, and ligated. The tibial, superficial peroneal, and deep peroneal nerves are transected under traction so that they will retract upward, away from the end of the residual limb, so as to minimize the risk of subsequent neuroma formation. The tourniquet is deflated, any bleeding small vessels are electrocauterized or sutured, and hemostasis is restored. The beveled anterior tibia is smoothed with a rasp. The surgical site is then irrigated with sterile saline and antibiotic solutions in preparation for wound closure (see Figure 19-15, *A*).[191,192]

When the residual limb is short, much of the syndesmosis between tibia and fibula will have been lost. The surgeon may opt to use an osteoplastic procedure using preserved periosteum before closure in an effort to stabilize the ends of the transected bones. This, theoretically, minimizes the likelihood of dislocation of the fibular head during subsequent activity and prosthetic use. For mid-length and longer residual limbs, closure begins with suturing of the deep fascia and gastrocnemius tendon in the posterior flap to the fascia of the anterior compartment. A closed suction drain can be positioned in the posterior flap toward the medial leg above the incision to reduce the risk of hematoma formation within the residual limb. The limb is then irrigated again with saline and antibiotics, and staples or sutures are used to approximate and close the wound, with the goal of uniform tension across the incision.

A nonadherent dressing is laid along the incision, covered with a fluffed-gauze bulky dressing, and then a conforming gauze bandage is applied evenly in a distal to proximal figure-of-eight. At this point the surgeon may apply a layer of Ace wrap for slight compression of the residual limb, use an Unna bandage to create a semirigid postoperative dressing, use a prefabricated adjustable thermoplastic rigid dressing, or apply a plaster or fiberglass cast (with the knee in extension). The reader is referred to Chapter 20 for further discussion of the indications and limitations of each type of postoperative bandaging.

The drain is typically pulled 24 to 48 hours after surgery. The operative dressing remains in place for 3 to 5 days unless signs of infection suggest earlier dressing change (Figure 19-18). In the first postoperative days the individual with new transtibial amputation is encouraged to keep the knee of the residual limb in full extension; elevation over a pillow leads to hip and knee flexion contracture that will be problematic later in rehabilitation. The individual is referred for rehabilitation services on postoperative day 2 or 3 to begin out-of-bed activity, transfers, and single-limb ambulation with a walker or crutches. Bedside commodes and wheelchairs with removable armrests assist self-care and mobility and reduce the risk of falls.

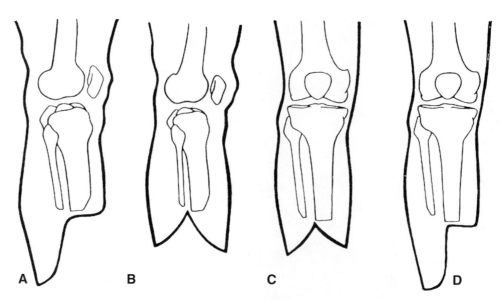

FIGURE 19-17 Examples of transtibial amputation techniques: **A,** This lateral view of the residual limb illustrates the trim line of a traditional posterior flap transtibial amputation. The flap of Bruckner approach would be slightly less full because of the excision of muscles of anterior compartment and more proximal trimming of the soleus. In both approaches, the suture line would run across the anterior surface of the residual limb, distal to the cut end of the tibia. **B,** In this lateral view there are equal anterior and posterior flaps, with the resulting suture line in the frontal plane, running medial-laterally on the underside of the residual limb. **C,** When equal medial and lateral sagittal flaps are used, the suture line lies in the sagittal plane, front to back across the distal inferior residual limb. **D,** When a long lateral flap is used, the suture line will be on the distal medial aspect of the residual limb. (Modified with permission from Singer JM. *Hershey Board Certification Review Outline Study Guide*. Camp Hill, PA: Philadelphia College of Podiatric Medicine, 1993. p. 640.)

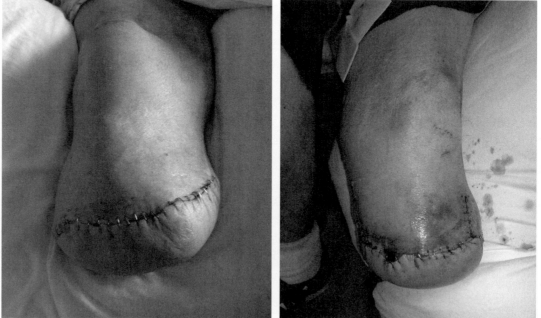

FIGURE 19-18 A, An anterior view of a posterior flap transtibial residual limb is healing well but has a slightly bulbous in shape at postoperative day 5. **B,** An anterior view of a posterior flap transtibial residual limb 3 days postoperatively in a patient with recent failed revascularization. Note the flow of the incision from the previous bypass incision into the new posterior flap, the serosanguineous drainage medially, and ecchymosis laterally over the tibial tubercle. (Courtesy Algis Maciunas, CPO, FAAOP, Hanger Orthotics and Prosthetics, Wethersfield, Conn.)

Staples or sutures typically remain in place for 3 weeks; if there are indications of delayed healing, the surgeon may opt to leave every second or third staple in place longer, reinforcing the incision with Steri-Strips when staples have been removed. Gentle mobilization of soft tissue begins to prevent adherence of the incision scar to underlying fascia and bone. Casting for initial prosthesis occurs only when there has been adequate closure of the surgical wound and the circumference of the distal and proximal portions of the residual limb below the knee is nearly equal. For some individuals this may occur within 3 weeks; for others it may require several months.

Modified Bruckner Procedure

The modified Bruckner procedure is based on the premise that, for individuals with significant PAD, risk of postoperative muscle necrosis will be less likely if the muscles most susceptible to ischemia are removed during surgery.[185,186] For that reason, anterior and lateral compartment muscles, as well as the lateral gastrocnemius, are excised. In addition, the soleus and its large venous plexus are removed to reduce risk of postoperative thrombosis.[194] The fibula is also removed, especially if the residuum is short, to create a limb that will be more tolerant of pressure within the prosthetic socket.

Preparation of the limb with tourniquet and skin incision is essentially the same as for a traditional posterior flap surgery. The tibia is transected 10 to 12 cm distal to the knee joint line, the edges beveled and smoothed. The fibula is disarticulated and completely removed. Muscles of the anterior and lateral compartments are dissected away from their attachments and removed. The soleus is completely resected, leaving the medial and, if necessary to achieve full coverage, lateral portions of the gastrocnemius muscle as the posterior flap. Arteries and veins are ligated, and nerves resected as in the traditional posterior flap surgery. A surgical drain is placed in the space where fibula has been removed, and the surgical construct is closed as described for traditional posterior flap surgery (see Figure 19-15, *B*).

Modified Ertl Procedure

One problematic complication after trauma-related amputation is the development of heterotopic ossification; the modified Ertl procedure theoretically reduces the likelihood of this complication by closing the intramedullary canal, supporting appropriate tension across the interosseous membrane between tibia and fibula, and stabilizing position of the fibula. This is achieved by using a bony strut harvested from the amputated segment of the fibula supported by a periosteal flap dissected from the tibia prior to resection of this long bone.[195] In many instances, more bony length can be preserved, resulting in a cylindrical residual limb with some end-bearing capacity for prosthetic use.[196] This procedure is most typically used in young, healthy individuals expected to be very active using their prosthesis, especially for those in the military.[196,197]

Initial preparation of the limb is similar to that of a posterior flap procedure. After initial skin incision, tibial periosteum is harvested from both medial and lateral surfaces of the bone, and prepared to be a "sling" to hold the subsequent bone graft in place.[187] Long bones are then transected with an amputation saw. A segment of bone is harvested from the amputated fibular shaft, sized to bridge the space between tibia and fibula of the residual limb. The inner edges of the tibia and fibula may be notched to allow the bone bridge to fit securely between them. The bone bridge may be secured in place in a number of ways; for example, use of compression screws, or running a "TightRope" (Anthrex Inc, Naples FL) suture through a hole drilled in the fibula, then through the shaft of the bone bridge, then through a hole drilled in the tibia.[196] The preserved tibial periosteum is then wrapped under the bone bridge and secured to fibular periosteum. The tourniquet is released, and hemostasis is achieved by ligating arteries and veins. Nerves (tibial, superficial and deep peroneal, saphenous, and sural) are injected with an anesthetic, put under tension, resected, and allowed to retract into the residual limb. The posterior flap is pulled up and over the end of the residual limb, and anchored to the anterior tibia, proximal to the bone bridge (see Figure 19-16). Muscle of the flap is sutured to anterior fascia with nonabsorbable suture, and then subcutaneous and skin layers are closed with either silk suture or with staples. Immediate postoperative care, focusing on management of pain and of edema, is the same as for the modified Burgess and modified Bruckner procedures.

Because of the extensive dissection required, this procedure uses more operative time (and more time under anesthesia and with tourniquet in place) than the modified Burgess and Bruckner surgeries. Because of this, it may not be the surgery of choice for persons with multiple comorbidities or those who are medically frail.[198] If performed prior to skeletal maturity, there is risk of development of a progressive varus deformity of the tibia likely to require surgical correction for functional prosthetic use.[199]

KNEE AND TRANSCONDYLAR AMPUTATION

In previous centuries, before development of surgical anesthesia and antibiotics, simple knee disarticulation surgery often had a much more favorable outcome than transtibial amputation.[200] Because this surgery does not transect major muscle mass, it can be done in less time and with significantly less blood loss than transtibial or transfemoral amputation. Additionally, simple disarticulation through the knee joint disrupts only the tissue compartment of the joint itself, making postoperative infection in fascia, muscle, or bone much less likely. The femoral condyles, with their cartilaginous covering, are designed to tolerate weight bearing, and preservation of the entire femur provides mechanical advantage to the prosthetic wearer.

The residual limb heals without much atrophy, requiring less socket replacement or revision early on, allowing fitting with a definitive prosthesis in less time than the typical transtibial or transfemoral residual limb. Additionally, this surgery preserves the growth plate of the distal epiphysis, an important consideration for children with neoplasm or traumatic injury of the proximal tibia.[201] For individuals with severe bilateral vascular disease who are nonambulatory before surgery, the extra length of the femurs provides a larger base of support in sitting, enhancing postural control.[202]

The length of an intact femur, along with the anatomy of the condyles, creates several important challenges to prosthetic fit and function in terms of choice and placement of the prosthetic knee unit, which affects energy cost, as well as efficiency of prosthetic gait. The bony, bulbous residual limb of those who undergo a simple knee disarticulation also creates a challenge regarding donning and doffing the prosthesis (Figure 19-19). Surgical techniques developed by Mazet and Hennessy in the 1960s removed the patella and trimmed the medial and lateral condylar surfaces to address the problems associated with bulbous distal anatomy.[203] In 1977, Burgess recommended removal of 1.5 to 2 cm of distal condyles to permit placement of a newly developed four-bar prosthetic knee unit closer to what had been the anatomical axis of the knee.[204,205] Some surgeons advocate modifying the patella and then fusing it to the intercondylar notch of the femur to create a flat, weight-bearing surface.[206]

Many current transcondylar surgical procedures combine these two approaches to form a residual limb that resembles a long transfemoral limb (Figure 19-20). Typically either equal sagittal flaps or a long posterior flap are used to provide additional "cushion" for weight bearing through the distal residual limb.[207,208] Proponents of simple knee disarticulation, without

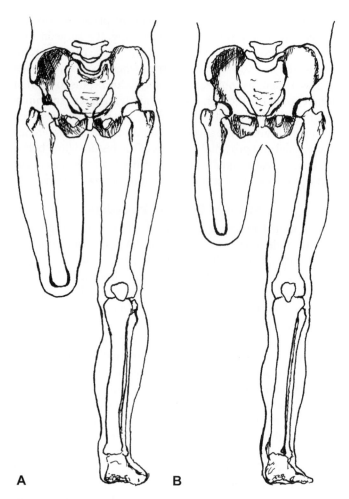

FIGURE 19-20 Comparison of amputations through the femur. **A,** Knee disarticulation transects the knee joint, while transcondylar amputation modifies the distal femur and condyles. **B,** Traditional transfemoral amputation preserves 50% to 66% of femoral length. A long transfemoral residual limb (>66% of femoral length) and knee disarticulation provide a mechanical advantage for prosthetic use but problems with prosthetic cosmesis as a result of incorporation of a knee unit distal to the socket. A short transfemoral limb (<50% of femoral length) may challenge prosthetic fit and suspension.

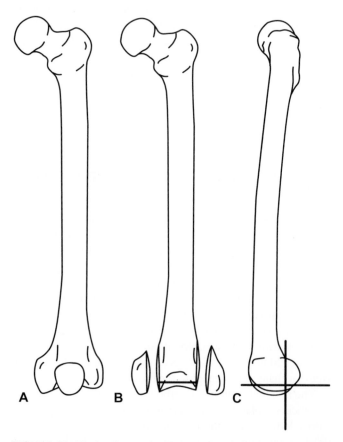

FIGURE 19-19 A, The residual bony architecture in a simple knee disarticulation, in which no modification of the patella or femur is done. **B,** Anterior view. **C,** Lateral view of transcondylar amputation, which shapes the residual femur to resemble a long transfemoral residual limb.

modification of the distal femur, suggest that the combination of reduced rates of infection, better primary healing, larger surface areas for weight bearing, and advances in prosthetic design and technology lead to better functional outcome and higher rates of prosthetic use.[208,209]

The preparation for knee disarticulation or transcondylar amputation is similar to that of transtibial amputation. The anesthesiologist selects spinal, epidural, or general anesthesia as determined by the health and physiological condition of the person undergoing disarticulation. After application of a tourniquet, the surgeon outlines the incision to guide creation of equal mediolateral flaps (Figure 19-21) approximately half of the anteroposterior diameter of knee in length; some surgeons prefer a long posterior flap as described in the discussion of transtibial surgery (see "Transtibial Amputation" above). After careful incision of skin and subcutaneous tissue and reflection of the skin flaps, the surgeon transects the patellar tendon at the

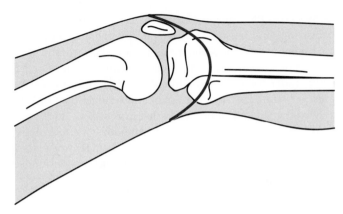

FIGURE 19-21 A lateral view of the guideline for incision creating equal lateral and medial flaps during knee disarticulation.

tibial tubercle, as well as the medial and lateral collateral ligaments just above the menisci. Next, the knee is slightly flexed and the infrapatellar fold is cut. This provides access to the cruciate ligaments, allowing the surgeon to free them from their attachment to the tibia. The posterior joint capsule is carefully cut, with attention to keeping neurovascular structures in the popliteal fossa intact, while exposing the femoral attachment of the gastrocnemius muscle. The popliteal artery and vein and saphenous vein are clamped and ligated, and the medial and common peroneal and saphenous nerves are transected under traction and allowed to retract into the residual limb. The surgeon then cuts through the gastrocnemius at the distal edge of the wound, and the lower leg is removed.

For a simple disarticulation the wound is irrigated with saline and antibiotics and prepared for closure at this point. When transcondylar modification is desired, an oscillating saw is used to trim the edges of the condyles before irrigation. The tourniquet is removed, and hemostasis is ensured. In preparation for closure the patellar tendon is sutured to the anterior and posterior ligaments, and the cut edge of the gastrocnemius muscle is sutured to the anterior joint capsule (myoplasty). The hamstring tendons are transected high and allowed to retract. The lateral tendons of the biceps femoris and the iliotibial band are transected low and reconstructed at the time of wound closure to provide muscle stability. The lateral and medial flaps are positioned with approximated edges, and subcutaneous tissues are sutured closed. Finally, the outer layer of skin is closed using staples or external sutures.

A nonadherent gauze is placed over the wound edges, followed by a layer of gauze fluff and a figure-of-eight gauze wrap. The surgeon may choose to apply an Ace wrap, an Unna dressing, a prefabricated adjustable removable rigid dressing, or a plaster or fiberglass cast as the final layer of bandage. The dressing is typically changed at day 5 unless there are indications of infection. Mobility training begins on postoperative day 1, with single-limb ambulation with crutches or walker the next day. A bedside commode and wheelchair allow the individual with new disarticulation who is capable to manage much of the individual's own self-care. Some or all of the staples or external sutures are removed at 2 to 3 weeks, depending on the condition of the incision. Readiness for a training

prosthesis is determined by full healing of the surgical construct, typically between 3 and 8 weeks after surgery.

TRANSFEMORAL AMPUTATION

Amputation through the femur is chosen when there has been significant trauma to the proximal tibia and knee, when there is a tumor in the proximal tibia or distal femoral condyles that cannot be replaced by allograft or a total joint, when there is infection or failure to heal following transtibial amputation, following failed revascularization of the lower leg, and at times for intractable infection following total knee arthroplasty.[210-213] For persons with PAD, the level of choice (if there is adequate circulation for wound healing) is transtibial because functional prosthetic ambulation is most likely when the knee joint has been preserved; some individuals, however, have serious enough circulatory impairment that amputation at transfemoral levels is necessary.[214] Morbidity and mortality following transfemoral amputation is high among older persons with concurrent diabetes and PAD.[215,216]

Considering not only vascular status, but also muscle attachment and biomechanics of the residual limb in gait, is important when deciding on the precise length of the residual femur. For those needing transfemoral surgeries, function and prosthetic control improves as length of residual femur increases. Preservation or reattachment of the adductor brevis, adductor longus, and especially adductor magnus provides sufficient power for stabilization of the residual limb in adduction in stance so that the abductors can work to keep the pelvis level during prosthetic gait (Figure 19-22).[217-219]

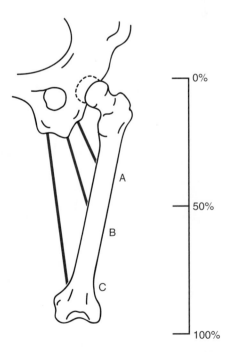

FIGURE 19-22 Diagram of point of attachment and line of pull for the (**A**) adductor brevis, (**B**) adductor longus, and (**C**) adductor magnus, as they relate to femoral length. As the length of the residual femur decreases, power and efficiency of adductor muscles groups are more and more compromised.

Preservation of femoral length and of muscle mass via myoplasty or myodesis, rather than trisection through muscle belly, results in a stronger residual limb that is more easily fit and has better prosthetic control.[219,220] It also reduces the risk of developing hip abduction and flexion contracture during rehabilitation and over the individual's lifetime. The surgeon must work with the viable thigh tissue to create a residual limb that is balanced in muscular power, provides a long enough lever to allow hip extensors to control prosthetic knee stability in stance, and has as smooth and sensate a skin surface as possible.[214,221]

Traditional Transfemoral Surgery

In preparation for surgery the patient is placed in a three-quarters supine position, lying on the side of the body opposite the limb to be amputated. The surgeon may or may not choose to use a tourniquet depending on the etiology of amputation. The surgeon may opt to use equal anteroposterior flaps, equal mediolateral flaps, or a long flap from any one limb surface that will be approximated to the opposite limb surface at closure (Figure 19-23).[214,222] The skin is opened, followed by subcutaneous tissue, according to the flap pattern chosen. The lower leg may be disarticulated at this point to provide a less cumbersome operative area for subsequent revision. The fascia and muscle of the quadriceps and adductors are transected as far distally as possible, and the femur is scored at the desired level of amputation. The periosteum is elevated and reflected upward and will be used during myoplasty later in the procedure. The femur is cut with an oscillating saw, and the distal bone is retracted (pulled) ante-

riorly so that the surgeon can access posterior structures. The hamstrings and tensor fascia lata are incised and transected as distally as possible. Major vessels are clamped and then sutured or ligated. The sciatic nerve is sutured or ligated, cut while under traction, and allowed to retract into hamstring muscle tissue. The sharp edges of the residual distal femur may be shaped and smoothed with a rasp or file. The wound is irrigated with sterile saline and antibiotics, the tourniquet is released, and hemostasis is restored. A drain may be placed, at the surgeon's discretion, as residual tissues are positioned for wound closure.

Some surgeons perform a multiple-layer myoplasty to close the surgical wound, suturing medial and lateral soft tissue and muscle groups together as a deep first layer, anterior and posterior soft tissue and muscle groups as a second layer, and then the skin for an outer layer (Figure 19-24). Others prefer myodesis, first pulling the adductor magnus under the distal femur medially to laterally and suturing it to the lateral surface of the femur, and then pulling the quadriceps under the distal femur in an anterior-to-posterior direction over the repositioned adductor, attaching it to the posterior surface of the femur, before closing the skin with staples or removable sutures. An alternative closure places multiple single sutures from the deep posterior subcutaneous tissue, through hamstrings, posterior and anterior periosteum, quadriceps, and finally anterior subcutaneous tissue, and finishing by stapling the skin surface closed.[222] The goal is to create a tapered, cylindrical residual limb with few "dimples" or redundant tissues.

A nonadherent dressing is placed over the suture line, followed by fluffed gauze and a figure-of-eight and spica gauze bandage. A layer of microporous tape may be applied at this joint to keep the wound clean and decrease the risk of contamination by urine or feces. The outer dressing may be by Ace wrap or Unna bandage for a semirigid dressing. The first dressing change occurs 3 to 5 days postoperatively unless there are indications of infection or excessive bleeding. If a drain has been placed, it is usually pulled at the first dressing change (Figure 19-25).

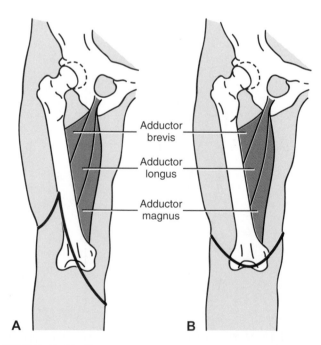

FIGURE 19-23 Illustration of incision guidelines for **(A)** a long medial flap and **(B)** equal anterior and posterior flaps for transfemoral amputation surgery. Note that both preserve as much of the adductor magnus as possible for later myoplasty or myodesis when the wound is closed.

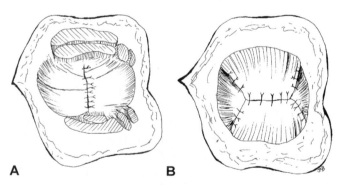

FIGURE 19-24 Myodesis of the muscles of the thigh is used to stabilize soft tissue after transfemoral amputation. The initial layer **(A)** attached medial adductor muscles to the vastus lateralis and iliotibial band. The second layer **(B)** connected anterior quadriceps to the posterior hamstrings, covering the first layer. Finally, the two layers are sutured together to stabilize the muscular sling that has been created across the bottom of the residual limb.

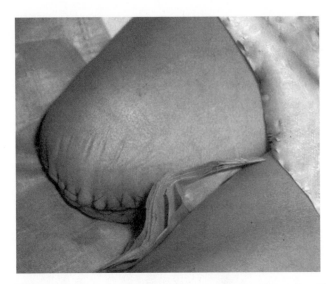

FIGURE 19-25 Postoperative appearance of a transfemoral residual limb before bandaging. An equal anteroposterior flaps approach has been used, placing the surgical incision in the frontal plane on the underside of the residual limb. (Courtesy Algis Maciunas, CPO, FAAOP, Hanger Prosthetics and Orthotics, Wethersfield, Conn.)

Mobility training and early preprosthetic positioning exercises (to encourage positioning of the residual limb in hip extension and adduction) are optimally initiated the day after surgery, and single-limb gait training with an appropriate assistive device follows as soon as the individual can tolerate increasing activity. The environment must be set up to minimize the risk of falls; a prefabricated, thermoplastic, adjustable, removable rigid dressing might be used to protect the healing residual limb. Strategies for consistent gentle soft tissue compression are initiated as soon as possible using an Ace wrap, elasticized stockinette, and eventually a commercially available "shrinker." External staples or sutures remain in place for 3 weeks or more, perhaps being removed in successive stages to ensure a solid wound closure. Fitting for initial prosthesis is, as in all other levels of amputation, determined by the condition of the suture line; for some patients this may occur as early as 3 or 4 weeks postoperatively, and for others several months after surgery.

Osseo-Integrated Transfemoral Amputation

An alternative to traditional transfemoral amputation for otherwise healthy individuals with traumatic injury or osteosarcoma has been used since 1990 by a group of surgeons and prosthetists at Sahlgrenska University Hospital in Sweden (Osseointegrated Prosthesis for Rehabilitation of Amputees [OPRA], Inegrum AB, Goeborg, Sweden).[223] This approach is an application of principles of successful endodontic implants to persons with trauma or tumor-related need for transfemoral amputation. In the OPRA approach, a titanium fixture is inserted into the shaft of the femur at time of amputation, and is permitted to heal in place for 6 months. During this time, a traditional prosthetic socket is often prescribed. A second surgery then screws a titanium rod (abutment) through the skin and into the fixture (Figure 19-26). This provides a mechanism to attach the prosthesis directly to the residual limb, without need for a

socket. Six weeks after the second surgery, once adequate soft tissue healing has occurred, rehabilitation begins with limited, protected weight bearing in standing and then while ambulating with the prosthesis. Over the next 6 months, the individual gradually increases both the weight bearing and the intensity of activity.[224] The overall goal of the procedure is to provide a comfortable and effective limb–prosthesis interface, enhancing the overall level of function with the prosthesis.[225]

There are two problems reported for osseointegrated systems: bone failure at the stem–bone interface resulting in pain, loosening of the implant, and possible fracture,[226] and infection (incidence approximately 5% to 18%).[227] The source of infection is typically normal flora of the skin; if treated effectively, few of these infections require removal of the implant. Both qualitative and quantitative studies suggest that the osseointegrated prosthesis option improves quality of life and level of function for the carefully selected group of individuals offered this option.[228,229] This approach has expanded to the United Kingdom[230,231] and the United States.[232]

HIP DISARTICULATION AND HEMIPELVECTOMY

Amputation at the level of the hip or pelvis is an extreme surgery that is undertaken to preserve life in the presence of extreme infection or damage of proximal structures: recurrent deep decubitus ulcers in individuals with paralysis, necrotizing wounds with wet gangrene and risk of systemic sepsis, severe crush or shrapnel injury damaging blood vessels in the groin when revascularization is not possible, or invasive tumor of the proximal femur or pelvis when limb-sparing strategies are not possible.[233–236] With these surgeries, significant body mass is removed and there is the likelihood of significant blood loss; careful monitoring of hydration and electrolytes is necessary during surgery and the immediate postoperative period.[237,238] These are complex surgeries best performed in facilities with an experienced interdisciplinary team available for preoperative, perioperative, and postoperative care.

In the operating room the patient is placed in a three-quarters supine position, with the limb to be amputated uppermost. The limb is prepped and draped for surgery, and a racquet-shaped guideline for incision is traced on the skin, with the goal of creating a large posterior flap of skin, subcutaneous tissue, and gluteal muscle mass for wound closure (Figure 19-27). The incision begins at the medial edge of the anterior superior iliac spine, continues along the inguinal ligament to just below the ischial tuberosity and gluteal crease, and then arches upward over the greater trochanter and anterior thigh back to the anterior superior iliac spine. The surgeon must carefully free and then stabilize neurovascular structures in the inguinal region, as well as detach each of the many surface and deeper muscles that cross the hip joint, starting with the anterior and medial groups, then moving laterally and posteriorly.

The gluteal muscles are detached from the greater trochanter but kept in place on the pelvis to be part of the posterior flap. The head of the humerus is forcefully dislocated from the acetabulum. The wound is irrigated with saline and antibiotics,

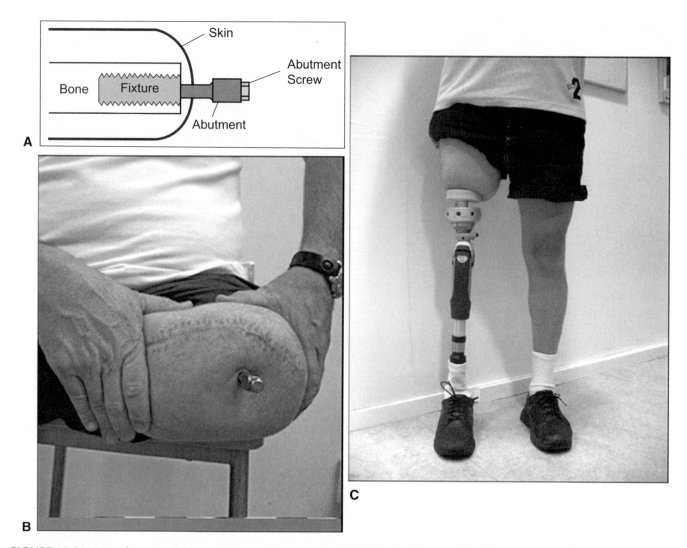

FIGURE 19-26 A, A schematic of the osseointegrated fixture embedded within the femur, and the abutment protruding through the skin of the residual limb. **B,** A healed transfemoral residual limb with the abutment that will be attached directly to the prosthesis. **C,** The platform of the prosthesis supports the tissue of the residual limb, once the abutment screw is attached. (From Hagberg K, Branemark R. One hundred patients treated with osseointegrated transfemoral prostheses—rehabilitation perspective. *J Rehabil Res Dev.* 2009;46:331-344.)

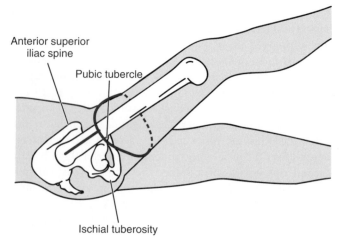

FIGURE 19-27 An example of the location of incision for a hip disarticulation, creating a posterior flap that will be used when the wound is closed.

and hemostasis is secured. Pairs of antagonistic muscles may be sutured together in myoplasty or to periosteum of the pelvis in myodesis as wound closure begins. Drains are placed; the posterior flap is positioned against anterior, medial, and lateral edges of the wound; subcutaneous closure is secured by a series of sutures; and skin is closed with staples.

The wound is dressed with a layer of nonadherent gauze; then fluff; and then a spica wrap of gauze and elastic bandage, directing soft tissue in a posterior-to-anterior medial direction consistent with the line of the posterior flap. Dressings are changed every 3 or so days, more frequently if there is significant drainage. There is considerable risk of deep venous thrombosis of the intact limb during the immediate postoperative period; low-dose heparin or Coumadin (warfarin) may be used as prophylactics. Limited periods of sitting, mobility, and transfer training, as well as ambulation on the remaining limb using a walker or crutches, begins as soon as the patient is medically stable and able to tolerate increasing levels of activity, optimally within 2 to 3 days after surgery. Special attention must be paid to the sitting posture, with minimal time spent in a posteriorly tilted "sacral sitting" position, to ensure skin integrity. Staples or external sutures remain in place for 2 to 3 weeks postoperatively. Patient and family education must include efforts to carefully protect the surgical site during movement and activities of daily living. An early referral to the prosthetist for fabrication of a custom thermoplastic removable rigid dressing may occur in the week immediately following surgery. Fitting for initial prosthesis, as in amputation at all other levels, is determined by rate and adequacy of healing of the surgical site.

Hemipelvectomy (transpelvic amputation) is a more aggressive and invasive surgery that leaves the individual without a bony case to support abdominal contents on one side of the body. Postoperatively, there is significant risk of developing ileus; many individuals with hemipelvectomy are ill enough to require nasogastric tube and limited feeding in the immediate postoperative period. Mobilization and transfer training may need to be deferred until the individual is well enough and nutritionally supported enough to tolerate increased levels of activity. Typically, prosthetic support of the soft tissue and abdominal contents of the residuum is necessary for functional sitting.[239]

SUMMARY

This chapter has presented the strategies used to examine a vascularly compromised or traumatically injured lower extremity and discussed the surgeon's evaluative process when making decisions about limb revascularization, thrombolytic intervention, limb salvage, disarticulation, or amputation. Several factors must be carefully considered: the likelihood of successful healing of the surgical construct; the preservation of the ankle and knee (if possible) to minimize the impact on energy cost of gait and postural control; and the creation of a residual limb with adequate skin surface (pressure tolerance), length (lever arm), and dimension for prosthetic fitting and function. The most common approaches for surgery at each level of amputation were discussed so that rehabilitation professionals could appreciate the manipulation of tissues and postoperative wound healing process. The authors explored the commonalities and differences in amputations performed because of dysvascular/neuropathic disease, bone infection, lower-extremity trauma, neoplasm, or revision in children with congenital limb deficiency. The authors hope that readers developed an appreciation of the complexity and challenges presented to the surgeon and the rehabilitation team when an individual undergoes amputation.

REFERENCES

1. Coffey L, Gallagher P, Horgan O, et al. Psychosocial adjustment to diabetes-related lower limb amputation. *Diabet Med.* 2009;26(10):1063–1067.
2. Stansbury LG, Lalliss SJ, Branstetter JG, et al. Amputations in U.S. military personnel in the current conflicts in Afghanistan and Iraq. *J Orthop Trauma.* 2008;22(1):43–46.
3. Anthony T, Roberts J, Modrall JG, et al. Transmetatarsal amputation: assessment of current selection criteria. *Am J Surg.* 2006;192(5):e8–e11.
4. Ryer EJ, Trocciola SM, DeRubertis B, et al. Analysis of outcomes following failed endovascular treatment of chronic limb ischemia. *Ann Vasc Surg.* 2006;20(4):440–446.
5. Grimer RJ. Surgical options for children with osteosarcoma. *Lancet Oncol.* 2005;6(2):85–92.
6. Aronow W. Management of peripheral arterial disease of the lower extremities in elderly patients. *J Gerontol.* 2004; 59A(2):172–177.
7. Singh R, Ripley D, Pentland B, et al. Depression and anxiety symptoms after lower limb amputation: the rise and fall. *Clin Rehabil.* 2009;23(3):281–286.
8. Chen MC, Lee SS, Hsieh YL, et al. Influencing factors of outcome after lower-limb amputation: a five-year review in a plastic surgical department. *Ann Plast Surg.* 2008;61(3):314–318.
9. Howe EG. Increasing consensus with patients and their loved ones. *J Clin Ethics.* 2009;20(1):3–12.
10. Ploeg AJ, Lardenoye JW, Vrancken Peeters MP, et al. Contemporary series of morbidity and mortality after lower limb amputation. *Eur J Vasc Endovasc Surg.* 2005;29(6):633–637.
11. Aragón-Sánchez J, Hernández-Herrero MJ, Lázaro-Martínez JL, et al. In-hospital complications and mortality following major lower extremity amputations in a series of predominantly diabetic patients. *Int J Low Extrem Wounds.* 2010;9(1):16–23.
12. Stineman MG, Kwong PL, Kurichi JE, et al. The effectiveness of inpatient rehabilitation in the acute postoperative phase of care after transtibial or transfemoral amputation: study of an integrated health care delivery system. *Arch Phys Med Rehabil.* 2008;89(10):1863–1872.
13. McCollum PT, Raza Z. Vascular disease: limb salvage versus amputation. In: Smith DG, Michaels JW, Bowker JH, eds. *Atlas of Amputation and Limb Deficiencies. Surgical Prosthetic and Rehabilitation Principles.* 3rd ed. Rosemont, IL: American Academy of Orthopaedic Surgeons; 2004:31–45.
14. Jude EB, Eleftheriadou I, Tentolouris N. Peripheral arterial disease in diabetes—a review. *Diabet Med.* 2010;27(1):4–14.
15. Chiriano J, Bianchi C, Teruya TH, et al. Management of lower extremity wounds in patients with peripheral arterial disease: a stratified conservative approach. *Ann Vasc Surg.* 2010; 24(8):1110–1116.
16. Nael K, Fenchel MC, Kramer U, et al. Whole-body contrast-enhanced magnetic resonance angiography: new advances at 3.0 T. *Top Magn Reson Imaging.* 2007;18(2):127–134.
17. Mwipatayi BP, Naidoo NG, Jeffery PC, et al. Transmetatarsal amputation: three-year experience at Groote Schuur Hospital. *World J Surg.* 2005;29(2):245–248.
18. Younger AS, Awwad MA, Kalla TP, et al. Risk factors for failure of transmetatarsal amputation in diabetic patients: a cohort study. *Foot Ankle Int.* 2009;30(12):1177–1182.
19. Taylor SM, Kalbaugh CA, Cass AL, et al. "Successful outcome" after below-knee amputation: an objective definition and influence of clinical variables. *Am J Surg.* 2008;74(7):607–612.
20. Jelic M, Eldar R. Rehabilitation following major traumatic amputation of lower limbs—a review. *Crit Rev Phys Med Rehabil Med.* 2003;15(3/4):235–253.
21. Allison MA, Ho E, Denenberg JO, et al. Ethnic-specific prevalence of peripheral arterial disease in the United States. *Am J Prev Med.* 2007;32(4):328–333.
22. Meadows TA, Bhatt DL, Hirsch AT, et al. Ethnic differences in the prevalence and treatment of cardiovascular risk factors

in US outpatients with peripheral arterial disease: insights from the reduction of atherothrombosis for continued health (REACH) registry. *Am Heart J.* 2009;158(6):1038–1045.

23. Ostchega Y, Paulose-Ram R, Dillon CF, et al. Prevalence of peripheral arterial disease and risk factors in persons aged 60 and older: data from the National Health and Nutrition Examination Survey 1999–2004. *J Am Geriatr Soc.* 2007; 55(4):583–589.

24. Aronow WS, Ahmed MI, Ekundayo OJ, et al. A propensity-matched study of the association of peripheral arterial disease with cardiovascular outcomes in community-dwelling older adults. *Am J Cardiol.* 2009;103(1):130–135.

25. Gregg EW, Sorlie P, Paulose-Ram R, et al. Prevalence of lower-extremity disease in the U.S. adult population ≥40 years of age with and without diabetes. *Diabetes Care.* 2004;27(7):1591–1597.

26. Bates B, Stineman MG, Reker DM, et al. Risk factors associated with mortality in veteran population following transtibial or transfemoral amputation. *J Rehabil Res Dev.* 2006; 43(7):917–928.

27. Jaff MR, Cahill KE, Yu AP, et al. Clinical outcomes and medical care costs among medicare beneficiaries receiving therapy for peripheral arterial disease. *Ann Vasc Surg.* 2010;24(5):577–587.

28. Regensteiner JG, Hiatt WR, Coll JR, et al. The impact of peripheral arterial disease on health-related quality of life in the Peripheral Arterial Disease Awareness, Risk, and Treatment: New Resources for Survival (PARTNERS) Program. *Vasc Med.* 2008;13(1):15–24.

29. Bahebeck J, Sobgui E, Loic F, et al. Limb-threatening and life-threatening diabetic extremities: clinical patterns and outcomes in 56 patients. *J Foot Ankle Surg.* 2010;49(1):43–46.

30. Harrison DK, Hawthorn IE. Amputation level viability in critical limb ischaemia: setting new standards. *Adv Exp Med Biol.* 2005;566:325–331.

31. Debus ES, Lohrenz C, Diener H, et al. Surgical reconstructions in peripheral arterial occlusive disease. *Vasa.* 2009; 38(4):317–333.

32. Goodney PP, Beck AW, Nagle J, et al. National trends in lower extremity bypass surgery, endovascular interventions, and major amputations. *J Vasc Surg.* 2009;50(1):54–60.

33. van den Berg JC. Thrombolysis for acute arterial occlusion. *J Vasc Surg.* 2010;52(2):512–515.

34. Lawall H, Bramlage P, Amann B. Treatment of peripheral arterial disease using stem and progenitor cell therapy. *J Vasc Surg.* 2011;53(2):445–453.

35. Sprengers RW, Moll FL, Verhaar MC. Stem cell therapy in PAD. *Eur J Vasc Endovasc Surg.* 2010;39(suppl 1):S38–S43.

36. Cavanagh PR, Bus SA. Off-loading the diabetic foot for ulcer prevention and healing. *J Vasc Surg.* 2010;52(3 suppl): 37S–43S.

37. Löndahl M, Katzman P, Nilsson A, et al. Hyperbaric oxygen therapy facilitates healing of chronic foot ulcers in patients with diabetes. *Diabetes Care.* 2010;33(5):998–1003.

38. Noble-Bell G, Forbes A. A systematic review of the effectiveness of negative pressure wound therapy in the management of diabetes foot ulcers. *Int Wound J.* 2008;5(2):233–242.

39. Kosinski MA, Lipsky BA. Current medical management of diabetic foot infections. *Expert Rev Anti Infect Ther.* 2010; 8(11):1293–1305.

40. Kanade RV, van Deursen RW, Price P, Harding K. Risk of plantar ulceration in diabetic patients with single-leg amputation. *Clin Biomech (Bristol, Avon).* 2006;21(3):306–313.

41. Smith DG, Assal M, Reiber GE, et al. Minor environmental trauma and lower extremity amputation in high-risk patients with diabetes: incidence, pivotal events, etiology, and amputation level in a prospectively followed cohort. *Foot Ankle Int.* 2003;24(9):690–695.

42. Armstrong DW, Tobin C, Matangi MF. The accuracy of the physical examination for the detection of lower extremity peripheral arterial disease. *Can J Cardiol.* 2010;26(10):346–350.

43. Abul-Khoudoud O. Diagnosis and risk assessment of lower extremity peripheral arterial disease. *J Endovasc Ther.* 2006; 13(suppl 2):II10–II18.

44. Ferreira AC, Macedo FY. A review of simple, non-invasive means of assessing peripheral arterial disease and implications for medical management. *Ann Med.* 2010;42(2):139–150.

45. Bueno A, Acín F, Cañibano C, et al. Diagnostic accuracy of contrast-enhanced magnetic resonance angiography and duplex ultrasound in patients with peripheral vascular disease. *Vasc Endovascular Surg.* 2010;44(7):576–585.

46. Nielsen YW, Eiberg JP, Løgager VB, et al. Whole-body magnetic resonance angiography with additional steady-state acquisition of the infragenicular arteries in patients with peripheral arterial disease. *Cardiovasc Intervent Radiol.* 2010;33(3):484–491.

47. Falconer TM, Eikelboom JW, Hankey GJ, Norman PE. Management of peripheral arterial disease in the elderly: focus on cilostazol. *Clin Interv Aging.* 2008;3(1):17–23.

48. Fontain R, Bubost C, eds. *Les Greffes Vascularies.* Paris: Brodard et Taupin; 1954.

49. Norgren L, Hiatt WR, Dormandy JA, et al. Inter-Society Consensus for the Management of Peripheral Arterial Disease (TASC II). *J Vasc Surg.* 2007;45(suppl S):S5–S67.

50. Myers SA, Johanning JM, Stergiou N, et al. Claudication distances and the Walking Impairment Questionnaire best describe the ambulatory limitations in patients with symptomatic peripheral arterial disease. *J Vasc Surg.* 2008;47(3):550–555.

51. Dormandy JA, Rutherford RB. Management of peripheral arterial disease (PAD). TASC Working Group. TransAtlantic Inter-Society Consensus (TASC). *J Vasc Surg.* 2000;31(1 Pt 2):S1–S296.

52. McCulloch JM, Kloth L, eds. *Wound Healing: Evidence-Based Management.* 4th ed. Philadelphia: Davis; 2010.

53. Bus SA, Maas M, de Lange A, et al. Elevated plantar pressures in neuropathic diabetic patients with claw/hammer toe deformity. *J Biomech.* 2005;38(9):1918–1925.

54. Feng Y, Schlösser FJ, Sumpio BE. The Semmes Weinstein monofilament examination as a screening tool for diabetic peripheral neuropathy. *J Vasc Surg.* 2009;50(3):675–682.

55. Gandhi RA, Marques JL, Selvarajah D, et al. Painful diabetic neuropathy is associated with greater autonomic dysfunction than painless diabetic neuropathy. *Diabetes Care.* 2010;33(7):1585–1590.

56. Botek G, Anderson MA, Taylor R. Charcot neuroarthropathy: An often overlooked complication of diabetes. *Cleve Clin J Med.* 2010;77(9):593–599.

57. Cournot M, Boccalon H, Cambou JP. Accuracy of the screening physical examination to identify subclinical atherosclerosis and peripheral arterial disease in asymptomatic subjects. *J Vasc Surg.* 2007;46(6):1215–1221.

58. Andersen CA. Noninvasive assessment of lower extremity hemodynamics in individuals with diabetes mellitus. *J Vasc Surg.* 2010;52(3 suppl):76S–80S.

59. Eiberg JP, Grønvall Rasmussen JB, Hansen MA, Schroeder TV. Duplex ultrasound scanning of peripheral arterial disease of the lower limb. *Eur J Vasc Endovasc Surg.* 2010;40(4):507–512.

60. Ziegler RE, ed. *Strandness's Duplex Scanning in Vascular Disorders.* 4th ed. Philadelphia: Lippincott Williams & Wilkins; 2009.

61. Baker JD. The vascular laboratory. In: Moore WS, ed. *Vascular Surgery: A Comprehensive Review.* 6th ed. Philadelphia: Saunders; 2002:235–250.

62. Kaufman JA. Vascular imaging with x-ray, magnetic resonance, and computed tomography angiography. In: Coffman JD, Eberhardt RT, eds. *Peripheral Arterial Disease Diagnosis and Treatment.* Totowa, NJ: Humana Press; 2002:75–92.

63. Chan D, Anderson ME, Dolmatch BL. Imaging evaluation of lower extremity infrainguinal disease: role of the noninvasive vascular laboratory, computed tomography angiography, and magnetic resonance angiography. *Tech Vasc Interv Radiol.* 2010;13(1):11–22.

64. Menke J, Larsen J. Meta-analysis: Accuracy of contrast-enhanced magnetic resonance angiography for assessing steno-occlusions in peripheral arterial disease. *Ann Intern Med.* 2010;153(5):325–334.

65. Met R, Bipat S, Legemate DA, et al. Diagnostic performance of computed tomography angiography in peripheral arterial disease: a systematic review and meta-analysis. *JAMA.* 2009;301(4):415–424.

66. Weadock WJ, Chenevert TL. *Emerging Concepts in MR Angiography, An Issue of Magnetic Resonance Imaging Clinics.* Philadelphia: Saunders; 2009.

67. Flieshman D, Hellinger JC, Nappolli A. Multidetector-row CT angiography of peripheral arteries: imaging upper and lower extremity vascular disease. In: Passariello R, Baert AL, eds. *Multidetector-Row CT Angiography.* New York: Springer; 2005:187–198.

68. Pomposelli F. Arterial imaging in patients with lower extremity ischemia and diabetes mellitus. *J Vasc Surg.* 2010;52 (3 suppl):81S–91S.

69. Mills JL. Surgical treatment. In: Cronenwett JL, Johnson W, eds. *Rutherfords's Vascular Surgery.* 7th ed. New York: Saunders; 2010:1682–1703.

70. Sadek M, Farles PL. Endovascular treatment. In: Cronenwett JL, Johnson W, eds. *Rutherfords's Vascular Surgery.* 7th ed. New York: Saunders; 2010:1704–1719.

71. Byrne J. Etiology and natural history: diagnosis and evaluation. In: Hallett JW, Mills JL, eds. *Comprehensive Vascular and Endovascular Surgery.* St. Louis: Mosby; 2009:243–260.

72. Agle SC, McNally MM, Powell CS, et al. The association of periprocedural hypertension and adverse outcomes in patients undergoing catheter-directed thrombolysis. *Ann Vasc Surg.* 2010;24(5):609–614.

73. Hodgson KJ, Hood DB. Endovascular diagnostic. In: Cronenwett JL, Johnson W, eds. *Rutherfords's Vascular Surgery.* 7th ed. New York: Saunders; 2010:1262–1276.

74. Working Party on Thrombolysis in the Management of Limb Ischemia. Thrombolysis in the management of lower limb peripheral arterial occlusion—a consensus document. *J Vasc Interv Radiol.* 2003;14(9 Pt 2):S337–S349.

75. Giannini D, Balbarini A. Thrombolytic therapy in peripheral arterial disease. *Curr Drug Targets Cardiovasc Haematol Disord.* 2004;4(3):249–258.

76. Lyden SP. Endovascular treatment of acute limb ischemia: review of current plasminogen activators and mechanical thrombectomy devices. *Perspect Vasc Surg Endovasc Ther.* 2010;22(4):219–222.

77. Robertson I, Kessel DO, Berridge DC. Fibrinolytic agents for peripheral arterial occlusion. *Cochrane Database Syst Rev.* 2010;Mar 17;(3): CD001099.

78. Kim CK, Schmalfuss CM, Schfield RS, et al. Pharmacological treatment of patients with peripheral arterial disease. *Drugs.* 2003;63(7):637–647.

79. Dorffler-Melly, Koopman MM, Prins MH, et al. Antiplatelets and anticoagulant drugs for prevention of restenosis/reocclusion following peripheral endovascular treatment. *Cochrane Database Syst Rev.* 2005;(1). Cochrane AN:CD002071.

80. Rasmussen TE, Clouse WD, Tonnessen GH. *Handbook of Patient Care in Vascular Diseases.* Philadelphia: Wolters-Kluwer; 2008.

81. Barmparas G, Inaba K, Teixeira PG, et al. Epidemiology of post-traumatic limb amputation: a National Trauma Databank analysis. *Am Surg.* 2010;76(11):1214–1222.

82. Stansbury LG, Lalliss SJ, Branstetter JG, et al. Amputations in US military personnel in the current conflicts in Afghanistan and Iraq. *J Orthop Trauma.* 2008;22(1):43–46.

83. Tintle LS, Keeling CJ, Shawen LS, et al. Traumatic and trauma-related amputations: part I: general principles and lower-extremity amputations. *J Bone Joint Surg.* 2010;92(17):2852–2868.

84. Armstrong MB. *Lower Extremity Trauma.* New York: Informa Healthcare; 2006.

85. Shawen SB, Keeling JJ, Branstetter J, et al. The mangled foot and leg: salvage versus amputation. *Foot Ankle Clin.* 2010;15(1):63–75.

86. Durrant CA, Mackey SP. Orthoplastic classification systems: the good, the bad, and the ungainly. *Ann Plast Surg.* 2011;66(1):9–12.

87. Higgins TF, Klatt JB, Beals TC. Lower Extremity Assessment Project (LEAP)—the best available evidence on limb-threatening lower extremity trauma. *Orthop Clin North Am.* 2010; 41(2):233–239.

88. MacKenzie EJ, Jones AS, Bosse MJ, et al. Health-care costs associated with amputation or reconstruction of a limb-threatening injury. *J Bone Joint Surg Am.* 2007;89(8):1685–1692.

89. MacKenzie EJ, Bosse MJ. Factors influencing outcome following limb-threatening lower limb trauma: lessons learned from the Lower Extremity Assessment Project (LEAP). *J Am Acad Orthop Surg.* 2006;14(10 Spec No.):S205–S210.

90. Archer KR, Castillo RC, MacKenzie EJ, et al. Gait symmetry and walking speed analysis following lower extremity trauma. *Phys Ther.* 2006;86(12):1630–1640.

91. Harris AM, Althausen PL, Bosse MJ, et al. Complications following limb-threatening lower extremity trauma. *J Orthop Trauma.* 2009;23(1):1–6.

92. Chung KC, Shauver MJ, Saddawi-Konefka D, et al. A decision analysis of amputation versus reconstruction for severe open tibial fracture from the physician and patient perspectives. *Ann Plast Surg.* 2011;66(2):185–191.

93. Lerner A, Reis D, Soudry M, eds. *Severe Injuries to the Limbs: Staged Treatment.* Berlin, Germany: Springer Verlag; 2007.

94. Archdeacon MT, Saunders R. Trauma: limb salvage versus amputation. In: Smith DG, Michael JW, Bowker JH, eds. *Atlas of Amputation and Limb Deficiencies.* 3rd ed. Rosemont, IL: American Academy of Orthopaedic Surgeons; 2005:69–75.

95. Reiber GE, McFarland LV, Hubbard S, et al. Service members and veterans with major traumatic limb loss from Vietnam War and OIF/OEF conflicts: survey methods, participants, and summary findings. *J Rehabil Res Dev.* 2010;47(4):275–298.

96. Mnaymneh W, Temple HT. Tumor: limb salvage versus amputation. In: Smith DG, Michael JW, Bowker JH, eds. *Atlas of Amputation and Limb Deficiencies.* 3rd ed. Rosemont, IL: American Academy of Orthopaedic Surgeons; 2005:55–67.

97. Khurana JC, McCarthy EF. Tumors and tumor-like lesions of bone. In: Khurana JS, McCarthy EF, Zhang PJ, eds. *Essentials in Bone and Soft Tissue Pathology.* New York: Springer; 2010:69–158.

98. Mirabello L, Troisi RJ, Savage SA. Osteosarcoma incidence and survival rates from 1973 to 2004: data from the Surveillance, Epidemiology, and End Results Program. *Cancer.* 2009;115(7):1531–1543.

99. Coleman RE. Clinical features of metastatic bone disease and risk of skeletal morbidity. *Clin Cancer Res.* 2006;12(20 Pt 2):6243s–6249s.

100. Nakashima Y. Metastasis involving bone. In: Folpe AL, Inwards CY, eds. *Bone and Soft Tissue Pathology.* Philadelphia: Saunders; 2010:446–454.

101. Major P. Optimal management of metastatic bone disease. *Eur J Oncol Nurs.* 2007;11(suppl 2):S32–S37.

102. Mortimer JE, Schulman K, Kohles JD. Patterns of bisphosphonate use in the United States in the treatment of metastatic bone disease. *Clin Breast Cancer.* 2007;7(9):682–689.

103. Trinkaus M, Simmons C, Myers J, et al. Skeletal-related events (SREs) in breast cancer patients with bone metastases treated in the non-trial setting. *Support Care Cancer.* 2010;18(2):197–203.

104. Nakashima H, Katagiri H, Takahashi M, et al. Survival and ambulatory function after endoprosthetic replacement for metastatic bone tumor of the proximal femur. *Nagoya J Med Sci.* 2010;72(1–2):13–21.

105. Davidson AW, Hong A, McCarthy SW, et al. En-bloc resection, extracorporeal irradiation, and re-implantation in limb salvage for bony malignancies. *J Bone Joint Surg Br.* 2005;87(6):851–857.

106. Jeys LM, Kulkarni A, Grimer RJ, et al. Endoprosthetic reconstruction for the treatment of musculoskeletal tumors of the appendicular skeleton and pelvis. *J Bone Joint Surg Am.* 2008;90A(6):1265–1271.

107. Muscolo DL, Ayerza MA, Aponte-Tinao LA, et al. Use of distal femoral osteoarticular allografts in limb salvage surgery. Surgical technique. *J Bone Joint Surg Am.* 2006;88(suppl 1 Pt 2):305–321.

108. Ebeid W, Amin S, Abdelmegid A. Limb salvage management of pathologic fractures of primary malignant bone tumors. *Cancer Control.* 2005;12(1):57–61.

109. Puri A, Agarwal M. Facilitating rotationplasty. *J Surg Oncol.* 2007;95(4):351–354.

110. Lahl M, Fisher VL, Lashinger K. Ewing's sarcoma family of tumors: an overview from diagnosis to survivorship. *Clin J Oncol Nurs.* 2008;12(1):89–97.

111. Papageloupoulos PJ, Mavrogenis AF, Savvidou OD, et al. Pathological fractures in primary bone sarcomas. *Injury.* 2008;39(4):395–403.

112. Scully SP, Ghert MA, Zurakowski D, et al. Pathologic fracture in osteosarcoma: prognostic importance and treatment implications. *J Bone Joint Surg Am.* 2002;84-A(1):49–57.

113. Bacci G, Balladelli A, Palmerini E, et al. Neoadjuvant chemotherapy for osteosarcoma of the extremities in preadolescent patients: the Rizzoli Institute experience. *J Pediatr Hematol Oncol.* 2008;30(12):908–912.

114. Lietman SA, Joyce MJ. Bone sarcomas: overview of management, with a focus on surgical treatment considerations. *Cleve Clin J Med.* 2010;77(suppl 1):S8–S12.

115. Yasko AW. Surgical management of primary osteosarcoma. *Cancer Treat Res.* 2009;152:125–145.

116. Graci C, Maccauro G, Muratori F, et al. Infection following bone tumor resection and reconstruction with tumoral prostheses: a literature review. *Int J Immunopathol Pharmacol.* 2010;23(4):1005–1013.

117. Ottaviani G, Robert RS, Huh WW, et al. Functional, psychosocial and professional outcomes in long-term survivors of lower-extremity osteosarcomas: amputation versus limb salvage. *Cancer Treat Res.* 2009;152:421–436.

118. Bekkering WP, Vliet Vlieland TP, Koopman HM, et al. Functional ability and physical activity in children and young adults after limb-salvage or ablative surgery for lower extremity bone tumors. *J Surg Oncol* 2011;103(3):276–282.

119. Bekkering WP, Vliet Vlieland TP, Koopman HM, et al. Quality of life in young patients after bone tumor surgery around the knee joint and comparison with healthy controls. *Pediatr Blood Cancer.* 2010;54(5):738–745.

120. Davies AM, Sundraram M, James SJ, eds. *Imaging of Bone Tumors and Tumor-Like Lesions: Techniques and Application.* Berlin, Germany: Springer Verlag; 2009.

121. Ilaslan H, Schils J, Nageotte W, et al. Clinical presentation and imaging of bone and soft-tissue sarcomas. *Cleve Clin J Med.* 2010;77(suppl 1):S2–S7.

122. Raymond AK, Jaffe N. Osteosarcoma multidisciplinary approach to the management from the pathologist's perspective. *Cancer Treat Res.* 2009;152:63–84.

123. Man TK, Chintagumpala M, Visvanathan J, et al. Expression profiles of osteosarcoma that can predict response to chemotherapy. *Cancer.* 2005;65(18):8142–8150.

124. Gibbs CP, Lewis VO, Peabody T. Beyond bone grafting: techniques in the surgical management of benign bone tumors. *Instr Course Lect.* 2005;54:497–503.

125. Yamaguchi U, Honda K, Satow R, et al. Functional genome screen for therapeutic targets of osteosarcoma. *Cancer Sci.* 2009;100(12):2268–2274.

126. So TY, Lam YL, Mak KL. Computer-assisted navigation in bone tumor surgery: seamless workflow model and evolution of technique. *Clin Orthop Relat Res.* 2010;468(11):2985–2991.

127. Ruggieri P, Kasimatis G, Errani C, et al. Desarthrodesis and prosthetic reconstruction of the knee after resection of bone tumors. *J Surg Oncol.* 2010;102(7):832–837.

128. Musculoskeletal practice pattern 4J: Impaired motor function, muscle performance, range of motion. gait, locomotion and balance associated with amputation. In: *Guide to Physical Therapist Practice.* Available at: http://guidetopractice.apta.org/content.

129. Klika RJ, Golik KS, Drum SN, et al. Comparison of physiological response to cardiopulmonary exercise testing among cancer survivors and healthy controls. *Eur J Appl Physiol.* 2011;111(6):1167–1176.

130. Campos MP, Hassan BJ, Riechelmann R, et al. Cancer-related fatigue: a review. *Rev Assoc Med Bras.* 2011;57(2):211–219.

131. Ramini SK, Brown R, Buckner EB, et al. Embracing changes: adaptation by adolescents with cancer. *Pediatr Nurs.* 2008;34(1):72–79.

132. Andrews EE, Williams JL, Vandecreek L, et al. Experiences of parents of children with congenital limb differences with health care providers: a qualitative study. *Rehabil Psychol.* 2009;54(2):217–221.

133. Kahle AL. Psychological issues in pediatric limb deficiency. In: Smith DG, Michaels JW, Bowker JH, eds. *Atlas of Amputation and Limb Deficiencies. Surgical Prosthetic and Rehabilitation Principles.* 3rd ed. Rosemont, IL: American Academy of Orthopaedic Surgeons; 2004:801–812.

134. Fisk JR, Smith DG. The limb deficient child. In: Smith DG, Michaels JW, Bowker JH, eds. *Atlas of Amputation and Limb Deficiencies. Surgical Prosthetic and Rehabilitation Principles.* 3rd ed. Rosemont, IL: American Academy of Orthopaedic Surgeons; 2004:773–777.

135. Edelstein JE. Developmental kinesiology. In: Smith DG, Michaels JW, Bowker JH, eds. *Atlas of Amputation and Limb Deficiencies. Surgical Prosthetic and Rehabilitation Principles.* 3rd ed. Rosemont, IL: American Academy of Orthopaedic Surgeons; 2004:783–788.

136. Watts H. Surgical modification of residual limbs. In: Smith DG, Michaels JW, Bowker JH, eds. *Atlas of Amputation and Limb Deficiencies. Surgical Prosthetic and Rehabilitation Principles.* 3rd ed. Rosemont, IL: American Academy of Orthopaedic Surgeons; 2004:931–943.

137. Nelson VS, Flood KM, Bryant PR, et al. Limb deficiency and prosthetic management. 1. Decision making in prosthetic prescription and management. *Arch Phys Med Rehabil.* 2006;87 (3 suppl 1):S3–S9, S28–S33, S103–S105.

138. Westberry DE, Davids JR. Proximal focal femoral deficiency (PFFD): management options and controversies. *Hip Int.* 2009; 19(suppl 6):S18–S25.

139. Tellisi N, Fragomen AT, Ilizarov S, Rozbruch SR. Lengthening and reconstruction of congenital leg deficiencies for enhanced prosthetic wear. *Clin Orthop Relat Res.* 2008;466(2):495–499.

140. Courvoisier A, Sailhan F, Thevenin-Lemoine C, et al. Congenital tibial deficiencies: treatment using the Ilizarov's external fixator. *Orthop Traumatol Surg Res.* 2009;95(6):431–436.

141. Westberry DE, Davids JR. Proximal focal femoral deficiency (PFFD): management options and controversies. *Hip Int.* 2009;19(suppl 6):S18–S25.

142. Glancy GL. Fibular deficiencies. In: Smith DG, Michaels JW, Bowker JH, eds. *Atlas of Amputation and Limb Deficiencies. Surgical Prosthetic and Rehabilitation Principles.* 3rd ed. Rosemont, IL: American Academy of Orthopaedic Surgeons; 2004:889–896.

143. Schmitz ML, Biavendoin BJ, Coulter-O'Berry C. Tibial deficiencies. In: Smith DG, Michaels JW, Bowker JH, eds. *Atlas of Amputation and Limb Deficiencies. Surgical Prosthetic and Rehabilitation Principles.* 3rd ed. Rosemont, IL: American Academy of Orthopaedic Surgeons; 2004:897–904.

144. Stanitski DF, Shahcheraghi H, Nicker DA, et al. Results of tibial lengthening with the Ilizarov technique. *J Pediatr Orthop.* 2003;16(2):168–172.

145. Dudkiewicz I, Schwarz O, Heim M, et al. Trans-metatarsal amputation in patients with a diabetic foot: reviewing 10 years' experience. *Foot (Edinb).* 2009;19(4):201–204.

146. Andersen CA. Diabetic limb preservation: defining terms and goals. *J Foot Ankle Surg.* 2010;49(1):106–107.

147. Levin AZ. Functional outcome following amputation. *Top Geriatr Rehabil.* 2004;20(4):253–261.

148. Esway J, Boyer M, Shereff M, et al. Lisfranc injuries: what have we learned since Napoleon's era. *Oper Tech Orthop.* 2006;16(1):60–67.

149. Condie DN, Bowers R. Amputations and disarticulations within the foot: prosthetic management. In: Smith DG, Michaels JW, Bowker JH, eds. *Atlas of Amputation and Limb Deficiencies. Surgical Prosthetic and Rehabilitation Principles.* 3rd ed. Rosemont, IL: American Academy of Orthopaedic Surgeons; 2004:449–457.

150. Carlson T, Reed JF. A case-control study of the risk factors for toe amputation in a diabetic population. *Int J Low Extrem Wounds.* 2003;2(1):19–21.

151. Caputo WJ. Surgical management of the diabetic foot. *Wounds.* 2008;20(3):74–83.

152. Barnes RW, Cox B. Toe amputation: phalangectomy and transmetatarsal. In: *Amputations: An Illustrated Manual.* Hanley & Belfus: Philadelphia; 2000:15–26.

153. Bowker JH. Amputations and disarticulations within the foot: surgical management. In: Smith DG, Michaels JW, Bowker JH, eds. *Atlas of Amputation and Limb Deficiencies. Surgical Prosthetic and Rehabilitation Principles.* 3rd ed. Rosemont, IL: American Academy of Orthopaedic Surgeons; 2004:429–448.

154. Laborde JM. Neuropathic plantar forefoot ulcers treated with tendon lengthenings. *Foot Ankle Int.* 2008;29(4):378–384.

155. Mueller MJ, Lott DJ, Hastings MK, et al. Efficacy and mechanism of orthotic devices to unload metatarsal heads in people with diabetes and a history of plantar ulcers. *Phys Ther.* 2006;86(6):833–842.

156. Roukis TS. Minimum-incision metatarsal ray resection: an observational case series. *J Foot Ankle Surg.* 2010;49(1):52–54.

157. Oznur A, Roukis TS. Minimum-incision ray resection. *Clin Podiatr Med Surg.* 2008;25(4):609–622.

158. Paola LD, Faglia E, Caminiti M, et al. Ulcer recurrence following first ray amputation in diabetic patients: a cohort prospective study. *Diabetes Care.* 2003;26(6):1874–1878.

159. Roukis TS, Singh N, Andersen CA. Preserving functional capacity as opposed to tissue preservation in the diabetic patient: a single institution experience. *Foot Ankle Spec.* 2010; 3(4):177–183.

160. Mwipatayi BP, Naidoo NG, Jeffery PC, et al. Transmetatarsal amputation: three-year experience at Groote Schuur Hospital. *World J Surg.* 2005;29(2):245–248.

161. Pollard J, Hamilton GA, Rush SM, Ford LA. Mortality and morbidity after transmetatarsal amputation: retrospective review of 101 cases. *J Foot Ankle Surg.* 2006;45(2):91–97.

162. Anthony T, Roberts J, Modrall JG, et al. Transmetatarsal amputation: assessment of current selection criteria. *Am J Surg.* 2006;192(5):e8–e11.

163. Attinger CE, Meyr AJ, Fitzgerald S, et al. Preoperative Doppler assessment for transmetatarsal amputation. *J Foot Ankle Surg.* 2010;49(1):101–105.

164. Krause FG, deVries G, Meakin C, et al. Outcome of transmetatarsal amputations in diabetics using antibiotic beads. *Foot Ankle Int.* 2009;30(6):486–493.

165. Schweinberger MH, Roukis TS, Schweinberger MH, et al. Balancing of the transmetatarsal amputation with peroneus brevis to peroneus longus tendon transfer. *J Foot Ankle Surg.* 2007;46(6):510–514.

166. Roukis TS. Flexor hallucis longus and extensor digitorum longus tendon transfers for balancing the foot following transmetatarsal amputation. *J Foot Ankle Surg.* 2009;48(3):398–401.

167. Schweinberger MH, Roukis TS. Intramedullary screw fixation for balancing of the dysvascular foot following transmetatarsal amputation. *J Foot Ankle Surg.* 2008;47(6):594–597.

168. La Fontaine J, Brown D, Adams M, et al. New and recurrent ulcerations after percutaneous Achilles tendon lengthening in transmetatarsal amputation. *J Foot Ankle Surg.* 2008;47(3):225–229.

169. Bowker JH, San Giovanni TP. Amputations and disarticulations. In: Myerson MS, ed. *Foot and Ankle Disorders.* Philadelphia: Saunders; 2000:466–503.

170. Roukis TS, Singh N, Andersen CA. Preserving functional capacity as opposed to tissue preservation in the diabetic patient: a single institution experience. *Foot Ankle Spec.* 2010;3(4):177–183.

171. Condie DN, Bowers R. Amputations and disarticulations within the foot; prosthetic management. In: Smith DG, Michaels JW, Bowker JH, eds. *Atlas of Amputation and Limb Deficiencies. Surgical Prosthetic and Rehabilitation Principles.* 3rd ed. Rosemont, IL: American Academy of Orthopaedic Surgeons; 2004:449–457.

172. Marks RM, Long JT. Exten EL Gait abnormality following amputation in diabetic patients. *Foot Ankle Clin.* 2010;15(3):501–507.

173. Barnes RW, Cox B. Syme amputation. In: *Amputations: An Illustrated Manual*. Philadelphia: Hanley & Belfus; 2000:49–66.

174. Frykberg RG, Abraham S, Tierney E, et al. Syme amputation for limb salvage: early experience with 26 cases. *J Foot Ankle Surg*. 2007;46(2):93–100.

175. Siev-Ner I, Heim M, Warshavski M, et al. A review of the aetiological factors and results of trans-ankle (Syme) disarticulations. *Disabil Rehabil*. 2006;28(4):239–242.

176. Ebrahimzadeh MH, Hariri S. Long-term outcomes of unilateral transtibial amputations. *Mil Med*. 2009;174(6):593–597.

177. Johannesson A, Larsson GU, Ramstrand N, et al. Outcomes of a standardized surgical and rehabilitation program in transtibial amputation for peripheral vascular disease: a prospective cohort study. *Am J Phys Med Rehabil*. 2010;89(4):293–303.

178. Bowker JH. Transtibial amputation: surgical management. In: Smith DG, Michaels JW, Bowker JH, eds. *Atlas of Amputation and Limb Deficiencies. Surgical Prosthetic and Rehabilitation Principles*. 3rd ed. Rosemont, IL: American Academy of Orthopaedic Surgeons; 2004:481–501.

179. Arwert HJ, van Doorn-Loogman MH, Koning J, et al. Residual-limb quality and functional mobility 1 year after transtibial amputation caused by vascular insufficiency. *J Rehabil Res Dev*. 2007;44(5):717–722.

180. Chuah KH, Thong CL, Krshnan H, Chan L. Low dose unilateral spinal anaesthesia for lower limb amputation in critically ill patients. *Med J Malaysia*. 2007;62(1):81–82.

181. Ong BY, Arneja A, Ong EW. Effects of anesthesia on pain after lower-limb amputation. *J Clin Anesth*. 2006;18(8):600–604.

182. Assal M, Blanck R, Smith DG. Extended posterior flap for transtibial amputation. *Orthopedics*. 2005;28(6):542–546.

183. Bruckner L. A standardized transtibial amputation method following chronic occlusive arterial disease. *Prosthet Orthot Int*. 1992;16:157–162.

184. Yurttas Y, Kurklu M, Demiralp B, Atesalp A. A novel technique for transtibial amputation in chronic occlusive arterial disease: modified Burgess procedure. *Prosthet Orthot Int*. 2009;33(1):25–32.

185. Tintle SM, Keeling JJ, Forsberg JA, et al. Operative complications of combat-related transtibial amputations: a comparison of the modified burgess and modified Ertl tibiofibular synostosis techniques. *J Bone Joint Surg Am*. 2011;93(11):1016–1021.

186. Deol PS, Lee TH, Berlet GC. Evolution and modification of the Ertl osteomyoplastic transtibial amputation. *Oper Tech Orthop*. 2008;18(4):293–298.

187. Anderson CD, Stewart JD, Unger DV. Recent advances in lower extremity amputations. *Curr Opin Orthop*. 2007;18:137–144.

188. Tisi PV, Callam MJ. Type of incision for below knee amputation. *Cochrane Database Syst Rev*. 2004:CD003749.pub2.

189. Jain SK. Skew flap technique in trans-tibial amputation. *Prosthet Orthot Int*. 2005;29(3):283–290.

190. Choksy SA, Chong PL, Smith C, et al. A randomised controlled trial of the use of a tourniquet to reduce blood loss during transtibial amputation for peripheral arterial disease. *Eur J Vasc Endovasc Surg*. 2006;31:646–650.

191. Heck RK, Carnesale PG. General principles of amputations. In: Canale ST, ed. *Campbell's Operative Orthopedics*. 10th ed. St. Louis: Mosby; 2003:537–554.

192. Carnesale PG. Amputations of lower extremity. In: Canale ST, ed. *Campbell's Operative Orthopedics*. 10th ed. St. Louis: Mosby; 2003:575–586.

193. Rasmussen S, Kehlet H. Management of nerves during leg amputation—a neglected area in our understanding of the pathogenesis of phantom limb pain. *Acta Anaesthesiol Scand*. 2007;51(8):1115–1116.

194. Stahel PF, Oberholzer A, Morgan SJ, et al. Concepts of transtibial amputation: modified burgess technique versus modified Bruckner procedure. *ANZ J Surg*. 2006;76(10):942–946.

195. DeCoster TA, Homedan S. Amputation osteoplasty. *Iowa Orthop J*. 2006;26:54–59.

196. Stewart JD, Anderson CD, Unger DV. The Portsmouth modification of the Ertl bone-bridge transtibial amputation: the challenge of returning amputees back to active duty. *Oper Tech Sports Med*. 2006;13:222–226.

197. Taylor BC, French B, Poka A, et al. Osteomyoplastic and traditional transtibial amputations in the trauma patient: perioperative comparisons and outcomes. *Orthopedics*. 2010; 33(6):390.

198. Granata JD, Philbin TM. Distal tibiofibular bone bridging in transtibial amputation. *Curr Orthop Pract*. 2010;21(3):264–267.

199. Segal LS, Crandal RC. Tibial vara deformity after below knee amputation and syntosis formation in children. *J Pediatr Orthop*. 2009;29:120–123.

200. Pinzur MS. Knee disarticulation: surgical management. In: Smith DG, Michaels JW, Bowker JH, eds. *Atlas of Amputation and Limb Deficiencies. Surgical Prosthetic and Rehabilitation Principles*. 3rd ed. Rosemont, IL: American Academy of Orthopaedic Surgeons; 2004:517–523.

201. Kauzlaric N, Kauzlaric KS, Kolundzic R. Prosthetic rehabilitation of persons with lower limb amputations due to tumour. *Eur J Cancer Care (Engl)*. 2007;16(3):238–243.

202. Ziewner I, Heim M, Wershavski M, et al. Why knee disarticulation (through knee amputation) is appropriate for nonambulatory patients. *Disabil Rehabil*. 2000;22(18):862–864.

203. Mazet R, Hennessy CA. Knee disarticulation: a new technique and a new knee joint mechanism. *J Bone Joint Surg Am*. 1966;48(1):129–139.

204. Burgess EM. Disarticulation of the knee: a modified technique. *Arch Surg*. 1977;112(10):1250–1255.

205. Pinzur MS, Bowker JH. Knee disarticulation. *Clin Orthop Relat Res*. 1999;361:23–28.

206. Duerksen F, Rogalsky RJ, Cochrane IW. Knee disarticulation with intercondylar patello-femoral arthrodesis, an improved technique. *Clin Orthop*. 1990;256:50–56.

207. Bowker JH, San Giovanni PT, Pinsur MS. North American experience with knee disarticulation with the use of a posterior myofasciocutaneous flap: healing rate and functional results in 77 patients. *J Bone Joint Surg Am*. 2000;82(11):1571–1574.

208. Barnes RW, Cox B. Through-knee amputation (knee disarticulation). In: *Amputations: An Illustrated Manual*. Philadelphia: Hanley & Belfus; 2000:87–102.

209. Jensen JS. Surgical techniques of knee disarticulation and femoral transcondylar amputation. In: Murdock G, Wilson AB, eds. *Amputation: Surgical Practice and Patient Management*. Oxford, UK: Butterworth-Heinemann; 1996:127–134.

210. Yip VS, Teoi NB, Johnstone F, et al. An analysis of risk factors associated with failure of below knee amputations. *World J Surg*. 2006;30:1081–1087.

211. Van Niekirk LJ, Steward CP, Jain AS. Major lower extremity amputation following failed infrainguinal vascular bypass study, a prospective study on amputation levels and stump complications. *Prosthet Orthot Int*. 2001;25(1):29–33.

212. Gottschalk F. Traumatic amputation. In: Bucholz RW, Heckman JD, eds. *Rockwood and Green's Fractures in Adults*. 5th ed. Philadelphia: Lippincott Williams & Wilkins; 2001:391–414.

213. Fedorka CJ, Chen AF, McGarry WM, et al. Functional ability after above-the-knee amputation for infected total knee arthroplasty. *Clin Orthop Relat Res.* 2011;469(4):1024–1032.

214. Gottschalk F. Transfemoral amputation, surgical management. In: Smith DG, Michaels JW, Bowker JH, eds. *Atlas of Amputation and Limb Deficiencies. Surgical Prosthetic and Rehabilitation Principles.* 3rd ed. Rosemont, IL: American Academy of Orthopaedic Surgeons; 2004:533–540.

215. Subramaniam B, Pomposelli F, Talmor D, et al. Perioperative and long-term morbidity and mortality after above-knee and below-knee amputations in diabetics and nondiabetics. *Anesth Analg.* 2005;100(5):1241–1247.

216. Remes L, Isoaho R, Vahlberg T, et al. Major lower extremity amputation in elderly patients with peripheral arterial disease: incidence and survival rates. *Aging Clin Exp Res.* 2008;20(5):385–393.

217. Gottschalk FA, Stills M. The biomechanics of transfemoral amputation. *Prosthet Orthot Int.* 1994;18(1):12–17.

218. Majeski J. Supracondylar amputation of the femur. *Am Surg.* 2004;70(3):265–267.

219. Jaegers SM, Arendzen JH, deJongh HJ. Changes in hip muscles after above knee amputation. *Clin Orthop.* 1995;Oct.(319):278–284.

220. Jaegers SM, Arendzen JH, deJongh JH. Prosthetic gait of unilateral transfemoral amputees: a kinematic study. *Arch Phys Med Rehabil.* 1995;76(8):736–743.

221. Met R, Janssen LI, Ville J, et al. Functional results after through knee and above knee amputations: does more length mean better outcome? *Vasc Endovascular Surg.* 2008;42(5):456–461.

222. Barnes RW, Cox B. Above-knee amputation. In: *Amputations: An Illustrated Manual.* Philadelphia: Hanley & Belfus; 2000:103–117.

223. Branemark R, Branemark PI, Rydevick B, et al. Osseointegration in skeletal reconstruction and rehabilitation: a review. *J Rehabil Res Dev.* 2001;38:175–181.

224. Hagberg K, Branemakr R. One hundred patients treated with osseointegrated transfemoral amputation prostheses-rehabilitation perspective. *J Rehabil Res Dev.* 2009;46(3):331–344.

225. Lundberg M, Hagberg K, Bullington J. My prosthesis as a part of me: a qualitative analysis of living with an osseointegrated prosthetic limb. *Prosthet Orthot Int.* 2011;35(2):207–214.

226. Tomaszewski PK, Verdonschot N, Bulstra SK, et al. A comparative finite-element analysis of bone failure and load transfer of osseointegrated prostheses fixations. *Ann Biomed Eng.* 2010;38(7):2418–2427.

227. Tillander J, Hagberg K, Hagberg L, et al. Osseointegrated titanium implants for limb prostheses attachments: infectious complications. *Clin Orthop Relat Res.* 2010;468(10):2781–2788.

228. Hadberg K, Branemark R, Guterberg G, et al. Osseointegrated transfemoral prosthesis: prospective results of general and condition-specific quality of life in 18 patients at 2 year follow-up. *Prosthet Orthot Int.* 2008;32(1):29–41.

229. Frossard L, Hagberg K, Haggstrom E, et al. Functional outcome of transfemoral amputees fitted with an osseointegrated fixation: temporal gait characteristics. *J Prosthet Orthot.* 2010;22(1):11–20.

230. Sullivan J, Uden M, Robinson KP, et al. Rehabilitation of the transfemoral amputee with an osseointegrated prosthesis: the United Kingdom Experience. *Prosthet Orthot Int.* 2003;27:114–120.

231. Robinson KP, Branemark R, Ward D. Future developments; osseointegration in transfemoral amputees. In: Smith DG, Michael JW, Bowker JH, eds. *Atlas of Amputations and Limb Deficiencies: Surgical, Prosthetic, and Rehabilitation Principles.* 3rd ed. Rosemont, IL: American Academy of Orthopaedic Surgeons; 2004:673–681.

232. Aschoffm HH, Kennon RE, Keggi JM, et al. Transcutaneous, distal femoral intramedullary attachment for above-the-knee prostheses: an endo-exo device. *J Bone Joint Surg.* 2010;92A(suppl 2):180–186.

233. Zalavras CG, Rigopoulos N, Ahlmann E, et al. Hip disarticulation for severe lower extremity infections. *Clin Orthop Rel Res.* 2009;467(7):1721–1726.

234. Correa GI, Calderón WO, Burnier LA, et al. Proximal amputation of inferior extremity secondary to recurrent pressure ulcers in patients with spinal cord injuries. *Spinal Cord.* 2008;46(2):135–139.

235. Daigeler A, Lehnhardt M, Khadra A, et al. Proximal major limb amputations—a retrospective analysis of 45 oncological cases. *World J Surg Oncol.* 2009;7:15.

236. Schnall BL, Baum BS, Andrews AM. Gait characteristics of a soldier with a traumatic hip disarticulation. *Phys Ther.* 2008;88(12):1568–1577.

237. in SJ, Oliver CW, Kaufman MH. Hip disarticulation-the evolution of a surgical technique. *Injury.* 2004;35(3):299–308.

238. Chansky HA. Hip disarticulation and transpelvic amputation: surgical management. In: Smith DG, Michaels JW, Bowker JH, eds. *Atlas of Amputation and Limb Deficiencies. Surgical Prosthetic and Rehabilitation Principles.* 3rd ed. Rosemont, IL: American Academy of Orthopaedic Surgeons; 2004:557–564.

239. Carroll KM. Hip disarticulation and transpelvic amputation: prosthetic management. In: Smith DG, Michaels JW, Bowker JH, eds. *Atlas of Amputation and Limb Deficiencies. Surgical Prosthetic and Rehabilitation Principles.* 3rd ed. Rosemont, IL: American Academy of Orthopaedic Surgeons; 2004:565–573.

20

Postoperative and Preprosthetic Care

Michelle M. Lusardi

LEARNING OBJECTIVES

On completion of this chapter, the reader will be able to do the following:

1. Plan a comprehensive examination for an individual with recent lower extremity amputation, selecting appropriate tests and measures and documentation strategies.
2. Use information gathered in the examination, evidence from the clinical research literature, and knowledge of postoperative care to evaluate individuals with recent lower extremity amputation.
3. Formulate an appropriate physical therapy (PT) movement dysfunction diagnosis and prognosis for rehabilitation for individuals with recent lower extremity amputation.
4. Develop appropriate short-term goals and long-term goals and estimate duration, frequency, and intensity of care in the postoperative, preprosthetic care of an individual with recent lower extremity amputation.
5. Develop an appropriate PT plan of care for single limb mobility, residual limb care and wound healing, and preprosthetic rehabilitation.
6. Describe strategies to monitor progress and to adapt and advance the plan of care during the preprosthetic period of rehabilitation.
7. Describe strategies to evaluate outcomes of postoperative, preprosthetic rehabilitation.

PATIENT-CLIENT MANAGEMENT AFTER AMPUTATION

Individuals with New Amputation

In the early days following surgery, the person with a new amputation is likely to experience acute surgical pain and is likely to be grieving the loss of his or her limb. The immediacy of pain combined with a sense of loss may make it difficult for those with recent amputation to recognize their potential for a positive rehabilitation outcome.[1] Older persons with dysvascular or neuropathic limb loss may have had time to physically and psychologically prepare for an elective amputation after a prolonged period of managing a poorly vascularized foot or nonhealing neuropathic ulcer, and therefore may be somewhat less distressed about the loss of their limb than younger persons who have suddenly lost a limb in

a traumatic accident or other medical emergency. Whatever the circumstances leading to amputation, however, the loss of one's limb requires significant psychological adjustment.[2] Early education and discussion about the process of rehabilitation and the person's ultimate goals are extremely important.[3]

Patient-Centered Care and Multidisciplinary Teams

In response to the numbers of military personnel with traumatic amputation and to older veterans with dysvascular amputation, the Departments of Defence and of Veterans Affairs have adopted interdisciplinary, patient-centered care as the ideal model for rehabilitation of persons with amputation.[4,5] The physical therapist and prosthetist, as members of the rehabilitation team, will interact with surgeons, patients, and family members as decisions about surgical levels, plans for postoperative care, potential for prosthetic use, and prosthetic rehabilitation plans are made. For persons facing elective amputation because of dysvascular disease, a period of PT intervention prior to surgery can positively impact on postoperative outcomes.[6]

In the days immediately after amputation, this initial stage of acute care and early rehabilitation sets the stage for eventual return to functional mobility, ability to return to valued activities, and participation in key family and social roles.[4] Although the immediate goals of each member of the interdisciplinary team vary, all ultimately lead toward the person with a newly amputated limb's independence and return to his or her preferred lifestyle. To accomplish this, the team must use an holistic and comprehensive approach to address the person's comorbid burden of illness and psychological and developmental needs, as well as his or her long-term functional, vocational, and leisure goals. Surgical and medical members of the team are most concerned about the healing suture line and overall health status, especially for individuals with vascular insufficiency and for those at risk of infection after traumatic amputation.[7] Nursing professionals provide general medical and wound care as the suture line heals, and administer medications for pain management.[8] Registered dieticians assess the patient's nutritional needs related to wound healing and exercise demands.[9] Physical and occupational therapists focus on enhancing the patient's early single limb mobility, self-care, assessment of the potential for prosthetic use, control of edema and pain management, optimal shaping of the residual limb for prosthetic wear, and prevention of secondary complications.[10]

The prosthetist may fabricate an immediate or early postoperative prosthesis or semirigid dressing and begins to consider which prosthetic components and suspension systems will ultimately be most appropriate, given the individual's characteristics and functional needs.[11] The person with new amputation and his or her family are often most concerned about pain management and what life will be like without the lost limb.[12] A psychologist, social worker, vocational counselor, or school counselor is involved as needed to help with psychological adjustment and to organize long-term rehabilitation care or community resources in preparation for discharge.[13] A clergyman can also be a valuable resource for the person with new amputation, the family, and the team.

Although the multidisciplinary team can vary in size, depending on patient needs and practice settings, the members at the center are the individual with new amputation and his or her caregivers.[14] Communication among all team members, especially the opportunity for the person and family members to ask questions and voice concerns, is more important in this early postoperative and preprosthetic period than it is during the process of prosthetic prescription and training later in the rehabilitation process. This early period sets the stage for the individual's expectations, and ultimately success, as a person with an amputation.[14]

The unique training, clinical expertise, and individual roles of each team member contribute, in a collaborative process, to the development of a plan for rehabilitation that best meets the needs and optimizes the potential of the individual who has lost a limb.[6] The team must come to agreement on the timing and prioritization of specific rehabilitative interventions to meet the goals defined for each patient. Effective communication and strong relationships among the surgeons, orthopedists, or trauma teams who perform the majority of amputations and the rehabilitation team substantially improve the quality of patient care and assist the rehabilitation process.

This chapter focuses on the roles of rehabilitation professionals who work with persons with new amputation in the days and weeks immediately after surgery. It explores how surgical pain and phantom sensation are managed, strategies for controlling postoperative edema, and methods to assess a patient's readiness for prosthetic fitting. Interventions that help a person with new amputation gain competence with single limb mobility tasks and exercises that provide the foundation for successful prosthetic use are identified. The strategies for patient management are organized around the model outlined in the American Physical Therapy Association's Guide to Physical Therapist Practice (Figure 20-1).[15]

EXAMINATION

Ideally, for those undergoing a "planned" or "elective" amputation, the rehabilitation team will meet with the individual and caregivers before surgery to begin collecting information that will be used to guide intervention and provide information about the rehabilitation process. In some instances, input from rehabilitation professionals may be sought by trauma

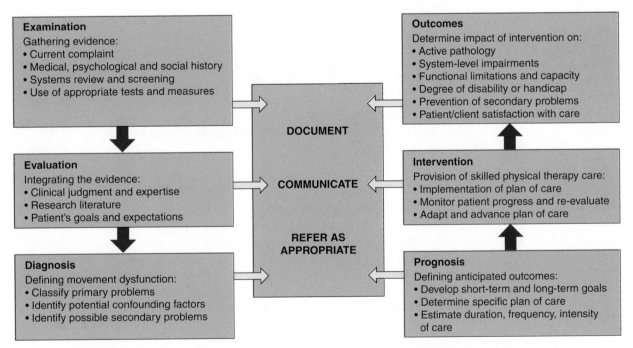

FIGURE 20-1 The components of a systematic and effective patient-client management process. (Modified from American Physical Therapy Association. *Who are Physical Therapists? Guide to Physical Therapist Practice*. Alexandria, VA: American Physical Therapy Association. http://guidetoptpractice.apta.org.)

surgeons to assist patients and families in making informed decisions when faced with amputation after severe injury of the limb. Preoperative interaction may not always be possible, especially when amputation occurs subsequent to failed revascularization, acute and severe limb ischemia, severe infection, or civilian or combat-related traumatic injury. If preoperative assessment is not possible, referral to rehabilitation should be made as soon after surgery as possible; delaying referrals often leads to contracture formation, further cardiovascular and musculoskeletal deconditioning, delayed prosthetic fitting and training, a greater risk of dependency, and a higher risk of reamputation, institutionalization, and mortaltity.[16,17] Box 20-1 summarizes the components of a comprehensive assessment for persons with lower extremity amputation.

BOX 20-1 *Comprehensive Assessment for Patients with Lower extremity Amputation*

HISTORY (DATA COLLECTED FROM CHART REVIEW AND INTERVIEW)

Demographics	Age, gender, primary language, race/ethnicity
Social history	Family and caregiver resources, other social support systems
Occupational history	Employment or retirement status, typical work and leisure activities
Developmental status	Physical/motor, perceptual, cognitive, and emotional dimensions
Living environment	Characteristics and accessibility of "home" environment, projected discharge destination
Current condition	Reason for referral, current concerns/needs, previous medical/surgical interventions for current condition
Past medical history	Prior hospitalizations and surgeries; smoking, alcohol, or drug use (past and present)
Family history	Health risk factors for vascular and cardiac disease
Medications	Prescription medication for current and other medical conditions
	Over-the-counter medications typically used
Functional status	Current and prior abilities and functional limitations (ADLs/IADLs)

SYSTEMS REVIEW (CONCURRENT/COMORBID DISEASE AND IMPAIRMENT RELATED TO PROGNOSIS FOR AND PARTICIPATION IN REHABILITATION)

Cardiopulmonary and cardiovascular systems
Endocrine and metabolic systems
Musculoskeletal system
Neuromuscular system
Gastrointestinal and genitourinary systems

TESTS AND MEASURES (AREAS FOR SPECIFIC ASSESSMENT)

Pain	Presence of phantom limb sensation or pain
	Postoperative pain and pain management strategies
	Muscle soreness related to altered movement patterns
	Joint pain related to motion or comorbid arthritis, etc.
Anthropomorphic characteristics	Residual limb length (bone length, soft-tissue length)
	Residual limb girth, redundant tissue ("dog ears," adductor roll)
	Residual limb shape (bulbous, cylindrical, conical)
	Assessment of type and severity of edema
	Effectiveness of edema control strategy being used
	Overall height, weight, body composition
Skin/integument	Assessment of surgical wound healing
	Assessment/management of adhesions and existing scar tissue
	Other skin problems (other incisions, grafts, psoriasis, cysts, etc.)
	Integrity of remaining foot/limb, especially if neuropathic or dysvascular etiology of amputation
Circulation	Palpation/auscultation of lower extremity pulses, residual and intact limbs
	Skin temperature and presence of trophic changes, residual and intact limbs
	Skin color and response to elevation or dependent position, residual and intact limbs
	Claudication time and distance, impact on function
Range of motion/muscle length	Range of motion, soft-tissue length, and joint contracture

BOX 20-1 *Comprehensive Assessment for Patients with Lower extremity Amputation—cont'd*

Joint integrity	Ligamentous integrity or joint instability
	Structural alignment or joint deformity
	Integrity or inflammation of synovium, bursae, cartilage
Muscle performance	Current muscle strength of upper extremity, trunk, lower extremity
	Muscular power for functional activity
	Muscular endurance for functional activity
	Potential for improvement
Motor function	Motor control, including dexterity, coordination, agility, tone
	Motor learning, including previous use of ambulatory aids, prostheses
Upper extremity function	Power and strength of upper extremity and of trunk
	Ability to use upper extremity in functional activities
Aerobic capacity	Blood pressure, heart rate, respiratory rate (at rest, as well as during and following activity)
	Perceived exertion, dyspnea, angina, during functional activity
	Overall level of physical fitness and functional capacity
Attention/cognition/ emotion	
	Level of consciousness, sleep patterns
	Ability to learn and preferred learning style
	Cognitive dysfunction screening (delirium, depression, dementia)
	Motivation, attention/distractibility, learning styles
Sensory integrity	Protective sensation of residual and remaining limb
	Superficial sensation: light touch, sharp/dull, pressure, temperature
	Proprioception: kinesthesia, position sense
Mobility	Changing position in bed (rolling, scooting, coming to sitting)
Postural control	Static, anticipatory, reactionary balance, in sitting, standing, during functional activities
Transfers	Ability to transfer to/from bed, toilet, wheelchair, mat, tub/shower
Assistive/adaptive equipment	Assistive devices/adaptive equipment currently being used
Ambulation and locomotion	
	Ability to use ambulatory aid safely for single limb gait
	Ability to use wheelchair safely
	Adaptations/equipment necessary for patient's living environment
Gait and balance	Assessment of postural control in quiet standing, reaching, ability to stop/start, change direction, and alter velocity while walking
	Reaction to unexpected perturbation, at rest and during activity
	Observational gait assessment, identification of gait deviations
	Kinematic gait assessment (e.g., speed, stride length, cadence)
	Energy cost or efficiency of locomotion/gait, perceived exertion and dyspnea
	Ability/safety to manage uneven terrain, stairs, ramps, etc.
Posture	Resting posture in sitting, standing, other positions
	Alteration in posture due to loss of limb segment
Self-care	Ability to perform basic ADLs
	Ability to perform IADLs
	Availability of assistance and preparation of caregivers
Community/work reintegration	
	Analysis of roles/activities/tasks
	Functional capacity analysis, determination of essential functions
	Analysis of environment, safety assessment
	Assessment of need for adaptation
Prosthetic requirements	Potential for functional prosthetic use
	Readiness for prosthetic fitting/prescription
	Appropriate prosthetic design, components, suspension

ADLs, Activities of daily living; *IADLs*, instrumental activities of daily living.
Modified from *Phys Ther* 2001;77(11):1354-1367.

Whenever the first contact with the individual and family occurs, the rehabilitation team begins by gathering baseline information that will guide planning for and implementing of the rehabilitation process. This initial information is gathered in three ways: developing a complete patient–client history, performing a review of physiological systems to identify important comorbidities that will affect the rehabilitation process, and using appropriate tests and measures to identify impairments and functional limitations to be addressed in the rehabilitation plan of care.[18] The volume and complexity of information needed to guide planning for prosthetic rehabilitation means that information gathering is a somewhat continuous process and must be integrated with early mobility training in preparation for the individual's discharge from the acute care setting. Examination in the acute care setting likely focuses on four priorities: initial healing of the surgical site, pain management and volume control of the residual limb, bed mobility and transfers, and readiness for single limb ambulation. Examination later in the preprosthetic period (in an outpatient, home care, or subacute setting) would add more detail to determine potential for prosthetic prescription.

Patient-Client History and Interview

Rehabilitation professionals use several strategies to gather information about an individual's medical history. In the acute care setting, the process usually begins with a review of the individual's current medical record or chart, as well as previous medical records (if available). The chart review process provides a broad overview of the individual's health, comorbidities, current medications, previous and current functional status, as well as details about the surgical procedure. Data that other members of the health care team have generated in their examination and evaluative processes are quite relevant to PT care, not only to avoid redundancy in examination but also in planning what additional information will be necessary to collect during subsequent interviews and discussion with the individual and family caregivers.

The interview process provides key information about the individual's priorities and concerns so that they can be appropriately integrated into the plan of care. The physical therapist may also choose to gather supplementary information from the clinical research literature at this point to assist in the subsequent development of prognosis and plan or care, especially if the individual's situation is unusual or complex.[19]

Demographic and Sociocultural Information

The information gathered when reviewing history often begins with basic demographics such as age, gender, race/ethnicity, primary language, and level of education. These data help us to appropriately target communication during our interaction with an individual with recent amputation. It is also important to build an understanding of the individual's sociocultural history including beliefs, expectations and goals, preferred behaviors, and family and caregiver resources, as well as access to and quality of informal and formal support systems.[20-22] Each of these is a potentially important influence on the individual's engagement in the rehabilitation process.

Rehabilitation professionals also gather information about the individual's employment status and task demands, roles and responsibilities within the family system, and leisure interests and hobbies, as well as previous and preferred involvement in the community (access, transportation, and key activities). Additionally, information about smoking, alcohol intake, and other previous substance use/abuse, as well as the individual's coping style and preferred coping strategies help the team to better understand how the individual may behave in the postoperative period. This information is important in developing a prognosis and plan of care; it helps rehabilitation professionals to better define the long-term goals and anticipated outcomes of rehabilitation.

Developmental Status

Another piece of information that informs an appropriate rehabilitation plan of care is the physical, cognitive, perceptual, and emotional developmental status of the individual and his or her caregivers, as well as an understanding of the family system as an organization.[23-25] Although the relevance of developmental status is most obvious when the individual being examined is a child, the perspective afforded by understanding of life span development is valuable for individuals with recent amputation of any age. Examples of factors that evolve over the life span that affect an individual's participation in rehabilitation include postural control, motor abilities, perceptual abilities, willingness to take risks, problem solving, coping styles and strategies, and limb dominance. Observation and interchange during the interview process help the therapist to determine if further clinical examination of developmental status will be necessary.

Living Environment

Rehabilitation professionals gather information about the characteristics of an individual's physical living environment.[26] They ask about getting into and out of the house (e.g., how far is it from the car to the house? What kind of surfaces will be encountered moving from the car to the house? Are there steps and railings at the entry? What are the distances between the major living areas that the person will have to navigate? How accessible and functional are each of the major living areas in the home for those using ambulatory aids or a wheelchair for mobility? Is it possible to adapt the home if necessary? What adaptive equipment is already available? What type of assistance is likely to be routinely available? What type of equipment is likely to be acceptable for the individual and family?).

Asking about the individual's ability to drive, access public transportation, or plans for alternatives for transport once discharged from the acute care setting is important. This may determine what services will be necessary and where they will be provided. Will the individual be returning to his or her home environment on discharge from acute care? If so, will he or she require home care or is transportation available for follow-up appointments with physicians and for outpatient rehabilitation? Alternatively, will the individual have an interim stay in another health care facility for further rehabilitation?

This information will help set rehabilitation priorities and begin the process of discharge planning.

Health, Emotional, and Cognitive Status

During the interview the rehabilitation professional's impression of the individual's general health status that initially developed during chart review broadens. The rehabilitation professional asks questions to discern how the person perceives his or her health and his or her ability to function in self-care, family, or social roles. They assess the individual's understanding of the current situation and prognosis, as well as expectations about the rehabilitation process. They may explore the person's coping style and response to stress, as well as preferred coping skills and strategies.[27,28] This conversation also provides an indication about the individual's current emotional status, ability to learn, cognitive ability, and memory functions.

Because rehabilitation involves physical effort, it is important to understand the person with recent amputation's usual level of activity and fitness, as well as his or her readiness to be involved in exercise. Is physical activity a regular part of the preamputation lifestyle? Has there been a period of prolonged inactivity prior to surgery?[29] Will any additional health habits, such as smoking and use of alcohol or other substances, affect the individual's ability to do physical work and ability to learn or adapt?[30]

Medical, Surgical, and Family History

Potentially important medical conditions that may influence the postoperative/preprosthetic rehabilitation include diabetes, cardiovascular disease, cerebrovascular disease, obesity, neuropathy, renal disease, congestive heart failure, uncontrolled hypertension, and preexisting neuromuscular or musculoskeletal pathologies or impairments, such as stroke or osteoporosis.[31-33] Each of these has a potential impact on wound healing, functional mobility, and exercise tolerance during rehabilitation. Healing and risk of infection are also concerns for those with compromised immune system function, whether from diseases such as human immunodeficiency virus (HIV)/acquired immunodeficiency syndrome (AIDS), those on transplantation medications, those involved in chemotherapy or recent stem cell transplantation, or those using medical steroids.[34] Wound healing, skin condition, and endurance may be issues for persons who are currently undergoing chemotherapy or radiation treatments for cancer.[35,36]

Review of the individual's past surgical history provides additional information that helps rehabilitation professionals anticipate what the individual's response to physical activity might be like. Has the individual had a cardiac pacemaker or defibrillator implanted? Has there been previous amputation of toes or part of the foot of either the newly amputated or "intact" limb? Are there recent surgical scars to be aware of (e.g., following revascularization before amputation)? Has there been total joint replacement or lower extremity fracture that might affect rehabilitation activities and prosthetic component selection?

The "laundry list" of comorbidities and previous surgeries identified in chart review does not necessarily mean that the individual is in poor health.[37] Many individuals manage chronic illnesses and conditions quite effectively, and although they may have less functional reserve than those without pathology, they have the potential for positive rehabilitation outcomes.[38]

Physical therapists must also be aware of the results of tests and diagnostic procedures that other team members have undertaken as part of their examination and evaluation. These might include preoperative cardiac or peripheral vascular studies, electrocardiogram (ECG), stress tests, pulmonary function tests, radiographs, CT, MRI, urinalysis, and laboratory tests for various components of blood (e.g., hemoglobin, cell counts, cultures). Comparison of the individual's test results to established norms provides an index of overall health status and tolerance of levels of activity. Monitoring laboratory test values (e.g., white blood cell [WBC], hematocrit [HCT], hemoglobin [Hb], platelet, international normalized ratio [INR], partial prothrombin time [PPT], glycosylated hemoglobin [HbA1c], and blood glucose levels) and oxygen saturation levels provide ongoing information about general health status and exercise/activity tolerance, allowing the therapist to adapt intervention to the individual's potentially changing condition.[39,40]

Because many of the medications used to manage postoperative pain affect thinking and learning, it is important to understand what pain management strategies are in place and when medication is typically administered.[41,42] Given the likelihood of cardiovascular comorbidity in older adults with vascular disease and diabetes, it is also important to understand what cardiac medications are being administered and how these medications affect response to physical activity and position change.[43-45] It is not unusual for persons who have been immobile or on bed rest to be at risk of postural (orthostatic) hypotension, especially if they are taking medications to manage hypertension.[46] Additionally, given the stress of the surgery and hospital environment, especially if the amputation was performed under general anesthesia, there is the possibility of a temporary postoperative delirium or difficulty with learning and memory.[47] If confusion is observed it is important to clarify typical preoperative cognitive status by speaking with family and caregivers.

Current Condition

Review of the operating room report in the medical record provides information about surgical procedure, drain placement, method of closure, and planned postoperative wound and limb-volume strategies being used (Chapter 19 provides an overview of the most common surgical procedures at the transtibial and transfemoral levels). This information, when combined with knowledge of pain management strategies and demographic information, guides early postoperative/preprosthetic care. Physical therapists use this information to identify potential issues with healing, determine educational needs for the person with new amputation, develop strategies for early positioning of the residual limb, identify potential issues affecting prosthetic fit, and prepare the residual limb for wearing a prosthesis. Determining how comorbidities and injuries are being actively managed is also important, as these affect readiness for early mobility, learning, and memory. Impressions of the individual's psychological state, fears, and expectations round out the baseline with which the person will begin early rehabilitation.

Systems Review

In the acute care setting, there has likely been a fairly comprehensive review of physiological systems as a component of preoperative workup (or emergency care in the case of traumatic injury). Rehabilitation professionals find the results of such review in the physician notes and intake forms in the medical record. The therapist may choose to screen or evaluate in more detail if the information in the record is insufficient in depth or detail as it relates to functional status and response to increasing activity and exercise. Review of systems must include anatomical and physiological status of the cardiovascular, cardiopulmonary, integumentary, musculoskeletal, and neuromuscular systems, as well as communication, affect, cognition, language, and learning style.[48]

Ongoing screening as rehabilitation progresses will help to identify the onset of secondary problems and postoperative complications that require medical intervention or referral to other members of the team. Deterioration in cognitive status or onset of new confusion over a relatively short period of time is especially important to watch for, as it is often the first indication of dehydration, adverse drug reaction, or infection (e.g., pneumonia, urinary tract infection, infection of surgical construct) in older adults.[49]

Test and Measures

In the postoperative, preprosthetic period, physical therapists employ a variety of objective tests and measures to determine the severity of impairment and functional limitation and to establish a baseline that will be used to determine PT movement-related diagnosis, determine prognosis, and assess outcomes of the rehabilitation process.[50] Table 20-1 lists examples of tests and measures appropriate for the postoperative, preprosthetic period. Although most strategies are similar to those used in general PT practice, some may need to be adapted to accommodate the condition or length of the residual limb (e.g., the point of application of resistive force

TABLE 20-1   *Examples of Tests and Measures Important in the Postoperative-Preprosthetic Period*

Category	Examples of Test or Measurement Strategy
Pain	Description of nature or type of pain Visual analog scale for intensity of pain Body chart for location of painful areas Description of factors to increase/decrease discomfort
Anthropometric characteristics	Residual limb length Residual limb circumference Description of edema type and location
Integumentary integrity	Condition of the incision Nature and extent of drainage Condition of "intact" limb Skin color, turgor, temperature
Circulation	Palpation of peripheral pulse Skin temperature
Arousal, attention, cognition	Mini-Mental State Examination, Mini-Cog Delirium scales Depression scales (e.g. Geriatric Depression Scale, Centers for Epidemiologic Studies Depression scale)
Sensory integrity	Protective sensation (Semmes-Weinstein filament) Proprioception and kinesthesia Visual acuity, figure-ground, light/dark accommodation Vestibuloocular function during position change Hearing impairment (acuity, sensitivity to background noise)
Aerobic capacity, endurance	Heart rate at rest, % maximal attainable in activity Arm ergometry, single limb bicycle ergometry, combined upper extremity/lower extremity ergometry Respiratory rate at rest, during activity Ratings of perceived exertion or dyspnea
Mobility	Observation of bed mobility (e.g., rolling) Observation of transitions (e.g., supine–sit) Observation of description of level of assistance, cueing required transfers (various surfaces, heights)

TABLE 20-1 *Examples of Tests and Measures Important in the Postoperative-Preprosthetic Period—cont'd*

Category	Examples of Test or Measurement Strategy
Balance	Static postural control (various functional positions) Anticipatory postural control in functional activity Reaction to perturbation Specific balance tests (e.g., Berg, Functional Reach)
Gait and locomotion	Use of assistive devices Level of independence, cuing or assistance required Time and distance parameters (velocity, cadence, stride) Pattern and symmetry Perceived exertion and dyspnea
Joint integrity and mobility	Manual examination of ligamentous integrity Documentation of bony deformity
Neuromotor function	Observation of quality of motor control in activity Observation of efficiency of motor planning Determination of stage of motor learning with new or adapted tasks Muscle tone Reflex integrity
Muscle performance	Strength: manual muscle test, handheld dynamometer Power: isokinetic dynamometer, manual resistance through range at various speeds of contraction Endurance: 10 repetitions maximum, or maximum number contractions, time to fatigue
Range of motion/muscle length	Goniometry Functional tests (e.g., Thomas test, straight-leg raise)
Self-care and home management	Observation of BADLs and IADLs BADL and IADL rating scales

Abbreviations: BADLs, Basic activities of daily living; IADLs, instrumental activities of daily living.

during manual muscle testing of knee extension strength after transtibial amputation). Whenever measurement technique is altered, however, the reliability and validity of the data collected may be questionable and the data generated less precise. Therapists often begin with examination at the level of impairment and then move into functional assessment.

Assessing Acute Postoperative Pain

The individual with new amputation is likely to be coping with significant acute postoperative pain and may be distressed by the sense that the limb is still in place (phantom sensation) after amputation. Pain is a subjective sensation; each person defines his or her own level of tolerance. Physical therapists have a number of strategies available to document the nature of pain, location of pain, and the intensity of discomfort that the individual is experiencing. These include descriptors generated by the individual with recent amputation or circled on a pain checklist, body maps, visual analog scales, provocation tests, or specific pain indices or questionnaires developed for postsurgical patients (Figure 20-2).[51,52] It is also important to assess how severely that pain interferes with functions, what activities or conditions increase the pain, and what positions or strategies have been helpful in managing the postoperative pain. Documentation of pain management strategies is also important: narcotic and opioid medications potentially impact on attention, ability to learn, and response time during movement and balance activities.[53,54]

Phantom Sensation and Phantom Pain

Commonly, persons with recent amputation experience a sense that the amputated limb remains in place in the days and weeks after surgery.[55] Research reports indicate that from 54% to 99% of persons with new amputation have noticeable *phantom limb sensation*.[56-59] Phantom sensations are typically described as a sense of numbness, tingling, tickling, or pressure in the missing limb, and some complain of itchy toes or mild muscle cramps in the foot or calf.[56] In contrast, *phantom pain* is described as shooting pain, severe cramping, or a distressing burning sensation that may be localized in the amputated foot or present throughout the missing limb. A smaller percentage (46% to 63%) to of those with new amputation experience phantom pain.[56-59] Fortunately, fewer than 15% of those experiencing phantom pain rate it as severe or constant; most experience transient mild to moderate discomfort that does not interfere with usual activity. Phantom pain is more likely in those with longstanding and severe preoperative dysvascular pain, and for those requiring amputation after severe traumatic injury.[56,59]

In most cases, if the individual reports significant phantom sensation or pain, careful inspection of the residual limb helps to rule out other potential sources of pain, such as a neuroma or an inflamed or infected surgical wound. Phantom limb sensation and pain tend to decrease over time whether the amputation was the result of a dysvascular/neuropathic

McGill Pain Questionnaire

Part 1: Where is Your Pain?

Please mark, on the drawings below, the areas where you feel pain.
Put "E" if the pain is external
Put "I" if the pain is internal
Put "EI" if the pain is both internal and external

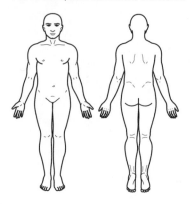

Part 2: What Does Your Pain Feel Like?

Some of the words below describe your PRESENT pain. Circle ONLY those words that best describe your pain right now. Leave out any category that is not suitable. Use only a single word in the appropriate category—the one that applies the best.

1	2	3	4
Flickering	Jumping	Pricking	Sharp
Quivering	Flashing	Boring	Cutting
Pulsing	Shooting	Drilling	Lacerating
Throbbing		Stabbing	
Beating		Lancinating	
Pounding			

5	6	7	8
Pinching	Tugging	Hot	Tingling
Pressing	Pulling	Burning	Itchy
Gnawing	Wrenching	Scalding	Smarting
Cramping		Searing	
Crushing			

9	10	11	12
Dull	Tender	Tiring	Sickening
Sore	Taut	Exhausting	Suffocating
Hurting	Rasping		
Aching			
Heavy			

13	14	15	16
Fearful	Punishing	Wretched	Annoying
Frightful	Grueling	Blinding	Troublesome
Terrifying	Cruel		Miserable
	Vicious		Intense
	Killing		Unbearable

17	18	19	20
Spreading	Tight	Cool	Nagging
Radiating	Numb	Cold	Nauseating
Penetrating	Drawing	Freezing	Agonizing
Piercing	Squeezing		Dreadful
	Tearing		Torturing

Part 3: How Does Your Pain Change With Time?

1. Which word or words would you use to describe the *pattern* of your pain?

1	2	3
Continuous	Rhythmic	Brief
Steady	Periodic	Momentary
Constant	Intermittent	Transient

2. What kind of things *relieve* your pain?

3. What kind of things *increase* your pain?

Part 4: How Strong is Your Pain?

People agree that the following five words represent pain of increasing intensity.
They are:

1	2	3	4	5
Mild	Discomforting	Distressing	Horrible	Excruciating

To answer each question below, write the number of the most appropriate word in the space beside the question.

1. Which word describes your pain right now?   _____
2. Which word describes your pain at its worst?   _____
3. Which word describes it when it is least?   _____
4. Which word describes the worst toothache you ever had? _____
5. Which word describes the worst headache you ever had?   _____
6. Which word describes the worst stomach-ache you ever had? _____

A

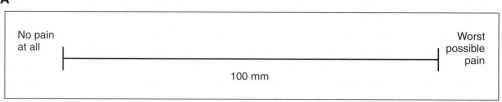

B

FIGURE 20-2 Examples of tools used to document pain and discomfort. **A,** McGill Pain Questionnaire. Descriptor groups: sensory (1 to 10), affective (11 to 15), evaluative (16), and miscellaneous (17 to 20). (Modified from Melzack R. The McGill pain questionnaire; major properties and scoring methods. *Pain.* 1975;1(3):280-281.) **B,** The visual analog scale. (From Bijur PE, Silver W, Gallagher EJ. Reliability of the visual analog scale for measurement of acute pain. *Acad Emerg Med.* 2001;8(12):1153-1157.)

extremity or a traumatic injury.[56-59] A variety of medications (e.g., amitriptyline, tramadol, carbamazepine, ketamine, morphine) have can be used if phantom pain is disabling, however efficacy appears to be low.[60] Use of epidural anesthesia during surgery and/or perineural infusion of local anesthetic for several days following surgery may help reduce development of phantom pain.[61,62] Although a number of models or theories for phantom limb sensation and phantom pain have been proposed, the neurophysiological mechanism that underlies this phenomenon is not well understood.[63,64]

The likelihood of postoperative phantom limb sensation must be discussed with the individual and family before amputation surgery, as well as in the days immediately after operation. Phantom limb sensation is quite vivid; its realistic qualities can be disturbing and frightening to those with recent amputation. Candid discussion about phantom limb sensation as a normally anticipated occurrence helps to reduce an individual's anxiety and distress should phantom sensation occur. It also alerts the individual to issues of safety in the immediate postoperative period. Individuals with recent amputation are at significant risk of falling when they awaken from sleep and attempt to stand and walk to the bathroom in the middle of the night, thinking in their semialert state that both limbs are intact. Ecchymosis or wound dehiscence sustained during a fall can lead to major delays in rehabilitation and prosthetic fitting; some fall-related injuries require surgical revision or closure.

Assessing Residual Limb Length and Volume

The length and volume of the residual limb are important determinants of readiness for prosthetic use, as well as socket design and components chosen for the training prosthesis.[65-67] Initial measurements can be made at the first dressing change. Changes in limb volume are tracked by frequent remeasurement during the preprosthetic period of rehabilitation.

The two components of *residual limb length* are the actual length of the residual tibia or residual femur and the total length of the limb including soft tissue. Measurements are taken from an easily identified bony landmark to the palpated end of the long bone, the incision line, or the end of soft tissue. In the transtibial limb the starting place for measurement is most often the medial joint line of the knee; an alternative is to begin measurement at the tibial tubercle (Figure 20-3, *A*). In the transfemoral limb the starting place for measurement can be the ischial tuberosity or the greater trochanter (Figure 20-3, *B*). Clear notation must be made about the proximal and distal landmarks that are used for the initial measurement to ensure consistency in the subsequent measurement process. Table 20-2 presents a descriptive classification schema for residual limb lengths.

Residual limb volume is typically assessed by serial circumferential girth measurements with a tape measure.[68] For persons with transtibial amputation, circumferential measurement begins at either the medial tibial plateau or the tibial tubercle and is repeated at equally spaced points to the end of the limb (Figure 20-4). For those with transfemoral amputation, measurement begins at either the ischial tuberosity or the

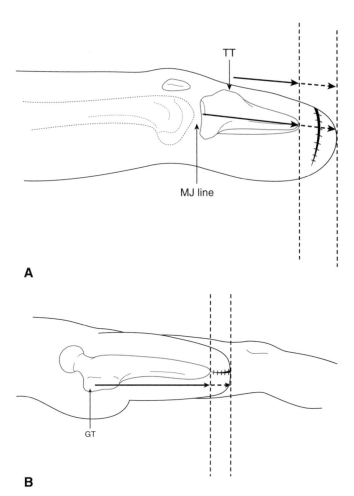

FIGURE 20-3 A, Medial view of a left transtibial residual limb. Limb length is measured to the end of the tibia (*solid arrow*) and to the end of soft tissue (*dotted arrow*) from a bony landmark such as the medial joint (*MJ*) line or tubercle of the tibia (*TT*). **B,** Lateral view of a right transfemoral residual limb. Limb length is measured from the greater trochanter (*GT*) or ischial tuberosity to the end of bone (*solid arrow*) and to the end of soft tissue (*dotted arrow*).

greater trochanter and is also repeated at equally spaced points to the end of the residual limb. The interval between measurements should be clearly documented (i.e., every 5 cm or every inch) for consistency and reliability in future measurement. Prosthetists use a variety of technology-based volumetric measurement strategies to digitally capture residual limb anthropomorphic characteristics to guide socket fabrication.[68-70]

One determinant of readiness for prosthetic fitting is comparison of the proximal and distal circumference of the limb. Often, referral for prosthetic fit is made when the distal limb circumference measurement is equal to or no more than ¼-inch greater than proximal limb circumference. Ideally, with effective control of edema and compression, the transtibial residual limb will mature into a tapered cylindrical shape with distal circumference slightly less than proximal circumference. The transfemoral limb typically matures into a more conical shape, with distal circumference significantly less than proximal circumference. A smaller distal circumference is desirable

TABLE 20-2   *Residual Limb Lengths and Associated Prosthetic Consequences*

Segment	Level	Preserved	Inches	Centimeters	Functional Outcome
Adult tibia[65]	Intact	100%	14.5 ± 1.2	36.9 ± 3.0	Effective walking ability
Transtibial residual limb[66,67]	Short	<35%	<5 especially if <3	<12.7 especially if <7.6	Insufficient knee extension strength and power for prosthetic control; intolerance of weight-bearing pressures applied to skin and soft tissue by a prosthetic socket
	Standard	35% to 50%	5 to 7	12.7 to 17.8	Effective prosthetic control for safe and energy efficient gait; relatively comfortable prosthetic fit[66,67]
	Long	>50%	>7	>18	Distal anterior discomfort and skin irritation in sitting and during swing limb advancement related to high socket pressure at limb-socket interface.[66,67]
Adult femur[65]	Intact	100 %	17.1 ± 1.1	43.5 ± 2.8[65]	Effective walking ability
Transfemoral residual limb[66,67]	Short	<35%	<5	<15.2	Insufficient hip extension and abduction strength and power for stance control when using prosthesis
	Standard	35% to 50 %	5 to 8.5	15.2 to 21.8	Effective prosthetic control for safe and energy efficient gait; relatively comfortable prosthetic fit
	Long	>50%	>8.5	>21.8	Long lever arm enhances prosthetic control in stance; but may limit choice of prosthetic knee units (if residual limb length and knee unit length exceeds femur length of intact limb)

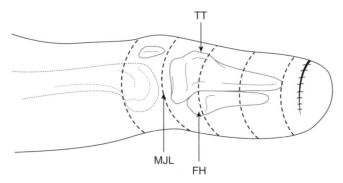

FIGURE 20-4 Limb volume and shape of a transtibial residual limb is assessed by taking successive circumferential measures (*dotted lines*) from a bony landmark such as the medial joint line (*MJL*) to the suture line. *FH*, Fibular head; *TT*, tibial tubercle.

so that shear forces on soft tissue will be minimal when the prosthesis is donned and used.

Assessing Integumentary Integrity and Wound Healing

Assessment of skin condition and the vascular, sensory, and motor status of both of the patient's limbs is imperative. During assessment there is an opportunity to introduce the individual with new amputation and family to strategies that are likely to be used for compression/edema control after surgery. Instructing the individual and family about proper positioning of the residual limb is also important, as well as the need to maintain knee extension and neutral hip alignment to minimize soft tissue tightness and joint contracture.

In most settings, the surgeon who performed the amputation assesses the condition of the surgical site at the initial dressing change. This can occur as early as the first postoperative day, when soft dressings and elastic wraps have been used, or on the third postoperative day, if the residual limb has been casted in a rigid dressing.[71] After this initial appraisal the status of the surgical wound is assessed by the nurse or physician at each dressing change. In some settings, the physical therapist is charged to inspect the residual limb to monitor the stage of healing of the incision and the limb's shape, length, sensory integrity, and volume; the therapist works closely with the surgeon in postoperative wound management and timing of prosthetic replacement.

With each dressing change, the wound is carefully examined and the quantity and quality of drainage from the wound are documented. Initially, drainage will be sanguinous (primarily bloody); typically, as the surgical wound begins to heal over the next few days, drainage transitions to serosanguineous, and eventually to serous exudate. Much of this early drainage is absorbed by the wound dressing. Significant amounts of bright red arterial blood (hemorrhage) or darker venous blood (draining hematoma) should be reported to the surgeon for further assessment. Although pre-, peri-, and postoperative antibiotic administration is becoming the standard of care,[72,73] the incidence of postoperative infection involving the incision following amputation is relatively high: as many as one in four patients will develop infected wounds.[74] Increasing amounts of drainage, as well as thickening, discolored exudate, may signal infection of the wound; this must be immediately reported to the physician, especially if it occurs in persons who are immunocompromised or whose limbs may have been environmentally contaminated during traumatic injury.[74] Infection can significantly delay healing, increase length of acute care stay, require revision of the surgical construct or reamputation to a more proximal level, increase risk of deconditioning and contracture development associated with bed rest, and compromise rehabilitation outcomes.[75,76]

In the first several postoperative days, signs of inflammation (erythema, edema and elevated tissue temperature surrounding the incision) are likely present along the incision line secondary to tissue trauma sustained during surgery.[77] The edges of the wound should be closely approximated for effective primary healing; any areas of wound separation (dehiscence), scab or eschar formation, ecchymosis, or other signs of tissue fragility or decreased viability must be carefully documented and monitored. Clinicians watch for signs of epithelial resurfacing across the incision, as well as development of a healing ridge along the incision, signal of collagen deposition signals progression into the proliferative stage of wound healing.[77] Prolonged edema delays wound healing because the associated pressure compromises angiogenesis; which, in turn, increases risk of wound ischemia, tissue necrosis, infection, and need for revision to a higher level.[78] Risk of residual limb osteomyelitis should be suspected when delayed healing and residual limb pain persist in the weeks and months following amputation.[79] Persons with recent or current history of smoking are more likely to experience significantly delayed healing following amputation.[80]

Many persons with traumatic or other nondysvascular amputation have achieved sufficient healing and limb volume control within 2 weeks to use a prefabricated adjustable prosthesis or to be casted for their initial (preparatory, training) prosthesis (Figure 20-5).[81] Those with amputation secondary to vascular disease often require 4 to 8 weeks or more to achieve adequate healing and limb shaping to allow for prosthetic casting; this is greatly influenced by the strategy used to manage edema in the immediate postoperative period.[82] The surgeon may begin to remove sutures or staples from the incision as early as 10 to 14 days after surgery. Initially, every other or every third suture/staple can be left in place to guard against wound dehiscence; remaining sutures or staples are removed over successive days. The surgical wound is often reinforced with Steri-Strips when sutures or staples are removed to protect the incision from shearing forces during preprosthetic activity and early prosthetic training. The Steri-Strips can remain on the limb for 2 or more additional weeks after the sutures/staples have been removed. Gait training with a prosthesis can cautiously begin, with the approval of the surgeon, when clear evidence of primary healing is found, even if several sutures have been left in place to protect an area along the incision line that has been slow in closing.

Delayed healing of the surgical wound may postpone prosthetic use. Older persons with diabetes and vascular insufficiency, as well as those who smoke, are particularly at risk for delayed healing.[80] The healing process can also be delayed as a consequence of infection, immunosuppression, or traumatic damage sustained during activity or in a fall in the days or weeks after surgery.[83] Nutritional status is another important determinant of wound healing in the early postoperative and preprosthetic period; individuals with compromised nutritional status are more likely to experience delayed wound healing and are at greater risk of postoperative infection, as well as cardiopulmonary and septic complications.[84] When transcutaneous oxygen and carbon dioxide

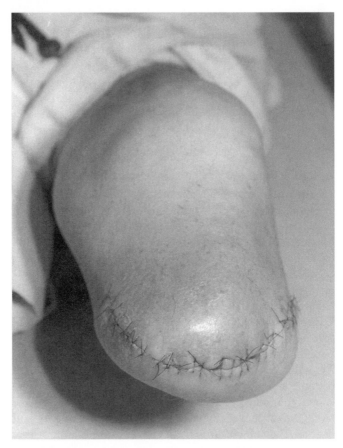

FIGURE 20-5 A well-healed, transtibial residual limb with equal anterior posterior flaps 14 days after amputation. The edges of the wound are approximate, and although several small scabs have formed between sutures, primary healing is well established. Strategies for control of edema and initial limb shaping have been successful as well; this residual limb could be described as cylindrical, with little redundant tissue present.

are carefully monitored, persons with small nonhealing incisional wounds (1 cm × 1 cm) can safely use a pneumatic prosthesis to preserve/improve mobility and endurance before being fit with a prosthesis.[80]

Assessing Circulation

Because so many amputations are associated with the dyad of vascular insufficiency and polyneuropathy, it is particularly important to examine and monitor vascular status and skin integrity of the remaining (intact) limb, as well as of the residual limb. One criterion for determining the level of amputation is the likelihood of healing of the surgical construct.[7] Surgeons caring for persons with dysvascular limbs typically determine the status of peripheral circulation using both noninvasive and invasive tests before amputation; however, delayed healing or failure of the suture line to close sometimes occurs even with careful preoperative evaluation. In the days and weeks after amputation surgery, members of the team watch for signs of vascular compromise that might threaten adequate closure of the surgical wound.

The remaining limb becomes much more vulnerable to skin and soft-tissue damage because of increased biomechanical stress associated with single limb mobility following amputation surgery.[85,86] Noninvasive strategies to assess the adequacy of blood flow (described in detail in Chapter 18) include skin temperature and turgor, skin color at rest and after position change, palpation or auscultation of pedal and popliteal pulses, segmental blood pressures, and calculation of an ankle-brachial index. A thorough baseline assessment enables the team to identify and respond to any circulatory problems that might develop as rehabilitation continues.

Assessing Range of Motion and Muscle Length

Having near-normal range of motion (ROM) in the remaining joints of the residual limb is essential for effective prosthetic use.[87] Persons with recent amputation are much at risk for developing soft tissue contracture at the joint proximal to amputation during the preprosthetic period. The risk of hip and knee flexion contracture formation is associated with spending long periods of time sitting in a wheelchair or resting in bed, before and after amputation surgery. Other factors that contribute to the risk of flexion contracture formation include the protective flexion withdrawal pattern associated with lower extremity pain, muscle imbalances that result from loss of distal attachments, and the loss of tonic sensory input generated by weight bearing on the sole of the foot.[88,89] Because limitation in the lower extremity ROM can have a significant impact on the quality and energy efficiency of prosthetic gait, it is essential to assess and monitor ROM.[68] Equally important is implementing strategies to prevent or minimize contracture development as early in the postoperative, preprosthetic period as possible.[68,82]

For persons with transtibial amputation, definitive measurement of hip ROM is possible with standard goniometric techniques. With the loss of the malleolus as a distal reference point, accurate measurement of knee extension ROM can be challenging, especially when there is a short residual limb (Figure 20-6). Familiarity with the normal anatomy of the tibia improves the therapist's positioning of the mobile arm of the goniometer and the accuracy of measurement. For individuals with transtibial and transfemoral amputation, the Thomas test may be an effective tool for determining the severity of hip flexion contracture (Figure 20-7). Full hip extension is critical for prosthetic knee stability when walking with a transfemoral prosthesis.[87] The accuracy of standard goniometric measurement of hip adduction and abduction

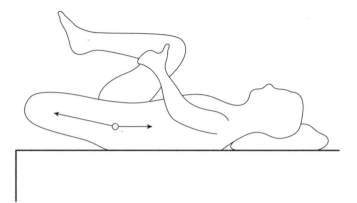

FIGURE 20-7 The Thomas test can be used to assess the tightness or contracture of hip flexors for patients with transtibial and transfemoral residual limbs. The patient is positioned in supine with both limbs flexed toward the chest and the pelvis in slight posterior tilt. While the opposite limb is supported in place, the residual limb is gently lowered toward the support surface. Tightness or contracture of hip flexors causes the pelvis to move into an anterior tilt before the limb is fully lowered.

decreases as residual limb length decreases. There is no effective way to assess rotation of the transfemoral residual limb.

Hip flexor tightness is likely to result in increased lumbar lordosis when standing and walking with a prosthesis later in the rehabilitation process. Attempts to achieve an upright posture over the prosthesis in the presence of hip flexion contracture can lead, over time, to excessive mobility of the lumbosacral spine and the development of low back pain when walking with a prosthesis.[90] Individuals with bilateral transtibial amputation, as well as those who wear a transfemoral prosthesis, are much at risk for this problem: Secondary spinal dysfunction and low back pain can be more disabling than the original amputation.[90,91] Attention to the importance of achieving near-normal joint ROM and soft tissue excursion early in the preprosthetic period has a powerful impact on effective prosthetic use over the long run.

When sitting or lying in bed, the natural tendency is for the lower limb to roll outward into a slightly flexed, abducted, and externally rotated position. Excursion of the hip is important to assess; tightness of external rotators may be masked by apparent tightness of hip flexors or abductors. The functional length of two-joint muscles is also important to consider. Adequate hamstring length is essential if the person with recent transtibial amputation is to maintain a fully extended knee when seated. If the knee is held in extension by a rigid dressing or thermoplastic splint, hamstring tightness will pull the pelvis into a marked posterior tilt. Instead of sitting squarely on the ischial tuberosities, the person with hamstring tightness sits in a kyphotic position with weight shifted onto the sacrum. This compromised postural alignment increases the risk of spinal dysfunction and of skin irritation and decubitus ulcer formation. Tightness in the rectus femoris, sartorius, and tensor fascia latae can interfere with advanced mobility skills such as the ability to kneel while transferring to and from the floor.

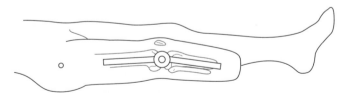

FIGURE 20-6 Measurement of knee extension for persons with transtibial amputation requires an understanding of the normal anatomy of the tibia to compensate for loss of the distal malleolus as a point of reference for the mobile arm of the goniometer.

Assessing Joint Integrity and Mobility

For individuals with transtibial residual limbs, the alignment and ligamentous integrity of the knee will be an important determinant of socket design, suspension strategy, and eventually the dynamic alignment of the prosthesis. Specific assessment of joint function of the residual limb is often deferred to later in the preprosthetic period when there has been primary healing of the surgical site; however, history of previous ligament injury or tear of the meniscus and concurrent degenerative joint disease or existing bony deformity (e.g., genu recurvatum, genu valgus, genu varum) should be noted during initial assessment.

The special tests used to assess knee function in those with amputation are the same as those used to assess joint integrity in individuals with musculoskeletal dysfunction in intact limbs. They include joint play, medial and lateral gap tests to assess the integrity of the collateral ligaments, anterior and posterior draw test to assess cruciate integrity, and the various tests for meniscus tear.[92] The techniques, however, must be adapted to the length of the residual limb; the loss of the foot means that the examiner's distal point of stability is moved upward on the limb, compromising the biomechanical advantage, as well as the accuracy, of the examiner. It may be helpful to first examine the knee of the intact limb using traditional hand placement to get a sense of the individual's baseline, then move the distal hand upward on the intact limb and repeat the examination using hand placement appropriate for the residual limb. Comparison of distal and proximal test results of the intact limb provides a frame of reference for subsequently testing the knee of the residual limb.

Assessing Muscle Performance and Motor Control

Although assessment of strength and muscle function is a key component of preprosthetic and prosthetic rehabilitation, definitive strength assessment beyond active, nonresisted antigravity motion at the joint just proximal to the amputation is usually postponed until there is adequate healing of the surgical site, so as to protect the new incision from sheer forces associated with testing. Strength of key muscle groups at the next most proximal joints can be specifically assessed with standard manual muscle testing or handheld dynamometry techniques.[93] Given time constraints during initial assessment, the therapist may opt to use functional antigravity activities to screen for impairments of strength and power of the remaining limb and trunk, specifically testing strength of particular muscles if functional problems are identified.

For those with transtibial amputation, observation of active knee flexion and extension strength is used to determine if at least fair (a rating of 3 out of 5) full antigravity strength is present until the physician determines sufficient wound healing has been accomplished. For those with transfemoral amputation, assessment of hip muscle strength beyond active antigravity fair muscle grade must also be postponed pending incisional healing.

Once the surgeon and rehabilitation team are confident that enough healing has occurred so that the incision cannot be compromised by externally applied resistance, definitive strength testing can be implemented at the joint proximal to amputation. Because of the length of the residual limb, the examiner must apply the resistive force at a more proximal position on the extremity than is defined by the standard manual muscle test technique. With an altered manual contact, the mechanical advantage of the examiner is reduced and the subjective sense of strength grade may be somewhat inflated. This altered point of force application affects the validity of test results. Many therapists attempt to maximize validity by first testing the intact or remaining limb (assuming similarity of strength between the patient's limbs), using standard technique to assign a muscle grade (Figure 20-8, *A*). The intact limb is then retested with a more proximal hand placement, simulating the position for testing of the residual limb (Figure 20-8, *B*). This grade serves as a point of reference when the residual limb is then tested (Figure 20-8, *C*). For persons with transtibial amputation, the functional strength of hip extensors can be assessed with the individual lying in supine, a small bolster or towel roll positioned under the lower thigh of the residual limb and the intact limb held flexed against the trunk (Figure 20-9, *A*). The ability to lift the pelvis (bridge) up from the supporting surface by pushing downward into the bolster suggests functional hip extensor strength. Similarly, hip abduction can be tested in side-lying position (residual limb down) against a bolster, asking the individual to push downward to raise the pelvis up off of the supporting surface (Figure 20-9, *B*) These positions can also be used as strengthening exercises to repeatedly lift body weight in concentric, holding (at the top), and eccentric (controlled lowering) contraction.

Because a healing transtibial suture line is vulnerable to resistive forces applied during strength testing and strengthening exercise, resistance to knee extension should only be applied if and when the suture line can be observed. Resistance must not be applied through a soft dressing or compressive garment during the first several weeks of the preprosthetic program. Unless healing has been delayed, most surgeons consider

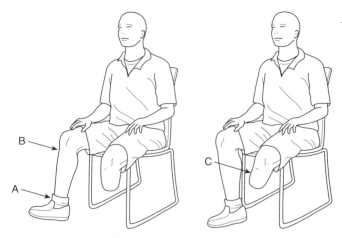

FIGURE 20-8 Suggested points of force application for to improve accuracy of manual muscle test (MMT) for knee extension strength in a transtibial residual limb. **A,** Standard MMT position on the remaining limb. **B,** Moving the point of force application proximally on the intact limb provides a frame of reference for subsequent testing (**C**) of the residual limb.

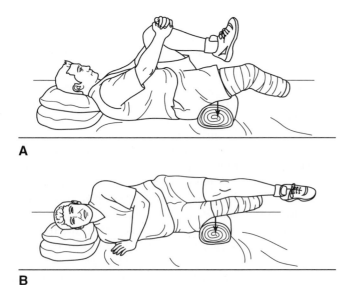

A

B

FIGURE 20-9 Strategies for functional testing of hip extensor (**A**) and hip abductor (**B**) muscle strength following transtibial amputation. A small bolster or firm towel roll is positioned at the distal thigh, and the individual attempts to lift the pelvis from the supporting surface. In persons with transfemoral amputation, these positions can be used once sufficient healing of the surgical construct has occurred. These positions can later be used, with body weight as resistance, for concentric (lifting), isometric (holding), and eccentric (controlled lowering) strengthening exercises.

initiation of conservative resistive exercise a few days after sutures have been removed. Surgeon preference, tissue integrity, and the individual's cardiovascular condition must be factored into strength assessment and strengthening exercise programs.

Function is influenced not only by the maximal force that the individual can generate (as examined in standard manual muscle test), but it also depends on the rate and efficiency at which the individual can generate force (power); the ability of the individual to grade and sustain an effective contraction during activity (endurance); and the ability to control muscle length in concentric (shortening), isometric (holding), and eccentric (lengthening) contractions. Observation of functional activities can identify if there are impairments of these types of muscle function. More specific testing of power can be accomplished using an isokinetic apparatus set at varying speeds or by asking the person to move at varying speeds against manual resistance.

Assessment of the ability to switch between types of muscle contraction can be accomplished by providing manual resistance while asking the individual to "contract," "hold," and "let go slowly" for key muscle groups. An example of a key functional activity in which this type of control is important is the task of rising from sitting to standing and then returning to a seated position. Many persons can generate adequate force in the intact lower extremity to stand up, but have difficulty controlling their descent back to sitting—"plopping" back into their seat. This is especially true for individuals who have been inactive or on prolonged bed rest.[94,95]

If there is any indication of previous or current neuromuscular dysfunction, examination of tone and motor control is also important. Assessment of muscle tone includes deep tendon reflexes (DTR), response to passive movement of limbs and trunk (hypotonicity or hypertonicity, rigidity), placement and drop tests, coordination and fine-motor tests (e.g., rapid alternating movement; fine, quick tapping or clapping), as well as observation of any abnormal synergy pattern, tremors, or involuntary movement.[96] Qualitative assessment of the individual's ability to initiate, sustain, and terminate movement during functional activities will help the therapist identify issues of motor control that may need to be addressed as part of the plan of care.

Assessing Upper Extremity Function

Because most individuals use an ambulatory aid (e.g., four-wheeled walker, standard walker, crutches) for single limb ambulation until they are ready for prosthetic training, it is important to screen for deformity or other musculoskeletal or neuromuscular impairments involving the upper extremity. Many of those with dysvascular- and neuropathic-related lower extremity amputation have age-related degenerative joint disease that might make use of a walker or crutches challenging. Screening for functional strength and muscle endurance of muscles that stabilize the shoulder and elbow identifies individuals who would benefit from a progressive resistive exercise program targeting the upper extremity to enhance their ability to transfer, as well as ambulate.

Polyneuropathy, in a "stocking-glove" distribution, is the most common neuromuscular impairment encountered in those with diabetes who have undergone lower extremity amputation. Diabetic polyneuropathy affects all extremities—not only the sensory system, but also the voluntary motor and autonomic systems.[97,98] For this reason, it is important to at least screen for distal upper extremity sensory loss, weakness of intrinsic muscles of the hand, and autonomic impairment (e.g., postural hypotension) during the preprosthetic period. Compromised upper extremity sensation and functional strength may affect the type of assistive device used for mobility; compression strategy for the residual limb; and, eventually, selection of a suspension strategy for the prosthesis.

Assessing Aerobic Capacity and Endurance

Determining baseline (resting) vital signs (e.g., pulse, blood pressure, respiratory rate, blood oxygen levels via pulse oximetry) is the first step in assessment of aerobic capacity and endurance. Screening for orthostatic (postural) hypotension is important for any individual who has sustained a period of inactivity and bed rest, especially if the individual is older, is on medications that blunt blood pressure response, or has a history of autonomic dysfunction from peripheral or systemic pathology.[99] Change in vital signs during transfers or early mobility training and the time to return to resting baseline values provide information about responsiveness to exercise. Importantly, soon after surgery, anxiety about pain or risk of injury during activities may contribute to a physiological "fight-or-flight" response, influencing vital signs.[100] A calm and focused demeanor on the part of the therapist, as well as explanation and education about what will happen and the reason for the assessment, can help an individual with recent amputation better manage fears and concerns.

Ratings of perceived exertion and dyspnea are useful assessment strategies in the postoperative/preprosthetic period, both to assess how the person with new amputation is tolerating increasing activity and to help the individual target an appropriate level of activity.[101,102] Upper extremity ergometry, single-leg cycling tests, or combined upper and lower limb ergometry tests have been used as indexes of aerobic capacity for those who have recently lost a limb if definitive testing is indicated.[103–105]

Given the similarities in etiology and impact of peripheral vascular, cardiovascular, and cerebrovascular disease, many persons with dysvascular amputation are likely to be at risk for, or have even had, heart attack (myocardial infarction [MI]) or brain attack (stroke).[106–108] The rehabilitation team must be alert for early signs and symptoms of cardiac compromise as the person with new amputation begins transfer and single limb mobility training. Individuals who have had previous cardiac rehabilitation following MI, angioplasty, or coronary artery bypass may better understand the importance of conditioning exercise as part of their preprosthetic program. Assessment of quality of motor control and tone is important if there is history of stroke.

Assessing Attention and Cognition

The tool most commonly used to assess cognitive status in the acute care setting is the Mini-Mental State Examination (MMSE)[109] (Figure 20-10). Typically, scores of 24 of 30 or less indicate some form of cognitive impairment; however, the MMSE does not identify the etiology or type of cognitive dysfunction. In older adults, the most common form of cognitive

The Mini-Mental State Exam

Patient ______________ Examiner ______________ Date ________

Maximum	Score	
		Orientation
5	( )	What is the (year) (season) (date) (day) (month)?
5	( )	Where are we (state) (country) (town) (hospital) (floor)?
		Registration
3	( )	Name 3 objects: 1 second to say each. Then ask the patient all 3 after you have said them. Give 1 point for each correct answer. Then repeat them until he/she learns all 3. Count trials and record. Trials ________
		Attention and Calculation
5	( )	Serial 7's. 1 point for each correct answer. Stop after 5 answers. Alternatively spell "world" backward.
		Recall
3	( )	Ask for the 3 objects repeated above. Give 1 point for each correct answer.
		Language
2	( )	Name a pencil and watch.
1	( )	Repeat the following "No ifs, ands, or buts"
3	( )	Follow a 3-stage command: "Take a paper in your hand, fold it in half, and put it on the floor."
1	( )	Read and obey the following: CLOSE YOUR EYES
1	( )	Write a sentence.
1	( )	Copy the design shown.

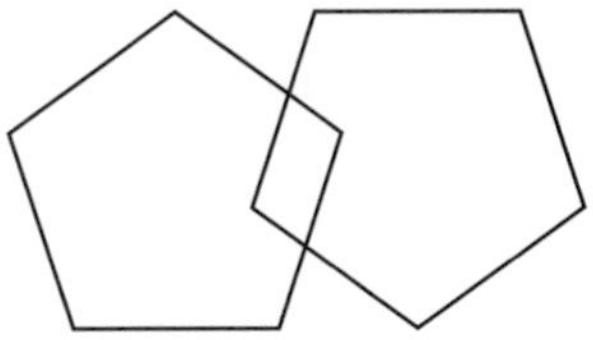

_____ Total Score

ASSESS level of consciousness along a continuum ______________

Alert Drowsy Stupor Coma

FIGURE 20-10 The Mini-Mental State Examination. (From Folstein MF, Folstein SE, McHugh. "Mini-mental state." A practical method for grading the cognitive state of patients for the clinician. *J Psychiatr Res.* 1975;12(3):189-198.)

impairment is a delirium, a temporary and typically reversible problem that is associated with physiological stressors (e.g., clearing from anesthesia, psychotropic effects of narcotic pain medications, stress of hospitalization, dehydration, onset of infection).[109-111] Table 20-3 presents risk factors for, signs and symptoms of, and measures used to screen for and quantify severity of delirium.

Cognition and the ability to learn may also be compromised by depression associated with mourning the loss of one's limb.[22,112] Perception of acute surgical pain and phantom pain tend to increase in persons with significant depression following amputation, as well as in those who view amputation as a catastrophic event.[113,114] Persons whose amputation was traumatic (accident related, combat related, or work related) often must also contend with significant anxiety, anger, or posttraumatic stress disorder, and may require psychiatric referral for posttraumatic stress disorder symptoms that hamper rehabilitation.[115-117] Measures commonly used to evaluate depression in the preprosthetic period include the Geriatric Depression Scale,[118] the Beck Depression Inventory,[119] and the Center for Epidemiological Studies Depression Scale.[120] Anxiety following amputation can be assessed using the Hospital Anxiety and Depression Scale,[121,122] and the Geriatric Anxiety Inventory.[123] Scores indicating moderate to high levels of delirium, depression, or anxiety should prompt referral to mental health services for further evaluation and intervention. Participation in rehabilitation often reduces levels depression and anxiety[112]; it can be more informative to track how scores change over a period of time than to interpret a single value.

It is important to note that, for those with amputation as a result of dysvascular problems, the underlying mechanism for peripheral arterial disease (PAD), cardiovascular disease, and cerebral vascular disease is the same; in population studies, persons with severe PAD tend to have more cognitive impairment than those without PAD.[124] There is a positive relationship between level of cognitive resources (e.g., memory, executive function, problem-solving ability), the ability to walk with a prosthesis, and postamputation adjustment and quality of life.[125-127] Cognitive impairment should not preclude postoperative rehabilitation and prosthetic prescription: supervised use of ambulatory assistive devices and eventually prostheses may improve safety during self-care and reduce overall caregiver burden.[128]

TABLE 20-3   *Risk Factors for, Signs/Symptoms of, and Screening Tools for Delirium*

Risk factors for delirium[332,333]	Patient-related predisposing	Advanced age
		Dementia
		Previous stroke or head injury
		Parkinson disease
		Multiple comorbid diseases
		Impaired vision and/or hearing (nonuse of typical glasses or hearing aids)
		History of alcohol or other substance abuse
		Functional impairment
		Male gender
	Patient-related precipitating	Dehydration, electrolyte imbalance, hypo- or hyperglycemia, other metabolic abnormalities
		Onset of acute medical problem, especially infection (pneumonia, urinary tract infections)
		Exacerbation of chronic medical problem
		Sepsis
		Polypharmacy (>3 medications) and adverse drug reaction
		Recent surgery and anesthesia
		Pain with or without opioid/narcotic pain medication
		Severe illness
		Sleep deprivation
		Urinary catheter use
		Constipation or fecal impaction
		Malnutrition
		Hepatic or renal dysfunction or failure
		Trauma
		Head injury
		Alcohol or other substance withdrawal
		Hypo or hyperthermia
		Fearfulness, loss of self-determination, altered self-esteem
	Environment related	Transition to new or unfamiliar environment
		Lack of privacy
		Differences in noise (type, loudness) and lighting
		Isolation
		Physical or chemical restraint use

TABLE 20-3 *Risk Factors for, Signs/Symptoms of, and Screening Tools for Delirium—cont'd*

Signs and symptoms of delirium[332,333]	Hypoactive and hyperactive behaviors	Change from usual cognition over hours or several days
		Confusion and disorientation
		Difficulty concentrating, poor attention span, distractibility
		Altered perception (illusion, delusion, visual and auditory hallucination)
		Inability to multitask or parallel process
		Impaired learning and memory
		Noncompliance with interventions
		Disorganized speech (rambling or inarticulate)
		Emotional lability
		Paranoia
		Disordered sleep pattern (sundown syndrome)
		Fearfulness
		Aggressiveness and anger
		Alternating lethargy and hyperactivity
Measures for diagnosis of delirium	Cognitive screening	Mini-Mental State Exam[334]
		Mini-Cog[335]
	Delirium-specific	Confusion Assessment Method (CAM)[336]
		One Day Fluctuation Scale[337]
		Delirium Index[338]
		Neelon and Champagne Confusion (NEECHAM) Scale[339]
		Delirium Observation Screening Scale[340]
		Delirium Rating Scale (DRS)[341]
		Memorial Delirium Assessment Scale (MDAS)[342]

Readers are referred to the excellent chapter on motivation and patient education by Resnik and Avers in *Geriatric Physical Therapy* as a resource on assessment of learning styles and readiness to change health behaviors (as well as on facilitation of learning).[129]

Assessing Sensory Integrity

Early in the postoperative period, screening of sensory function (vision, hearing, and somatosensation) is aimed at determining if strategies for enhancing communication may be necessary and if the individual has sufficient "data-collection" mechanisms in place to monitor the surgical wound condition, to inspect the condition of the remaining foot and limb, and to scan the environment in preparation for and during functional activities.[130-132] Sensory integrity is also a factor influencing selection of prosthetic components and suspension method.

Given the age and common morbidities of those with vascular and neuropathic etiology of amputation, it is quite likely that some degree of visual impairment will be present in this group (Box 20-2).[133,134] If the individual typically wears glasses for daily function, glasses should be worn during examination and subsequent intervention as well. Simple strategies to reduce glare, increase contrast (e.g., handgrips on walkers), and enhance acuity (e.g., large, simple, bold type on written instructions) can be used to help those with common age-related visual changes be more functional during the postoperative/preprosthetic period.[135]

Similarly, there are cumulative age-related changes in structure, physiology and function of the auditory system to be aware of (see Box 20-2) when interacting with older persons with recent amputation.[136] Attention to the ability to hear and interpret sound is especially important when examining persons with concurrent confusion caused by postoperative delirium or acquired brain injury after trauma who may have impairment of attention as well. Simple strategies to enhance the ability to listen and hear include dropping the pitch of the speaking voice; speaking more slowly and projecting the voice without shouting; maintaining direct eye contact; interacting in as quiet an environment as possible; and augmenting what is said with directive gestures, simple diagrams, or brief written instruction in large print.[137] Ensuring that hearing aids are in place and functional is especially important during interviews and for patient/family education. Importantly, hearing aids typically amplify all sound; attention to volume and complexity of background noise must always be considered.

In examining somatosensation the therapist is screening for areas of diminished sensation and areas of hypersensitivity or dysthesias on the surface of the residual limb, as well as on the remaining limb.[138] Box 20-2 also summarizes age- and pathology-related changes in sensation. For those with neuropathic-dysvascular disease, it is especially important to ascertain if there is adequate protective sensation (ability to consistently perceive the 5.07 Semmes-Weinstein filament) on weight-bearing surfaces of the intact limb, which will be subject to repeated loading during single limb ambulation.[139] Standard sensory testing protocols for light touch, point and generalized pressure (am I touching you? yes/no), the ability to localize (where am I touching you?), and temperature discrimination (hot/cold) are employed and often documented on a body chart.[140]

BOX 20-2 *Age-Related and Pathological Conditions of the Sensory Systems in Later Life*

VISUAL SYSTEM

Age-Related Changes

Diminished visual acuity

Diminished ability to accommodate between near/far visual targets

Delayed dark–light adaptation, especially sudden changes in lighting

Diminished contrast sensitivity and figure–ground discrimination

Diminished color discrimination

Diminished depth perception and visual–spatial sensitivity

Slowed pupillary light responses

Diminished corneal reflex

Diminished ability to converge eyes

Decreased ability to gaze upward/diminished upper visual field

Diminished lateral peripheral field

Increased likelihood of ptosis

Diminished efficiency of vestibular–ocular reflexes

Functional Consequences

Susceptibility to glare

Increasing need for sharp contrast (in text style and color)

Difficulty recognizing and responding to subtle changes in the visual environment

Need for gradual transition from dark-to-light environments

Need to keep directional signs at eye level

Use of bifocals/trifocals to improve visual clarity at near/far distances

Pathologies Affecting the Visual System

Cataract

Age-related maculopathy/macular degeneration

Diabetic retinopathy

Glaucoma

Homonymous hemianopsia consequent to cerebrovascular accident

AUDITORY SYSTEM

Age-Related Changes

Gradual progressive bilateral hearing loss, beginning with high frequencies

Diminished sensitivity to low-volume sounds

Increasing pure tone auditory threshold

Diminished ability to screen background noise

Diminished discernment of speech sounds

Diminished word and sentence recognition

Decreased ability to accommodate to rapid speaking rates

Distortion of sound/sensitivity to shouting and emotional cues

Functional Consequences

Less efficient listening, especially in noisy environments

Compensation by watching facial expression, movement of mouth

Need for adaptation of learning/listening environment:
  Lower tone speech
  Slower rate of speaking
  Higher volume (loudness) without shouting

Use of hearing aids (most effective is conductive hearing loss)

Pathologies Affecting the Auditory System

Buildup of cerumen in the external auditory canal

Traumatic hearing loss from exposure to excessively loud sounds

Acoustic neuroma

Vascular insufficiency in the brainstem auditory system

Cerebrovascular accident affecting auditory cortex function

Ototoxic medications

SOMATOSENSORY SYSTEM

Age-Related Changes

Decrease in number and distribution of receptors for discriminatory touch

Loss of afferent nerve fibers in peripheral nerves

Degeneration of dorsal columns (central sensory discriminatory pathway)

Increased latency for sensory stimulation (diminished conduction velocity)

Increased threshold of stimulation and decreased sensitivity
  Point localization
  Vibration (toe and ankle > upper extremity)
  Two-point discrimination
  Cutaneous pain
  Temperature detection
  Passive movement/joint position sense (lower extremity > upper extremity)

Functional Consequences

Reduced ability to monitor environmental conditions

Less-efficient postural responses

Increased risk of tissue damage under low-load, repetitive conditions

Pathologies Affecting Somatosensory Systems

Diabetic neuropathy

Entrapment neuropathy (e.g., carpal tunnel syndrome)

Toxic neuropathy (e.g., chronic alcoholism)

Sensory and perceptual impairment consequent to cerebrovascular accident

---

This information is used to guide patient–family education about skin inspection and wound care, as well as decisions about appropriate socket–limb interface for prosthetic prescription. Screening for proprioceptive send kinesthetic awareness at intact joints provides information that will be useful when designing interventions for postural control and, eventually, prosthetic gait training.

Sensory testing requires that the individual be able to concentrate and focus so as to respond when a stimulus is presented. The reliability of sensory testing is diminished in individuals with confusion or delirium or if the examiner uses a consistent (predictable) pattern or rhythm during testing.[141] To minimize the likelihood of "lucky guesses" in those with suspected sensory impairment, it may be helpful to test specific sites multiple times, in random order and uneven timing, documenting the number of accurate responses versus number of times stimulated (e.g., 0/3 1/3, 2/3, or 3/3) at each testing site.

Noting how the individual with new amputation perceives the residual limb is also important; is the individual willing to look at the limb, watch it during dressing changes, touch it, or freely move it? One challenge in the preprosthetic period is to assist the incorporation of this "different" limb in the person's body image and self-perception.[21,22,142] Some individuals with dysvascular-neuropathic disease continue to perceive their limb as fragile and needing protection. Those with traumatic amputation may become emotionally distressed when confronted with the real evidence of their loss. These situations may interfere with readiness to wear and use a prosthesis effectively. Awareness of the person's emotional response to his or her altered body guides the therapist in patient education and intervention activities aimed to accomplish adaptation of body image necessary for effective prosthetic use.

Assessing Mobility, Locomotion, and Balance

An individual with recent amputation may find that simple mobility tasks (rolling over, coming to sitting/returning to supine, transitioning from sitting to standing) are more difficult than anticipated following surgery. With the reduction of body mass that results from lower extremity amputation, for example, the individual's functional center of mass (COM) shift slightly upward and to the opposite side of the body; the degree of the shift is directly related to the amount of body mass removed during amputation surgery.[143] When this alteration in body mass is paired with deconditioning associated with bed rest, performance of mobility tasks degrades. It is important to document baseline functional status, and to discern how much that altered body mass, altered muscle performance, and even fear of pain or of falling may be contributing to difficulty in moving. These alterations in COM may require adaptation of strategies used before surgery for postural control; most persons with recent amputation can effectively adapt their postural control mechanisms by practicing activities that require them to anticipate or respond to postural demands.

One of the most functionally important aspects of preoperative assessment is determination of the person with new amputation's usual (previous) and current (postoperative) ambulatory status. The therapist is interested in the individual's familiarity with the use of assistive devices (e.g., walker, crutches, canes), need for assistance to assume standing and while walking, typical distances walked before surgery, the overall effort (energy cost) of walking, the frequency of walking, any other factors or comorbidities that limit walking, and the type of walking environment that the person is most likely to encounter after discharge from acute care (e.g., level inside, uneven outside, stairs and ramps). Self-reports and direct observation of walking provide this information.

Preamputation ambulatory status is a very strong predictor of functional postoperative prosthetic use.[144,145]

At this early point in rehabilitation the priority is safety and functionality of walking, rather than quality and preciseness of the gait pattern. Detailed observational gait analysis is typically deferred until training with the prosthesis begins. Quantitative kinematics (e.g., cadence, gait speed, step or stride length) and ratings of perceived exertion can be used to establish a baseline early in the postoperative period, as a benchmark for progression and readiness for discharge. Individuals with new amputation must be able to use a step-to or swing-through gait pattern with the type of walker or crutches that provides adequate stability and energy efficiency with the least activity restriction.[146]

In acute care settings, initial examination and training of gait is likely to focus on level, predictable surfaces in a relatively closed environment. The ability to manage on a variety of surfaces in active and open environments is examined as care progresses; discharge from acute care approaches; and preprosthetic rehabilitation continues at home, in subacute settings, or on an outpatient basis. The individual with recent amputation using an assistive device in single limb ambulation must be able to walk forward, sideways, backward, change direction, and turn, in addition to managing stairs and inclines so as to be safe and functional in the home environment. Familiarity with and effectiveness of propulsion and maneuverability of a wheelchair are likely to be important in the preprosthetic period for both the individual and family caregivers.

Determining the effectiveness of the individual's postural control is also important. This includes stability in quiet sitting and standing; anticipatory postural adjustments in reaching, transitions from sitting to standing as well as during locomotion; and reactionary postural adjustments when there is unexpected perturbation or unpredictable environmental conditions (e.g., a wet area on the floor, an area rug that may shift when stepped on). Although testing protocols such as functional reach, Tinetti Performance Oriented Mobility Assessment, and measures of balance confidence are used clinically for persons with recent amputation, the reliability, validity, and norms for safe or impaired performance are not well documented in the research literature.[147-149] Subjective assessment of postural control (poor, fair, good, excellent) is somewhat influenced by the therapist's level of experience and comfort with allowing an individual to move toward his or her limits of stability.[150] The Amputee Mobility Predictor (Figure 20-11) may be a useful tool to establish baseline preprosthetic balance and walking abilities, as well as an outcome measure for preprosthetic rehabilitation.[151] Minimal detectable change for the Amputee Mobility Predictor is reported to be 3.5 points.[152] Providing an opportunity for the individual to practice moving from sitting to standing and ambulation with an appropriate assistive device allows the therapist to identify potential problems with balance and postural control. This also helps the individual anticipate what mobility will be like while the residual limb heals and while awaiting the prosthesis.

AMPUTEE MOBILITY PREDICTOR ASSESSMENT TOOL – AMPnoPRO

Initial instructions: Testee is seated in a hard chair 40-50cm height with arms. The following maneuvers are tested without the prosthesis. Advise the person of each task or group of tasks prior to performance. Please avoid unnecessary chatter throughout the test and no task should be performed if either the tester or testee is uncertain of a safe outcome. One attempt only per item
Maximum of 2 days allowed to complete assessment

The right limb is:☐ PF ☐ TT ☐ KD ☐ TF ☐ HD ☐ intact   The left limb is: ☐ PF ☐ TT ☐ KD ☐ TF ☐ HD ☐ intact

NAME: ASSESSOR: DATE: TIME:

			COMMENTS
1.Sitting Balance Sit forward without backrest, with arms folded across chest for 60s.	Cannot sit upright independently for 60s Can sit upright independently for 60s	=0 =1	
2.Sitting reach Reach forwards and grasp the ruler using preferred arm (Tester holds ruler 26cm beyond extended arm midline to the sternum, or against the wall, intact foot midline)	Does not attempt Cannot grasp or required arm support Reaches forward and successfully grasps item	=0 =1 =2	
3.Chair to chair transfer 90° Chair height between 40-50cm , allowed to use aid but no armrests	Cannot do or requires physical assistance Performs task but unsteady or needs contact guarding Performs independently	=0 =1 =2	
4.Arises from chair–single effort Chair height between 40-50cm, tester asks patient to cross arms over chest. If unable, uses arms or assistive device	Unable without physical assistance Able, uses arms/assistive device to help Able without arms	=0 =1 =2	
5.Arises from chair-multiple effort Chair height between 40-50cm, multiple efforts allowed without penalty	Unable without physical assistance Able but requires >1attempts Able to rise in one attempt	=0 =1 =2	
6. Immediate standing Balance(1st 5 secs) Standing on one leg, timing commences at initial hip extension	Unable Able, but requires use of arms for support Able without arm support	=0 =1 =2	
7. Standing balance :30seconds 1st attempt do not use arm support, if unable, may use arm support on 2nd attempt	Unable Able, but requires use of arms for support Able without arm support	=0 =1 =2	
8. (Amypro only)			
9. Standing balance: standing reach Reach forward and grasp the ruler 26cm beyond preferred arm midline to the sternum or against a wall	Unable Able, but requires use of arms for support Able without arm support	=0 =1 =2	
10. Standing balance: nudge test Standing on one leg, tester gently pushes on subjects sternum with palm of hand 3 times (ONLY if safe to do so)	Begins to fall, needs catching catches self using arms for support Steady, toes come up for equilibrium reaction	=0 =1 =2	
11. Standing balance: eyes closed 30sec.	Unsteady or uses arm support Steady without arm support	=0 =1	
12. Standing balance: picking object off the floor Object is placed 30cm in front of patient, midline	Unable Able, but requires use of arms for support Able without arm support	=0 =1 =2	
13. Stand to sit Patient is asked to sit in chair with arms crossed over chest. If unable, allow use of hands	Unable, or falls into chair Able, but uses arms for support Able, without use of arms	=0 =1 =2	
14. Initiation of gait Patient is asked to hop with an aid and observed for hesitancy	Any hesitancy or multiple attempts to start No hesitancy	=0 =1	
15. Hopping 8 meters a) Step length b) Foot clearance (discourage deviations incl. Circumduction, foot sliding or shuffling	a) Does not advances 30cm on each hop Advances minimum of 30cm each hop b) Unable to clear foot without deviations Clears foot on every step	=0 =1 =0 =1	
16. Step continuity	Stopping or discontinuity between hops Hops appear continuous	=0 =1	
17. Turning 180° turn to sit in chair	Unable to turn without physical assistance No assistance, 4 or more hops to turn No assistance, 3 or less hops to turn	=0 =1 =2	
18. Variable cadence Patient is asked to hop 4 metres, and repeat a total of 4 times. Speeds are to vary from slow, fast, fast and then slow (ONLY if safe to do so)	Unable to vary cadence Able to vary cadence, but asymmetrical step lengths used or balance compromised Able without asymmetry or balance compromise	=0 =1 =2	

FIGURE 20-11 Items of the Amputee Mobility Predictor scale. (Modified from Gailey RS, Roah KE, Applegate EB, et al. The Amputee Mobility Predictor: an instrument to assess determinants of the lower limb amputee's abilty to ambulate. *Arch Phys Med Rehabil.* 2002;83(5):613-627.)

Assessing Posture, Ergonomics, and Body Mechanics

In the assessment of symmetry of alignment in sitting and standing, it is important to differentiate habitual or preferred postures from fixed postures, malalignments, and deformities.[153] This might be accomplished by noting whether a particular postural orientation is maintained during different functional activities, as well as whether the individual with new amputation can change position or alignment when so directed. Quantitative measures to document abnormalities in posture and alignment include comparison with vertical and horizontal using plumb line and grids, goniometry and angle assessment, and passive movement.

Given the typical age group of persons with dysvascular-neuropathic etiology of amputation, there may be kyphosis associated with osteoporosis, especially if there is history of pathological compression fractures of the spine.[153] Assessing the health and function of the lumbar spine in standing and during reaching and lifting activity (including excursion of hamstrings and flexibility of hip flexors and adductors) is important because of the likelihood of developing low back pain with the use of a prosthesis if there is contracture. This is especially true for individuals with a transfemoral or any bilateral amputation level.[154] Considering back health early in the preprosthetic program is a health promotion/wellness activity that is a worthwhile investment in time and effort. It is also important to note that, over time, persons with amputation are likely to develop osteopenia or osteoporosis of the residual limb; those with transfemoral amputation may be at increased risk of pathological hip fracture as they age.[155,156]

Assessing Self-Care and Environmental Barriers

In the acute care setting and in many acute rehabilitation centers the Functional Independence Measure (FIM) is commonly used to determine how much assistance an individual with new amputation requires for self-care and toileting, transfers and locomotion, and with cognition-related aspects of task performance[157,158] (Table 20-4). Each item on the FIM is rated between 1 (complete dependence) to 7 (complete independence); possible FIM scores range between 18 and 126 points, with low scores indicating that greater assistance is required. It is important to note that because the FIM was designed to measure burden of care in hospital settings, many of the criteria used to indicate independence for mobility items do not necessarily represent level of function required for community living. In the early postoperative, preprosthetic period, use of the FIM is appropriate; later during preprosthetic care or during prosthetic care, there is likely to be a ceiling effect that makes it less sensitive to change in functional status.[159,160] FIM scores may not be particularly useful as indicators of improvement once an individual has reached relative modified independence, especially on the locomotion and mobility subscales.[161]

Whether using the FIM or other measures of function, the individual's ability to transfer to and from the toilet, in and out of the shower or bathtub, and in and out of a car, bus, or subway; to manage stairs, elevators and escalators; and to get up from the floor (in case of a fall) should be examined as the preprosthetic period advances. This is part of the assessment

TABLE 20-4 *Dimensions of the Functional Independence Measure*

Self-Care Subscale (8 to 56 points)	1.	Eating
	2.	Grooming
	3.	Bathing
	4.	Dressing the upper body
	5.	Dressing the lower body
	6.	Toileting
	7.	Bladder management
	8.	Bowel management
Mobility Subscale (5 to 35 points)	9.	Transfers: bed to chair or wheelchair
	10.	Transfers: to and from toilet
	11.	Transfers: in and out of bathtub or shower
	12.	Locomotion: walking or wheelchair propulsion
	13.	Stairs
Cognition Subscale (5 to 35 points)	14.	Communication: comprehension (auditory and visual)
	15.	Communication: expression (verbal and nonverbal)
	16.	Social interaction
	17.	Problem solving
	18.	Memory
Total FIM Score	**Range 18 to 126 points**	

NOTE: The FIM is a proprietary measurement tool of the Uniform Data System for Medical Rehabilitation (270 Northpointe Parkway, Suite 300, Amherst, NY 14228, www.info@udsmr.org). Readers are encouraged to contact the UDSMR for detailed information about administering, scoring, and interpreting the tool.

of readiness to return to the home environment or determine the need for continued rehabilitation. The rehabilitation team must also consider the individual's ability to dress, perform self-care and grooming activities, inspect his or her residual and remaining limbs, and function in typical food preparation roles and other instrumental activities of daily living (ADLs).

The team assesses the family caregiver's ability to provide appropriate and effective assistance at home if the individual needs help or guarding during functional activities. Discussion about what work and leisure activities are important for the individual to resume once home will guide selection of appropriate adaptive equipment and adaptive movement strategies necessary to carry out important tasks and roles before receiving the prosthesis.

Finally, information about the accessibility of person's living environment must be gathered, to determine whether it is feasible to return home to function on a single limb during the preprosthetic period. The therapist may ask family members to measure doorway widths, determine whether there is adequate space for maneuvering a wheelchair, and consider the need for installation of ramps to make entering/exiting the home both less effortful and safer. Readers are referred to Chapter 35: Environmental Assessment: Home, Community, and Work in M. Cameron and L. Monroe (eds.), Physical Rehabilitation: Evidence-Based Examination, Evaluation, and Intervention, St. Louis, MO: Elsevier Saunders, 2007 for more information.

Monitoring for Postoperative Complications

Many individuals undergoing amputation, whether related to an infected diabetic foot wound, peripheral vascular disease, or traumatic injury, carry a high comorbid burden of illness. It is important to be aware of potentially life-threatening and rehabilitation-delaying complications in the postoperative, preprosthetic period. In-hospital mortality following amputation is estimated to be 7.5% to 12.5%.[162-166] Predictors of mortality during this vulnerable time include significant renal disease, chronic obstructive pulmonary disease and congestive heart failure (CHF), previous MI or ischemic stroke, liver dysfunction, and an age of 75 years or older.[161-166] Patients who require blood transfusion during or following surgery tend to have both more postoperative complications and a greater risk of mortality.[167]

There is high risk of morbidity during the immediate postoperative period as well. The stress of surgery may contribute to problematic hyperglycemia and need for insulin in persons with diabetes, even those who had not previously required insulin.[168] Cardiac complications for persons with diabetes, PAD, and coronary artery disease in the postoperative period include arrhythmia (with associated risk of cerebral embolism), exacerbation of CHF, and new MI or stroke.[162-166] Bed rest and inactivity are associated with risk of deep venous thrombosis and associated pulmonary embolism, risk of developing pneumonia, and risk of developing decubitus (pressure) ulcer on the heel of the intact limb or sacrum.[169,170] Placement of catheter for collection of urine increases risk of urinary tract infection.[171] Infection of the surgical wound has been reported to be between 10% and 26% in dysvascular disease and 34% in those with amputation as a consequence of trauma.[170,172,173] Pneumonia, urinary tract infection, or infection of the wound may contribute to development of sepsis and eventual multisystem organ failure.[174,175]

CASE EXAMPLE 1A

An 89-Year-Old Facing "Elective" Transtibial Amputation for Severe Arterial Occlusive Disease of Her Right Foot

---

N. H. is a slight but energetic woman who is referred to your interdisciplinary team for preoperative examination and education about the rehabilitation program she will be involved in after her planned transtibial amputation. She stands 5 ft 2 in tall with slight kyphosis and weighs 101 lb. She rises to standing by scooting to the edge of her wheelchair (used for community mobility), then rocking back and forth several times to build momentum. She tells you that she spends her days reading the *New York Times*, writing to grandchildren and the few long-term friends still alive, cooking (with help to assemble ingredients and take things in and out of the oven), and talking to other "shut ins" from her church on the phone. N. H. lives in the home of her youngest son, a 67-year-old who has recently undergone quadruple coronary artery bypass grafting and is recovering from an embolic stroke that left him with mild left hemiparesis. Grandchildren and great-grandchildren visit fairly often. According to her chart, N. H. has hypertension controlled by β-blockers, had a mild MI 15 years ago, has never smoked cigarettes, and enjoys a glass of wine with her evening meal. She had lens implants for cataracts bilaterally but still wears glasses to read. Over the past year, claudication has become an increasing problem, making it uncomfortable for her to walk from her bedroom at one end of the ranch-style home to the kitchen and family room at the other. When presented with the choice of revascularization versus amputation, she decided that, in the long run, she would rather take her chances with amputation surgery with spinal anesthesia than bypass graft with general anesthesia. She expresses concern that she is "very out of shape" because her walking has been so limited by ischemic pain. She has a good friend whose husband used a transtibial prosthesis for many years after losing his foot in a lawnmower accident; this has assured her that a prosthesis will allow her adequate mobility and function once she heals after surgery. She tells you she has come through many difficult times during her long life, and although sad at the prospect of losing her leg, she looks forward to being free of claudication pain and anticipates she will muster the determination necessary to get back on her feet.

Questions to Consider

- What additional data might you want to gather from the medical record to build your understanding of her current condition and medical prognosis?
- What are the most important questions to ask during your interview with N. H. and her son as you begin to formulate her PT diagnosis and plan of care?
- Given her age and general health status, what additional review of physiological systems would be important to carry out before surgery? Why have you chosen these systems? How might they affect her ability to participate in rehabilitation?
- What specific tests and measures, at an impairment level, will be important to do during your physical examination? How long do you think the assessment might take? How might you prioritize if your time with N. H. is limited? How reliable are the strategies that you have chosen? How precise does the information you are collecting at this preoperative visit need to be?
- What functional activities would you choose to assess before her surgery? What tests and measures will you use to document her functional status?
- What information would be important for you to share with N. H. and her son about the first few days after her surgery? Before discharge from acute care? During the preprosthetic period until she is ready to be casted for her initial prosthesis?
- Given the limited information currently available to you, what impression or expectations do you have about her postoperative care? How might this be different if she had a medical diagnosis of type 2 diabetes?

A 25-Year-Old with Bilateral Traumatic Transtibial Amputations Sustained in a Construction Accident

P. G. is a construction worker who was pinned between the fenders of two vans when the driver of one van put the vehicle in reverse as P. G. was walking between them. He sustained severely comminuted and open fractures of the mid tibia and fibula and significant damage to soft tissue and neurovascular structures. Tourniquets were placed on his limbs by emergency medical technicians responding to the 911 call. In the emergency department trauma surgeons determined that neither of P. G.'s limbs met criteria for limb salvage. Because the limbs were contaminated by dirt and debris from the job site, the surgeon performed bilateral open transtibial amputations to allow for frequent wound inspection. P. G. was placed on intravenous antibiotics. Three days after the operation, there is no sign of infection in either limb. Revision and closure of his residual limbs is scheduled for tomorrow, using an equal anterior and posterior flaps closure, leaving approximately 5 inches of residual tibia in length. Adjustable polypropylene, removable, semirigid dressings are planned for compression and protection of the wound postoperatively.

Review of the medical record indicates that P. G. was in generally good health before his injury, although he has been a pack-per-day smoker since the beginning of high school. He was 6 ft 4 in tall, weighing 210 lb before his injury. His only previous hospitalization was at age 17, for open-reduction, internal fixation of a midshaft right femoral fracture sustained in a motorcycle accident. P. G. has been married for slightly more than 1 year, and his wife is 7 months' pregnant. They live on the third floor of a three-family home in the ethnic city neighborhood in which they grew up. Extended family members have kept vigil at the hospital since the accident to support P. G. and his wife. When not working, P. G. is an avid motorcycle and quad rider, competing locally in both speed and distance events. He also participates in an intracity adult basketball league.

Pain management has been via a morphine pump; even with this, P. G. reports typical pain levels of five to six out of 10, increasing in severity during dressing changes. When you come to discuss his postoperative rehabilitation with him, he is in a semireclined position in bed, with both lower limbs abducted and externally rotated at the hip, resting in apparent 20 degrees of knee flexion. He is anxious and quite angry over the situation, stating that he "can't believe this has happened" and "doesn't want to end up in a wheelchair" unable to work. The only experience he has with persons with amputation is an uncle with poorly controlled diabetes who had successive amputations of multiple toes as a consequence of vascular insufficiency, subsequently revised to transmetatarsal because of osteomyelitis of a neuropathic wound, and then to transtibial because of delayed healing. P. G.'s uncle's rehabilitation was complicated by a significant stroke a week after transtibial

amputation, and although he wears a prosthesis, his mobility limitations keep him homebound.

Questions to Consider

- What additional data might you want to gather from the medical record to build your understanding of P. G.'s current condition and medical prognosis?
- What are the most important questions to ask during your interview with P. G. and his family as you begin to formulate his PT diagnosis and plan of care?
- What additional review of physiological systems would be important to carry out before surgery? Why have you chosen these systems? How might they affect his ability to participate in rehabilitation?
- What specific tests and measures, at an impairment level, will be important to do during your physical examination? How long do you think the assessment might take? How might you prioritize if your time with P. G. is limited? How reliable are the strategies that you have chosen? How precise does the information you are collecting at this preoperative visit need to be?
- What functional activities would you choose to assess before his surgery? What tests and measures will you use to document his functional status?
- What information would be important for you to share with P. G. and his family about the first few days after the next surgery? Before discharge from acute care? During the preprosthetic period until he is ready to be casted for his initial prostheses?
- Given the limited information currently available to you, what impression or expectations do you have about his postoperative care? How might P. G.'s care be similar to or different from that of his uncle and the older woman in the previous case?

THE PROCESS OF EVALUATION, DIAGNOSIS, AND PROGNOSIS

Understanding an individual's rehabilitation needs emerges as baseline data are collected and integrated with health professionals' clinical expertise and judgment, as well as evidence from the clinical research literature. As part of the evaluative process, the team weighs factors that are likely to influence the rehabilitation program and begins to formulate a plan of care to address the individual's specific needs. The team identifies key problems that will need to be addressed, formulates a PT (rehabilitation) movement dysfunction diagnosis, estimates the level of function that will likely be reached and the time and intensity of intervention necessary to reach it, specifies measurable goals that will be used to judge progression over time, and prioritizes interventions to be carried out as part of the rehabilitation program. Readers are referred to the *Guide to Physical Therapist Practice* to review for details about the patient-client management process and the practice patterns applicable to PT care of persons with recent amputation (http://www.apta.org/Guide/) (Box 20-3).

BOX 20-3   *Guide to Physical Therapist Practice Patterns Relevant for Individuals with Amputation*

MUSCULOSKELETAL SYSTEM

Impaired motor function, muscle performance, range of motion, gait, locomotion, and balance associated with amputation

NEUROMUSCULAR SYSTEM

Impaired motor function and sensory integrity associated with acute or chronic polyneuropathies

CARDIOVASCULAR/CARDIOPULMONARY SYSTEM

Primary prevention/risk reduction for cardiovascular/pulmonary disorders or

Impaired aerobic capacity/endurance associated with deconditioning

INTEGUMENTARY SYSTEM

Primary prevention/risk reduction for integumentary disorders

Impaired integumentary integrity associated with skin involvement extending into fascia, muscle, or bone and scar formation

Physical Therapy Diagnosis

The PT diagnosis reflects the problems with body structure and function (impairments) and activity (functional limitations) that the person with recent amputation encounters as a consequence of their surgery and current health status. The PT diagnosis differs from the medical diagnosis in that it focuses on the functional consequences of a condition at the level of the system and, more importantly, at the level of the whole person.[7]

The models used to frame the rehabilitation process has evolved from the process of disablement[176] to a focus on enablement, based on the World Health Organization's (WHO) International Classification of Functioning, Disability and Health (ICF).[177-179] The models provide a way of organizing information collected in the patient-client interview and examination process, to facilitate development of a PT movement diagnosis, prognosis and goals, and plan of care. For students and new therapists, it may be helpful to complete an organizational table on the basis of the ICF model that lists all relevant descriptors of active disease/comorbidity, the impairments and resources of body structures and function, and the activity and participation level issues that need to be addressed during the episode of care (Table 20-5). The entries in each column in the table can be prioritized, with notations about which issues are likely to improve or change and which will require adaptive equipment or alternative strategies. The statement of PT diagnosis for the particular individual begins with a prioritized list of activities to be addressed during the episode of care, followed by the contributing impairments of body systems and structures elated to or result from the individual's constellation of active pathologies and comorbidities.

Formulating the PT diagnosis in this way clearly guides establishment of goals and appropriate interventions.

Plan of Care: Prognosis

Forecasting the length of the proposed episode of PT care and the potential for prosthetic replacement and rehabilitation can be challenging. Decisions must be informed by several factors:

1. The overall health, cognitive, and preamputation functional status of the individual;
2. The level of amputation as it affects prosthetic control and the energy cost of walking;
3. The likely contribution of prosthetic use to perform basic and instrumental ADLs, for the individual or for the caregivers who will be assisting and managing daily function;
4. The resources (financial and instrumental) available to the individual during the entire rehabilitation process; and
5. Knowledge of typical length of stay for patients with amputation in the setting in which care if being provided (acute care, inpatient rehabilitation, subacute care, home care, or outpatient care).

The premorbid factors that tend to predict successful prosthetic use (i.e., rehabilitation potential) include the ability to walk functional distance in the months prior to surgery, overall level of physical fitness, requiring little assistance in ADLs, and the ability to maintain single limb stance without assistance.[180] Persons of advanced age often require a longer period of rehabilitation, but eventually become functional prosthetic users. Delayed wound healing (which delays prosthetic fitting), as well as knee and hip flexion contracture, reduce the likelihood of successful prosthetic use.[181] A long list of past or chronic illnesses does not predict poor rehabilitation potential: Approximately 75% of persons with amputation are able to return to independent living, managing multiple chronic conditions effectively to become highly functional prosthetic users.[182] Premorbid health conditions what make prosthetic use less likely (odds ratio >2.0) include moderate to severe dementia, end-stage renal disease, and advanced coronary artery disease.[183] Persons with very low body mass (underweight) may have more difficulty with prosthetic ambulation and functional independence than those who are overweight and obese, given a similar comorbid burden of illness.[182] Hip extensor strength is a powerful contributor to overall function with a prosthesis for persons with both transtibial and transfemoral amputation.[184] Difficulty learning has more of an impact during the postoperative and preprosthetic period than does depression or anxiety.[185] The sooner an individual is fit for a prosthesis and begins rehabilitation following amputation, the more likely the individual will become a functional prosthetic user.[186]

Long-term outcome of function and survivorship following amputation is more difficult to forecast: The relatively high morbidity and mortality for patients with amputation secondary to vascular disease have been well documented.[187-189] Unless there is clear evidence that ambulation will not be possible and that provision of prosthesis will not improve the patient's mobility (e.g., reducing the amount of assistance that is necessary to transfer), prosthetic replacement should and must be considered.

TABLE 20-5 Application of the WHO International Classification of Functioning, Disability and Health (ICF) Model, Completed Postoperatively, for Case Example 1: N. H., an 89-Year-Old, Following with Elective Transtibial Amputation Secondary to Severe Peripheral Arterial Disease

	Overall Health Status	Body Structure and Function (Physiological Systems)	Activity (Overall Functional Status)	Participation (Ability to Engage in Social Roles)	Buffers or Confounding Factors
Resources (preoperative)	Effective management of chronic conditions prior to surgery Intact cognitive status and effective executive function preoperatively Self-rated health "good" other than claudication	Effective vision and hearing Effective communication Highly motivated: determined to eventually return to own home	Previous use of walker and wheelchair Able to ambulate independently with assistive device functional (in home) distances Self-selected walking speed .85 m/s preoperatively Independent in self-care (toileting, bathing with tub seat and handheld shower, dressing) Independent in stair management, step up to step pattern, with rail	Active and engaged in community (church) Able to manage food preparation and cleanup with minimal assistance	Knowledge of successful prosthetic use by friend Understanding of the rehabilitation process: previous participation in cardiac rehabilitation Lives in 1 story home, with ramp at entry Significant emotional and instrumental support available by a number of family caregivers
Active problems (examination findings)	Medical diagnosis: Peripheral arterial disease with critical limb ischemia Status post right transtibial amputation, posterior flap (2/15/12) Removable rigid dressing 2" square ecchymosis suture line Moderate amount of serosanguineous drainage at mid suture line Postoperative pain (morphine pump) Comorbid conditions Hypertension (β blockers) Status post MI (1997) Cataract (lens implants 6/12/07) Recent fall in hospital bathroom (2/17/12) Mild postoperative delirium with sundown syndrome Stress incontinence Possible osteoporosis Possible sarcopenia	Postoperative pain (4/10 VAS) Phantom sensation (cramping) Potential for delayed healing because of injury to surgical site sustained in fall Postoperative edema Limited excursion right knee flexion and hip extension ROM Less than 3/5 muscle strength right knee extension, hip abduction, hip extension Diminished functional core and upper extremity muscle strength Limited muscular endurance Limited cardiovascular endurance Limited short-term memory and distractibility (MMSE preoperation 28/30, postoperation 18/30) Hypersensitivity to touch and pressure bordering suture line Inadequate protective sensation left forefoot Impaired postural control in single limb support (static and dynamic)	Difficulty with transitions Effortful but functional rolling side to side Minimal assistance to shift upward in bed (difficulty sustaining "bridge" position) Minimal assistance supine to/from sitting with directional cuing Moderate assistance sit to stand, with directional cuing Maximal assistance stand to sit with poor eccentric control upper extremity and left lower extremity Inability to ambulate functionally Moderate assist of 1, hop to pattern in parallel bars, requires consistent cueing Step length 6 inches, perceived exertion 7/10, distance 10ft Diminished exercise and activity tolerance Difficulty with toileting, dressing, and other self-care activities Quickly becomes frustrated and agitated when encounters difficulty with mobility and self-care tasks Possible difficulty with carryover of new learning from session to session until delirium clears Difficulty self-monitoring status of residual limb and remaining limb	Inability to function in typical premorbid roles in interactions with family at home Inability to function in premorbid roles in interactions with members of her communities (church, friends, extended family)	Left lower extremity claudication may limit activity

Physical Therapy Diagnosis: N. H. has difficulty with functional activity (mobility and transfers, ambulation, and self-care activities) secondary to postoperative dysfunction of body structure and systems (transient cognitive impairment, pain, impaired muscle strength and motor control, diminished endurance, limited range of motion of at key lower extremity joints, impaired postural control) related to recent transtibial amputation, postoperative delirium, and various comorbidities.

A key component of prognosis is delineation of the frequency, intensity, and duration of the episode of care. In the acute care setting, hospitalization for an uncomplicated amputation may be 4 to 7 days and PT may occur for 30 to 45 minutes, once or twice daily. For frail or chronically ill older adults coping with multiple comorbidities, length of stay often increases to 21 or more days. For individuals with amputation as a result of trauma affecting multiple systems, the period of hospitalization depends on the severity of damage across all systems, so that duration of care may be longer. Postacute care occurs in inpatient rehabilitation settings (approximately 55%), subacute rehabilitation settings (approximately 21%), or by discharge to home with referral for in-home nursing and rehabilitation services (approximately 24%).[190] Discharge location is determined by overall health status and need for care, availability and capacity of family caregivers, the type of rehabilitation settings or care that is available in the area, as well as by insurance and financial considerations. In subacute settings, for those on Medicare, the rehabilitation stay may be for a month or more and care is much more intense, with PT typically occurring twice daily with an hour of more of PT and occupational therapy planned each day. Care provided at home and in outpatient settings may be somewhat less intense, occurring three times a week for an hour or more, but is certainly supplemented by an active home program.

CASE EXAMPLE 2B

Determining a Physical Therapy Diagnosis for P. G. Following Revision of Bilateral Transtibial Amputations

You have collected the following information in your chart review, interview, and brief initial examination:
- *Surgery:* Underwent revision and closure of bilateral open amputation 2 days ago (under general anesthesia) with equal anterior and posterior flaps closures; 5.25-inch residual tibia on left, 4.75-inch residual tibia on right. Placed in bulky dressing and Ace wrap for compression, then into bilateral adjustable prefabricated semirigid dressings to hold knees in full extension and protect surgical construct. Moderate serosanguineous drainage noted at first dressing change. Wound edges slightly inflamed consistent with operative trauma. No dehiscence noted. Proximal circumference at joint line 10.25 inches bilaterally, distal circumference (4 inches below) of right residual limb 11.25 inches and of left residual limb 11 inches.
- *Postoperative health:* Elevated temperature postoperatively, with diminished breath sounds in posterior bases of lungs bilaterally. Radiograph suggests early pneumonia. Cough nonproductive.
- *Cognition/affect:* Signs of agitation and distress in recovery room, being mildly sedated for combination of pain relief and calming. Currently lethargic and somewhat distractible, requiring consistent cueing to stay on task during examination.

- *Pain/phantom sensation:* Reports postoperative pain at seven out of 10 level. Complains of shooting pains in phantom right lower extremity and is distressed by "itchy" toes on phantom left lower extremity. Currently IV narcotics every 3 hours for pain management.
- *ROM/muscle length:* Reports "pulling" behind knees when head of bed elevated into long sitting position. Requests time out of semirigid dressing to allow knee flexion and be more comfortable.
- *Muscle performance/motor control:* Able to actively extend both knees to approximately 10 degrees from full extension, stops because of "pulling" behind knee.
- *Upper extremity function and transfers:* Able to "push up" to lift body weight when assisted to bedside chair, requiring contact guard/minimal assist, using a sliding board to transfer.
- *Aerobic capacity/endurance:* Reports transfer effort six out of 10 on perceived exertion scale. Reports dyspnea five out of 10 immediately following transfer.
- *Rolls independently:* Able to come to sitting from side-lying with minimal assistance.
- *Postural control:* Maintained static sitting balance on edge of bed 2 minutes. Able to reach forward 7 inches, sideward more than 10 inches bilaterally, reluctant to turn and reach behind because of discomfort. Effective postural responses to mild perturbations forward and backward, moderate perturbations sideways.

Questions to Consider
- List all of the active pathologies and comorbidities that will influence P. G.'s postoperative/preprosthetic care.
- List and prioritize the impairments, across physiological systems and from a psychological perspective, that should be directly addressed or considered in his rehabilitation plan of care.
- List and prioritize the functional limitations that will be addressed during his acute care stay. Suggest additional functional limitations that will be addressed as his rehabilitation progresses at home or at a subacute or rehabilitation facility.
- List and prioritize disabilities that P. G. is likely to be concerned about and that the rehabilitation team will be attempting to minimize over the course of his care.
- Develop a definitive PT diagnosis for P. G. on the basis of the disablement model.
- Develop a rehabilitation prognosis for P. G. and explain or justify your expectations.
- Develop a list of prioritized goals for P. G. for the next 2 weeks in the acute care hospital. Expand these goals as if care would continue after discharge in a rehabilitation center, at home, or on an outpatient basis. What will frequency, duration, and intensity of his rehabilitation sessions be? How will you judge if he is making progress toward achieving these goals?

Plan of Care: Determining Appropriate Goals

Goals to be achieved during a particular episode of care are influenced by the setting in which care is provided. Although the overall goal of the preprosthetic period is to prepare the individual for prosthetic fitting and training, the specific goals of the acute care setting may be to achieve primary wound closure, initiate an effective strategy for compression, and achieve supervision or minimal assist in transfers and in locomotion using a wheelchair or ambulatory device on level surfaces during the days or week that the person is hospitalized. In subsequent subacute, home care, and outpatient settings, goals expand to include strengthening of core and key muscle groups; ensuring adequate ROM for prosthetic use; improving cardiovascular fitness; and achieving more advanced ADLs, instrumental activities of daily living (IADLs), and mobility skills over a longer period of intervention.[191] An effective goal is directly linked to the impairments and functional limitation identified in the PT diagnosis and is stated in measurable terms so that progression can be assessed as postoperative and preprosthetic care continues (Box 20-4).

BOX 20-4   *Acute Care Goals for Case Example 1A*

N. H. is an 89-year-old woman with recent transtibial amputation secondary to peripheral arterial disease. By the conclusion of this episode of care (projected 4 to 5 days), N. H. will be able to do the following:

- Actively participate in inspection of her surgical wound during dressing changes and of her remaining limb.
- Describe and recognize signs of inflammation, dehiscence, ecchymosis, and infection along her incision site and of inflammation or developing neuropathic or vascular ulceration of her remaining extremity.
- Direct caregivers in the proper application of her compressive dressing and removal of her rigid dressing.
- Safely perform rolling and bridging activities, without assistance, for effective bed mobility with perceived exertion of no more than three out of 10.
- Demonstrate active contraction into full-knee extension in supine and seated positions.
- Demonstrate understanding of proper stretching and flexibility for knee extension and hip extension in multiple functional positions.
- Safely rise and return from sitting to standing position from a standard arm chair or wheelchair with minimal assistance and occasional verbal cues, with perceived exertion of four out of 10.
- Ambulate with contact guard and occasional cues, using a hop-to pattern using a standard walker for 25 feet, with a perceived exertion of four out of 10.
- Direct caregivers in assisting her with toilet transfers and clothing management during toileting and other self-care activities

---

INTERVENTIONS FOR PERSONS WITH RECENT AMPUTATION

After amputation surgery the focus shifts to preparation for prosthetic use.[192] Strategies for control of edema, pain management, and facilitation of wound healing are implemented. The person with a new amputation and his or her caregivers receive instruction and the opportunity to practice single limb mobility with an appropriate assistive device. For persons with dysvascular or diabetes-related amputation, condition of the remaining foot must be carefully monitored as single limb mobility training begins.[193] Handling of the residual limb during dressing changes and skin inspection, as well as the consistent use of compression devices, helps to desensitize the residual limb, enhancing readiness for prosthetic use. Exercises to strengthen key muscle groups in the residual and remaining limb and to assist effective postural responses are implemented to assist function and prepare for prosthetic gait. Functional training in self-care and transfers begins in the acute care setting and is followed up in home care, subacute, or outpatient settings. The therapist may employ a combination of manual therapy, therapeutic exercise, facilitation techniques, physical agents, and mechanical or electrotherapeutic modalities to help manage pain, assist healing, minimize risk of soft tissue contracture, and enhance mobility. A rigid dressing or temporary socket may be fabricated or adapted to protect the residual limb while it heals.

Postoperative Pain Management

In addition to reducing acute discomfort, effective postoperative pain management is important for several other reasons. Pain is a significant physiological stressor that affects homeostasis, as well as the patient's ability to concentrate and learn.[8,9,113] In the early postoperative period persons with recent amputation are faced with learning how to care for their new residual limb including monitoring for signs of infection, using strategies to control edema, and appropriate positioning to minimize the risk of contracture formation. They must also learn a variety of new motor skills including exercises to preserve strength and ROM and how to protect their healing suture while moving around with crutches or a walker on their remaining limb. If postoperative discomfort and pain are kept to a minimum, they can better learn and retain these new cognitive and motor skills.

Pain can also be fatiguing and demoralizing; those with significant pain may be reluctant to participate fully in active rehabilitation programs because they fear that movement will only increase their pain. Individuals with significant pain may be erroneously labeled as unmotivated or uncooperative, when their primary goal is to find a way to escape their discomfort. Importantly, although certain types of pain medications (opioid and narcotic analgesics) are effective in providing relief, they may compromise cognitive function or increase the risk of postural hypotension.[53] Therapists must be aware of the actions and side effects of the pain medication being used.

In the days immediately after amputation the goal is to minimize the severity of acute postoperative pain. Because prevention is more effective than reduction of significant pain, those with recent amputations are encouraged to request pain medication before pain becomes severe.[54] Preoperative and intraoperative pain management also affects postoperative pain: In patients undergoing amputation due to vascular insufficiency who receive epidural analgesia before surgery, problematic phantom limb pain after amputation may be less likely to develop.[61,62] Effective management of postoperative edema is an important element in the control of postoperative pain as well.

Dealing with Phantom Limb Sensation and Phantom Pain

A variety of pharmacological and nonpharmacological interventions have been used for individuals with significant phantom limb sensation or pain, although management of phantom pain is often challenging and frustrating for all involved.[55,60,64,194,195] Table 20-6 summarizes the results of a recent Cochrane Review focused on efficacy of pharmacological management of phantom limb pain.[196] Current best evidence is, at best, limited as a result of differences in study methodology and design, insufficient control groups, and acuity/chronicity of the pain. Readers are encouraged to follow developing evidence from future randomized controlled trials of pharmacological agents in the management of phantom limb pain. One strategy designed to impact development

of phantom limb pain in the postoperative period is continuous analgesic infusion to control the severity of phantom limb pain in the immediate postoperative period; the success of this intervention varies with pharmacological agents and the rate of their administration.[62,63,197] Pulse radiofrequency ablation[198] and botulinum toxin type A injection[199] are being investigated as possible interventions for severe longstanding phantom limb pain that has not been responsive to more conservative approaches. Sympathetic blocks appear to reduce pain intensity over the short-term (up to 1 week) but not over the long-term (up to 8 weeks).[200] Implantation of spinal cord stimulators has been explored for persons with severe, intractable phantom limb pain, however results appear to be equivocal, and complications of the implantation worrisome.[201]

Physical Therapy for Postoperative and Phantom Pain

The success of early rehabilitation is influenced by the effectiveness of postoperative pain management; for this reason, physical therapists must be aware of medications being used and be involved in assessing the effectiveness of the pain management strategy and its impact on patient learning and function.[202] When epidural anesthesia has been used during surgery or in the immediate postoperative period, it is imperative that the patient's cognitive, autonomic, sensory, and motor function is carefully evaluated before transfer training

TABLE 20-6   *Results of a Cochrane Review of Prescription Medications Used in the Management of Moderate to Severe Phantom Limb Pain and Their Side Effects*

Medication	Class	Primary and Secondary Outcomes*	Adverse Effects Reported
Oral or IV morphine	Opioid	Short-term decrease in pain intensity Better sleep No impact on mood Satisfaction higher in oral vs. IV	Sedation, fatigue, dizziness/vertigo, constipation, sweating, difficulty voiding, itching, respiratory depression
Ketamine or dextromethorphan	N-methyl-D-aspartate (NMDA) receptor antagonists	Short-term decrease in pain intensity Better sleep Better sense of well-being No impact on functional status	Sedation, hallucinations, loss of consciousness, hearing impairment, balance problems, insobriety
Gabapentin	Anticonvulsant	Trend toward short-term decrease in pain intensity No impact on mood No impact on functional status No impact on sleep	Somnolence, dizziness, headache, nausea
Amitriptyline	Tricyclic antidepressant	No impact on pain intensity No impact on mood No impact on functional status Negative impact on sleep	Dry mouth, drowsiness, blurred vision, dizziness, constipation, altered sleep, nausea/vomiting/diarrhea, tinnitus, urinary retention
Calcitonin infusion	Polypeptide hormone	Trend toward decreased intensity and frequency of phantom limb pain in persons with recent amputation	Facial flushing, nausea, sedation, dizziness
Lidocaine; bupivacaine	Anesthetics	No different than morphine	Stinging sensation at injection site

*Primary outcomes: change in phantom limb pain intensity; possible secondary outcomes: changes in mood (depression), functional status, quality of sleep, patient satisfaction with intervention, severity of adverse effects.

Adapted from Alviar MJ, Hale T, Dungca M. Pharmacologic interventions for treating phantom limb pain. *Cochrane Database Syst Rev.* 2011;(12):CD006380.

and single limb mobility activities are begun. In whatever setting PT care is provided, it is important that administration of medications be timed so that pain control is optimal during PT activities. If the patient is experiencing phantom sensation or pain, the physical therapist plays an important role in educating the patient and family about these sensations. Noninvasive alternatives such as relaxation techniques, imagery, desensitization, hypnosis, or therapeutic touch may be effective adjuncts for pharmacological interventions aimed at pain reduction.[203,204]

Transcutaneous electrical nerve stimulation (TENS) is an effective adjunct for pain management for patients with acute postsurgical pain.[205-207] TENS may also play a role in the management of troubling phantom sensation or pain in the immediate postoperative period; however, its efficacy in the prevention or management of phantom limb pain over time is not well supported in the clinical research literature.[208-210]

Additional PT interventions that have been used to manage on postoperative pain include mechanical stimulation (massage, vibration, percussion) and superficial heat (ultrasound, hot packs, cryotherapy) or cold; although there are clinical reports of short-term pain relief, there are few studies that have carefully evaluated their efficacy.[210] For any PT intervention in the postoperative/preprosthetic period, it is imperative to pay careful attention to the healing status of the wound: wound closure must not be compromised by any intervention that is aimed at reducing discomfort or pain.

Energy-based medicine therapies (e.g., mind–body connection approaches, therapeutic touch, eye-movement reprocessing and desensitization, and motor imagery) may be alternative approaches to the management of acute and chronic phantom limb pain, although there are few well-designed and well-controlled studies of their efficacy.[211,212] Mirror box therapy is being investigated as a strategy to minimize the development and severity of phantom pain after amputation.[213,214] This approach attempts to facilitate cortical reorganization by accessing the mirror motor and sensory neuron systems and prefrontal cortex in the brain.[215-217] In the most commonly used paradigm, persons with amputation attempted to move their "missing" limb while simultaneously moving and observing reflected image of the movement of the intact limb.[218] Although preliminary evidence suggests that this strategy may be helpful,[218-221] more carefully designed and controlled studies are necessary before it can be widely adopted for clinical use. Mirror therapy is not without adverse effects: Some individuals experience dizziness and disorientation, or sense of irritation in their residual limb, or do not tolerate the intervention, especially if mirror therapy is concurrent with traditional prosthetic training.[222]

Limb Volume, Shaping, and Postoperative Edema

The management of postoperative edema is important for four reasons: Edema control strategies are essential components of pain control, enhance wound healing, protect the incision during functional activity, and assist preparation for prosthetic replacement by shaping and desensitizing the residual limb.[7] A variety of postsurgical dressing and edema control strategies are available. These include soft dressings with or without Ace wrap compression, semirigid dressings, various removable rigid dressings (RRDs) applied over soft dressings, or the application of a rigid cast dressing in the operating room.[223,224] An immediate or early postoperative prosthesis (IPOP or EPOP) is a rigid dressing with an attachment for a pylon and prosthetic foot.[225,226] Pneumatic IPOP/EPOP options are also available for early ambulation. Each option contributes to pain control, wound healing and protection, and preparation for prosthetic use in a significantly different way. The choice of strategy is determined by the etiology and level of amputation, the condition of the skin, the medical and functional status of the patient, access to prosthetic consultation and care, the preference and experience of the surgeon, and established institutional protocol. Table 20-7 compares characteristics of the most commonly used postoperative/preprosthetic options.[223-225]

Soft Dressings and Compression

The traditional postoperative edema-control and wound-management strategy is a soft dressing with or without compression wrap. A nonadherent dressing is placed over the suture line, sterile absorbant gauze fluff is then placed over this, and one or more rolls of gauze is loosely overwrapped in figure-of-eight pattern around the residual limb. A compressive Ace bandage wrap may then be used in an effort to control some of the postsurgical edema. Although this method continues to be the most frequently used immediate postsurgical option for patients with transfemoral amputation, or when significant wound drainage and a high risk of infection are present, soft dressings with Ace wraps are ineffective for limiting postoperative edema.[107,223,224] Soft dressings cannot protect a healing incision from bumps, bruising, or shearing during activity, or from fall-related injury. The other practical disadvantage of elastic Ace bandage compression of the residual limb is the need for frequent reapplication: Movement during daily activities quickly loosens the bandages, compromising the effectiveness of the compression. Most rehabilitation professionals suggest that Ace bandages should be removed and reapplied every 4 to 6 hours and should never be kept in place for more than 12 hours without rebandaging.[227]

Effective application of an Ace wrap requires practice, manual dexterity, and attention to details if the desired distal-to-proximal pressure gradient is to be achieved (Figures 20-12 and 20-13).[67,227,228] It may be difficult for patients with limited vision, arthritis of the hands and wrist, limited trunk mobility, or compromised postural control to master this technique for independence in control of edema. Nurses, residents, surgeons, therapists, prosthetists, and family members (and anyone else who may be taking down the soft dressing to care for the wound) must be consistent and effective in reapplication of the Ace bandage if maximal control of edema is to be achieved. Ineffectively applied elastic wraps can lead to a bulbous, poorly shaped residual limb, which is likely to delay prosthetic fitting.[228] Tight circumferential wrapping can significantly compromise blood flow, compromising healing of the incision and even leading to skin breakdown.[228]

TABLE 20-7   *Comparison of Various Postoperative Options for Management of New Transtibial Residual Limbs Following Amputation*

STRATEGY	Cost	Ease of Application	Wound Healing	OUTCOMES				
				Protection from Trauma	Degree of Postoperative Edema	Postoperative Pain	Knee Flexion Contracture Risk	Time to First Prosthetic Fitting
Soft gauze dressing without Ace	Inexpensive	Not difficult	Little impact on primary or secondary healing	None	Significant	Often severe	Very high	Prolonged
Soft gauze with Ace wrap	Inexpensive	Figure-of-eight wrap requires skill, frequent reapplication	Little impact on primary or secondary healing	None	Significant	Often severe	Very high	Prolonged
"Shrinker" garment	Low to moderate cost	Requires UE strength, dexterity	Used after primary healing has occurred	Minimal	Moderate	Somewhat less	Very high	Slightly shortened
Rigid dressing (above knee cast)	Low cost	Requires training; MD or CP	Reduces time to primary healing	Excellent	Minimal	Minimized	Extremely low	Shortened
RRD (below knee) Plaster/custom	Low to moderate cost	Requires training; PT or CP	Reduces time to primary healing	Very good	Minimal	Minimized	Moderate	Shortened
RRD Prefabricated (thigh level)	Moderate cost	CP custom fits	Reduces time to primary healing	Very good	Minimal if worn consistently	Minimized if worn consistently	Extremely low	Shortened
IPOP Rigid dressing Plaster/custom	Low to high cost	CP applies in the OR, or fabricates	Reduces time to primary healing if protected WtB only	Very good when worn, protected WtB only	Reduced if worn consistently	Minimized if worn consistently	Low if worn consistently	Shortened
IPOP: pneumatic	Moderate to high cost	PT uses as part of rehabilitation	Less evidence about impact on healing available	Very good when worn, protected WtB only	Reduced if shrinker worn between IPOP use	Depends on options in place between IPOP use	Moderate if not in thigh RRD between use	Shortened

CP, Certified prosthetist; *IPOP*, immediate postoperative prosthesis; *MD*, physician; *OR*, operating room; *PT*, physical therapist; *UE*, upper extremity; *ROM*, range of motion; *RRD*, removable rigid dressing; *WtB*, weight-bearing.

Data from Nawijn SE, van der Linde H, Emmelot CH, Hofstad CJ. Stump management after transtibial amputation: a systematic review. *Prosthet Orthot Int.* 2005;29(1):13-26; Smith DG, McFarland LV, Sangeorzan BJ, et al. Addendum 1: Post-operative dressing and management strategies for transtibial amputations: a critical review. *J Prosthet Orthot.* 2004:16(S3):15-25; and Walsh TL. Custom removable immediate postoperative prosthesis. *J Prosthet Orthot.* 2003;15(4):158-161.

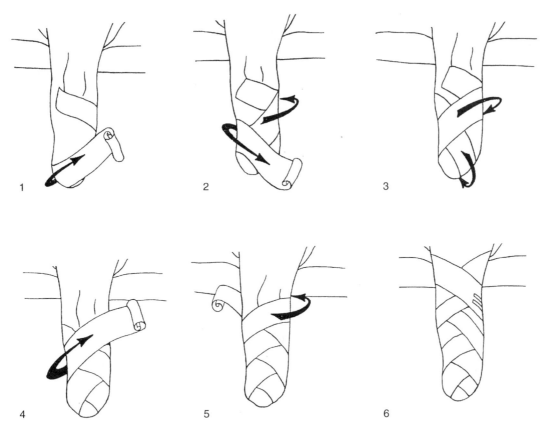

FIGURE 20-12 The application of an effective Ace wrap to a transtibial residual limb uses successive diagonal figure-of-eight loops between the distal residual limb and thigh to create a distal-to-proximal pressure gradient. This creates a distal-to-proximal, tapering, cylindrical residual limb with minimal excess distal soft tissue. (Modified from Karacollof LA, Hammersley CS, Schneider FJ. *Lower Extremity Amputation*. Gaithersburg, MD: Aspen, 1992. pp. 16-17.)

Some patients with bulbous or pressure-sensitive residual limbs do not tolerate Ace wrap for compressions. An alternative to these patients, as well as for those with limited dexterity, is application of a elasticized stockinet or Tubigrip sock (Seton Health Care Group TLC, Oldham, England). Both materials are available with various levels of elasticity; minimal to significant compression can be achieved, depending on the patient's tolerance of pressure. The double-layer method starts with careful application of a long piece of elastic stockinet or Tubigrip over the transtibial residual limb to midthigh level (Figure 20-14). The remaining length of elastic stockinet or Tubigrip is turned or twisted 180 degrees (to minimize pressure over the new incision) and rolled over the residual limb as a second layer of compression. As residual limb volume decreases and the limb becomes more pressure tolerant, stockinet or Tubigrip with progressively narrower diameters is used to increase compressive forces and assist limb shrinkage and maturation. These materials are relatively inexpensive, but they are not as durable as commercially available elastic shrinker socks.

Pressure Garments: "Shrinkers"

Once the suture line has healed sufficiently, many prosthetists and therapists recommend the use of a commercially manufactured elasticized "shrinker" pressure garment whenever the prosthesis is not being worn (Figure 20-15).[82,228] These garments are designed to apply significant distal to proximal graded compressive force to the residual limb, and it may be difficult for individuals with limited manual dexterity or upper extremity strength to apply them. Patients with recent amputation must be careful to minimize or avoid excessive shear forces over the incision as the shrinker is being applied. Although shrinkers are effective for control of edema and limb volume, it is not possible to create "relief" for bony prominences or pressure-vulnerable areas on the residual limb. As with other soft dressings, commercial shrinkers cannot protect the residual limb from trauma during daily activities or in the event of a fall. It is not unusual for patients to continue to use a shrinker for limb volume control, whenever they are not wearing their prosthesis, for 6 months to a year after amputation.[82]

Although a number of edema control options are available for persons with transtibial amputation, those with transfemoral residual limbs have fewer strategies from which to choose. Commercially manufactured shrinkers are more convenient to don and are more likely to remain in place than the more cumbersome Ace wraps, but those who choose this option must be just as careful to capture all the soft tissue high in the groin within the shrinker to avoid the development of an adductor roll, redundant tissue that may make prosthetic

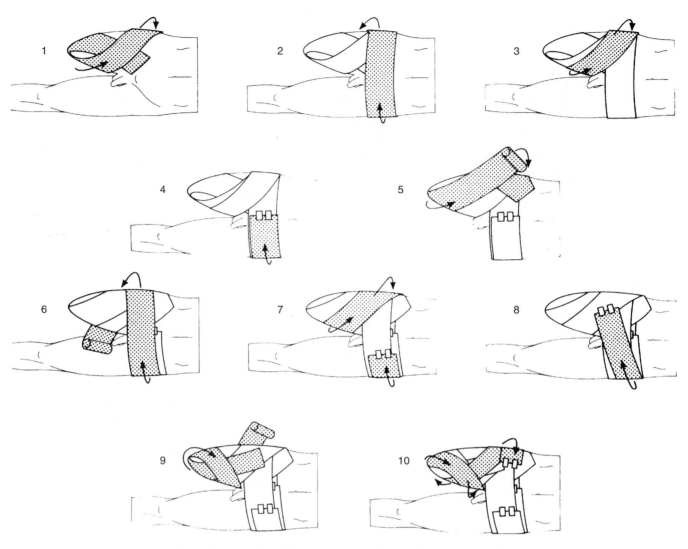

FIGURE 20-13 The application of an effective Ace wrap to a transfemoral limb also strives to create a distal-to-proximal pressure gradient using a modified figure-of-eight pattern. For patients with transfemoral amputation, the wrap is anchored around the pelvis and applied to pull the hip toward hip extension and adduction. Note the importance of capturing soft tissue high in the groin within the Ace wrap, to reduce the risk of developing an adductor roll of noncompressed soft tissue. (From May BJ. *Amputation and Prosthetics: A Case Study Approach.* Philadelphia, PA: F. A. Davis, 1996. p. 84.)

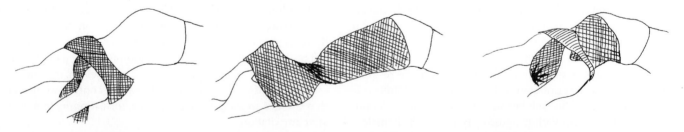

FIGURE 20-14 One strategy to control edema and manage limb volume is to use a double layer of an elastic stockinet or Tubigrip to apply compressive forces to the limb. After the initial layer (**A**) has been smoothly applied, the stockinet is twisted closed (**B**) at the end of the limb and the excess is applied (**C**) as a second layer of compression.

fitting more challenging. Another alternative for those with transfemoral amputation is a custom-fit Jobst pressure garment. Jobst garments can be fabricated either as a half-pant or full pant garment; the full pant garment achieves a more consistent suspension and compression, especially for patients

who are obese. A Jobst garment may be the only effective alternative for patients with short transfemoral amputation.

Because shrinkers, Tubigrip, and prosthetic socks worn over a healing residual limb are permeable, they absorb perspiration from the skin of the residual limb, as well as any

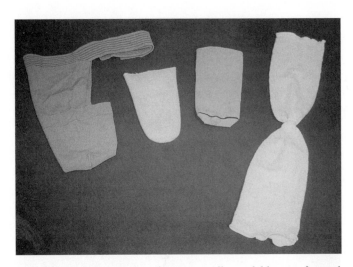

FIGURE 20-15 Examples of commercially available transfemoral (*left*) and transtibial shrinkers used for edema control and shaping of the residual limb.

drainage from the suture line. For this reason they must be laundered daily in warm water and a mild soap. Cotton, wool, or elasticized materials do not tolerate the heat and turbulence of a clothes dryer; most prosthetists recommend that shrinkers and socks be smoothed out on a flat surface to dry. The person wearing the garment must have a sufficient number available in order to apply compression around the clock.

Nonremovable Rigid Dressings

Many surgeons opt to use a cylindrical plaster or fiberglass cast placed on the new transtibial residual limb in the operating room immediately after amputation (Figure 20-16).[71,82,229] Rigid dressings accomplish three very important postoperative goals: (a) control of immediate postoperative edema (and subsequently, reduction of postoperative pain); (b) protection of the vulnerable newly sutured residual limb from inadvertent trauma during bed mobility, transfers, and single limb ambulation; and (c) prevention of postoperative knee flexion contracture. All three of these goals help to reduce time to initial prosthetic fitting.[88,229,230]

A rigid dressing is a simple postoperative cast applied in the same way as a cast that is used to immobilize a fracture of the proximal tibia or distal femur. The newly sutured surgical construct is dressed with gauze, and a cottonette or Tubigrip "sock" is pulled over the residual limb. A layer of

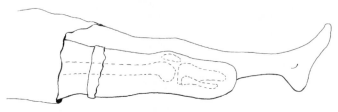

FIGURE 20-16 A plaster or fiberglass cast, applied immediately after amputation in the operating room, is an effective method of edema control, protection of the residual limb, and prevention of knee flexion contracture.

cast padding is applied smoothly over the stockinette, and extra cushioning is placed to protect the patella and femoral condyles. The knee is placed in as close to a fully extended position as possible, and fast drying plaster of paris or fiberglass casting material is wrapped around the limb, at least to the level of upper thigh (2 to 4 inches below the perineum). The stockinette is then folded over the proximal edge of the newly applied cast, and is incorporated into one or two addition wraps of casting material to finish the proximal border of the cast.

Modifications of the cast as it is setting or drying, such as molding it fit closely over the supracondylar thigh are used to aide suspension. A strip of webbing may be incorporated on the anterior surface for attachment to a waist belt to further aide to suspension. If the cast is to be used as the base for an immediate postoperative prosthesis (discussed in more detail below), the prosthetist modifies the cast as in a patellar tendon bearing socket to insure that weight-bearing forces are directed to pressure tolerant areas of the limb and that bony prominences and the suture line are well protected.

The initial rigid dressing stays in place on the residual limb for 2 to 5 days postoperatively (or more), depending on the patient's condition and the surgeon's preference.[82,88,223,224] When the cast is removed, the status of the wound is carefully inspected. If the wound is healing well, the physician may opt for reapplication of the cast for an additional period, which varies by protocol used, of between 5 and 21 days. If the status of the wound is questionable or risk of infection high, an alternative method of edema control that allows more frequent wound inspection and care must be used. Some physicians opt to replace a thigh-encasing rigid dressing with a removable rigid dressing after the first cast is taken off, regardless of wound status.

Application of a rigid cast, especially if it is the base of an immediate postoperative prosthesis (discussed below) requires careful attention to anatomy and alignment, well-developed manual skills, and a clear understanding of prosthetic principles. A poorly applied or inadequately suspended rigid dressing can lead to skin abrasions or pressure-related ulcerations over bony prominences, delaying prosthetic fitting until wound healing occurs. Pistoning or rotation of the rigid dressing on the residual limb can apply distracting forces over the suture line, compromising healing and increasing the risk of ecchymosis or dehiscence.

A major criticism of thigh-level nonremovable rigid dressings is that the cast prevents visual inspection and monitoring of the new surgical wound, and limits access for wound care.[229] For this reason a nonremovable rigid dressing may not be appropriate for those with significant risk of infection, especially if wounds were potentially contaminated during traumatic injury. Wound status can only be monitored indirectly, using body temperature, white blood cell count, size and color of drainage stains on the cast, and patient reports of increasing discomfort and pain as indicators of a developing infection.

There are several strategies that physicians and prosthetists have to address access to the healing while providing the protection and other benefits of nonremovable rigid dressing.

One is to bivalve the cast, so that it can be removed for short periods to allow wound care (Figure 20-17). Prefabricated rigid dressings, custom fit by the prosthetist to the individual with new amputation, are also available.[231]

Removable Rigid Dressings

The RRD is a "cap" cast worn over a soft or compressive dressing (Figure 20-18).[232] This edema-control strategy effectively protects the healing residual limb and helps to limit the development of edema. RRDs are used in three circumstances. For some individuals managed with a nonremovable rigid dressing applied in the operating room, the next step in postoperative edema control may be fabrication of an RRD. For others the RRD is applied instead of a cylindrical cast in the operating room. The RRD can also be fabricated after surgery for those initially managed with soft dressings and elastic bandages. The physical therapist may be responsible for fabrication of the RRD, working in collaboration with the surgeon, surgical nurse, or prosthetist.

One of its major advantages, when compared with a cylindrical cast, is the ability to doff (remove) and don (apply) the RRD quickly and easily to monitor wound healing and provide daily wound care. Use of an RRD also assists residual limb shaping and shrinkage; patients who wear RRDs are often ready for prosthetic fitting more quickly than those managed with soft dressings or Ace wraps alone.[233,234] Because the RRD limits the development of edema, it is an important adjunct in the management of postsurgical pain. The protective cap limits shearing across the incision site as the person recovering from amputation surgery moves around in bed or during therapy; this soft tissue immobilization can assist wound healing.

The RRD is not as likely to become displaced or dislodged during activity when compared to Ace wrap compression. The ease of donning and doffing means that individuals with new amputation can quickly become responsible for this task

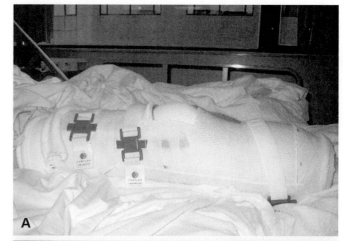

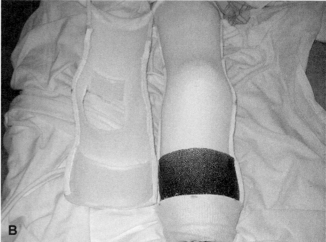

FIGURE 20-17 Example of a custom, removable, immediate postoperative cast **(A)** bivalved at first dressing change and held closed with Velcro straps. **B,** Interior view of the immediate postoperative prosthesis with gel pads placed to protect the distal anterior tibia and patella. (From Walsh TL. Custom removable immediate postoperative prosthesis. *J Prosthet Orthot.* 2003;15(4):160.)

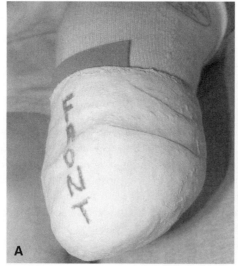

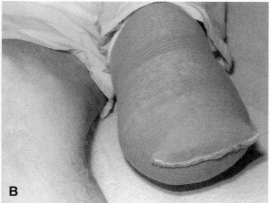

FIGURE 20-18 **A,** This removable rigid dressing has been donned over a nylon sheath and five-ply wool prosthetic sock, with an additional foam pad at the proximal anterior edge for comfort and protection of the skin. Marking the anterior midline of the cast ensures that it will be applied in optimal alignment. **B,** The removable rigid dressing is held onto the limb by application of an elasticized Tubigrip, sewn closed at one end and pulled up to midthigh level for a sleeve suspension. A Velcro-closing thermoplastic or woven supracondylar strap is applied over the sleeve to ensure suspension.

component of caring for their residual limb. Because the RRD is removed and reapplied several times a day for wound care, the residual limb quickly becomes desensitized and tolerant of pressure, which assists transition to prosthetic wear. Fabrication and use of an RRD provide the opportunity to educate those new to prosthetic use about the fabrication of a preparatory prosthesis and the use of prosthetic socks to obtain and maintain socket fit.

The RRD is most appropriate for patients whose transtibial incision appears to be in the initial stages of healing. Although the wound may be inflamed secondary to the trauma of surgery, no signs of infection, significant ecchymosis, or large areas of wound dehiscence should be present. Those with substantial drainage from their surgical wound requiring bulky soft dressings and frequent dressing changes are not good candidates for RRD; it is difficult to accommodate distally placed bulky dressings within the RRD shell. Those with fluctuating edema secondary to CHF or dialysis can be managed with an RRD if it is fabricated when limb volume is high: Layering prosthetic sock ply over the limb before putting on the RRD accommodates for volume loss. The RRD works best if distal residual limb circumference is no more than 0.5 inch larger than its proximal circumference. Compressive dressings may be more appropriate for patients with extremely bulbous residual limbs.

The residual limb is prepared for casting by first placing a protective layer of gauze fluff over the suture line.[232,235] The limb can be loosely wrapped in plastic wrap to assist removal of the completed RRD after casting. Next, a "sock" made from elasticized cotton stockinet or Tubigrip is applied over the limb, with particular care to avoid shearing across the suture line. Pieces of Webril or a similar filler material are layered around the limb to create reliefs within the RRD for bony prominences (tibial crest, fibular head, distal tibia) and the hamstring tendons. When the distal residual limb has a larger circumference, additional padding is added proximally to ensure that the RRD will be cylindrical and easily donned. A long sock made from regular cotton stockinet is carefully donned over the padding; this will be the inner layer of the finished RRD. The outline of the patella marked on the stockinet will serve as a guide for trim lines after the cast has dried. Typically, two rolls of fast-setting plaster cast material are sufficient for an RRD. The residual limb is supported in full knee extension, and successive layers of plaster are smoothed into place, building a cast with an anterior trim line at midpatella and a slightly lower posterior trim line to allow knee flexion without tissue impingement.

The cotton stockinet sock is then folded down over the cast at the knee, and several additional circumferential layers of plaster are used to finish and reinforce the proximal brim (to ensure that the RRD can subsequently withstand repeated donning/doffing). An Ace wrap can be applied to provide additional compression while the plaster sets. Once the RRD has hardened sufficiently, the patient is asked to flex the knee slightly and the cast is carefully removed from the residual limb. The extra Webril or padding is pulled out of the RRD, and the inner surface is inspected for potentially problematic rough areas or ridges. Because the RRD is almost cylindrical, it is helpful to mark the front of the cast to ensure that it is correctly donned.

Before the completed RRD is applied, one or two gauze pads are placed over the suture line for protection. A prosthetic sock, Tubigrip, elasticized stockinet sock, or commercially manufactured "shrinker" is carefully donned, with minimal shear stress across the suture line. Additional ply of prosthetic socks are used as needed to ensure a snug fit within the RRD. A small amount of Webril or other fluffy padding is placed in the distal anterior RRD to protect the distal tibia and suture line; then the RRD is carefully slipped onto the residual limb, aligning the markings on the front of the RRD with the patella for optimal fit (see Figure 20-18, *A*). A small foam filler or cushion can be placed between the anterior brim and residual limb to minimize the risk of friction during activity. The outer Tubigrip or stockinet suspension sleeve is then rolled over the RRD and onto the thigh, the supracondylar strap is secured in place, and the sock is folded back down over the strap to minimize the risk of loss of suspension. The skin must be inspected within the first 60 to 90 minutes of initial fitting with an RRD to assess skin integrity and identify potential pressure-related problems. If no skin problems develop, routine wound inspection once per nursing shift is usually adequate.

The RRD is designed to be worn continuously, even when sleeping, except during routine wound care or bathing. If the individual with recent amputation is expecting to be out of the RRD for more than several minutes, another form of compression such as a shrinker or several layers of Tubigrip must be available to minimize the development of edema. The individual wearing an RRD must be encouraged to report any localized pain or discomfort as signs of potential problems with RRD fit or function. Layers of prosthetic sock are added, over time, as the residual limb "shrinks." There is some evidence polymer gel socks worn under a removable rigid dressing may help to control edema and associated pain, and reduce the time to prosthetic fitting.[236] Sometimes short distal socks are necessary to provide for distal compression without excessive proximal bulkiness that can prohibit donning. The consistent use of 12- to 15-ply socks to achieve appropriate fit usually indicates the need for fabrication of a smaller RRD. Significant change in the shape or configuration of the residual limb also requires fabrication of a new RRD.

The referral for fabrication of the initial (preparatory or training) prosthesis can occur within 12 to 17 days of surgery if the incision has healed sufficiently. Many individuals continue to use their RRD in conjunction with a shrinker for control of edema and limb protection whenever they are not wearing their prosthesis for as long as 6 months after surgery.

Removable Polyethylene Semirigid Dressings

An alternative to a plaster RRD is a removable polyethylene semirigid dressing (SRD; Figure 20-19).[237] Like the RRD, the SRD is an effective strategy for control of edema, protection of the healing incision, and shaping of the residual limb.[238] Unlike the RRD, however, the SRD requires the skill of a

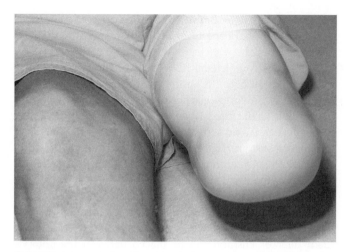

FIGURE 20-19 A flexible, polyethylene semirigid dressing is fabricated by a prosthetist over a positive model of the patient's residual limb. This ensures an intimate fit for effective control of edema, protection of the healing incision, and optimal "shaping" of a new residual limb.

prosthetist for fabrication. The prosthetist may take a negative mold of the patient's residual limb while in the operating room or when the rigid dressing is removed on the third or fourth postoperative day. A positive model is created using the negative mold and is modified to incorporate reliefs for pressure-intolerant areas of the residual limb. The polyethylene is heated and vacuum molded over the positive model in the same way that a thermoplastic socket would be. The polyethylene SRD is often ready for delivery in 2 or 3 days after casting. When someone is initially casted for a polyethylene SRD in the operating room before being placed in a plaster or fiberglass cast, the SRD may be delivered on the day that the rigid plaster dressing is removed.

The polyethylene SRD has several advantages when compared with the plaster of Paris RRD. First, polyethylene is easier to clean; as a result, hygiene of the residual limb may be improved. The polyethylene SRD is lighter in weight and somewhat more durable than a plaster RRD; it does not melt if exposed to liquids. The flexibility of the material makes it easier to don and doff than the stiff plaster RRD. Because the polyethylene SRD closely resembles a transtibial socket, greater carryover about proper use of prosthetic socks for optimal fit in the socket of the initial (preparatory, temporary, or training) prosthesis is likely.

The major disadvantage of a polyethylene SRD is the cost associated with casting and fabrication. Because most residual limbs become progressively smaller with maturation in the weeks and months after amputation, several successfully smaller SRDs may need to be fabricated as the limb shrinks. In some settings plaster RRDs are used until the initial prosthetic fitting. At that point the prosthetist makes a polyethylene SRD in addition to the socket for the training prosthesis. Some companies now offer a prefabricated adjustable SRD

with Velcro closures as an alternative to the custom-molded polyethylene SRD.

Zinc Oxide Impregnated Semirigid Dressing

Another postoperative strategy is the fabrication of a SRD using a zinc oxide impregnated Unna bandage. Unna is most often used in the management of chronic venous stasis ulcers (Unna boot)[239]; because it appears to enhance healing, it has been also been used as a strategy to control edema and facilitate healing following transtibial amputation.[240] As the unna dressing dries, it provides nonelastic external support to the residual limb, preventing development of edema. The Unna dressing is, basically, a roll of gauze impregnated with zinc oxide, triglycerine, calamine, and gelatin. This pasty dressing easily adheres to the skin on application, drying to a semirigid leathery consistency within 24 hours. Typically, an Unna dressing would be applied to the residual limb immediately after wound closure in the operating room.[240] Although not as rigid and protective as a RRD or SRD, Unna paste dressings are more effective in limiting postoperative edema than are soft dressings and Ace wrapping.[240] An Unna SRD can be left on for as long as 5 to 7 days; if more frequent wound inspection is desired, it can be easily removed with bandage scissors. Because the Unna dressing remains in place for an extended period, fewer opportunities are available for limb desensitization and patient education about socket fit compared with those for the RRD and polyethylene SRD.

Pneumatic Compression for Early Ambulation

The deconditioning associated with inactivity is a particular concern in the postoperative and preprosthetic periods. Ambulation on a single limb, however, can be quite challenging for persons with a high comorbid burden of illness. Although pneumatic compression (such as the air splints use for immobilization following acute fracture) is relatively inexpensive and can be quickly removed and reapplied for wound inspection, the compression tends to be uneven, so shaping of the residual limb is not as effective as other methods. The splint can be uncomfortably hot if worn for more than 20 to 30 minutes. Its major benefit, however, is that it allows early protected weight bearing on the residual limb; this is especially beneficial for individuals who are physically or functionally frail.[241] The air splint provides limited mobility for patients who would not otherwise be ambulatory and may be a useful means of assessing the potential for prosthetic rehabilitation. Several air-filled early prosthetic options exist for compression in the postoperative and preprosthetic periods (Figure 20-20).[242–245]

When donning a pneumatic compression device for early ambulation, the suture line is covered with smooth gauze pads for protection. Prosthetic socks, stockinet, or Tubigrip is then applied over the residual limb before the air splint is inflated. Felt pads are strategically placed over the residual limb's soft dressing, or a shrinker loads pressure-tolerant areas (medial tibial flare and patellar tendon) while protecting pressure-sensitive

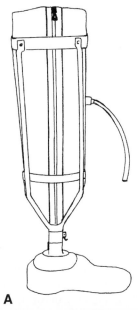

A

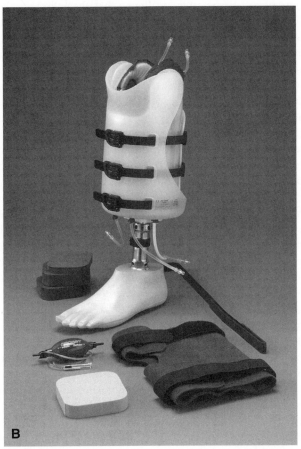

B

FIGURE 20-20 A, An air splint and prosthetic frame may provide limited ambulation for patients who are unable to accomplish single limb gait with an assistive device. The splint is inflated within the frame to 35 to 40 mm Hg, allowing toe touch to partial weight bearing, with minimal risk to the healing incision. **B,** The Aircast Airlimb, an example of a commercially available, noncustom, pneumatic, immediately postoperative prosthesis. (Courtesy Aircast Inc., Summit, N.J.)

areas (crest of the tibia and fibular head) after inflation of the air splint. The sleeve is zipped into place around the limb, and the limb is positioned in the frame before inflation. The sleeve is inflated with a hand or foot pump to an air pressure of 35 to 40 mm Hg. This low pressure sustains toe touch to partial weight without compromising capillary blood flow to the healing suture line. Recently a variety of prefabricated pneumatic immediate postoperative prostheses, with inflatable air bladders within an adjustable closure polyethylene "socket," has become available.[246-249]

Rigid Dressing as a Base for Immediate Postoperative Prosthesis

When a nonremovable rigid dressing is to be used as an IPOP, a prosthetist joins the surgical team in the operating room during cast application to incorporate the features of a patellar tendon-bearing socket and an attachment for a pylon into the cast (Figure 20-21).[250] Several felt or gel pads are positioned on the limb to direct and distribute weight-bearing forces more effectively onto pressure-tolerant areas (e.g., medial tibial flare, anterior muscle compartment, patellar tendon). The residual limb is then supported with the knee extended, and several layers of elastic or nonelastic plaster of Paris or fiberglass casting material are applied. The proximal edges of the cast are finished at the upper thigh (2 to 4 inches below perineum) level. Modifications of the cast (as it is setting) are used to aid suspension or, for an IPOP, to ensure that weight-bearing forces are directed to pressure-tolerant areas. Pressure applied to the outside of the cast just above the femoral condyles captures normal femoral anatomy to create supracondylar suspension. For an IPOP, the prosthetist incorporates a patellar tendon bar, a broad "shelf" for the medial tibial flare, and a stabilizing popliteal bulge by applying manual pressure to these areas as the cast begins to set. The prosthetist also incorporates a point of attachment and alignment into the distal cast for subsequent attachment of a pylon and prosthetic foot. Finally, the prosthetist or surgeon can incorporate a suspension attachment, which will connect to a waist belt, into the proximal anterior surface of the cast.

The early mobility afforded by application of an IPOP may be important for individuals with new amputation who would otherwise be unable to achieve single limb ambulation with a walker or crutches, especially those who are at significant risk

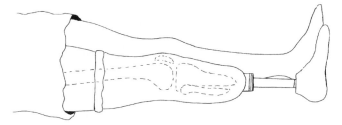

FIGURE 20-21 Incorporation of a pylon and features of a patellar tendon–bearing socket in an immediate postoperative prosthesis (IPOP) can facilitate early mobility in selected patients.

of functional decline, physiological deconditioning, or atelectasis and pneumonia secondary to inactivity and immobilization. Although an IPOP replaces the amputated limb with a pylon and prosthetic foot, limited and protected weight bearing is essential in the early postoperative period: most physicians suggest toe-touch or partial weight bearing. Shearing forces that result from excessive weight shift and repeated loading of the residual limb in an IPOP can compromise or delay wound healing.[250] Because of this risk, an IPOP is inappropriate for frail or confused individuals who are likely to be unreliable about limiting weight bearing. Many proponents of IPOP suggest that gradual controlled application of mechanical stress to healing connective tissues actually assists tissue modeling for better tolerance of the mechanical stresses of prosthetic wear and ambulation. Although the early application of mechanical stresses is apparently well tolerated by wounds with adequate blood supply, ischemic wounds tolerate only minimum stress in their healing phase.

Selecting the Appropriate Compression Strategy

In deciding which edema control and limb-shaping strategy is most appropriate, the rehabilitation team should consider the following questions:

1. Can the person don/doff the device independently? If not, is a family member available who can assist with this task?
2. Given the individual's physical characteristics and likely level of activity, will the device remain securely in place on the residual limb?
3. Will the device apply enough compression for effective progressive limb shrinkage?
4. Will the device apply enough compression for symmetric shaping of the residual limb?
5. Will the device protect the skin and healing suture line during daily activities, and does use of the device carry any risk of skin irritation or breakdown?
6. Is the device comfortable for the patient to use or wear over the long periods of time that are required for effective control of edema and limb shaping?
7. Is the device relatively cost-effective in terms of fabrication, modification, and replacement?

Monitoring tissue tolerance and potential areas of pressure closely in whatever edema control method is chosen is very important, especially in the first few days and weeks after amputation. Although rigid dressings, IPOPs, and Unna dressing remain on the limb for extended periods, each other method of edema control and shaping should be removed and reapplied a minimum of three times each day to assure appropriate fit and tissue tolerance in the acute phase of healing. When a rigid cast or IPOP is removed, it must be quickly replaced with an alternative compression device so that limb volume does not increase substantially. Individuals with recent amputation must wear the compression device at all times unless walking in a training prosthesis (even time out of compression during bathing should be as short as possible). Most people find that a compression device is necessary to maintain the desired limb volume for 6 months to a year after surgery. Some persons with mature residual limbs who have fluctuation in volume because of concurrent medical conditions continue to require compression well beyond the first postoperative year.

Many people with amputation experience a transient increase in residual limb volume after a shower or bathing; they often choose to bathe in the evening so that volume change does not interfere with prosthetic use. Those who prefer to bathe in the morning may need to use a compression device immediately after bathing to achieve optimal prosthetic fit and suspension, especially if suction suspension (which requires consistent limb volume) is used. Those who use prosthetic socks may require a few less ply of sock immediately after bathing but need to add a few more ply after a few hours as limb volume decreases.

Skin Care and Scar Management

It is important that the healing incision move without adherence to underlying deep tissue or bone as healing progresses. There must be sufficient gliding between skin and underlying layers of soft tissue after healing so that shear forces will be minimal while the prosthesis is donned and used for function. An adherent scar at the distal tibia can be quite problematic: If a point of adherence is present along an incisional scar, the mobility of tissues will be compromised. The resulting traction and shear forces are likely to lead to discomfort, skin irritation, and often recurrent breakdown of soft tissues with prosthetic use. Once primary healing has been established, the person with recent amputation learns to use gentle manual massage to enhance tissue mobility in preparation for prosthetic use. At first, this is performed above and below, but not across, the incision to minimize the risk of dehiscence.

When the wound is well closed and Steri-Strips are no longer necessary to support and protect the incision, gentle mobilization of the scar itself can begin. Handling of the limb during soft tissue mobilization and massage not only minimizes adhesion formation but also helps the individual to adapt his or her body image to include the postamputation residual limb and prepare for the sensory experience of prosthetic use.[251,252]

Persons with new amputation may have surgical scars from previous vascular bypass or from harvesting veins for coronary artery bypass surgery. These may require carefully applied soft tissue mobilization or friction massage to free adhesions and restore the mobility of the skin. Those with traumatic amputation may have healing skin grafts or abrasions from road burn, thermal injury, or electrical burn. In such cases wound care and debridement are important components of preprosthetic rehabilitation. For individuals with healing burns or skin graft, the use of an appropriate compression garment or shrinker assists healing and maturation of skin, controls postoperative edema, and shapes the residual limb.

Once the sutures have been removed, normal bathing resumes and a routine for daily skin care is established. Most physicians, prosthetists, and therapists recommend daily cleansing of the residual limb with a mild, nondrying soap. Patting or gently rubbing the limb with a terry cloth towel until it is fully dry also helps to desensitize it in preparation for prosthetic use. A small amount of moisturizer or skin cream can be applied if the skin of the residual limb is dry or flaky. A limb with soft, healthy pliable skin is much more tolerant of prosthetic wear than a limb with tough, dry, easily irritated skin. Persons with new amputation and their caregivers are taught to inspect the skin of the entire residual limb carefully, using a mirror if necessary to visualize difficult-to-see areas. Areas over bony prominences that may be vulnerable to high pressure within the socket are especially important to assess.

Persons with amputation are as likely to have other dermatological conditions such as eczema or psoriasis as the general population.[253-255] Those with hairy limbs or easily irritated skin may be more at risk of folliculitis and similar inflammatory skin conditions once the prosthesis is worn consistently. Effective early management of skin irritation or other skin problems is important: Serious skin irritation or infection precludes prosthetic use until adequate healing has occurred.

Some persons with new amputation mistakenly assume that something must be used to "toughen" the skin in preparation for prosthetic use. They may opt to rub the skin with alcohol, vinegar, salt water, or even gasoline, erroneously thinking that this will make the skin thicker and more pressure tolerant. In fact, these "treatments" can damage the skin, making it more susceptible to pressure-related problems. Patient and family education about effective cleansing and skin care strategies is essential in the early postoperative/preprosthetic period.

Range of Motion and Flexibility

Persons with transtibial amputation are at significant risk of developing both knee and hip flexion contractures. Those with transfemoral amputation are very likely to develop hip flexion and external rotation contracture. Such contractures cause substantial problems for prosthetic fit and alignment, as well as on efficiency of walking with a prosthesis. Impairment of extensibility of two joint muscles, such as the hamstrings and rectus femoris, may not be obvious when an individual is seated, but may have profound impact on comfort when wearing a prosthesis during functional activities. For this reason, proper positioning is a key component of preprosthetic rehabilitation.

Prolonged dependence of the residual limb held in knee flexion when sitting also leads to development of distal edema, which can delay readiness for prosthetic fitting. Persons with transtibial amputation must maintain the knee in as much extension as possible, whether in bed, sitting in a wheelchair or lounge chair, or during exercise and activity. Although it may be comfortable to place a pillow under the knee when sitting or lying in bed, a more effective strategy is to position a small towel roll under the distal posterior residual limb to encourage knee extension (Figure 20-22). Use of a wheelchair with elevating leg rests on the side of the amputation helps to keep the residual limb in an extended position, although a "bridge" between the seat and calf support may be necessary for those with short residual limbs. In some settings the therapist fabricates a posterior trough splint from low-temperature thermoplastic materials; this splint supports the limb in knee extension when the individual with recent amputation is resting in bed or sitting in a wheelchair.

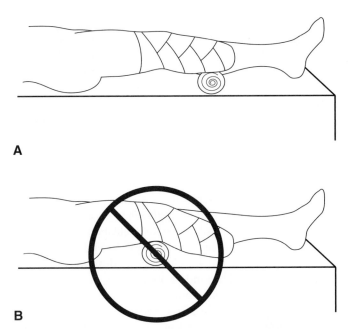

A

B

FIGURE 20-22 The optimal position for individuals with recent transtibial amputation is in full extension. **A,** A small rolled towel, bolster, or pillow placed under the distal posterior residual limb encourages knee extension, while (**B**) support under the knee makes development of knee flexion contracture more likely.

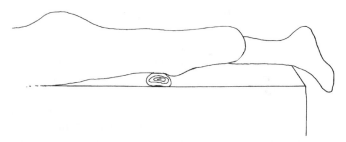

FIGURE 20-23 Prone positioning for stretching of the posterior soft tissue and prevention of knee flexion contracture. A small towel roll placed just above the patella elevates the residual limb from the surface of the mat or bed. The therapist can use hold–relax or contract–relax techniques, or the patient can actively contract the quadriceps to assist elongation of the hamstrings and posterior soft tissues.

If the individual is able to assume prone position, the weight of the limb can be used to assist elongation of the hamstring muscles and soft tissue of the posterior knee (Figure 20-23). A small towel roll positioned just above the patella effectively positions the limb for elongation. Although there is little conclusive evidence in the research literature about contracture management in persons with recent lower limb amputation, evidence from studies of soft tissue contracture following total knee arthroplasty suggest that prolonged stretching, dynamic splinting, and manual therapy may be effective following amputation as well.[256-258] Stretching programs also have a positive impact on the quality and efficiency of gait in older adults.[259] What is not well understood is the intensity necessary if stretching is to prevent or minimize degree of contracture formation, especially if there is also evidence of central nervous system dysfunction.[260-262] Intervention strategies currently used to target joint ROM and flexibility include proprioceptive neuromuscular facilitation hold-relax or contract-relax[263,264] and myofascial release.[265] Although the strength of the clinical research evidence on interventions for stretching and flexibility following lower limb amputation is low, the consequences of not attending to risk of contracture development are substantially negative. Converging recommendations by experts strongly support that interventions aimed at contracture prevention or minimization are essential in the postoperative/preprosthetic period.[266-270] Readers are referred to *Stretching and Strengthening for Lower Extremity Amputees* (Miami, FL: Advanced Rehabilitation Therapy Inc.) and to *Facilitated Stretching* (Champaign, IL: Human Kinetics), for more detailed information about designing exercise programs for stretching and flexibility.

Persons with recent amputation are instructed how to perform exercises (done at the bedside while an inpatient or at home while an outpatient) that are designed to elongate muscles and soft tissue to counteract the tendency to develop tightness, especially in two-joint muscles. Performed independently or with the assistance of a family member or caregiver several times a day, these stretching exercises are as important as individualized PT sessions during preprosthetic and prosthetic rehabilitation.

Significant hip flexion contracture can render a person with transfemoral amputation ineffective in controlling a prosthetic knee unit and walking with a prosthesis. Persons with recent transfemoral amputation tend to hold their residual limb diagonally outward when seated, unconsciously and automatically increasing their seated base of support to enhance postural stability. If they spend significant amounts of time in a seated position, development of hip flexor, abductor, and external rotator tightness is almost inevitable. PT interventions that elongate these soft tissues, including manual stretching, active exercise, and functional postural training, are used to counteract the tendency for tightness to develop.[266-272] Resting in a prone position with a towel roll under the distal anterior residual limb provides prolonged elongation for tight hip flexors. Care must be taken, however, to maintain a neutral pelvis or slight posterior tilt when lying prone. Excessive hip flexor tightness leads to lordosis of the lumbosacral spine.

Muscle Performance

Strengthening programs have two goals: (a) remediation of specific weaknesses detected in the examination and (b) maximization of overall strength and muscular endurance for safe, energy-efficient prosthetic gait. Because functional activities require use of muscles at varying lengths and types of contraction, effective preprosthetic exercise programs include activities that require concentric, holding (isometric), eccentric, and cocontraction in a variety of positions and muscle lengths.[266-272] In the immediate postoperative period the specific strengthening program is often a combination of isometric and active isotonic exercise within a limited ROM

of the joint just proximal to the amputation.[266-272] This strategy minimizes stress or tension across the incision while preserving and improving the strength of key muscle groups. It is as important to include strengthening exercise for the intact (nonamputated limb) as for the residual limb. Core stability also needs to be addressed.

Incorporation of controlled exhalation during isometric contraction minimizes the risks to cardiac function and fluctuations of blood pressure that are associated with the Valsalva maneuver.[273] For persons with transtibial amputation, exercises to strengthen knee extension that are initiated within the first week of amputation might include "quad sets" in the supine position or "short arc quads" performed in the supine or sitting position. For those with transfemoral amputation, "glut sets" in the prone or supine position or "short arc" hip extension and abduction in a gravity-eliminated position would be initiated. Gailey[269] recommends an exercise strategy of slow, steadily controlled, 10-second muscular contraction, followed by 5 to 10 seconds of rest, for 10 repetitions as one that is easily learned and physiologically sound. As wound healing is accomplished, exercises can be progressed to include active exercises through larger arcs of motion, active resistive exercise (using weights or manual resistance), or isokinetic training. Application of manual resistance during functional activities, as in proprioceptive neuromuscular facilitation, allows the therapist to provide appropriate resistance as muscle strength varies throughout the active ROM while providing facilitation and augmented sensory feedback to the patient.[274,275] Progressive resistive exercise for strength development (low repetition-high load) as well as muscular endurance (high repetition-low load) are key should also be included.[276-279] Readers are referred to *ACSM's Exercise Management for Persons with Chronic Disease and Disability* (Champaign, IL: Human Kinetics, 2002), *Therapeutic Exercise: Foundations and Techniques* (Philadelphia, PA: F.A. Davis, 2007) and *Essentials of Strength Training and Conditioning* (Champaign, IL: Human Kinetics, 2008) for information on designing progressive resistive exercise programs of adequate intensity and duration.

Isokinetic exercise, involving both concentric and eccentric contraction, allows the patient to develop muscle strength and control at a variety of movement velocities and has a marked positive impact on functional ability.[278-282] Isokinetic exercise, if prescribed properly, is well tolerated by older adults, even at speeds of 180 degrees per second angular velocity.[283]

For individuals with transtibial amputation, attachments of the quadriceps and hamstrings are typically intact, and preprosthetic strengthening exercises emphasize control of the knee, as well as hip extensor and abductor strength for stability in stance. There is evidence that older men who are unable to develop knee extension force above 1.13 Newton-meters(Nm)/kg (measured by handheld isokinetic dynamometer, normalized by body weight) and older women who are unable to develop knee extension force above 1.01 Nm/kg have a high risk for functional decline, morbidity, and mortality.[284]

These strength values may represent the minimum threshold for community function and could serve as evidence-based functional goals for persons recovering from transtibial amputation (both limbs) and transfemoral amputation (remaining limb). Those with transtibial amputation are also very likely to have deficits in muscle performance around the hip; strengthening programs must include hip abductors (for stance phase stability) and hip extensors,[285] much like those who are receiving rehabilitation following total knee arthroplasty.[286,287]

Persons with transfemoral amputation must develop strong hip extension capabilities to control the prosthetic knee unit. They must also have effective hip abduction power if the pelvis is to remain level during stance.[285] It is important to recognize that the distal attachments of the hamstrings, rectus femoris, sartorius, tensor fasciae latae/iliotibial band, adductor longus, and adductor magnus are relocated by myodesis or myoplasty or are lost entirely (for patients with short residual limbs) during transfemoral surgery. The combination of an altered line of pull and loss of muscle mass often creates an imbalance of muscle action around the hip.[288-290] The gluteus maximus, gluteus medius, and iliopsoas, with their intact distal attachments, are more powerful in determining resting hip position than the altered adductor group. If the tensor fasciae latae/iliotibial band and gluteus maximus become secondarily shortened, function of the adductor group is further compromised. Because of this imbalance, it is important to include activities that strengthen the remaining hip adductors, as well as hip extensors and hip abductors, to prepare the patient for effective postural control in sitting and standing and stance phase stability in prosthetic gait.[290] Readers are referred to *Stretching and Strengthening for Lower Extremity Amputees* (Miami, FL: Advanced Rehabilitation Therapy) for more examples of postoperative, preprosthetic strengthening activities.

General strengthening exercises for the trunk and upper extremities are also essential components of an effective preprosthetic exercise program. Back extensors and abdominal muscles play an important role in postural alignment and postural control. Activities that involve trunk rotation or diagonal movements activate trunk and limb girdle muscles in functional patterns, addressing strength and flexibility for functional activities and enhancing reciprocal arm swing and pelvic control in gait. Upper extremity strengthening, targeting shoulder depressor and elbow extensors, enhances the patient's ability to use an assistive device for single limb ambulation before prosthetic fitting.

Endurance

Many older adults with dysvascular amputation begin rehabilitation with compromised cardiopulmonary endurance because of the effects of comorbid cardiac and pulmonary diseases, and on deconditioning associated with inactivity and bed rest.[291] In persons with significant peripheral vascular disease without amputation, endurance training on treadmill improved endurance (6-minute walk distance) and physical function (SF-36 physical functioning values).[292] Although treadmill training is not appropriate in the preprosthetic period, other strategies, such as cycle ergometer driven by the intact limb, upper extremity ergometer, or cycle/recumbent combined upper- and lower extremity ergometers (e.g., NuStep Inc, Ann Arbor, MI) (Figure 20-24) can be safely and successfully used for persons with lower limb amputation.[293-295] Endurance and physical conditioning are predictors of prosthetic use: the ability to exercise at or above 50% of age-predicted VO_{2max} differentiated between persons with amputation able to walk functional distances (100 m) with a prosthesis and those who were unable to do so.[296-298] Because energy cost of walking with a prosthesis increases as limb

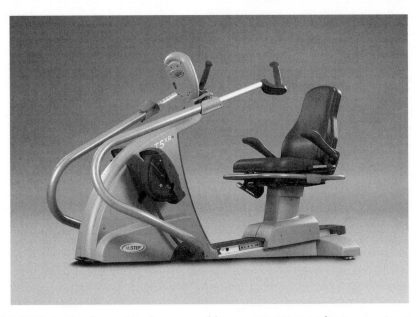

FIGURE 20-24 Example of a combined upper- and lower extremity recumbent ergometer appropriate for endurance exercise as part of the preprosthetic program for persons with amputation. (Courtesy of NuStep Inc., Ann Arbor, MI.)

length decreases, endurance training is particularly important for persons with transfemoral amputation.[299] Persons with amputation can substantially improve level of fitness (VO_{2max}) and with that, their potential for physical activity and prosthetic use.[300] Readers are referred to the ACSM's *Guidelines for Exercise Testing and Prescription,* 8th edition (Philadelphia, PA: Wolters Kluwer, Lippincott Williams & Wilkins, 2009)[301] and ACSM's *Exercise Management for Persons with Chronic Disease and Disabilities*, 3rd edition (Champaign, IL: Human Kinetics, 2009) for additional information about exercise testing and endurance exercise prescription.

Postural Control

Loss of a limb shifts the position of the body's COM, moving it slightly upward, backward, and toward the remaining or intact extremity; the magnitude of this shift is determined by the extent of limb loss. The shift may have relatively little impact on postural control and functional ability in patients with partial foot or Syme amputation. It may, however, have a significant impact on sitting balance, transitions between sitting and standing, and single limb ambulation for persons with transtibial, transfemoral, or hip disarticulation amputation. An effective preprosthetic program incorporates activities that challenge patients to improve core stability, postural control, and equilibrium responses, learning how to control the repositioned COM effectively over an altered base of support. In sitting, this can be accomplished using a variety of reaching tasks including forward reaching, diagonal reaching across and away from the midline, reaching down to a lower surface or objects, reaching up and away from their center, and turning to reach behind them. Anticipatory and reactive postural responses can also be practiced by throwing and catching games that require an automatic weight shift as part of the activity. The difficulty of the task can be advanced by progressively shifting the location of the catch or toss away from the midline of the patient's trunk; alternating locations from side to side or upward or downward; increasing the speed of the activity; increasing the weight of the object or ball that is being used; or performing the activity on a less stable seating surface (e.g., theraball, large bolster, or air-filled balance cushion). Similar activities can be implemented in single limb stance, initially within the parallel bars with physical guarding to insure safety. Such opportunity to practice anticipatory and reactionary postural control in single limb stance lays the foundation for the postural control necessary for single limb ambulation with an assistive device, as well as for eventual prosthetic use. Readers are referred to *Balance, Agility and Coordination for Lower Extremity Amputees* (Miami, FL: Advanced Rehabilitation Therapy) for more activities that can be used to enhance postural control.

The effectiveness of postural responses is influenced by efficiency of the somatosensory system and visual systems, flexibility and strength of the trunk and limb girdles, as well as the length and power of the residual limb.[184,302,303] The prosthetic replacement of a missing limb increases the functional base of support in sitting; for some individuals the weight of the prosthesis serves as a stabilizing anchor during functional activity. For those with limited flexibility or strength, such a replacement might be essential for effective postural responses and the ability to reach, even if the potential for functional ambulation is small.

Wheelchairs, Seating, and Adaptive Equipment

Many patients with amputation rely on a wheelchair for at least some of their mobility needs during the postoperative, preprosthetic period.[304] Some patients with short transfemoral amputation, hip disarticulation, or bilateral amputation prefer the relative energy efficiency of wheelchair mobility to ambulation with or without a prosthesis.[305,306] For others, comorbid cardiovascular or cardiopulmonary dysfunction precludes ambulation and the wheelchair becomes their primary mode of locomotion.[307] The shift in COM after amputation has important implications in choice of wheelchairs.

The design of many standard or traditional wheelchairs is based on the anthropomorphic characteristics of an "average" adult male with intact lower extremities. With the loss of a limb, the COM shifts in a posterior and lateral direction; when the patient is seated in a wheelchair, this moves the COM closer to the axis of rotation of the chair's wheels. If the patient with lower extremity amputation turns or reaches backward during a functional activity, the COM shifts even farther toward, or even beyond, the wheel axis, and the chair may tip backward. The provision of simple antitip devices reduces the risk of posterior tipping during functional activities. For those with transfemoral or bilateral amputation, a wheelchair with wheels that can be offset posteriorly is recommended. Patients with recent amputation must also be aware of altered dynamics when they reach forward while sitting in a wheelchair: High downward pressure on the wheelchair foot plate by the intact limb when reaching forward is likely to lead to anterior tipping.

Specific wheelchair assessments and prescription are warranted for all individuals who will be using a wheelchair as their primary means of locomotion and mobility (see Chapter 16). This individual evaluation and prescription process ensures that the wheelchair will provide adequate support of the thighs to increase seating stability and reach, effective seating with an appropriate cushion for pressure distribution, and configuration of components that provides ease of wheelchair locomotion.

Wheelchair skills to be mastered by persons with new amputation and their caregivers include effective propulsion over level, carpeted, and uneven ground; turning and backing up; positioning of the wheelchair for safe bed, toilet, bathtub, furniture, and car transfers; ascending and descending thresholds, curbs and ramps, and getting the wheelchair into and out of the family's motor vehicle. In addition, practice getting to and from the floor and opportunity to react to a controlled fall (lowering backward to the ground) may allay concerns about aftermath of falls. Readers are referred to textbooks on spinal cord injury rehabilitation, which contain chapters on wheelchair skill development that can be applied to persons with amputation.[308,309]

Along with a wheelchair, many persons with new amputation would benefit from provision of adaptive equipment for their homes (e.g., tub benches, grab bars, toilet frames, raised toilet seats, handheld shower adapter) and installation of temporary (or permanent) ramps to entrance/egress to the home. Consideration must also be given to access to sinks, as well as to using insulated coverings of exposed hot water and drain pipes. In some cases, if the individual is likely to use the wheelchair for a long period of time as primary means of mobility, modification of the home may be recommended for both safety and efficiency of function. Although these concerns are more typically addressed in inpatient and subacute rehabilitation settings, many patients with new amputation may be discharged to home to await sufficient healing prior to beginning prosthetic rehabilitation. Therapists in acute care must consider referral to home care services if there is insufficient time to address wheeled mobility and accessibility during hospitalization. Once again, textbooks on spinal cord injury are good sources of information about durable medical equipment and home modifications for accessibility.[310,311]

Bed Mobility and Transfers

In the acute care setting, PT intervention at the bedside includes instruction about optimal positioning of the residual limb and activities to assist the patient's ability to change position in bed and move to or from a seated position. Early mobility and activity significantly reduce the risk of atelectasis, pneumonia, and further physiological deconditioning.[312] The therapist must, however, be aware of the risk of postural hypotension and of postoperative complications including deep venous thrombosis and pulmonary embolism. Assessment and monitoring of the patient's vital signs (pulse, respiratory rate, blood pressure, pulse oximetry) are recommended as bed mobility and out-of-bed activity begin.[313] Care must also be taken to minimize the risk of trauma to the newly amputated limb during activity, exercise, or transfers.

Many individuals with recent amputation can roll from supine to or from the prone position without great difficulty, although those with transfemoral amputation of the dominant limb may need to develop an adapted movement pattern or sequence. The strategies for transition into sitting are not substantially different from preferred preoperative strategies; however, efficiency of postural responses may be challenged by the alteration in body mass after amputation. Those who have become deconditioned by inactivity in the days and weeks before amputation may find bed rails, a trapeze, bed ladders, or other devices helpful early in rehabilitation. Strategic placement of a bed table or walker near the bedside at night serves as a reminder of the amputation for individuals who are likely to get up during the night to go to the bathroom (without otherwise fully awakening), reducing the risk of falling.

An important goal of postoperative preprosthetic rehabilitation is development of the ability to move between seating surfaces or from sitting to standing as safely and independently as possible. The majority of falls for persons with new amputation in acute care settings occur during self-transfer between wheelchair and bed or toilet.[314] Depending on the individual's preamputation level of activity, transferring between seating surfaces may require some degree of assistance or use of adaptive devices or may be accomplished relatively smoothly and easily. Those who are deconditioned or who have previous neuromuscular-related postural impairment may require a mechanical lifting aid, multiperson lifting, or some level of assistance in the early postoperative period. Others may benefit from a strategically placed transfer board as they develop their ability to perform a pivot transfer on their remaining limb.

Some persons require a walker or crutches for extra stability in single limb stance in the midst of their pivot transfers. Still others quickly master scooting in sitting and pivoting on their remaining limb to become independent in transfers. Persons with single limb amputation initially prefer transferring toward their remaining limb, but should be encouraged to master moving in either direction. Individuals with bilateral limb loss or injury that precludes weight bearing on the remaining limb can scoot across a sliding board to a wheelchair or commode that is positioned diagonally from the bed. Those with bilateral transfemoral amputation (and those with bilateral transtibial amputation who have sufficient hamstring excursion) may prefer the surface-to-surface stability that is provided when the entire anterior edge of the wheelchair seat abuts the side of the bed, allowing them to scoot directly forward. Some individuals who require significant assistance to transfer without a prosthesis become nearly independent in pivot transfers when a prosthesis is worn: The sensory feedback that is provided to the residual limb within the socket when there is contact between the prosthetic foot and the floor enhances sitting balance during sliding board or pivot transfers. Persons with transfemoral amputation must learn that, although they can wear a prosthesis when seated, the prosthesis cannot be counted on for stability during transfers. Readers are referred to *Patient Care Skills*, 6th edition (Upper Saddle River, NJ: Prentice-Hall, 2010)[315] for suggestions about interventions to enhance bed mobility, transfers, and ambulation with assistive devices.

Mastery of single limb or non–weight-bearing transfers in the postoperative period is the foundation for functional transfers whenever the person with amputation is not wearing his or her prosthesis. At times in the future, mechanical problems with the prosthesis, skin problems on the residual limb, or a medical problem (e.g., CHF or renal failure) may affect socket fit, temporarily precluding prosthetic use. Providing opportunities for patients to practice transferring between surfaces at different levels (e.g., wheelchair to stool to floor) in the postoperative preprosthetic period is very important, especially if delayed prosthetic fitting is anticipated.

Ambulation and Locomotion

Single limb ambulation with an appropriate assistive device provides an opportunity to enhance postural control and to build strength and cardiovascular endurance, in addition to allowing patients with recent amputation to move about in their environment. A number of factors (e.g., safety, balance and postural control, endurance, lower extremity muscle performance, fear of falling) must be considered in recommending an ambulator assistive device.[315,316] Although use of a standard or rolling walker may be appropriate in the initial PT sessions, many individuals with new amputation quickly master a two- or three-point swing-through pattern with crutches on level surfaces and are ready to build advanced gait skills on uneven surfaces, inclines, and stairs. Others are fearful of using crutches, preferring the stability provided by a walker to the mobility of crutches. A walker may be appropriate for patients with limited endurance and balance impairment who would otherwise be limited to wheelchair use.

Therapists must be aware, however, of the potential long-term limitation in gait patterns imposed by walkers: The halting hop-to gait pattern interrupts forward progression of the COM. Individuals who have adapted to this pattern of motion before receiving a prosthesis may have difficulty developing a smooth step-through pattern or becoming comfortable with a less supportive ambulation aid once they are using their prosthesis. Walkers are also more difficult to use on inclines and are dangerous to use on stairs. Whenever possible, patients are encouraged to use crutches.[315,316] Table 20-8 summarizes the progressive single limb ambulation skills for preprosthetic rehabilitation.

TABLE 20-8   *Progressive Strategies for Preparing for and Mastering Single limb Mobility After Amputation*

Phase	Purpose	Target	Examples of Activity Progression
Preparation	Strengthening		All activities: concentric, holding, eccentric contraction
			All activities: intact limb and residual limb
		Hip extensors	Bridging; uniplanar, diagonal antigravity, with resistance
		Hip interior and exterior rotators	Gluteal sets
			Hip extension in prone, in standing, adding resistance, open chain, closed chain
		Hip abductors	Hip abduction side-lying, in standing, adding resistance, open chain, closed chain
		Knee extensors	Quad sets, short arc quads
			Sit to stand at varying heights and speeds
			Progressive resistive exercise
			Low load, high repetition (endurance)
			High load, low repetition (strength)
		Ankle dorsiflexors	Toe raises in standing
			Manual resistance of active movement
	Flexibility	Hip flexor tightness	Prolonged passive stretching, positioning antigravity
		Knee flexor tightness	Thomas test position or prone
		Tensor fascia lata/ iliotibial band	Proprioceptive neuromuscular facilitation: hold-relax/contract-relax followed by concentric exercise in new ROM
		Plantarflexor tightness	Active stretching in various positions
Stability in standing	Rising to standing	Control of COM during transition	Part-to-whole practice progressing to serial practice of sit-to-stand transition
			Scooting to edge of seating surface
			Forward lean with trunk extension (anterior weight shift)
			Weight transfer onto foot
			Extension into upright position
			Achieving stability in upright position
			Controlled lowering back into sitting position
			Practice with varying speeds
			Adding appropriate resistance for sensory feedback and/or strengthening
			Practice with higher to lower seating surfaces
			Practice with various seating surfaces (firm to soft chair, toilet seat, tub seat)
			Practice with transfers into/out of car
	Postural control in single limb stance	Discovering limits of stability Developing postural control	Static: standing in parallel bars
			Bilateral upper extremity support, single upper extremity support, no upper extremity support
			Anticipatory: directional reaching
			Forward, diagonal toward stance limb, diagonal away from stance limb
			Throwing activities: lightweight to heavier weighted balls; forward to diagonal directions; various distances
			Reactionary: gentle unexpected perturbations; catching activities; lightweight to heavier weighted balls; toward body center, away from body center; various speeds and distances
			All activities: initially standing on firm surface, progressing to compliant surface

TABLE 20-8 *Progressive Strategies for Preparing for and Mastering Single limb Mobility After Amputation—cont'd*

Phase	Purpose	Target	Examples of Activity Progression
Mobility	Ambulation	Forward progression	In parallel bars to overground with appropriate assistive devices
		Changing direction	Over simple (tile) surface to more challenging (carpet, grass, etc.)
		Backing up	surfaces
		Sideward stepping	In closed (predictable) environment, to open (unpredictable) environment
			Over level surfaces, inclines (ascend and descend)
		Stair management	Bilateral railings, to railing and one crutch
			Low to standard height steps
			Provide opportunity for family caregiver to practice guarding
		Managing environmental challenges	Opening doors: away from self, toward self, weighted doors, revolving doors
			Managing thresholds
			Managing curbs
			Environmental scanning: avoiding obstacles in walking path
			Home safety evaluation
			Crossing the street at times crosswalks
		Fall management	At least: demonstration/observation of chair to floor, stand to floor transition
			Discussion of risk factors for falls from wheelchair, from standing, on stairs
			Develop plan of action should fall occur
			Practice chair-to-floor and stand-to-floor transitions in controlled circumstances

Individuals with limited endurance or poor balance spend much time practicing a hop-to or swing-through gait in the parallel bars before they acquire the confidence and motor skill necessary to move out of the parallel bars with a walker or crutches. Importantly, single limb ambulation with an assistive device is often more energy intensive than walking with a prosthesis.[317] Achievement of functional single limb ambulation is not a prerequisite for prosthetic fitting.[318] All individuals who can stand and use an assistive device to walk should be encouraged to ambulate as much as possible, even if they are walking for aerobic exercise rather than to accomplish a functional task. For those with single limb amputation, wheelchair use should be reserved for long-distance transportation unless ambulation is not medically advisable. Wheelchairs are appropriate for patients with bilateral amputation; self-propulsion provides some aerobic conditioning, as well as an energy-efficient means of locomotion.[319]

Patient and Family Education: Care of the Remaining Limb

Patient and family education begins in the initial interview process and continues throughout the acute hospital stay, as illustrated in the preceding discussions of positioning, residual limb care, remaining/intact limb care, and enhancing motor performance and functional training.

Patient education about the risk of decubitus ulceration and strategies to reduce this risk are also important components of early postoperative care. Individuals with vascular disease and neuropathy are particularly at risk, with the heel and lateral border of the remaining foot most vulnerable.[320] Those with dysvascular limbs may have barely enough circulation to support tissue health in an intact or noninjured foot; once a wound has occurred, circulation may be inadequate for tissue healing. An open wound on the remaining limb would preclude single limb ambulation, increasing the risk of inactivity-related postoperative complications and making prosthetic rehabilitation even more challenging. Pressure-related wounds significantly delay rehabilitation, increase disability, and multiply health care costs for patients with amputation. Vulnerability to pressure increases with sensory impairment; altered mechanical characteristics of injured, calcified, or scarred tissues; poor circulatory status; microclimate of the skin; and (in combination with these factors) advanced age.[321] For those who have limited ability to change position, a pressure-distributing mattress and well-designed, carefully applied heel protectors can reduce the risk of decubitus ulcer formation. A routine of frequent position change, weight shifting, and exercise reduces weight-bearing pressures and enhances circulation to vulnerable tissues.

Before discharge, the rehabilitation team must ascertain how close to functional independence the individual and caregivers are in a variety of self-care activities, in mobility and locomotion, and in performance of preprosthetic exercises (Figure 20-25). As the program progresses, the ability of the individual and family in these areas is a key determinant of discharge readiness and placement (home with home care, home with outpatient follow-up, or to a rehabilitation or subacute facility).

ACTIVITY	INDICATOR
Wound Inspection ____	Individual or caregiver is able to independently inspect status of incision and residual limb
____	Individual or caregiver is able to describe signs of inflammation, infection, dehiscence, bleeding, orecchymosis requiring contact/visit with health professional
____	Individual or caregiver is able to effectively inspect and care for intact limb
____	Supervision or assistance by a health professional is necessary for wound inspection and care of either residual limb or intact limb
Residual Limb Care ____	Individual or caregiver is able to change wound dressings effectively, maintaining clean environment
____	Individual or caregiver is able to appropriately cleanse and care for residual limb
____	Individual or caregiver is able to safely effectively self-mobilize skin around incision site
____	Individual or caregiver is able to apply appropriate compression strategy (circle: Ace wrap, RRD or SRD, commercial shrinker garment, other)
____	Individual with transtibial amputation is able to maintain limb in extended knee position
Mobility ____	Individual is able to move around in bed as needed Level of assistance_____ Equipment used _____
____	Individual is able to transition from supine to sitting and return Level of assistance _____ Equipment used _____
____	Individual is able to transfer from bed or chair to wheelchair and return Level of assistance _____ Equipment used _____
____	Individual is able to transfer sit to single limb standing and return Level of assistance _____ Equipment used _____
____	Individual is able to transfer to toilet and return Level of assistance _____ Equipment used _____
____	Individual is able to transfer to shower or tub and return Level of assistance _____ Equipment used _____
Locomotion ____	Individual is able to ambulate on level surfaces using appropriate assistive device Level of assistance _____ Assistive/ambulatory device used _____ Gait pattern _____ Distance _____ Perceived exertion _____
____	Individual is able to ascend/descend stairs using railing and appropriate assistive device Level of assistance_____ Assistive/ambulatory device used_____ Gait pattern_____ Number of steps_____ Perceived exertion_____
____	Individual is able to ambulate on inclines and outdoor surfaces Level of assistance_____ Assistive/ambulatory device used_____ Gait pattern_____ Distance_____ Perceived exertion_____

FIGURE 20-25 Example of checklist of key patient and family knowledge and skills after lower limb amputation.

_____ Individual is able to ambulate on inclines and outdoor surfaces
    Level of assistance_____
    Assistive/ambulatory device used_____
    Gait pattern_____
    Distance_____
    Perceived exertion_____
_____ Individual/caregiver is able to safely propel wheelchair functional distances
    Level of assistance_____
    Distance_____
    Perceived exertion_____

Self-Care Activities _____ Individual is able to manage clothing during ADL and dressing activities
    Level of assistance_____
    Positions_____
    Adaptive equipment needs_____
    Perceived exertion_____
_____ Individual is able to manage bathing and grooming activities
    Level of assistance_____
    Positions_____
    Adaptive equipment needs_____
    Perceived exertion_____
_____ Individual is able to manage key IADL activities
    Level of assistance_____
    Types of activities_____
    Adaptive equipment needs_____
    Perceived exertion_____
_____ Sufficient and safe transportation is available
    Type of transportation_____
    Level of assistance_____
    Equipment used_____
    Perceived exertion_____

Exercise Program _____ Individual and caregiver demonstrate mastery of stretching/flexibility component of program
    Positions/activities_____
    Assistance required_____
    Equipment used_____
    Repetitions and frequency_____
_____ Individual and caregiver demonstrate mastery of strengthening component of program
    Positions/activities_____
    Assistance required_____
    Equipment used_____
    Repetitions and frequency_____
_____ Individual and caregiver demonstrate mastery of aerobic conditioning component of program
    Positions/activities_____
    Assistance required_____
    Equipment used_____
    Repetitions and frequency_____
_____ Individual and caregiver demonstrate mastery of balance/coordination components of program
    Positions/activities_____
    Assistance required_____
    Equipment used_____
    Repetitions and frequency_____

Follow-Up Care _____ Plans for return to surgeon for post-op visit are in place
_____ Plans for continued rehabilitation care are in place
_____ Additional services are in place as appropriate
    Nursing_____
    Dietician_____
    Counseling_____
    Home health_____
    Others_____

FIGURE 20-25—cont'd

CASE EXAMPLE 1B

Interventions for N. H., an 89-Year-Old with "Elective" Transtibial Amputation

N. H. is now 4 days postsurgery, and her delirium is clearing. She is conversing with her typical sense of humor with family and staff. Her casted fiberglass rigid dressing was removed yesterday; the surgical wound is draining moderate amounts of serosanguineous fluid; edges are closely approximate. An area of pressure-related abrasion and inflammation at the anterior distal tibia was noted when the cast was removed; granulation is now evident. N. H. can transfer to a bedside chair with moderate assistance of one person, with noted moderate impairment of postural control. N. H. tolerates being up in a bedside chair for 45 minutes. She rates her postoperative pain as four out of 10, except at dressing change, when it increases to six out of 10. She laughs but feels concern that she feels mild cramping in the instep of the limb that is no longer there, wanting to stretch her foot and toes into dorsiflexion to relieve her discomfort. She is somewhat reluctant to look at or to touch her residual limb, but does not mind if nurses, physicians, or PT staff handle it during dressing changes or functional activities. She transferred sitting to standing with a walker at bedside with moderate assistance of one person, complaining of dizziness after standing for more than a minute and requesting to return to sitting. She tells you that she is "ready to get going" and wants to return to her own home to use her wheelchair as soon as possible.

Questions to Consider

- Given her postoperative pain and phantom sensation, what PT interventions would be appropriate at this time for N. H.? Why would these be most appropriate from among available options? What are the pros and cons of each, with respect to attention, memory, and ability to learn?
- Given the status of her wound and condition of her residual limb, what strategies for management of edema and limb shaping would you recommend? What are the pros and cons that you considered when deciding among options for compression and residual limb protection? Why do you think the option you selected is the most appropriate? How would this be similar or different if her amputation was at the transfemoral level?
- What strategies for intervention and patient–family education would you implement for skin care and scar management for N. H.? What issues or factors will assist or inhibit her ability to take responsibility for her skin care?
- What specific strategies for intervention and patient–family education aimed at ROM and flexibility do you recommend for N. H.? What impairments or functional limitations are you particularly concerned about for N. H.? What activities will you engage her in? What positions? For what period of time? With what equipment? What would you emphasize if her amputation was at a transfemoral level? What issues or factors will assist or inhibit her ability to take responsibility for exercises aimed at ensuring adequate ROM and flexibility in preparation for prosthetic use?
- What specific strategies for intervention and patient–family education aimed at improving muscle performance do your recommend for N. H.? How do you address strengthening of key muscle groups of extremities and trunk? How do you address power and muscle endurance? How do you address concentric, isometric, and eccentric control and performance? What issues or factors must be considered regarding exercise tolerance, intensity, frequency, and duration during her acute care stay? How will you address her concerns about her low level of aerobic fitness and conditioning?
- What specific strategies for intervention and patient–family education aimed at improving static, dynamic, and reactionary postural control during functional activities do you recommend for N. H.? During which activities is postural control most likely to be problematic? What apparatus, equipment, and activities might you use to assist her postural control?
- What are your concerns about seating and wheelchair mobility for N. H.? Do you think that a standard wheelchair will adequately meet her needs? Do you think she will be able to propel her chair? What tasks does she need to master if the wheelchair will be her primary source of mobility during the preprosthetic period?
- What types of bed mobility and transfer activities are important for N. H. and her family caregivers to master? What specific intervention and patient–family education strategies will you use to help her move toward safe and, hopefully, independent performance of bed mobility and transfer activities? How will you vary environmental conditions and task demands to ensure that she can adapt her strategies and skills?
- What strategies for intervention and patient–family education will you use to get her up and walking? What assistive or ambulatory device do you feel would be most appropriate? Why have you chosen this particular device from among available options? What gait pattern will she use? For what other dimensions or ambulatory skills (in addition to walking forward) will you provide instruction and opportunity for N. H. to practice? How will you address the likelihood that she will experience a fall at some point in her preprosthetic period? What is "functional distance" for ambulation for N. H. and her family?
- Are there any additional interventions that would be appropriate for N. H. at this point in her postoperative, preprosthetic rehabilitation?
- How will you determine her readiness for prosthetic fitting?

Interventions for P. G., an Individual with Recent Amputation of Both Lower Extremities Following a Construction Accident

Now 3 days postoperation, P. G. is beginning his rehabilitation in preparation for discharge to home until there is adequate healing for prosthetic fitting and prosthetic training. Pain continues to be a serious concern, generally reported as five or six out of 10 on the visual analog scale. Postoperative agitation has cleared, although P. G.'s wife reports he is more subdued in affect than usual, and she is concerned about possible depression. Low-grade temperature persists, but white cell counts are within normal limits. P. G. can actively flex and extend both knees to within 10 degrees of full ROM, with effort and a "tight pulling sensation" behind the knee, when out of his SRD for dressing changes and wound inspection. Although he reports feeling "weak as a baby" and is quickly fatigued, P. G. can use upper extremity and body strength for contact guard sliding board transfers to and from bed to a bedside chair. Moving between sitting and supine is effortful and fatiguing, but P. G. manages these transitions with occasional standby assistance. He was previously involved in both aerobic and strengthening exercise at the local YMCA, but he is not sure how to use the weights and equipment now that he has lost his limbs. Plans are being made to move temporarily to his parent's home, on the first floor of a three-family house (although there are six steps to reach a front porch and entryway), as it is more accessible than his third-floor walk-up apartment. In the meantime, family and friends are apartment hunting for housing that will be less challenging for P. G. in the months ahead. P. G.'s major goal is to achieve independent mobility with a wheelchair before the birth of his child.

Questions to Consider

- Given his postoperative pain and phantom sensation, what PT interventions would be appropriate at this time for P. G.? Why would these be most appropriate from among available options? What are the pros and cons of each, with respect to attention, memory, and ability to learn?
- Given the status of his wound and condition of his residual limb, what strategies for management of edema and limb shaping would you recommend? What are the pros and cons that you considered when deciding among options for compression and residual limb protection? Why do you think the option you selected is the most appropriate? How would this change if his amputations were at the transfemoral level?
- What strategies for intervention and patient–family education would you implement for skin care and scar management for P. G.? What issues or factors will assist or inhibit his ability to take responsibility for his skin care?
- What specific strategies for intervention and patient–family education aimed at ROM and flexibility do you recommend for P. G.? What impairments or functional limitations are you particularly concerned about for P. G.? What activities will you engage him in? What positions? For what period of time? With what equipment? How would these be similar or different if his amputations were at the transfemoral level? What issues or factors will assist or inhibit his ability to take responsibility for exercises aimed at insuring adequate ROM and flexibility in preparation for prosthetic use?
- What specific strategies for intervention and patient–family education aimed at improving muscle performance do you recommend for P. G.? How do you address strengthening of key muscle groups of extremities and trunk? How do you address power and muscle endurance? How do you address concentric, isometric, and eccentric control and performance? How would this be similar or different if his amputations were at the transfemoral level? What issues or factors must be considered regarding exercise tolerance, intensity, frequency, and duration during his acute care stay? How will you address his concerns about low level of aerobic fitness and conditioning?
- What specific strategies for intervention and patient–family education aimed at improving static, dynamic, and reactionary postural control during functional activities do you recommend for P. G.? During which activities is postural control most likely to be problematic? What apparatus, equipment, and activities might you use to assist his postural control?
- What are your concerns about seating and wheelchair mobility for P. G.? Do you think that a standard wheelchair will adequately meet his needs? Do you think he will be able to propel his chair? What tasks does he need to master if the wheelchair will be his primary source of mobility during the preprosthetic period?
- What additional bed mobility and transfer activities do you think are important for P. G. and his family caregivers to master? What specific intervention and patient–family education strategies will you use to help him move toward safe and, hopefully, independent performance of bed mobility and transfer activities? How will you vary environmental conditions and task demands to ensure that he can adapt his strategies and skills?
- How will you address the likelihood that he will experience a fall at some point in his preprosthetic period?
- Are there any additional interventions that would be appropriate for P. G. at this point in his postoperative, preprosthetic rehabilitation to assist with his coping and adjustment to his limb loss?
- How will you determine his readiness for prosthetic fitting?

TABLE 20-9   *Examples of Outcome Measures for Preprosthetic Rehabilitation*

Tool	Purpose	Level of Measurement	Comments
Activity Measure for Post-Acute Care (AM-PAC)	Assess limitations in three ICF Activity domains: 1. Physical and Movement 2. Personal Care and Instrumental 3. Applied Cognitive	Ordinal (raw score) Interval (standardized score) Paper and computerized instruments available	Physical and Movement and Personal Care and Instrumental subscales have minimal ceiling effect as compared to Functional Independence Measure[323,343,344]
Amputee Mobility Predictor–no prosthesis (AMP-noPro)[157-161]	Sitting balance, transfers, standing balance, gait, stairs, use of assistive device	Ordinal scale 21 items in 6 domains Score range: 0 to 42 Performance-based MDD = 3.4	Predicts likelihood of prosthetic use; also used as outcome measure in preprosthetic period[151,161,345]
Barthel Index (BI)	Activities of Daily Living	Ordinal 10 items; weighted ratings 0 to 100 range Performance based or by interview (self-report)	Developed initially for persons with neurological problems; applied to those with amputation. Ceiling effect possible as rehabilitation progresses[346,347]
Functional Independence Measure (FIM)[157-161]	Burden of care, activities of daily living	Ordinal 18 items for 6 categories Score range: 18 to 126 Performance based or self-report (interview)	Marked ceiling effect; does not reflect community function. May be more appropriate in acute care than for intensive rehabilitation[159,323,348-350]
Office of Population Consensus and Surveys Scale (OPCS)	WHO International Classification of Impairments, Disabilities, Handicaps–based measure of functional capacity	Ordinal 108 items over 13 disability categories Weighted overall "Disability Score" (requires computer)	Developed for assessment community-living individuals with disability; useful for inpatient rehabilitation[351]
Patient Generated Index (PGI)	Impact of amputation (or other medical event) on quality of life	Ordinal Respondents identify 5 activities impacted by amputation, rate severity and importance of impact on quality of life Overall score (0 to 10) mathematically derived Patient Specific Functional Scale: rate current ability to	Can be challenging for patients to understand[352,353]
Patient Specific Functional Scale (PSFS)	Impact of amputation (or other medical event) on functional performance of important activities	Ordinal Respondents identify 3 to 5 activities impacted by amputation then rate their ability to perform (0 to 10) Mean of items used as PSFS score MDD: 3 to 4.5 per item	Effective measuring change for the individual patient[345,354,355]
Prosthetic Profile of the Amputee (PPA)	Assesses predisposing, enabling, and facilitating factors for eventual prosthetic use	Nominal and ordinal data 38 questions in 6 sections Self-report or interview Requires training to score (computer)	For adults with unilateral amputation Recommended for use in research, rather than clinical settings[346,356,357]

Instrument	Construct	Details	Comments
Rivermead Mobility Index (RMI)	Capacity to perform mobility activities	Ordinal; 15 Items; Forced choice format; Self-report or interview	Ceiling effects in late preprosthetic and prosthetic rehabilitation[358-360]
Short Form-36 or Short-Form-12	Health-related quality of life	Ordinal; 8 subscales over 2 domains (physical and mental functioning); Self-report or interview; MDD for SF-36 Health: 17.1; MDD for SF-36 Physical Functioning: 34.2; MDD for SF-36 Physical Role: 26.3	Designed for general population; has not been specifically evaluated for use with persons with amputation[345,346,361,362]
Function Component of the Late Life Function and Disability Instrument (LLFDI)	Function and disability in community-living older adults	Ordinal; Interview or self-report; 32 questions: rated 1 to 5; 8 additional questions if assistive device is routinely used; Raw score transformed to scaled score (0 to 100); Overall function score; Upper extremity subscale; Basic lower extremity subscale; Advanced lower extremity subscale	High scores = better function; Has been used for a variety of conditions and health care settings but not fully evaluated for persons with amputation[363-366]
Walking Speed (self-selected and/or fast)	Overground mobility; Proxy for overall health/functional status	Continuous; Performance based; MDD range: 0.10 to 0.2 m/s for most medical diagnoses	Minimal equipment: stopwatch and hallway; Use of assistive device during testing possible; 4-m walk protocol effective (6 to 8 m total walkway) comparable to 10 m (20 m total walkway)[367]; Norms available for healthy adults by decade of age and gender[368]
2-Minute Walk Test (Brooks)	Cardiovascular endurance	Continuous; Performance based; Distance (m) covered in 2-minute period	Developed as alternative to exercise stress test for persons with CHF; applied to wide variety of medical diagnoses[369,370]
Wheelchair Skills Test Version 4.1	Assessment of performance and safety of manual wheelchair use	Ordinal; Performance or questionnaire; 32 items; Indoor use; Community use; Advanced skills; Scoring: performance: pass/fail; Safety: safe/unsafe	Used to assess ability of users of manual wheelchair, caregivers, and power chairs[371,372]

ICF, International Classification of Functioning, Disability, and Health; *MDD,* minimal detectable difference.

PREPROSTHETIC OUTCOME ASSESSMENT

Current models of health care practice (and reimbursement) require assessment of the efficacy of intervention that has been provided, often by comparing information collected at initial and discharge examinations. A number of tools and measures can be used to assess outcome of intervention in the pre-prosthetic period; Table 20-9 provides examples of such measures. The selection of the most appropriate tools from among those available can be challenging.[322] The first consideration is to determine which "population" the tool has been designed and validated for. Some measures have been evaluated for use with older adults who are hospitalized, others specifically for persons with lower limb amputation.[323,324] The next concern is the domain that the tool evaluates: outcomes can be assessed at the level of body structure and function (e.g., wound healing, limb volume); activity ability or limitation (e.g., ability to ambulate, complete ADLs); or at the level of participation (e.g., quality of life, ability to participate in meaningful social roles).[325,326] It is also important to understand the level of measurement of the tool, so as to be able to interpret findings.[327] The various scales and tools may provide *descriptive/categorical* information (e.g., Medical Functional Classification Levels), *ordinal* information (e.g., ranking, severity, FIM scores) or robust *continuous* data (e.g., walking speed, limb circumference, functional reach distances). How the information is collected is also a factor: tools may be based on self-report, observation of performance, or require use of precise measurement tools. Given all of these aspects of measurement, it becomes obvious that there is no single "perfect" outcome measure for preprosthetic rehabilitative care; instead the rehabilitation team should collectively select those measures that best meet the needs of the patient, therapeutic goals, and expectations of the practice environment.[328–330] Although it would be wonderful to have professional consensus of the type and scope of data that should be routinely collected, the reality is that outcome measurement in rehabilitation, although not in its infancy, is at least in its troubling teenage years! We have a lot of growing up to do.

What makes a good outcome measure for preprosthetic rehabilitation? The selection of measures should be based on the primary goals of the setting in which care is provided and the specific patient-centered goals that have been defined for the individual: What concepts, function, or attribute needs to be measured? In choosing an outcome measurement tool, we look for evidence of

- *Reliability:* Can we trust the numbers that the tool provides? Is the tool consistent in measurement over time? Do different raters tend to come up with similar scores? How much measurement error might be present in the "score"?
- *Validity:* How well does the tool measure what it intends to measure? Is it designed for patients like the ones that we provide care for? How well do scores on the measure

discriminate between persons with and without the problem that the measure attempts to examine?
- *Responsiveness:* How well can this measure capture change? What is the minimal change in status or function that it can predict (minimal detectable difference [MDD] or minimal detectable change [MDC])? Do we understand what a clinically meaningful change might be (minimal clinically important difference)?[331]

Readers are referred to Portney LG, Watkins MP. *Foundations of Clinical Research: Applications to Practice*, 3rd ed. (Upper Saddle River, NJ: Prentice Hall, 2009) for more information on the process of measurement, and to Stokes EK, *Rehabilitation Outcome Measures* (Philadelphia, PA: Elsevier/Churchill Livingstone, 2011) as a resource for evaluating and selecting outcome measures.

SUMMARY

Early rehabilitation in the postoperative preprosthetic period lays the foundation for prosthetic rehabilitation. Initial emphasis is placed on wound healing and control of edema, essential prerequisites for prosthetic use. Early in the process, the individual with new amputation and family caregivers become actively involved in the rehabilitation process and decision making, assuming responsibility for limb compression, skin care, and desensitization. The therapist is alert for postoperative medical complications such as postural hypotension or deep venous thrombosis, as early mobility begins. The therapist implements strategies to prevent secondary impairments and functional limitations such as further deconditioning and contracture formation. Strengthening exercises, targeting the residual limb and overall fitness, begin in the acute or subacute setting and continue as an aggressive home program to prepare the individual for prosthetic training. Persons with new amputation are encouraged to become as independent as possible in transfers, single limb gait, and wheelchair mobility, depending on their medical status and functional capability. As the wound heals and edema subsides, the individual with new amputation, family caregivers, therapist, prosthetist, and physician begin discussion about future prosthetic rehabilitation. The postoperative, preprosthetic period is a time of transition in which many individuals mourn the loss of their limb and question their future yet are challenged and encouraged by the possibilities offered by prosthetic replacement of their limb. If the consensus is that prosthetic fitting is not viable, emphasis shifts to development of wheelchair mobility skills and adaptation of the patient's environment as rehabilitation continues. If the consensus is that prosthetic fitting is likely, rehabilitation during this time focuses on building the physical and psychological resources that will ensure the person with new amputation will become a successful prosthetic user.

REFERENCES

1. Robinson V, Sansam K, Hirst L, Neumann V. Major lower limb amputation—what, why and how to achieve the best results. *Orthopaed Trauma.* 2010;24(4):276–285.

2. Kratz AL, Williams RM, Turner AP, et al. To lump or to split? Comparing individuals with traumatic and nontraumatic limb loss in the first year after amputation. *Rehabil Psychol.* 2010;55(2):126–138.

3. Livingstone W, Van de Mortel TF, Taylor B. A path of perpetual resilience: Exploring the experience of a diabetes-related amputation through grounded theory. *Contemp Nurse.* 2011;39(1):20–30.

4. Sigford BJ. Paradigm shift for VA amputation care. *J Rehabil Res Dev.* 2010;47(4):xv–xix.

5. Pasquina PF. DOD paradigm shift in care of service members with major limb loss. *J Rehabil Res Dev.* 2010;47(4):xi–xiv.

6. Hakimi KN. Pre-operative rehabilitation evaluation of the dysvascular patient prior to amputation. *Phys Med Rehabil Clin N Am.* 2009;20(4):677–688.

7. Smith DG. General principles of amputation surgery. In: Smith DG, Michael JW, Bowker JH, eds. *Atlas of Amputation and Limb Deficiencies: Surgical, Prosthetic, and Rehabilitation Principles.* 3rd ed. Rosemont, IL: American Academy of Orthopaedic Surgeons; 2004:21–30.

8. Richardson C. Nursing aspects of phantom limb pain following amputation. *Br J Nurs.* 2008;17(7):422–426.

9. Melsom H, Danjoux G. Perioperative care for lower limb amputation in vascular disease. *Contin Educ Anaesth Crit Care Pain.* 2011;11(5):162–166.

10. Goldberg T. Postoperative management of lower extremity amputations. *Phys Med Rehabil Clin N Am.* 2006;17(1):173–180.

11. Bowker JH. The art of prosthesis prescription. In: Smith DG, Michael JW, Bowker JH, eds. *Atlas of Amputation and Limb Deficiencies: Surgical, Prosthetic, and Rehabilitation Principles.* 3rd ed. Rosemont, IL: American Academy of Orthopaedic Surgeons; 2004:739–744.

12. McFarland LV, Choppa AJ, Betz K, et al. Resources for wounded warriors with major traumatic limb loss. *J Rehabil Res Dev.* 2010;47(3):1–13.

13. Dillingham TR, Yacub JN, Pezzin LE. Determinants of post-acute care discharge destination after dysvascular lower limb amputation. *PM R.* 2011;3(4):336–344.

14. Gajewski D, Granville R. The United States Armed Forces Amputee Patient Care Program. *J Am Acad Orthop Surg.* 2006;14(10 Spec No):S183–S187.

15. *Who are physical therapists? Guide to Physical Therapist Practice.* Alexandria, VA: American Physical Therapy Association. http://guidetoptpractice.apta.org; Accessed 04.08.11.

16. Dillingham TR, Pezzin LE. Rehabilitation setting and associated mortality and medical stability among persons with amputations. *Arch Phys Med Rehabil.* 2008;89(6):1038–1045.

17. Stineman MG, Kwong PL, Kurichi JE, et al. The effectiveness of inpatient rehabilitation in the acute postoperative phase of care after transtibial or transfemoral amputation: study of an integrated health care delivery system. *Arch Phys Med Rehabil.* 2008;89(10):1863–1872.

18. Basics of Patient/Client Management: The Five Elements of Patient/Client Management. *Guide to Physical Therapist Practice.* Alexandria, VA: American Physical Therapy Association. http://guidetoptpractice.apta.org. Accessed 18.08.11.

19. Strauss SE, Richardson WS, Glaszious P, Haynes RB. *Evidence-Based Medicine: How to Practice and Teach EBM.* 3rd ed. Philadelphia, PA: Churchill Livingstone; 2005.

20. Spector RE. *Cultural Diversity in Health and Illness.* 7th ed. Saddle River, NJ: Prentice-Hall; 2008.

21. Horgan O, MacLachlan M. Psychosocial adjustment to lower limb amputation: a review. *Disabil Rehabil.* 2004; 26(14/15):837–850.

22. Coffey L, Gallagher P, Horgan O, et al. Psychosocial adjustment to diabetes-related lower limb amputation. *Diabet Med.* 2009;26(10):1063–1067.

23. Arnett JJ. *Human Development: A Cultural Approach.* New York, NY: Pearson; 2012.

24. Lusardi MM. Older adults and their families. In: Guccione AA, Avers D, Wong RA, eds. *Geriatric Physical Therapy.* 3rd ed. St. Louis, MO: Elsevier Mosby; 2012:207–227.

25. Anderson SA, Sabatelli RN. *Family Interaction: A Multigenerational Developmental Perspective.* 5th ed. Upper Saddle River, NJ: Prentice Hall; 2010.

26. Ainsworth E, de Jonge D. *An Occupational Therapist's Guide to Home Modification Practice.* Thorofare, NJ: Slack; 2011.

27. Couture M, Desrosiers J, Caron CD. Cognitive appraisal and perceived benefits of dysvascular lower limb amputation: a longitudinal study. *Arch Gerontol Geriatr.* 2011;52(1):5–11.

28. Martz E, Livneh H. *Coping with Chronic Illness and Disability: Theoretical, Empirical, and Clinical Aspects.* New York, NY: Springer; 2007.

29. Gillis A, MacDonald B. Deconditioning in the hospitalized elderly. *Can Nurse.* 2005;101(6):16–20.

30. Cohen B, Vittinghoff E, Whooley M. Association of socioeconomic status and exercise capacity in adults with coronary heart disease. *Am J Cardiol.* 2008;101(4):462–466.

31. Kurichi JE, Stineman MG, Kwong PL, et al. Assessing and using comorbidity measures in elderly veterans with lower extremity amputations. *Gerontology.* 2007;53(5):255–259.

32. Landry GJ, Silverman DA, Liem TK, et al. Predictors of healing and functional outcome following transmetatarsal amputations. *Arch Surg.* 2011;146(9):1005–1009.

33. Aragón-Sánchez J, Hernández-Herrero MJ, Lázaro-Martínez JL, et al. In-hospital complications and mortality following major lower extremity amputations in a series of predominantly diabetic patients. *Int J Low Extrem Wounds.* 2010;9(1):16–23.

34. Neil JA. Perioperative care of the immunocompromised patient. *AORN J.* 2007;85(3):544–564.

35. Shih T, Lindely C. Bevacizumab: an angiogenesis inhibitor for the treatment of solid malignancies. *Clin Ther.* 2006;28(11):1779–1802.

36. Olascoaga A, Vilar-Compte D, Poitevin-Chacon A, Contreras-Ruiz J. Wound healing in radiated skin: pathophysiology and treatment options. *Int Wound J.* 2008;5(2):246–257.

37. Remes L, Isoaho R, Vahlberg T, et al. Predictors for institutionalization and prosthetic ambulation after major lower extremity amputation during an eight-year follow-up. *Aging Clin Exp Res.* 2009;21(2):129–135.

38. Richardson J, Letts L, Chan D, et al. Rehabilitation in a primary care setting for persons with chronic illness—a randomized controlled trial. *Prim Health Care Res Dev.* 2010;11(4):382–395.

39. Wells CL, Walker M. Evaluation of the acute, medically complex patient. In: Guccione AA, Avers D, Wong RA, eds. *Geriatric Physical Therapy.* St. Louis, MO: Mosby; 2012:153–182.

40. Billek-Sawhney B, Wells CL. Oncology implications for exercise and rehabilitation. *Acute Care Perspect.* 2009;18(4):12–19.

41. Chapman S. Pain management in patients following limb amputation. *Nurs Stand.* 2011;25(19):35–40.

42. Ketz AK. Pain management in the traumatic amputee. *Crit Care Nurs Clin North Am.* 2008;20(1):51–57.

43. Derman W. Antihypertensive medications and exercise. *Int Sport Med J.* 2008;9(1):32–38.

44. Di Stasi SL, MacLeod TD, Winters JD, Binder-Macleod SA. Effects of statins on skeletal muscle: a perspective for physical therapists. *Phys Ther.* 2010;90(10):1530–1542.

45. Green S, Askew CD, Walker PJ. Effect of type 2 diabetes mellitus on exercise intolerance and the physiological responses to exercise in peripheral arterial disease. *Diabetologia.* 2007;50(4):859–866.

46. Knight J, Nigam Y, Jones A. Effects of bedrest 1: cardiovascular, respiratory and haematological systems. *Nurs Times.* 2009;105(21):16–20.

47. Mason SE, Noel-Storr A, Ritchie CW. The impact of general and regional anesthesia on the incidence of post-operative cognitive dysfunction and post-operative delirium: a systematic review with meta-analysis. *J Alzheimers Dis.* 2010;22(suppl 3):67–79.

48. Boissonnault WG, Umphred DA. Differential diagnosis phase 1: medical screening for the therapist. In: Umphred DA, ed. *Neurological Rehabilitation.* 5th ed. St. Louis, MO: Mosby; 2007:149–163.

49. Marcantonio ER. In the clinic. Delirium. *Ann Intern Med.* 2011;154(11): ITC61–ITC6-15.

50. *What are tests and measures? Guide to Physical Therapist Practice.* Alexandria, VA: American Physical Therapy Association. http://guidetoptpractice.apta.org/content/1/SEC5.body. Accessed 04.08.11.

51. Institute for Clinical Systems Improvement. *Assessment and Management of Acute Pain.* 6th ed. http://www.icsi.org/pain_acute/pain__acute__assessment_and_managementof__3.html; 2008. Accessed 15.12.11.

52. Pasero C, McCaffrey M. *Pain Assessment and Pharmacologic Management.* St. Louis, MO: Mosby; 2011.

53. Ciccone CD. Opioid analgesics. In: Ciccone CD, ed. *Pharmacology in Rehabilitation.* 4th ed. Philadelphia, PA: FA Davis; 2007:183–198.

54. Ciccone CD. Patient-controlled analgesia. In: Ciccone CD, ed. *Pharmacology in Rehabilitation.* 4th ed. Philadelphia, PA: FA Davis; 2007:237–249.

55. Casale R, Alaa L, Mallick M, Ring H. Phantom limb related phenomena and their rehabilitation after lower limb amputation. *Eur J Phys Rehabil Med.* 2009;45(4):559–566.

56. Richardson C, Glenn S, Nurmikko T, Horgan M. Incidence of phantom phenomena including phantom limb pain 6 months after major lower limb amputation in patients with peripheral vascular disease. *Clin J Pain.* 2006;22(4):353–358.

57. Schley MT, Wilms P, Toepfner S, et al. Painful and nonpainful phantom and stump sensations in acute traumatic amputees. *J Trauma.* 2008;65(4):858–864.

58. Probstner D, Thuler LC, Ishikawa NM, Alvarenga RM. Phantom limb phenomena in cancer amputees. *Pain Pract.* 2010;10(3):249–256.

59. Rayegani SM, Aryanmehr A, Soroosh MR, Baghbani M. Phantom pain, phantom sensation, and spine pain in bilateral lower limb amputees: results of a national survey of iraqiran war victims' health status. *J Prosthet Orthot.* 2010;22(3):162–165.

60. Wolff A, Vanduynhoven E, van Kleef M, et al. Phantom pain. *Pain Pract.* 2011;11(4):403–413.

61. Wilson JA, Nimmo AF, Fleetwood-Walker SM, Colvin LA. A randomized double blind trial of the effect of pre-emptive epidural ketamine on persistent pain after lower limb amputation. *Pain.* 2008;135(1/2):108–118.

62. Borghi B, D'Addabbo M, White PF, et al. The use of prolonged peripheral neural blockade after lower extremity amputation: the effect on symptoms associated with phantom limb syndrome. *Anesth Analg.* 2010;111(5):1308–1315.

63. Subedi B, Grossberg GT. Phantom limb pain: mechanisms and treatment approaches. *Pain Res Treat.* 2011;2011:864605.

64. Giummarra MJ, Moseley GL. Phantom limb pain and bodily awareness: current concepts and future directions. *Curr Opin Anaesthesiol.* 2011;24(5):524–531.

65. Shultz SJ, Nguyen A. Bilateral asymmetries in clinical measures of lower extremity anatomic characteristics. *Clin J Sports Med.* 2007;17(5):357–361.

66. Arwert HJ, van Doorn-Loogman MH, Koning J, et al. Residual-limb quality and functional mobility 1 year after transtibial amputation caused by vascular insufficiency. *J Rehabil Res Dev.* 2007;44(5):717–722.

67. *Standard of Care: Lower Extremity Amputation.* Boston, MA: The Brigham and Women's Hospital, Department of Rehabilitation Services; 2011.

68. Sanders JE, Fatone S. Residual limb volume change: Systematic review of measurement and management. *J Rehabil Res Dev.* 2011;48(8):949–986.

69. de Boer-Wilzing VG, Bolt A, Geertzen JH, et al. Variation in results of volume measurements of stumps of lower limb amputees: a comparison of 4 methods. *Arch Phys Med Rehabil.* 2011;92(6):941–946.

70. Geil MD. Consistency, precision, and accuracy of optical and electromagnetic shape-capturing systems for digital measurement of residual-limb anthropometrics of persons with transtibial amputation. *J Rehabil Res Dev.* 2007;44(4):515–524.

71. Bowker JH. Transtibial amputation: surgical management. In: Smith DG, Michaels JW, Bowker JH, eds. *Atlas of Amputation and Limb Deficiencies: Surgical, Prosthetic, and Rehabilitation Principles.* 3rd ed. Rosemont, IL: American Academy of Orthopaedic Surgeons; 2004:481–501.

72. McIntosh J, Earnshaw JJ. Antibiotic prophylaxis for the prevention of infection after major limb amputation. *Eur J Vasc Endovasc Surg.* 2009;37(6):696–703.

73. Sadat U, Chaudhuri A, Hayes PD, et al. Five day antibiotic prophylaxis for major lower limb amputation reduces wound infection rates and the length of in-hospital stay. *Eur J Vasc Endovasc Surg.* 2008;35(1):75–78.

74. Tintle SM, Forsberg JA, Keeling JJ, et al. Lower extremity combat-related amputations. *J Surg Orthop Adv.* 2010;19(1):35–43.

75. Lim TS, Finlayson A, Thorpe JM, et al. Outcomes of a contemporary amputation series. *ANZ J Surg.* 2006;76(5):300–305.

76. Carney ML, Ullrich P, Esselman P. Early unplanned transfers from inpatient rehabilitation. *Am J Phys Med Rehabil.* 2006;85(5):453–462.

77. Bates-Jensen BM, Woolfolk N. Acute surgical wound management. In: Sussman C, Bates-Jensen BM, eds. *Wound Care: A Collaborative Practice Model.* 3rd ed. Philadelphia, PA: Wolters Kluwer–Lippincott Williams & Wilkins; 2007:322–335.

78. Stasik CN, Berceli SA, Nelson PR, et al. Functional outcome after redo below-knee amputation. *World J Surg.* 2008;32(8):1823–1826.

79. Smith E, Ryall N. Residual limb osteomyelitis: A case series from a national prosthetic centre. *Disabil Rehabil.* 2009;31(21):1785–1789.

80. VanRoss ER, Johnson S, Abbott CA. Effects of early mobilization on unhealed dysvascular transtibial amputation stumps: a clinical trial. *Arch Phys Med Rehabil.* 2009;90(4):610–617.

81. Kapp SL, Fergason JR. Transtibial amputation: prosthetic management. In: Smith DG, Michaels JW, Bowker JH, eds. *Atlas of Amputation and Limb Deficiencies: Surgical, Prosthetic, and Rehabilitation Principles.* 3rd ed. Rosemont, IL: American Academy of Orthopaedic Surgeons; 2004:503–515.

82. Smith DG, Berke GM. Standards of care in post operative management of the lower extremity amputee: Proceedings of the Clinical Standards of Practice Consensus Conference. *J Prosthet Orthot.* 2004;16(3 S):6–12.

83. Yu JC, Lam K, Nettel-Aguirre A, et al. Incidence and risk factors of falling in the postoperative lower limb amputee while on the surgical ward. *PM R.* 2010;2(10):926–934.

84. Eneroth M, Apelqvist J, Larsson J, Persson BM. Improved wound healing in transtibial amputees receiving supplementary nutrition. *Int Orthop.* 1997;21(2):104–108.

85. Robertshaw D, Robertshaw L. What role do we play post-amputation? *Diabetic Foot J.* 2003;6(1):43–44 46–77.

86. Evans KK, Attinger CE, Al-Attar A, et al. The importance of limb preservation in the diabetic population. *J Diabetes Complications.* 2011;25(4):227–231.

87. Perry J. Amputee gait. In: Smith DG, Michaels JW, Bowker JH, eds. *Atlas of Amputation and Limb Deficiencies: Surgical, Prosthetic, and Rehabilitation Principles.* 3rd ed. Rosemont, IL: American Academy of Orthopaedic Surgeons; 2004:367–384.

88. van Velzen AD, Nederhand MJ, Emmelot CH, Ijzerman MJ. Early treatment of trans-tibial amputees: retrospective analysis of early fitting and elastic bandaging. *Prosthet Orthot Int.* 2005;29(1):3–12.

89. Gottschalk F. Transfemoral amputation: surgical management. In: Smith DG, Michaels JW, Bowker JH, eds. *Atlas of Amputation and Limb Deficiencies: Surgical, Prosthetic, and Rehabilitation Principles.* 3rd ed. Rosemont, IL: American Academy of Orthopaedic Surgeons; 2004:533–540.

90. Gailey R, Allen K, Castles J, Kucharik J, Roeder M. Review of secondary physical conditions associated with lower limb amputation and long-term prosthesis use. *J Rehabil Res Dev.* 2008;45(1):15–29.

91. Uellendahl JE. Bilateral lower limb prosthesis. In: Smith DG, Michaels JW, Bowker JH, eds. *Atlas of Amputation and Limb Deficiencies: Surgical, Prosthetic, and Rehabilitation Principles.* 3rd ed. Rosemont, IL: American Academy of Orthopaedic Surgeons; 2004:621–632.

92. Magee DJ. Knee. In: Magee DJ, ed. *Orthopedic Physical Assessment.* 5th ed. St. Louis, MO: Saunders; 2008:727–843.

93. Kendall FP, McCreary EK, Provance PG, et al. *Muscles: Testing and Function.* 5th ed. Philadelphia, PA: Lippincott Williams & Wilkins; 2005.

94. Krebs DE, Scarborough DM, McGibbon CA. Functional vs. strength training in disabled elderly outpatients. *Am J Phys Med Rehabil.* 2007;86(2):93–103.

95. Marimuthu K, Murton AJ, Greenhaff PL. Mechanisms regulating muscle mass during disuse atrophy and rehabilitation in humans. *J Appl Physiol.* 2011;110(2):555–560.

96. O'Sullivan SB. Assessment of motor function: motor control and motor learning. In: O'Sullivan SB, Schmitz TJ, eds. *Physical Rehabilitation: Assessment and Treatment.* 5th ed. Philadelphia: F.A. Davis; 2007:227–271.

97. Bales JG, Meals R. Peripheral neuropathy of the upper extremity: medical comorbidity that confounds common orthopedic pathology. *Orthopedics.* 2009;32(10):758–765.

98. May O, Arildsen H. Long-term predictive power of simple function tests for cardiovascular autonomic neuropathy in diabetes: a population-based study. *Acta Diabetol.* 2011;48(4):311–316.

99. Pop-Busui R. Cardiac autonomic neuropathy in diabetes: a clinical perspective. *Diabetes Care.* 2010;33(2):434–441.

100. Umphred DA. The limbic system: influence over motor control and learning. In: Umphred DA, ed. *Neurological Rehabilitation.* 5th ed. St. Louis, MO: Mosby; 2007:71–118.

101. Borg G, Domserius M, Kaijser L. Psychophysical scaling with applications in physical work and the perception of exertions. *Scand J Work Environ Health.* 1990;16(suppl 1):55–58.

102. Borg GA. Psychosocial bases of perceived exertions, basis of perceived exertion. *Med Sci Sports Exerc.* 1982;14(5):377–387.

103. Erjavec T, Presern-Strukelj M, Burger H. The diagnostic importance of exercise testing in developing appropriate rehabilitation programmes for patients following transfemoral amputation. *Eur J Phys Rehabil Med.* 2008;44(2):133–139.

104. Vestering MM, Schoppen T, Dekker R, et al. Development of an exercise testing protocol for patients with a lower limb amputation: results of a pilot study. *Int J Rehabil Res.* 2005;28(3):237–244.

105. Chin T, Sawamura S, Fujita H, et al. %VO2max as an indicator of prosthetic rehabilitation outcome after dysvascular amputation. *Prosthet Orthot Int.* 2002;26(1):44–49.

106. Yosefy C. Diabetic heart and the cardiovascular surgeon. *Cardiovasc Hematol Disord Drug Targets.* 2008;8(2):147–152.

107. Belmont PJ, Davey S, Orr JD, et al. Risk factors for 30-day postoperative complications and mortality after below-knee amputation: a study of 2,911 patients from the national surgical quality improvement program. *J Am Coll Surg.* 2011;213(3):370–378.

108. Aragon-Sanchez J, Hernandez-Herrero MJ, Lazaro-Martinez JL, et al. In-hospital complications and mortality following major lower extremity amputations in a series of predominantly diabetic patients. *Int J Low Extrem Wounds.* 2010;9(1):16–23.

109. Avers D, Williams AK. Cognition in the aging adult. In: Guccione AA, Avers D, Wong RA, eds. *Geriatric Physical Therapy.* 3rd ed. St. Louis, MO: Elsevier Mosby; 2012:121–152.

110. Schulte OJ, Stephens J, Ann J. Brain function, aging, and dementia. In: Umphred DA, ed. *Neurological Rehabilitation.* 5th ed. St. Louis, MO: Mosby; 2007:902–930.

111. Balasundaram B, Holmes J. Delirium in vascular surgery. *Eur J Vasc Endovasc Surg.* 2007;34(2):131–134.

112. Singh R, Ripley D, Pentland B, et al. Depression and anxiety symptoms after lower limb amputation: the rise and fall. *Clin Rehabil.* 2009;23(3):281–286.

113. Ide M. The association between depressive mood and pain amongst individuals with limb amputations. *Eur J Trauma Emerg Surg.* 2011;37(2):191–195.

114. Vase L, Nikolajsen L, Christensen B, et al. Cognitive-emotional sensitization contributes to wind-up-like pain in phantom limb pain patients. *Pain.* 2011;152(1):157–162.

115. Copuroglu C, Ozcan M, Yilmaz B, et al. Acute stress disorder and post-traumatic stress disorder following traumatic amputation. *Acta Orthop Belg.* 2010;76(1):90–93.

116. Cheung E, Alvaro R, Colotla VA. Psychological distress in workers with traumatic upper or lower limb amputations following industrial injuries. *Rehabil Psychol.* 2003;48(2):109–112.

117. Cavanagh SR, Shin LM, Karamouz N, Rauch SL. Psychiatric and emotional sequelae of surgical amputation. *Psychosomatics.* 2006;47(6):459–464.

118. Friedman B, Heisel MJ, Delavan RL. Psychometric properties of the 15-item geriatric depression scale in functionally impaired, cognitively intact, community-dwelling elderly primary care patients. *J Am Geriatr Soc.* 2005;53(9):1570–1576.

119. Schoppen T, Boonstra A, Groothoff JW, et al. Physical, mental, and social predictors of functional outcome in unilateral lower limb amputees. *Arch Phys Med Rehabil.* 2003;84(6):803–811.

120. Behel JM, Rybarczyk B, Elliott TR, et al. The role of perceived vulnerability in adjustment to lower extremity amputation: a preliminary investigation. *Rehabil Psychol.* 2002;47(1):92–105.

121. Pritchard MJ. Using the Hospital Anxiety and Depression Scale in surgical patients. *Nurs Stand.* 2011;25(34):35–41.

122. Desmond DM, MacLachlan M. The factor structure of the hospital anxiety and depression scale in older individuals with acquired amputations: a comparison of four models using confirmatory factor analysis. *Int J Geriatr Psychiatry.* 2005;20(4):344–349.

123. Pachana NA, Byrne GJ, Siddle H, et al. Development and validation of the Geriatric Anxiety Inventory. *Int Psychogeriatr.* 2007;19(1):103–114.

124. Rafnsson SB, Deary IJ, Fowkes FG. Peripheral arterial disease and cognitive function. *Vasc Med.* 2009;14(1):51–61.

125. Phelps LF, Williams RM, Raichle KA, et al. The importance of cognitive processing to adjustment in the 1st year following amputation. *Rehabil Psychol.* 2008;53(1):28–38.

126. O'Neill BR, Evans JJ. Memory and executive function predict mobility rehabilitation outcome after lower limb amputation. *Disabil Rehabil.* 2009;31(13):1083–1091.

127. Sansam K, Neumann V, O'Connor R, Bhakta B. Predicting walking ability following lower limb amputation: a systematic review of the literature. *J Rehabil Med.* 2009;41(8):593–603.

128. Taylor SM, Kalbaugh CA, Blackhurst DW, et al. Preoperative clinical factors predict postoperative functional outcomes after major lower limb amputation: an analysis of 553 consecutive patients. *J Vasc Surg.* 2005;42(2):227–235.

129. Resnik B, Avers D. Motivation and patient education. In: Guccione AA, Avers D, Wong RA, eds. *Geriatric Physical Therapy.* St. Louis, MO: Mosby; 2012:183–206.

130. Dhital A, Pey T, Stanford MR. Visual loss and falls: a review. *Eye (Lond).* 2010;24(9):1437–1446.

131. Tideiksaar R. Sensory impairment and fall risk. *Generations.* 2002–2003;26(4):22–27.

132. Lord SR, Menz HB, Tiedemann A. A physiological profile approach to falls risk assessment and prevention. *Phys Ther.* 2003;83(3):237–252.

133. Servat JJ, Risco M, Nakasato YR, Bernardina CR. Visual impairment in the elderly: impact on functional ability and quality of life. *Clin Geriatr.* 2011;19(7):49–56.

134. Dillon CF, Gu Q, Hoffman HJ, Ko CW. Vision, hearing, balance, and sensory impairment in Americans aged 70 years and over: United States, 1999–2006. *NCHS Data Brief* 2010; Apr:1–8 .

135. Wharton MA. Environmental design: accommodating sensory changes in the older adult. In: Guccione AA, Avers D, Wong RA, eds. *Geriatric Physical Therapy.* St. Louis, MO: Mosby; 2012: 104–120.

136. Pratt SR, Kuller L, Talbott EO. Prevalence of hearing loss in black and white elders: results of the cardiovascular health study. *J Speech Lang Hear Res.* 2009;52(4):973–989.

137. Middleton A, Niruban A, Girling G, Myint PK. Communicating in a healthcare setting with people who have hearing loss. *BMJ.* 2010;341(7775):726–729.

138. Mold JW, Vesely SK, Keyl BA, et al. The prevalence, predictors, and consequences of peripheral sensory neuropathy in older patients. *J Am Board Fam Pract.* 2004;17(5):309–318.

139. Andrews KL. The at-risk foot: What to do before and after amputation. *J Vasc Nurs.* 2011;29(3):120–123.

140. Schmitz TJ. Examination of sensory function. In: O'Sullivan SB, Schmitz TJ, eds. *Physical Rehabilitation.* 5th ed. Philadelphia, PA: FA Davis; 2007:121–156.

141. Fuller G. *Neurological Examination Made Easy.* Edinburgh, UK: Churchill Livingstone; 2008.

142. Hamill R, Carson S, Dorahy M. Experiences of psychosocial adjustment within 18 months of amputation: an interpretative phenomenological analysis. *Disabil Rehabil.* 2010;32(9):729–740.

143. Ward SR. Biomechanical applications to joint structure and function. In: Levangie PK, Norkin CC, eds. *Joint Structure and Function.* 5th ed. Philadelphia, PA: FA Davis; 2011.

144. Munin MC, Espejo-DeGuzman MC, Boninger ML, et al. Predictive factors for successful early prosthetic ambulation among lower limb amputees. *J Rehabil Res Dev.* 2001;38(4): 379–384.

145. Sansam K, Neumann V, O'Connor R, Bhakta B. Predicting walking ability following lower limb amputation: a systematic review of the literature. *J Rehabil Med.* 2009;41(8):593–603.

146. May BJ. Amputation. In: O'Sullivan SB, Schmitz TJ, eds. *Physical Rehabilitation.* 5th ed. Philadelphia, PA: FA Davis; 2007:1031–1055.

147. McGuire TL. Performance-based measures following transtibial amputation: a case report. *Top Geriatr Rehabil.* 2004;20(4):262–272.

148. Burger H, Marincek C. Functional testing of elderly subjects after lower limb amputation. *Prosthet Orthot Int.* 2001;25(2):102–107.

149. Miller WC, Deathe AB, Speechley M. Psychometric properties of the Activities Specific Balance Confidence Scale among individuals with a lower limb amputation. *Arch Phys Med Rehabil.* 2003;84(5):656–661.

150. Alghwiri AA, Whitney SL. Balance and falls. In: Guccione AA, Avers D, Wong RA, eds. *Geriatric Physical Therapy.* 3rd ed. St. Louis, MO: Mosby; 2012:331–353.

151. Gailey RS, Roach KE, Applegate EB, et al. The amputee mobility predictor: an instrument to assess determinants of the lower limb amputee's ability to ambulate. *Arch Phys Med Rehabil.* 2002;83(5):613–627.

152. Resnik L, Borgia M. Reliability of outcome measures for people with lower limb amputations: distinguishing true change from statistical error. *Phys Ther.* 2011;91(4):555–565.

153. Lindsey C. Impaired posture. In: Guccione AA, Avers D, Wong RA, eds. *Geriatric Physical Therapy.* 3rd ed. St. Louis, MO: Mosby; 2012:292–315.

154. Gailey R, Allen K, Castles J, et al. Review of secondary physical conditions associated with lower limb amputation and long-term prosthesis use. *J Rehabil Res Dev.* 2008;45(1):15–29.

155. Smith CC, Comisky RN. A study of bone mineral density in lower limb amputees at a national prosthetics center. *J Prosthet Orthot.* 2011;1:14–20.

156. Sherk VD, Bemben MG, Bemben DA. BMD and bone geometry in transtibial and transfemoral amputees. *J Bone Miner Res.* 2008;23(9):1449–1457.

157. Granger CV, Hamilton BB, Linacre JM, et al. Performance profiles of the functional independence measure. *Am J Phys Med Rehabil.* 1993;72(2):84–89.

158. Masedo AI, Hanley M, Jensen MP, et al. Reliability and validity of a self-report FIM (FIM-SR) in persons with amputation or spinal cord injury and chronic pain. *Am J Phys Med Rehabil.* 2005;84(3):167–179.

159. Passalent LA, Tyas JE, Jaglal SB, Cott CA. The FIM as a measure of change in function after discharge from inpatient rehabilitation: a Canadian perspective. *Disabil Rehabil.* 2011;33(7):579–588.

160. Franchignoni F, Orlandini D, Ferriero G, Moscato TA. Reliability, validity, and responsiveness of the locomotor capabilities index in adults with lower limb amputation undergoing prosthetic training. *Arch Phys Med Rehabil.* 2004;85(5):743–748.

161. Gailey RS. Predictive outcome measures versus functional outcome measures in the lower limb amputee. *J Prosthet Orthot.* 2006; Proceedings 6: P51–P60.

162. Belmont PJ, Davey S, Orr JD, et al. Risk factors for 30-day postoperative complications and mortality after below-knee amputation: a study of 2,911 patients from the national surgical quality improvement program. *J Am Coll Surg.* 2011;213(3):370–378.

163. Aragón-Sánchez J, Hernández-Herrero MJ, Lázaro-Martínez JL, et al. In-hospital complications and mortality following major lower extremity amputations in a series of predominantly diabetic patients. *Int J Low Extrem Wounds.* 2010;9(1):16–23.

164. Bates B, Stineman MG, Reker DM, et al. Risk factors associated with mortality in veteran population following transtibial or transfemoral amputation. *J Rehabil Res Dev.* 2006;43(7):917–928.

165. Kobayashi L, Inaba K, Barmparas G, et al. Traumatic limb amputations at a level I trauma center. *Eur J Trauma Emerg Surg.* 2011;37(1):67–72.

166. Harris AM, Althausen PL, Kellam J, et al. Complications following limb-threatening lower extremity trauma. *J Orthop Trauma.* 2009;23(1):1–6.

167. D'Ayala M, Huzar T, Briggs W, et al. Blood transfusion and its effect on the clinical outcomes of patients undergoing major lower extremity amputation. *Ann Vasc Surg.* 2010;24(4):468–473.

168. Rizvi AA, Chillag SA, Chillag KJ. Perioperative management of diabetes and hyperglycemia in patients undergoing orthopaedic surgery. *J Am Acad Orthop Surg.* 2010;18(7):426–435.

169. Huang ME, Johns JS, White J, Sanford K. Venous thromboembolism in a rehabilitation setting after major lower extremity amputation. *Arch Phys Med Rehabil.* 2005;86(1):73–78.

170. Ploeg AJ, Lardenoye JW, Vracken-Peeters MP, Breslau PJ. Contemporary series of morbidity and mortality after lower limb amputation. *Eur J Vasc Endovasc Surg.* 2005;29(6):633–637.

171. Nicolle LE. Catheter-related urinary tract infection. *Drugs Aging.* 2005;22(8):627–639.

172. Lim TS, Finlayson A, Thorpe JM, et al. Outcomes of a contemporary amputation series. *ANZ J Surg.* 2006;76(5):300–305.

173. Tintle SM, Keeling JJ, Forsberg JA, et al. Operative complications of combat-related transtibial amputations: a comparison of the modified Burgess and modified Ertl tibiofibular synostosis techniques. *J Bone Joint Surg Am.* 2011;93-A(11):1016–1021.

174. Goodman CC, Peterson C. Infectious disease. In: *Pathology: Implications for the Physical Therapist.* 5th ed. St. Louis, MO: Elsevier Saunders; 2009:298–347.

175. Awad SS. State-of-the-art therapy for severe sepsis and multisystem organ dysfunction. *Am J Surg.* 2003;186(5A):23S–30S.

176. Jette AM. Physical disablement concepts for physical therapy research and practice. *Phys Ther.* 1994;74(5):380–386.

177. Masala C, Petretto DR. From disablement to enablement: conceptual models of disability in the 20th century. *Disabil Rehabil.* 2008;30(17):1233–1244.

178. Roush SE, Sharby N. Disability reconsidered: the paradox of physical therapy. *Phys Ther.* 2011;91(12):1715–1727.

179. Jette AM. Toward a common language for function, disability, and health. *Phys Ther.* 2006;86(5):726–734.

180. Sansam K, Neumann V, O'Connor R, Bhakta B. Predicting walking ability following lower limb amputation: a systematic review of the literature. *J Rehabil Med.* 2009;41(8):593–603.

181. Munin MC, Espejo-De Guzman MC, Boninger ML, et al. Predictive factors for successful early prosthetic ambulation among lower limb amputees. *J Rehabil Res Dev.* 2001;38(4):379–384.

182. Kalbaugh CA, Taylor SM, Kalbaugh BA, et al. Does obesity predict functional outcome in the dysvascular amputee? *Am Surg.* 2006;72(8):707–713.

183. Taylor SM, Kalbaugh CA, Blackhurst DW, et al. Preoperative clinical factors predict postoperative functional outcomes after major lower limb amputation: an analysis of 553 consecutive patients. *J Vasc Surg.* 2005;42(2):227–235.

184. Raya MA, Gailey RS, Fiebert IM, Roach KE. Impairment variables predicting activity limitation in individuals with lower limb amputation. *Prosthet Orthot Int.* 2010;34(1):73–84.

185. Larner S, Van Ross E, Hale C. Do psychological measures predict the ability of lower limb amputees to learn to use a prosthesis? *Clin Rehabil.* 2003;17(5):493–498.

186. Wasiak K. Analysis of prognostic factors for locomotion in patients after amputation of the tibia performed due to atherosclerotic critical limb ischemia. *Ortop Traumatol Rehabil.* 2005;7(4):411–417.

187. Icks A, Scheer M, Morbach S, et al. Time-dependent impact of diabetes on mortality in patients after major lower extremity amputation: survival in a population-based 5-year cohort in Germany. *Diabetes Care.* 2011;34(6):1350–1354.

188. Faglia E, Clerici G, Caminiti M, et al. Mortality after major amputation in diabetic patients with critical limb ischemia who did and did not undergo previous peripheral revascularization Data of a cohort study of 564 consecutive diabetic patients. *J Diabetes Complications.* 2010;24(4):265–269.

189. Moxey PW, Hofman D, Hinchliffe RJ, et al. Epidemiological study of lower limb amputation in England between 2003 and 2008. *Br J Surg.* 2010;97(9):1348–1353.

190. Dillingham TR, Yacub JN, Pezzin LE. Determinants of post-acute care discharge destination after dysvascular lower limb amputation. *PM R.* 2011;3(4):336–344.

191. Gailey RS, Clark CR. Physical therapy. In: Smith DG, Michaels JW, Bowker JH, eds. *Atlas of Amputation and Limb Deficiencies: Surgical, Prosthetic, and Rehabilitation Principles.* 3rd ed. Rosemont, IL: American Academy of Orthopaedic Surgeons; 2004:589–619.

192. Uustal H. Prosthetic rehabilitation issues in the diabetic and dysvascular amputee. *Phys Med Rehabil Clin N Am.* 2009;20(4):689–703.

193. Kanade RV, van Deursen RW, Price P, Harding K. Risk of plantar ulceration in diabetic patients with single-leg amputation. *Clin Biomech (Bristol, Avon).* 2006;21(3):306–313.

194. Halbert J, Crotty M, Cameron ID. Evidence for the optimal management of acute and chronic phantom pain: a systematic review. *Clin J Pain.* 2002;18(2):84–92.

195. Hanley MA, Ehde DM, Campbell KM, et al. Self-reported treatments used for lower limb phantom pain: descriptive findings. *Arch Phys Med Rehabil.* 2006;87(2):270–277 310–311.

196. Alviar MJ, Hale T, Dungca M. Pharmacologic interventions for treating phantom limb pain. Dec 7 *Cochrane Database Syst Rev.* 2011;(12): CD006380.

197. Grant AJ, Wood C. The effect of intra-neural local anaesthetic infusion on pain following major lower limb amputation. *Scott Med J.* 2008;53(1):4–6.

198. West M, Wu H. Pulsed radiofrequency ablation for residual and phantom limb pain: a case series. *Pain Pract.* 2010;10(5):485–491.

199. Kollewe K, Jin L, Krampfl K, et al. Treatment of phantom limb pain with botulinum toxin type A. *Pain Med.* 2009;10(2):300–303.

200. Cohen SP, Gambel JM, Raja SN, Galvagno S. The contribution of sympathetic mechanisms to post-amputation phantom and residual limb pain: a pilot study. *J Pain.* 2011;12(8):859–867.

201. Viswanathan A, Phan PC, Burton AW. Use of spinal cord stimulation in the treatment of phantom limb pain: case series and review of the literature. *Pain Pract.* 2010;10(5):479–484.

202. Kuiken T. Perioperative rehabilitation of the transtibial and transfemoral amputee. *Phys Med Rehabil State Art Rev.* 2002;16(3):521–537.

203. Leskowitz ED. Phantom limb pain treated with therapeutic touch: a case report. *Arch Phys Med Rehabil.* 2000;81(4):522–524.

204. Department of Veterans Affairs/Department of Defense. *VA/DoD Clinical Practice Guideline for Rehabilitation of Lower Amputation.* Washington, DC: Department of Veterans Affairs, Department of Defense; 2007. Available at: http://www.guideline.gov/content.aspx?id=11758&search=amputation. Accessed 29.12.11.

205. Freynet A, Falcoz PE. Is transcutaneous electrical nerve stimulation effective in relieving postoperative pain after thoracotomy? *Interact Cardiovasc Thorac Surg.* 2010;10(2):283–288.

206. Gregorini C, Cipriano G, Aquino LM, et al. Short-duration transcutaneous electrical nerve stimulation in the postoperative period of cardiac surgery. *Arq Bras Cardiol.* 2010;94(3):325–331, 345–351.

207. Desantana JM, Santana-Filho VJ, Guerra DR, et al. Hypoalgesic effect of the transcutaneous electrical nerve stimulation following inguinal herniorrhaphy: a randomized, controlled trial. *J Pain.* 2008;9(7):623–629.

208. Halbert J, Crotty M, Cameron ID. Evidence for the optimal management of acute and chronic phantom pain: a systematic review. *Clin J Pain.* 2002;18:84–92.

209. Mulvey MR, Bagnall AM, Johnson MI, Marchant PR. Transcutaneous electrical nerve stimulation (TENS) for phantom pain and stump pain following amputation in adults. *Cochrane Database Syst Rev.* 2010 May 12;(5): CD007264.

210. Casale R, Alaa L, Mallick M, Ring H. Phantom limb related phenomena and their rehabilitation after lower limb amputation. *Eur J Phys Rehabil Med.* 2009;45(4):559–566.

211. Leskowitz E. Energy medicine perspectives on phantom-limb pain. *Alternative and Complementary Therapies.* 2009;15(2):59–63.

212. Moseley GL. Graded motor imagery for pathologic pain: a randomized controlled trial. *Neurology.* 2006;67(12):2129–2134.

213. Diers M, Christmann C, Koeppe C, et al. Mirrored, imagined and executed movements differentially activate sensorimotor cortex in amputees with and without phantom limb pain. *Pain.* 2010;149(2):296–304.

214. Rothgangel AS, Braun SM, Beurskens AJ, et al. The clinical aspects of mirror therapy in rehabilitation: a systematic review of the literature. *Int J Rehabil Res.* 2011;34(1):1–13.

215. Weeks SR, Anderson-Barnes VC, Tsao JW. Phantom limb pain: theories and therapies. *Neurologist.* 2010;16(5):277–786.

216. Egsgaard L, Petrini L, Christoffersen G, Arendt-Nielsen L. Cortical responses to the mirror box illusion: a high-resolution EEG study. *Exp Brain Res.* 2011;215(3/4):345–357.

217. Diers M, Christmann C, Koeppe C, et al. Mirrored, imagined and executed movements differentially activate sensorimotor cortex in amputees with and without phantom limb pain. *Pain.* 2010;149(2):296–304.

218. Chan BL, Witt R, Charrow AP, et al. Mirror therapy for phantom limb pain. *N Engl J Med.* 2007;357(21):2206–2207.

219. Hanling SR, Wallace SC, Hollenbeck KJ, et al. Preamputation mirror therapy may prevent development of phantom limb pain: a case series. *Anesth Analg.* 2010;110(2):611–614.

220. Murray CD, Pettifer S, Howard T, et al. The treatment of phantom limb pain using immersive virtual reality; three case studies. *Disabil Rehabil.* 2007;29(18):1465–1469.

221. MacLachlan M, McDonald D, Waloch J. Mirror treatment of lower limb phantom pain. *Am J Phys Med Rehabil.* 2004;26(14–15):901–904.

222. Casale R, Damiani C, Rosati V. Mirror therapy in the rehabilitation of lower-limb amputation: are there any contraindications? *Am J Phys Med Rehabil.* 2009;88(10):837–842.

223. Nawijn SE, van der Linde H, Emmelot CH, Hofstad CJ. Stump management after transtibial amputation: a systematic review. *Prosthet Orthot Int.* 2005;29(1):13–26.

224. Smith DG, McFarland LV, Sangeorzan BJ, et al. Addendum 1: post-operative dressing and management strategies for transtibial amputations: a critical review. *J Prosthet Orthot.* 2004;16(S3):15–25.

225. Walsh TL. Custom removable immediate postoperative prosthesis. *J Prosthet Orthot.* 2003;15(4):158–161.

226. Tang PC, Ravji K, Key JJ, et al. Let them walk! Current prosthesis options for leg and foot amputees. *J Am Coll Surg.* 2008;206(3):548–560.

227. Seymour R. Clinical use of dressings and bandages. In: Seymour R, ed. *Prosthetics and Orthotics: Lower Limb and Spinal.* Philadelphia, PA: Lippincott Williams & Wilkins; 2002:123–142.

228. Broomhead P, Dawes D, Hancock A, et al. *Clinical Guidelines for the pre and post operative management of adults with lower limb amputation.* London: Chartered Society of Physiotherapy; 2006.

229. Woodburn KR, Sockalingham S, Gilmore H, et al. A randomised trial of rigid stump dressing following transtibial amputation for peripheral arterial insufficiency. *Prosthet Orthot Int.* 2004;28(1):22–27.

230. Vermeulen H, Ubbink DT, Goossens A, et al. Dressings and topical agents for surgical wounds healing by secondary intention. *Cochrane Database Syst Rev.* 2004;(1): CD003554.

231. Ladenheim E, Oberti-Smith K, Tablada G. Results of managing transtibial amputations with a prefabricated polyethylene rigid removable dressing. *J Prosthet Orthot.* 2007;19(1):2–6.

232. Wu Y, Krick H. Removable rigid dressing for below-knee amputees. *Clin Prosthet Orthot.* 1987;11(1):33–44.

233. Deutsch A, English RD, Vermeer TC, et al. Removable rigid dressings versus soft dressings: a randomized, controlled study with dysvascular, trans-tibial amputees. *Prosthet Orthot Int.* 2005;29(2):193–200.

234. Taylor L, Cavenett S, Stepien JM, Crotty M. Removable rigid dressings: a retrospective case-note audit to determine the validity of post-amputation application. *Prosthet Orthot Int.* 2008;32(2):223–230.

235. Wu Y. Removable rigid dressings for residual limb management. Appendix D. In: Karacoloff LA, Hammersley CS, Schneider FJ, eds. *Lower Extremity Amputation: A Guide to Functional Outcomes in Physical Therapy Management.* Rehabilitation Institute of Chicago Procedure Manual. Gaithersburg, MD: Aspen; 1992: 241–248.

236. Graf M, Freijah N. Early trans-tibial oedema control using polymer gel socks. *Prosthet Orthot Int.* 2003;27(3):221–226.

237. Johannesson A, Larsson GU, Oberg T, Atroshi I. Comparison of vacuum-formed removable rigid dressing with conventional rigid dressing after transtibial amputation: similar outcome in a randomized controlled trial involving 27 patients. *Acta Orthop.* 2008;79(3):361–369.

238. Tsai P, Geffen S. Use of a polyethylene removable rigid dressing in a transtibial amputee. *J Australasian Rehabil Nurs Assoc.* 2007;10(1):22–23.

239. Bergan JJ, Sparks SR. Non-elastic compression: an alternative in management of chronic venous insufficiency. *J Wound Ostomy Continence Nurs.* 2000;27(2):83–89.

240. Wong CK. Unna and elastic post-operative dressings: comparison of their effects on function of adults with amputation and vascular disease. *Arch Phys Med Rehabil.* 2000;81(9): 1191–1198.

241. Vanross ER, Johnson S, Abbott CA. Effects of early mobilization on unhealed dysvascular transtibial amputation stumps: a clinical trial. *Arch Phys Med Rehabil.* 2009;90(4):610–617.

242. Scott H, Condie ME, Treweek SP, Sockalingham S. An evaluation of the Amputee Mobility Aid (AMA) early walking aid. *Prosthet Orthot Int.* 2000;24:39–46.

243. De Noordhout BM, Brogniez LPA. Early fitting of artificial limbs to amputated lower limbs. *Acta Chir Belg.* 2004;104: 393–395.

244. Boucher HR, Low C, Schon MD, et al. A biomechanical study of two postoperative prostheses for transtibial amputees: a custom molded and a prefabricated adjustable pneumatic prosthesis. *Foot Ankle Int.* 2002;23(5):452–456.

245. Mazari FA, Mockford K, Barnett C, et al. Hull early walking aid for rehabilitation of transtibial amputees—randomized controlled trial (HEART). *J Vasc Surg.* 2010;52(6):1564–1571.

246. Walsh TL. Custom removable immediate postoperative prosthesis. *J Prosthet Orthot.* 2003;15(4):158–161.

247. Sathishkumar S, Manigandan C, Asha T, et al. A cost-effective, adjustable, femoral socket, temporary prosthesis for immediate rehabilitation of above-knee amputation. *Int J Rehabil Res.* 2004;27(1):71–74.

248. Schon LC, Short KW, Soupiou O, et al. Benefits of early prosthetic management of transtibial amputees: a prospective clinical study of a prefabricated prosthesis. *Foot Ankle Int.* 2002;23(6):509–514.

249. Pinzur MS, Angelico J. A feasibility trial of a prefabricated immediate postoperative prosthetic limb system. *Foot Ankle Int.* 2003;24(11):861–864.

250. Folsom D, King T, Rubin JR. Lower extremity amputation with immediate postoperative prosthetic placement. *Am J Surg.* 1992;164(4):320–322.

251. Benetato BB. Post-traumatic growth among operation enduring freedom and operation Iraqi freedom amputees. *J Nurs Scholarsh.* 2011;43(4):412–420.

252. Atherton R, Robertson N. Psychological adjustment to lower limb amputation amongst prosthetic users. *Disabil Rehabil.* 2006;28(19):1201–1209.

253. Uustal H. Prosthetic rehabilitation issues in the diabetic and dysvascular amputee. *Phys Med Rehabil Clin N Am.* 2009;20(4):689–703.

254. Rossbach P. Skin care. Some do's and don'ts. *InMotion.* 2006;16(2):10–11.

255. Highsmith JT, Highsmith MJ. Common skin pathology in LE prosthesis users. *JAAPA.* 2007;20(11):33–36.

256. Bonutti PM, Marulanda GA, McGrath MS, et al. Static progressive stretch improves range of motion in arthrofibrosis following total knee arthroplasty. *Knee Surg Sports Traumatol Arthrosc.* 2010;18(2):194–199.

257. Bonutti PM, McGrath MS, Ulrich SD, et al. Static progressive stretch for the treatment of knee stiffness. *Knee.* 2008;15(4):272–276.

258. Slif U. Focused rehabilitation treatment of poorly functioning total knee arthroplasties. *Clin Orthop Relat Res.* 2007;464(1):138–145.

259. Cristopoliski F, Barela JA, Leite N, et al. Stretching exercise program improves gait in the elderly. *Gerontology.* 2009;55(6): 614–620.

260. Harvey LA, Glinsky JA, Katalinic OM, Ben M. Contracture management for people with spinal cord injuries. *NeuroRehabilitation.* 2011;28(1):17–20.

261. Swanton R, Kinnear B. There is robust evidence that stretch interventions do not prevent or reverse joint contractures in people with neurological conditions. *Aust Occup Ther J.* 2011;58(2): 134–135.

262. Katalinic OM, Harvey LA, Herbert RD. Effectiveness of stretch for the treatment and prevention of contractures in people with neurological conditions: a systematic review. *Phys Ther.* 2011;91(1):11–24.

263. Ryan EE, Rossi MD, Lopez R. The effects of the contract-relax-antagonist-contract form of proprioceptive neuromuscular facilitation on postural stability. *J Strength Cond Res.* 2010;24(7):1888–1894.

264. Ferber R, Osternig LR, Gravelle DC. Effect of PNF stretch techniques on knee flexor muscle EMG activity in older adults. *J Electromyogr Kinesiol.* 2002;12(5):391–397.

265. Dommerholt J, Bron C, Franssen J. Myofascial trigger points: an evidence-informed review. *J Man Manip Ther.* 2006;14(4):203–221.

266. May BJ, Lockard MA. *Prosthetics & Orthotics in Clinical Practice: A Case Study Approach.* Philadelphia, PA: FA Davis; 2011.

267. Edelstein J, Moroz A. *Lower Limb Prosthetics and Orthotics: Clinical Concepts.* Thorofare, NJ: Slack; 2010.

268. Carroll K, Edelstein J. *Prosthetics and Patient Management: A Comprehensive Clinical Approach.* Thorofare, NJ: Slack; 2006.

269. Gailey RS, Gailey AM. *Stretching and Strengthening for Lower Extremity Amputees.* Miami, FL: Advanced Rehabilitation Therapy; 1994.

270. McAtee R, Charland J. *Facilitated Stretching.* 3rd ed. Champaign IL: Human Kinetics; 2007.

271. Burgess EM, Rappoport A. *Physical Fitness: A Guide for Individuals With Lower Limb Loss.* Darby, PA: Diane Publishing; 1993.

272. Karacoloff LA, Mannersley CS, Schneider FJ, eds. *Lower Extremity Amputation: A Guide to Functional Outcomes in Physical Therapy Management.* 2nd ed. Austin, TX: Pro-Ed; 2005.

273. Huggett DL, Elliott ID, Overend TJ, et al. Comparison of heart-rate and blood-pressure increases during isokinetic eccentric

versus isometric exercise in older adults. *J Aging Phys Act.* 2004;12(2):157–169.

274. Gailey RS, Clark CR. Physical therapy. In: Smith DG, Michael JW, Bowker JH, eds. *Atlas of Amputation and Limb Deficiencies: Surgical, Prosthetic, and Rehabilitation Principles.* 3rd ed. Rosemont, IL: American Academy of Orthopaedic Surgeons; 2004:589–620.

275. Adler SS, Beckers D, Buck M. *PNF in Practice: An Illustrated Guide.* 3rd ed. New York, NY: Springer; 2007.

276. Kinser C, Colby L. *Therapeutic Exercise: Foundations and Techniques.* 5th ed. Philadelphia, PA: FA Davis; 2007.

277. Baechle T, Earle RW. *Essentials of Strength Training and Conditioning.* 3rd ed. National Strength and Conditioning Association. Champaign, IL: Human Kinetics; 2008.

278. Durstine JL, Moore GE, Painter PL, Roberts SO. *ACSM's Exercise Management for Persons with Chronic Diseases and Disabilities.* 3rd ed. American College of Sports Medicine. Champaign, IL: Human Kinetics; 2009.

279. Galvão DA, Taaffe DR. Resistance exercise dosage in older adults: single versus multiset effects on physical performance and body composition. *J Am Geriatr Soc.* 2005;53(12):2090–2097.

280. Murray DP, Brown LE, Zinder SM, et al. Effects of velocity-specific training on rate of velocity development, peak torque, and performance. *J Strength Cond Res.* 2007;21(3):870–874.

281. Salli A, Sahin N, Baskent A, Ugurlu H. The effect of two exercise programs on various functional outcome measures in patients with osteoarthritis of the knee: a randomized controlled clinical trial. *Isokinet Ex Sci.* 2010;18(4):201–209.

282. Symons TB, Vandervoort AA, Rice CL, et al. Effects of maximal isometric and isokinetic resistance training on strength and functional mobility in older adults. *J Gerontol A Biol Sci Med Sci.* 2005;60A(6):777–781.

283. Malliou P, Fatouros I, Beneka A, et al. Different training programs for improving muscular performance in healthy inactive elderly. *Isokinet Ex Sci.* 2003;11(4):189–195.

284. Manini TM, Visser M, Seok WP, et al. Knee extension strength cutpoints for maintaining mobility. *J Am Geriatr Soc.* 2007;55(3):451–457.

285. Nadollek H, Brauer S, Isles R. Outcomes after trans-tibial amputation: the relationship between quiet stance ability, strength of hip abductor muscles and gait. *Physiother Res Int.* 2002;7(4):203–214.

286. Piva SR, Teixeira PE, Almeida GJ, et al. Contribution of hip abductor strength to physical function in patients with total knee arthroplasty. *Phys Ther.* 2011;91(2):225–233.

287. Bhave A, Mont M, Tennis S, et al. Functional problems and treatment solutions after total hip and knee joint arthroplasty. *J Bone Joint Surg Am.* 2005;87(suppl 2):9–21.

288. Burger H, Valencic V, Marincek C, et al. Properties of musculus gluteus maximus in above-knee amputees. *Clin Biomech (Bristol, Avon).* 1996;11(1):35.

289. Lewis CL, Sahrmann SA, Moran DW. Effect of position and alteration in synergist muscle force contribution on hip forces when performing hip strengthening exercises. *Clin Biomech (Bristol, Avon).* 2009;24(1):35–42.

290. Croisier JL, Noordhout B Maertens de, Maquet D, et al. Isokinetic evaluation of hip strength muscle groups in unilateral lower limb amputees. *Isokinet Ex Sci.* 2001;9(4):163–169.

291. van Velzen JM, van Bennekom CA, Polomski W, et al. Physical capacity and walking ability after lower limb amputation: a systematic review. *Clin Rehabil.* 2006;20(11):999–1016.

292. Gupta S. Endurance and strength training have different benefits for people with peripheral arterial disease, but both improve quality of life. *Aust J Physiother.* 2009;55(1):63.

293. Simmelink EK, Wempe JB, Geertzen JH, Dekker R. The combined arm-leg (Cruiser) ergometer: a suitable instrument to measure physical fitness? *Clin Rehabil.* 2008;22(12):1135–1136.

294. Chin T, Sawamura S, Fujita H, et al. Effect of endurance training program based on anaerobic threshold (AT) for lower limb amputees. *J Rehabil Res Dev.* 2001;38(1):7–11.

295. Chin T, Sawamura S, Fujita H, et al. Physical fitness of lower limb amputees. *Am J Phys Med Rehabil.* 2002;81(5):321–325.

296. Hamamura S, Chin T, Kuroda R, et al. Factors affecting prosthetic rehabilitation outcomes in amputees of age 60 years and over. *J Int Med Res.* 2009;37(6):1921–1927.

297. Chin T, Sawamura S, Shiba R. Effect of physical fitness on prosthetic ambulation in elderly amputees. *Am J Phys Med Rehabil.* 2006;85(12):992–996.

298. Chin T, Sawamura S, Fujita H, et al. %VO2max as an indicator of prosthetic rehabilitation outcome after dysvascular amputation. *Prosthet Orthot Int.* 2002;26(1):44–49.

299. Göktepe AS, Cakir B, Yilmaz B, Yazicioglu K. Energy expenditure of walking with prostheses: comparison of three amputation levels. *Prosthet Orthot Int.* 2010;34(1):31–36.

300. Chin T, Sawamura S, Fujita H, et al. Effect of endurance training program based on anaerobic threshold (AT) for lower limb amputees. *J Rehabil Res Dev.* 2001;38(1):7–11.

301. *ACSM's Guidelines for Exercise Testing and Prescription.* 8th ed. Philadelphia, PA: Wolters Kluwer–Lippincott Williams & Wilkins; 2009.

302. Quai TM, Brauer SG, Nitz JC. Somatosensation, circulation and stance balance in elderly dysvascular transtibial amputees. *Clin Rehabil.* 2005;19(6):668–676.

303. Mayer A, Tihanyi J, Bretz K, et al. Adaptation to altered balance conditions in unilateral amputees due to atherosclerosis: a randomized controlled study. *BMC Musculoskelet Disord.* 2011;12(1):118–124.

304. Stokes D, Curzio J, Berry A, et al. Pre prosthetic mobility: the amputees' perspectives. *Disabil Rehabil.* 2009;31(2):138–143.

305. Chin T, Oyabu H, Maeda Y, Takase I, Machida K. Energy consumption during prosthetic walking and wheelchair locomotion by elderly hip disarticulation amputees. *Am J Phys Med Rehabil.* 2009;88(5):399–403.

306. Laferrier JZ, McFarland LV, Boninger ML, et al. Wheeled mobility: factors influencing mobility and assistive technology in veterans and service members with major traumatic limb loss from Vietnam war and OIF/OEF conflicts. *J Rehabil Res Dev.* 2010;47(4):349–360.

307. Karmarkar AM, Collins DM, Wichman T, et al. Prosthesis and wheelchair use in veterans with lower limb amputation. *J Rehabil Res Dev.* 2009;46(5):567–575.

308. Somers MF. Wheelchair and wheelchair skills. In: Somers MF, ed. *Spinal Cord Injury: Functional Rehabilitation.* 3rd ed. Upper Saddle River, NJ: Pearson; 2010:230–296.

309. Koontz A, Shea M. Wheelchair skills. In: Sisto S, Druin E, Sliwinski MM, eds. *Spinal Cord Injuries: Management and Rehabilitation.* St. Louis, MO: Mosby; 2009:351–379.

310. McCarthy S, Nead C. Accessible home modification and durable medical equipment. In: Sisto S, Druin E, Sliwinski MM, eds. *Spinal Cord Injuries: Management and Rehabilitation.* St. Louis, MO: Mosby; 2009:326–350.

311. Somers MR. Architectural adaptations. In: Somers MF, ed. *Spinal Cord Injury: Functional Rehabilitation.* 3rd ed. Upper Saddle River, NJ: Pearson; 2010:381–399.

312. Gosselink R, Bott J, Johnson M, et al. Physiotherapy for adult patients with critical illness: recommendations of the European Respiratory Society and European Society of Intensive Care Medicine Task Force on Physiotherapy for Critically Ill Patients. *Intensive Care Med.* 2008;34(7):1188–1199.

313. Schmitz TJ. Vital signs. In: O'Sullivan SB, Schmitz TJ, eds. *Physical Rehabilitation.* 5th ed. Philadelphia, PA: FA Davis; 2007:81–120.

314. Dyer D, Bouman B, Davey M, Ismond KP. An intervention program to reduce falls for adult in-patients following major lower limb amputation. *Healthc Q.* 2008;11(3 Spec No).117–121.

315. Duesterhaus Minor MA, Duesterhaus Minor D, Minor SR. *Patient Care Skills.* 6th ed. Upper Saddle River, NJ: Prentice Hall; 2010.

316. Schmitz TJ. Locomotor training. In: O'Sullivan SB, Schmitz TJ, eds. *Physical Rehabilitation.* 5th ed. Philadelphia, PA: FA Davis; 2007:523–560.

317. Waters RL, Mulroy SJ. Energy expenditure of walking in individuals with lower limb amputations. In: Smith DG, Michael JW, Bowker JH, eds. *Atlas of Amputation and Limb Deficiencies: Surgical, Prosthetic, and Rehabilitation Principles.* 3rd ed. Rosemont, IL: American Academy of Orthopaedic Surgeons; 2004:395–407.

318. Condie ME, McFadyen AK, Treweek S, Whitehead L. The trans-femoral fitting predictor: a functional measure to predict prosthetic fitting in transfemoral amputees—validity and reliability. *Arch Phys Med Rehabil.* 2011;92(8):1293–1297.

319. Wu Y, Chen S, Lin M, et al. Energy expenditure of wheeling and walking during prosthetic rehabilitation in a woman with bilateral transfemoral amputations. *Arch Phys Med Rehabil.* 2001;82(2):265–269.

320. Baumgarten M, Margolis DJ, Localio A, et al. Pressure ulcers among elderly patients early in the hospital stay. *J Gerontol A Biol Sci Med Sci.* 2006;61A(7):749–754.

321. Brem H, Tomic-Canic M, Tarnovskaya A, et al. Healing of elderly patients with diabetic foot ulcers, venous stasis ulcers, and pressure ulcers. *Surg Technol Int.* 2003;11:161–167.

322. Roach KE. Measurement of health outcomes: reliability, validity and responsiveness. *J Prosthet Orthot.* 2006;18(1 S):8–12.

323. Coster WJ, Haley SM, Jette AM. Measuring patient-reported outcomes after discharge from inpatient rehabilitation settings. *J Rehabil Med.* 2006;38(4):237–242.

324. Deathe B, Miller WC, Speechley M. The status of outcome measurement in amputee rehabilitation in Canada. *Arch Phys Med Rehabil.* 2002;83(7):912–918.

325. Hebert JS, Wolfe DL, Miller WC, et al. Outcome measures in amputation rehabilitation: ICF body functions. *Disabil Rehabil.* 2009;31(19):1541–1554.

326. Kohler F, Xu J, Silva-Withmory C, Arockiam J. Feasibility of using a checklist based on the international classification of functioning, disability and health as an outcome measure in individuals following lower limb amputation. *Prosthet Orthot Int.* 2011;35(3):294–2301.

327. Deathe AB, Wolfe DL, Devlin M, et al. Selection of outcome measures in lower extremity amputation rehabilitation: ICF activities. *Disabil Rehabil.* 2009;31(18):1455–1473.

328. Hefford C, Haxby AJ, David Baxter G, Arnold R. Outcome measurement in clinical practice: practical and theoretical issues for health related quality of life (HRQOL) questionnaires. *Phys Ther Rev.* 2011;16(3):155–167.

329. Beattie P. Measurement of health outcomes in the clinical setting: applications to physiotherapy. *Physiother Theory Pract.* 2001;17(3):173–185.

330. Huijbregts MPJ, Myers AM, Kay TM, Gavin TS. Systematic outcome measurement in clinical practice: challenges experienced by physiotherapists. *Physiother Can.* 2002;54(1):25–31.

331. Resnik L, Borgia M. Reliability of outcome measures for people with lower limb amputations: distinguishing true change from statistical error. *Phys Ther.* 2011;91(4):555–565.

332. Caring for the delirious patient, part 1 of 2: assessing for risk factors and signs of delirium. *Joint Commission Perspectives on Patient Safety.* 2009;9(12):5–7.

333. Brown S, Fitzgerald M, Walsh K. Delirium dichotomy: a review of recent literature. *Contemp Nurse.* 2007;26(2):238–247.

334. Cockrell JR, Folstein MF. Mini-Mental State Examination (MMSE). *Psychopharmacol Bull.* 1988;24(4):689–692.

335. Alagiakrishnan K, Marrie T, Rolfson D, et al. Simple cognitive testing (Mini-Cog) predicts in-hospital delirium in the elderly. *J Am Geriatr Soc.* 2007;55(2):314–316.

336. Wei LA, Fearing MA, Sternberg EJ, Inouye SK. The confusion assessment method: a systematic review of current usage. *J Am Geriatr Soc.* 2008;56(5):823–830.

337. Walker MP, Ayre GA, Cummings JL, et al. The clinician assessment of fluctuation and the one day fluctuation assessment scale. Two methods to assess fluctuating confusion in dementia. *Br J Psychiatry.* 2000;177(3):252–256 C.

338. McCusker J, Cole MG, Dendukuri N, Belzile E. The Delirium Index, a measure of the severity of delirium: new findings on reliability, validity and responsiveness. *J Am Geriatr Soc.* 2004;52(10):1744–1749.

339. Matsushita T, Matsushima E, Maruyama M. Early detection of postoperative delirium and confusion in a surgical ward using the NEECHAM confusion scale. *Gen Hosp Psychiatry.* 2004;26(2):158–163.

340. Scheffer AC, van Munster BC, Schuurmans MJ, de Rooij SE. Assessing severity of delirium by the delirium observation screening scale. *Int J Geriatr Psychiatry.* 2011;26(3):284–291.

341. Chakrabarti S, Shah R, Kumar V, Grover S. A factor analytic study of the Delirium Rating Scale-Revised-98 in untreated patients with delirium. *J Psychosom Res.* 2011;70(5):473–478.

342. Shyamsundar G, Raghuthaman G, Rajkumar AP, Jacob KS. Validation of memorial delirium assessment scale. *J Crit Care.* 2009;24(4):530–534.

343. Haley SM, Coster WJ, Andres PL, et al. Activity outcome measurement for post-acute care. *Med Care.* 2004;42(suppl 1):49–61.

344. Haley SM, Andres PL, Coster WJ, et al. Short form activity measure for post-acute care. *Arch Phys Med Rehabil.* 2004;85(4):649–660.

345. Resnik L, Borgia M. Reliability of outcome measures for people with lower limb amputations: distinguishing true change from statistical error. *Phys Ther.* 2011;91(4):555–565.

346. Condie E, Scott H, Treweek S. Lower limb prosthetic outcome measures: a review of the literature 1995 to 2005. *J Prosthet Orthot.* 2006;18(1 S):13–45.

347. Treweek SP, Condie ME. Three measures of functional outcome for lower limb amputees: a retrospective review. *Prosthet Orthot Int.* 1998;22(3):178–185.

348. Stineman MG, Shea JA, Jette A, et al. The Functional Independence Measure: tests of scaling assumptions, structure, and reliability across 20 diverse impairment categories. *Arch Phys Med Rehabil.* 1996;77:1101–1108.

349. Masedo AI, Hanley M, Jensen MP, et al. Reliability and validity of a self-report FIM (FIM-SR) in persons with amputation or spinal cord injury and chronic pain. *Am J Phys Med Rehabil.* 2005;84:167–176.

350. Panesar BS, Morrison P, Hunter J. A comparison of three measures of progress in early lower limb amputee rehabilitation. *Clin Rehabil.* 2001;15(2):157–171.

351. McPherson K, Sloan RL, Hunter J, Dowell CM. Validation studies of the OPCS scale—more useful than the Barthel Index? Office of Population Census's and Surveys. *Clin Rehabil.* 1993;7(2):105–112.

352. Callaghan BG, Condie ME. A post-discharge quality of life outcome measure for lower limb amputees: test-retest reliability and construct validity. *Clin Rehabil.* 2003;17(8):858–864.

353. Martin F, Camfield L, Rodham K, et al. Twelve years' experience with the Patient Generated Index (PGI) of quality of life: a graded structured review. *Qual Life Res.* 2007;16(4):705–715.

354. Stratford PW, Gill C, Westaway M, Binkley J. Assessing disability and change on individual patients: a report of a patient specific measure. *Physiother Can.* 1995;47:258–263.

355. Kowalchuk Horn K, Jennings S, Richardson G, et al. The patient-specific functional scale: psychometrics, clinometrics, and application as a clinical outcome measure. *J Orthop Sports Phys Ther.* 2012;42(1):30–42.

356. Streppel KR, Vries J, Van Harten WH. Functional status and prosthesis use in amputees, measured with Prosthetic Profile of the Amputee (PPA) and the short version of the Sickness Impact Profile (SIP68). *Int J Rehabil Res.* 2001;24(3):251–256.

357. Gauthier-Gagnon C, Grise M. Tools to measure outcome of people with a lower limb amputation: update on the PPA and LCI. *J Prosthet Orthot.* 2006;18(1 S):61–67.

358. Ryall NH, Eyres SB, Neumann VC, et al. Is the Rivermead Mobility Index appropriate to measure mobility in lower limb amputees? *Disabil Rehabil.* 2003;25(3):143–152.

359. Gardiner MD, Faux S, Jones LE. Inter-observer reliability of clinical outcome measures in a lower limb amputee population. *Disabil Rehabil.* 2002;24:219–225.

360. Franchignoni F, Brunelli S, Orlandini D, et al. Is the Rivermead Mobility Index a suitable outcome measure in low limb amputees?—A psychometric validation study. *J Rehabil Med.* 2003;35(3):141–144.

361. Pezzin LE, Dillingham TR, Mackenzie EJ. Rehabilitation and the long term outcomes of persons with trauma-related amputations. *Arch Phys Med Rehabil.* 2000;81(3):292–300.

362. de Godoy JM, Braile DM, Buzatto SH, Longo O, Fontes OA. Quality of life after amputation. *Psychol Health Med.* 2002;7(4):397–400.

363. Jette A, Haley S, Coster W, et al. Late life function and disability instrument: I. Development and evaluation of the disability component. *J Gerontol A Biol Sci Med Sci.* 2002;57A:M209–M216.

364. Haley S, Jette A, Coster W, et al. Late life function and disability instrument: II. Development and evaluation of the function component. *J Gerontol A Biol Sci Med Sci.* 2002;57A:M217–M222.

365. Denkinger MD, Igl W, Coll-Planas L, et al. Evaluation of the Short Form of the Late-Life Function and Disability Instrument in geriatric inpatients-validity, responsiveness, and sensitivity to change. *J Am Geriatr Soc.* 2009;57(2):309–314.

366. Jette AM, Haley SM, Kooyoomjian JT. *Late Life FDI Manual.* Boston, MA: Roybal Center for the Enhancement of Late Life Function, Boston University; 2006.

367. Peters DM, Fritz SL, Krotish DE. PT. Assessing the reliability and validity of a shorter walk test compared to the 10 meter walk test for measurements of gait speed in healthy, older adults. *J Geriatr Phys Ther.* 2012 Mar 11. [Epub ahead of print].

368. Chui KK, Lusardi MM. Spatial and temporal parameters of self-selected and fast walking speeds in healthy community-living adults aged 72–98 years. *J Geriatr Phys Ther.* 2010;33(4):173–183.

369. Brooks D, Hunter JP, Parsons J, et al. Reliability of the two-minute walk test in individuals with transtibial amputation. *Arch Phys Med Rehabil.* 2002;83(11):1562–1565.

370. Miller WC, Deathe AB, Harris J. Measurement properties of the Frenchay Activities Index among individuals with a lower limb amputation. *Clin Rehabil.* 2004;18(4):414–422.

371. *Wheelchair Skills Test Manual: Version 4.1.* www.wheelchairskillsprogram.ca; 2008. Accessed 19.01.12.

372. Lindquist NJ, Loudon PE, Magis TF, et al. Reliability of the performance and safety scores of the Wheelchair Skills Test Version 4.1 for manual wheelchair users. *Arch Phys Med Rehabil.* 2010;91(11):1752–1757.

21

Understanding Prosthetic Feet

KEVIN CARROLL, JOHN RHEINSTEIN, AND ELICIA POLLARD

LEARNING OBJECTIVES

On completion of this chapter, the reader will be able to:
1. Define the Medicare functional levels.
2. Explain key factors analyzed when prescribing a prosthetic foot.
3. Define the fundamental characteristics of the different types of prosthetic feet.
4. Formulate a prescription recommendation for a prosthetic foot based on the patient's needs.

Just as every person is unique, every person with an amputation presents a different set of characteristics that should be considered when selecting a prosthetic foot. This selection should be made carefully as safety, performance, and patient satisfaction can be impacted if the foot is not well matched to the patient.[1] To make an effective selection among the multitude of choices offered by prosthetic foot manufacturers and to succeed in matching the right foot to the right recipient, it is important to thoroughly consider each individual's current and potential abilities and needs. The rehabilitation team should carefully review a patient's medical and prosthetic history while keeping in mind the performance features, specifications, and appearance of available feet. Past research studies offered data concerning foot performance and patient preferences, but studies have not yet provided pathways to successful foot selection based on clinical evidence.[2-4]

The aim of providing a prosthetic foot is to maximize every patient's rehabilitation potential so that they may return to their daily activities and work at a level comparable to their peers. Ideally, the function of a prosthetic foot should match that of an anatomical human foot.[5] It should offer shock absorption, compliance to uneven terrain, push-off, and shortening during the appropriate points in the gait cycle, all in a lightweight, low-maintenance package. In reality, no prosthetic foot available today matches the human foot in all these characteristics. The final choice is always a compromise, as no single prosthetic foot performs optimally for all activities and conditions. The most appropriate foot is one that best serves the user's unique needs at the time of selection.

Once a specific foot design is selected it must be ordered to meet the specific weight and activity level of each person.

If patients experience physical or lifestyle changes, the foot should be replaced to match their new functional needs. For example, a weight gain of 20 or more pounds or substantial increase in activity or loads carried may result in the catastrophic failure of the structural element of a foot. All the parts of a prosthetic system, especially feet, should be checked regularly for wear and tear and replaced immediately if any cracks or other signs of structural failure occur. It is difficult to predict the useful life span of a foot because of the wide range of users and the way they are used.

FACTORS IN SELECTING A PROSTHETIC FOOT

When working with a patient to design an appropriate prosthesis, the rehabilitation team (physiatrist, surgeon, primary care physician, physical therapist, and prosthetist) should assess and consider a number of factors that influence component selection. In addition, explaining the function and features to the user and why a foot was selected can enhance their satisfaction.

Functional Level

- Medicare guidelines describe functional levels into which all persons with lower-limb amputation fall and are widely accepted by most payers.[6] This classification system determines the medical necessity for components such as feet and other additions to the prosthesis and is based on the patient's current and potential functional abilities

Medicare policy states, "A lower limb prosthesis is covered when the patient: (1) Will reach or maintain a defined functional state within a reasonable period of time; and (2) is motivated to ambulate." Clinical assessments of patient rehabilitation potential must be based on the following classification levels:

Level 0: Does not have the ability or potential to ambulate or transfer safely with or without assistance and a prosthesis does not enhance their quality of life or mobility.

Level 1: Has the ability or potential to use a prosthesis for transfers or ambulation on level surfaces at fixed cadence. Typical of the limited and unlimited household ambulator.

Level 2: Has the ability or potential for ambulation with the ability to traverse low-level environmental barriers such as curbs, stairs or uneven surfaces. Typical of the limited community ambulator.

Level 3: Has the ability or potential for ambulation with variable cadence. Typical of the community ambulator who has the ability to traverse most environmental barriers and may have vocational, therapeutic, or exercise activity that demands prosthetic utilization beyond simple locomotion.

Level 4: Has the ability or potential for prosthetic ambulation that exceeds basic ambulation skills, exhibiting high impact, stress, or energy levels. Typical of the prosthetic demands of the child, active adult, or athlete."

Note: Persons with bilateral amputation are not strictly bound by the functional level classification requirement.

Potential functional ability is based on the reasonable expectations of the prosthetist, and treating physician, considering factors including, but not limited to the following:

- the patient's past history (including prior prosthetic use if applicable);
- the patient's current condition including the status of the residual limb and the nature of other medical problems; and
- the patient's desire to ambulate.

Ideally, the rehabilitation team examines and interviews the patient and reaches a consensus as to the potential functional level each patient is most likely to achieve. The key word in reaching such a decision is "potential," which challenges the team to predict future outcomes based on past performance and other unknowns. This decision has real implications for patients as it determines what type of foot they will receive. Therefore, if the rehabilitation team believes that a person currently performing at K2 level will at some future date achieve K3 category, the patient should receive a K3-level prosthesis immediately. Not only will this allow the person to work toward achieving the K3 performance with an appropriate foot, but it will save cost over the long run by eliminating the need to purchase two different feet. In addition to the factors mentioned below, the Amputee Mobility Predictor instrument, designed to measure ambulatory potential of lower-limb amputees, can also help to determine future potential.[7]

Activities of Daily Living and Work Requirements

No single foot can meet a person's needs in all situations. By determining the most frequent and important activities a balance of performance features can be achieved. For example, someone who works in an office and who also plays golf on weekends should be provided with a multiaxial ankle to accommodate uneven terrain.

Patient's Weight

Sizes and strengths are available for patients ranging from a baby to those adults weighing more than 500 pounds (Figure 21-1). Weight should be recorded at every patient encounter to insure that a foot is still appropriately matched

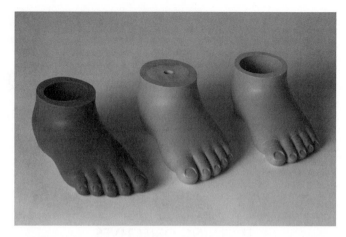

FIGURE 21-1 Very small children's feet. (Courtesy of Hanger Clinic, Austin, TX.)

to the patient. The assumption that an extremely heavy patient cannot be fitted with a prosthesis is no longer true. Because a growing population of patients is overweight, manufacturers are offering prosthetic feet for heavier patients. A prosthetic foot expected to support heavier weights must be specially crafted for increased strength and durability; consequently, the prosthesis itself is larger and heavier because of the additional material included in the foot, pylon, and socket.

Obesity makes prosthetic fitting more difficult; however, the results achieved by overweight people can be very inspirational. Even patients weighting more than 300 pounds should not give up hope. Although initially confined to a nursing home bed, rehabilitation teams that work with overweight patients can fit them with a prosthesis, assist them with standing, begin therapy, and within just a few months have the same bedridden patients walking in and out of the prosthetist's office on their own. It is not uncommon for functional K1-level patients to progress to K2 level with appropriate care and therapy. Patients are often deconditioned from the illnesses that precipitated their amputation and can make great strides as long as they are motivated.

Amputation Level and Residual Limb Characteristics

Foot selection can bear directly on the health of the person's residual limb. Ground reaction forces that are transmitted through a person's body can be damaging to the person's residual limb, knee, hip, or back. Choosing a foot with compliant heel action can reduce these impact forces. The foot and pylon may also offer vertical shock absorption features, which reduce impact on the residual limb. In general, short or painful residual limbs are fit with feet that are softer to attenuate ground force transmission through the prosthesis. To benefit from feet that store and return energy, a user must walk with a minimum velocity to load the foot so that energy can be returned. If this is not possible because of physical restrictions in strength, range of motion, or balance, a lower-functional-level foot should be provided.

Comorbidities

The deflection dynamics of a foot can have an effect on the health and well-being of a person's joints. Excessive toe stiffness can cause hyperextension of the knee. The contralateral limb should also be taken into consideration as too soft of a prosthetic toe can cause increased impact on the sound side.

Environmental Stresses and Durability

People exposed to extreme environments need a foot that will not deteriorate under those conditions. If conditions are very harsh, a separate prosthesis may be required. Any foot that is not properly maintained or not dried after getting wet can fail prematurely.

Shoe Choices (Heel Heights and Shoe Shape)

A heel height-adjustable foot (Figure 21-2) can make a significant difference for someone who wants to wear high heels or switch between different heel-height shoes, depending on the formality of the occasion or work requirements.

Although a heel-height adjustable foot can flatten for barefoot walking, the prosthetic foot shell will wear out quickly if it is used without a shoe. Seasonal aspects are also important; providing a split between the big toe and its neighbor may not seem important in the fall or winter, but is very noticeable in the summer when the user wants to wear thong sandals (Figure 21-3).

Feet that are too wide may prove difficult to get into a shoe and a foot that is too narrow may move around in the shoe causing instability. Asking the patient to bring the shoes they intend to wear to clinic can reduce uncertainty about foot size and shape. Patients who have been prescribed a diabetic shoe should be encouraged to wear only those shoes.

Interaction with Other Prosthetic Components

The foot is part of a closed chain in which ground reaction forces are transmitted through the prosthesis. The characteristics of the foot will affect the way a prosthetic knee and hip joint respond to ground forces. For example, a foot with a stiff heel will send more flexion force to the knee at heel strike.

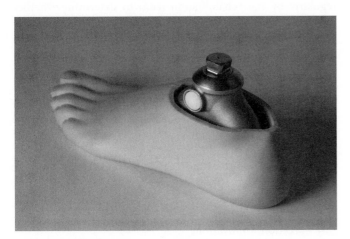

FIGURE 21-2 Heel height-adjustable foot. (Courtesy of Hanger Clinic, Austin, TX.)

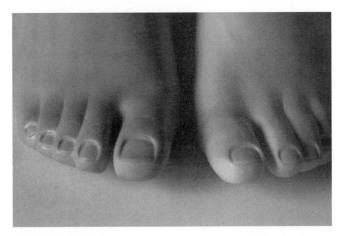

FIGURE 21-3 Feet with split toes. (Courtesy of Hanger Clinic, Austin, TX.)

Prior Prosthetic Feet and Gait Habits

Patients who have become accustom to the characteristics of a foot over many years may have difficulty adapting to a new foot. If a change is warranted, the patient should understand that a period of adjustment is required of any new foot. Therapy is recommended anytime a new prosthesis or component is provided.

Psychological Influences and Personality Traits

The wearer's age has less to do with the choice of prosthesis than the wearer's attitude. For example, an 80-year-old might be running marathons, while a 45-year-old with less determination remains wheelchair-bound. The difference may lie solely in their state of mind. A prosthesis wearer's personal preferences, practical goals, and lofty ambitions should all be considered when selecting a foot. Many people are able to expand their capabilities and motivation dramatically once they are fitting with an appropriate prosthesis that allows them to improve range of activities.

Skin Tone

Each of the feet described in this chapter is available with a protective cover or foot shell that gives the appearance of a foot in addition to protecting the structural element of the foot. Today's foot shells have a more natural appearance and greater durability than did their predecessors. Most have toes and are available in three basic flesh tones. Flexible skins can be added that closely approximate the patient's skin tone.

Cost

Foot choices may be limited by insurance coverage and the patient's ability to pay. In general, higher-functional-level feet cost more.

All of the factors mentioned above should be considered when narrowing the selection of appropriate prosthetic choices for your patient. It is important to thoroughly discuss with the patient all aspects of the choices available to them, and ensure that everyone on the rehabilitation team understands the patient's wishes and his plans for future or potential activities. Each person has different values as to what is important to them. Ideally, more than one foot can be tried so that an individual can make a choice based on actual performance as well as the considerations mentioned above.

PERFORMANCE FEATURES AND APPEARANCE OF AVAILABLE PROSTHETIC FEET: A COMPACT GUIDE

K1 Feet

The solid-ankle, cushion-heel (SACH) (Figure 21-4) foot is the most basic prosthetic foot available. It is recommended only for those with limited functional ability and potential to ambulate. The SACH foot is provided primarily for transfers and limited ambulation. This foot's immovable ankle and soft heel give it the ability to absorb the impact of heel strike but provides minimal energy return. There are numerous manufacturers who produce a version of the SACH foot, simply crafted from a wooden or plastic block with a soft cushion under the heel segment and rubber toes. Because the SACH foot has no moving parts, little maintenance is required until the foot is worn out, at which time it should be replaced. No device is indestructible, however, and with our increasingly overweight society, care should be taken to provide a foot with the appropriate weight category to avoid damage or failure. A carbon composite foot (see "K3 Feet" below) may be required if a SACH foot cannot be made strong enough to support an extremely obese patient.

K2 Feet

Some of the of prosthetic feet used for persons with amputation who are at the K2 functional level are as follows:

- Ossur Flex-Foot K-2 Balance (Figure 21-5, *A*)
- Otto Bock 1M10 Adjust (Figure 21-5, *B*)
- Endolite Navigator
- Trulife Kinetic
- Dycor FMA
- College Park Celsus

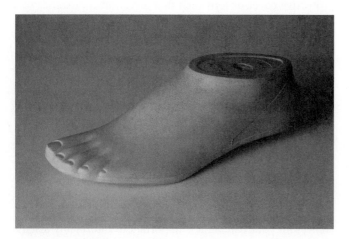

FIGURE 21-4 K1 foot: the solid-ankle, cushion-heel (SACH) foot. (Courtesy of Hanger Clinic, Austin, TX.)

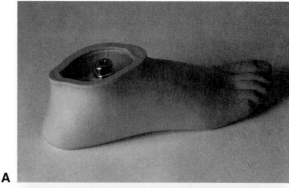

A

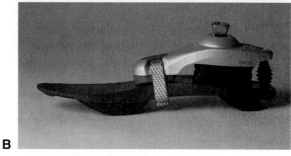

B

FIGURE 21-5 Prosthetic feet for persons with amputations at the K2 functional level. **A,** Flex-Foot Balance. **B,** Otto Bock 1M10 Adjust. (Courtesy of Hanger Clinic, Austin, TX.)

There is an array of different feet suited for persons with amputation at function level K2 who are able to walk inside their homes and outside in the community at a slow pace. Most K2 feet are lightweight, have a flexible keel, a multiaxial ankle, and provide some energy return. A full-length toe mechanism lends stability while providing smooth transitioning from heel strike to toe-off. These feet have foam-rubber cushions that assist the wearer with soft plantarflexionby providing a smooth transition from heel strike to mid-stance. The feet also allow for some transverse rotation. The flexibility of the ankle on most of these feet can be softened or stiffened by changing the rubber cushions. More features and adjustments also mean that more attention and maintenance must be provided. Function level K2 patients should be reassessed regularly by the rehabilitation team to determine whether they can progress to function level K3. Additional therapy and motivation may be all that is need to push them to the next level.

K-3 Feet

Many of the manufacturers of prosthetic feet for persons with amputation at the K3 functional level are as follows. Each offers a number of different foot configurations within this category:

- Carbon fiber composite feet with energy-storing dynamic response:
  - Ossur Flex-Foot
  - Otto Bock
  - Freedom Innovations
  - Ohio Willow Wood
  - Endolite

- Microprocessor feet:
  - Ossur
  - Endolite
  - Fillauer
  - iWalk

Functional level K3 feet are appropriate for patients with the ability or potential to do all daily activities and walk with variable cadence. They are fabricated from lightweight flexible carbon fiber, which is very responsive and extremely durable. Compared to a SACH foot, they reduce energy consumption; offer increased ankle motion; reduce sound side loading; and store and return more energy.[3] There are nearly 100 different designs available in this category, which vary based on the shape of the carbon fiber and the addition of other materials to absorb shock and rotational forces. They can be fitted with or without an integrated pylon. Because they are designed with no moving parts, they offer low-maintenance but should be checked semiannually for wear and to determine if they still meet the needs of the patient.

The integrated pylon foot (Figure 21-6) is the lightest of all foot prostheses. It is one continuous carbon fiber composite material unit from the toe to the top of the pylon, including a heel segment that allows significant plantarflexion/dorsiflexion. Some of these feet also provide inversion/eversion and rotation through a longitudinal split that bisects the foot, a urethane cushion, or a floating sole plate. Alignment capabilities are somewhat limited by the integrated pylon as adjustments must be made just below the socket rather than at the ankle. Wedges can be added at the foot to compensate for this shortcoming.

Energy-storing feet without the integrated pylon offer the same features as those described above but also allow the

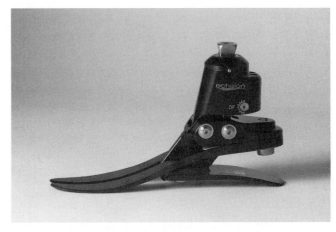

FIGURE 21-7 K3 foot with hydraulic ankle—Endolite Echelon. (Courtesy of Hanger Clinic, Austin, TX.)

prosthetist to perform alignment adjustments at the ankle where the foot is joined to a separate pylon. This permits greater alignment flexibility; however, it adds slightly more weight than the integrated pylon prostheses. These feet can also be matched with a separate ankle joint that provides plantarflexion/dorsiflexion and eversion/inversion by adding a flexible link between the prosthetic foot and the pylon. Although add-on ankles add weight to the prosthesis and require regular maintenance, many patients consider it a small price to pay for the more natural feel of an ankle moving as they ambulate.

Another advantage an ankle joint can offer is the ability for users to adjust their own heel height (Figure 21-7). Patients who enjoy a versatile shoe wardrobe can switch from a tennis shoe or casual slipper into a dressy high-heeled shoe easily, by pushing a button on the side of the ankle, concealed by the cosmetic covering. The ankle is allowed to bend into the desired position and then safely locked. The foot still provides normal gait and energy-storing capability in any height position.

Other beneficial functions include shock and torsion absorption that are designed into the foot or added in the pylon. These features are especially important for high-activity people and those performing repetitive motions. They reduce the vertical and sheer forces that are transmitted to the residual limb by allowing these motions to take place in the component rather than inside the socket. Hydraulic damping is another ankle add-on that permits increased fluidity of sagittal plane movement (Figure 21-8).

Microprocessor feet (Figure 21-9) are the latest development in prosthetic foot technology, and have opened an exciting new spectrum of possibilities for many persons with lower-extremity amputation. In contrast to traditional prosthetic feet that are passive, microprocessor feet actively respond to changes in the environment. If the wearer ascends an incline, the foot automatically provides dorsiflexion, and continues to do so for the extent of the incline. Similarly, the foot automatically responds with plantarflexion during the descent on a downhill grade. The Endolite Élan, Fillaurer Raize, and Ossur Proprio all perform these functions.

The newly introduced BiOM foot is designed to replace the propulsive function of the gastroc-soleus muscles; its use

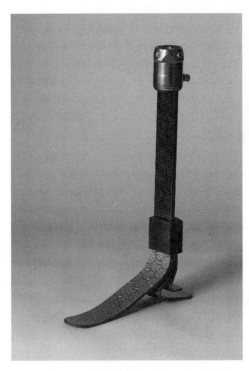

FIGURE 21-6 K3 foot with integrated pylon—Freedom Innovations Silhouette. (Courtesy of Hanger Clinic, Austin, TX.)

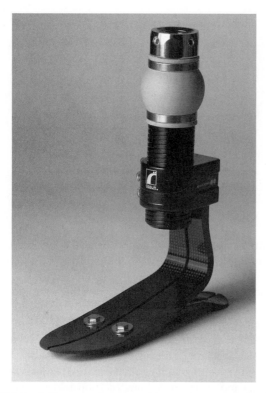

FIGURE 21-8 Dynamic Response Foot with Vertical Shock and Torque Absorbing Pylon-Flex-Foot Re-Flex Rotate with EVO. (Courtesy of Hanger Clinic, Austin, TX.)

results a near-normalized gait for persons with transtibial amputation. The BiOM generates power during plantar flexion, propelling the prosthesis forward. The the first published research study demonstrated a significant reduction in metabolic cost, which allows persons with amputation to walk with greater economy and symmetry.[8] The BiOM generates its powered plantarflexion by using a combination of microprocessors, sensors, motors, and springs. It reacts in real time to changes in speed and terrain.

Microprocessor feet are heavier than most traditional feet. They are powered by an onboard battery that requires nightly recharging. The range of motion of microprocessor feet is thus far limited to this single axis capability, but inversion and eversion flexibility are likely to be available in the future. Contraindications for microprocessor feet are exposure to water, dirt, and extreme heat.

K-4 Feet: High Activity

A number of specialized prosthetic feet (Figure 21-10) are available for the serious athlete and weekend runner. Different configurations are available for sprinting and running. The sprinting foot, with a stiffer, springy character, is designed for powerful bursts of speed, such as a 100-meter or 200-meter race. The running foot combines stiffness that is gentler and serves as a distance running foot for marathon or half-marathon challenges. Choice of design depends on

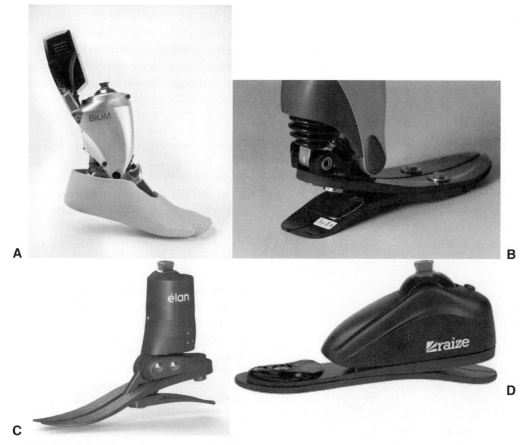

A

B

C

D

FIGURE 21-9 Microprocessor foot. **A,** BiOM. **B,** Ossur Proprio. **C,** Endolite Élan, Miamisburg, OH. **D,** Fillauer Raize, Chattanooga, TN. (Courtesy of Hanger Clinic, Austin, TX.)

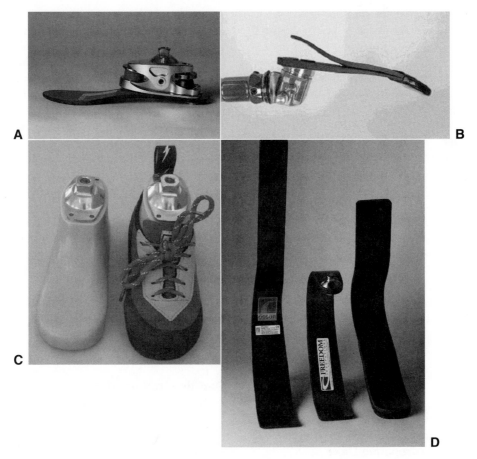

FIGURE 21-10 Specialized prosthetic feet. **A,** K3 foot with multiaxial ankle and rotation (College Park Venture, Fraser, MI). **B,** Swim foot with moveable ankle. **C,** Adult climbing foot. **D,** Running feet. (A, B, and D Courtesy of Hanger Clinic, Austin, TX; C, courtesy TRS, Inc, Boulder, CO.)

the patient's activity and special interest. Their unique design makes them appropriate for running or sprinting but they are not recommended for everyday wear.

Specialized activity feet are available for sportsmen and athletes. Multiaxis feet are recommended for golfers and hikers who traverse uneven terrain. A swim foot is available that can be locked in plantarflexion for use with a swim fin. Swim ankles that offer additional flexibility may also be added to a waterproof foot for added efficiency in the water. A short, rock climbing foot is sold with a specialized climbing shoe.

SUMMARY

Selecting the most appropriate prosthetic foot can be a complex clinical decision because of a variety of factors, including a patient's current and potential functional level patient's specific needs, the wide array of choices available, and cost. A small oversight in the selection process can make a significant difference in the level of success the patient achieves. Rehabilitation team professionals, together with the patient family members, and caregivers, should analyze and evaluate the best prosthetic options for advancing mobility that is functional, efficient, practical, and safe in persons with lower-extremity amputation. Advances in energy-storing materials and microprocessor technology offer persons with

lower-extremity amputation improved function in daily activites as well as high-activity-performance in sports such as running, swimming, golfing, biking, and hiking.

CASE EXAMPLE 1

An Individual with a Transtibial Amputation

A. J., a former marine soldier, was 20 years old when he endured traumatic injuries after driving his motor vehicle over a landmine. He was one of three people who survived the explosion. A. J. was flown to Germany for emergency surgery and later transferred to a military medical center in Washington, DC. He severely injured his left leg, incurred damage to his right tympanic membrane, and lost his left thumb. After multiple surgeries, bone infection in his left leg, and months of rehabilitation, doctors decided to amputate his leg below the knee. A. J. was offered honorable discharge because of his injuries. He accepted the discharge and returned to his hometown where he continued rehabilitation.

In high school A. J. had been a competitive athlete for his track team and he maintained an average weight of 180 pounds. One year after the accident, the 5-foot 11-inches-tall former soldier weighs 206 pounds and is ambulating independently with a transtibial prosthesis. A. J. has accepted the loss of his left leg and is ready to return to a "normal" life. He is determined to run again and plans to enroll at a local college. A. J. currently lives with his mother in a small one-story house in a rural community and has not driven a vehicle since the accident.

Questions to Consider

- To what extent would A. J.'s age, height, weight, and lifestyle impact the selection and maintenance of a prosthetic foot?
- What prosthetic foot design would be most appropriate for athletic challenges?
- What environmental challenges might A. J. encounter on a college campus? What environmental challenges might he encounter in a rural community?
- How does a prosthetic foot simulate the functional characteristics of a human foot?
- What social issues might A. J. face as he enters college? How would a prosthetic foot affect his psychosocial health?
- What specific recommendations should be given to meet A. J.'s needs and assist him in meeting his goals?

CASE EXAMPLE 2

An Older Adult with Amputation due to Infected Non-healing Neuropathic Ulcer

Mrs. R. T. is a 79-year-old with long-standing diabetes and peripheral arterial disease who developed a neuropathic ulcer at the first metatarsal head of her right forefoot 6 months ago. Despite conservative attempts to heal the wound using a total contact cast, and subsequent vascular bypass surgery to restore blood flow to the distal extremity, the wound failed to heal and osteomyelitis developed. Mrs. R. T. underwent standard transtibial amputation 2 months ago, managed postoperatively with removable rigid dressing to protect the surgical site and control postoperative edema. Although the surgical incision was slow to heal, her surgeon has determined that it is now safe to begin prosthetic training, and she has been referred for prosthetic prescription.

Until the development of her neuropathic ulcer, Mrs. R. T. lived independently in a second-floor apartment of an urban retirement community in a small city, drove her own car to a nearby park to walk for exercise at least 3 times each week, and participated in many activities at her local senior center. Since her surgery, she has been living with her daughter in a nearby suburb, using a wheelchair (propelling it herself) for mobility, and receiving home care physical therapy to build her strength and endurance. She reports that she is able to transfer between bed and wheelchair independently but requires assistance to get into and out of the car. She is anxious to receive a prosthesis, but wonders if she has the ability to return to community ambulation without the need of an assistive device.

Mrs. R. T. is 5 feet, 3 inches tall and weighs 150 pounds. She admits that her memory "is not what it used to be" and has recently been diagnosed with mild cognitive impairment, but she has no clinical signs of dementia. She has significant osteoarthritis of her fingers and wrists, as well as in both of her hips.

Questions to Consider

- To what extent would Mrs. R. T.'s age, height, weight, and lifestyle impact the selection and maintenance of a prosthetic foot?
- What K-level best reflects Mrs. R. T.'s functional potential? Why have you selected this K-level?
- What prosthetic foot design would be most appropriate for Mrs. R. T.'s first prosthesis?
- What environmental challenges might Mrs. R. T. encounter if she is able to resume her pre-ulcer activities? How might the challenges be similar or different in an urban versus suburban community?
- How does the prosthetic foot that you have chosen simulate the functional characteristics of a human foot?
- What are the effects of a prosthetic foot on gait? How does a prosthetic foot's function during gait differ during running?
- What specific recommendations should be given to meet Mrs. R. T.'s needs and assist her in meeting her goals?

REFERENCES

1. Powers CM, Torburn L, Perry J, et al. Influence of prosthetic foot design on sound limb loading in adults with unilateral below-knee amputations. *Arch Phys Med Rehabil.* 1994;75(7):825–829.
2. van der Linde H, Hofstad CY, Geurts AC, et al. A systematic literature review of the effect of different prosthetic components on human functioning with a lower-limb prosthesis. *J Rehabil Res Dev.* 2004;41:555–570.
3. Cummings DR, Kapp S. *State-Of-The-Science Conference on prosthetic feet and ankle mechanisms.* Available at: http://www.oandp.org/jpo/library/index/2005_04S.asp.
4. Czerniecki JM. Research and clinical selection of foot-ankle systems. *J Prosth Orthot.* 2005;17(4S):358.
5. Perry J. *Gait Analysis: Normal and Pathological Function.* Thorofare, NJ: Slack; 1992.
6. DMERC Region A Lower Limb Prostheses Policy #LLP20030401, The DME MAC Jurisdiction, A Supplier Manual. Available at: http://www.medicarenhic.com/dme/medical_review/mr_lcds/mr_lcd_archived/L11464_2003-04-01.pdf.
7. Gailey RS, Roach KE, Applegate EB, et al. The amputee mobility predictor: an instrument to assess determinants of the lower-limb amputee's ability to ambulate. *Arch Phys Med Rehabil.* 2002;83(5):613–627.
8. Herr HM, Grabowski AM. Bionic ankle–foot prosthesis normalizes walking gait for persons with leg amputation. *Proc Royal Soc B.* 2012;279(1728):457–464.

22

Postsurgical Management of Partial Foot and the Syme Amputation

EDMOND AYYAPPA AND HEATHER WORDEN

LEARNING OBJECTIVES

On completion of this chapter, the reader will be able to do the following:

1. Differentiate among the various disarticulation and transaction surgeries used when amputation of the forefoot, midfoot, or rearfoot is necessary.
2. Describe usual gait performance and limitations of individuals with a partial foot and with the Syme amputation.
3. Compare the advantages and disadvantages of prosthetic options for individuals with partial foot amputation.
4. Compare the advantages and disadvantages of the various prosthetic designs for persons with the Syme amputation, including donning and pressure tolerance.
5. Compare how the various nonarticulating and dynamic response Syme prosthetic feet mimic the three rockers of gait.
6. Describe typical static and dynamic alignment variables or issues affecting gait for patients with a Syme or partial foot prosthesis.
7. Use knowledge of prosthetic options to suggest prosthetic prescriptions and plans of care for patients with partial foot and Syme amputation.

Partial foot and Syme-level amputations present advantages and challenges to the patient and the rehabilitation team. Preservation of the ankle and heel (in partial foot amputation) and most of the length of the lower limb (in Syme amputation) has an important advantage of distal weight-bearing capability: The individual with partial foot or Syme-level amputation is often able to ambulate without a prosthesis if necessary. The prosthesis, however, provides protection for the vulnerable distal residual limb for patients with vascular compromise and neuropathy.

The length and shape of the residual limb present three challenges for successful fitting and prosthetic training for patients with partial foot or Syme amputation: suspension of the prosthesis on the residual limb, distribution of weight-bearing forces within the prosthesis, and attachment and alignment of the prosthetic foot. This chapter defines the most common partial foot and Syme amputations, and

reviews the prosthetic management options currently available. Also identified are specific indications and contraindications for the various prosthetic designs.

PARTIAL FOOT AMPUTATIONS

Until the advent of antibiotics, disarticulation through the joints of the foot reduced the risk of sepsis and shock and improved the prognosis for healing compared with amputations that transected bone. The earliest partial foot amputation was recorded in 434 BC by the Greek historian Herodotus,[1] who told of a Persian warrior who escaped death while in the stocks by disarticulating his own foot. He hobbled 30 miles to a nearby town, where he was nursed to health until he could construct a prosthesis for himself. Later he became a soothsayer for the Persian army but ultimately was recaptured by the Spartans and killed.

At present, partial foot amputations include a wide variety of ray resections, digit (phalangeal) amputations, and metatarsal transections (Figure 22-1). Midfoot amputations include surgical ablation at the Chopart and Lisfranc levels (Figure 22-2).[2] Chopart disarticulation involves the talocalcaneonavicular joint and separates the talus and navicular as well as the calcaneus and cuboid.[3] Lisfranc disarticulation separates the three cuneiform bones and the cuboid bone from the five metatarsal bones of the forefoot.

The three hindfoot amputations are the Pirogoff, Boyd, and Syme. The Pirogoff amputation is a wedging transection of the calcaneus, followed by bony fusion of the calcaneus and distal tibia with all other distal structures removed. In a Boyd amputation, the calcaneus remains largely intact rather than being wedged before arthrodesis with the tibia. Today these amputations are infrequently performed on adult patients. Neither provides an easy fit with a prosthesis. The Boyd amputation has received positive clinical reviews when used in the management of congenital limb deficiencies in children in which the amputated limb is shorter than the sound limb.[4,5] In this case, there are usually fewer postoperative complications, such as scarring and heel pad migration, and less susceptibility to the bony overgrowth common in children with congenital limb deficiencies. The Syme amputation is performed more frequently in adults because of the ease of prosthetic management

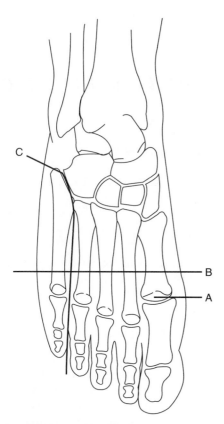

FIGURE 22-1 Examples of amputations involving the forefoot. **A,** This digit (phalangeal) amputation involves disarticulation at the tarsal–metatarsal joint. More distal digit amputations remove either the distal phalanx or the middle and distal phalanges. **B,** In this complete transmetatarsal amputation, transaction occurred just proximal to all five metatarsal heads. **C,** Ray resections involve disarticulation of one or more metatarsals and their phalanges from the tarsal and neighboring metatarsals. Ray resections often require skin graft to achieve adequate tissue closure.

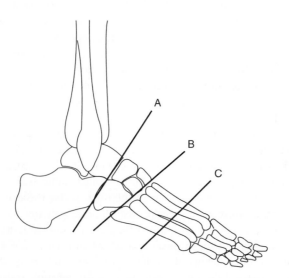

FIGURE 22-2 In a Chopart amputation **(A)** there is disarticulation of the midfoot from the forefoot at the level of the talus and calcaneus. In a Lisfranc amputation **(B)** there is disarticulation of the forefoot (metatarsals) from the midfoot (tarsals). **(C)** In a transmetatarsal amputation, there is transaction through the length of one or more metatarsals, usually just proximal to the metatarsal heads.

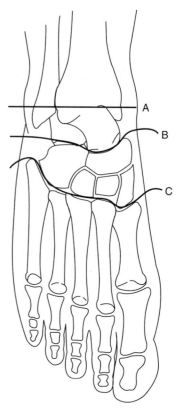

FIGURE 22-3 A, The Syme amputation involves removal of the inferior projections of the tibia and fibula and all bone structures distally while preserving the natural weight-bearing fat pad of the heel. **B,** The Chopart amputation preserves the talus and calcaneus. **C,** The Lisfranc amputation has disarticulation of metatarsals from the midfoot.

at this level (Figure 22-3). Because of the length of the residual limb in Pirogoff and Boyd amputations, the attachment of a prosthetic foot lengthens the limb when a prosthesis is worn. A heel lift on the contralateral sound limb is usually necessary to counteract this artificially long prosthetic limb.

Proximal partial foot amputations often result in equinus deformities because of muscular imbalance created by severed dorsiflexors and intact triceps surae.[6-8] Nevertheless, many individuals with a partial foot amputation function extremely well. In one survey, physicians and prosthetists reported that patients with partial foot amputation function better than those with the Syme amputation.[9] Although surgeons and prosthetists have long supported the Syme amputation in preference to the Lisfranc or Chopart amputations, many patients with midfoot amputation achieve high levels of function. For example, Jack Dempsey, a professional football player with a midfoot amputation, set several all-time field goal records wearing a custom-designed kicking boot.[10]

Gait Characteristics After Partial Foot Amputation

A person with a partial foot amputation typically has vascular insufficiency, is usually between the ages of 60 and 70 years, has compromised proprioception and sensation, and has weak lower limb musculature. After a Syme or partial foot amputation a patient may be able to ambulate without a prosthesis but has a loss of the anterior lever arm in ambulation and an inefficient, somewhat dysfunctional gait. The primary need immediately after amputation is to protect the remaining tissue, which is vulnerable to vascular or neuropathic disease. The neuropathic walker developed at Rancho Los Amigos Medical Center locks the ankle in a custom-molded, foam-lined, thermoplastic ankle-foot orthosis (AFO) (Figure 22-4). A rocker bottom is contoured to promote a smooth rollover as a substitute for the second and third rockers of gait, and the orthosis provides optimum protection for the insensate residual foot. For patients with adequate protective sensation, the risk of tissue breakdown is less and a custom shoe insert with in-depth or postoperative shoes often provides adequate protection.

A review of gait in partial foot case histories showed variations in single-limb support time directly related to the reduction of the forefoot lever arm of a partial foot and subsequent increase in the force concentration on the distal end during terminal stance, reflected as reduced time in single-limb support on the limb with amputation (Figure 22-5).[11]

In a person with a whole foot, a fully intact anterior lever arm preserves elevation of the center of mass at terminal stance. With normal quadriceps strength and eccentric control, slight knee flexion (15 to 20 degrees) provides shock absorption as weight is rapidly transferred onto the

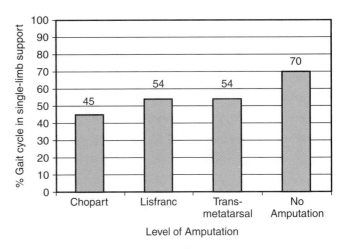

FIGURE 22-5 Percent of the gait cycle spent in single-limb support for patients with midfoot Chopart or Lisfranc amputations and forefoot transmetatarsal amputation. Healthy older adults with intact feet typically spend between 65% and 75% of their gait cycle in single-limb support.

limb during loading response (Figure 22-6). Most people with dysvascular partial foot and a Syme amputation demonstrate significant weakness of the quadriceps. This functional weakness threatens eccentric control of the usual knee flexion angle that occurs during loading response. To compensate, the patient may keep the knee extended during loading response. This strategy shifts the ground reaction force vector to a position anterior to the knee joint axis, thus reducing the workload of the quadriceps. Although this compensatory strategy enhances early stance phase stability, it sacrifices the shock absorption mechanism at the knee and hip joints, increasing the likelihood of cumulative joint trauma at both joints (see Figure 22-6, *B*). Neuropathic impairment of proprioception and sensation may further complicate control of the knee in early stance. In addition, compromised forefoot support increases center of gravity displacement. A penalty of higher energy cost results.

A recent study of the gait of persons with partial foot amputation included 18 patients with transmetatarsal amputations, 11 with one or more metatarsal amputations, 15 with ray resections, and two with either a Lisfranc or a Chopart amputation.[11-13] One portion of the analysis focused on the mechanics of the residual limb rockers. Partly because of a delay in the forefoot rocker, patients with all types of partial foot amputations walked with a significantly slower velocity than control subjects with healthy, intact feet (Figure 22-7). Peak ankle dorsiflexion was also significantly delayed for all three partial foot groups compared with those with intact feet. Although the control group with intact lower limbs reached peak ankle dorsiflexion at a point 43% into the gait cycle, patients with partial foot amputation did not reach peak dorsiflexion angle until nearly the halfway point of the gait cycle (Figure 22-8). This delay in reaching peak dorsiflexion subsequently delays forward progression over the shortened stance limb and the transition to double-limb support.

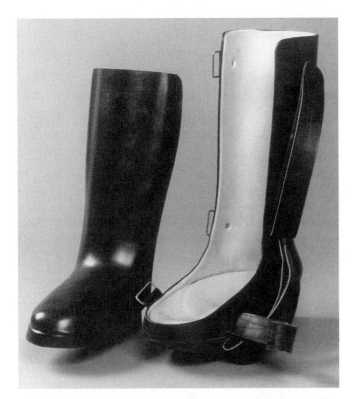

FIGURE 22-4 The neuropathic walker provides maximum protection for the denervated foot at risk for amputation. The combination of custom-molded multidurometer liner, locked neutral ankle, and rocker bottom permits a rollover with minimal plantar pressure and shear.

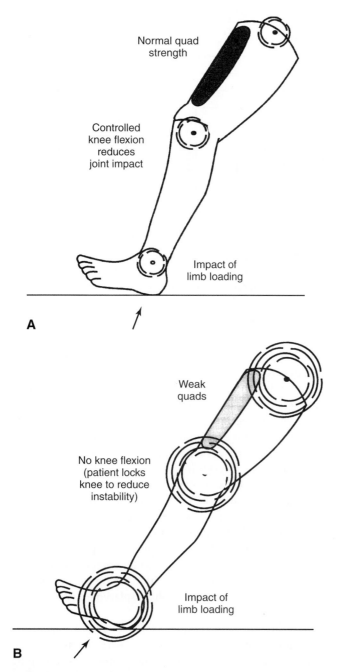

A, Normal quad strength

Controlled knee flexion reduces joint impact

Impact of limb loading

A

Weak quads

No knee flexion (patient locks knee to reduce instability)

Impact of limb loading

B

FIGURE 22-6 A, During loading in normal gait, knee flexion provides a significant shock absorption mechanism to protect the proximal joints. **B,** The patient with weakness associated with dysvascular disease avoids knee flexion to increase stability, with a penalty of increased trauma to the proximal joints as a consequence of repeated higher impact loading.

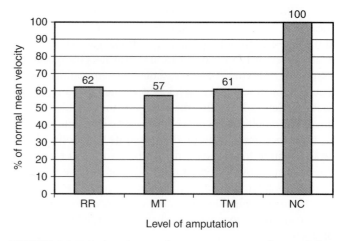

FIGURE 22-7 Reduced gait velocity in patients with partial foot amputations. On average, patients walked at 62% of gait velocity of control subjects with intact lower limbs. *MT,* Metatarsal amputation of one to four rays; *NC,* normal control subjects; *RR,* ray resection; *TM,* complete transmetatarsal amputation.

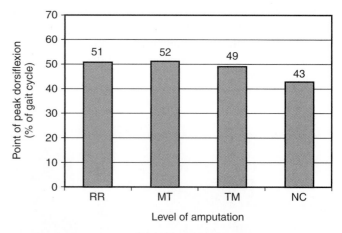

FIGURE 22-8 For persons with partial foot amputations, maximum dorsiflexion is delayed during stance phase of the gait cycle. Although control subjects with intact feet achieved a maximum dorsiflexion angle at a point 43% into the gait cycle, those with partial foot amputation did not reach the maximum dorsiflexion angle until halfway through the cycle. The consequence of this delay is a slowed forward progression of the body's center of mass and transition to the subsequent period of double-limb support. *MT,* Metatarsal amputation of one to four rays; *NC,* normal control subjects; *RR,* ray resection; *TM,* complete transmetatarsal amputation.

The rise rate of the vertical ground reaction force is the amount of force that occurs in 1% of the gait cycle and can be expressed as Newtons divided by the percent of the gait cycle. After controlling for variation in velocity, the rise rate of the vertical ground reaction force from mid to terminal stance (as the force pattern nears its F2 peak) was significantly lower for all three amputation groups compared with the control group (Figure 22-9). Peak vertical ground reaction forces

were significantly higher for the sound limb than the affected limb, likely reflecting an abrupt unloading of the partial foot amputation limb.

The forefoot lever arm of the trailing limb typically provides anterior support and results in adequate terminal stance support time (Figure 22-10). This results in appropriate step length of the advancing limb. By contrast, inadequate anterior support of the trailing limb of the partial foot amputee reduces the lever arm, resulting in premature toe break and forefoot collapse. The step length of the advancing limb may be correspondingly reduced (Figure 22-10, *B*).

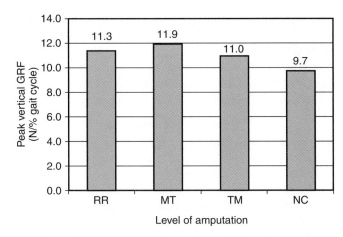

FIGURE 22-9 Comparison of peak vertical ground reaction force (*GRF*) of the intact limbs of patients with partial foot amputations and persons without amputation, expressed as Newton divided by % of gait cycle. *MT,* Metatarsal amputation of one to four rays; *NC,* normal control subjects; *RR,* ray resection; *TM,* complete transmetatarsal amputation.

An inverse relation exists between surface area and peak pressure when body weight is loaded on the foot during stance. This relation is especially important for individuals with partial foot amputation during terminal stance. As the plantar surface area of the supporting forefoot is reduced, the magnitude of the pressure is increased.[11-13] The reduced forefoot lever arm also creates abrupt weight transfer to the contralateral side and can reduce step length, stride length, and velocity. Without prosthetic support, the advancing sound-side step length diminishes. Fear, insecurity, and pain aggravated by increased pressure near the amputation site collectively create an abrupt transfer of weight to the sound side, thus increasing the magnitude of the initial vertical force peak.[14]

In normal gait, the weight line is positioned more and more anterior to the knee joint as the gait cycle moves from midstance into terminal stance and preswing phases (Figure 22-11). As a result, the limb is held in a passive, energy-efficient extended knee position, effectively supporting body weight and increasing stability in late stance. The length of the forefoot lever arm is one of the key determinants of this support. For persons with partial foot amputation, the lever arm of the foot is greatly reduced, leading to a less-effective, premature loss of support at the end of stance phase. This shorter lever places the ground reaction force closer to or behind the knee in late stance (Figure 22-11, *B*). Because much of the passive stability provided by a normal forefoot lever in late stance is absent, the quadriceps must contract to maintain stance phase stability, contributing to an increased energy cost of walking for persons with partial foot amputation.

Pinzur and colleagues[15] described a functional relation between gait velocity and the level of amputation at the foot. As the amputation level becomes more proximal (as the length of the residual foot decreases), changes in temporal and kinetic gait characteristics include reduced sound-side step length, decreased velocity, increased energy cost, and increased vertical load on the sound side. An inverse relation exists between

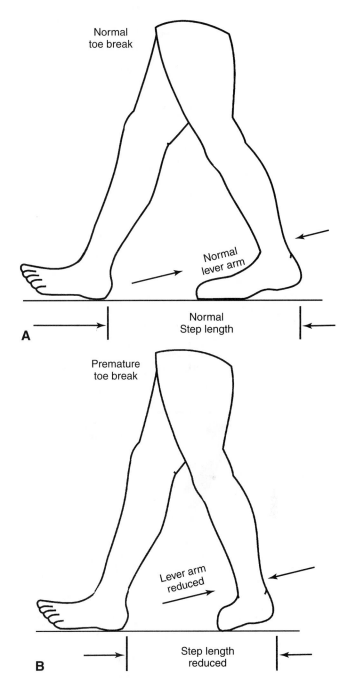

FIGURE 22-10 A, The forefoot lever arm contributes to a normal step length. **B,** Reduction of the forefoot support after partial foot amputation produces a consequent reduction in contralateral step length.

the length of the remaining portion of the forefoot and the time spent in single-limb support on the amputated side.[14] When the level of amputation is proximal to the metatarsal heads, medial support is lost at loading response. This may require orthotic "posting" to limit resultant valgus deformity. Patients with partial foot amputation frequently have plantar flexion contracture develop from muscle imbalance. Any plantar flexion contracture, in turn, increases pressure at the distal residual limb during terminal stance, causing discomfort, pain, and risk of ulceration.[16] A contracture is even more problematic for individuals with Hansen disease

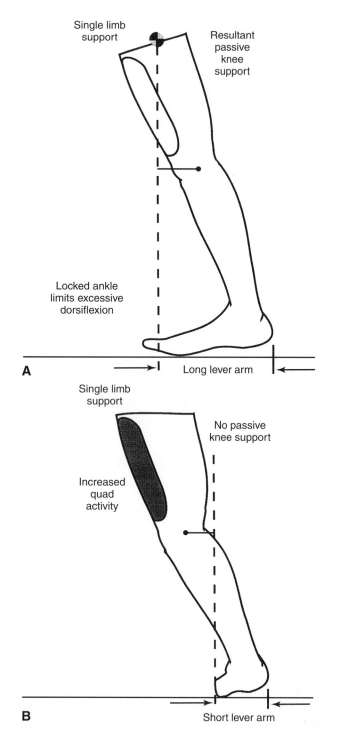

FIGURE 22-11 A, Normal energy-efficient passive knee support in late stance relies on a locked or rigid forefoot that limits further dorsiflexion at the ankle and a normal forefoot lever arm to maintain the ground reaction force anterior to the knee during late stance. **B,** After partial foot amputation, the reduced forefoot lever arm often leads to increased quadriceps activity to compensate for reduced passive knee support and ensure stability in late stance.

or diabetic neuropathy because they already have compromised sensation.[17,18] Shoes worn without prosthetic replacement of the missing forefoot quickly become disfigured, collapsing at a displaced toe break, further endangering the vulnerable areas of the residual limb.[19] The areas of the

residual foot most vulnerable to tissue damage during walking include the distal end, first and fifth metatarsal heads, navicular, malleoli, and tibial crest. The longitudinal and transverse arches, the heel pad, and the area along the pretibial muscle belly are pressure-tolerant areas for loading in a custom shoe or prosthesis.

Prosthetic Management

During the 1800 s, digit amputations were fitted by a wood or cork sandal with a leather ankle lacer.[20,21] Partial foot amputations were sometimes fitted with a socket and keel fashioned from one piece of carefully chosen root wood, the grain of which followed the curve of the ankle. This was referred to as the *natural crook technique*. Another commonly used historical design incorporated steel-reinforced leather sockets.[22]

In recent decades, a wide variety of prosthetic options for individuals with partial foot amputation have emerged. The prescribing physician and patient care team must familiarize themselves with the broad array of options available in prosthetic components and design so that prescription considerations can best accommodate the special needs of each patient. Because of variability in level of amputation, sensitivity or insensitivity of the residual limb, concurrent foot deformity, and patient activity, no single prosthetic prescription can be used for all patients with foot amputation.[23] As the amputation level becomes more proximal and the length of the residual foot decreases, prostheses are more likely to incorporate supramalleolar containment or more superior support. This is especially true as a patient's activity level increases. Commonly used prosthetic approaches include toe fillers placed inside the shoe, a foot orthosis or an arch support, the University of California Biomechanics Laboratory (UCBL) orthosis to control heel position, and a boot or slipper made of flexible urethane resin (Smooth-On, Easton, PA). Cosmetic restoration of silicone and several variations of AFOs are also in common use.

The length and degree of flexibility of the prosthetic forefoot affect the anterior lever arm and consequently foot and ankle motion. The biomechanical goal is to allow anterior support in the area of the lost metatarsals as well as a controlled fulcrum of forward motion as the foot-ankle complex pivots over the area of the lost metatarsal heads in the third rocker of late stance. An additional goal is to minimize pressure at the amputated distal end within the socket or shoe.

Toe Fillers and Modified Shoes

If a simple filler is prescribed, an extended steel shank or band of rigid spring steel should also be placed within the sole of the shoe, extending from the calcaneus to the metatarsal heads. The challenge that faces the prosthetist is to match the appropriate degree of forefoot flexibility to the needs of each patient. For an energy-efficient and cosmetic gait, relative plantar rigidity should give way to at least 15 degrees of forefoot flexibility distal to the metatarsal heads. The extended steel shank is helpful in providing a limited degree of buoyancy that substitutes for the lost anterior support of the foot.[24] Stiffening the sole with a spring steel shank increases the lever arm support, but often at the expense of additional pressure on the distal end of the residual limb.[25]

For a patient with a more complex partial foot amputation, a rocker bottom shoe modification distributes force over a greater area and advances stance more quickly and efficiently. A curved roll or buildup on the plantar surface of the shoe encourages tibial advancement while minimizing weight-bearing pressures on the distal amputated end (Figure 22-12). For optimal function the plantar contour of a rocker bottom should follow a radius originating from the knee joint center but break or roll more abruptly just distal to the metatarsal heads. Although a rocker bottom assists rollover, it also compromises symmetry of gait. It is often prescribed for individuals with chronic pain or in conjunction with a custom-molded accommodative interface for those with a neuropathy-related risk of reamputation. Extra-depth shoes have 6 to 8 mm or more of space inside the shoe on the plantar surface to accommodate an orthotic insert or prosthesis and may be useful for patients with digit or ray amputations.[23]

Custom-molded shoes, when used in conjunction with a filler and shank, improve the comfort level and reduce the risk of ulceration in many dysvascular patients with amputation. They are not as subject to forefoot collapse, provide major protection to the endangered foot, and may last longer than stock shoes.[26]

Custom Shoe Inserts and Toe Fillers

A custom-molded, flexible, plantar shoe insert is one of the options for individuals with amputation of the hallux or first ray. This orthotic approach is typically used in combination with extra-depth shoes. The goal is to provide a flexible ante-rior extension to compensate for a missing or shortened first ray to improve the third rocker and yet support and protect the amputation site during the simulated metatarsophalangeal hyperextension in late stance and preswing.[27] This provides some relief for metatarsal head pressure, supports the arch, and probably assists in normalizing the ground reaction force pattern during terminal stance and preswing. It may incorporate a toe filler to prevent premature forefoot shoe collapse.[28-30] Toe fillers consist of soft foam material such as room-temperature vulcanized elastomer, which fills the voids in the toe box of the shoe. They provide limited extension of the shoe life and a moderate degree of cosmesis. They also act as spacers, keeping adjoining toes properly positioned and reducing abnormal motion that can otherwise lead to ulceration. The toe filler alone provides limited mechanical advantage. A spring steel shank within the sole of the shoe and extending from mid-calcaneus to the metatarsal heads can further improve gait. An alternative to the spring steel shank is a longitudinal support built into a flexible custom insole. Either support device must end at the metatarsal heads to allow hyperextension of the metatarsophalangeal joints. A foot orthotic with arch support and filler is preferable to the simple filler because it can be used in different shoes and because it provides plantar support to an already compromised weight-bearing surface.[31] Custom insoles can also be made from a sawdust and epoxy resin instead of foams and thermoplastics.

The UCBL orthosis, a foot orthosis that encapsulates the calcaneus, was developed at the UCBL during the 1960s and was comprehensively described in 1969.[32,33] The UCBL orthosis is designed to provide better control of subtalar and forefoot position than are custom-made shoe inserts, reducing motion and thus friction with a closer fit or purchase over the calcaneus and forefoot (Figure 22-13).[34] The UCBL orthosis design can be effectively incorporated into a custom orthosis and filler for persons with partial foot amputation.

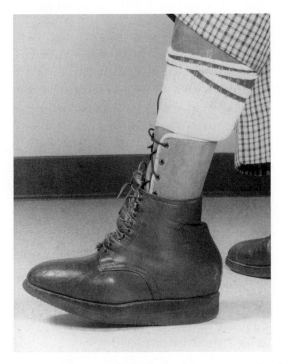

FIGURE 22-12 A supramalleolar leather lacer, worn inside a high-top extra-depth shoe with toe filler and rocker bottom, is an effective prosthetic choice for this patient with a Chopart amputation.

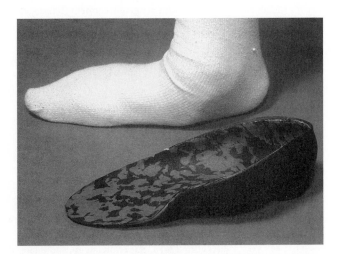

FIGURE 22-13 The custom-molded University of California Biomechanics Laboratory orthosis attempts to obtain a purchase over the os calcis and is thought to influence alignment of the subtalar joint. This patient has ray resection of the hallux and first metatarsal.

CASE EXAMPLE 1

A Patient with a Unilateral Hallux Amputation

B. B. is a 49-year-old male with a 14-year history of diabetes. He has controlled his diabetes and has never had any complications secondary to his diabetic condition. B. B. noticed that he had stepped on a tack which he removed approximately 3 to 4 days after the incident. He noted there that was no pain but he did notice that when he manipulated the great toe, the nail bed looked different than usual, slightly irritated, and the skin did not behave like the skin on his other toes. He neglected to receive medical attention because he was already taking antibiotics for a preexisting infection. Ten days after the initial incident B. B. underwent an amputation involving a disarticulation of the first metatarsophalangeal joint of the right foot, resulting in a hallux amputation (Figure 22-14).

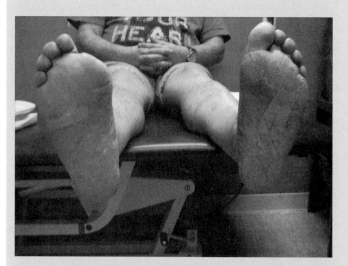

FIGURE 22-14 The patient was seen for an initial evaluation postoperatively. Patient came to the clinic after seeing podiatry, where his feet were examined and routine maintenance and care was performed. Note the significant bilateral callusing of the heels, as well as over metatarsals 2, 3, and 5 with areas of treatment (bandages).

Questions to Consider

- Considering his medical situation and awareness of his diabetic condition, what concerns might exist about the residual foot? Which part of the foot is most vulnerable to future complications?
- What is the primary mechanism for an increase in energy consumption with any digit amputation, and what is particularly concerning about a great toe (hallux) amputation?
- How will his shortened foot affect progression throughout the gait cycle with respect to each phase of gait and the specific three rockers of the foot?
- What would be the most optimal prosthetic recommendation? What are the primary goals of the prosthesis? How should the rehabilitation team assist him in caring for his new amputation as well as in prevention of future proximal amputations?

Recommendations

After obtaining all additional information from B. B. and from all medical sources concerning B. B., it was noted that the he had medically significant bilateral callusing of the heels, as well as over metatarsals 2, 3, and 5. He had a Morton toe on the left foot, as well as tight Achilles tendon bilaterally. He was wearing a size 11 wide shoe but measured for a size 11.5. It was noticed overall that his right foot was considerably swollen relative to his left foot. After reviewing his condition the treatment team recommended extra-depth diabetic shoes with bilateral custom foot orthoses. The custom foot orthoses consisted of a hallux filler for the right, bilateral deep heel cups, a metatarsal bar on the left, and bilateral relief at the second metatarsal head (Figure 22-15). After fitting him with his new shoes and foot orthoses, he was able to ambulate free of any pain or discomfort. He stated he felt like he was able to "walk faster compared to before the orthoses" as a consequence of the increased stability, positioning and comfort that the prescription provided in comparison to walking without foot orthoses.

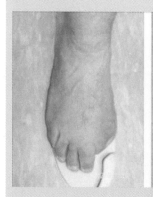
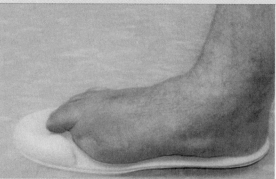
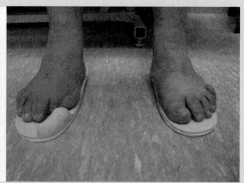

FIGURE 22-15 Superior, lateral, and bilateral images of a foot orthosis with the toe filler. The patient was able to ambulate without pain and stated that with the foot orthoses, as well as his correct fitting shoes, he was able "to walk faster compared to before the orthoses."

Cosmetic Slipper Designs

The slipper, one variation of which has been referred to as the *slipper-type elastomer prosthesis*, is fabricated from semi-flexible urethane elastomer.[35] A similar design in silicone may not provide adequate forefoot support without the addition of an extended steel shank in the patient's shoe. Another similar variation is made from a combination of silicone Silastic (Dow Corning, Midland, MI), polyester resin, and prosthetic (polyurethane) foam. These designs provide much of the support and control of the UCBL approach but with added cosmesis. These designs may be appropriate for individuals with transmetatarsal amputations or disarticulations. They are ideal for swimming or water sports because most are water impervious, cosmetic, and capable of providing a flexible whip action, which is useful with swim fins.

Some slipper-type prostheses are cosmetic restorations made of silicone or vinyl and based on a "life cast," or an alginate impression of a human model (Figure 22-16). This prosthesis is made for patients who consider cosmesis paramount. This custom prosthesis is most often produced in special manufacturing centers and frequently requires a considerable amount of time for delivery. It can be ordered with hair, freckles, and in a large variety of skin tones; however, it is most often a less-than-perfect match when compared with the intact contralateral foot. The patient should always share responsibility in the color swatch selection. The material itself is easily stained and changes color with time when exposed to sunlight. The cosmetic restoration provides little ambulation advantage but does increase shoe life. It may be appropriate for patients with transmetatarsal amputations who place a premium on cosmesis.

Prosthetic Boots

The prosthetic boot, with laced or hook-and-loop material ankle cuff closures, has greater proximal encompassment to reduce distal motion and increase control (Figure 22-17). This design is appropriate for individuals with a Lisfranc or transmetatarsal disarticulation or amputation. One variation, the Chicago boot, or Imler partial foot prosthesis, combines

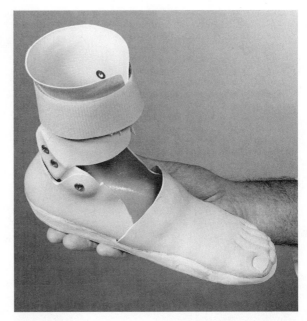

FIGURE 22-17 A prosthetic boot, composed of epoxy-modified acrylic resin combined with supramalleolar containment and free motion, single-axis ankle joints may be helpful at the transmetatarsal level. Without the circumferential containment above the ankle, patients often report joint pain toward the end of the day.

a thermoplastic UCBL-type heel cup with a flexible urethane prosthetic forefoot.[36,37] Other designs incorporate urethane with a modified solid-ankle, cushion-heel foot; some are fabricated from leather, laminated plastic, or Silastic elastomer (Dow Corning), Plastazote (Bakelite Xylonite Ltd, London, UK) combinations, as an insert for a boot, or as an outer boot with inner filler to accommodate bony prominences.[38-41] Such boots often have an anterior or medial tongue and laces or some other means of obtaining a firm purchase above the ankle.[42-45] Some variation of the prosthetic boot may be the general prosthesis of choice for most patients with midfoot amputations.

Ankle-Foot Orthoses

The AFO is another option for persons with partial foot amputation. The polypropylene or copolymer shell supports the plantar aspect of the foot, incorporates the heel, and extends up the posterior leg to the belly of the gastrocnemius (Figure 22-18). A circumferential anterior strap stabilizes the limb in the AFO. As an alternative metal uprights may be attached to a shoe but have obvious cosmetic drawbacks. The AFO, whether metal or plastic, provides advantages of the arch support/UCBL orthosis and boot with maximum containment and a lever arm for support and substitution of the rocker mechanism. It offers enhanced stability and control because of its high proximal trim line. It has been an excellent solution for many patients with partial foot amputation and may be the prosthesis of choice for the active patient with a Chopart or Lisfranc amputation. Supramalleolar thermoplastic or laminated versions are fit with Tamarack (Blaine, MN) or Gillette (Gillette Children's Specialty Healthcare, St. Paul, MN)

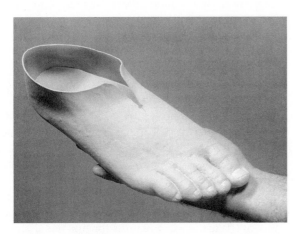

FIGURE 22-16 The life cast prosthesis provides excellent cosmesis with little or no biomechanical assistance. Without additional reinforcement a silicone slipper-style prosthesis does not provide adequate forefoot support.

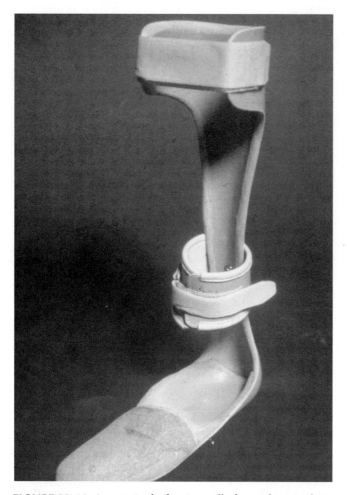

FIGURE 22-18 A posterior leaf spring andle-foot orthosis with toe filler and anterior strap is successful for many patients with partial foot amputation.

joints to provide free plantar and dorsiflexion motion. This biomechanical solution is popular for the higher activity level of midfoot amputations. In the presence of acute ankle pain, a patient with a Chopart amputation was successful with a rear-entry ground reaction force AFO with rigid ankle.

CASE EXAMPLE 2

An Individual with a Bilateral Chopart Amputation

A. E. is a 64-year-old man with a 23-year history of peripheral vascular disease, diabetes, and recurring foot ulcers. He underwent a Chopart amputation of his left lower extremity 7 years ago and has since successfully worn an orthopedic shoe with a toe filler. When needing to walk for long distances, A. E. uses a straight cane on the right to reduce distal anterior discomfort of his residual limb. Twelve months ago a neuropathic ulcer developed on his right plantar forefoot. Despite conservative management with felted foam and a Darco heel wedge shoe, the ulcer failed to heal and ultimately became infected and developed into osteomyelitis. He underwent the Chopart amputation without

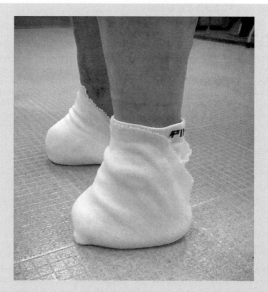

FIGURE 22-19 An individual with bilateral the Chopart amputation is able to stand steadily. Because of the short forefoot lever, however, the "sway envelope" for dynamic postural control is likely narrowed. Plantar flexion contracture, if present, would compromise stability and increase pressure at the distal plantar surface of the residual limb. In this illustration, the patient is wearing several layers of socks before putting on his prostheses.

complication, healed successfully, and now is able to stand unsupported without shoes or orthosis (Figure 22-19). He is able to ambulate in shoes with prosthetic fillers; however, he walks with a remarkably slow velocity and an observable shortened step length.

Questions to Consider
- Given his medical history, what concerns exist about the condition of his residual feet? What areas are most vulnerable to pressure from repetitive loading during walking in Chopart residual limbs?
- Are there muscle imbalances as a result of a Chopart amputation that place him at risk for development of contracture? How should joint excursion of his shortened feet be examined? What indicators of muscle performance are important to assess? What measures should be used to assess muscle function and strength? How should any impairments be addressed?
- How will his shortened feet affect his progression through the gait cycle? Will he have compromise of the first rocker from initial contact through loading response? Of the second rocker from loading response through midstance to terminal stance? Of the third rocker in terminal stance into preswing? Why will there be shortened step and stride length of the opposite swing limb?
- What are the major goals for prosthetic intervention for A. E.? What specific recommendations should be made and why? What is his prognosis for functional ambulation? Should an assistive device be recommended for long-term use? Why or why not? How should the efficacy of intervention be assessed?

Recommendations

After reviewing his overall gait performance and discussing his functional needs, the team recommends bilateral rocker bottom walking boots (Figure 22-20). (Walking boots are most often recommended for individuals with a single-limb Chopart amputation.) After prosthetic fitting with bilateral rocker boots, temporal parameters significantly improved over orthopedic shoes. Although A. E. had identical cadence with both conditions (shoe and boot), his step length dramatically increased and single-limb support time decreased when wearing the rocker boots. The overall result is a significantly higher gait velocity. Although he initially used a straight cane on the left for balance and to reduce anterior distal pressures of his newly amputated limb, A. E. is now able to ambulate functional distances without assistive devices. He uses his cane only when in crowds to "buy himself more space" and reduce the likelihood he will be bumped or jostled by others.

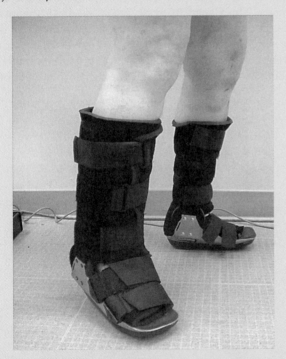

FIGURE 22-20 This individual with a bilateral Chopart amputation has been fit with bilateral rocker bottom walkers. The rocker bottom mimics second and third rockers of the gait cycle, whereas the extension of the anterior lever provides additional dynamic stability in gait. These combine to increase stride and step length for improved functional mobility and a more energy-efficient gait.

SYME AMPUTATION

In 1867, E. D. Hudson, the surgeon general of the United States, described the Syme amputation with a litany of superlatives: "No amputation of the inferior extremity can ever compare in value with that of the ankle joint originated by Mr. Syme. Twelve years of experience with that variety of operation have afforded me assurance that it is a concept which is complete in itself and not capable of being improved in its general character."[46]

The Syme, or tibiotarsal, amputation is a disarticulation of the talocrural joint. The forefoot is completely removed, but the fat pad of the heel is preserved and anchored to the distal tibia. This allows distal end bearing and some degree of ambulation without a prosthesis (Figures 22-21 and 22-3).[47] It gained popularity during the late 1800 s primarily because the likelihood of survival with this technique was substantially greater than with other surgical choices, given the reduced degree of sepsis and shock that occurred when bone was not severed.[48]

Two possible problems exist in amputations at the Syme level: migration of the distal heel pad (which may be surgically avoidable) and poor cosmetic result (which can sometimes be partially addressed by removal of the malleoli). For a positive outcome, the vascular supply must be adequate to ensure healing. The resurgence of popularity of the Syme amputation today is from an increased awareness of its energy efficiency in gait compared with transtibial levels as well as improved vascular evaluation techniques and medical procedures that increase the likelihood of more distal primary wound healing.[49,50] In addition, the dramatic weight-bearing potential of

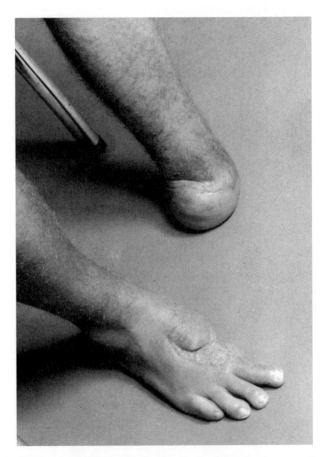

FIGURE 22-21 This individual has had a Syme-level amputation of the left lower extremity and a first ray (hallux) resection in the right lower extremity. Early weight-bearing before prosthetic fitting can aggravate migration of the heel pad after the Syme amputation, even though migration is primarily a function of surgical technique.

a well-performed Syme surgery (with or without a prosthesis) has always been considered.[51] Pressure-sensitive areas of the Syme residual limb include the tibial crest, lateral tibial flair, fibula head, and the bony prominence around the distal expansion.[52,53] Pressure-tolerant areas include the midpatella tendon, medial tibial flair, and anterior tibialis.

Postoperative Care: Walking Casts

To avoid medial migration of the heel pad in the postoperative period, gait training and other therapy that involve weight bearing should be encouraged only after delivery of the prosthesis. The prosthesis is designed to hold the ankle and bulbous distal residual in an appropriate relation. A fully mature residual limb is less likely to displace. Early prosthetic fitting may involve a definitive prosthesis or a temporary walking cast with a patten bottom (Figure 22-22). The temporary walking cast may be especially preferred if the patient has edema, is obese, or has other medical conditions in which significant volume loss is anticipated. The initial walking cast should be applied as soon as the sutures have been removed, usually within 2 weeks of surgery. The successful application of the Syme walking cast requires a more thorough knowledge base in prosthetics than might be readily appreciated. Application of a walking cast should be done by a clinician with a solid prosthetic background.

Prosthetic Management

The prosthesis for the Syme amputation must be strong enough at the ankle section to withstand the forces of tension and compression that are produced by the long tibial lever arm throughout the gait cycle and at the same time provide an acceptable degree of cosmesis over the bulbous expansion at the ankle. All prosthetic designs strive to encompass

the tibial section above the distal expansion firmly and still permit donning and doffing. Although prostheses designed for Syme amputations may be appropriate for Pirogoff and Boyd amputations, use of such prostheses requires that a lift be placed on the contralateral shoe to achieve bilateral limb length symmetry.

Before World War II, most patients with Syme amputations were fit with anterior lacing wooden sockets or leather sockets supported by a superstructure of heavy medial and lateral steel sidebars.[53,54] The prostheses most frequently fabricated today include the Canadian, medial opening, sleeve suspension, and flexible wall (bladder) designs.

Canadian Syme Prostheses

The *Canadian Syme prosthesis* design was introduced during the 1950s as the first major improvement over the traditional steel-reinforced leather (Figure 22-23).[55-58] When viewing the ankle in the coronal plane, no obvious build-ups, windows, or hardware is present to increase the ankle diameter. The Canadian Syme prosthesis has a removable posterior panel to facilitate donning and doffing. This donning window extends from the apex of the distal expansion, moving proximal as far as necessary to provide clearance for the bulbous end.[59] Breakage may be higher than with other

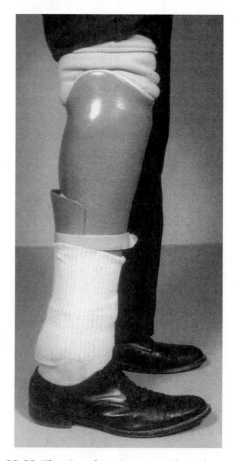

FIGURE 22-23 The Canadian Syme prosthesis has a posterior opening access panel that diminishes its strength at the ankle. It may be inappropriate for heavy-duty wearers.

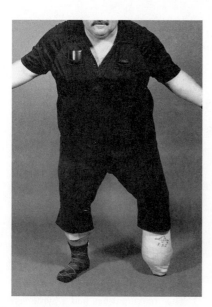

FIGURE 22-22 The patten bottom in a walking cast is used when the clinic team anticipates gross volume changes in a patient with a Syme amputation.

Syme prostheses because the ankle area, which undergoes the most compression and tension during ambulation, is weakened by the window cutout around the ankle in the posterior region. Modern carbon fiber and acrylic lamination materials and techniques have aided in meeting this challenge.[60,61] The Canadian prosthesis is a relatively cosmetic approach, but more recent options have limited its use.

Medial Opening Syme Prostheses

The *medial opening Syme prosthesis,* also known as the *Veterans Administration Prosthetic Center Syme prosthesis,* followed the introduction of the Canadian Syme prosthesis. Developed at the New York City Veterans Administration Medical Center in 1959,[62] it has a removable donning door that extends proximally from the distal expansion to a level approximately two thirds of the height of the tibial section on the medial side (Figure 22-24).[63] Like the Canadian design, the medial opening prosthesis is relatively cosmetic at the ankle and compares favorably with the Canadian design. The medial placement of the donning panel provides much more opportunity for anteroposterior strengthening of the prosthesis. All other factors being equal, this design is stronger than the Canadian and is the approach of choice for many patients with The Syme amputation.

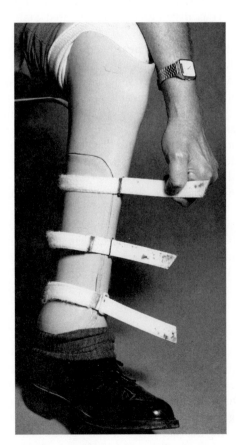

FIGURE 22-24 The Veterans Administration Prosthetic Center Syme prosthesis has a medial opening window, and has long been a popular approach to fitting the the Syme amputation.

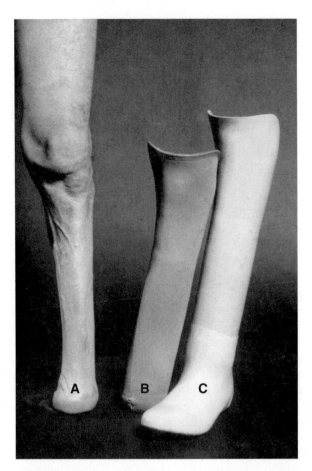

FIGURE 22-25 A, A mature Syme residual limb. The sleeve suspension Syme prosthesis has a full-length liner (**B**) that slips into the prosthetic socket (**C**). This design accommodates adjustments well. It offers excellent strength at the cost of cosmesis and is an excellent option for the obese or heavy-duty wearer.

Sleeve Suspension Syme Prostheses

The *sleeve suspension Syme prosthesis* is sometimes referred to as the *stovepipe Syme prosthesis* because of the cylindrical appearance of its removable liner (Figure 22-25). It is constructed with an inner flexible insert or sleeve that has filler material in the areas just proximal to the distal expansion.[64,65] Before slipping into the outer shell or socket, the wearer first pulls on the flexible liner.[66] The outside sleeve then telescopes within the outer prosthetic shell. In another version the leather and foam inner sleeve does not cover the entire residual limb but wraps around the leg and fills up the void areas above the expansion.[67] The sleeve suspension prosthesis is bulky and not very cosmetic, but its strength is significantly better because no window is present to create a structural weakness. It is often chosen for the obese or very heavy-duty wearer or for the patient with recurring prosthetic breakage with other designs. It is more adjustable and forgiving than the other Syme designs and is often chosen when major fitting problems are anticipated.

Expandable Wall Prostheses

The *flexible,* *expandable wall,* and *bladder Syme prostheses,* of which several varieties are available, vary more by materials used than by mechanism of action. All are based on the concept of an inner socket wall just proximal to the distal expansion that is elastic or expandable enough to allow entry of the limb into the prosthesis and still provide a level of total contact around the ankle once donned.[68,69] This design normally requires a double prosthetic wall. The original bladder Syme prosthesis, described by Marx[70] in 1969, obtained expansion by using flexible polyester resin in the neck area. The more recent Rancho Syme prosthesis uses a flexible inner socket, supported by a frame or superstructure of laminated thermosetting plastic. The use of flexible thermosetting plastics and silicone elastomer for expandable wall sockets has gradually eclipsed the use of Surlyn (DuPont, Wilmington, DE) and other thermoplastics as a material of choice for the inner liner. Expandable wall Syme prostheses are slightly bulkier and less cosmetic at the ankle than their Canadian or medial opening counterparts because they require a flexible inner socket and a rigid exterior superstructure. The fabrication process is more involved, and fitting adjustments to the flexible inner socket can be difficult. Creating either a silicone elastomer or a Surlyn inner socket flexible enough for comfortable donning and doffing may significantly limit its durability. The Syme residual limb presents greater pressure distribution challenges to a prosthetist than do other types of lower-limb prosthetics. A test socket is especially recommended for all Syme prostheses. Because the act of donning and doffing with this system is relatively simple, it may be the prosthesis of choice for patients with upper limb dysfunction or cognitive impairment.

Tucker-Winnipeg Syme Prostheses

The *Tucker-Winnipeg Syme prosthesis*, rarely seen in the United States, ignores the traditional requirement of comprehensive total contact by introducing lateral and medial donning slots.[71] The design is well suited for children. It is contraindicated for patients with severe vascular disease and for others who are prone to window edema. A loss of total contact can also affect proprioception and control of the prosthesis. In general, the method permits a prosthesis that is relatively cosmetic, easy to don, and not prone to the noises that are sometimes created by rubbing at the window covers of the medial opening and Canadian Syme prostheses.

Prosthetic Feet for Syme Prostheses

One of the challenges in selecting prosthetic components for patients with a Syme amputation is fitting a prosthetic foot and ankle bolt within the very limited space under the residual limb while still maintaining equal leg lengths and a level pelvis. The rare exception to this is when bilateral ankle disarticulation has occurred; Syme bilaterality fits many more choices of foot designs. When there is unilateral Syme amputation, great care must be given to the minimal amount of space available between the distal end and shoe so that a heel lift on the contralateral side would not be necessary.

Determining the Prosthetic Clearance Value

In determining whether a particular Syme's foot can accommodate a patient, the available space between the distal end of the residual limb and the floor is measured with the pelvis level, and the anatomical clearance value is derived. Most Syme feet are attached to the socket by a foot bolt screwed upward from below the prosthetic heel into a Syme nut, a threaded disk that is laminated into the socket. The nut, shaped to approximately match the contours of the distal residual limb, is approximately ⅝ inches tall, and this height must be considered when constructing the prosthesis. In addition, the typical Syme foot has a liner with distal end thickness which is ⅛- to ¼-inch thick. To determine the applicability of a particular foot for a patient the space between the bottom of the heel of the foot and the top of the foot is added to height of the Syme nut and the liner and end-pad thickness. This measurement is the prosthetic clearance value.

Nonarticulating Syme Feet

Many prosthetic feet used for transtibial amputation have been adapted for the Syme amputation. The first was the *solid-ankle, cushion-heel* (SACH) foot, patented in 1863 by Marks and further developed at the University of California at Berkeley after World War II. It was introduced as a component of the Canadian Syme prosthesis in the 1950s. The Syme SACH is distributed in the United States primarily by Kingsley (Kingsley, Costa Mesa, CA). It is available in a regular men's shoe heel height and a running shoe heel height.

The SACH foot design simulates plantar flexion as the patient rolls over a compressible heel, but because of a rigid wooden (typically maple) keel, it is neither flexible nor elastic in late stance. The SACH-type Syme foot was the historical foot of choice for patients with a Syme amputation in previous decades, and remains a highly durable, cost-effective foot design today.

The *stationary-ankle flexible-endoskeletal* (SAFE) Syme foot has the advantage of providing a modest inversion and eversion component of motion, through elasticity of the forefoot, and is useful for uneven terrain ambulation. Not including the thickness of the Syme's nut, the SAFE II (Campbell-Childs, White City, OR) Syme foot requires 1⅜ inches of space between the distal end and the floor or shoe with pelvis leveled.

Dynamic Response Syme Feet

In the last decade a variety of dynamic response foot designs have emerged for more active Syme walkers. The Impulse Syme's Foot (Ohio Willow Wood, Mt. Sterling, OH) has a Kevlar (DuPont, Wilmington, DE) keel with carbon deflection toe-spring plates and a weight limit of up to 250 lb (113 kg). The toe spring is a carbon-epoxy composite. A unique manufacturing technique allows carbon fibers to be optimal oriented and avoid wrinkling, buckling, and deformation. The most interesting part of the foot is alignment adjustability. Ohio Willow Wood also has a Carbon Copy II Syme foot available in two heel heights and with all the toe resistances and sizes of the standard (non-Syme) Carbon Copy II. The Carbon Copy II is available with a medium heel density for patient weights up to 250 lb (113 kg).

The Steplite Foot (Kingsley) provides a compressible heel design with the buoyancy of a carbon keel. It is quite durable and applicable to almost every patient with a Syme amputation because it requires only 1⅝ inches of prosthetic clearance value. That accounts for 1 inch for the foot itself and ⅝ inch for the nut and socket thickness. The low-profile version accommodates a typical man's heel height. The "Strider" is made for a man's running shoe, and "Flattie" is a narrow foot for females that accommodates a flat heel. The Steplite provides a buoyant elastic forefoot but, like many Syme feet, is limited in its heel compression.

Ossur (Aliso Viejo, CA) offers a low-profile carbon Syme foot version for a very active prosthetic wearer weighing up to 285 lb (129 kg). The same foot can be worn by a low-activity amputee weighing up to 365 lb (165.5 kg). The Ossur Low Profile requires 2 inches of clearance from the floor to the distal end of the socket and is designed with a flexible double-spring keel. It uses a fenestrated heel that allows greater compression, thus reducing shock. The upper spring bumper is coated with Teflon (DuPont), which reduces squeaks, a characteristic not uncommon to feet with more than one keel in the forefoot. Another Syme foot that may be used for patients up to 500 lbs (227 kg) is the Vari-Flex (Ossur) which requires only 1¾ inches of space under the socket and is attached using epoxy filler and lamination.

Another dynamic elastic foot choice for the active individual is the Seattle Light Foot (Seattle Orthopedic Group, Seattle, WA).

Almost all prosthetic feet for Syme prostheses have ankles that are essentially locked. This characteristics results in increased work for the quadriceps for controlled knee flexion during loading response. Incorporation of several degrees of adjustable articulated plantar flexion (at the risk of increasing the weight of the prosthesis) might improve function for certain patients.

Alignment Issues

With most prosthetic feet, the small area between the distal residual limb and floor limits the prosthetist's ability to refine the special relation between the socket and foot in the dynamic alignment phase. Adjustable alignment devices, similar to those available for transtibial prostheses, have historically not been compact enough to fit in the available space between the prosthetic foot and the end of the socket. Two component options have been introduced with the goal of addressing this limitation.

A novel functional alignment device for the Impulse Syme available from Ohio Willow Wood permits some degree of dynamic alignment by enabling the prosthetist to adjust the angular positions of the foot during the fitting process. This Impulse Syme socket adapter kit (Figure 22-26) allows angular adjustments during the dynamic alignment phase of between 4 and 8 degrees,

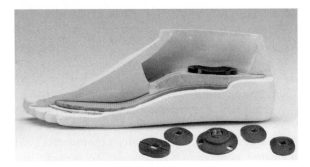

FIGURE 22-26 The Impulse Foot is a dynamic response foot system for Syme prostheses. This foot is particularly useful when prosthetic clearance value is limited. The adaptable design allows the prosthetist to fine tune during the dynamic alignment process to achieve a gait pattern that is energy efficient and cosmetic. (Photo courtesy Ohio Willow-Wood, Inc., Mt. Sterling, Ohio.)

depending on the direction. In addition, ⅛-inch carbon spacers allow for length additions up to ⅜ inch. It is used with a 1-inch Syme "dished" nut contoured to interface with the distal end of the limb.

The SL Profile and the Lo Rider Syme feet (Otto Bock, Minneapolis, MN) provide angular adjustability by a pyramid. Unfortunately, the height of the pyramid may preclude their use on many patients with a Syme amputation. The newest and very promising addition is the 1 C20 ProSyme's (Otto Bock), which can be fit on most patients and is a moderately dynamic urethane carbon fiber foot for Syme amputees up to 275 lb (125 kg) (Figure 22-27). It has a wide range of alignment adjustability as well as heel height changes.

Placing the Syme foot in slight dorsiflexion relative to the shin section mimics normal gait patterns, encourages a smooth cosmetic and energy-efficient rollover during stance phase, and optimizes the weight-bearing potential of the socket contours. For individuals with quadriceps weakness, the dorsiflexion angle can be reduced to minimize excessive

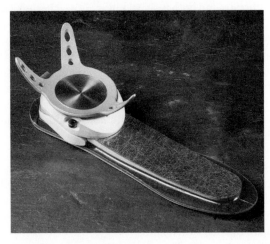

FIGURE 22-27 The IC20 Pro Symes, similar to the Impulse, is unique in its alignment adjustability. Angular and linear alignment as well as heel height adjustments make it an exceptional choice. (Photo courtesy Otto Bock, Minneapolis, Minn.)

demands on the quadriceps. The telltale clinical sign of excessive demand is trembling of the knee during midstance. Although early alignment recommendations placed optimal initial dorsiflexion up to 12 to 15 degrees, current practice is to set the foot at a smaller angle of approximately 5 degrees.[72] The long Syme residual limb does not easily accommodate itself, cosmetically or functionally, to more than 5 degrees of dorsiflexion.

Alignment can be significantly compromised when knee flexion contracture is present. To prevent breakage and premature wear from the anterior lever arm, the degree of anterior (linear) displacement of the socket over the foot is generally reduced from that of a transtibial prosthesis.

The Syme socket is positioned in an angle of adduction that matches the anatomical adduction angle of the tibia. The adduction of the socket should be positioned to create as smooth a transition as possible at the ankle and knee so that the prosthetic foot rolls over with the sole flat on the floor. The optimal spatial relation in the coronal plane is one that creates a slight varus moment. Socket adduction angle, foot eversion angle, and linear displacement affect the external varus moment at the knee during midstance. For an efficient and cosmetic gait, the knee must displace approximately 12 mm laterally at midstance. Insufficient displacement implicates malalignment, most often at an inadequate eversion angle. Excessive displacement may be the result of malalignment or lateral collateral ligament laxity at the knee. The most successful strategy to address chronic weight-bearing ulceration at the knee that has not responded to a silicone liner, or to address major laxity of the collateral ligaments, is the addition of orthotic components (external knee joints and a thigh lacer) to provide extra support and protection.

CASE EXAMPLE 3

A Patient with Bilateral Dysvascular Syme Amputation

H. P. is a 56-year-old man with an 18-year history of insulin-controlled diabetes. Eight years ago, a left hallux ray resection failed to heal and became infected, necessitating a left Syme amputation. After healing, he became proficient with a Syme prosthesis, ambulating functional distances without assistive devices. One year ago a large neuropathic wound developed under the second through fourth metatarsal heads of his right foot. The wound failed to heal despite several trials of total contact casting. H. P. and his vascular surgeon agreed that a Syme amputation on the right would improve his functional status and allow him to return to work as a junior high school teacher and baseball coach. Amputation occurred 7 months ago, and both residual limbs are well healed. He has Rancho-style expandable wall Syme prostheses with SACH feet (Figure 22-28). He has been on an exercise program and is walking 2 miles per day. He ambulates at a relatively high speed (120 steps/min) and can walk long distances (more than 1 mile) at that velocity. He has poor socket fit wearing 10-ply socks. Stress cracks can be seen on the foot. The team agrees that a change in prosthetic design and components would improve his function and satisfaction.

Questions to Consider
- Given his medical history, what concerns exist about the condition of his residual feet? What areas are most vulnerable to pressures from repetitive loading during walking in Syme residual limbs?
- What types of muscle performance at his knee and hip are important to assess? What measures should be used to assess muscle function and strength? How will any impairments be addressed?

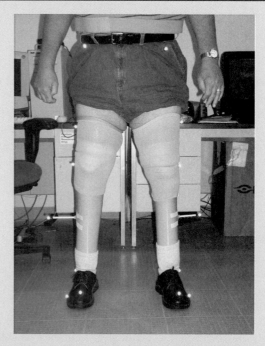

FIGURE 22-28 This patient is wearing bilateral Rancho-style expandable wall Syme prostheses with solid-ankle, cushion-heel feet. Note the wide diameter at the ankle, necessary to accommodate the bulbous distal residual limb during donning. His prostheses incorporate a patellar tendon-bearing design at the knee, and he wears neoprene suspension sleeves as auxiliary suspension. Note also the widened base of support that he has adopted to enhance stability in quiet standing. Reflective markers have been placed at the pelvis, greater trochanter, lateral lower thigh, lateral prosthesis, lateral malleolus, and the shoe in preparation for comprehensive gait analysis.

- How does the Syme amputation affect progression through the gait cycle? How might a prosthesis substitute for compromise of the first rocker from initial contact through loading response? Of the second rocker from loading response through midstance to terminal stance? Of the third rocker in terminal stance into preswing? How might the Syme amputation affect step and stride length of the opposite swing limb?
- What are the major goals for prosthetic intervention for H. P.? What specific recommendations should be made for socket design, suspension, and prosthetic feet? What options should be chosen from among those available? What is his prognosis for functional ambulation? Is an assistive device recommended for long-term use? Why or why not? How should the efficacy of intervention be assessed?

Recommendations

The clinical team determines H. P. is a candidate for a dynamic response foot and a design consistent with an active lifestyle. The paying agency will want to know the item description as well as the associated Medicare code. For example, this amputee is provided with a Syme's prosthesis (L5050), test socket (L5618), acrylic socket (L5629), medial opening window (L5636), expandable wall (Rancho style) (L5630), extended patellar-tendon bearing brim design socket (L5632), total contact (L5637), suspension sleeve (L5685), ultralight construction (L5940), Freedom Innovation FS-2000 Low Profile Foot (L5981) and alignable system (L5910), and six prosthetic socks for each limb (Figure 22-29). After delivery of the limbs, H. P. reports immediate improvement of long-distance walking.

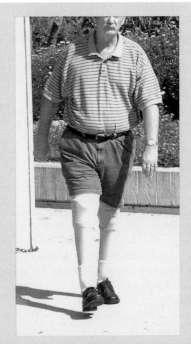

FIGURE 22-29 The same individual as in Figure 22-28 after receiving his new prostheses with dynamic response feet. Distance between heels has been reduced in both standing and walking, stride length has increased substantially, and he reports greater comfort and ease in walking long distances required for his job and leisure activities.

SUMMARY

This chapter explored the options for prosthetic management for patients with partial foot and Syme amputations. Because of the variability in surgical procedures, condition of the residual limb, and altered biomechanics of the residual limb in gait, no single best option exists for prosthetic design. Instead, the characteristics of each patient (weight, skin condition, desired activity level, and length of residual limb) must be carefully considered in prosthetic prescription. The goal is to find the best match of the person's status and needs from the growing array of prosthetic design options for the partial foot and Syme amputations. This places an increasing demand on the knowledge base of medical professionals. More than ever, the physician, physical therapist, and prosthetist are challenged to function as a cohesive team, drawing on each other's strengths to achieve the best possible outcome for each patient.

REFERENCES

1. Herodotus. *Library IX, 37, Loeb Classical Edition*. Vol 4. London: Heinemann; 1924.
2. Bowker JH. Partial foot and Syme amputations—an overview. *Clin Prosthet Orthot*. 1988;12(1):10–13.
3. Bahler A. The biomechanics of the foot. *Clin Prosthet Orthot*. 1986;10(1):8–14.
4. Frankovitch KF, Farrell WJ. Syme and Boyd amputations in children. *ICIB J Assoc Childrens Prosthet Orthot Clin*. 1984;19(3):61.
5. Oglesby DG, Tablada C. The child amputee: lower limb deficiencies: prosthetic and orthotic management. In: American Academy of Orthopaedic Surgeons, eds. *Atlas of Limb Prosthetics*. 2nd ed. St. Louis: Mosby; 1992:837.
6. Burgess EM. Prevention and correction of fixed equinus deformity in mid-foot amputations. *Bull Prosthet Res*. 1966;10(5):45–47.
7. Pritham CH. Partial foot amputation—a case study. *Clin Prosthet Orthot*. 1977;1(3):5–7.
8. Wagner FW. Partial Foot Amputations. In: American Academy of Orthopaedic Surgeons, eds. *Atlas of Limb Prosthetics*. St. Louis: Mosby; 1981:315–325.
9. Wilson AB. Partial foot amputation results of the questionnaire survey. *Newsletter Prosthet Orthot Clin*. 1977;1(4):1–3.
10. Kay HW. Limb deficits no bar to record performance. *Int Clin Info Bull*. 1970;10(3):17.
11. Dorostkar M, Ayyappa E, Perry J. *Gait Mechanics of the Partial Foot Amputee, Rehabilitation Research & Development Final Report*. Project #A861-RA -2000. Long Beach, CA: VA National Prosthetic Gait Laboratory; July 11, 1999.
12. Dorostkar M, Ayyappa E, Perry J. *Gait Mechanics of the Partial Foot Amputee*, Project #A861-RA. JRRD Progress Reports. Vol 35. Long Beach, CA: VA National Prosthetics Gait Laboratory, July 1998:17–18.
13. Dorostkar M, Ayyappa E, Perry J. *Gait Mechanics of the Partial Foot Amputee*. Project #A861-RA. JRRD Progress Reports. Vol 36. Long Beach, CA: VA National Prosthetics Gait Laboratory, July 1999.

14. Ayyappa E, Moinzadeh H, Friedman J. Gait Characteristics of the Partial Foot Amputee. In: *Proceedings of the 21st annual meeting and scientific symposium of the American Academy of Orthotists and Prosthetists*. New Orleans, March 21–25, 1995.

15. Pinzur MS, Gold J, Schwartz D, et al. Energy demands for walking in dysvascular amputees as related to the level of amputation. *Orthopedics*. 1992;15(9):1033–1037.

16. New York University Post Graduate Medical School. *Lower Limb Prosthetics*. New York: New York University; 1979.

17. Enna CD, Brand PW, Reed JK, Welch D. The orthotic care of the denervated foot in Hansen's disease. *Orthot Prosthet*. 1976;30(1):33–39.

18. Menon PBM. A new type of protective footwear for anesthetic feet. *Int Soc Prosthet Orthot Bull*. 1976;18:4.

19. Veterans Administration Prosthetics Center. Semiannual report of the VA Prosthetics Center. *Bull Prosthet Res*. 1965;10(3):142–146.

20. Marks AA. *Manual of Artificial Limbs*. New York: AA Marks; 1931.

21. Marks GE. *A Treatise on Artificial Limbs with Rubber Hands and Feet*. New York: AA Marks; 1888.

22. American Academy of Orthopaedic Surgeons. *Orthopedic Appliance Atlas. Vol 2: Artificial Limbs*. Ann Arbor, MI: J.W. Edwards; 1960.

23. Cestaro JM. Comments on partial foot amputations. *Newslett Prosthet Orthot Clin*. 1977;1(3):7.

24. Levy SE. Total contact restoration prosthesis for partial foot amputations. *Orthot Prosthet*. 1961;15(1):34–44.

25. Lunsford T. Partial foot amputations: prosthetic and orthotic management. In: American Academy of Orthopaedic Surgeons, eds. *Atlas of Limb Prosthetics*. St. Louis: Mosby; 1981:320–325.

26. Staros A, Peizer E. Veterans Administration Prosthetic Center research report. *Bull Prosthet Res*. 1969;10(12):340–342.

27. Zamosky I. Shoes and their modifications. In: Light S, Kampuetz H, eds. *Orthotics Etcetera*. 2nd ed. Baltimore: Williams & Wilkins; 1980:368–431.

28. Potter JW, Stockwell JE. Custom foamed toe filler for amputation of the forefoot. *Orthot Prosthet*. 1974;28(3):57–60.

29. Young RD. Functional positioning toe restoration. *Orthot Prosthet*. 1985;39(3):57–59.

30. Young RD. Special Chopart prosthesis with custom molded foot. *Orthot Prosthet*. 1984;38(1):79–85.

31. Platts RGS, Knight S, Jakins I. Shoe inserts for small deformed feet. *Prosthet Orthot Int*. 1982;6(2):108–110.

32. Henderson WH, Campbell JW. UC-BL shoe insert, casting and fabrication. *Bull Prosthet Res*. 1969;10(11):215–235.

33. Inman VT. UC-BL dual axis ankle control system and UC-BL shoe insert; biomechanical considerations. *Bull Prosthet Res*. 1969;10(11):130–145.

34. Quigley MJ. The present use of the UCBL foot orthosis. *Orthot Prosthet*. 1974;28(4):59–63.

35. Stills M. Partial foot prosthesis/orthosis. *Clin Prosthet Orthot*. 1988;12(1):14–18.

36. Imler CD. Imler partial foot prosthesis IPFP—the Chicago boot. *Orthot Prosthet*. 1985;39(3):53–56.

37. Imler CD. Imler partial foot prosthesis IPFP "Chicago boot." *Clin Prosthet Orthot*. 1988;12(1):24–28.

38. Wilson MT. Clinical application of TRV elastomer. *Orthot Prosthet*. 1979;33(4):23–29.

39. Fillauer K. A prosthesis for foot amputation near the tarsal-metatarsal junction. *Orthot Prosthet*. 1976;30(3):9–12.

40. Pullen JJ. A low profile pediatric partial foot. *Prosthet Orthot Int*. 1987;11(3):137–138.

41. Rubin G, Danisi M. A functional partial-foot prosthesis. *ISPO Bull*. 1972;3(7):6.

42. Collins JN. A partial foot prosthesis for the transmetatarsal level. *Clin Prosthet Orthot*. 1988;12(1):19–23.

43. Rubin G, Danisi M. Functional partial-foot prosthesis. *Bull Prosthet Res*. 1971;10(16):149–152.

44. Staros A, Goralnik B. Lower limb prosthetic systems. In: American Academy of Orthopaedic Surgeons, eds. *Atlas of Limb Prosthetics*. St. Louis: Mosby; 1981:293–295.

45. LaTorre R. The total contact partial foot prosthesis. *Clin Prosthet Orthot*. 1987–1988;12(1):29–32.

46. Hudson ED. *Mechanical Surgery; Artificial Limbs, Apparatus for Resections, by U.S. Soldiers*. New York: Commission of the Surgeon-General; 1867 (Library of Congress Call No. RD 756.H86).

47. Jansen K. Amputation—principles and methods. *Bull Prosthet Res*. 1965;10(4):19–20.

48. Harris RI. *The History and Development of the Syme's Amputation: Selected Articles from Artificial Limbs*. Huntington, NY: Krieger; 1970.

49. Burgess EM, Romano RL, Zettl JH. *The Management of Lower-Extremity Amputations*. Washington, DC: U.S. Government Printing Office; 1969.

50. Wagner FW. The Syme amputation: surgical procedures. In: American Academy of Orthopaedic Surgeons, eds. *Atlas of Limb Prosthetics*. St. Louis: Mosby; 1981:326–334.

51. Quigley M. The Rancho Syme prosthesis with the Regnell foot. *Clin Prosthet Orthot*. 1988;12(1):33–40.

52. Hanger HB. *The Syme and Chopart Prostheses*. Chicago: Northwestern University Prosthetic-Orthotic Center; 1965.

53. Wilson AB. Prostheses for Syme amputation. *Artif Limbs*. 1961;61(1):52–75.

54. Leimkuehler J. Syme's prosthesis—a brief review and a new fabrication technique. *Orthot Prosthet*. 1980;34(4):3–12.

55. Foort J. The Canadian type Syme prosthesis. *UCBL Technical Reports*. 1956;30:75–76.

56. Murphy EF. Lower extremity components. In: American Academy of Orthopaedic Surgeons, eds. *Orthopedic Appliance Atlas. Vol 2*. Ann Arbor, MI: J.W. Edwards; 1960:212–217.

57. Voner R. The Syme amputation: prosthetic management. In: American Academy of Orthopaedic Surgeons, eds. *Atlas of Limb Prosthetics*. St. Louis: Mosby; 1981:334–340.

58. Boccius CS. The plastic Syme prosthesis in Canada. *Artif Limbs*. 1961;6(1):86–89.

59. Department of Veterans Affairs. *Syme Amputation and Prosthesis*. Toronto: Department of Veterans Affairs, Prosthetic Services Centre; 1954.

60. Dankmeyer CH, Doshi R, Alban CR. Adding strength to the Syme prosthesis. *Orthot Prosthet*. 1974;28(3):3–7.

61. Radcliffe CW. *The Biomechanics of the Syme Prosthesis: Selected Articles from Artificial Limbs*. Huntington, NY: Krieger; 1970.

62. Schwartz RE, Bohne WO, Kramer HE. Prosthetic management of below knee amputation with flexion contracture in the child. *J Assoc Childrens Prosthet-Orthot Clin*. 1986;21(1):8–10.

63. Iuliucci L, Degaetano R. *V.A.P.C. Technique for Fabricating a Plastic Syme Prosthesis with Medial Opening*. New York: New York University Medical School; 1969.

64. Byers JL. Fabrication of Cordo, Plastizote, or Pelite removable liner for closed Syme sockets. *Bull Prosthet Res*. 1972;10(18):182–188.

65. Warner R, Daniel R, Lesswing A. Another new prosthetic approach for the Syme's amputation. *Int Clin Info Bull*. 1972;12(1):7–10.

66. Byers JL. The closed Syme socket with removable liner. *ISPO Bull.* 1973;7:4–5.

67. McFarlen JM. The Syme prosthesis. *Orthot Prosthet.* 1966; 20(3):23–27.

68. Eckhardt AL, Enneberg H. The use of a Silastic liner in the Syme's prosthesis. *Int Clin Info Bull.* 1970;9(6):1–4.

69. Meyer LC, Bailey HL, Friddle D. An improved prosthesis for fitting the ankle-disarticulation amputee. *Int Clin Info Bull.* 1970;9(6):11–15.

70. Marx HW. An innovation in Syme prosthetics. *Orthot Prosthet.* 1969;23(3):131–141.

71. Lyttle D. Tucker-Syme prosthetic fitting in young people. *Int Clin Info Bull.* 1984;19(3):62.

72. Hanger of England. *Prosthesis for Below-Knee Amputation—Roelite Instruction Manual.* Bath, UK: Trowbridges; 1982.

23

Transtibial Prosthetics

DAVID KNAPP

LEARNING OBJECTIVES

On completion of this chapter, the reader will be able to do the following:

1. Describe the principles underlying current transtibial socket design.
2. Discuss the pros and cons of the various options for prosthetic suspension.
3. Identify key weight-tolerant and pressure-intolerant surfaces of a typical transtibial residual limb.
4. Identify key determinants of appropriate transtibial prosthetic alignment.
5. Recognize and differentiate the various factors that may lead to transtibial prosthetic gait deviations.
6. Suggest appropriate strategies to address transtibial gait deviations.

PROSTHETIC EVALUATION

When evaluating a candidate for transtibial prosthesis, a comprehensive physical examination that includes a detailed history interview is essential. The typical physical examination includes: inspection, palpation, evaluation of muscle performance—manual muscle testing (MMT); and active and passive range of motion (ROM) testing—sensory testing, and skin integrity assessment. The interview assesses the individual's cognitive level, age, health history, vocation, avocation, and home living status. This is also an ideal time to discuss rehabilitation goals with the individual and the rest of the clinical team. Setting realistic goals that are challenging but offer opportunities for incremental victories can go a long way toward reaching a successful outcome. Each member of the clinical team—therapist, physician, person with amputation, and prosthetist—has information and input that is useful in the rehabilitation process. The best outcome will be the result of a collaborative endeavor involving all the team members. There are no hard-and-fast rules that determine the rehabilitation potential; the decision to move ahead with prosthetic fitting is made on an individual basis.

When determining prosthetic candidacy, the individual's motivation and belief that they are capable of walking are determinant factors. The rehabilitation process will require both physical and mental effort, and sometimes involve working through pain and discomfort. When persons with amputation have the desire and drive to walk again, there is very little the team can do to dissuade them. Likewise, if the person does not believe that walking might be possible, efforts to enhance recovery may be in vain. Involving the person with recent amputation in an amputee support group, or requesting a peer visitor from a local prosthetist, can provide some inspiration and encouragement that therapists, family members, or prosthetist's who have not experienced amputation simply cannot offer. Peer visitors are individuals of similar age, gender, and amputation level that have been through the rehabilitation process and have successfully reintegrated into the communities (work, leisure, social) that are important to them. Peer visitors are available to spend time with those with recent amputation and share their first-hand experiences. The Internet hosts a variety of organizations that provide support and information for persons new to amputation and prosthetic use, and is a good resource to find local groups that may be beneficial.

Because amputation is often the result of trauma or disease, there are often comorbidities that complicate the overall management of the person with amputation. There are a variety of options available to the prosthetist to provide a functional prosthesis, even when presented with a residual limb that is not ideal. Mild to moderate knee flexion contractures and weakness, for example, may be accommodated for by altering the alignment of the prosthesis. Skin issues, such as adherent scarring and eczema, can be addressed by selecting the appropriate interface material., Pressure on skin and soft tissue over prominent bones can be relieved by altering the socket shape. There are also prosthetic options for those with severe upper-limb dysfunction that will enable the individual to don and doff his or her prostheses independently. It is only with careful consideration of the person's complete profile that the clinical team can recommend the components and design that will lead to the most optimal prosthetic outcomes.

This clinical analysis includes choosing the features that are most appropriate for the individual's current status and their anticipated level of function. The most appropriate prosthesis is the prosthesis that suits the person's individual requirements. One size does not fit all: the ideal prosthesis for one person may be completely useless to another.

Prosthetic design is often a compromise of weight versus function. Adding features that may seldom be used will increase the weight and maintenance requirements of the device. Increased weight leads to increased energy expenditure and premature fatigue.[1] On the other hand, exclusion of features that the person will need on a regular basis may lead to excessive stresses on the limb, premature component wear or breakdown, and inefficient gait. The clinical team should agree on the indivdual's functional goals so that the prosthesis can be designed to meet them. With the materials and fabrication techniques that are available to contemporary prosthetists, those using a prosthesis can walk farther, with greater a energy efficiency than ever before.

Generally speaking, persons who undergo transtibial amputations are likely to return to their previous level of function.[2] Those with dysvascular disease, or those who have additional comorbidities because of injury or disease need special consideration when developing their rehabilitation goals and anticipated level of function. The Center for Medicare Services created a hierarchical system to classify the functional potential of persons with lower limb amputations. This system, referred to by "K-levels," is summarized in Table 23-1.[3] Note that each functional level uses the phrase "has the ability or potential" in the description. This highlights the fact that individuals cannot reach their full potential until their prosthesis is provided and rehabilitation has been successful. For certain benefits to be covered under Medicare, the individual must be certified by his or her prosthetist and physician with the appropriate K-level. This is to prevent prescription of prosthesis with costly components that person will not be able to manage or use effectively.

EARLY PROSTHETIC MANAGEMENT

Goals for postoperative management of the transtibial amputee include (a) to maintain full ROM of the hip and knee, (b) to facilitate rapid healing of the suture line, (c) to maintain or improve cardiovascular and pulmonary conditioning, (d) to enhance static and dynamic balance; and (e) to faciltiate functional strength in the remaining musculature.[4] Table 23-2 breaks the lifelong rehabilitation of the amputee down into nine distinct stages and summarizes the goals for each stage.

TABLE 23-1 *Classification of Functional Potential of Patients with Lower-Limb Amputations*

K-Level	Medicare Functional Classification Level
K0	The patient does not have the ability or potential to ambulate or transfer safely with or without assistance and a prosthesis does not enhance quality of life or mobility.
K1	The patient has the ability or potential to use a prosthesis for transfers or ambulation on level surfaces at fixed cadence. Typical of the limited and unlimited household ambulator.
K2	The patient has the ability or potential for ambulation with the ability to traverse low-level environmental barriers such as curbs, stairs, or uneven surfaces. Typical of the limited community ambulator.
K3	The patient has the ability or potential for ambulation with variable cadence. Typical of the community ambulator who has the ability to traverse most environmental barriers and may have vocational, therapeutic, or exercise activity that demands prosthetic utilization beyond simple locomotion.
K4	The patient has the ability or potential for prosthetic ambulation that exceeds basic ambulation skills, exhibiting high impact, stress, or energy levels. Typical of the prosthetic demands of the child, active adult, or athlete.

From Centers for Medicare and Medicaid Services. Medicare Region C Durable Medical Equipment Prosthetic Orthotic Supplier (DMEPOS) Manual. Columbia, SC: Palmetto GBA, 2005.

TABLE 23-2 *Phases of Rehabilitation for Persons with Amputation*

Phases	Hallmarks
1. Preoperative	Medical and body condition assessment, patient education, surgical-level discussion, functional expectations, phantom limb discussion
2. Amputation surgery and wound dressing	Residual limb length determination, myoplastic closure, soft-tissue coverage, nerve handling, rigid dressing application, limb reconstruction
3. Acute postsurgical	Residual limb shaping, shrinking, increasing muscle strength, restoring patient's sense of control
4. Preprosthetic	Wound healing, pain control, proximal body motion, emotional support, phantom limb discussion
5. Prosthetic prescription and fabrication	Team consensus on prosthetic prescription
6. Prosthetic training	Prosthetic management and training to increase wearing time and functional use
7. Community integration	Resumption of family and community roles; regaining emotional equilibrium; developing healthy coping strategies, recreational activities
8. Vocational rehabilitation	Assessment and training for vocational activities, assessment of further education needs or job modification
9. Followup	Lifelong prosthetic, functional, and medical assessment; emotional support

From Esquenazi A, DiGiacomo RD. Rehabilitation after amputation. *J Am Podiatr Med Assoc.* 2001;91(1):13-22.

One common complication of transtibial amputation surgery is a loss of full knee extension. Failure to promote full extension of the tibiofemoral joint can lead to delays in prosthetic fitting while ROM is restored. If the lack of knee extension remains, a permanent joint contracture can alter the prosthetic fitting process. The clinical team generally encourages rigid dressings that extend well above the knee and hold the knee in full extension. It has been shown that rigid removable dressings (RRDs) provide more favorable outcomes than elastic bandages when used to control postoperative edema and to provide protection to the surgical site.[5] In some regions, persons with new amputation are fitted with immediate postoperative prostheses (IPOP) in the operating room or soon after surgery. The immediate postoperative prosthesis is intended to serve the same purpose as the RRD with the additional feature of allowing supported weight bearing for early mobility. Because of the gross changes to the limb that are anticipated in the first few days after amputation, the IPOP sockets are designed to allow some weight-bearing forces direct to the medial tibial flare and patellar tendon because these structures are far from the surgical site and are not likely to be impacted by post operative edema. It is important to note that weight bearing while in an IPOP should be at the level of toe touch partial weight bearing: Full weight bearing is discouraged as there is generally not enough area to distribute the full body weight in a manner that the skin will tolerate for extended periods of time. Full weight bearing through an IPOP carries risk of damage to the healing surgical construct, and subsequent delayed healing and prosthetic fitting. Assistive devices should be used to encourage partial weight bearing while allowing functional use of the remaining muscles.

The limb will change rapidly throughout the early rehabilitation process and the prosthetist and therapist should closely monitor the fit and alignment of the IPOP. Adding extra layers of socks to the residual limb will accommodate early changes in limb volume. Eventually this will become counterproductive and a replacement socket should be ordered. Immediate postoperative prostheses are fabricated with modular components that allow changes to be made easily.

The surgeon may decide that an IPOP is not an option for the individual because of factors including excessive soft-tissue damage or delayed wound healing, a RRD should be utilized.[6] One variant of the RRD is a custom-molded plaster socket with a prefabricated plastic collar that encapsulates the indivdual's limb from the distal end up to approximately two-thirds of the thigh. There also are other variants, including a completely prefabricated plastic socket that is adjustable or a custom-molded plastic socket that is made from a digital scan of the limb.[7] Regardless of the variation of RRD chosen, the goals are the same: the RRD (a) keeps the knee in full extension to prevent contracture, (b) protects the limb from exterior trauma, and (c) controls swelling through total contact. This removable device is worn over at least one layer of cotton sock and is held in place with Velcro straps (Figure 23-1). It is also fenestrated to allow airflow and release moisture. The

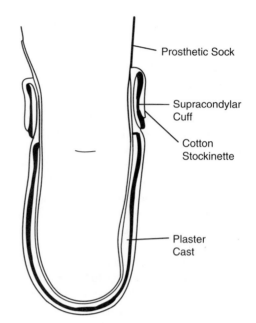

FIGURE 23-1 Cross sectional diagram of a Rigid dressing for transtibial amputation. Cotton stockinette is placed over the residual limb, and padding is placed over vulnerable areas (i.e., suture line, bony prominences). The residual limb is then wrapped with several layers of plaster-of-Paris impregnated gauze. Rigid dressings can be used until the suture line closes. They have been shown to reduce postoperative complications and accelerate the rehabilitation process. (Reprinted with permission from: *Below Knee Prosthetics*, Prosthetics-Orthotics Program, University of Texas Southwestern Medical Center at Dallas, TX, 1988, p. 7-7).

device can be worn 23 hours a day and can be removed easily for dressing changes and bathing.

PROSTHETIC PRESCRIPTION

A prosthetic prescription is a detailed description of all the features of the completed prosthesis: (a) socket design, (b) skin-socket interface, (c) suspension strategy, and (d) additional modular components. For transtibial prostheses, the components are limited to feet, shock absorbers, torque absorbers, and dynamic pylons.

The socket is the interface between the residual limb and the prosthesis; all the forces from the ground during gait are transferred to the limb through the socket. All the forces from the limb needed to control the motion of the prosthesis are transferred to the prosthesis through the socket. Much care and time should be spent on socket design and fitting, as a less than ideal fit can quickly lead to pain, injury, and lack of function. The socket design, interface, and suspension need to be considered together as their functions are often interrelated and interdependent upon one another. A soft liner, for example, can function both as an interface and as the suspension for the prosthesis. In the same way, a socket that is designed with a different interface may contraindicate certain suspension options. Forethought regarding how those three design elements intermingle will increase the probability of producing a comfortable and functional prosthesis for the indivdual.

SOCKET DESIGNS

Early transtibial prostheses were fashioned by hollowing out a block of wood and attaching metal single-axis knee joints and a leather thigh corset. The sockets were referred to as "plug-fit" sockets because they were open-ended and the limb fit into the socket like a plug fits in a drain. The attached thigh corsets took advantage of the conical shape of the thigh to transfer weight proximally and transmit mediolateral forces to and from the limb. Although many persons with amputation were quite functional with this system, the lack of contact on the distal end of the residual limb often led to painful edema in that area. Additionally, the joints and corset added bulk and weight to the prosthesis and unnecessarily restricted knee motion.[8]

Patellar Tendon-Bearing Socket

By the end of World War II, the large number of veterans who suffered limb loss during combat inspired prosthetists to experiment with new materials and techniques to improve prosthetic comfort and function. In 1959, a symposium was held at the University of California Biomechanics Laboratory to promote the development of transtibial socket fitting. The result was the patellar tendon-bearing (PTB) socket design. This design has been used successfully over the past five decades to strategically load the limb in areas that are more pressure tolerant, namely the patellar tendon and medial tibial flare, and relieve the tissue over bony prominences like the tibial crest and head of the fibula. In most cases, this eliminated the need for proximal weight bearing.[9]

The main goal of the PTB socket design was to increase the surface area on the residuum that is available for weight bearing so as to eliminate the need for the knee joints and thigh corset. The PTB socket was described as "total contact," which meant that there were supposed to be no voids or air pockets between the limb and socket. This design allowed weight bearing to occur in any area that capable of supporting a load. The term *patellar tendon-bearing* originates from the use of a patellar "bar" that is built into the socket at the level of the center of the patellar ligament, midway between the patella and the tibial tubercle (Figure 23-2). The socket is aligned in approximately 5 degrees of knee flexion, which allows the bar to act as a weight-bearing surface within the socket. The proximal trim line of the posterior wall is located just proximal to the patellar bar to stabilize the limb in the anteroposterior direction and to prevent the limb from sliding to far down into the socket. The posterior trim line should be lower on the medial side to accommodate the insertion of the medial hamstring during knee flexion.

The other major weight-bearing surface in the PTB socket is the medial flare of the tibia. The proximal end of the tibia broadens out medially and, when stabilized by pressure from the lateral wall of the socket, can effectively accept loading. It is necessary to simultaneously create a relief for the fibular head, which is at the same level, to avoid any pressure on that bony structure. Filling the distal end of the socket with a compliant foam material provides the slight pressure during full

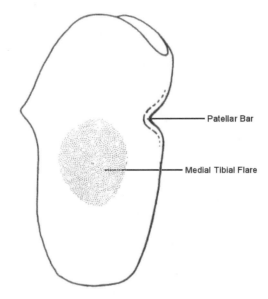

FIGURE 23-2 The patellar tendon bar and medial tibial flare are the major weight-bearing areas of the PTB socket; this total-contact socket design has been used for more than 60 years for a comfortable prosthetic fit persons with transtibial amputation. (Reprinted with permission from: *Below Knee Prosthetics Manual*, Prosthetics-Orthotics Program, University of Texas Southwestern Medical Center at Dallas, TX, 1988, p. 4-2).

weight bearing, which is necessary to control distal edema. The medial and lateral walls of the PTB socket extend up to the level of the adductor tubercle to provide lever arms for mediolateral stability. The PTB technique is still used successfully today, and many modern fitting techniques incorporate at least some of the attributes of the original PTB design.

Total Surface-Bearing Socket

The total surface-bearing (TSB) socket strives to further distribute the weight-bearing load over the entire surface of the limb, even in areas that had been traditionally considered to be pressure intolerant. Strategic compression of soft tissue and relief for bony prominences are the tools used to direct more force into areas of the limb that can tolerate it, and less force into areas that are prone to skin breakdown. The intent in designing a TSB socket is to distribute uniform pressure over the entire surface of the limb.[10] It is expected however, that during a typical step while walking, the pressure in any given location will change from a negative pressure during swing phase to high pressure in stance that, if sustained, would cause tissue damage. Because the forces on the limb change quite dramatically throughout the gait cycle, that dynamic pattern must be anticipated so as to use those forces to design the reliefs for pressure-intolerant areas; larger forces means more tissue compression, which require larger reliefs. The other factor to consider is the density and structure of the tissues comprising the limb. Tissue properties vary widely, and there are temporal effects too; muscle tissue, for example, behaves one way while relaxed and very differently while contracting. Once they are accommodated, the relative locations of these tissues within the socket must be preserved;

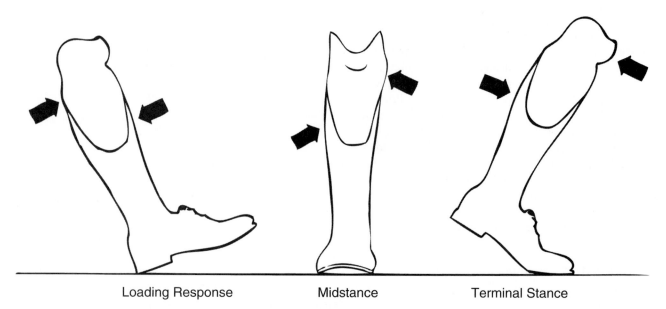

Loading Response   Midstance   Terminal Stance

FIGURE 23-3 The magnitude and direction of the forces on the socket change throughout stance phase, concentrating pressure in predictable areas. At initial contact and loading response there is an anterior force at the proximal posterior knee and distal anterior residual limb. At midstance weight bearing forces create proximal-medial and distal-lateral pressures. At the end of stance phase the anterior force moves to the proximal anterior knee and distal-posterior residual limb. (Adapted with permission from: *Below Knee Prosthetics Manual*, Prosthetics-Orthotics Program University of Texas Southwestern Medical Center at Dallas, TX, 1988, p. 5-5).

this not only provides a good environment for the tissues, but also allows accurate control of the prosthesis.

To fully accommodate the dynamic tissue loading that occurs in a prosthetic socket, the prosthetist must consider both the *shear* and the *normal* forces on the limb. Shear forces run parallel to the limb surface and are best mitigated through the use a socket interface. Interface materials, such as socks, sheaths, flexible liners, and gel liners, offer a continuum of shear reduction on the skin surface. The best materials to minimize shear are those found in gel liners. Normal forces are those that are applied perpendicular to the surface of the limb. The socket walls should be contoured according to the type of tissue in the area and the anticipated loading patterns. Because there is no way to reduce the force on the limb without restricting the inidividual's activities, the best way to reduce pressure is to distribute the forces over as broad a surface as possible. The actual forces on the limb are a combination of shear and normal forces that occur together in various proportions.

Ambulation is a dynamic event in which the forces on the limb are continually changing; for this reason the prosthetic socket must be designed to function under a variety of loading patterns. The socket must be designed and fitted under physiologic conditions that match that of the intended use. Soft-tissue compression will vary with load; the socket contours must reflect the anticipated load so as to prevent excessive loading on bony prominences. Throughout the gait cycle the forces and moments on the socket and limb change continuously. There is a flexion moment during loading response, a varus moment throughout midstance, an extension moment

in terminal stance, and a flexion moment again in preswing (Figure 23-3). The forces on the limb range from a compressive force of 1.2 times body weight in stance, to a distractive force slightly higher than the weight of the prosthesis in swing phase.[11] A well-fitting prosthesis must provide tolerable pressure distribution in all of those varied loading conditions. Soft tissue, muscle tissue, and bone contours must each be accounted for in a specific way to achieve a good fit. Soft tissue can tolerate moderate compression so the prosthetist will precompress that tissue in the socket. Muscles can tolerate mild compression but should be encouraged to contract with each step so less precompression should be applied. The shape of muscle tissue changes when it contracts. Flexible materials can be used over muscle bellies that allow for the geometric variability. Finally, bony prominences must be given extra volume within the socket so that when the tissue around them compresses during loading, the pressure will not exceed the tolerable limit.

The load-bearing capabilities of the limb can also be affected by the surgical technique used for the amputation. The Ertl procedure, named after Dr. Janos Ertl Sr., is a surgical procedure that involves creating a bone bridge between the distal end of the tibia and fibula, as shown in Figure 23-4 (see Chapter 19 for more detail). The goal of this procedure is to create a tougher, more force-tolerant limb. One problem that this technique aims to solve is nerve impingement. Transtibial amputees are prone to nerve compression between the long bones of the lower leg.[12] Forces within the socket push the tibia and fibula together and compress anything in between. If the tibial nerve is trapped between the bones,

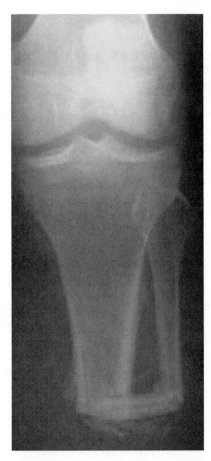

FIGURE 23-4 In the Ertl procedure, a weight-tolerant transtibial residual limb is constructed by joining the distal ends of the tibia and fibula with a bone bridge that is constructed from a piece of the fibula. Radiograph of a healed bone bridge (tibia–fibula synostosis) several months following a transtibial amputation using the Ertl approach. (Reprinted with permission from Dionne CP, Ertl WJ, Day JD. Rehabilitation for those with transtibial osteomyoplastic amputation. *J Prosthet Orthot*. 2009;21[1]:64-70.)

pain can result. By fusing the bones together at the distal end, the relative motion between them is minimized thereby protecting the soft tissues that are located between them. Many individuals who have had this type of surgical procedure can bear weight directly on the distal end of their limb. This end-bearing capability allows the prosthetist to distribute the person's weight differently and potentially provide a prosthesis that does not extend as far proximally; this can increase comfort over standard weight-bearing areas and increase the range of knee flexion available to the individual. However, the increased surgical time and subsequent increase in infection risk are often cited as reasons to forgo the Ertl procedure surgical technique.[13]

INTERFACE MATERIALS

The material that separates the limb from the socket is referred to as an interface. Interfaces play an important role in lower-limb prosthetics. Interfaces can offer shock absorption, they can mimic soft tissue to provide an extra layer of cushioning for those who are bony, and they can help to mitigate shear forces on the limb. Interfaces influence the hygiene, ease of donning, and maintenance requirements of the prosthesis as well. With new materials being developed continuously, there are many interface options for the prosthetist; a discussion of commonly used interface materials is presented here.

Hard Socket

Early prostheses were made from hard materials like wood, which did not offer much cushioning. Persons with amputation used layers of cotton or wool socks to provide a soft interface between their limb and the hard socket. There are several advantages to this system: the socket is relatively thin, so the it is easily concealed under clothing; a clean sock can be used each day, or changed times throughout the day if needed; the number and ply of socks can be adjusted to accommodate for limb volume fluctuation during the day; and the socket itself is very durable. Because there are no compressible surfaces, the fit is reliable; it will not become "packed down" in high pressure areas. It is nonporous, easy to clean, and relatively maintenance free. It also does a fair job of eliminating shear as the coefficient of friction between the socks and socket is relatively low compared to that between the socks and skin.[14] This type of socket is most challenging to fit and is not recommended for mature limbs that have lost much of their soft-tissue protection over bony prominences. It is also more difficult to adjust than other socket styles.

Socks and Sheaths

Prosthetic socks can be made from various combinations of cotton, nylon, wool, Lycra, polyester, and spandex. Some manufacturers have recently started using silver fibers in their socks as well to enhance the antimicrobial properties of their socks and sheaths (Figure 23-5). The prosthetic sock provides shock absorption, decreases the shear forces on the limb, and wicks away moisture. To further decrease friction, a nylon sheath is often recommended as the initial layer and the thicker socks would be donned over the sheath. The sock also provides the individual with a method to control socket fit; as the residual limb matures and shrinks, additional sock ply may be required to restore the fit and comfort of the socket.

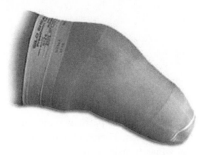

FIGURE 23-5 Prosthetic sheaths are very thin stocking-like garments worn between the skin and prosthetic sock or socket liner. They are used to reduce friction, disperse moisture, and control bacterial growth. (Reprinted with permission from Kingsley Manufacturing Co, Costa Mesa, CA)

Prosthetic socks come in various ply thicknesses for convenience to the prosthetic wearer; for example, a person can wear one five-ply sock rather than having to don five individual single-ply socks. New prosthetic wearers are typically provided an assortment of one-, three-, and five-ply socks from which they can select. The socks can be layers one on top of the other to achieve the appropriate number of ply.

Soft Inserts

Closed cell foam, used because they do not absorb moisture, can be molded over a model of the limb to create a soft insert. This insert lines the entire socket and terminates just proximal to the socket trim lines (Figure 23-6). For increased protection, a distal end-pad, which is an extra layer of soft material at the

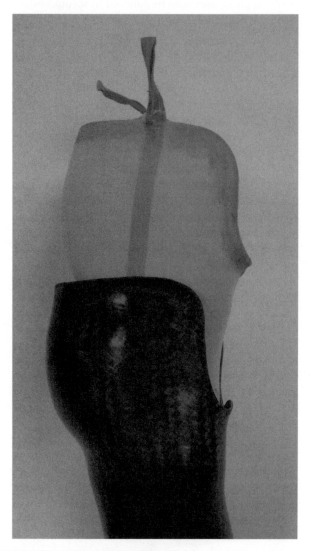

FIGURE 23-6 This soft insert is partially removed from the supracondylar suprapatellar socket. There are pull loops mounted on the medial and lateral wings to help with doffing the prosthesis. Once inserted into the rigid socket, the thicker portions of the insert lock over the femoral condyles and suspend the prosthesis. To remove the prosthesis, the user must pull up on the insert while pushing down on the socket. (Photo courtesy of David A. Knapp, CPO, Hanger Prosthetics & Orthotics, Inc., North Haven, CT)

bottom of the insert, can be used to cushion the distal end of the tibia. Soft inserts provide an extra layer of cushioning that is needed for more mature limbs that lack adequate soft-tissue thickness. They can be worn over a nylon sheath, which is a very thin nylon stocking similar to women's stocking, or over any number of sock ply. Wearing the insert directly over the skin without a sock may lead to excessive shear and skin breakdown because of the relative motion between the limb and insert. Single durometer inserts provide a uniform compression profile whereas multidurometer inserts, made from layers of different materials with varied properties, can take advantage of the force-altering characteristics of each layer. For example, a material that has high plastic deformation might offer good shock absorption but would wear out very quickly if used alone. Mating that material with one that has low compression resistance would prevent some of the plastic deformation and extend the useful life of the insert. Soft inserts that can deform during the donning process can be used to accommodate anatomic irregularities that would not be able to slide directly into a rigid socket. For example, an insert for a limb with a bulbous distal end can be made thicker in the narrow area above the bulge so that the diameter of the finished socket would not impede donning. Another example is the wedge needed for supracondylar suspension; this wedge can be integrated as part of the soft insert to facilitate ease of donning.

Flexible Inner Socket

If PTB theory is to direct weight bearing into specific areas of the limb and away from others, then the flexible inner socket is the incarnation of that idea. With this system, an inner socket is made over a model of the limb from a flexible material that will stretch upon the application of force. Then a rigid frame is built around the inner socket, corresponding to areas of the residual limb where weight bearing is desirable. The result is a socket that flexes away from forces in non–pressure-tolerant areas, but remains rigid in the force-tolerant areas. Because flexible sockets in rigid frames can eliminate compressive forces in any specific area, this system is useful for persons with particularly bony residual limbs and those with severe localized sensitivity. They are not recommended for residual limbs with adherent scarring, however, because pressure differentials created by the frame tend to amplify the shear forces on the limb.

Expandable Wall Socket

When the limb is amputated at or below the ankle, the resulting long residual limb present an interesting challenge to the prosthetist. The proximal trim lines of the prosthesis can be lowered to a more distal position on the limb because there is a long lever arm for prosthetic control during ambulation. However the distal residual limbs is larger in diameter than they are in the more proximally because the malleoli are still present. The prosthetist can accommodate for a larger distal size by creating a removable wall in the socket that is replaced after the prosthesis is donned, by using a specially designed soft liner, or by creating an expandable wall socket. The expandable wall socket is made from an elasticized material that stretches enough for the individual to push his or her limb through in weight bearing, and tightens up over the malleoli to provide suspension. This socket is too flexible to attach a foot to, so a rigid frame is made over the flexible socket with a small space between them in which the expansion can occur. This is a self-suspending socket that can be very comfortable for the person. It is difficult to fabricate this style socket, and it is even more difficult to make adjustments to the fit once it is fabricated. More information on these designs can be found in Chapter 22.

Gel Liner

The term *gel liner* is loosely used in the field to describe a liner that is made from a material that exhibits gel-like properties. There are three basic varieties of these liners: (a) silicone elastomers, which are highly cross-linked at the molecular level; (b) silicone gels that have a relatively low amount of crosslinking; and (c) urethanes. The properties of these materials vary and are relevant to the prosthetist and person with amputation because they directly affect the forces that are transmitted through them to the residual limb. Of particular interest are certain properties of gel liners including: coefficient of friction, compressive stiffness, and shear stiffness. Silicone gels have the lowest compressive and shear stiffness values; this makes them useful in reducing compressive loading and eliminating shear forces on the limb. Lower shear stiffness would be beneficial for a bony limb, but might compromise stability by creating excessive motion on a limb that has more biological soft tissue. Silicone elastomers present the highest compressive stiffness values, so they are best suited to supporting loading without deformation. Elastomers would be beneficial for use on a limb that has a high proportion of soft tissue. Urethanes show the highest coefficient of friction with skin, a property that is useful for preventing localized skin tension and shear.[15] Understanding these properties, allows the prosthetist to choose a material that is complementary to the socket design and effectively leverages the force transmission properties of the material against the soft-tissue characteristics of the limb.

Gel liners are a key component of TSB sockets. Gel liners are designed to be worn directly on the skin or over a thin liner referred to as "liner liners." Liner liners are thin nylon sheaths with silver fibers that are meant to be worn between the skin and gel liner to prevent skin irritation caused by the warm moist environment of the gel. Although great effort is made to eliminate relative motion between the limb and socket, a small amount of motion is unavoidable. Gel liners have a high-friction inner surface, where it is in contact with the limb, and a low friction outer surface where it meets the socket. This encourages whatever small amount of motion is present to occur on the outer surface of the liner and minimizes motion at the liner–skin interface. The colloidal nature of the gel absorbs the shear that is not dissipated by the liner–socket interface so that only a small percentage reaches the skin (Figure 23-7).

Incorporation of a locking pin at the distal end of the gel liner allows the liner to be used for suspension as well. This type of liner is referred to as a "locking liner" as opposed to a "cushion liner" that has no pin. The pin mates with a locking mechanism built into the socket to suspend the prosthesis.

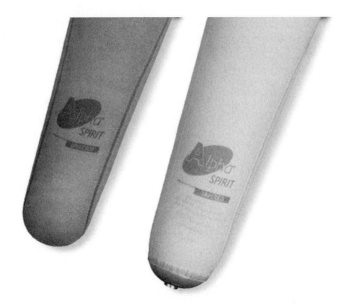

FIGURE 23-7 A cushion liner *(left)* provides shock absorption and a low shear interface, the distal connector found on a locking liner *(right)* adds a means of suspension as well. (Reprinted with Permission from Ohio Willow Wood Company, Mount Sterling, OH).

Roll-on liners should fit snugly, but not tightly. As the liner is stretched, a shear profile is established on the limb. A tighter fit creates higher frictional forces and if the pressure distribution is not equal, the frictional forces on the skin will be uneven, leading to blisters and skin problems. This can occur with a very bony limb, unless the liner is custom made for the individual. Custom made gel liners are created over a mold of the residual limb. This is indicated for unusually shaped limbs, those with deep invaginations, or those that need specifically located reliefs or cushions.

SUSPENSION

Another important consideration when designing a prosthesis is the method by which the prosthesis is held to the limb; this is referred to as the "suspension." When prosthesis is suspended perfectly, there is no relative motion between the socket and the limb. When motion occurs because of a faulty or inadequate suspension system, the limb is subjected to an entirely different loading pattern. This motion is referred to as "pistoning" as it bears some resemblance to the motion of a piston in the cylinder of an internal combustion engine. Pistoning can lead to pain, skin breakdown, and reduced control of the prosthesis. Great care should be taken to minimize motion within the socket. There are several strategies for suspension, they can be used individually as the primary mode of suspension or more than one technique can be used simultaneously to provide auxiliary suspension.

Waist Belt

A waist belt connected by an elastic strap to the thigh corset was used to suspend early transtibial sockets. Waist belts encircle the pelvis between the iliac crests and the greater trochanters. These adjustable belts have buckles on the anterior aspect that mated with an inverted Y-strap that is attached to the socket; this allows them to be donned separately and then joined together. Because this system crosses the hip and knee joints, flexion and extension of these joints must be accommodated by an elastic component. Further accommodation of knee flexion is accomplished by the inverted Y-strap (Figure 23-8). The Y-strap is fitted over the patella so that the two arms of the Y move posteriorly during knee flexion to reduce elongation of the elastic strap. The person can adjust tension in the strap based upon individual comfort. Pistoning in the socket is controllable with enough tension in the elastic. Tension in the strap decreases with hip flexion so that the strap has slack while the person is seated. Hip extension produces tension in the strap and will aid in limb advancement as it assists hip flexion in preswing.

Joints and Corset

The joints and corset feature (first discussed in the section on Socket Design) provides suspension as well as a weight-bearing element if the thigh corset is properly fitted over the femoral condyles. A skillfully molded corset can gain purchase over the smaller circumference of the thigh just proximal to the knee joint. The stiff leather corset is fabricated with either straps or laces that can be tightened as the wearer dons the prosthesis. This permits the limb to pass through the corset and then be held securely in position once the corset

is tightened. The knee joints, which are typically made from steel, provide a secure connection to the socket. When the condyles are prominent, this can serve as the primary means of suspension and a waist belt is not needed. As the prosthetic knee joints are positioned slightly posterior to the anatomical knee joint center, tension in the cuff to decreases over the condyles as knee flexes, thereby enhancing sitting comfort (Figure 23-9). The joints and corset system can also include a posterior check strap that limits full knee extension. This can be used to eliminate the terminal impact at the end of swing phase, which can be audible, and to prevent excessive wear on the prosthetic knee joints. The thigh cuff allows for full functional range of knee flexion but will cause binding in the popliteal fossa when the knee is flexed beyond approximately 110 degrees. Joints and corset may be the suspension of choice for persons with ligamentous instability of the knee.

Cuff Strap

A cuff strap is a flexible leather cuff that attaches to the medial and lateral walls of the socket at the same point that orthotic knee joints would attach, that is, just posterior and proximal to anatomic knee center (Figure 23-10). The cuff has an adjustable strap that completely encircles the thigh just

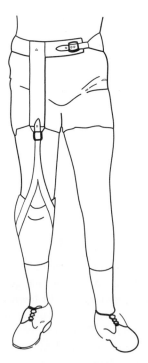

FIGURE 23-8 Waist belt and inverted Y-strap suspends the prosthesis through tension in the elastic strap between the belt and Y-strap. The strap is fitted to allow hip and knee flexion during swing phase. The elastic recoil of the strap during swing phase assists swing limb advancement of the prosthesis. (Reprinted with permission from: *Below Knee Prosthetics Manual*, Prosthetics-Orthotics Program, University of Texas Southwestern Medical Center at Dallas, TX, p. 5-15)

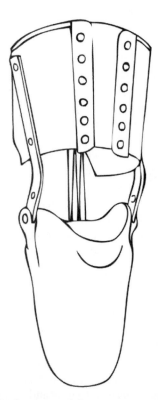

FIGURE 23-9 Thigh corset with knee joints is used when the residual limb is not capable of supporting the full weight of the patient, for example, for someone with a very short residual limb, or with significant scarring or fragile skin over traditional weight bearing surfaces. It may also be used for persons with mechanically unstable knee joints secondary to ligamentous insufficiency. (Reprinted with permission from: *Below Knee Prosthetics Manual*, Prosthetics-Orthotics Program, University of Texas Southwestern Medical Center at Dallas, TX, 1988, p. 4-7)

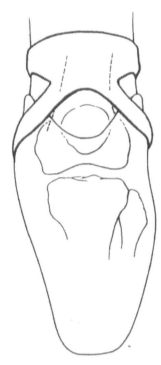

FIGURE 23-10 The cuff strap suspension uses the proximal aspect of the patella as well as the femoral condyles to achieve suspension of the prosthesis on the residual limb. (Reprinted with permission from: *Below Knee Prosthetics Manual*, Prosthetics-Orthotics Program, University of Texas Southwestern Medical Center at Dallas, TX, 1988, p. 4-7)

proximal to the patella. After the person dons the socket, the cuff is secured in place so that prosthesis will hang from the cuff while standing and walking. The anatomic structures that provide the suspension are the patella and the femoral condyles. To create a strong hold, the medial and lateral walls of the socket need to be lower than the standard height; because this reduces mediolateral stability, cuff strap suspension it is not a good choice for short residual limbs. An elastic component may be added to the strap over the patella to increase sitting comfort. This system is simple, quick to fabricate, and provides a secure suspension for the prosthesis while accommodating an unencumbered angle of knee flexion. The cuff does not provide any weight-bearing or mediolateral stability. Cuff strap suspension may be problematic for Persons with much muscle or adipose tissue arounp the lower thigh

Supracondylar Suspension

Suspension can be achieved by incorporating the femoral condyles completely within the rigid transtibial socket. By extending the medial and lateral trim lines of the socket approximately 2 cm proximal to the adductor tubercle, the medial–lateral dimension of the top of the socket can be made narrower than the knee joint; this prevents the knee joint from moving upward out of the socket by capturing the femoral condlyes. Supracondylar suspension also adds significant medial–lateral stability to the prosthesis by increasing the length of the lever arm proximal to knee center. This technique, when combined with a PTB-style socket, is collectively referred to as "PTB-SC."

This type of socket can be difficult to don because the width of the proximal opening is smaller than the width of the condyles. This problem can be addressed in two ways: either by making the medial wall detachable, or by including the supracondylar wedge in a soft insert. The first method uses a steel bar that is formed into the prosthesis. The entire medial wall of the prosthesis, along with the steel bar, can be removed for donning. Once the limb is in the socket, the bar slides back into a channel in the distal portion of the socket and locks into position with a ball detent (Figure 23-11). The second method uses a flexible liner that has a wedge built into it proximal to medial condyle. The rigid socket is fabricated over the liner such that the medial–lateral dimension of the proximal end of the socket is equal to the widest dimension of the knee. This allows donning of the flexible liner first, then with slight compression of the liner, the limb and liner together slide into the socket and are locked in pace through pressure and friction (Figure 23-12).

It is necessary to have at least a 1-cm difference between the medial–lateral dimension of the knee joint and that of the thigh just proximal to the adductor tubercle so as to provide a secure supracondylar suspension. Widening the socket in the region just posterior to the condyles serves to loosen the grip over the condyles while seated in 90 degrees of knee flexion. It is noteworthy to mention that the high medial and lateral walls of this type of socket are apparent even through long pants when the knee is flexed. Some individuals might find this unsightly and unacceptable.

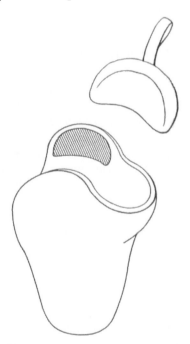

FIGURE 23-11 One option to ease the process of donning a supracondylar or supracondylar/suprapatellar socket is to remove a thick medial wedge when the residual limb is pushed into the socket. This wedge is repositioned once the limb is within the socket. A ridge in the socket along the proximal edge of the wedge holds it in place during ambulation. (Reprinted with permission from: *Below Knee Prosthetics Manual*, Prosthetics-Orthotics Program, University of Texas Southwestern Medical Center at Dallas, TX, 1988, p. 4-6)

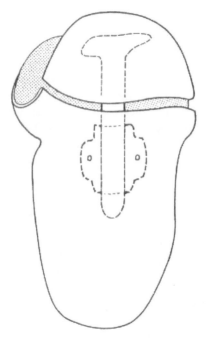

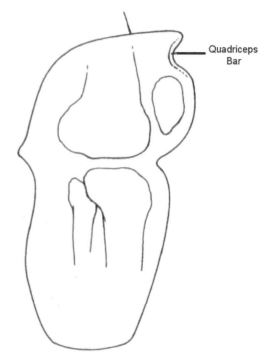

FIGURE 23-12 Another option for donning supracondylar or supracondylar/suprapatellar sockets is removal of the medial wing of the socket. This allows the wide condyles to pass through the narrow proximal dimension of the socket. The medial wing is repositioned after donning; the metal flange holds the medial wing in place, to achieve the proximal purchase over the femoral condyles used to suspend the prosthesis. (Reprinted with permission from: *Below Knee Prosthetics Manual*, Prosthetics-Orthotics Program, University of Texas Southwestern Medical Center at Dallas, TX, 1988, p. 4-6)

FIGURE 23-13 The quadriceps bar of the patellar tendon-bearing–supracondylar/suprapatellar socket resists knee hyperextension and enhances suspension. It also stiffens the wings to improve purchase over the condyles, further enhancing suspension of the prosthesis on the residual limb. (Reprinted with permission from: *Below Knee Prosthetics Manual*, Prosthetics-Orthotics Program, University of Texas Southwestern Medical Center at Dallas, TX, 1988, p. 4-4)

Supracondylar/Suprapatellar

By extending the trim line of the anterior aspect of the PTB-SC socket up to the level of the medial and lateral walls, the proximal surface of the patella also can be used to assist suspension (Figure 23-13). The patellar tendon-bearing–supracondylar/suprapatellar (PTB-SCSP) socket allows the formation of a quadriceps "bar" above the patella that provides suspension and resists hyperextension. The continuous trim line at the proximal brim also increases the rigidity of the medial and lateral walls, further enhancing suspension. The advantages and disadvantages of this variation match those of the PTB-SC with the exception that it is even more visible under clothing when the knee is flexed.

Sleeve

One of the most versatile means of suspending a prosthesis is with a knee sleeve. A suspension sleeve provides suspension through two biomechanical principles: friction and vacuum. The sleeve extends approximately 20 cm proximal and distal to knee center, and is fitted over the proximal end of the prosthetic socket (Figure 23-14). The sleeve should fit snugly but not hinder circulation. Sleeves can be made from a variety of materials, depending upon the goals of the prosthetic design. Neoprene and elastic fabric are common materials used for sleeves because they contour nicely to the anatomy and provide a high coefficient of friction with the skin. These sleeves

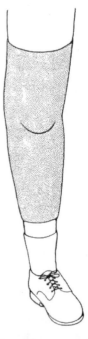

FIGURE 23-14 Roll on knee sleeves provide a fairly cosmetic, low profile, versatile means of suspension. Sleeves use friction against the shell of the prosthetic socket distally and the wearer's skin proximally to suspend the prosthesis on the residual limb. (Reprinted with permission from: *Below Knee Prosthetics Manual*, Prosthetics-Orthotics Program, University of Texas Southwestern Medical Center at Dallas, TX, 1988, p. 4-9)

use friction only to suspend the prosthesis because they allow for air to flow through them, in and out of the socket. This is useful for dissipating perspiration and keeping the limb cooler, but it also allows undesirable motion to occur between the socket and the limb. Over time, this can lead to pain and skin breakdown. The sleeve can be worn over a sock, which can be good for hygiene; however, this will affect the coefficient of friction between the sleeve and the limb, which could lead to suspension failure. Sleeves permit functional ROM for the knee, but because they bunch up in the popliteal fossa, they can restrict knee flexion beyond approximately 100 degrees.

Suction

Modern sleeves are referred to as "sealing sleeves" because they are made from nonporous materials that seal the proximal end of the socket against the skin so that no air can flow into, or out from, the socket. This creates a suction suspension. One-way air valves are commonly used in conjunction with sealing sleeves to allow air that is trapped during donning to escape from the socket. Sealing sleeves provide excellent suspension when combined with a TSB socket style. Once the socket is sealed, very little pistoning can occur because there are no voids between the limb and socket. For the sleeve to seal, the sleeve must touch the skin directly for at least the top 5 cm. The skin must be free from deep scars or invaginations in that area, as they would provide a path for air to enter under the sleeve. Because the sealing sleeves rely on an airtight seal to function, they are highly susceptible to failure as a consequence of leaks. Even a small hole in the sleeve can allow air to flow into the socket, defeating the vacuum and impairing suspension. Although sleeves are not very durable, they can be replaced without any special tools or equipment.

The soft tissue of the residual limb behaves like a incompressible fluid. For the limb to move within the sealed volume of the socket, the volume of the limb itself would have to change. This can only happen if fluid moves into or out from the limb through the bloodstream, a process that is too slow to be accomplished within the short interval of swing phase. Therefore, the cyclic alteration between compression in stance and tension in swing slowly draws fluid into the limb and pushes it back out, assisting normal circulation. Suction suspension may provide a means for improving healthy circulation in the residual limb and controlling limb volume.

Locking Liners

The first references to locking liners involve the use of a roll-on silicon liner, referred to as an "Icelandic roll-on suction socket" (Iceross).[16,17] The use of the term *suction* for this type of suspension is incorrect, however. The liner is primarily held on by friction because it is not possible to maintain a vacuum within a flexible structure. If friction is eliminated through the use of a lubricant, the liner can be pulled off the limb. It is more accurate to describe this type of suspension as a locking mechanism. These roll-on gel liners are compliant

enough to contour nicely to the shape of the residual limb and include a threaded hole at the distal end. This hole serves as a point of attachment for the suspension hardware.

There are three basic options for the hardware:
1. Early sockets *used a ring* that was screwed into the distal end of the liner. When the ring came through a special opening in the distal end of the socket, the prosthetic wearer could pass a thin bar through the ring so that it could be retracted back into the socket. This system is still good for individuals who have difficulty doffing the prosthesis because it allows them to remove the bar and then use both hands to push the socket off. This system requires additional clearance under the limb to accommodate the diameter of the ring and the associated attachment fixture. The bar is also a separate component, so it can easily get lost. The individual should be instructed to store the bar in the prosthesis and take it out only during the donning process.
2. Difficulties with the ring gave rise to *using a strap* that is manually fed through a hole in the distal end of the socket and then secured to the outside of the socket (Figure 23-15). The strap must be of sufficient length to be put through the hole before the limb enters the socket. This eliminates the need to carefully align the sleeve during donning as the limb will be drawn down into the socket by tension in the strap. It also eases donning force required to push into the socket because the limb elongates and decreases in girth under tension. As no locking mechanism is mounted on the distal end, no additional clearance is needed, leaving precious space for other components. One variant of this system uses a lanyard and a special lock mechanism to secure the lanyard in the distal end of the socket, the lanyard is permanently attached to the locking mechanism so it needs to be disconnected from the liner each time the liner is taken off.
3. Most modern sockets use a *pin-and-lock mechanism*. This pin can range from approximately 3 to 10 cm in length. It works in conjunction with a locking mechanism built into the distal end of the socket that engages when the individual dons the prosthesis. Some wearers experience frustration with this as it can be difficult to align the pin so that it engages with the locking mechanism. To remove the prosthesis, the prosthetic wearer must disengage the pin manually while pushing the socket off with the other hand. There are several variants of locking mechanisms: some offer an audible "click" to indicate that the pin has engaged but will only lock in a limited number of positions, others use a clutch mechanism or a smooth pin that allow for an infinite number of locking positions. Ideally, only one position should be needed, that is when the limb is positioned correctly in the socket. However, as an individual's limb volume varies throughout the day, it is not uncommon for there to be an additional "click" or two as they spend more time weight-bearing in the prosthesis (Figure 23-16).

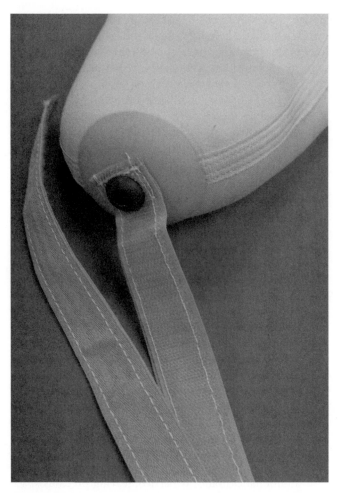

FIGURE 23-15 An example of a distally mounted strap or lanyard that can be used to pull the limb, within its liner, into the socket. (photo courtesy of David A. Knapp, CPO, Hanger Prosthetics & Orthotics, Inc., North Haven, CT)

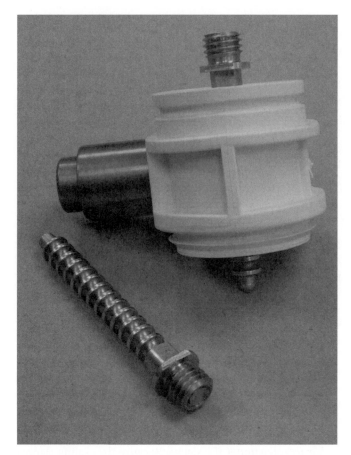

FIGURE 23-16 An example of the pin that is attached to the liner, and the locking receptacle incorporated into the distal socket for a pin lock suspension system. Pin locks are extremely popular because of their effectiveness and relative ease of use. (Photo courtesy of David A. Knapp, CPO, Hanger Prosthetics & Orthotics, Inc., North Haven, CT)

Locking liners allow some pistoning to occur.[18] The amount of motion can be dramatic when loose tissue is present at the distal end of the residual limb. As the limb is lifted off the ground in swing phase, the weight of the prosthesis pulls on the pin causing the liner and limb to elongate in length and contract in girth. This effect is most apparent at the distal end. This "milking" motion creates unnecessary stress on the distal end of the limb and can lead to pain, edema, and skin breakdown.[19] This is especially problematic for limbs with adherent scar tissue as the liner will attempt to pull the tissue away from the bone. This type of suspension is not ideal for a newly amputated limb as the distal end is not fully healed. This problem can be averted if suction, rather than the pin, is used to hold the liner to the socket wall.

Semirigid Locking Liner

A semirigid locking liner is used to combine the convenience of a locking liner with the benefits of full suction suspension. The indivdual first dons an interface, which can be a sheath, sock, or cushion gel liner that the prosthesis was designed to fit over; then puts on a thin flexible custom molded socket that has a locking liner rolled over it; and finally steps into the rigid

frame to engage the locking mechanism. The locking liner seals the limb in the flexible socket and virtually eliminates pistoning of the limb within the socket. Because the locking liner is under the rigid frame rather than stretched over it, the life of the locking liner is greatly extended. Having the socket under the liner prevents deformation of the locking liner so that pistoning is virtually eliminated and the distal tissue is protected. To further enhance the suction of this system, an expulsion valve can be incorporated into the flexible socket; this allows any air that is trapped in the socket during donning to be removed (Figure 23-17). This one-way valve provides a path for air to move from inside the socket to the outside of the locking liner. Wearing a sock or a liner that has a fabric exterior helps any remaining air to migrate toward the valve and out of the socket.

Elevated Vacuum

As the advantages of suction suspension are clearly documented in the literature,[20,21] there has been considerable interest in using external vacuum pumps to increase the level of suction (decrease the pressure) within the socket. These systems are referred as "elevated vacuum." Pumps can be either electric (battery-operated), or mechanical. The mechanical pumps use the natural cycle of compression during stance

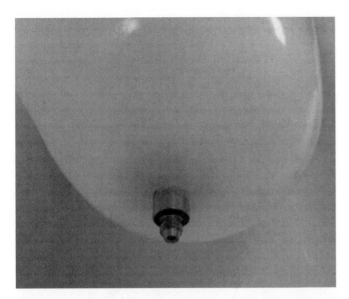

FIGURE 23-17 Close-up of valve on the distal end of flexible socket of the semirigid locking liner system. This system takes advantage of the benefits of full suction and the convenience of a locking mechanism. (Photo courtesy of David A. Knapp, CPO, Hanger Prosthetics & Orthotics, Inc., North Haven, CT)

and distraction during swing to pull air from the socket during gait. Electric pumps have the added benefit of being able to accurately control the level of vacuum within the socket by turning on and off at preset thresholds (Figure 23-18). Elevated vacuum maintains limb volume by preventing fluid loss that occurs during prolonged weight bearing.[22] The elevated vacuum environment within the socket leads to decreased motion, and therefore to fewer skin problems, improved prosthetic control, better balance, and enhanced comfort.[18] It has also been shown that elevated vacuum sockets have lower peak pressures and lower impact forces than traditional suction sockets.[23] To achieve elevated vacuum, a sealing sleeve is required to prevent air from entering through the proximal end of the socket. Some wearers report a decrease in the amount of available knee flexion once the air has been evacuated from the socket; this is likely caused by tension in the sealing sleeve as it spans the entire knee joint.

IMPRESSION TECHNIQUES

The first step in creating a well-fitting socket is capturing an accurate impression of the residual limb. This can be done in a variety of ways ranging from plaster bandages to noncontact optical scanners. Each technique has its own set of advantages and disadvantages and there is no one best method for every limb. All methods share the common goal of capturing a model of the limb that accurately represents the location and geometry of each aspect of the limb. Capturing a static impression of the limb is quite simple and any method will suffice if done properly. The challenging task is to capture the dynamic nature of the biological tissue by compressing the soft tissues during the process to simulate the conditions that will be on the limb during weight-bearing.

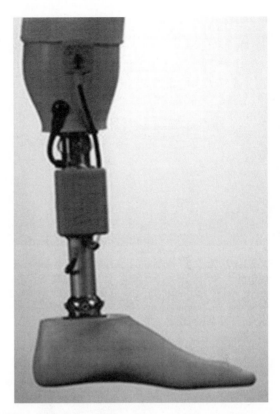

FIGURE 23-18 This figure shows a microprocessor controlled device that draws air out of the socket to maintain elevated vacuum necessary for effective suspension of the prosthesis on the residual limb. Electronic vacuum pumps are reliable and can accurately maintain specified levels of vacuum. (Reprinted with permission, Hanger Prosthetics & Orthotics, Inc., Austin, TX)

Hand Casting

During hand casting, the limb is gently wrapped with a plaster bandage and the prosthetist pushes in key weight-bearing areas while the plaster is setting up. How much compression is needed and which areas to compress are determined based on the prosthetist's individual knowledge, skill, and experience. Multistage casting procedures involve molding specific regions of the limb individually and then joining them together once the individual sections are set up. This allows the prosthetist to position the limb in multiple postures during casting to capture unique features; for example, the insertion of the hamstrings can be molded during active knee flexion when they are most prominent (Figure 23-19). For more details about casting, the reader is referred to Chapter 6.

Pressure Casting

Another way to precompress the tissue is to use a pressurizing technique.[24] This involves placing the limb into a vacuum or pressure chamber while the plaster is setting up (Figure 23-20). A vacuum chamber is typically a latex bladder that is pulled over the wet cast and sealed on the thigh. A vacuum pump attached to the distal end removes all the air between the cast and bladder; this allows the atmospheric pressure to compress the limb up to approximately 14 psi. Alternatively, a pressure chamber is a clear cylinder with a

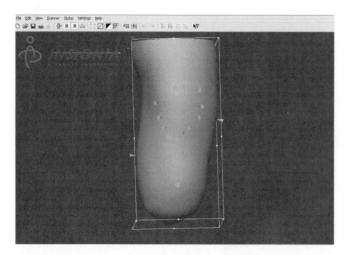

FIGURE 23-19 Three-dimensional image of a limb captured with optical scanner during the prosthetic prescription process. This computer model of the limb's surface is accurate to within 1 mm. (photo courtesy of David A. Knapp, CPO, Hanger Prosthetics & Orthotics, Inc., North Haven, CT)

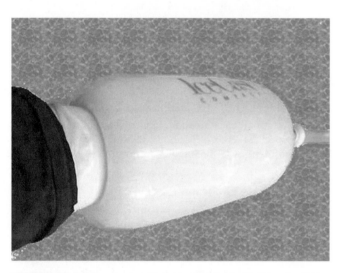

FIGURE 23-20 Pressure casting provides an isobaric environment to pre-compress the tissue and achieve an optimal socket fit. This figure shows the flexible pressure chamber and the pump that is used to increase the pressure during casting. (Reprinted with permission from Ossur Americas, Foothill Ranch, CA)

latex bladder attached. The limb, with the unset plaster wrap, is placed in the bladder and air is pumped into the space between the cylinder and bladder; pressure in the cylinder can be increased to 30 to 40 psi, providing additional compression. In either method, the differential pressure between the limb and the environment serves to apply uniform pressure over the entire surface of the limb. This leads to the most tissue compression in the softest areas and the least amount of tissue compression in the bony areas. The amount of differential pressure required will vary with the indivdual's weight, and the prosthetist will use the least amount of pressure required to achieve the optimal fit. Once the plaster has hardened, the pressure is released and the limb is removed from the chamber.

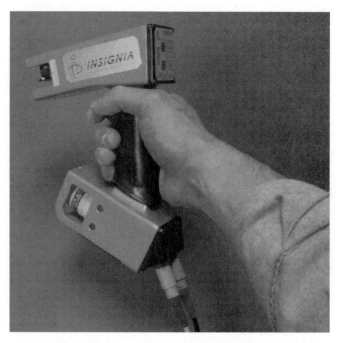

FIGURE 23-21 An example of a noncontact optical scanner uses a laser to capture a three-dimensional image of the surface of the limb. It is particularly useful in applications where casting is contraindicated. (Photo courtesy of David A. Knapp CPO, Hanger Prosthetics & Orthotics, Inc., North Haven, CT)

Optical Scanning

Optical scanners can be used to capture the three-dimensional external shape of the limb to within 1 mm of accuracy (Figure 23-21).[25] They are quite useful in situations when casting is impossible or impractical such as immediately following surgery or with bulbous limbs that cannot be removed from a plaster cast without cutting or distorting the cast. Digital markers and alignment lines can be attached to the virtual model to reference the location of bony landmarks and pressure sensitive areas. Although it is not possible to compress the skin by hand while scanning because the hand would block the view of the surface, the isobaric techniques described in the previous paragraph can be used to precompress the soft tissue.

ALIGNMENT

Alignment refers to the spatial orientation of the prosthetic socket relative to the foot. This alignment will influence the magnitude and direction of the ground reaction force throughout the gait cycle. There are four goals in prosthetic alignment: (1) facilitating heel strike at initial contact; (2) providing adequate single limb stability during stance phase; (3) creating smooth forward progression (rollover) during the transition from early to late stance phase; and (4) insuring adequate swing phase toe clearance.[26] These goals are reached through dynamic alignment of the prosthesis, during which the person walks on a prosthesis that is fitted with an adjustable device that allows for alignment changes in all three planes. Although "normal" gait is not a goal, modern components do allow many persons with transtibial amputations to evade detection of gait abnormalities or deviations by all but the most skillful gait observers. Prosthetic alignment can also be used in conjunction with socket fit to address pressure issues within the socket. Because of this socket fitting and dynamic alignment must occur simultaneously. Effective fitting and alignment requires an iterative process as changing one aspect can affect many others. The end result is often a compromise. For example, the foot may require excessive dorsiflexion in order for the person to achieve sufficient swing clearance, even though this may contribute to an higher than optimal knee flexion moment during loading response. The prosthetist must understand biomechanics of the limb and gait cycle and weigh these factors appropriately to make the best decisions.

The modular components that connect the socket, pylon, and foot allow the prosthetist to make angular changes to the alignment. Socket flexion or socket extension refer to tilting the proximal end of the socket forward or backward in the anteroposterior direction respectively. Socket abduction moves the proximal end of the socket medially while socket adduction moves it laterally. Adjustments around the ankle can be described with standard anatomic terminology: inversion, eversion, plantarflexion, and dorsiflexion. Changes to the alignment can refer to the motion of the socket relative to the foot, or vice versa. Dorsiflexing the foot for example, causes socket flexion, while everting the foot leads to the same motion as adducting the socket.

The socket can also be shifted medially or laterally in the frontal plane and anteriorly or posteriorly in the sagittal plane, these are referred to as *linear* changes. These, too, are relative changes; a lateral shift of the socket for example, is equal to a medial shift of the foot. This type of adjustment is useful during static alignment to ensure that the foot is directly under the indivudal's knee. Linear adjustments can be made by either using a special component that permits this type of shift, or by using a pair of standard pyramid connectors and making equal but opposite angular adjustments (Figure 23-22).

Bench Alignment

The first step in the alignment of a transtibial prosthesis is to position the socket in what is known as "bench alignment." This is the alignment that serves as the starting point for the dynamic alignment process. Standard bench alignment has the socket in 5 degrees of flexion and 5 degrees of adduction while the top of the prosthetic foot is level in both the frontal and sagittal planes and the medial border of the foot is parallel to the line of progression. When viewed in the sagittal plane, a plumb line should fall from anatomic knee center and pass through the foot at a point one-third of the foot length from the back of the heel. In the frontal plane, the line should go from midpatella through the center of the heel. The reason for the 5 degrees of socket flexion is to elongate quadriceps, muscles slightly so that they are better prepared to accept the full weight of the body and to aid in shock absorption during loading response. The 5 degrees of adduction ensures that the foot is sufficiently inset to create the appropriate varus moment during stance; this properly loads the proximomedial and distolateral aspects

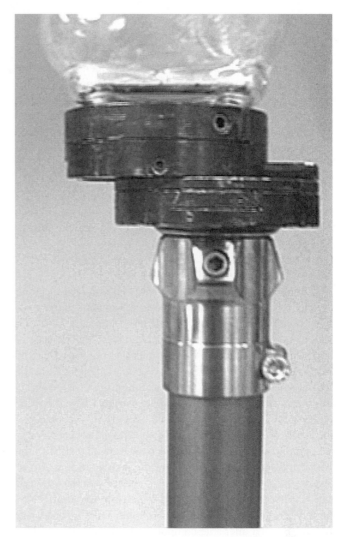

FIGURE 23-22 The adapter under the socket allows the prosthetist to slide the socket anteriorly/posteriorly, and medially/laterally, with respect to the prosthetic foot position, during dynamic alignment. This socket in this image is shifted approximately 1.5 cm anteriorly (left). (Photo courtesy of David A. Knapp, CPO, Hanger Prosthetics & Orthotics, North Haven, CT)

of the limb that are best able to carry those forces. Standard bench alignment is not used when joint contracture or deformity is present; instead, the actual limb alignment is marked during the casting procedure and that alignment is used as the starting point in the dynamic analysis.

Height

Once the prosthesis is bench aligned, the person dons the prosthesis, and stands with equal weight bearing on both lower extremites. The first measurement examines the length of the prosthesis. The goal is to achieve relatively equal leg length, comparing the intact and prosthetic limbs There are two accepted ways to assess the height: statically and dynamically. In a static assessment, the individual is asked to stand with feet shoulder-width apart, knees fully extended, and bearing equal weight on either limb. The distances from each iliac crest to the floor can be measured and compared.

An alternative is to evaluate whether left and right iliac crests appear to be level. The measurement should not be taken in the supine position because the length of the prosthesis changes during weight bearing as a consequence of flexion of the dynamic components and compression of the interface material. In a dynamic assessment, the person is asked to walk and the entire body is observed, especially the head and torso. Many factors will affect the motion of the head and torso so it is best to focus only on gross asymmetries that can be corrected by changing the length of the prosthesis. When the static and dynamic height measurements are different, a clinical decision is made to determine the optimal length for the prosthesis to provide the best function for the individual. It is not uncommon for the prosthesis to be up to 1 cm shorter than the sound limb under static conditions.

Dynamic Alignment

Alignment changes can be made with the standard modular connectors that are used to fasten the components of the prosthesis together. A standard pyramid connector (Figure 23-23) can be set anywhere within an approximately 20 degree arc of adjustability. This means, for example, that the socket can be flexed up to 10 degrees or extended up to 10 degrees from the neutral starting position. This is accomplished by loosening one screw and then tightening the opposite screw the same amount. Each pyramid permits adjustment in two orthogonal planes. For simplicity, the prosthetist will typically rotate the pyramid so that the adjustable planes are aligned with the frontal and sagittal planes. Transverse plane rotation is almost always infinitely adjustable; the standard connectors can accommodate any foot position. When the dynamic alignment differs greatly from bench alignment, it may be necessary to add a special alignable component to the prosthesis. This component will accommodate a larger window of adjustment and allows for linear changes in addition to angular changes.

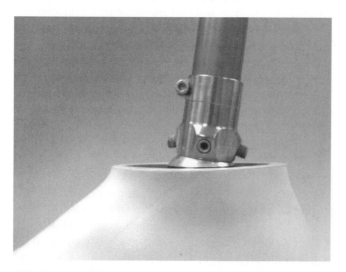

FIGURE 23-23 An example of the component that attaches the prosthetic foot to the pylon. This pyramid is set to its maximum limit of approximately 10 degrees of plantarflexion. (Photo courtesy of David A. Knapp, CPO, Hanger Prosthetics & Orthotics, North Haven, CT)

For example, the foot can be inset relative to the socket simply by sliding the foot medially and retightening the connector. This device is to be used during the dynamic alignment only and then removed during the final fabrication procedure. Small linear adjustments can also be made without that special component by performing equal but opposite angular adjustments on two adjacent pyramid connectors; however, this method will simultaneously affect the height of the prosthesis.

During the dynamic analysis, the prosthetist will ask the individual to walk in a safe environment, typically within the parallel bars, and observe the motion of the prosthesis throughout the gait cycle. Adjustments are made to minimize gait deviations and create a smooth and stable gait pattern. The prosthetist will attempt to create an energy efficient stride by minimizing the horizontal and vertical excursion of the center of mass. Goals for the optimal alignment are stance stability, swing clearance, equal step length, and energy efficiency. Socket fit and suspension play an important role in providing stability, so final adjustments to both of those aspects are included as part of the dynamic analysis. Although dynamic alignment is typically done on a flat, level surface, many prosthetists will also attempt to simulate other terrains that an individual will encounter in their daily lives. Ramps, stairs, and uneven surfaces all require slightly different alignments for optimal performance. Final alignment is often a compromise of function on the varied terrain that an amputee will encounter.

As the question of whether or not the alignment of the prosthesis is "good" or not is ultimately answered by the function and contentedness of the person wearing the prosthesis, there is a fairly broad range of alignments that can be considered acceptable.[27] In an effort to standardize what is ultimately a subjective estimate of proper alignment, the concept of vertical alignment axis and alignment reference center has been proposed. The vertical alignment axis is a vertical line that passes through the geometric center of the socket at the level of the midpatellar tendon. The alignment reference center is the point along the line from the center of the foot through the tip of the shoe, one-third of the way forward from the back of the heel. To align the prosthesis, the individual is asked to fully weight bear on the socket while the socket is supported on a padded stand. The person determines the socket axis based upon the most comfortable weight-bearing position. When the socket is aligned with the socket axis in the most comfortable position and the vertical alignment axis goes directly through the alignment reference center (Figure 23-24), the prosthesis is generally accepted to be "well-aligned."

Electronic Alignment

Technology has been developed to assist the prosthetist in objectifying the alignment process and thereby making prosthetic alignments more repeatable and predictable. Electronic sensors imbedded in the prosthetic components are capable of transmitting real-time gait data to a nearby computer. The computer processes these data and superimposes a graph of the actual forces and moments for one complete gait cycle over a set of "normal" data (Figure 23-25).[28] Displaying the otherwise invisible forces and moments on the prosthesis cues

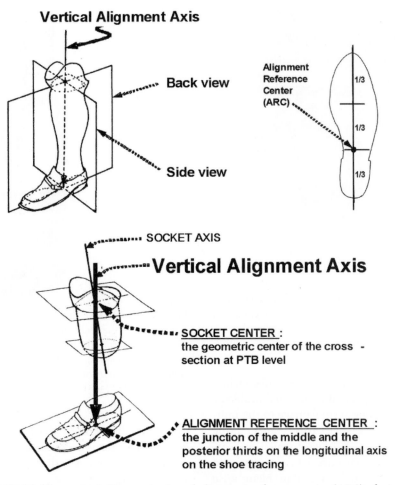

FIGURE 23-24 The vertical alignment axis and alignment reference center (ARC) of a transtibial prosthesis. Note that the socket axis is set in slight flexion from vertical. The center of the socket should be at the center of the cross section of the socket at the level of the patellar tendon bar. The alignment reference center is one-third the distance from the posterior edge of the shoe worn on the prosthetic foot. (Reprinted with permission from Lin C, Wu YC, Edwards M. Vertical alignment axis for transtibial prostheses: a simplified alignment method. *J Formos Med Assoc*. 2000;99[1]:39-44.)

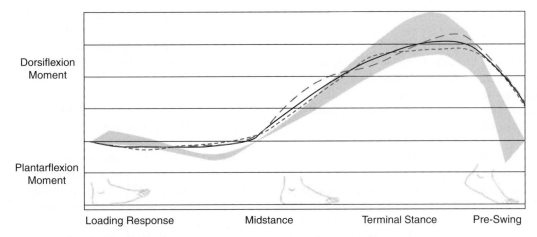

FIGURE 23-25 This graph shows sagittal plane moment data collected for three cycles of stance phase by an individual walking with a prosthesis as compared with the typical pattern of walking by persons with intact lower extremities (shaded area). (Reprinted with permission from Orthocare Innovations, Oklahoma City, OK; http://www.orthocareinnovations.com/caffeine/uploads/files/Compas-Mastery-Lesson-2-Excessive-Valgus.pdf)

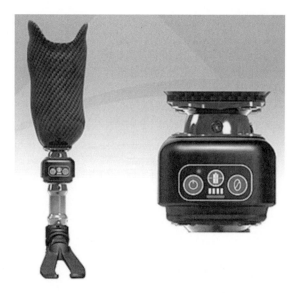

FIGURE 23-26 The prosthesis is fitted with an electronic sensor that can capture real-time gait data and transmit them to the clinician's computer. (Reprinted with permission from College Park Inc., Frasier, MI; http://www.hellotrade.com/college-park-industries/product.html)

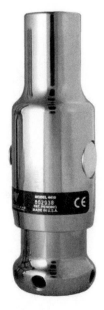

FIGURE 23-27 An example of a extra component that is mounted directly under the socket to reduce amount of torque and shock that is transferred from the ground to the limb. It replaces all or part of the pylon, depending on available length. (Reprinted with permission from Ossur Americas, Foothill Ranch, CA; http://www.ossur.com/?PageID=13468)

the prosthetist to focus in on specific variances and consider their possible causes. This can prevent undetected problems with alignment from causing long-term damage to the indivdual's limb. For example, an excessive varus moment at the knee can lead to premature medial compartmental osteoarthritis over a long period. These objective data can be printed and kept in the person's file to be referenced if problems arise or changes are necessary in the future (Figure 23-26).

ADDITIONAL FEATURES

There is an assortment of modular components that can be added to a prosthesis between the socket and the foot to enhance certain features and function of the prosthesis. These include shock absorbers, torque absorbers, and dynamic pylons. The downside of such components are that they weight and require sufficient clearance between the socket and foot. They may limit foot choices for that reason and are typically used in cases where excessive shock is expected or when an acceptable gait pattern is not attainable with existing feet alone. Care should be taken to mount these components as proximal as possible on the prosthesis to minimize the inertial effects of the additional weight during swing phase.

Torque Absorber

When rotational motion in the socket is causing discomfort or excessive stress on the skin, a torque absorber can be used to decrease the rotational torque from the ground reaction force. A torque absorber is a component that uses a viscoelastic bumper to allow a limited amount or rotation to occur at the foot without displacing the socket. The amount of rotation is proportional to the torque and can range up to 30 degrees in either direction. This is especially useful in sports applications, such as golf and tennis, that require a wide range

of rotation during the activity. Torque absorbers may also be beneficial for turns encountered in normal daily ambulation, especially for persons with fragile skin (Figure 23-27).

Shock Absorber

Although much of the functional shock absorption needed for gait is attainable with controlled knee flexion in loading response, some individual's benefit from additional vertical excursion afforded by the addition of a shock absorber.[29] This component uses a viscoelastic spring to dampen the ground reaction forces by slowing down their transmission to the limb. As weight is transferred to the prosthesis, the shock absorber compresses relative to the magnitude of the ground reaction force. This reduces impact by spreading the force out over a longer time interval. This compression leads to a reduction of the overall prosthesis height during early stance.

Dynamic Pylon

Typical prosthetic pylons are rigid and only function as an attachment between the socket and foot to establish the correct overall height. Dynamic pylons allow for energy to be stored as spring tension as they flex through midstance and terminal stance. This energy is released in preswing to assist with hip and knee flexion and promote toe clearance and limb advancement. This energy return allows the individual to walk with less energy consumption and increased efficiency, meaning that they can walk farther and longer. The angle of flexion in a dynamic pylon is small and is difficult to observe during casual ambulation. The effects are more readily apparent during jogging or running (Figure 23-28).

A Man with Traumatic Transtibial Amputation

Prosthetic Prescription

Let us consider the case of J. W., a 37-year-old male whose left leg was amputated below the knee following a motorcycle accident. He has since recovered from all his injuries and is now medically stable. He was recently approved for weight-bearing as tolerated on his left limb. He is 5′8″ tall, weighs 175 lb (79.5 kg), and his residual limb measures approximately 20 cm from knee center to distal end. He has significant amounts of scar tissue on the surface of the residual limb including a skin graft from his thigh. The skin on the distal end of the limb is adhered to the distal end of the tibia. He was very active prior to his injury and would like to return to that lifestyle as soon as possible. He arrives at the clinic on crutches.

Questions to Consider

- Is the individual a good prosthetic candidate?
- What type of interface, suspension, and socket design are appropriate?
- What other components are recommended?

Recommendations

The first decision is to determine whether or not J. W. is a prosthetic candidate. His entry into the clinic on crutches indicates that his balance, upper extremity strength, and contralateral limb are all sufficient for gait. The only factor that jeopardizes his prosthetic candidacy is the condition of the soft tissue of his residual limb. In the past, that might prevent successful use of the prosthesis, but with modern techniques and materials, a successful fitting is likely.

The interface with the skin should be determined next. Two conditions need to be considered: the adherent tissue on the distal end; and the fragile skin graft. Gel liners are most efficient at eliminating shear forces on the limb. This will be a major factor in preventing skin breakdown of the adherent skin. The skin graft would benefit from a soft durometer gel, rather than a silicone elastomer or urethane liner. The selection of the right interface will be critical to J. W.'s outcome. The decision to use an off-the-shelf size or a custom-made liner will depend upon the shape of the limb and how well he could be fitted with a standard liner size.

The suspension for J. W. should be the system that will lead to the least amount of pistoning. Elevated vacuum will maintain the limb volume by drawing fluid back into the tissues between weight-bearing cycles. This is important for J. W. because the tissues of his limb will be subjected to a large amount of strain once he reaches his goal of readopting an active lifestyle.

Prosthetic Fitting and Alignment: Visit 1

J. W. is seen today for the initial fitting of his first prosthesis. The gel liner is donned directly on the skin and a single-ply

sock is worn over the liner. The limb is then placed into the socket and a sealing sleeve is rolled up to midthigh to seal off the proximal edge of the socket. J. W. is then asked to stand up in the parallel bars, keeping all his weight on the sound limb. As tolerated, J. W. will then slowly transfer weight over to the prosthesis. Once he is comfortable bearing his full weight on the prosthesis, he can begin to take his first steps.

As he begins to walk and feel more confident in the prosthesis, J. W. begins to let go of the bars and walk hands-free. Once he does this, his knee begins to rapidly flex during loading response and the foot starts slapping the floor.

Questions to Consider

- Is the alignment of the prosthesis adjusted properly? Is the foot making an appropriate heel strike? Has the heel height of the shoe been properly accommodated?
- Is the socket stable on his limb? Are there signs of pistoning? Is there excessive medial shift of the prosthesis during stance?
- Are his knee extensors strong enough to eccentrically control knee flexion during full weight-bearing?

Recommendations

A plumb bob through the midline of the socket falls between the posterior one-third and anterior two-thirds of the foot when the shoe is donned, and the top of the foot shell is level with the ground. This is indicative that the alignment is appropriate. Muscle strength testing reveals that the quadriceps of the residual limb are 2two of +/5five. Due toBecause of his lack of quadriceps strength, he is unable to regulate knee flexion during loading response. A rehabilitation protocol for quadriceps strengthening should be implemented that includes ambulation with the prosthesis. At the same time, the prosthesis can be altered to improve his gait pattern as he regains his strength. The foot should be moved anteriorly, relative to the socket. This will decrease the mechanical advantage of ground reaction force to flex the knee by shortening the heel lever. It will simultaneously increase the length of the toe lever which will provide more stability in midstance. The potential downside is that the knee extension moment in terminal stance will also be increased so there is potential for the knee to hyperextend. The indivudal should be asked to monitor posterior knee pain and report any as soon as it is recognized.

Because his muscle weakness is expected to resolve relatively quickly, the alignment of the prosthesis should be monitored on a regular basis so that the foot can be gradually shifted back to the appropriate position and normal gait can be restored.

Prosthetic Fitting and Alignment: Visit 2

J. W. has done well with rehabilitation and use of his lower-extremity prosthesis. His limb has healed well and his

Continued

strength is generally good. He has good balance and endurance for walking with the prosthesis. He has gradually increased his prosthesis wear time and activity level. He works a 5-hour day in agriculture. Today he returns to therapy for a scheduled followup appointment. He complains of discomfort in the distal end and loss of stability in the socket. As you observe his gait, the prosthesis appears to be a little short. Assessment of the residual limb reveals erythema on the distal end and on the distal aspect of the patella.

Questions to Consider

- What changes have occurred since his last visit? Has he made changes to sock ply or footwear? Has he gained or lost weight?
- Is this an alignment- or fit-related issue? When does the pain occur in the gait cycle? Does the pain increase throughout the day?
- Is the interface worn out? How old is the interface now? How long should it be expected to last? Are there thin areas in the interface that might indicate excessive pressure and premature wear?

Recommendations

You find that his weight and footwear have not changed. He is wearing the same single-ply sock with which he began his prosthetic use. His gel liner is still in excellent condition and should be expected to last for about a year of constant wear. Consideration of all the information indicates that the limb has changed since the initial fitting. As his pain is worst at midstance and increases proportionally with his time spent weight bearing, the conclusion is that the limb is too far distal in the socket. He should increase the number of socks that he is wearing by one ply until the limb is seated correctly in the socket. This will also address the length of the prosthesis which had appeared too short.

In experimenting with sock ply, J. W. went from initially wearing a single sock to six plies, but he found this number of socks created a new set of problems. He was then feeling excessive pressure on the tibial tubercle and proximal aspect of the fibular head. During loading response he was unable to regulate his knee flexion because of pain on the anterodistal aspect of the tibia. Despite good suspension, he was also starting to scuff his toe during swing phase. All these symptoms indicate that he is now too far out of the socket. This position decreases the control of the tibia and allows the socket to flex and extend beyond the position of the limb, leading to excessive pressure on the ends of the bones. It also positions the bony prominences of the limb in areas that do not have adequate reliefs. Removal of several sock plies is the correct intervention, as this will allow him to seat further in the socket and increase comfort and stability. When J. W. wore four-ply socks, the comfort and control of the prosthesis were restored.

CASE EXAMPLE 2

An Older Woman with Amputation Related to Vascular Disease

Prosthetic Prescription

G. R. is a 76-year-old woman with type 2 diabetes and peripheral vascular disease. G. R. sustained an abrasion at the lateral malleolus of the right leg. The skin abrasion failed to heal and developed into a stage 4 nonhealing wound. Circulation at the lower leg was markedly impaired. After several months of multiple failed therapies to improve circulation and promote wound healing, the right leg was amputated below the knee 2 months ago. G. R. is 5′4″ tall and weighs 204 lb (92.5 kg). Prior to the problems with her leg, she was living independently and caring for her husband, who is significantly disabled. The transtibial amputation wound site is completely healed. Her physician is recommending that she begin bearing weight on the limb as tolerated. She has been using a wheelchair for mobility in the house, but she is able to stand on her left leg with support of a standard walker. She is concerned that she will not be able to do her chores around the house and the shopping even after she receives her prosthesis.

Questions to Consider

- What are the G. R.'s goals for the prosthesis? Will she be a functional ambulator? Will the prosthesis be used only for standing and transfers?
- Will she require assistance with activities of daily living and care for her husband?
- What are the main design goals for her prosthesis? What system will allow her to don the prosthesis independently? Which will require the least maintenance and most reliable function?

Recommendations

Evaluating G. R.'s candidacy for a prosthesis will involve assessing her risk-to-benefit ratio as a bipedal ambulator against the negative health effects of prolonged sitting. Her motivation to ambulate is clear in her expressed desire to continue to care for her husband. Her ability to stand on one leg is a fortuitous sign, even if her balance is impaired at this point. Her knee ROM is within normal limits. If her skin integrity is good and her right knee extensors are four of five, she will likely be a good prosthetic candidate.

Her prosthesis should be easy to put on, as she will not have assistance available. Her limb has ample soft tissue based on her weight and etiology, although her diabetes puts her at risk for fragile skin and delayed healing. The most appropriate interface for her will be one that most effectively reduces shear. A silicone elastomer cushion liner in a TSB socket will work well for her. A sealing sleeve and expulsion valve will utilize suction as a means of suspension, thus minimizing pistoning. This prosthesis should allow her to wear a cotton sock that is easily laundered as she loses limb volume. The trim lines should be set higher proximally to gain as much control as possible for her prosthesis.

Prosthetic Alignment and Fitting: Visit 1
G. R. is seen for delivery of her preparatory prosthesis. She is instructed on donning the device and she is able to roll on the gel liner and place her limb into the socket, with moderate effort. Her limb is seated correctly all the way in the socket. After she rolls the sealing sleeve into position, she stands at her walker and slowly begins to load the prosthesis. She is comfortable in the socket and a small amount of air is heard as it is expulsed from the socket through the valve. The sleeve is rolled down so that a corset stay can be inserted between the gel liner and the socket. As no areas were found to have excessive pressure, the corset stay is removed and the sleeve is rolled back up. Her first steps are tentative and she is bearing the majority of her weight through her arms during stance on the prosthetic side. After some guidance from her therapist, she begins to bear more weight through the prosthesis. Her strides are asymmetric, with a very large step on the prosthetic side and a truncated step on the sound side.

Questions to Consider
- Why is her step length shorter on the sound side? Is the prosthesis aligned properly? Is her range of hip flexion and extension within functional limits? Is she stable in stance?
- What are her goals for ambulation? Does she have sufficient stance stability? Does she have adequate clearance in swing? Is her gait pattern energy efficient?

Recommendations
The gait pattern she uses is typical of the individual with recent amputation who is uncertain about weight bearing through a mechanical device. The feeling of instability on the prosthesis causes the her to limit stance time on that side, thereby shortening swing phase on the sound side. Alternately, the individual is accustomed to bearing weight unilaterally on the sound side, so the stance time is increased allowing the prosthesis to move ahead excessively. Weakness of the quadriceps and gluteus minimus and medius will also impair stance stability. She should be encouraged to take smaller steps with the prosthesis and larger steps with her sound limb. She may need further conditioning of her knee extensors and hip abductors to completely eliminate this asymmetry.

Excessive socket flexion can increase prosthetic step length, but it also tends to increase the step length on the sound side as well. Extending the socket makes it more difficult to advance over the foot during stance and will tend to shorten step length on the contralateral side.

Prosthetic Fitting and Alignment: Visit 2
G. R. returns for therapy and is complaining about discomfort in her socket. Inspection of her skin reveals excessive pressure, as evidenced by erythema, on her femoral condyles and fibular head. She has been doing a good job managing her sock ply and is now seated correctly in the socket wearing eight ply. She explains that the tightness she feels does not get worse during weight bearing.

Questions to Consider
- What changes may have taken place since her last visit? As her activity level increases, what is the effect on limb volume? Which areas of the limb are most susceptible to volume loss?
- What is the source of the erythema? Is there swelling of the knee? Does the redness appear anywhere else on the limb? Does it appear to be an allergic reaction like contact dermatitis? Is her liner clean and in good condition?

Recommendations
After discussing good hygiene and prosthetic care with G. R., it is clear that she is washing her gel liner daily with a mild soap and then rinsing it thoroughly, and that she is washing her limb every day and patting in dry. She is not using any lotions that may create buildup in the liner or an allergic reaction when confined in the warm moist environment of the liner. The fit of the socket is assessed next by probing between the liner and socket with a thin metal corset stay. This is done in the non–weight-bearing state as that is when the pressure is occurring. The corset stay encounters great resistance when passing over the fibular head and is completely stuck when trying to pass over the femoral condyles. This indicates excessive pressure over those bony structures. Although she is wearing the appropriate number of socks, they are creating the extra bulk that makes the socket too tight in those areas. A referral should be made to her prosthetist so that the socket can be modified. It is likely that pads can be added in strategic areas that are more prone to volume loss, such as the area over the calf muscle and on either side of the tibia. This will take up volume in the socket and require her to reduce the number of sock ply that she wears. Following that adjustment, G. R. is feeling more comfortable in the socket and her skin is free from irritation.

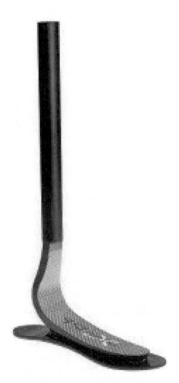

FIGURE 23-28 An example of an energy-return foot with an integrated dynamic pylon. (Courtesy of Otto Bock Healthcare, Minneapolis, MN; http://en.red-dot.org/2796.html?&cHash=20236 b03d8cbbe4dd8ba7acc74ae67aa&detail=3950)

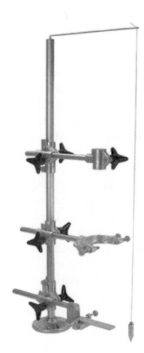

FIGURE 23-29 A prosthetist uses this device to preserve the relative positions of the foot and socket during fabrication. This allows the exact alignment of the diagnostic prosthesis to be transferred to the definitive prosthesis. (From Hosmer/Fillauer, Campbell CA; http://www.cascade-usa.com/products/TOOLS%20@@26%20 EQUIPMENT/ALIGNMENT%20AND%20FITTING%20AIDS/ VERTICAL%20FABRICATING%20JIG.aspx)

Diagnostic Sockets

Because the fit of the socket is the single most critical factor in providing a functional prosthesis, great care is taken to ensure that the fit is optimal. One tool used by prosthetists is a clear plastic socket that is used during the fitting process and then discarded, often destroyed, during the fabrication process. The diagnostic socket or "check socket" is made from a translucent plastic so that the prosthetist can inspect the limb during loading and see the blanching of the skin as the person goes through various activities of weight bearing. The plastic is also very amenable to changes in shape and volume simply by heating the area and deforming the plastic. Extended fittings, during which the individual takes the diagnostic socket home for a day or more, must be conducted carefully as some of the materials used for diagnostic sockets are brittle and can fracture under normal loading conditions. Extended fittings can be quite useful though as the prosthesis will be used under more realistic conditions and some problems will only become apparent after spending several hours in the socket.

FINISHING TECHNIQUES

After the prosthetist and the prosthetic wearer are both satisfied with the fit and alignment, the final prosthesis can be fabricated. The exact finishing technique varies based on the components that were selected, but the main goal is to preserve the alignment and create a lightweight prosthesis with a cosmetic appearance. The foot is removed and the remainder

of the prosthesis is secured in a vertical alignment jig (Figure 23-29). The socket is filled with plaster and a pipe that is held in place by the alignment jig is set into the wet plaster. After the plaster hardens, the alignment has been captured and the prosthesis can be removed from the jig. The jig preserves the alignment until the final prosthesis is reassembled. The prosthetic technician will determine the best method of fabrication to create the lightest weight prosthesis without sacrificing structural integrity. Extra alignment devices are removed during this process. The final limb is assembled with either endoskeletal or exoskeletal components based on the individual individual's needs.

Endoskeletal

The term *endoskeletal* implies that the structure of the prosthesis is located deep inside the prosthetic limb. The exterior of the prosthesis may consist of passive foam rubber or latex that gives the prosthesis a realistic appearance and protects the structural and functional parts that are hidden underneath (Figure 23-30). This type of prosthesis provides two distinct advantages: adjustability and realistic appearance. Endoskeletal design allows for the use of modular components that can be adjusted or replaced quickly and easily when needed. If a single component were to fail, repair would involve simple removal and replacement of that component, the same way a tire can be changed on a car. These modular components can be easily procured as they are not custom made for the individual. The appearance of the endoskeletal limb can be quite realistic. Virtually any size and

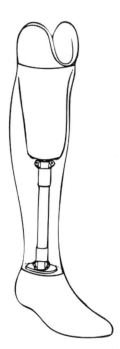

FIGURE 23-30 A diagram of an endoskeletal prosthesis, in which the socket and pylon are concealed to within a cosmetic cover. (Reprinted with permission from: *Below Knee Prosthetics*, Prosthetics-Orthotics Program, University of Texas Southwestern Medical Center at Dallas, TX, 1988, p. 4-11)

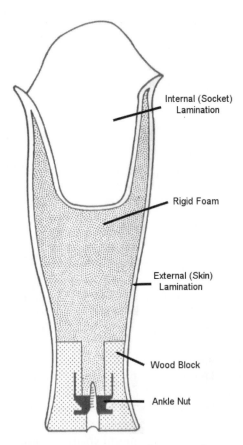

FIGURE 23-31 A cross-sectional diagram of an exoskeletal prosthesis that transmits weight bearing forces through the external lamination. The lamination gets its shape from the rigid foam interior. (Reprinted with permission from: *Below Knee Prosthetics*, Prosthetics-Orthotics Program, University of Texas Southwestern Medical Center at Dallas, TX, 1988, p. 4-10)

shape can be created by shaping soft lightweight foam over the components. The foam can be coated with a variety of finishes that provide color and texture and may include lifelike details such as moles, freckles, pores, and even hair. Premium restorations are nearly indistinguishable from the sound limb.

Exoskeletal

When a more durable and easily cleanable prosthesis is desired an exoskeletal prosthesis can be fabricated. The socket of an exoskeletal prosthesis is attached to the foot through an external composite lamination that is custom shaped for the individual (Figure 23-31). To create this shape, a wooden ankle block is first bonded to the socket with rigid foam in the vertical alignment jig. The foam is rigid enough to maintain the alignment between the socket and foot that was preserved in the jig. The foam and ankle block are then shaped by hand to match the contralateral side, only a little bit smaller to accommodate the thickness of the final lamination. The final step is to seal the foam and laminate the exterior; this final composite covering provides the structure of the prosthesis as well as the cosmesis. Exoskeletal prostheses are often heavier than their endoskeletal counterparts, and are always less adjustable. The advantage of the exoskeletal system is the durability. The hard surface that covers the prosthesis is nonporous, chemically inert, and waterproof, making it easy to clean and virtually indestructible.

GAIT DEVIATIONS

Gait deviations can be caused by improper socket fit, misalignment of the prosthesis or by weakness or other musculoskeletal pathologies of the individual. Careful evaluation

is essential to determine the cause of the deviations and what can be done to correct them (Readers are referred to Chapter 5 for a review of the biomechanics of normal gait). Variations in limb volume or shoe type can introduce deviations in a prosthetic wearer's gait that had not been exhibited before. It can be very productive to ask the person if there have been any changes in their routine recently. Changes in diet, medications, shrinker wear, or activity level can all effect limb volume. If a shoe with a higher or lower heel is placed on the prosthesis it will change the orientation of the socket to the ground. Unless there is a component that will accommodate the new heel height, the patent's gait will be adversely affected. Common gait deviations will be reviewed as they occur in the gait cycle in each individual plane.

Initial Contact

Sagittal

Initial contact should be made with the heel (Figure 23-32). If contact at the forefoot first there may be either excessive plantarflexion of the prosthetic foot or limitation of the person's knee extension range of motion (i.e. knee flexion contracture). Both of these circumstances contribute to a high knee

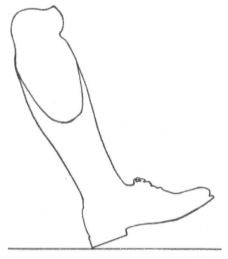

FIGURE 23-32 Ideally, initial contact of the prosthesis with the ground should be at the heel, followed by a controlled flexion of the knee and foot flat. (diagram courtesy of David A. Knapp, CPO, Hanger Prosthetics & Orthotics, North Haven, CT)

extension moment during loading response that causes the knee to move posteriorly. This motion, decimates efficiency and can damage the knee over time. Every effort should be made to create a heel strike at initial contact. This includes therapeutic exercises to increase knee ROM and knee extensor strength; prosthetic alignment changes to accommodate knee flexion contractures; and proper height and suspension of the prosthesis. If the prosthesis is too long or does not suspend well, the prosthesis may hit the ground prior to the end of swing phase.

Frontal

Excessive inversion or eversion of the foot at initial contact indicates misalignment of the prosthesis. The heel of the prosthetic foot should be level when it meets the ground.

The lateral border of the heel should contact the surface first; this is related to the transverse plane alignment of the foot to accommodate a normal toe-out angle of 5 to 10 degrees. This lateral heel contact sets up the standard progression of the ground reaction force up the lateral border of the foot and then crossing to the medial aspect of the forefoot during stance phase.

Transverse

The rotation of the prosthesis is fairly consistent throughout stance phase. The medial border of the foot should be parallel to the line of progression. Transverse plane rotation at initial contact is an indicator that the limb is fitting too loosely in the socket, or that the foot is not directly under the limb. External motion may be seen with an inset foot, while internal motion could be a result of an outset foot (Figure 23-33).

Loading Response

Sagittal

Excessive knee flexion moment during loading response is caused by a foot that is set too far posteriorly, is too dorsiflexed, or has a heel that is too rigid. The transition during loading response should be smooth and controlled, the knee should bend to approximately 20 degrees of flexion as the forefoot meets the ground; this moves the limb forward and aids in shock absorption. Insufficient knee flexion moment can be caused by a heel that is too soft or a foot that is positioned too far anteriorly. This can cause the knee to hyperextend leading to pain and inefficiency. Adjustment of the heel lever length, stiffness, and orientation should be made to provide the appropriate degree of knee flexion.

Frontal

Rapid loading of the foot during this phase would produce significant moments at the knee if the foot were not parallel to the ground at initial contact. The plantar surface of the

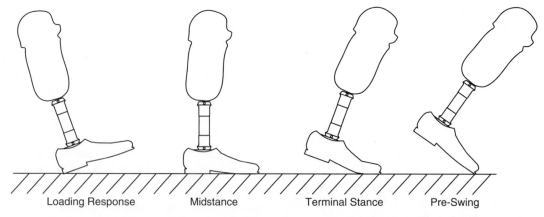

Loading Response   Midstance   Terminal Stance   Pre-Swing

FIGURE 23-33 The progression of the transfemoral prosthesis during stance phase. Initial contact is made at the heel, and compression of the prosthetic heel simulates controlled lowering of the foot during loading response. At midstance, weight bearing forces move anteriorly to the ball of the foot. In terminal stance, the anterior portion of the prosthetic foot simulates toe extension and the heel rises. In pre-swing, the individual rolls over the toe and moves into knee flexion for effective shortening of the limb for swing limb clearance. (Diagram courtesy of David A. Knapp, CPO, Hanger Prosthetics & Orthotics, North Haven, CT)

foot should be level during this phase as viewed in the frontal plane. Some modern prosthetic feet have rearfoot inversion and eversion capabilities and can adapt to the surface upon weight bearing, which is useful for uneven surfaces. Be sure to observe the motion as the loading occurs. When there is motion while ambulating on a flat surface, the alignment of the foot should be changed to eliminate that motion.

Transverse

Any rotation of the foot during loading may indicate a loose or faulty torsion adapter. Rotary moments can be generated by excessive toe-in or toe-out and the torsion adapters allow that motion to occur uncontrolled.

Midstance

Sagittal

A choppy or segmented midstance is caused by differences in the dynamic characteristics between the prosthetic heel and the prosthetic toe, indicating a lack of stability. The heel and toe lever arms are adjustable by shifting the socket anteriorly to shorten the toe or posteriorly to shorten the heel. The optimal foot position is one where the forward velocity of the knee is consistent between loading response and midstance. The prosthetic foot must accommodate smooth transition of the ground reaction force from the heel to the forefoot during midstance. Over this period, the moment at the knee changes from a flexion moment to an extension moment. A steady increase in dorsiflexion should be observed as the knee moves over the foot.

Frontal

There is a normal and desirable varus moment during midstance. This is because, in order to be most energy efficient while walking, the body's center of mass does not shift all the way over the stance foot. The knee should move laterally approximately 1 cm during midstance. Shift of the knee greater than 2 cm indicates an excessive varus moment and will lead to stress on the medial compartment and lateral ligaments of the person's knee. This can be reduced by adducting the socket or shifting it medially. If the socket does not move or shifts medially during midstance, the socket is too far inset (or the foot is too outset) or the socket excessively adducted. Lateral gapping is a condition where a large gap occurs during loading between the limb and the lateral wing of the socket. If a gap larger than 2 cm is observed, the socket may be too loose and an additional ply of sock should be added.

Transverse

Rotation that occurs during midstance is typically seen between the limb and socket and is almost always attributable to poor socket fit. If motion is occurring, the person may complain of patellar impingement on either the medial or lateral aspects of the patella. The remedy is often tightening the socket by adding a ply or two of socks. In cases in which the socks are insufficient to stabilize the rotation, the

socket should be adjusted by the prosthetist. Pretibial pads that provide pressure on either side of the tibial crest are an effective solution to stop rotation.

Terminal Stance

Sagittal

Drop off is the excessive descent of the center of mass during terminal stance caused by a toe lever that is either too short or too soft. It is often characterized by diminished heel rise. This compromises energy efficiency of walking. It occurs at a point when the body's center of mass is already near the bottom of its sinusoidal path. The toe lever of the prosthetic foot must have sufficient stiffness to resist dorsiflexion when the person's entire weight is placed on the ball of the foot. This is a critical phase of gait when it comes to energy efficiency. Proper loading of the forefoot promotes knee stability, maintains altitude (i.e., level pelvis), and stores energy in the ligaments that can be released during swing phase to assist with limb advancement (Figure 23-34).

Early heel off is an indication that the foot is too plantarflexed or the toe lever is too stiff. The heel should come off the ground at the point when the swing foot has already passed anterior to the stance limb. Forward momentum of the body is impeded by early toe-off and may force the individual into an anterior lean with the trunk to maintain forward progression. The ankle should be set to dorsiflex until the swing limb reaches terminal swing so that the heel remains on the ground until the center of mass has progressed sufficiently forward. This will preserve step length and enhance stability.

Frontal

The heel should rise off the ground with the knee breaking over the point on the foot between the first and second toes. Any large variance from this position will create instability and consequently shorten step length. The knee should travel in a straight line as it flexes; any lateral motion during this phase will lead to a whip in swing.

Transverse

The toe load is highest during this phase of gait, therefore there is potential for rotation of the prosthesis due to suboptimal alignment. External rotation can be caused by a foot that is too far outset or had excessive too toe-out. Internal rotation is caused by an excessively inset or internally rotated foot.

Preswing

Sagittal

As the body weight transfers rapidly to the contralateral limb, the prosthesis should roll forward over the toe and lift off the ground. Toe-drag may be a result of a foot that is excessively plantarflexed or a faulty suspension.

Frontal

The knee should not move medially or laterally during preswing. An externally rotated foot can cause a valgus moment that pushed the knee medially as the weight is transferred off

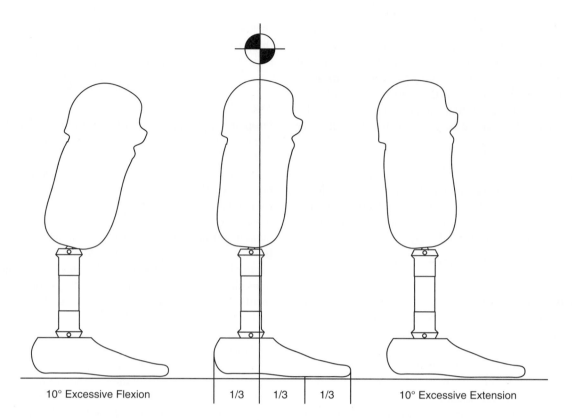

10° Excessive Flexion   1/3 | 1/3 | 1/3   10° Excessive Extension

FIGURE 23-34 Socket angle will affect the magnitude and timing of the ground reaction force through the knee during stance phase. Optimal alignment (center) varies with specific foot design but will be approximated by the centerline of the socket falling through the posterior one-third and anterior two thirds of the foot. (Diagram courtesy of David A. Knapp, CPO, Hanger Prosthetics & Orthotics, North Haven, CT)

the prosthesis. This can also be caused by an outset foot or an excessively adducted socket. Lateral motion during preswing can be caused by an internally rotated foot, an excessively inset foot, or an excessively abducted socket.

Transverse

Many of the same factors that lead to instability in the frontal plane can lead to instability in the transverse plane as well. Appropriate attention to transverse plane alignment throughout stance phase should help to avoid issues in preswing as well.

Swing Phase

Sagittal

The transtibial prosthesis swings passively forward during swing phase. If sufficient ground clearance is not obtained the amount of knee flexion should be noted. In cases where appropriate knee flexion is observed, the suspension of the prosthesis should be evaluated. A faulty suspension or a plantarflexed foot will reduce swing clearance. The amount of pistoning varies with the type of suspension used. Motion exceeding 1 cm should be considered excessive. If knee flexion is observed during swing phase, active and passive motion should be assessed. Weakness or contracture of the knee can limit knee motion, as can a tight suspension sleeve or an aggressive supracondylar wedge. Although suspension and

knee flexion are often adversarial, a balance should be attainable that permits enough foot clearance for safe ambulation. Otherwise, the prosthesis may require shortening.

Frontal

Socket instability during swing is typically caused by either a faulty suspension or a loose-fitting socket. The weight of the socket pulls the prosthesis into varus during swing if the limb is not well seated in the socket. Increasing sock ply and implementing an improved suspension should remedy any swing phase instability.

Transverse

Rotation during swing phase is often caused by what is known as a "whip." When the heel of the prosthetic foot moves medially in initial swing and then laterally during midswing, it is referred to as a medial whip. A lateral whip follows the opposite pattern. Whips can be caused by misalignment of the knee axis at the onset of swing or by irregular loading of the limb in terminal stance. Alignment of the knee axis in a person using a transtibial prosthesis is determined by the function of the hip, and should be addressed by strengthening and ROM exercises. Prosthetic remedies must examine the loading of the prosthesis. Medial whips can be caused by a foot that is too far inset or externally rotated. Both medial and lateral whips can be caused by a foot that is too plantarflexed.

TROUBLESHOOTING

A common problem encountered by individuals with recent transtibial amputation is application of too few or too many sock ply. Sock-ply management is a skill that develops as the indivudal wears the prosthesis more and is conscientious about examining the limb after doffing the prosthesis. The number of socks will eventually become consistent, but early in the process of limb maturation, a large degree of variability is common. The correct number of socks may vary from day to day, or even from hour to hour. There are a few basic cues that the those new to prosthetic use must consider to ensure that the limb is in the correct position within the socket.

The first cue is during donning—the limb should slide into the socket with some resistance. Although this is a subjective determination, after a short time the person should recognize the amount of force needed to fully don the prosthesis with the correct number of socks. Too few socks allows the limb to "bottom out" in the socket, where most of the weight-bearing will occur on the distal end. This leads to pain, instability, and increased pistoning. Conversely, too many socks prevents the limb from fully entering the socket; this leads to loss of control and pressure on bony prominences.

The second cue to the prosthetic wearer is increased pistoning, anteroposterior, or medial–lateral motion within the socket when walking. This can be caused by an insufficient number of socks.

The final cue is found upon doffing the prosthesis. The skin should be checked for erythema. Erythema on the distal aspect of the fibular head or patella indicates that the limb is too far in the socket and extra ply of socks are needed. If too many socks are being used, the erythema will appear on the tibial tubercle or the proximal aspect of the fibular head, as the limb is not far enough into the socket. In this case, there may also be signs of verrucose hyperplasia on the distal end of the limb as a result of the lack of distal contact.

Another common problem that arises with prosthetic users is caused by inappropriate shoe wear. Although some prosthetic feet accommodate for the heel height of the shoe, most do not. Wearing a heel that is too high positions the limb such that there is a relative excessive flexion of the socket and actual of the knee joint during stance. A heel that is too low or going barefoot tends to hyperextend the knee. Proper foot wear is important for safe ambulation. The prosthesis can be checked by evaluating the top surface of the foot shell while the prosthesis is free standing on a level surface. If the top of the foot shell tilts posteriorly, the heel is too low (Figure 23-35).

In a well-fitting socket, the skin should appear uniform in color after wearing the prosthesis. Areas of erythema that fade after 20 minutes are not likely to be problematic. The skin should be soft and supple, especially on the distal end. Firm tissue associated with edema is a sign of poor contact and an effort should be made to create some contact in the

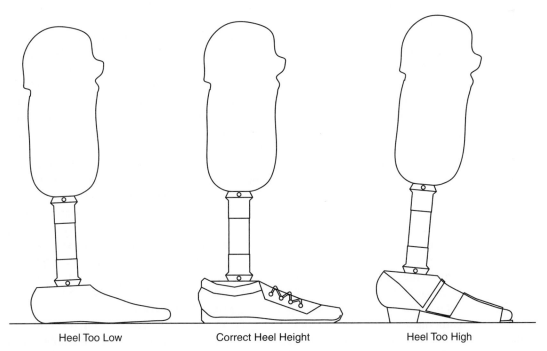

| Heel Too Low | Correct Heel Height | Heel Too High |

FIGURE 23-35 Heel height of the shoes affects the sagittal plane moments throughout stance. A heel that is too low for the prosthetic foot creates excessive extensor moment at the knee in midstance, hampering forward progression. A heel that is too high for the prosthetic foot creates a flexion moment at the knee at midstance, leading to early "drop off" and compromise of stance phase stability. (Photo courtesy of David A. Knapp, CPO, Hanger Prosthetics & Orthotics, North Haven, CT)

area of the firm tissue. The individual may not tolerate much pressure, but only a small amount of pressure is needed to push the extra fluid back into circulation. If erythema is observed over bony prominences, and the person's residual limb is properly seated in the socket, pressure in those areas needs to be relieved. Prosthetists can adjust fit of thermoplastic sockets by heating and reshaping the areas that need adjustment. Thermoset sockets, like composites, can only be adjusted by cutting out fenestrations or by adding padding to the area around the prominent bone to shift it away from the socket wall. It is important to note that addition of padding requires removal of some equivalent sock ply to maintain the same volume within the socket.

If skin irritation is present, especially over a bony prominence, placing a small mark on the affected areas with lipstick before donning the prosthesis will allow the lipstick to transfer to the socket during ambulation. Once the prosthetic wearer removes the prosthesis, the lipstick will mark the areas of excessive contact. Alternatively, a thin flexible steel probe (a corset stay works exceptionally well) can be inserted between the socket and the interface to act as a feeler gauge to find areas of high pressure. The individual should be putting some weight through the socket during this evaluation. To assess distal contact in a finished socket, a ball of soft clay, about the size of a blueberry, can be placed into the bottom of the socket prior to donning. After the person dons the prosthesis and walks a few steps, the prosthesis should be removed and the clay examined. The clay should appear compressed. Postcompression clay thickness of 3 to 5 mm is considered ideal. Total contact in the socket can be assessed by lightly powdering the interior surface of the socket with a fine powder like cornstarch and having the individual carefully don the prosthesis and walk a few steps. Any powder that remains on the socket's surface after walking indicates that those areas are not in contact with the residual limb.

The amount of pistoning that is present in a socket depends upon the socket design and the type of suspension that is used. If the person is complaining of discomfort while ambulating but is comfortable while standing, pistoning is the likely cause of the pain. Pistoning can be assessed by asking the individual to fully weight bear on the socket and then lift the prosthesis off the ground while the examiner is palpating the patella; motion of more than 1 cm should be considered excessive. Faulty suspension and/or loose socket fit are generally responsible for pistoning. Wearing the correct ply of sock and ensuring that the suspension is functioning well should minimize the motion in the socket to pain-free levels.

There are several patterns of erythema that indicate poor alignment of the prosthesis. Excessive varus moment on the limb is suspected when signs of pressure are observed on both the distolateral and the proximomedial aspects of the limb together. This pattern can be caused by excessive foot inset or too much socket adduction. When the erythema is observed on the distomedial and proximolateral aspects of the limb, an excessive valgus moment is likely. The foot may be too far outset or the socket may be excessively abducted. Anterior distal pressure accompanied by pressure in the posterior proximal

aspect of the socket may be a result of an excessively long heel lever arm, excessive dorsiflexion, excessive socket flexion, or a heel that is too firm. This pattern can also be observed when an individual wears a shoe that has a higher heel than the prosthesis can accommodate. Conversely, if the person goes barefoot, the opposite pattern of pressure will be observed; erythema on the posterior distal end and the anteroproximal end. This is the same pattern that can be caused by a toe lever arm that is too long, an overly plantarflexed foot, or an excessively extended socket.

SPECIALTY PROSTHESES

There are novel prosthetic designs that are intended for use in specialized activities such as water sports, running, and bicycling. The biomechanical goals of these prosthetic devices are different from those designed for everyday ambulation. They must take into account the unique loading and environmental exposure requirements that will be encountered. Running feet, for example, lack a heel spring because sprinting takes place on the toes only; a heel would interfere with limb motion and add unnecessary weight. Because knee flexion during a sprint may reach beyond 110 degrees, the posterior proximal trim line needs to be lower; and because there is a great deal more impact force at initial contact, more care should be given to ensuring that the person and prosthesis are capable of absorbing the impact slowly in a manner that will prevent damage to the skin and limb. Running also subjects the prosthesis to greater tension in swing phase, so the suspension system will be under increased strain. Runners often use an auxiliary suspension just in case their primary suspension fails at high speed.

A prosthesis that is designed for swimming includes a lot more than just the ability to get wet. Attention must be given to the buoyancy of the device. Neutral buoyancy is preferred because a prosthesis that floats may inhibit the individual's ability to keep his or her head above the water surface, and a prosthesis that sinks could drag the person down with it. Any water that gets inside the prosthesis should have a quick path to get back out once the person finishes swimming. A swimming prosthesis can also be fitted with an adjustable ankle that allows the swimmer to lock the ankle in approximately 70 degrees of plantarflexion, which accommodates the use of a swim fin. Waterproof components and materials that do not absorb water are the best choices when designing a swimming prosthesis so that the individual can also use the device on the way to and from the swimming area. Any time the prosthesis is used in salt water, it is advised that the the prosthesis be thoroughly rinsed with fresh water after swimming, even if it was designed for maritime use.

There are specialized feet for downhill skiing that clip directly into the ski binding, rock climbing feet that require no shoes, cycling feet that clip directly into the pedals, and many other specialized feet for sports and recreational activities. To save money and time and to avoid carrying several complete prostheses with them, active prosthetic wearers can use a quick disconnect adapter to keep one socket and rapidly switch between different specialty feet. The adapter ensures that the alignment of the prosthesis is optimal for each different activity that the specific foot is intended for. It also provides a light-weight secure and safe connection so the individual is confident that the prosthesis will not fail. Most insurance companies will pay for these types of prostheses when they are shown to be medically necessary.

SUMMARY

Persons with transtibial amputation have the opportunity to participate in a rehabilitation process that seeks to maximize function and minimize impairments so that they can participate as fully as they can in activities of daily living and instrumental activities of daily living. An interdisciplinary team is available to support medical, nursing, social, therapy, and prosthetic needs of the individual and the team develops a plan of care that addresses the goals of the persos, family, and caregivers. Standard and new advances in prosthetics for persons with transtibial amputation offer a wide array of options that range from prosthesis use for cosmesis and home-bound ambulator to community ambulator with variable cadence and intensive athletic involvement. The clinicians dedicated to enhancing the quality of life of persons with transtibial amputation evaluate the many variables that come into play when engaging in a postamputation rehabilitation program including (a) overall health, functional status, and mobility skills; (b) prosthetic componentry and technology to assure the most appropriate and best fitted prosthesis; and (c) materials and equipment that need to be tailored to the individual to optimize outcome in the prosthetic rehabilitation process. The Medicare K-level standards speak to "potential" to achieve a level of ambulation and community engagement. Persons with transtibial amputation should be scheduled for followup care to assure that the prosthetic prescription provided at one point in time meets the needs of the individual, as changes associated with skill progression and advancement occur over time. Therapists, prosthetists, and other health care providers should advocate on behalf of persons with amputation for a change in prosthesis as the need arises.

REFERENCES

1. Gailey R, Nash M, Atchley T, et al. The effects of prosthesis mass on metabolic cost of ambulation in non-vascular trans-tibial amputees. *Prosthet Orthot Int.* 1997;21(1):9–16.
2. Green VG. Transtibial amputation: Prosthetic use and functional outcome. *Foot Ankle Clin.* 2001;6(2):315–327.
3. Centers for Medicare and Medicaid Services, U.S. Department of Health and Human Services. *HCFA Common Procedure Coding System (HCPCS) 2001.* Springfield (VA): U.S. Department of Commerce, National Technical Information Service; 2001 [Chapter 5.3].
4. Esquenazi A, DiGiacomo R. Rehabilitation after amputation. *J Am Podiatr Med Assoc.* 2001;91(1):13–22.
5. Mueller MJ. Comparison of removable rigid dressings and elastic bandages in preprosthetic management of patients with below-knee amputations. *Phys Ther.* 1982;62(10):1438–1441.
6. Wu Y, Keagy RD, Krick HJ, et al. An innovative removable rigid dressing technique for below-the-knee amputation. *J Bone Joint Surg Am.* 1979;61(5):724–729.
7. Ladenheim E, Oberti-Smith K, Tablada G. Results of managing transtibial amputations with a prefabricated polyethylene rigid removable dressing. *J Prosthet Orthot.* 2007;19(1):2–4.
8. Witteck F. Some experience with patellar-tendon bearing below-knee prostheses. *Artif Limbs.* 1962;6:74–85.
9. Radcliffe CA. *The Patellar-Tendon-Bearing Below-Knee Prosthesis.* Berkeley: University of California Biomechanics Laboratory; 1961.
10. Staats T, Lundt J. The UCLA total surface bearing suction below-knee prosthesis. *Clin Prosthet Othot.* 1987;118–130.
11. Perry J. *Gait Analysis: Normal and Pathological Function.* 2 Thorofare, NJ: SLACK; 2010.
12. Pinzur MS, Beck J, Himes R, et al. Distal tibiofibular bone-bridging in transtibial amputation. *J Bone Joint Surg Am.* 2008;90:2682–2687.
13. Granata JD, Philbin TM. Distal tibiofibular bone bridging in transtibial amputation. *Curr Orthop Pract.* 2010;21:264–267.
14. Sanders JE, Greve JM, Mitchell SB, et al. Material properties of commonly-used interface materials and their static coefficients of friction with skin and socks. *J Rehabil Res Dev.* 1998;35:161–176.
15. Sanders J, Nicholson B, Zachariah S, et al. Testing of elastomeric liners used in limb prosthetics: classification of 15 products by mechanical performance. *J Rehabil Res Dev.* 2004;41:175–186.
16. Fillauer C, Pritham C, Fillauer K. Evolution and development of the silicone suction socket (3S) for below-knee prostheses. *J Prosthet Orthot.* 1989;1:92–103.
17. Kristinsson Ö. The ICEROSS concept: a discussion of a philosophy. The Journal of the International Society for Prosthetics and Orthoics. *J Prosthet Orthot.* 1993;17(1):49–55.
18. Ferraro C. Outcomes study of transtibial amputees using elevated vacuum suspension in comparison with pin suspension. *J Prosthet Orthot.* 2011;23:78–81.
19. Beil T, Street G. Comparison of interface pressures with pin and suction suspension systems. *J Rehabil Res Dev.* 2004;41(6A):821–828.
20. Roberts RA. Suction socket suspension for below-knee amputees. *Arch Phys Med Rehabil.* 1986;67(3):196–199.
21. Grevsten S. Ideas on the suspension of the below-knee prosthesis. *Prosthet Orthot Int.* 1978;2(1):3–7.
22. Board W, Street G, Caspers C. A comparison of trans-tibial amputee suction and vacuum socket conditions. *Prosthet Orthot Int.* 2001;25:202–209.
23. Biel TL, Street G, Covey S. Interface pressures during ambulation using suction and vacuum-assisted prosthetic sockets. *J Rehabil Res Dev.* 2002;39(6):693–700.
24. Goh J, Lee P, Chong S. Comparative study between patellar-tendon-bearing and pressure cast. *J Rehabil Res Dev.* 2004;41(3B):491–502.
25. Polhemus. Cobra_Scorpion_brochure.pdf. Available at: http://www.polhemus.com/polhemus_editor/assets/New%20FastSCAN%20Cobra&Scorpion%20brochure.pdf; 2008. Accessed 12.03.11.
26. Smith DG, Fergason JR. Transtibial amputations. *Clin Orthop Relat Res.* 1999;(361):108–115.
27. Lin C, Wu YC, Edwards M. Vertical alignment axis for transtibial prostheses: a simplified alignment method. *J Formos Med Assoc.* 2000;99(1):39–44.
28. *Compas Overview Pamphlet.* 2009. Available at: http://www.orthocareinnovations.com/uploads/files/Compas%20Overview%20Pamphlet_Low-res.pdf. Accessed 08.03.11.
29. Gard S, Konz R. The effect of a shock-absorbing pylon on the gait of persons with unilateral transtibial amputation. *J Rehabil Res Dev.* 2003;40(2):109–124.

24

Transfemoral Prostheses

RICHARD PSONAK

LEARNING OBJECTIVES

On completion of this chapter, the reader will be able to do the following:

1. Describe the indications for, functional characteristics of, and advantages and limitations of the most commonly used transfemoral components and suspension strategies.
2. Compare and contrast the design, fit, and function of the four most popular transfemoral socket designs: quadrilateral, ischial containment, Marlo Anatomical Socket (MAS), and subischial.
3. Describe the interaction among alignment stability, mechanical stability, and muscular stability on the control and function of the prosthetic knee in standing, during gait, and on uneven surfaces.
4. Describe the key influences that bench, static, and dynamic alignment have on fit and function of a transfemoral prosthesis.
5. Identify the nine items that will cause variations in socket fit and the quality of transfemoral gait.
6. Recognize and describe the intraindividual and extraindividual causes of the most common transfemoral gait deviations, and suggest appropriate corrective action.

ADVANCES IN TECHNOLOGY

Advances in technology, materials, and prosthetic components have had a considerable positive impact on the quality of life of individuals with transfemoral amputation. In the past, ambulation wearing a transfemoral prosthesis was labored and often painful. Only the most physically fit individuals attempted to run with their prostheses. Now socket designs better approximate anatomy of the lower limb, suspension systems enhance and maintain intimate residual limb contact within the socket, and dynamic prosthetic feet and knee components offer improved, energy-efficient function. The result has been a significant improvement in quality of gait, allowing more people with transfemoral amputation to walk comfortably and naturally with their prostheses. In addition, athletes with amputations can run in a natural "step-over-step" pattern with a higher degree of stability and comfort than previously possible.

This chapter presents information about current socket designs, suspension systems, and prosthetic knee components

available for individuals with transfemoral amputation. It also provides the reader with a strategy to assess fit and alignment of a transfemoral prosthesis as well as explaining the major user-errors and prosthetic-related reasons for commonly observed gait deviations.

PROSTHETIC MANAGEMENT AFTER KNEE DISARTICULATION OR TRANSFEMORAL AMPUTATION

An amputation proximal to the anatomical knee joint is referred to as a transfemoral (above knee) amputation. An amputation through the center of the anatomical knee joint is known as a knee disarticulation (Figure 24-1). Individuals with knee disarticulation present with prosthetic challenges and functional advantages when compared with those with transfemoral amputation. The disarticulation residual limb tends to be long and distally bulbous, a result of the preservation of the femur and its condyles. Prosthetically, this creates a challenge in donning the prosthesis and cosmetically finishing a knee component. The bulbous distal end does, however, enhance prosthetic suspension. The normal adduction angle of the lower extremity is more likely to be preserved, and the long lever arm of the femur facilitates control of the prosthetic knee. Also, as the proximal component of a weight-bearing joint, the distal femur tolerates end-bearing pressures within the socket.

In contrast, the transfemoral residual limb varies in length, depending on how much of the femur has been retained. The shape of the residual limb is likely to be a tapered cylinder so that donning a prosthesis is less difficult. Suspension can be challenging, however, as a result of this cylindrical shape of the residual limb. The fleshiness of the transfemoral residual limb presents an opportunity for suction suspension. As the length of the residual limb decreases, socket suspension and control of the prosthetic knee (especially stance stability) become more problematic.

The successful prosthetic management of individuals who have suffered an amputation above the knee involves providing a prosthesis that is comfortable in containing the residual limb, stable during the stance phase of gait, smooth in transition to the swing phase of gait, and acceptable in appearance.[1] In choosing components for an individual's transfemoral or knee disarticulation prosthesis, the prosthetic team must consider

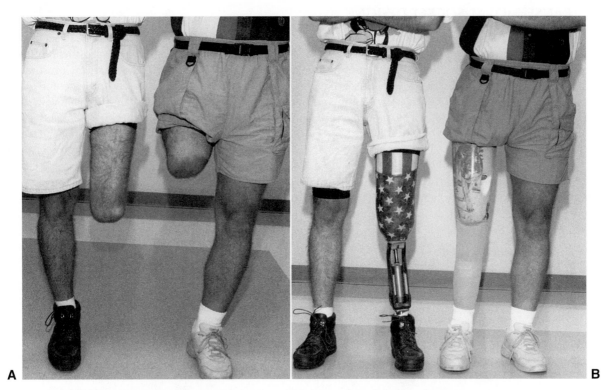

FIGURE 24-1 The similarities and differences in prosthetic fit and function between amputations at transfemoral and knee disarticulation levels are determined, to a large degree, by the length of the preserved femur. **A,** The knee disarticulation residual limb is long and bulbous, whereas the transfemoral residual limb is a tapered cylinder. **B,** In a knee disarticulation prosthesis, the center of the prosthetic knee is generally lower than that of the intact limb, whereas the knee center of most transfemoral prostheses matches that of the intact limb.

the interrelationships among the component's weight, function, cosmesis, comfort, and cost. Often the most functional or technologically sophisticated components are also the heaviest, most expensive, most likely to need maintenance, and least cosmetic. Because of the great variation in physical characteristics, health, and preferred activities of individuals with transfemoral amputation, no single material, component, or transfemoral design is appropriate for all persons with amputation. The preferences and needs of each individual must be considered carefully, in the context of weight, function, cosmesis, comfort, and cost, for the optimal prosthetic outcome.

ENERGY EXPENDITURE

An individual with a transfemoral amputation faces considerable energy expenditure when ambulating with a prosthesis (Box 24-1). The energy cost of gait increases significantly as the length of the residual limb decreases.[2-6] Fisher and Gullickson report the energy cost of walking for healthy individuals (mean gait speed: 83 m/min) as 0.063 kcal/min/kg (oxygen consumption/physical effort) and 0.000764 kcal/m/kg body weight (oxygen cost/energy required to ambulate).[6] Individuals with transtibial amputation walk 36% more slowly, expending 2% more kilocalories per minute and 41% more kilocalories per meter to cover a similar distance. For individuals with transfemoral amputation, gait speed is 43% slower, whereas energy

---

> **BOX 24-1** *Prosthetic Features That Affect Energy Expenditure*
>
> - Weight of the prosthesis
> - Quality of the socket fit
> - Accuracy of alignment of the prosthesis
> - Functional characteristics of the prosthetic components

cost is reflected as 5% less kilocalories per minute and 89% more kilocalories per meter. In other words, the individual ambulating on a transfemoral prosthesis walks more slowly to avoid an increase in energy consumption per minute and is dramatically less efficient in terms of energy expended over distance (per meter). This increase in energy cost is manifested as a higher rate of oxygen consumption, elevated heart rate, and notable reduction in comfortable (self-selected) walking speed.[2,5,6]

Because of this high energy cost, many older individuals with high-level transfemoral amputations may be limited in their ability to become functional community ambulators. Individuals who wear a prosthesis and have been diagnosed with vascular disease are often relegated to walking slowly, on flat terrain, with the assistance of a walker or cane.[5,6] Elderly individuals with bilateral transfemoral amputations rarely become community ambulators with prostheses, instead choosing a wheelchair for long-distance mobility.

TRANSFEMORAL SOCKET DESIGNS

Prior to the 1950s, prosthetists typically carved a "plug fit" socket from a block of wood, which, depending on the skill of the craftsman, was often uncomfortable and cumbersome while walking and sitting. The plug socket was crafted to contain the remnant thigh muscles, support body weight at the groin level (below the ischium), and was often open ended to eliminate distal limb contact.

Quadrilateral Socket

The traditional quadrilateral (quad) socket, developed at the University of California at Berkeley in the 1950s, offered a notable improvement in fit, total contact, function, and remained the socket design of choice until the mid-1980s. The quad socket, as its name implies, has four distinct walls fashioned to contain the thigh musculature. The quad socket was designed to be a complete above-the-knee prosthetic system that interfaces with the individual who wears the prosthesis. The socket's primary functions are to provide for weight-bearing during the stance phase of gait and to allow the hip and thigh muscles to function at maximum potential during the stance phase of gait (Figure 24-2, *A*).[1,7,8] A flat posterior shelf, the ischial seat, is the primary weight-bearing surface for the ischium and gluteal muscles. The anterior wall contours create a posterior-directed force at the anatomical Scarpa's triangle, which is intended to stabilize the ischium on its prosthetic seat. As a result, the socket is narrower in its anterior–posterior dimension than its medial–lateral dimension (Figure 24-3, *A*).

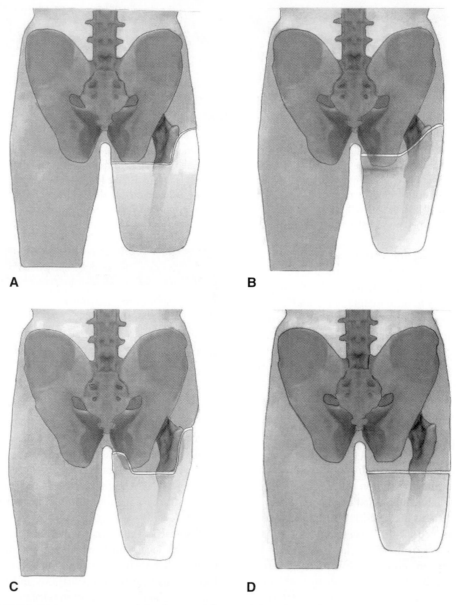

A   **B**

C   **D**

FIGURE 24-2 Comparison of the design of the quadrilateral (quad) socket (**A**), the ischial-ramal containment (IRC) socket (**B**), the Marlo Anatomical Socket (MAS) (**C**), and subischial socket (**D**) from a posterior perspective. The quad socket is designed to have the ischium sitting on the socket brim (seat). In the IRC socket and the MAS, the ischium sits inside the socket. With the subischial socket, as the name implies, the socket trim line is below the ischium.

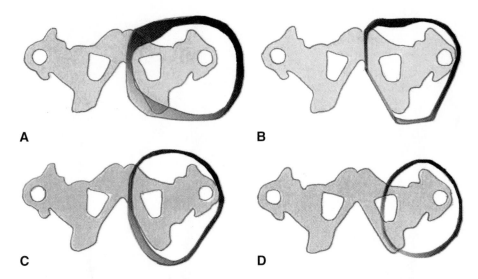

FIGURE 24-3 From a cross-section view of the four different transfemoral sockets designs it is noted that the quad socket has a narrow anteroposterior dimension **(A)**, the ischial-ramal containment (IRC) socket **(B)**, and Marlo Anatomical Socket (MAS) **(C)** have narrow mediolateral dimensions. The subischial socket **(D)** has a more oval shape which is consistent with the shape of the proximal thigh.

Evolution of Ischial Containment Sockets

The next stage of socket designs evolved in 1970s after prosthetist Ivan Long took part in a project that evaluated radiographically the femoral alignment of the transfemoral limb within a quad socket.[9] Long observed that many individuals who wear a quadrilateral socket walk with an extremely wide base and demonstrated a Trendelenburg or gluteus medius limp, causing the individual to lean to the amputated side. He also noted that in most cases the transected femur was aligned in abduction as opposed to the normal adduction angle of the sound side femur (Figure 24-4). The abnormal abduction angle of the femur was believed to be in part the result of the quad socket's unnaturally wide medial–lateral dimension and narrow anteroposterior dimension. The wide medial–lateral dimension of the quad socket allows the socket to displace laterally during midstance, thus increasing pressure to the perineal tissues and decreasing the efficiency of the gluteus medius muscle.[9,10]

Long's socket design was part of a frontal plane alignment procedure that became known as "Long's Line."[9,10] Long believed that by aligning the distal femur over the center of the knee and through the center of the foot, the wearer of the prosthesis could bring their residual limb into a normal anatomical position and walk more naturally. Long narrowed the medial–lateral dimension of his socket design and increased anteroposterior dimension in an attempt to support the femur and to prevent lateral shifting of the socket during weight bearing. According to Long,[9,11] an additional advantage of his design is that the wider anteroposterior dimension enhances muscle function by providing more room to accommodate muscle contraction than possible in the crowded anteroposterior dimension of the quad socket.

In the 1980s prosthetist John Sabolich expanded upon Long's concept and developed his contoured anterior trochanteric-controlled alignment method (CAT-CAM) socket (see Figure 24-2, *B*).[11-13] His design attempted to both maintain the femur in an adducted position and control socket rotation by containing the ischial tuberosity within the contours of the socket. Since the CAT-CAM design, a series of sockets have been developed that have become known as ischial containment or ischial-ramal containment (IRC) sockets, depending on what anatomy is contained within the socket.[12,13] When comparing the IRC socket with the quad socket, the most obvious difference is the narrow medial–lateral dimension that is highly contoured around the ischial–ramal complex (see Figure 24-3, *B*).[12]

Socket Configuration Influence on Femur Position

The degree to which the prosthetic socket design can influence the position of the transected femur has been hotly disputed. Orthopedic surgeon Frank Gottschalk developed a myodesis surgical technique to ensure proper femoral adduction in a transfemoral residual limb.[14] In the journal article, "Does socket configuration influence the position of the femur in above-knee amputation?," Gottschalk and colleagues concluded that the prosthetic socket cannot provide enough lateral pressure to change the position of the femur.[15] The authors indicated that proper anatomical adduction is achieved only through specific surgical techniques. Most practitioners would agree with Gottschalk when he suggests that "successful prosthetic fitting starts at the time of surgery."[14,15] However, there is also a consensus that indicates that an intimately contoured socket in optimal alignment enhances an individual's gait, decreases energy expenditure, increases socket comfort, and improves overall function.[16] Clearly more research is required to understand the relationship between alignment, socket design, and femoral adduction.

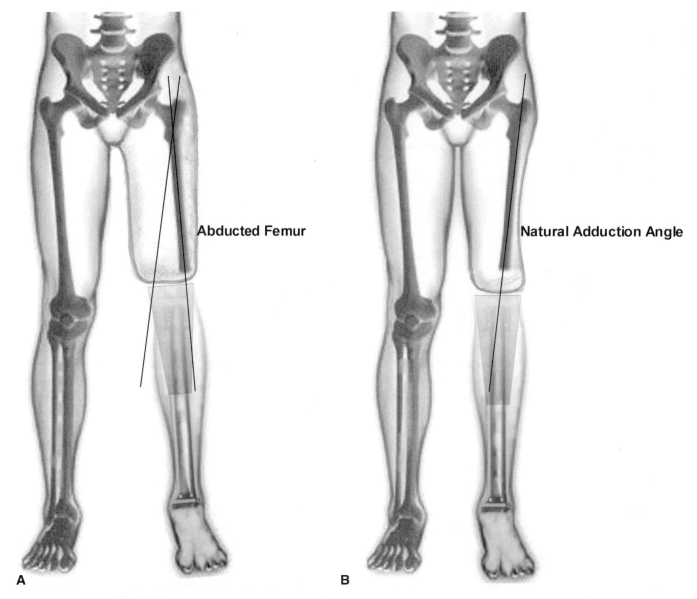

A   **Abducted Femur**

B   **Natural Adduction Angle**

FIGURE 24-4 Long noted that for many individuals who wear a quadrilateral socket the transected femur was aligned in abduction as opposed to the normal adduction angle of the sound side femur **(A)**. Quad socket wearers typically walk with an unnaturally wide base. Ischial-ramal containment (IRC) sockets **(B)** are more naturally designed and aligned to enhance an individual's gait, decrease energy expenditure, increase socket comfort, and improve function.

Marlo Anatomical Socket

In the late 1990s, Marlo Ortiz, an engineer-prosthetist from Mexico, developed a socket configuration that focuses on providing skeletal support along the medial ischial–ramal complex (IRC) (see Figure 24-3, *C*).[17] The socket design became known as the MAS socket (Marlo Anatomical Socket). The MAS socket attempts to encapsulate the ischial tuberosity, as well as portions of the ramus, with a distinguishable containment buttress that is designed to maximize socket stabilization (see Figure 24-2, *C*). The socket features a low posterior trim line that is said to facilitate the containment of the ischial–ramal complex without interference from the gluteus maximus trim lines. The low gluteal trim lines also allow the prosthetic user to sit directly on the gluteus

maximus instead of the posterior socket. External rotation at the hip is virtually unrestricted, minimizing the need for a transverse rotation unit (see Figure 24-18) proximal to the prosthetic knee joint.

Elevated Vacuum Sockets

The latest rendition of transfemoral socket designs has developed as a result of the ever expanding interest in elevated vacuum suspension, also referred to as subatmospheric suspension (see Figure 24-3, *D*).[18] This socket design is characterized by lower trim lines (subischial) in comparison to other transfemoral socket designs, resulting in substantially increased patient comfort and range of motion (see Figure 24-2, *D*). The proximal socket brim has been lowered as much as two-four inches below the ischial tuberosity level on transfemoral residual limbs greater than midlength.[19] By utilizing elevated negative pressure around the distal two-thirds of the residual limb, the socket no longer requires compression of the proximal residual limb anatomy to provide weight bearing and stabilization. As a result of less proximal compression, there is no longer a need for prominent flares, reliefs, and channels, thus allowing lower trim lines of the socket. The proximal roll on liner contains the soft tissue of the adductor muscles. Some have referred to this style of socket as brimless.[19]

Radcliffe[7] suggests that, regardless of socket design, the primary goals of the transfemoral prosthesis are to achieve comfort in weight bearing, to provide a narrow base of support in standing and walking, and to accomplish as close to normal swing phase function as possible. Mak and colleagues indicate that, "For all prosthetic socket designs, the optimal load distribution should be proportional to the ability of the body to sustain such stresses." The authors go on to summarize that, "The basic principles for socket design vary from either distributing most of the load over specific load-bearing areas or more uniformly distributing the load over the entire limb."[20]

RIGID AND FLEXIBLE SOCKET MATERIALS

Most transfemoral sockets are fabricated from various thermoplastic or thermosetting resin materials. A rigid socket consists of a resin-laminated or thermoformed plastic socket that is intended to have an intimate, total contact fit over the entire surface of the residual limb. The rigid socket is durable, easy to clean, and often less bulky and less expensive to produce than flexible sockets. The disadvantage , is that it more difficult to adjust the fit of a rigid socket, especially for individuals with "bony" or sensitive residual limbs.

The flexible socket is vacuum formed using any number of flexible thermoplastic materials.[21,22] It is encased in a rigid frame, which provides support during weight bearing and helps to maintain socket shape. The flexible socket accommodates to change in muscle shape during contraction and can be easily modified after initial fabrication to provide relief for bony prominences. Flexible sockets may also be more comfortable to wear, especially in sitting, because there are no hard edges at the brim to impinge on the groin. Flexible sockets are especially useful if suction suspension is desired. They are, however, somewhat less durable, more bulky to wear (requiring a socket and a frame), and more expensive to produce than rigid sockets.

TRANSFEMORAL SUSPENSION SYSTEMS

Keeping the prosthesis on in its optimal functional position is more challenging for individuals with transfemoral amputation than with transtibial amputation. The transfemoral residual limb is fleshy and cylindrical, lacking the bony prominences that aid in suspending the transtibial prosthesis. The weight of the transfemoral prosthesis with the addition of its knee unit creates an additional challenge for adequate suspension. Depending on the nature of the prosthetic wearer's normal activities, a single system or a combination of several systems may be chosen.

Traditional Pull-in Suction Suspension

Traditional pull-in suction suspension uses negative air pressure, skin-to-socket contact, and muscle tension to hold the socket onto the limb (Figure 24-5).[23] A suction prosthesis can be donned in several ways. One option uses donning sock (cotton stockinette or similar material), donning sleeve (parachute nylon or similar material), or elastic bandage to pull the residual limb down into the socket. Once the limb is well seated in the socket, the sock, sleeve, or elastic wrap is pulled through the valve housing at the distal socket, and the air expulsion valve is then screwed into place. This process requires considerable agility and balance on the part of the wearer. A second option is to add a lubricant to the skin to facilitate the residual limb sliding into the socket. The air-expulsion valve is then "burped," by pushing or pulling the valve button, to release any trapped air.

The intimate fit required for suction suspension has several additional benefits. The wearer often reports enhanced prosthetic control and a better proprioceptive sense of the prosthesis during walking. Because an intimate fit is essential, suction suspension is inappropriate for patients with recent

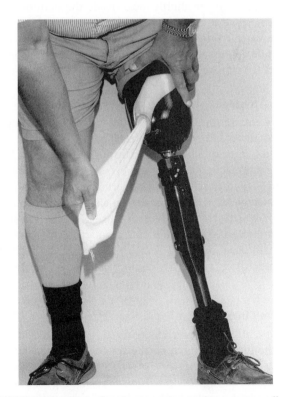

FIGURE 24-5 Patient donning a suction socket using a pull sock. The air expulsion valve has been removed so that the donning sock can be pulled completely out of the socket.

amputation who will continue to lose limb volume or for those with a history of fluctuating edema or unstable weight. The high shearing forces associated with donning a suction socket also may preclude its use for patients with fragile or sensitive skin, painful trigger points, significant scarring, or adhesions.

Roll-on Suspension Liners

Growing in popularity as a suspension system is the use of roll-on liners. These liners are available as an alternative to the standard suction suspension system. Roll-on liners are manufactured from various materials, including silicone, urethane, and elastomer. They are produced by several manufacturers in a variety of sizes, thicknesses, and tapers.[24] Worn against the skin, roll-on liners are donned by first being turned inside-out, then rolled directly over the residual limb. The roll-on suspension liner creates a negative atmospheric pressure and somewhat adhesive bond to the skin. The liner can be used for suspension in several different ways: in a shuttle lock system, as part of a lanyard system, as a cushion liner used with an air expulsion valve, or as a vital part of an elevated vacuum socket.

Shuttle Lock Systems

This liner is commonly called a locking liner. It is similar to the cushion liner except for a distal stabilizing matrix incorporated into the liner to prevent elongation. This liner also has an external distal cap, the center of which a serrated pin screws into and sticks out approximately 1½ inches. The pin engages into the shuttle lock, inside the bottom of the socket, when the individual stands and pushes his or her limb down into the socket. To remove the prosthesis, the individual depresses a release button on the medial aspect of the socket that disengages the serrated pin (Figure 24-6, *A*).

Lanyard System

This system uses the locking liner, but instead of a locking pin screwed into the liner's distal cap, a lanyard (strap or cord) is attached to the cap. This is routed through the distal socket to pull the residual limb into the socket (see Figure 24-6, *B*). The lanyard is then attached to the external lateral aspect of the socket using Velcro. Many designs maintain suspension and rotational control by providing suspension distally and stability laterally through an additional loop attached to the liner proximally (Figure 24-7). Some systems utilize a ratcheted strap much like a ski boot binding as a lateral suspension strap.

Cushion Liner with Air Expulsion Valve

This type of liner is generally referred to as a cushion liner. After the liner is donned on the residual limb, it is pushed into the socket, creating a negative pressure environment by expelling air through the expulsion valve (see Figure 24-6, *C*). This process is similar to the traditional skin suction socket method mentioned previously.

Elevated Vacuum

Elevated vacuum is different than suction suspension. Both methods use a difference in atmospheric pressure to suspend and secure the socket to the residual limb. Suction suspension requires a passive expulsion valve to allow air to exit from the socket, but only creates a negative pressure differential when the prosthetic limb is unweighted as when moving into swing phase. With vacuum suspension the residual limb is continuously under vacuum. A vacuum pump creates negative pressure to remove air from a sealed environment between the total surface bearing socket and a wicked-liner (see Figure 24-6, *D*). The vacuum created by a vacuum pump's removal of air holds the intimately fitting liner firmly to the walls of the socket.[25] This system does not depend on the limb position. An elevated vacuum of approximately 15 inches Hg between the limb liner and the socket controls volume fluctuations in the socket.[26,27]

Pistoning between the limb, liner, and socket is virtually eliminated within an elevated vacuum system. Individuals using vacuum-suspended prostheses report having greater proprioception and a sense that the prosthesis feels lighter when using vacuum suspension in comparison to other types of suspension.[25] It has also been suggested that an elevated vacuum system maintains the volume of the limb in the socket by improving circulation within the limb, and may help to heal wounds and improve limb health.[28]

The major advantage of roll-on suspension is a significant reduction in the amount of friction and shear on the residual limb.[29] The donning procedure is simple, and can be accomplished while seated. This suspension system has been useful for individuals with short residual limbs and those who have experienced discomfort using the traditional pull-in suction method. The disadvantages of this system include its expense and durability. Roll-on liners become worn or torn, and must be replaced two to three times a year depending on the wearer's activity level. These types of liners may also increase skin temperature and perspiration. Some wearers have experienced rashes or other types of skin irritation as a result. Wearers who choose this type of suspension must clean the liners daily to prevent the buildup of perspiration and bacteria.[30,31]

Silesian Belt Suspension

A Silesian belt is usually made from leather or lightweight webbing (Figure 24-8). It is attached to the lateral aspect of the socket, encircles the pelvis, and then runs through a loop or buckle on the anterior of the socket. The Silesian belt is most often used as an auxiliary (backup) for traditional suction suspension systems. The problem with choosing the Silesian belt as the sole means of suspension lies in its inability to control residual limb rotation within the socket. For individuals with long residual limbs who are not expected to be vigorous ambulators, the Silesian belt may provide adequate suspension.

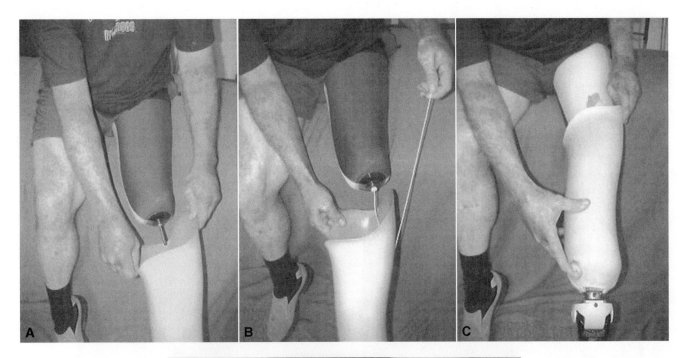

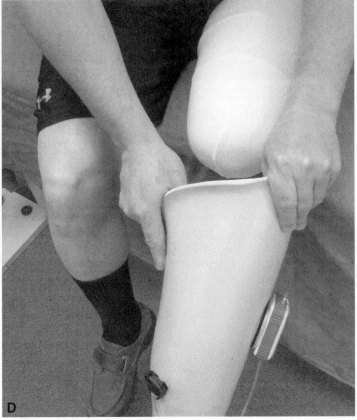

FIGURE 24-6 Roll-on liners are a popular suspension system. The liner can be used for suspension in at least four different ways. A shuttle lock system uses a pin that engages into the shuttle lock in the bottom of the socket (**A**). The lanyard system incorporates a strap or cord into the liner that is routed through the distal socket and used to pull the residual limb into the socket (**B**). An air expulsion valve system is similar to the traditional skin suction socket method. Once the liner is donned, the residual limb is pushed into the socket, expelling air through the expulsion valve, thus creating a negative pressure environment (**C**). A vacuum pump (attached to socket) creates negative pressure to remove air from a sealed environment between the socket and roll-on liner. The vacuum created by a vacuum pump's removal of air holds the intimately fitting liner firmly to the walls of the socket (**D**).

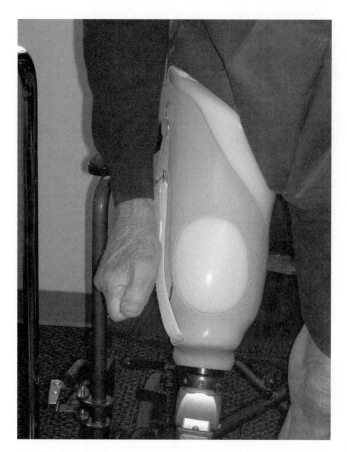

FIGURE 24-7 The lanyard suspension system often incorporates a lateral rotational control loop and strap positioned laterally on the socket.

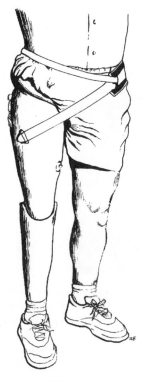

FIGURE 24-8 Example of Silesian belt suspension. Although the belt suspends the prosthesis to the pelvis, it cannot fully counteract rotary forces between limb and socket during vigorous walking.

Total Elastic Suspension Belt

The total elastic suspension (TES) belt is typically made of an elastic neoprene material. The distal sleeve of the TES belt fits snugly around the proximal half of the thigh section of the transfemoral prosthesis. The neoprene belt encircles the waist and attaches in front with Velcro (Figure 24-9). The TES belt is easy to don, comfortable to wear and is an excellent auxiliary suspension system. This system is generally not recommended as a sole source of suspension for prosthetic users who are active ambulators, because like the Silesian belt, the TES belt cannot control residual limb rotation adequately within the socket. The major disadvantages of the TES system include its limited durability, especially for active ambulators, and

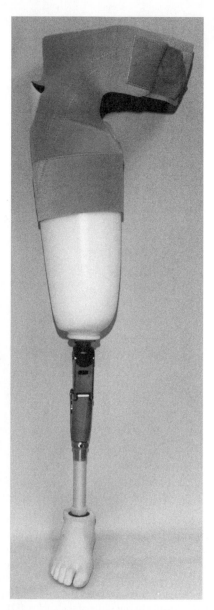

FIGURE 24-9 The total elastic suspension belt (TES) is a simple and comfortable suspension system that is often used as an auxiliary suspension.

its tendency to retain heat. It is often chosen for individuals with recent amputation whose residual limb has not yet matured to a stable size, for older patients who are unable to use the pull-in suction or roll-on liners because of upper-extremity weakness or pain, and for those with easily irritated skin or adhesions who cannot tolerate suction. It may also be used as a backup or secondary suspension system for individuals who use suction suspension when playing sports or engaging in high-activity leisure activities.

Pelvic Belt and Hip Joint

For some patients, a pelvic belt and hip joint are used as a means of suspension (Figure 24-10). Generally, the pelvic belt is made of leather and attached to the prosthesis by means of a metal hip joint. Recently, lighter-weight plastic materials have been used as an alternative to the metal joint. Whatever the material, the joint center should be positioned just superior and anterior to the anatomical greater trochanter. This system not only suspends the prosthesis but also helps to control rotation and increase medial-lateral stability of the residual limb within the socket. Traditionally, this has been the suspension of choice for those with short residual limbs. The major drawbacks of this type of suspension are its bulkiness under clothing, added weight, and tendency to be uncomfortable when sitting.

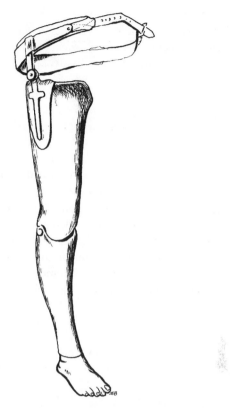

FIGURE 24-10 A pelvic belt with hip joint not only suspends the prosthesis but also helps to control rotation and increases medial lateral stability of the residual limb within the socket.

CASE EXAMPLE 1

A Grandmother Who Wants to Dance at Her Granddaughter's Wedding

T. F. is a 68-year-old grandmother who wants to attend her granddaughter's wedding, so she comes into her prosthetist's office asking for assistance with her 6-year-old transfemoral prosthesis. T. F. underwent elective amputation 6 years ago when she developed osteomyelitis and nonunion of a comminuted fracture of her left femur after being hit by a car. Although she was initially deconditioned, her rehabilitation was quite successful, and she returned to her home to live independently after a 2-month stay in a subacute rehabilitation setting. Previously, she smoked a half pack of cigarettes per day, but she has not smoked since her injury.

T. F.'s residual limb is relatively short: 4½ inches as measured from the perineum to the distal end of her residual limb. She currently wears an endoskeletal prosthesis with rigid socket and prosthetic socks, a polycentric knee, and single-axis foot, and ambulates functional distances by using a straight cane. For suspension she uses a pelvic band with a leather belt and hip joint, which is typical for those with her level of amputation. She complains that her prosthesis pistons on her residuum, is heavy and noisy, and pinches her when she sits. Her major goal is that she be able to "blend into the ceremony" such that her prosthesis will not be a distraction. She is also hoping to dance with her son and her new grandson-in-law at the wedding reception.

Her prosthetist consults with her physician and suggest the fabrication of a new flexible IRC socket in a rigid frame, but retaining the foot and knee that she has been wearing. For suspension, the prosthetist recommends using a roll-on sleeve with a shuttle locking device. This suspension system will eliminate the metal pelvic band with leather belt and hip joint as well as improve suspension and decrease pistoning by means of the locking pin and high coefficient of friction of the urethane sleeve. The new socket and suspension system give T. F. better control of her prosthesis, allowing her to participate in all of the wedding activities without her cane.

Questions to Consider

- Why was a pelvic band with leather belt and hip joint used for suspension in T. F.'s initial prosthesis? What are the pros and cons of this suspension system? Considering that roll on suspension was not commonly used at the time of her initial fitting 6 years ago, why did the team not recommend a TES belt, Silesian belt, or suction suspension?

- Why do you think the team decided to replace T. F.'s rigid socket with a flexible socket in a rigid frame? What are the advantages and disadvantages of each type of socket?
- Why do you think the team decided to retain the polycentric knee unit when they replaced her socket and suspension system? Are there other knee units that might

have been appropriate for someone of her age and activity level? Why or why not?
- Why do you think the team decided to retain the single axis prosthetic foot when they replaced her socket and suspension system? Would you have considered a different prosthetic foot? Why or why not?

Knee Disarticulation Considerations

When femoral condyles are not prohibitively bulbous, roll on sleeves can be used in combination with air expulsion. Although a pin is not recommended because of space limitations, a lanyard system can be effective. This creates a positive lock that is engaged even if limb volume changes. When the femoral condyles are prominent a removable door suspension design can be used to suspend the prosthesis. This suspension uses external straps, attached to a door, which can apply variable pressure proximal to the femoral condyles locking them in place (Figure 24-11). This suspension system is similar to the medial opening door occasionally used for Symes prosthesis.

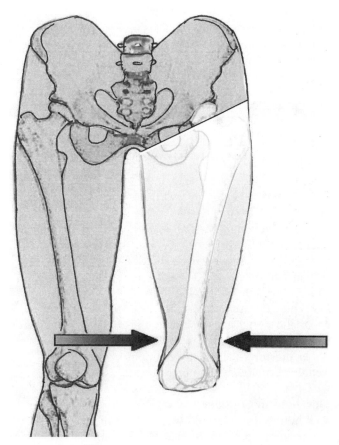

FIGURE 24-11 Generally, the residual limb of an individual with a knee disarticulation has prominent femoral condyles. When this is the case, a removable door suspension or stovepipe liner design can be used to suspend the prosthesis. This suspension applies variable pressure proximal to the femoral condyles locking the limb into the socket.

The stovepipe Pelite liner is another method of suspending a bulbous residual limb in the knee disarticulation prosthesis. This suspension method is also similar to a suspension system used for Symes amputations. This method, utilizes pads built up around the femoral condyles that are blended into the largest circumference of the liner until the limb is more cylindrical in shape (similar to a stovepipe). A slit is cut over the medial condyle area to allow the bulbous end of the residual limb to pass through the narrow section of the liner when donning.[32] This system is easy to fabricate and provides good suspension and comfortable padding, especially for more bony limbs.

PROSTHETIC SYSTEMS

A transfemoral prosthesis can be fabricated as either an exoskeletal or endoskeletal system. The weight-bearing strength and cosmetic shape of an exoskeletal prosthesis are provided by a laminated shell that incorporates the socket, knee–shin component, and ankle block (Figure 24-12, *A*). This system is durable and requires little maintenance but cannot be easily realigned or adjusted. In the endoskeletal system, weight-bearing strength comes from an internal pylon that connects the knee unit to the prosthetic foot (Figure 24-12, *B*). The cosmetic shape of the prosthesis is provided by a soft foam cover, carved to mirror the remaining limb, which is fit over the socket, knee unit, and pylon. This foam shell is, in turn, covered by cosmetic stockings or a silicone "skin" to achieve the desired skin color. The endoskeletal system has two distinct advantages: the prosthetist is quickly able to adjust prosthetic alignment, and easily interchange or replace modular components. This is particularly helpful as new prosthetic users become more competent in controlling their knee unit or when advancing mobility leads to different functional needs (e.g., involvement in athletic activities). The durability of the foam and cosmetic coverings may be an issue for some prosthetic users, especially when work or leisure activities are physically demanding or occur in harsh environments.

PROSTHETIC KNEE UNITS

The function of the human knee joint is difficult to replicate. Henschke Mauch, who developed hydraulic guidance systems for rockets during World War II, turned his considerable knowledge and creativity to designing a hydraulic prosthetic knee for veterans with amputations after the war.[33] He commented that it was far easier to design a large rocket with a

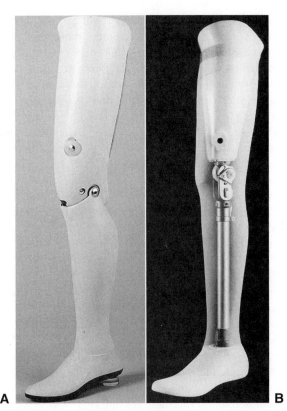

FIGURE 24-12 Comparison of the rugged exoskeletal **(A)** and the modular endoskeletal **(B)** transfemoral prosthetic systems. (Reprinted, with permission, from Otto Bock Health Care, Minneapolis, MN.)

guidance system capable of maneuvering hundreds of miles than to duplicate the human knee. The anatomical knee is a modified hinge-type synovial joint. The offset axis of the knee allows rotation in addition to flexion and extension, practically making it three joints rolled into one.[34] Because most prosthetic knees function in a single plane of motion, the action of the anatomical knee is difficult to fully replicate. As a result, it is more difficult for the individual who is using a transfemoral prosthesis to walk as efficiently and cosmetically as someone using a transtibial prosthesis.

Prosthetic knee mechanisms have two primary functions. First, to simulate normal gait, the prosthetic knee must smoothly flex and extend through the swing phase of gait. The speed or rate of shin advancement during swing is determined by the mechanical properties (friction or resistance) of the prosthetic knee unit. Second, the prosthetic knee must remain stable as body weight rolls forward over the prosthetic foot during the stance phase of gait. The major categories of commonly used prosthetic knee units vary with respect to how, and to what degree, they accomplish these two tasks. Various knee units are available in endoskeletal and exoskeletal versions.

Single-Axis Knee Units

The single-axis knee simulates a simple hinge and allows the prosthetic shin to swing freely in flexion and extension. Stance-phase knee stability is achieved by a combination of

positioning of the knee unit with respect to the weight line (alignment) and muscular control (activity of hip extensors). This knee is lightweight, durable, and low maintenance, but because of its unrestricted movement, it has no inherent mechanical stability. For this reason, it is not appropriate for individuals with relatively short residual limbs who lack the mechanical advantage of a long femoral lever for muscular control of the knee unit or for those whose stability is compromised for other reasons. Although the rate of advancement of the shin during swing phase (determined by the friction setting of the knee) can be individualized, cadence responsiveness is minimal once the resistance has been set. The shin of the prosthesis will swing forward at the same rate, regardless of gait speed. As a result, an audible terminal impact often occurs as the knee reaches full extension. To run with a single-axis knee, the individual must use a skipping pattern on the intact stance limb while waiting for the prosthesis to complete the swing phase and begin the initial heel contact. The single-axis knee is primarily for patients with long residual limbs who can voluntarily stabilize the knee through active hip extension against the posterior wall of the prosthesis.

Polycentric Knee Units

The single-axis knee has a fixed center of rotation, while the polycentric knee has a moving center of rotation. Like the human knee, the polycentric knee rotates around more than one axis through a four or more bar linkage system (Figure 24-13). A proximal and posterior location of the

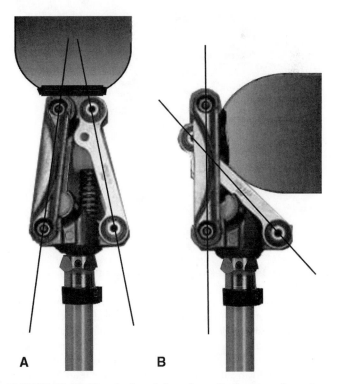

FIGURE 24-13 The single-axis knee has a fixed center of rotation, while the polycentric knee has a moving center of rotation. Like the human knee, the polycentric knee rotates around more than one axis through a four or more bar linkage system. **A,** The polycentric knee in the extended position. **B,** The knee fully flexed.

instantaneous center of rotation promotes knee stability during the stance phase of gait.[35]

As the knee unit flexes during swing phase, the polycentric axis of motion leads to relative "shortening" of the distal prosthesis (shin and foot components), which enhances toe clearance throughout swing phase.[36] It is especially helpful for individuals with long residual limbs or knee disarticulation because the changing center of rotation allows the shin to tuck under the thigh when sitting, resulting in a more natural and cosmetic appearance of thigh and shin lengths. The polycentric knee unit's inherent stance phase stability also makes it an option for individuals who have short residual limbs or significant weakness of hip extensors. The major disadvantage of the polycentric knee, with its multiple mechanical joints, is its durability.

WEIGHT-ACTIVATED STANCE CONTROL KNEE UNITS

The stance control knee has a braking mechanism that is activated when weight is applied through the knee during the stance phase of gait (Figure 24-14). The intent of the braking mechanism is to prevent (or at least reduce) unwanted knee flexion during stance. The sensitivity of the braking mechanism can be adjusted to match the individual's level of activity and ability to control the knee voluntarily. If initial contact is made when the knee is not completely extended, as when walking on uneven ground, the braking mechanism provides additional mechanical stability to keep the knee from rapidly buckling. During swing phase, the weight-activated stance control knee unit functions like a single-axis knee and has similar disadvantages. Advancement of the prosthetic shin occurs at the same rate regardless of changes in gait speed; minimal cadence responsiveness is present. This type of knee unit is most often prescribed for individuals who have recently undergone amputation, and who have short residual limbs or weakness of hip extensors and would otherwise have difficulty in actively stabilizing their prosthetic knees.

Manual Locking Knee Units

For patients who must rely on mechanical stability in stance, the knee of choice is often a manual locking knee. This unit is basically a single-axis knee with the addition of a locking pin mechanism (Figure 24-15). The pin automatically locks with a distinctive click when the knee is fully extended. Individuals who use a manual locking knee unit walk with their prosthetic knees locked in extension. Although a locked knee provides maximum mechanical stability in stance, it also significantly compromises mobility and toe clearance in swing. The prosthesis is often fit to be slightly shorter than the sound

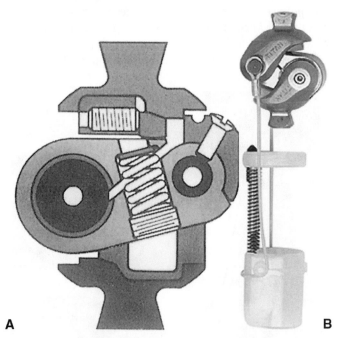

A   **B**

FIGURE 24-14 A "cut-away" diagram **(A)** and photo **(B)** of a stance control knee unit with extension assist for a transfemoral prosthesis. As body weight is shifted on the prosthesis in early stance, compression of the spring causes the cylindrical brake bushing to engage and resist the knee flexion moment associated with loading response. This braking mechanism provides stability even if the knee is slightly flexed during weight shift. When the knee is unloaded in late stance/preswing, decompression of the spring leads to "unlocking" of the brake, allowing free knee flexion for limb clearance during swing phase. (**A,** Reproduced, with permission, from Shurr DG, Michael JW. Prosthetics and Orthotics, 2nd ed. Englewood Cliffs, NJ: Prentice Hall, 2002. p. 111. **B,** Courtesy Otto Bock Orthopedic Industry, Inc., Minneapolis, MN.)

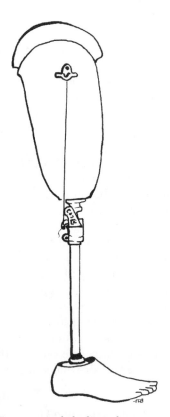

FIGURE 24-15 A manual locking knee provides maximum stability when the knee is in the locked position. The knee can be unlocked manually by manipulating a lever and cable system connected to the knee.

side limb to facilitate toe clearance during swing of the prosthesis. The prosthetic wearer can manually unlock the knee by manipulating a pulley or lever system attached to the outside of the socket. This unit is often used in the initial training prosthesis for patients when balance, endurance, or cooperation may be problematic.

Hydraulic Knee Units

Hydraulic knee units are cadence responsive; the forward progression of the prosthetic shin changes as gait speed changes. This is because the flow of hydraulic fluid through narrow channels within the prosthetic knee unit provides a frictional resistance, which increases with the speed of compression (Figure 24-16). This variable resistance permits a swing phase that more closely simulates normal gait. As gait speed increases, the shin of the prosthesis also extends more rapidly. Little swing-phase delay is experienced in knee extension as compared with strictly single-axis or polycentric knee units. This variable cadence characteristic has been helpful for both young, active individuals, and older adults with mobility impairment.[37] This enhanced function, however, is associated with increased weight, higher maintenance needs, and higher cost. Additionally, with colder temperatures the knee may initially be slow to respond to changes in cadence until the hydraulic fluid warms up from typical daily use.

Some manufacturers offer a variation of hydraulic knee units that allow both variable cadence in swing and mechanical stability in stance (swing and stance [SNS] control).[33] Stance control occurs as a result of hydraulic resistance to knee flexion during weight bearing or by a braking mechanism that is activated by weight bearing through the prosthesis. This feature allows the individual to ambulate with greater confidence over uneven surfaces and also permits the use of a more natural step-over-step pattern when negotiating hills and going down stairs.

Pneumatic Knee Units

Pneumatic knee units offer the prosthetic user a varied cadence capability, using air pressure dynamics in much the same way that fluid is used in the hydraulic knee. Because air is compressible, the channels within the knee can be adjusted to affect the rate of swing. Pneumatic knees usually weigh less and are less expensive than their hydraulic counterparts; however, they provide less precise cadence control and require just as much maintenance. This is because hydraulic fluid is denser and has a higher coefficient of viscosity than air.[38]

Microprocessor Technology

The initial theory of microprocessor knee control was developed in Japan in the early 1980s. Charles A. Blatchford & Sons, Ltd, the developer of the Endolite carbon composite prosthetic system, collaborated with a Japanese electronics company to produce the first commercial application of microprocessor control in a transfemoral prosthesis.[39] The microprocessor swing phase control knee is known as the Intelligent Prosthesis Plus (IP+). Since then the microprocessor knee technology has been further developed into well-known products such as C-Leg (Otto Bock Orthopedic Industry, Minneapolis, MN), Rheo (Ossur, Iceland), and Plie (Freedom Innovations, Irvine, CA). Microprocessor knees are typically equipped with sensors that monitor the knee position during swing and pressure sensors detecting and evaluating ground related forces during stance. Sensor technology is capable of measuring angles, moments, and pressures at the rate of 50 times per second. Customized adjustments are commonly made to microprocessor knees using a laptop or handheld computer (Figure 24-17). Unique software algorithms determine the phase of gait, then immediately adjust the knee functions to compensate during both the stance and swing phases of gait.[40] Most knee mechanisms provide a stumble recovery feature that limits unintentional bending of the knee that sometimes occurs when walking on uneven terrain. The microprocessor enables the patient with transfemoral amputation to move in a natural way, which makes it easier to navigate down stairs, slopes, and uneven terrain.[41,42] There is also a reported reduction in energy expenditure and mental concentration required for ambulation. Microprocessor knees are typically powered by

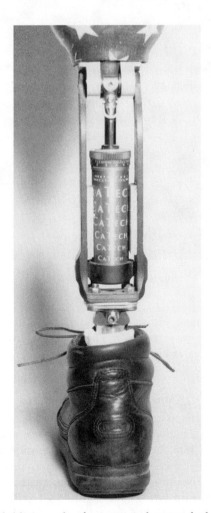

FIGURE 24-16 Example of a swing and stance, hydraulic, fluid-controlled knee unit. This type of hydraulic unit is fit inside the knee frame of an endoskeletal prosthesis or the shin section of an exoskeletal knee.

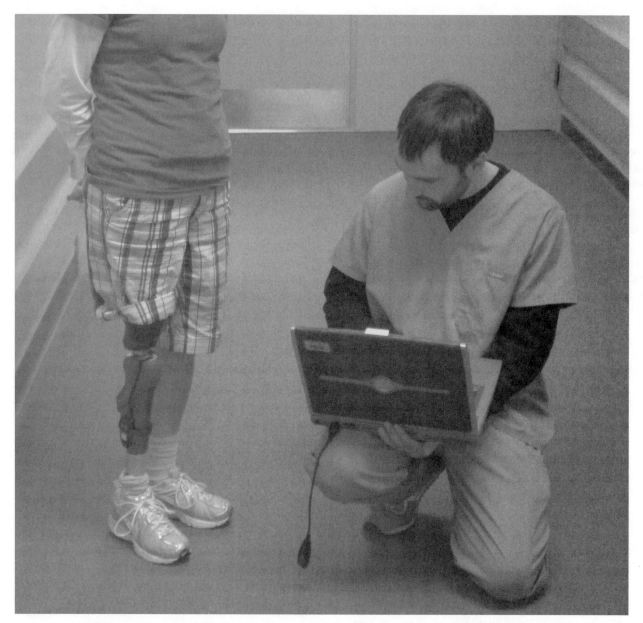

FIGURE 24-17 Customized stance and swing phase adjustments can be made to the microprocessor knee using a handheld or laptop computer.

rechargeable lithium-ion batteries. In most cases batteries can be fully charged in approximately 2 hours, and can last for up to 24 hours when fully charged.

The current disadvantage of microprocessor technology in prosthetics is the significant expense of such devices. The cost of an entire prosthesis that incorporates a computerized knee can be two to three times that of a prosthesis that features a hydraulic knee.

Next-Generation Knees

Prosthetic knee technology becomes more advanced each year. The next generation prosthetic knees feature actuators that actively lift and stimulate the users own muscles for walking up stairs, inclines and ramps. New microprocessor knees provide what is being called "artificial intelligence" features, which allow the systems to anticipate and direct movement within "the whole state of the respective human–machine interface."[43] These knees allow patients to walk with greater efficiency upstairs, backwards, and over obstacles.[44]

Additional Components

For individuals who require assistance to initiate knee extension in early swing phase, an extension aid can be incorporated into the prosthesis. An extension aid is usually an internal spring or an elastic strap that recoils from an elongated position to accelerate the prosthetic shin into extension during swing (see Figure 24-14, *B*). Extension aids may also be useful to control excessive heel rise in early swing phase.

Torque absorbers (axial rotation devices) are designed to simulate axial rotation during stance, which would normally occur in an intact anatomical limb. In the absence of the ankle and knee joint, significant shearing forces can occur at the socket–residual limb interface as the prosthetic user pivots on the prosthesis. Torque absorbers are effective in reducing shearing, and may be especially useful for individuals with fragile, sensitive skin, or adherent scars. They are also often indicated for those involved with sports or work that requires them to negotiate uneven ground. Although these units reduce shear to the residual limb and increase comfort during functional activities, they also add weight to the prosthesis and are susceptible to mechanical failure.

Transverse rotation units have been developed to allow prosthetic wearers to passively rotate the shin section of their prosthesis passively (Figure 24-18).[45] An external button is pushed to unlock the unit, allowing a full 360 degrees of rotation. The unit automatically locks once the knee is moved back into its natural position. This type of device allows the prosthetic wearer to sit in a crossed-legged position, change shoes without having to remove the prosthesis, and enter and exit automobiles with greater ease.

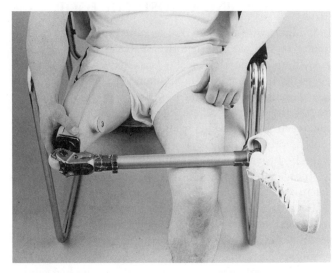

FIGURE 24-18 A transverse rotation unit is generally installed between the socket and the prosthetic knee. When the unit is unlocked, the individual can sit with legs crossed (e.g., to change shoes without having to remove the prosthesis). (Reprinted, with permission, from Otto Bock Health Care, Minneapolis, MN.)

CASE EXAMPLE 2

A Young Man with Multiple Trauma as a Result of a Motor Vehicle Accident

C. J. is a 23-year-old man who lost control of his motorcycle on an icy roadway 10 days ago, sustaining moderate head injury, traumatic amputation of the left lower extremity, and comminuted fracture of the right femur. On admission, he was taken to the operating room for debridement and closure of his amputated limb, and open reduction/internal fixation of his fractured femur. Initially responsive to pain and voice, C. J. now fluctuates between level 4 (confused and agitated) and 6 (confused and appropriate) on the Rancho Los Amigos Cognitive Scale. C. J. is extremely agitated and combative while in bed but calms somewhat when seated in a bedside chair. He repeatedly requests to be allowed to get up to walk but cannot comprehend the need to limit weight bearing on the fractured side and doesn't seem to understand that he has lost his left limb. The rehabilitation team wonders if his cognitive function will stabilize and advance if he can be upright. After much discussion and debate, the team decides that C. J.'s residual limb is healed sufficiently for early fitting with an IRC socket suspended by a TES belt, with a locking knee and solid-ankle, cushion-heel (SACH) foot. The team is hopeful that careful early mobilization into upright posture will reduce his combativeness without compromising his healing residual limb.

When elevated on a tilt table (with a 3-inch lift under the prosthetic side to maintain the non–weight-bearing status of the fractured extremity), C. J.'s cognitive function and behavior improve rapidly. Within several days, he can step off the tilt table and begin to ambulate, non–weight bearing on the right, using a walker for short distances with moderate assistance of one therapist. Over the next 3 weeks, he becomes independent with crutches and continues to use the locking knee until his fracture site heals enough to

safely tolerate full weight bearing safely. The team anticipates that his prosthetic prescription will be significantly modified as he recovers from his head injury and is better able to learn to use and control a more advanced knee unit, prosthetic foot, and methods of suspension.

Questions to Consider

- Why do you think that an ischial containment socket was selected for C. J.'s initial prosthesis? What are the advantages and disadvantages when compared with a traditional quadrilateral socket?
- Considering his current cognition and non–weight-bearing status, what are the advantages and disadvantages of the locking knee unit that the team recommends? Why do you think that they selected this option from among the other types of knee units that are available?
- Why do you think that the team recommended a SACH foot for C. J.'s initial prosthesis? What are the benefits and tradeoffs of SACH, articulating, and dynamic response feet for individuals with head injury in C. J.'s situation? (See Chapter 21 for detailed information about prosthetic feet.)
- Would an extension aide, torque absorber, or transverse rotational unit be appropriate at this point for C. J.? Why or why not?
- What are the implications for safety, energy cost, and cosmesis of gait when using a locked knee and a SACH foot?
- As C. J. regains cognitive function and the fracture of his right femur heals, what options might the rehabilitation team consider for his next prosthesis, in terms of socket design, suspension, knee unit, and prosthetic foot?

CHOOSING A PROSTHETIC FOOT

Individuals with transfemoral amputation and knee disarticulation can use the majority of the prosthetic feet and ankle options that are available (see Chapter 21). For someone with transfemoral amputation, one of the important considerations in choosing a prosthetic foot is its influence on stability of the prosthetic knee during stance. A foot that can reach foot flat quickly (e.g., single-axis or multiaxial foot) is preferable because it enhances stance phase knee stability. Reaching foot flat quickly is especially important for individuals who have a short residual limb or weak hip extensors.

For active individuals, dynamic response feet and those with flexible keels may have advantages. The energy-storing capabilities of these prosthetic feet at push-off promote rapid advancement of the shin section during swing phase. This enhances the ability of the individual who is using a transfemoral prosthesis to walk at faster speeds. Most of these feet are much lighter in weight than the articulating feet.

GAIT CHARACTERISTICS IN TRANSFEMORAL PROSTHETICS

Normal ambulation is a result of dynamic symmetric relationships of the head, spine, and upper and lower extremities. With a transfemoral amputation, an individual's gait pattern wearing a prosthesis becomes significantly asymmetric, regardless of the functional characteristics of the prosthetic components.[46] The more asymmetric the pattern and uneven the cadence, the greater the energy cost of walking. Asymmetry also increases the demand for postural adaptation and balance reactions. For patients with impairment of musculoskeletal and neuromuscular systems, which are common among those with diabetes or advanced age, the incidence of instability and falls increases significantly.

In normal gait, the muscles of the hip, knee, and ankle work in three ways. First, muscle contraction provides stability during stance by resisting the effects of gravity. Second, during push-off and early swing phase, they act to provide propulsion and accelerate the limb. Third, they also act to decelerate forward progression, especially in late swing in preparation for subsequent initial contact. The loss of ankle and knee musculature as a result of transfemoral amputation compromises energy efficiency and quality of gait.

Knee Stability

The most important goal in transfemoral prosthetics is to obtain optimum knee stability throughout the stance phase of gait. A prosthetic knee that is unstable or difficult to control during stance is a great danger, and could lead to a serious fall. Alternately, a knee that is difficult to flex can cause problems with swing phase clearance, increasing the relative length of the limb and the likelihood of tripping and falling.

Three variables influence knee stability during stance:
1. The individual's ability to voluntarily control the knee using muscular power;
2. The alignment of the knee unit with respect to the weight line (trochanter-knee-ankle [TKA] line); and,
3. The inherent mechanical stability of the knee unit.

Radcliffe introduced the "zone of voluntary stability" as an important element in the alignment of the transfemoral prosthesis.[47] Radcliff states that the prosthetic knee will be stable at the critical instant of heel contact if the knee center is positioned within this zone. Knee stability can be best understood by visualizing the TKA line,[48] representing body weight in stance (drawn from the greater trochanter to the ankle of the prosthetic foot), and considering the position of the knee with respect to the line (Figure 24-19). The most appropriate position of the socket, knee, and ankle components is the one that allows the individual to best use his or her muscle control with the minimum amount of alignment stability and still consistently stabilize the knee. If the prosthetic knee is positioned slightly behind the TKA line, so that the weight line passes anterior to the knee axis, the resulting extensor moment provides alignment stability during stance so that little muscular power is required. However, this alignment also increases the muscular effort and energy required to initiate knee flexion for the swing phase of gait. If the knee is positioned at or slightly in front of the TKA line, so that the weight line passes behind the knee, the resulting flexion moment decreases stance phase stability, making muscular power much more important. However, this alignment enhances the ability to flex the knee to initiate swing phase.

An individual's ability to voluntarily control the prosthetic knee is determined by the strength and endurance of muscles around the hip and by the length of the residual limb. If stance stability is provided primarily by voluntary control, hip extensors must be forcefully activated at heel strike to create an extensor moment at the knee. For an individual with a knee disarticulation or long residual limb, the long bony lever is a distinct advantage: An inverse relationship between length of residual limb and amount of muscular force necessary to control the prosthetic knee exists. With a long limb, less muscular power is necessary to control prosthetic knee extension or to initiate flexion in the early swing phase, and the prosthetic knee can be placed at or in front of the TKA line. For an individual with a short residual limb, much more muscular power is necessary to achieve the same level of control. For this reason, stance phase stability is provided by using a knee unit with high mechanical stability or by aligning the knee unit posterior to the TKA line. Voluntary control is also compromised for patients with hip flexion contracture, weakness of hip extensors, or physical frailty.

Prosthetists attempt to enhance muscular control by placing the transfemoral socket in a slight amount of flexion (in relation to the hip). Slight elongation of the hip extensors enhance their contractile ability just enough to develop an effective force (against the posterior wall of the socket) to keep

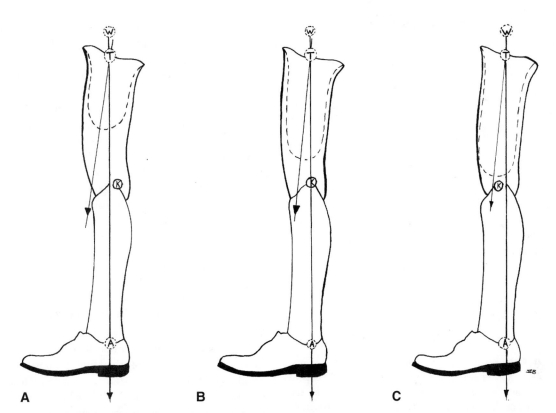

FIGURE 24-19 The imaginary trochanter-knee-ankle (TKA) line is a useful way to understand the components of stance phase stability at the knee. **A,** Alignment stability is at its maximum when the weight line (W) passes anteriorly to the knee axis. This is often important for prosthetic wearers with short residual limbs or weak muscles or when initial socket flexion is increased more than the typical five degrees of preflexion. **B,** Alignment stability is minimal when the weight line passes through the center of the knee axis, making additional muscular or mechanical stability necessary. Many prosthetic wearers with midlength residual limbs and good muscular power benefit from the enhanced initiation of swing that this alignment provides. **C,** No inherent alignment stability is present when the weight line passes behind the knee axis; all of the stance phase stability must be provided by the mechanical characteristics of the knee unit or by muscular activity, or both. Prosthetic wearers with long residual limbs can best manage this alignment.

the prosthetic knee extended (see Figure 24-19).[1,38] This also reduces the individual's tendency to substitute for the weakness of hip extensor muscles with excessive pelvic lordosis. The amount of initial socket flexion is determined by the initial available range of motion at the hip joint. In preparation for initial alignment (bench alignment), the prosthetist sets the socket in 5 degrees of flexion, in addition to the number of degrees of flexion contracture that may be present at the hip.

The stability or, conversely, the mobility of the knee is further influenced by the mechanical properties of the prosthetic knee itself. The degree of inherent stability of the knee varies greatly among the different designs of commercially available prosthetic knees. Because a manually locking knee offers ultimate mechanical stability, placement with respect to the weight line and muscular power is of lesser importance. At the other end of the continuum, a freely moving single-axis knee offers virtually no mechanical stability; stance phase stability must come from voluntary control, alignment, or a combination of the two. The mechanical stability provided by hydraulic swing and stance, and weight-activated stance control knee units fall between these extremes. Especially

important is consideration of the contribution of mechanical stability for individuals with short residual limbs and weak hip muscles and those who routinely negotiate uneven or rough terrain.

Pelvic Stability

Because of transfemoral amputation, the direct anatomical connection between the femur and the ground surface is lost and closed-chain, medial-lateral stability of the pelvis is significantly compromised.[49-51] The femur, without its distal attachment at the knee, is susceptible to marked lateral displacement within the socket during weight bearing in the stance phase. This lateral shift makes it impossible to maintain a horizontal pelvis, even for individuals with strong hip abductor muscles, and results in an apparent Trendelenburg sign and compensatory gait deviations (Figure 24-20). Pelvic stability is especially problematic for those with short residual limbs and those who have developed flexion, abduction, and external rotation contracture. The design of a quadrilateral socket primarily applies stabilizing forces in the anteroposterior plane so that there is little to keep the femur from drifting laterally

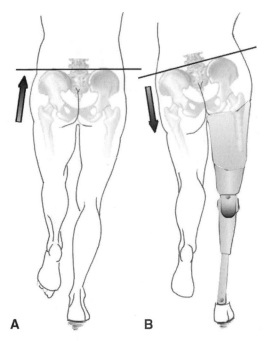

A   **B**

FIGURE 24-20 A, Normally, when weight is borne on the stance limb the pelvis dips to the swing side because of gravity. Excessive pelvic dip is prevented by contraction of the gluteus medius, on the stance side, which is anchored to a femur fixed to the floor through its distal attachment. **B,** The femur, without its distal attachment at the knee, is susceptible to lateral displacement within the socket during weight bearing. This displacement can make it difficult to maintain a horizontal pelvis and results in an apparent Trendelenburg sign and compensatory gait deviations. Pelvic stability is especially problematic for those with short residual limbs. Lateral stabilization of the pelvis is maintained by an anatomically aligned and shaped socket which mirrors the preamputation adduction angle of the femur.

within the socket. As a consequence, the pelvis drops when the intact limb is in swing phase. To compensate, the prosthetic wearer often leans or lurches laterally toward the prosthetic side. This strategy improves swing clearance but also results in a wide-based, energy-taxing gait. Because the femur is held in an abnormally abducted position, circumduction of the prosthesis during swing is likely to occur. In contrast, the design of the IRC socket attempts to hold the femur in its normal adducted position during stance with an upward and medially directed force along the length of the lateral femur. This strategy enhances the prosthetic wearer's ability to maintain a level pelvis and improves the quality of functional gait.

EVALUATION OF SOCKET FIT AND ALIGNMENT

Despite all the technological advances in prosthetic knee units, prosthetic feet, and materials, the single most important influence on functional outcome in prosthetics is the quality of socket fit. The socket is the interface between the wearer and the prosthesis. It must comfortably contain soft tissue when the patient is standing or sitting, furnish adequate relief for bony prominences, distribute stabilizing pressure to the femur and pelvis, and provide an adequate weight-bearing surface for the ischial gluteal region.

Transparent diagnostic sockets (test sockets) are routinely used to assess socket fit.[52] These thermoplastic sockets are molded over the modified positive model of the residual limb as an interim step in socket fabrication. In the case of skin suction suspension, the diagnostic socket is donned without a sock or over a thin nylon sheath so that contact with tissues and bony prominences can be clearly viewed (Figure 24-21). Areas of excessive or inadequate pressure can be detected according to the degree of skin blanching. To make necessary reliefs or to enhance total contact, corrections to the diagnostic socket are made by reheating the socket with a hot air gun or torch. The socket may be tried on and then modified several times before optimal fit and comfort are achieved. Once proper fit has been established, the diagnostic socket is filled with plaster or digitized to create a new, accurate positive model for fabrication of the definitive socket.

Donning Procedure

The first step in evaluation of socket fit is to ensure that the socket has been donned properly. If the socket is not positioned correctly on the residual limb because of being rotated or only partially donned , its fit cannot be accurately assessed. Optimally, the socket fits easily but snugly over the residual limb. If too many plies of prosthetic sock are worn, donning is difficult and the person will feel as if the residual limb is not fully down in the socket. If too few plies of sock are worn, the limb falls more deeply into the socket and the person will feel medial socket pressure at the pubic ramus as well as a high degree of distal end pressure.

When suction suspension is used, the socket is slightly more difficult to don because of the relatively tight total contact fit that is required to maintain suction. Whether elastic wrap, pull sock, or liquid powder is used, the donning procedure must be consistent each time the prosthesis is donned. Before the air-escape valve is screwed into place, total contact between skin and socket is evaluated. The skin should

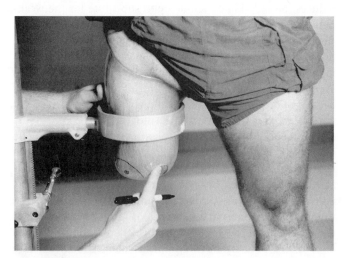

FIGURE 24-21 Transparent diagnostic sockets are used to visually evaluate the prosthetic socket fit. Inspection of the skin through the socket provides information about adequacy of residual limb containment.

protrude slightly into the valve housing; however, tissue should not be taut, bulging, painful, or discolored.

The size of the residual limb of individuals with recent amputation can vary if adequate volume management has not been maintained . Inconsistent use of elastic shrinkers or elastic wrapping (Ace wraps) can lead to increased limb circumference. Even small increases in limb size can compromise the ability to don a prosthetic socket correctly, and can significantly alter the quality of functional gait. The importance of the consistent use of a shrinker or elastic wrap whenever the prosthesis is not being worn cannot be overemphasized.

Total Contact Fit

Most prosthetic sockets are designed so that total contact is present between the skin of the residual limb, the socket interface (sock and/or roll-on-liner), and the walls of the socket. Total contact fit distributes socket pressure over the entire surface of the residual limb. Relief areas may be used to reduce pressure over bony prominences, bone spurs, neuromas, or other pressure-intolerant areas, but total contact is still the goal. Total contact also promotes venous return from the tissues of the residual limb and helps to reduce edema. Wherever contact is inadequate, the residual limb is likely to become edematous. Over time, secondary skin problems are likely to develop as well.

Once the socket has been donned, it may be difficult to determine if total contact has been achieved or to locate precise areas of discomfort or excessive pressure. Placing a small amount of clay or powder or a thin film of lipstick inside the socket before donning can assist with assessment of fit. The person dons the socket as usual and then walks (or, if too uncomfortable, stands) for several minutes. When the prosthesis is removed, relatively even traces of the substance should be found on the socks (or skin) of the residual limb. Alternatively, lipstick can be applied to the sock (or skin for suction suspension users) over the area of discomfort before the prosthesis is put on. After donning as usual and wearing for several minutes, the prosthesis is removed and the inside of the socket is inspected. Traces of lipstick identify the area of the socket that requires modification for pressure relief.

Sitting and Kneeling

Most people spend more time sitting than they do standing or walking. How the prosthesis feels when an individual using a prosthesis is seated is important. The sitting surface of the socket should be contoured so that the soft tissue of the upper posterior thigh is not impinged between the socket and the seat.[53] To be comfortable in sitting and in kneeling, individuals with transfemoral amputation must be able to reach at least 90 degrees of hip flexion. If the anterior wall of the socket is excessively high, the brim impinges on the abdomen and the anterior superior iliac spine. For those using pelvic belt and hip joint suspension, care should be taken to avoid painful pinching of flesh between the socket and belt.

Another important consideration that relates to standing and sitting is the suspension of the socket. When a person wearing a transfemoral prosthesis sits down or stands up,

gaps may occur between the posterior-lateral corner of the socket brim and the proximal residual limb.[53]

This lack of total contact causes a loss of the negative pressure environment required for maintaining proper suspension. One way to help prevent this problem is for the individual to maintain control of the prosthesis and not allow the muscles of the residual limb to go slack within the socket. The individual should expand the muscles of the residual limb, by an isometric contraction of the thigh, whenever going through the motions of sitting down or standing up.[54]

Evaluating Socket Fit and Brim Contours

The Quadrilateral Socket

For the quad socket, the brim shape is rectangular, with a narrow anteroposterior dimension (see Figure 24-3, *A*). The primary weight-bearing surface, the ischial seat, is located on the posterior–medial aspect of the brim. The seat should be widest at the posteromedial corner to adequately support the ischium and gluteal muscles. It should lie parallel to the ground. The overall height of the prosthesis is measured as the distance from this posteromedial corner to the ground with the knee in full extension. A channel for the adductor longus tendon is located at the anteromedial corner of the socket. The anterior brim is higher than the ischial seat as it moves toward the lateral wall. The contours of the anterior wall, at the Scarpa's (femoral) triangle, provide a posteriorly directed force to maintain the ischium on its seat.

The medial wall is a flattened surface that represents the line of forward progression. The height of the medial brim is usually the same as that of the ischial seat, fitting well into the groin. It should not, however, create undue pressure on the perineum or pubic ramus. For a person in whom an adductor roll has developed, the medial brim should be flared to accommodate the extra tissue but not lowered. Excessive lowering of the medial wall can exacerbate the problem. The primary function of the lateral wall is to maintain a "normal" femoral adduction angle. This is often difficult to achieve in the quad socket because of the wide mediolateral dimension of the design. Pressure is applied to the limb by flattening the socket along the femoral shaft. A relief area is usually necessary to accommodate pressure sensitivity of the distal lateral femur. The lateral wall completely encases the greater trochanter and fits snugly around the gluteal muscles as the socket wraps toward the posterior wall.[7,8,11]

The Ischial–Ramal Containment Socket

A proximal cross section of an IRC socket is more anatomically contoured in shape rather than rectangular, with a narrow mediolateral dimension (see Figure 24-3, *B* and *C*). This design more closely resembles the natural shape of the thigh. The brim of this socket captures more of the adductor muscle complex than does the quad socket. The ischial tuberosity and the pubic ramus are contained in a fossa well within the socket. This creates a bony lock that provides mediolateral stability and reduces the likelihood of socket rotation on the residual limb. The contour of the posterior socket captures gluteal muscles. No ischial seat is present because weight bearing occurs predominantly on the soft tissues of the thigh, gluteal region and medial aspect of the ischium.[9-13] Because stability is provided in the mediolateral plane, the concave pressure in the Scarpa triangle on the anterior wall is not as severe in comparison to the quad socket.

The medial wall of the IRC socket incorporates an adductor complex channel designed to contain all medial tissues. This minimizes problems with adductor roll pinching. The lateral socket wall is contoured in adduction, with additional pressure against the posterior shaft of the femur for added stability and rotational control. A pocket hollow or fossa is incorporated into the lateral wall posterior to the greater trochanter for a snug fit against the lateral gluteal muscles.

PROSTHETIC ALIGNMENT

The alignment of a prosthesis is defined as the orientation of the socket relative to the prosthetic components of the prosthesis.[55] The prosthetic alignment of a transfemoral prosthesis greatly impacts the comfort and functional characteristics of the prosthesis. Alignable endoskeletal prosthetic systems allow the prosthetist to alter the manner in which the prosthesis transmits the weight load between the residual limb and the ground. Optimal prosthetic alignment requires three steps: bench alignment, static alignment, and dynamic alignment.[56]

Bench Alignment

Bench alignment is the alignment in which the components of the prosthesis are assembled according to standards of practice and manufacturer's guidelines. This step is employed to ensure knee stability by aligning the prosthetic knee axis in a position that will promote stability. The load line should pass through the knee at a position dictated by the knee's kinematics and the manufacturer's recommendations. The prosthesis is often assembled in an alignment fixture using a plumb line or laser line projected on the lateral side of the socket, knee, and foot.

Static Alignment

Static alignment is the alignment that is obtained after an individual is comfortably fit in his or her socket and able to stand transmitting weight onto the prosthesis. Typically, this evaluation is performed with the patient standing within a set of parallel bars to provide upper extremity support and stability. In addition to evaluating socket fit, the static examination focuses on: a level pelvis (to check the height of the prosthesis), knee stability, and the width of the base of support. The LASAR (laser-assisted static alignment reference) Posture is a piece of equipment that can assist the practitioner in examining static alignment.

Height of the Prosthesis

Patients are encouraged to shift weight mediolaterally until they are comfortable with a symmetric standing position with relatively equal weight bearing on the prosthesis and intact limb. The prosthetist or therapist applies a firm downward force through the iliac crests to ensure equal distribution of body weight and then visually evaluates the position of the pelvis. Ideally the examiner's hands over the iliac crests will be in the same plane, and the pelvis will be level (Figure 24-22, *A*). Another way to evaluate this is by using a hip-leveling guide. This device, which has a bubble level at its center, is placed

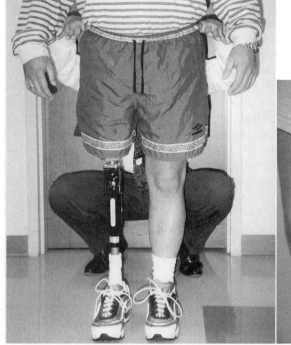
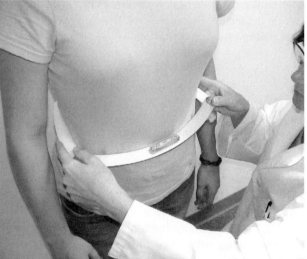

A   **B**

FIGURE 24-22 The height of the prosthesis should approximate that of the sound limb. **A,** One method of checking for adequate prosthetic height is to assess whether the pelvis is level, by comparing the height of the examiner's hands as they rest on the patient's iliac crests. **B,** A hip-leveling guide is a device that uses a bubble level to determine if the pelvis is level. If the hips are level, the bubble is centered. If the pelvis is not level, the bubble moves off center in the direction of the longer limb.

over the individual's iliac crests. If the hips are level, the bubble will be centered. If the pelvis is not level, the bubble will move off center in the direction of the longer limb (Figure 24-22, *B*).

The initial transfemoral prosthesis may be up to one-quarter inch shorter than the intact side to enhance toe clearance in swing phase. Leg-length discrepancy of more than one-quarter inch leads to back pain, gait deviation, and higher energy cost in gait. The examiner can place one or more shims or boards (cut in various increments of thickness) under the "short" limb to determine the extent of the discrepancy if the prosthesis appears to be too short or too long.

Evaluation of Knee Stability

When evaluating knee stability it must be quickly ascertained whether the prosthetic user has a sense of security with the prosthesis or fears that the knee will buckle under full weight bearing. The prosthetic user must be able to easily extend the prosthetic knee and maintain it in a stable position. Stability of the knee can be altered significantly if shoes other than those for which the prosthesis has been aligned are worn (Figure 24-23). Shoes with lower heels create an extension moment at the knee; the resulting stability is often excessive, and can interfere with the knee flexion that is necessary in late stance and early swing phase. Shoes with higher heels create a flexion moment at the knee, reducing stance stability and increasing the likelihood of the knee buckling at midstance. Accommodating higher heels is difficult unless the individual uses a prosthetic foot designed specifically for high heels.

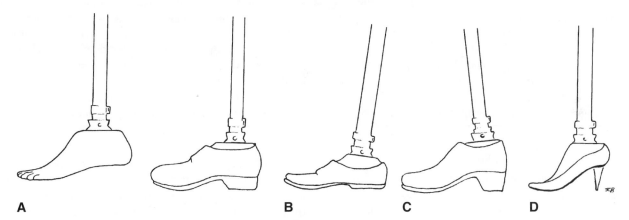

A   **B**   **C**   **D**

FIGURE 24-23 Shoes with differing heel heights affect knee stability for individuals who are using a transfemoral prosthesis. **A,** Most prosthetic feet are designed for a standard ¾-inch heel. **B,** Decreasing heel height creates an extension moment at the knee, leading to an excessively stable knee. **C,** Increasing heel height creates a flexion moment, leading to instability of the prosthetic knee. **D,** Special prosthetic feet are made for shoes with high heels.

CASE EXAMPLE 3

Why Should Changing Shoes Be an Issue?

P. O. is 21-year-old man who is learning the hard way about the effects of improperly changing heel heights. Having lost his leg just above the knee as the result of a motor vehicle accident 2 weeks ago, he is fitted with a transfemoral prosthesis, a flexible socket in a rigid frame, TES suspension, weight-activated stance-control knee unit, and dynamic-response foot while in the hospital. His knee unit is positioned at the TKA line because of the long lever and muscular control afforded by his residual limb.

After only a few days of inpatient therapy and education concerning his prosthesis, P. O. is able to ambulate by using a straight cane in a fairly symmetrical step-through pattern. He often attempts to ambulate without aids, but whenever he does, his physical therapist stops him immediately and cautions him against varying from the therapy program until his residual limb is sufficiently healed and tolerant of full weight bearing on the prosthesis. At this point, he is able to tolerate up to 3 hours at a time in his prosthesis and is anxious to begin full-time "all-day" wear.

Despite his need to complete a therapy program, P. O. discharges himself from the hospital against his physician's recommendations. Before discharge, he is instructed on the care of his prosthesis, the accommodation of limb volume fluctuation, the way to properly negotiate inclines and stairs, and the impact of changing heel heights. He is also cautioned to gradually increase his "in prosthesis" time to minimize risk of skin breakdown or dehiscence of his healing suture line. P. O. ignores the booklets and instructions he receives. He wants to "get back to life," and 2 days after discharge he wears his favorite pair of high-heeled cowboy boots to go out partying with his friends. While negotiating the first step out of his house, his prosthetic knee buckles and he falls down the next two steps, fracturing the femur of his residual limb and cracking the frame of his socket. He is readmitted to the hospital for open reduction internal fixation and eventually learns to ambulate with a swing-through pattern, using bilateral axillary crutches. He is discharged from the hospital after 1 week but is not able to return to prosthetic use for the next 3 months. He returns to physical therapy on an outpatient basis to begin the process of prosthetic training once again. This time, he is more cautious and attentive to the instruction and advice of his rehabilitation team. His story now serves as a warning about "what not to <u>do</u> when you go home" to everyone who attends the prosthetic clinic that assisted him.

Questions to Consider

- Describe the functional relationships among (a) mechanical stability of P. O's weight-activated stance control knee, (b) its alignment and position with respect to the TKA line, and (c) the length of his residual limb. How might the alignment of his knee unit be adjusted as his limb heals and is better able to tolerate forces generated during normal walking?
- What are the advantages of moving the axis of rotation of the knee unit forward with respect to the TKA line? Under what conditions would the prosthetist move the axis of rotation of the knee until it is behind the TKA line? What would you recommend for P. O. as he begins his outpatient rehabilitation after his fractured femur heals?

- Why would the rehabilitation team be concerned about the time P. O. spends in his prosthesis only 2 weeks after the amputation? What would be an appropriate wearing schedule for someone like P. O. who has been had an early prosthetic fitting? In what ways might the team's recommendation about in-prosthesis time be different as P. O. begins his second period of rehabilitation?
- Why did P. O.'s weight-activated stance control knee become unstable when he changed into his cowboy boots? What forces were acting at the knee at the time that it buckled? Is there anything he could have done to counteract the instability associated with higher heels?
- What would have happened if he had instead put on a pair of sandals with no heels at all? What types of functional problems might he have encountered during gait? How might he minimize the effect of changing to shoes with lower heels and preserve his functional abilities?
- What is the lesson from P. O.'s situation that should be conveyed to individuals new to prosthetic use?

Base of Support

The ideal distance between heels during comfortable stance is relatively narrow, approximating the normal base of individuals without amputation (2 to 3 inches). The prosthetic foot and shoe should lie flat on the ground with relatively equal weight bearing on medial and lateral borders. This can be assessed by slipping a piece of paper under both sides of the forefoot and rearfoot—the distances should be fairly equal. The individual must also be able to shift weight comfortably between the intact and prosthetic limbs. The adequacy of the suspension system is evaluated by asking the patient to lift the prosthetic foot off the ground using a hip-hiking motion. Minimal pistoning of the residual limb should occur within the socket.

LASAR Posture

The LASAR Posture is a laser platform apparatus used to visually identify the center of gravity line, or load line, while an individual is standing in their prosthesis (Figure 24-24).[56] The LASAR Posture consists of a platform containing pressure sensors and laser projection system. To measure the load line, an individual steps onto the force sensor platform with his or her prosthesis and places their contralateral leg on the leveling step plate. A laser line is then projected directly on the patient and prosthesis, whether in the frontal or sagittal plane, identifying alignment parameters that can be objectively documented.[57] The dynamic alignment of the prosthesis can then be optimized based on this static load line.

DYNAMIC ALIGNMENT

Dynamic alignment is the alignment made during basic ambulation while an individual walks with or without aids. According to Zahedi and colleagues, dynamic alignment is a progressive process in which a practitioner makes adjustments to the geometrical configuration of the prosthesis until an alignment is achieved that is acceptable to both the individual wearing the prosthesis and the prosthetist.[55] The goal is to achieve a gait pattern that is safe, comfortable, cosmetic, and energy efficient. The individual's ambulatory history, strength, endurance, activity level, concurrent medical conditions, previous experience in wearing prostheses, and current goals are just as important to consider as are the prescribed prosthetic components.

Dynamic alignment begins with a walk down the length of the parallel bars. Having an assistant or aid guard or assist new prosthetic users as they walk is helpful so that the examiner can focus on gait characteristics. For a complete understanding of the dynamic interaction of patient and prosthesis, gait must be observed from lateral–sagittal and anterior–posterior perspectives.

LATERAL–SAGITTAL VIEW

Four key areas evaluated from the lateral perspective are (a) knee stability throughout stance, (b) transition from initial heel contact to foot-flat position, (c) symmetry of step length and step duration, and (d) quality of knee flexion during late stance and swing phase.

Stability of the knee is the major determinant of safe ambulation. The new prosthetic wearer must learn to extend the hip at initial contact (heel strike) to stabilize the prosthetic knee adequately. Optimally, the knee will extend smoothly, with little hesitation.

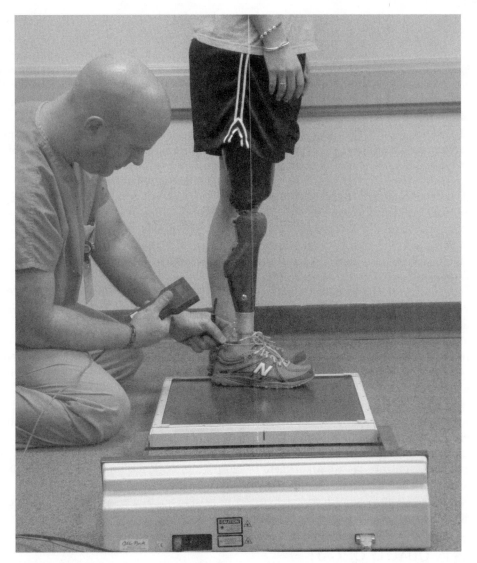

FIGURE 24-24 The LASAR (laser-assisted static alignment reference) Posture is a laser platform apparatus used to visually identify the center of gravity line, or load line, while an individual is standing in their prosthesis.

Initial contact (heel strike) is the most unstable point in prosthetic gait. Stability in stance increases significantly when a foot-flat position is reached. The transition from initial contact to foot-flat position should occur relatively quickly and smoothly, with the goal of reaching a position that promotes knee stability without obvious "foot slap." Quality of prosthetic gait and commonly occurring gait deviations are discussed later.

Optimally, the prosthesis and intact limb's step lengths are equal in distance, symmetric in pattern, and even in cadence. The individual should have little hesitation in initiation of swing on the prosthesis or intact limb. Asymmetry in step characteristics impedes the momentum necessary for energy-efficient forward progression, increasing the work of walking significantly.

Step length and swing phase function are influenced by knee flexion during late stance phase. As the patient moves from midstance into initial swing, a controlled and gradual knee flexion optimally occurs to provide adequate toe clearance during the swing phase of gait. Knee flexion that occurs too early compromises stance stability and excessive knee flexion during swing causes rapid heel rise.

ANTERIOR–FRONTAL VIEW

When viewing gait from an anterior or posterior perspective, the examiner is most interested in adequacy of suspension, width of the base of support, control of the pelvis during prosthetic stance, and quality and pattern of the prosthetic swing.

Suspension can be effective only if it is donned properly and fit adequately to the individual. The examiner must determine if the prosthesis remains in optimal orientation on the limb through all phases of the gait cycle. Pistoning or rotation of the prosthesis should be minimal on the residual limb at any point in the gait cycle, but especially during unweighted swing. Because the distal position of pistoning results in a relative lengthening of the prosthesis, wearers must use a compensatory strategy to achieve toe clearance. One of the most common gait deviations observed when suspension is incorrectly applied or inadequate is circumduction of the prosthetic limb during swing.

Optimally, a normal narrow base of support and swing path is present with a two-three inch separation between feet as they alternate between stance and swing. A wide base increases energy expenditure and results in a less cosmetic gait pattern.

The pelvis should remain relatively horizontal during the prosthetic stance phase with a maximum drop of 5 degrees on the intact swing side for optimal cosmetic and energy-efficient gait.[1,7] For those with short residual limbs or weakness of hip abductors, a level pelvis is a challenge to maintain. In these instances, the pelvis drops noticeably to the side of the intact swing limb during stance on the prosthesis. A compensatory pattern, such as lateral trunk bending, can be used to ensure adequate toe clearance of the intact swing limb. The frontal plane alignment of socket, knee, and foot plays a significant role in stabilizing the pelvis and trunk.

The line of progression of the prosthetic foot and knee during swing phase is also assessed. Ideally the foot and knee move forward in the same plane. If the prosthesis has been donned improperly, evidence of a medial or lateral whip may be seen with the foot circumscribing with an inward or outward arc during swing phase (see Figure 24-28). All of these factors should be considered by the prosthetist through diagnostic fittings and dynamic alignment sessions before delivery of the finished prosthesis.

VARIATIONS IN QUALITY OF GAIT

The pattern and quality of gait with a transfemoral prosthesis can vary a great deal between treatment sessions, especially for those new to their prosthesis or recently have had a change in prosthetic components. Most often, these variations in performance can be traced to intraindividual factors, rather than to malalignment or dysfunction of the prosthesis itself. If unrecognized, some of these quite controllable factors can significantly impede progress in gait training and functional mobility. The most common problems encountered include inadequate volume control and edema management, continued shrinkage of the residual limb as it matures, inappropriate number of sock ply, inappropriate heel heights, skin irritation from overuse of a new prosthesis, improper donning, inadequate suspension, worn or loose components, and "patient innovation." Effective patient education and communication between the prosthetic clinical team and the patient can solve many of these problems.[58]

Edema and Limb Volume

For a new prosthetic user who is having difficulty with prosthetic fit and donning, one of the first questions asked should concern compliance in wearing compression garments. An increase in limb circumference after only 15 to 30 minutes without wearing a shrinker or compressive elastic wrap is common. The importance of routine use of a compressive garment whenever the prosthesis is not being worn (including overnight while sleeping) cannot be overstated, especially for those within six months of amputation. Even in an experienced prosthetic wearer, limb volume can vary over the course of the day. Adding or subtracting one or more ply of prosthetic socks at some point during the day is not unusual. For those who need the snug fit of suction suspension, edema is a serious problem that can prevent donning the prosthesis and achieving suction. In this case, the compression garment or elastic wrap should be applied for 15 to 20 minutes before donning the prosthesis again.

Maturation and Shrinkage of the Residual Limb

New prosthetic users often experience rapid reduction of limb volume as their time in the prosthesis increases over the first few weeks and months after delivery of the prosthesis. Although this limb maturation may require several socket adjustments until limb size stabilizes, it is a natural and important process that should be supported by the use of compression whenever the prosthesis is not worn. The loss of limb volume is usually accommodated by the need to increase the number of ply of prosthetic socks being worn to a 15- to 20-ply maximum. When more than 20 plies of sock are worn, intimacy of fit is compromised and a new socket should be fabricated. Traditionally, the use of skin suction suspension is not recommended until limb volume has stabilized. For those using suction suspension who experience further reduction in limb size (e.g., because of weight loss, increased activity, time in the socket), the prosthetist can add padding to the socket to restore the intimate skin-socket fit necessary to restore suction.

Inappropriate Number of Sock Ply

Because of the normal fluctuation in limb volume, the number of prosthetic sock ply required for appropriate fit also can vary from day to day and within the same day. New and experienced prosthetic users often carry several one-ply socks with them during the day so that they are prepared should adjustment become necessary. Individuals wearing too many ply of sock lose total contact with the distal portion of the socket, complain of tightness at the proximal socket, and feel as if the prosthesis is excessively long (this may be manifested as difficulty with toe clearance in swing). Those who have too few ply of sock experience increasing distal end pressure or discomfort in the perineum because they are seated too far down in the socket. New prosthetic users should keep a record of the number of socks and overall ply (thickness) they wear, as well as the frequency with which they adjust ply during the day. This helps them to understand the dynamic nature of limb volume size and enhance proper care of the residual limb.

Problem Solving When the Prosthesis Suddenly Doesn't Fit

A physical therapist calls a prosthetist colleague one morning to warn him that T. M., a businessman who 3 years ago sustained a transfemoral amputation as the result of diabetes, has called complaining about his new prosthesis. T. M. had been comfortably fit with an IRC socket 9 weeks earlier without difficulty. However, he now reports that his socket is too small and he is not getting all the way down into his prosthesis. He is fearful that the tightness he is experiencing will cause skin breakdown, a frightening prospect for a person with diabetes. T. M. is wearing a transfemoral prosthesis with a stance control knee, dynamic response foot, and he is using a locking roll-on-liner for suspension.

The prosthetist and physical therapist set up an appointment with the patient for reevaluation in the physical therapy office the next morning. Their goal is to determine why T. M., who has been wearing his prosthesis in excess of 10 hours a day for 9 weeks, is just now complaining about the fit. When T. M. enters the clinic, he is obviously experiencing discomfort and is not shifting his weight equally over the prosthesis during the stance phase of gait. He has chosen to return to using bilateral axillary crutches in an effort to reduce his discomfort. The prosthetist and physical therapist ask T. M. to take his prosthesis off so that they can visually check whether any skin damage has occurred. They find proximal redness and tenderness over the hip adductors. The prosthetist inspects the prosthesis as the therapist examines her office notes from the man's last visit.

While watching the patient put on his socket, the physical therapist recognizes the source of the problem. During T. M's previous visit she had documented that he was wearing a single three-ply sock over a 3-mm roll-on liner. Today he is donning a five- and a three-ply socks over his roll-on liner. When asked why he has increased the sock ply, T.M. reports that since he had progressed from a liner-only fit to wearing an additional three ply in 3 weeks, he thought that by 9 weeks he should be wearing about eight to nine ply of sock. The prosthetist and therapist clarify with him the indicators of need to increase sock ply. The patient returns to using a three-ply sock over the liner and returns to the comfort he experienced before the arbitrary addition of socks. He is relieved to be able to ambulate once again without his crutches.

Questions to Consider

- What is the typical strategy for managing volume control and limb shrinkage in the first months following amputation? Is there a typical rate of maturation of limb volume that can be predicted? Why or why not? When might a new user expect that his or her limb will reach a stable size or volume?
- What are the indicators that an additional sock ply is necessary in the first months of prosthetic wear? What must a new prosthetic wearer understand to adjust sock ply appropriately? How can the therapist or prosthetist help a new prosthetic wearer master the art of changing sock ply to adjust prosthetic fit?
- How would T. M.'s complaints about fitting be different if he were wearing too few prosthetic socks?
- How many sock ply must a new user be wearing before it is time for the prosthetist to fabricate a new socket? What other indicators might there be that it is time for a change in socket or suspension?
- How might improper socket fit (whether too many or too few socks are worn) affect the prosthetic wearer's stability in stance and mobility during swing phase of gait?

Changing Footwear: Improper Heel Heights

All prosthetic feet are designed to be worn with shoes of a particular heel height (see Figure 24-23). They are available in various heel heights, ranging from a heel rise of 0 mm for sandals and flats to a 45-mm heel rise for women's high heels. Matching the heel rise of the prosthetic foot to the shoes most often worn by the patient is essential. A heel wedge placed inside the shoe can be used to accommodate shoes that have a lower heel than what the foot was designed for. Changing to shoes with significantly lower heels results in excessive knee stability in stance. Conversely, a change to shoes with much higher heels compromises alignment stability of the knee and places much greater demand on the patient for muscular control of knee position during stance.

Impact of Overuse

Whether learning to use a training prosthesis for the first time since amputation or being fit with a new definitive prosthesis, most prosthetic users benefit from a gradual break-in period. This strategy allows the skin, soft tissue, and musculature to grow accustomed to the forces acting on the residual limb. Failure to adhere to such a plan can lead to muscle soreness, skin irritation, and, in some cases, skin breakdown. New users should be advised to increase the length of time in their prosthesis gradually, carefully inspecting their skin each time the prosthesis is removed and wearing an appropriate compression garment when not in the prosthesis.

Improper Donning

When a prosthesis is not properly oriented on the residual limb as a result of improper donning technique or incomplete donning, it cannot operate efficiently. The wearer may experience discomfort within the socket or may exhibit various gait deviations. Emphasis on developing a careful systematic method of donning is essential when working with new prosthetic wearers. Attention to details when donning the prosthesis can minimize the frustration, inconvenience, and discomfort of having to reapply the prosthesis multiple times until the desired position is achieved.

Inadequate Suspension

Inadequately tightened or badly worn suspension straps, belts, or Velcro closures should be suspected when the wearer experiences pistoning of the residual limb within the socket. The prosthesis drops down slightly when it is unweighted during swing, resulting in a relatively longer swing limb and challenging toe clearance. Additionally, the prosthesis may rotate on the residual limb, leading to various compensatory gait deviations. New prosthetic users should be encouraged to assess the adequacy of suspension carefully and systematically each time they don the prosthesis. All prosthetic users must periodically inspect belts, straps, or Velcro closures for signs of fraying, stretching, or significant wear, and tear.

Worn or Loosened Components

As for any mechanical device subjected to daily use, the prosthesis should be periodically inspected for signs of excessive wear or loosening of the components. Periodic maintenance checkups with the prosthetist should be scheduled, especially if the prosthetic wearer is involved in physically demanding work or leisure activities. In some circumstances, the prosthesis may be misused or abused, increasing the likelihood of damage to prosthetic components. Fixing a small problem in the making is much less expensive than having to replace major components or fabricate a new prosthesis because of complete mechanical failure.

Patient Innovation

Prosthetic users who do not fully understand the intricate alignment and design specifics of their prostheses may attempt to modify them. If a patient who has been progressing well in gait training and compliant with compression strategies suddenly has difficulty with socket fit, patient innovation should be suspected. It may be that padding has been added or removed from inside the socket. If knee stability has suddenly changed without any change in footwear, the wearer may have attempted to fine-tune alignment or knee unit function. Individuals who have questions about alignment (including most physical therapists) should not make random alignment adjustments, but instead rely on the knowledge, equipment, and skilled experience of the prosthetist if adjustment is necessary.

QUALITY OF TRANSFEMORAL PROSTHETIC GAIT

The goal of a well-designed and accurately fit transfemoral prosthesis is an energy-efficient gait in as natural a pattern as possible. Quality of gait is inconsistent early in the gait-training phase but improves as the individual becomes more experienced with the prosthesis during therapy. If gait problems persist, especially if the risk of instability

and falls or skin irritation is present, the source of the problem should be identified, and an attempt made to correct it. A number of classic transfemoral prosthetic gait problems may be the result of prosthetic malalignment. Before changing alignment or adjusting mechanical settings of the prosthetic knee or foot, it is wise to rule out patient-related factors (e.g., hip flexion contracture, weakness, habit) as potential contributors.

Problems in Early Stance Phase

At initial contact, the prosthetic knee should be fully extended to position the prosthetic foot appropriately for smooth loading as body weight is transferred onto the prosthesis. As loading occurs, the prosthetic foot rolls smoothly into a foot-flat position. Problems with either of these functions increase the risk of instability and shorten the swing time and step length of the contralateral limb.

Knee Instability: Initial Contact to Midstance

If the prosthetic knee cannot maintain the necessary extension as the heel strikes the ground, and the prosthesis is loaded, several possible prosthetic and patient-related factors should be considered (Figure 24-25). The most common patient-related problems that lead to knee instability at initial contact include significant hip flexion contracture or weakness of hip extensor muscles, which compromise the patient's ability to stabilize the prosthetic knee by using

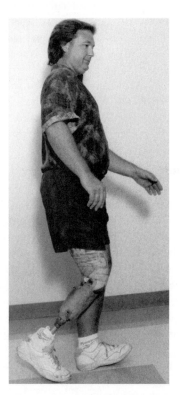

FIGURE 24-25 An unstable prosthetic knee during stance phase often results in a quick, short step taken by the sound limb. The problem may be caused by patient factors (e.g., hip extensor weakness, hip flexion contracture) or anterior alignment of the prosthetic knee.

active hip extension. If strength and range of motion are adequate, four different prosthetic factors might lead to knee instability:

1. The knee axis may be aligned too far anterior to the TKA line, promoting a flexion moment.
2. The socket may not have been set in the optimal pre-flexed position, which places the hip extensor muscles at a biomechanical advantage for stabilizing the knee.
3. The prosthetic foot may have been aligned in excessive dorsiflexion.
4. The plantar flexion bumper or SACH heel may be too stiff.

Foot Slap

The speed that the prosthetic forefoot descends to the floor at heel strike is determined by the stiffness of the heel or plantar flexion bumper and by how quickly or forcefully the individual loads the heel of the foot. If the prosthetic foot functions with an apparent foot slap, two factors should be considered. The heel cushion or plantar flexion bumper may be too soft for the user's weight and activity level. Alternatively, those prosthetic wearers fearful of instability in the early stance phase may be forcefully driving their heels into the ground to ensure complete knee extension. For those using a locking knee component, the ability to reach a foot-flat position quickly is essential for a smooth transition throughout the stance phase of gait.

External Rotation of the Prosthetic Foot

One of the gait deviations observed in the frontal plane is an external rotation of the prosthetic foot at initial contact and loading response as weight is transferred onto the prosthesis. This creates a rotary torque transmitted up the length of the prosthesis to the residual limb/socket interface, and can lead to skin irritation and discomfort. The most common prosthetic cause of this deviation is an excessively firm heel cushion or plantar flexion bumper. Inappropriate toe-out alignment of the prosthetic foot must first be ruled out. When girth of the residual limb is decreasing (for individuals in whom the whole limb is shrinking as it matures or in anyone who has recently lost weight), fit within the socket may be too loose so that the effect of even a small rotary torque is manifested. Three user-related factors must also be considered. First, if there is weakness of hip muscles, the wearer may be unable to maintain the limb in optimal alignment as transition to stance phase takes place. Second, a wearer who is fearful of knee instability in early stance may be extending the prosthetic knee too vigorously at heel strike to ensure full knee extension has been reached. Third, the shoe may be too tight for the prosthetic foot.

Problems in Midstance to Late Stance Phase

In early stance phase, the primary goal is to ensure sufficient stability of the knee while body weight is loaded onto the prosthesis. In midstance to late stance phase, two additional but equally important goals must be met: (a) smooth forward progression of the body over the prosthetic foot and (b) efficient preparation for the upcoming swing phase.

Pelvic Rise

Excessive pelvic elevation during the transition through midstance and terminal stance is often a compensatory strategy to achieve a smooth progression from foot-flat position to heel off. The prosthetic wearer may make the classic statement: "I feel as though I am walking up a hill." The individual must exert an extra effort, substituting a rise of the pelvis to roll over the toe-break area of the foot. This is most often a consequence of inappropriate alignment of the prosthetic foot, which may be excessively plantarflexed. Alternatively, the foot may be positioned too far anteriorly with respect to the knee and socket. Both conditions create a relative increase in foot length, moving the fulcrum of the third rocker of gait (toe rocker) farther forward.

Drop-off at Midstance

When relative shortening of the foot is present, the third rocker is reached prematurely and stability of late stance is compromised, just as relative lengthening of the prosthetic foot leads to delayed forward progression and difficulty in reaching the third rocker of gait. Prosthetic wearers may sense knee instability and report that they feel like they are stepping into a hole. A dropping off or lowering of the pelvis often occurs because rollover occurs too early in the transition between midstance and terminal stance, rather than during terminal stance to preswing. The stride of the swing limb must be shortened to compensate for lack of stability in late stance. Most often, this deviation is a consequence of inappropriate prosthetic alignment. The prosthetic foot may be positioned in too much dorsiflexion. If an articulating/axial foot is used, the dorsiflexion bumper may be worn out or excessively soft. The durometer of heel cushion on a SACH foot may be inappropriately soft for the patient's weight or activity level. Finally, the transfemoral socket may be positioned too far anteriorly (excessive alignment stability) so that the weight line falls toward the front of the foot at midstance. All of these conditions functionally decrease the length of the prosthetic foot, lead to premature rollover, and instability in later stance.

Lateral Trunk Bending

A common gait deviation observed in the frontal plane is lateral trunk bending toward the prosthetic side when the prosthetic limb is in stance phase. (Figure 24-26). If the lateral prosthetic wall is not contoured to stabilize the femur in a natural position of adduction, drift of the femur into an abducted position causes a drop of the pelvis on the swinging side. An exaggerated lateral lean toward the stance (prosthetic) side ensures adequate toe clearance. Lateral trunk bending is used to avoid discomfort or excessive pressure in the perineum. This may be a result of a medial wall that is excessively high or rigid. Excessive pressure occurs when fleshy tissue of an adductor roll gets pinched between the socket and the pubic ramus, or when too few prosthetic socks are worn and the residual limb is positioned too deeply in the prosthesis. Other possible explanations include a socket that is aligned in excessive initial abduction or a prosthetic foot excessively outset

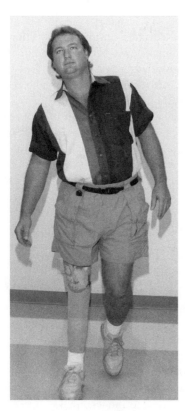

FIGURE 24-26 Lateral trunk bending over the prosthesis is typically the result of discomfort or excessive pressure in the perineum.

from the midline position. In both instances, the base of support is functionally wider than normal, and the only effective way to shift weight onto the prosthetic side is by leaning laterally. Finally, it is important to understand that it is difficult to provide lateral stabilization within the socket and align prosthetic components in the ideal narrow base of support for individuals with short residual limbs.

Problems in Swing Phase

The functional goal of swing phase is advancement of the unweighted limb. The prosthetic wearer has two tasks: (a) to initiate swing with enough hip flexion momentum to achieve the prosthetic knee flexion that is necessary for toe clearance and (b) to position the knee in extension in preparation for initial contact.

Excessive Lumbar Lordosis

Some prosthetic users move into excessive lumbar lordosis in late stance and into the early swing phase. This may be the result of an alignment problem: The transfemoral socket may not have been positioned in an appropriate amount of initial flexion, especially for patients with a hip flexion contracture. Patients with weakness of hip flexors or abdominal muscles may compensate by using exaggerated lumbar motion to initiate hip flexion necessary for a functional swing. Finally, lumbar lordosis may be a functional compensation for an ineffective femoral lever in those with short residual limbs.

Excessive Knee Flexion and Heel Rise

Excessive knee flexion/heel rise, a problem that occurs in initial swing phase, can be observed in the sagittal plane of motion (Figure 24-27). When the knee of the prosthesis flexes as swing phase begins, the prosthetic knee continues in flexion with the foot rising quickly away from the floor. If this heel rise is excessive, it delays extension of the prosthetic knee as the swing phase progresses. Prosthetic causes of this gait deviation include inadequate flexion resistance settings in the knee unit, or inadequate adjustment of the knee extension aid. Adjustment of friction or flexion resistance of the knee unit or replacement of worn extension aids generally solves the problem.

Medial and Lateral Whips

Optimally, forward progression of the prosthetic knee and foot occurs in the same line of progression, perpendicular to the floor. A whip occurs when forward progression of the distal parts of the prosthesis follows an oblique path. Whips differ from circumducted gait because the thigh advances in the expected, straight, forward line of progression, whereas the shin and foot travel in an arcing pattern. Whips are most easily observed while evaluating gait in the frontal plane. In a lateral whip (Figure 24-28, *A*), the prosthetic knee appears to rotate internally and the foot traces an arc of motion that moves away from the midline. The possible causes of a lateral whip are the exact opposite of those for a medial whip: The knee unit may be prepositioned in too much internal rotation, or the socket may have been positioned in a slightly internally rotated position during donning.

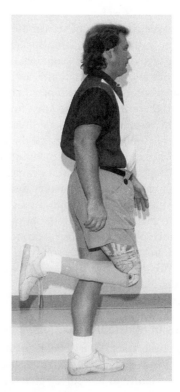

FIGURE 24-27 Excessive knee flexion/heel rise in early swing delays the extension of the knee, which is necessary to prepare for the next initial contact.

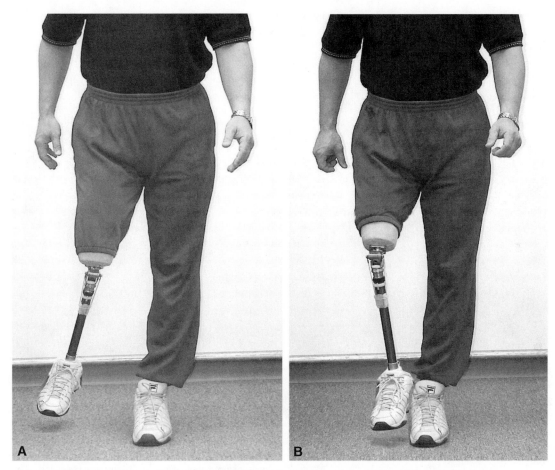

FIGURE 24-28 A, In a lateral whip, the shin and foot swing in a lateral arc, as opposed to proceeding straight in the line of progression. The cause of a lateral whip is that the knee is internally rotated. **B,** In a medial whip, the opposite occurs. The thigh moves forward as expected, whereas the shin and foot progress in a medial arc, typically the result of a knee set in excessive external rotation. Most whips are the consequence of improper donning or suspension.

In a medial whip (see Figure 24-28, *B*), the prosthetic knee appears to rotate externally so that the prosthetic foot moves in an arc of motion that carries the foot toward midline during swing. For some patients, the heels of the swing and stance limbs narrowly miss contact at midstance and midswing. Although this occurs when the prosthetic knee is aligned in too much external rotation, it also can be the result of several user-related factors. Medial whips occur when the prosthesis is donned incorrectly in too much external rotation or when the Silesian belt is worn too tightly and pulls the socket into external rotation. Medial whips may also be the consequence of poor purchase between skin and socket for individuals using suction suspension, especially those with "flabby" thigh tissue.

Terminal Impact

Excessive terminal impact is a gait deviation observed in the sagittal plane during terminal swing. The shin of the prosthesis moves forward so quickly that the fully extended position is reached early, often with an audible or visible impact against the proximal section of the prosthetic knee. Prosthetic factors that contribute to this deviation include insufficient resistance to extension of the knee unit, an excessively strong extension aid, or worn extension bumper. Prosthetic wearers fearful of knee instability in early stance may choose to flex the hip forcefully in initial swing to build momentum for knee extension, then forcefully extend the hip in terminal swing to snap the knee into full extension in preparation for initial contact.

Vaulting

If the prosthetic wearer must rise up on the toes during stance on the nonamputated limb to provide adequate clearance for the prosthesis through midswing (Figure 24-29), several possible prosthetic factors should be evaluated. First, the adequacy and correct application of suspension should be assessed. Second, if suspension is appropriate, adjustment of swing resistance in the prosthetic knee should be considered. Too much resistance to knee flexion and a foot set in excessive plantar flexion may relatively lengthen the prosthesis and compromise toe clearance in swing. Finally, if suspension and knee unit friction are appropriate, the height of the prosthesis should be double-checked to determine if the prosthesis is too long.

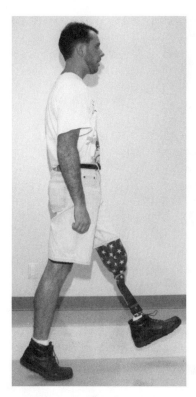

FIGURE 24-29 Vaulting is a common compensatory strategy for a prosthesis that is functionally too long. The prosthesis may actually be too long, have inadequate suspension, excessive friction of the knee unit, an excessively plantarflexed foot or could be the result of an acquired habit.

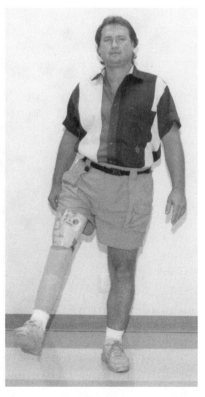

FIGURE 24-30 In a circumduction gait pattern, the entire prosthesis swings in a wide lateral arc (as opposed to a whip where only the shin section varies from the line of progression) to facilitate toe clearance in swing. Prosthetic causes of circumduction include inadequate suspension, a locked knee unit, or excessive friction in the knee unit.

Circumduction During Swing

Optimally, forward progression of the prosthesis during swing occurs in a straight line with enough knee flexion for adequate toe clearance (Figure 24-30). If the prosthetic knee is maintained in extension, one compensatory strategy would be to swing the limb in a wide lateral arc. In this strategy, the peak distance from midline occurs during midswing, and then the limb moves back toward midline during terminal swing, in preparation for a normal heel strike at initial contact. This deviation most easily observed from a position in front or behind the patient (frontal plane), is an attempt to compensate for a prosthesis that is functionally or actually too long. Circumstances that can lead to this compensation are similar to the vaulting deviation and include (a) inadequate suspension, in which the prosthesis pistons downward as a result of the force of gravity when unweighted during swing and (b) a prosthetic knee unit that is locked in extension or set with an excessive friction setting, preventing the knee flexion necessary during swing phase. The pattern is also adopted by prosthetic wearers who are nervous about catching their toe during swing or who are reluctant to use knee flexion because of anticipated instability in the subsequent early stance period. Circumduction also can be the result of a foot set in excessive plantar flexion, which makes the prosthesis functionally longer.

Other Issues

Ideally, an individual ambulating with a transfemoral prosthesis walks with a narrow base with minimal sway. There should be symmetry and evenness in stride length, cadence, and arm swing so that the gait pattern appears to be as natural as possible. Excessive side-to-side sway and asymmetry in place of fluid reciprocal movements increase the work and energy cost of walking and are obviously different from a normal gait pattern.

Abducted Gait Pattern

In an abducted gait pattern, the prosthesis is held away from the midline throughout the gait cycle. Functionally, this is most notable in the stance phase of gait. In initial contact, the prosthetic foot lands several inches lateral to the normal or ideal foot position, resulting in a wide base of support and requiring excessive side-to-side sway to accomplish weight transfer from one limb to the other. This deviation has a number of possible causes. The length of the prosthesis may need to be reduced. The socket may be aligned in a position of too much initial abduction. Uncomfortable or painful pressure may occur in the groin area (as in lateral leaning). An abducted gait pattern may be a compensatory strategy when pelvic instability is a result of inadequate lateral wall stabilization of the femur or weakness of hip abductors. The prosthetic wearer may be attempting to minimize lateral-distal femoral pain within the socket. Finally, for those fearful of falling, an abducted gait pattern may be a habitual movement strategy to minimize feelings of insecurity.

Uneven Step Length and Swing Time

Early in prosthetic training, new prosthetic wearers may be cautious and reluctant to use the prosthesis to its full capacity. The goal of equal step length and swing time must be emphasized. Patients gain confidence by practicing single-limb support on the prosthetic side and performing gait training exercises that provide appropriate visual, kinesthetic, and auditory feedback (e.g., equally spaced target marks on the floor, use of mirrors or videotape). Several possible patient-related issues or prosthetic problems, or both, should be considered if gait pattern asymmetry persists. First, the fit of the socket and condition of the skin should be examined carefully. Anyone would be reluctant to spend time in weight bearing if tissue is being pinched or irritated within the socket, if relief for bony prominences is inadequate, or if an inflamed or open area or unrecognized neuroma is present. Second, hip flexion contracture on the prosthetic side may limit excursion in hip extension in late stance, compromising forward progression of the opposite swing limb. If fit, skin condition, and range of motion are adequate, the mechanical and alignment stability of the knee unit should be reevaluated. A wearer who senses that the knee cannot provide adequate support in stance will compensate by shortening stance time to minimize the possibility of instability . Finally, individuals with impaired postural responses (poor balance) who are fearful of falling may decrease the time spent in single-limb support by reducing step length.

Uneven Arm Swing

Many individuals with amputations demonstrate diminished or absent reciprocal arm swing when walking with their prostheses. They may hold their arms on the prosthetic side stiffly and relatively still throughout the gait cycle. This is especially common in a new prosthetic user who has not yet developed confidence in the stability of the prosthesis as well as someone with a painful residual limb. This behavior is also observed in some proficient prosthetic users. The mechanism that underlies this alteration in motor behavior is not clearly understood, but it may be related to loss of sensation from the distal contact between the foot and the ground.

SUMMARY

Advances in technology and improved prosthetic components have greatly benefited individuals with transfemoral amputation. This chapter has explained that the successful functional outcome for individuals needing prosthetic care requires more than advanced technology. A prosthetic team in which the prosthetist and physical therapist are key contributors is necessary. A thorough understanding of the interrelationship between the prosthesis' weight, function, cosmesis, comfort, and cost is also required. Attention to socket design, knee biomechanics, and prosthetic alignment is important in provid-

ing optimal patient care. The prosthetic clinical team's goal is not merely to present an individual with a prosthetic product but to provide ongoing comprehensive care that focuses on the individual's needs, physical condition, and personal goals. In this way, patients who require a transfemoral prosthesis have an opportunity to reach their full functional potential.

REFERENCES

1. Radcliffe CW. Functional considerations in the fitting of above-knee prostheses. In: *Artificial Limbs*. New York: Krieger; 1970:35–60.
2. Huang CT, Jackson JR, Moore, et al. Amputation: energy cost of ambulation. *Arch Phys Med Rehabil.* 1979;60(1):18–24.
3. Waters RL. Energy expenditure. In: Perry J, ed. *Gait Analysis: Normal and Pathological Function.* Thorofare, NJ: Slack; 1992:443–487.
4. Waters RL. Energy cost of walking amputees: the influence of level of amputation. *J Bone Joint Surg.* 1976;58A:42–46.
5. Waters R, Yakura J. Energy expenditure of normal and abnormal ambulation. In: Smidt GL, ed. *Clinics in Physical Therapy: Gait in Rehabilitation.* New York: Churchill Livingstone; 1990:65–93.
6. Fisher SV, Gullickson G. Energy cost of ambulation in health and disability: a literature review. *Arch Phys Med Rehabil.* 1978;59(3):124–132.
7. Radcliffe CW. Prosthetics. In: Rose J, Gamble JG, eds. *Human Walking.* Baltimore: Williams & Wilkins; 1981:165–199.
8. Schuch CM. Report from the international workshop on above-knee fitting and alignment techniques. *Clin Prosthet Orthot.* 1988;12:81–98.
9. Long IA. Normal shape-normal alignment (NSNA) above knee prosthesis. *Clin Prosthet Orthot.* 1985;9:9–14.
10. Long IA. Allowing normal adduction of femur in above-knee amputations: technical note. *Orthot Prosthet.* 1975;29:53–54.
11. Pritham CH. Biomechanics and shape of the above-knee socket considered in light of the ischial containment concept. *Prosthet Orthot Int.* 1990;14:9–21.
12. Pritham CH. Workshop on teaching materials for above-knee socket variants. *J Prosthet Orthot.* 1988;1(1):51–67.
13. Sabolich J. Contoured adducted trochanteric-controlled alignment method (CAT-CAM): introduction and basic principles. *Clin Prosthet Orthot.* 1985;9:15–26.
14. Gottschalk F, Kourosh S, Stills M. The biomechanics of transfemoral amputation. *Prosthet Orthot Int.* 1994;18:12–17.
15. Gottschalk FA, Kourosh S, Stills M, et al. Does socket configuration influence the position of the femur in above-knee amputation? *J Prosthet Orthot.* 1989;2:94–102.
16. King C. Modern research and the forgotten prosthetic history of the Vietnam war. *J Rehabil Res Dev*.* 2009;46(9):xi–xxxvi.
17. Pike A. A new concept in AK socket design. *O&P Edge.* 2002;1(7):34.
18. Patterson S. Editorial: experiences with negative-pressure socket design. *Acad Today.* 2007;3(3):A7–A9.
19. Scussel R. Symmetry elevated vacuum systems. Instructional course. In: American Orthotic and Prosthetic Association, 93rd National Assembly. Orlando, FL; September 30, 2010.
20. Mak FT, Zhang M, Boone DA. State-of-the-art research in lower-limb prosthetic biomechanics-socket interface. *J Rehabil Res Dev.* 2001;38(2):161–174.
21. Jendrezejczk DJ. Flexible socket systems. *Clin Prosthet Orthot.* 1985;9:27–30.

22. Kristinsson O. Flexible above-knee socket made from low density polyethylene suspended by a weight transmitting frame. *Orthot Prosthet.* 1983;37:25–27.

23. Dietzen CJ, Harshburger J, Pidikiti RD. Suction sock suspension for above-knee prostheses. *J Prosthet Orthot.* 1991;3(2):90–93.

24. Ohio Willow Wood Company. *Advanced alpha solutions.* Presented at the Summit Seminars, Mt. Sterling, OH; 2002.

25. Street GM. Vacuum suspension and its effect on the limb. *Orthop Tech.* 2007;4:1–4.

26. Gerschutz M. Quantitative evaluation of elevated vacuum suspension system effectiveness under dynamic conditions. In: American Orthotic and Prosthetic Association, 93rd National Assembly. Orlando, FL; September 30, 2010.

27. Gerschutz MJ, Denune JA, Colvin JM, Schober G. Elevated vacuum suspension influence on lower limb amputee's residual limb volume at different vacuum pressure settings. *J Prosthet Orthot.* 2010;22(4):252–256.

28. Beil T, Street G, Covey S. Interface pressure during ambulation using suction and vacuum-assisted prosthetic sockets. *J Rehabil Res Dev.* 2002;39:693–700.

29. Covey SJ, Muonio J, Street GM. Flow constraint and loading rate effects on prosthetic liner material and human tissue mechanical response. *J Prosthet Orthot.* 2000;12(1):15–32.

30. Lake C, Supan TJ. The incidence of dermatological problems in the silicone suspension sleeve user. *J Prosthet Orthot.* 1997;9(3):97–106.

31. Haberman LJ, Bedotto RA, Colodney EJ. Silicone-only suspension (SOS) for the above knee amputee. *J Prosthet Orthot.* 1992;4(2):76–85.

32. Stark G. Overview of knee disarticulation. *J Prosthet Orthot.* 2004;16(4):130–137.

33. Mauch Laboratories. *Manual for the Henschke-Mauch Hydraulic Swing-N-Stance Control System.* Dayton, OH: Mauch Laboratories; 1976.

34. Moore KL. *Clinical Oriented Anatomy.* Baltimore: Williams & Wilkins; 1980:553.

35. Radcliffe CW. Four-bar linkage prosthetic knee mechanisms: kinematics, alignment and prescription criteria. *Prosthet Orthot Int*. 1994;18:159–173 36.

36. Gard SA, Childress DS, Uellendahl JE. The influence of four-bar linkage knees on prosthetic swing-phase floor clearance. *J Prosthet Orthot.* 1996;8(2):34–40.

37. Schuch CM. Prosthetic management. In: Bowker JH, Michael JW, eds. *Atlas of Prosthetics: Surgical, Prosthetic, and Rehabilitation Principles.* 2nd ed. St Louis: Mosby; 1992:528–529.

38. Mooney V, Quigley MJ. Above knee amputations: prosthetic management. In: Bowker JH, ed. *Atlas of Limb Prosthetics.* St Louis: Mosby-Year Book; 1981:381–401.

39. Datta D, Howitt J. Conventional versus microchip controlled swing phase control for transfemoral amputees: user's verdict. *Prosthet Orthot Int.* 1998;22:129–135.

40. Otto Bock Orthopedic Industry, Inc. *Manual for the 3c100 Otto Bock C-LEG.* Duderstadt, Germany: 1998.

41. Seymour R, Engbertson B, Kott K, et al. Comparison between C-Leg microprocessor-controlled prosthetic knee and nonmicroprocessor control prosthetic knees: a preliminary study of energy expenditure, obstacle course performance, and quality of life survey. *Prosthet Orthot Int.* 2007;31:51–61.

42. Kaufman KR, Levine JA, Brey RH, et al. Energy expenditure and activity of transfemoral amputees using mechanical and microprocessor-controlled prosthetic knees. *Arch Phys Med Rehabil.* 2008;89(7):1380–1385.

43. Ossur News. *Next Generation of the Power Knee in Early Release at Walter Reed Army Medical Center.* April 20 2009. Available at http://www.ossur.com/?PageID=13032&NewsID=2745. Accessed January 7, 2011.

44. Otto Bock Orthopedic Industry, Inc. *Otto Bock Microprocessor-Controlled Knees: Clinical Evidence and Background Information.* Available at: http://www.ottobock.com/cps/rde/xbcr/ob_us_en/10061933_MPKnee.ClinicalEvidence.pdf. Accessed January 7, 2011.

45. Otto Bock Orthopedic Industry, Inc. *Prosthetic Compendium: Lower Extremity Prostheses.* Duderstadt, Germany; 1994.

46. Padula PA, Friedman LW. Amputee gait. *Phys Med Rehabil Clin N Am.* 1991;2(2):423–432.

47. Radcliffe CW. The Knud Jansen lecture: above-knee prosthetics. *Prosthet Orthot Int.* 1977;37:146–160.

48. Radcliff CW. Biomechanics of above-knee prostheses. In: *Prosthetic and Orthotic Practice.* London: Edward Arnold; 1970:191–198.

49. Saunders JB, Inman M, Eberhart HD. The major determinants in normal and pathological gait. *J Bone Joint Surg.* 1953;35A:543–558.

50. Perry J. *Gait Analysis: Normal and Pathological Function.* Thorofare, NJ: Slack; 1992.

51. Gard SA, Childress DS. The effect of pelvic list on the vertical displacement of the trunk during normal walking. *Gait Posture.* 1997;5:233–238.

52. Quigley M. The role of test socket procedures in today's prosthetic practices. *Clin Prosthet Orthot.* 1985;9(3):11–12.

53. Carroll K. Getting down to basics: improving life with an above-knee prosthesis. *In Motion.* 2001;11(5):14–15.

54. Kahle JT, Highsmith JM. Isometric training helps prevent socket replacement. *In Motion.* 2003;13(3):66–67.

55. Zahedi MS, Spence WD, Solomonidis SE, Paul JP. Alignment of lower-limb prostheses. *J Rehabil Res Dev.* 1986;23(2):2–19.

56. Otto Bock Orthopedic Industry, Inc. *Alignment of Modular Leg Prostheses.* Available at: http://www.ottobock.com/cps/rde/xbcr/ob_us_en/08cat_5.pdf. Accessed January 7, 2011.

57. Breakey JW. Theory of integrated balance: the lower limb amputee. *J Prosthet Orthot.* 1998;10(2):42–44.

58. Nielsen CC, Psonak RP, Kalter TL. Factors affecting the use of prosthetic services. *J Prosthet Orthot.* 1989;1(4):242–249.

25

Prosthetic Options for Persons with High-Level and Bilateral Lower-Limb Amputation

JOHN W. MICHAEL AND MILAGROS JORGE

LEARNING OBJECTIVES

On completion of this chapter, the reader will be able to do the following:

1. Discuss the incidence and prevalence of high-level and bilateral lower-limb amputations.
2. Describe the etiology of high-level and bilateral lower-limb amputations.
3. Identify the two primary biomechanical limitations of hip disarticulation and higher-level prostheses.
4. Estimate the relative energy cost of ambulation with high-level or bilateral limb loss.
5. Describe the prosthetic and rehabilitation needs for persons with high-level and bilateral lower-limb amputation.

High-level transfemoral amputation and bilateral amputation of the lower extremity are the result of trauma or disease pathology such as peripheral vascular disease because of health conditions such as diabetes. The twenty-first century has started out to be a time of war in many nations around the globe. The United States and other North Atlantic Treaty Organization (NATO) countries have engaged in war and military conflicts. Traumatic amputation associated with war due to the use of landmines, improvised explosive devices (IEDs), and combat fire has resulted in an increase incidence and prevalence of high-level and bilateral lower-limb amputation.[1] Peripheral vascular disease either primary or diabetes related is the leading cause of bilateral amputation in the United States.[2] Such a significant limb loss presents a substantial challenge to the patient, the prosthetist, and other rehabilitation professionals. Successful prosthesis fitting is often time consuming and difficult; however, for many individuals with high-level or bilateral lower-extremity amputation, prostheses can enhance the ability to increase functional independence and mobility. This chapter summarizes key concepts for high-level transfemoral and bilateral lower-extremity prostheses prescription, fabrication, and rehabilitation based on clinical factors, research evidence, and expected outcomes.

HIGH-LEVEL LOWER-LIMB LOSS

The first part of this chapter focuses on options for patients with a unilateral high-level lower-limb absence, which is an amputation at or above the hip joint. Hip disarticulation and transpelvic and translumbar losses have been estimated to comprise fewer than 2% of all amputations in the United States.[3] As a result, only those clinicians associated with specialty centers, such as major trauma hospitals, have the opportunity to see significant numbers of such cases. Most prosthetists, therapists, and physicians see only a handful of patients with such high-level loss in a practice lifetime. One result of treating each high-level patient as one-of-a-kind is that many differing approaches can be found in the literature.

Etiology

Hip disarticulation is a relatively rare amputation. The incidence is reported at 0.5% to 3.0%.[3,4] There are three distinct causes of hip disarticulation: vascular disease, trauma, and malignancy. Vascular impairment, whether or not associated with diabetes mellitus, is the most common cause for lower-limb loss in the industrialized world. Dysvascular symptoms are generally most pronounced in the distal limb, leading to nonhealing ulceration, infection, gangrene, and ablation. The trunk and a portion of the upper thigh are usually spared even in the presence of severe peripheral vascular disease. Although rarely, vascular disease at times, leads to high-level amputation.[5] The assumptions about healing, cardiovascular limitations, and tolerance of activity derived from the experience with patients with dysvascular amputation do not apply to those with high-level amputation. Most patients with high-level amputation are relatively healthy and have reasonable cardiopulmonary reserves, excellent cognition, and a strong desire to attempt prosthetic fitting.

The more common cause for hip disarticulation or high-level lower-limb amputation today is a traumatic injury resulting in life-saving emergency medical services and surgical intervention. In civilian life, within the industrialized countries, motor vehicle accidents are the most common cause of lower-extremity amputation. The use of landmines in developing nations throughout the twentieth century contributed to high-level limb loss. Although the international community has banned the practice of placing landmines, many landmines still exist and continue to inflict trauma that results in high-level amputation. Military conflicts in Iraq and Afghanistan and the aggressive rebel tactic of use of IEDs has resulted in wounded warriors that survive the trauma and are transported to military hospitals for medical care and rehabilitation. Military hospitals are aggressively addressing the rehabilitation needs of soldiers with amputation. The Intrepid Center for Fallen Heroes Fund constructed the Center for the Intrepid at Brooke Army Medical Center in San Antonio, Texas. The Center for the Intrepid is a state-of-the-art rehabilitation facility for wounded warriors. Today, soliders with limb loss may be able to continue their military careers. The Center for the Intrepid rehabilitation programs work to maximize the functional abilities of men and women whether they plan to return to active duty or assume civilian life. Because of the prolonged U.S. involvement in the Iraq and Afghanistan wars, there are greater numbers of individuals with hip disarticulations.[6]

Many high-level amputations are performed for tumor of the femur, such as osteosarcoma. Fortunately, the frequency of tumor-related high-level amputation is decreasing with advances in limb-salvage procedures and more effective chemotherapy and radiation therapy.[7-9] Patients who require amputation because of tumor can be divided into two groups: those with benign or fully contained tumors who require no further oncological intervention and those undergoing chemotherapy and radiation after amputation. Persons with benign or fully contained tumors are typically in excellent physical condition after the amputation, eager to return to their former lifestyle as much as possible, and ready for early prosthetic fitting. The benefits of early prosthetic fitting are well established and are both physical and psychological.[10] Early mobilization and single-limb gait training on the contralateral limb with an appropriate assistive device is recommended to reduce the risk of deconditioning, which occurs even after a few days of hospitalization.[11,12] The rehabilitation and prosthetic management of patients requiring chemotherapy or radiation therapy may have to be adapted or delayed depending on the patient's physical condition, energy level, tolerance of activity, and healing of the surgical site.

Most patients with high-level amputation should be offered the opportunity for prosthetic fitting and rehabilitation. A multidisciplinary team rehabilitation team experienced in the management of persons with amputation is essential to assure the most desirable outcomes.[12]

Biomechanics

Although, historically, loss of the entire lower limb assumed the use of locked joints in the prosthesis, ample clinical evidence is available that locked prosthetic joints are seldom necessary. Since the 1950s, free-motion hip, knee, and ankle joints for hip disarticulation and transpelvic prostheses have become the norm. The Canadian design hip disarticulation prosthesis was introduced by Colin McLaurin,[13] and the biomechanics of this prosthesis were clarified by Radcliffe in 1957.[14]

These same biomechanical principles are also used in the functional design of prostheses for patients with higher level amputation.

In essence, the high-level prosthesis is stabilized by the ground reaction force (GRF), which occurs during walking.[15] For example, when standing quietly in the prosthesis, the person's weight-bearing line falls posterior to the hip joint, anterior to the knee joint, and anterior to the ankle joint. The resultant hip and knee extension moments are resisted by mechanical hyperextension stops of the prosthetic hip and knee joints, and the dorsiflexion moment is resisted by the stiffness of the prosthetic foot (Figure 25-1). This same principle permits the patient with paraplegia using bilateral Scott-Craig knee-ankle-foot orthoses to stand without external support.[16]

Ambulation with a high-level prosthesis also relies on the GRF (Figure 25-2). When an experienced prosthetic wearer walks with an optimally aligned hip disarticulation or transpelvic prosthesis, the dynamic gait is surprisingly smooth and consistent. Patients with hip disarticulation or transpelvic amputations who have sufficient balance and strength can learn to walk without any external aids, although the use of a cane is also common.

The basic functions of the GRF during ambulation with one type of high-level prosthesis can be summarized as follows.

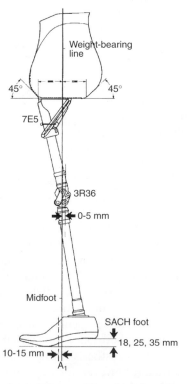

FIGURE 25-1 Static balance with a high-level lower-limb prosthesis is achieved when the GRF passes posterior to the hip joint and anterior to the knee and ankle joints. The resulting extensor moments at the hip and knee, and dorsiflexion moment at the ankle, make the prosthesis stable. Mechanical stops in the prosthetic joints prevent further movement, and the patient is able to stand without exertion. *SACH,* Solid-ankle, cushion-heel. (Courtesy Otto Bock Orthopedic Industry, Inc., Minneapolis, MN.)

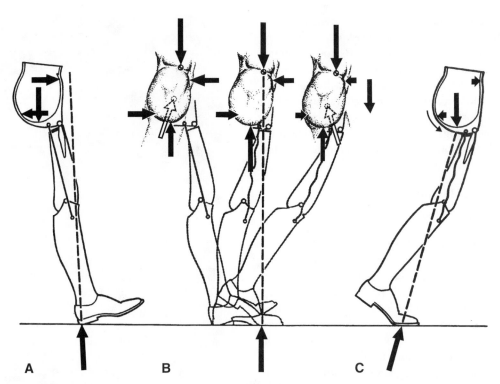

FIGURE 25-2 The GRF at initial contact. From loading response through midstance **(A)** and terminal stance **(B)** and just prior to preswing **(C)** of the gait cycle for patients using a unilateral high-level prosthesis. Once properly aligned, the prosthesis will move in a consistent, predictable fashion and permit slow but steady ambulation. The patient uses trunk motion to initiate and control prosthetic movements. (From Van der Waarde T, Michael JW. Hip disarticulation and transpelvic management: prosthetic considerations. In Bowker JH, Michael JW [eds], *Atlas of Limb Prosthetics: Surgical, Prosthetic, and Rehabilitation Principles*, 2nd ed. St. Louis: Mosby-Year Book, 1992. pp. 539-552.)

At initial contact, as the prosthetic heel touches the ground, the GRF passes posterior to the ankle axis, the heel cushion compresses, and the foot is lowered to the ground. At the same time, an extension moment is created at the prosthetic knee as the GRF passes anterior to the knee joint axis (see Figure 25-2, *A*). By midstance, alignment stability is maximal as the GRF passes posterior to the prosthetic hip joint axis and anterior to the prosthetic knee joint axis, just as it does during quiet standing (see Figure 25-2, *B*). As forward progression continues into preswing, the GRF moves posterior to the knee joint axis, allowing the knee to bend passively to facilitate swing phase foot clearance while weight is being shifted onto the opposite limb (see Figure 25-2, *C*).

Two major biomechanical deficits are inherent with hip disarticulation and transpelvic prostheses: First, the prosthetic limb is always fully extended at midswing because of the loss of active hip flexion. As a result, the length of the prosthesis is typically shortened slightly, compared with the remaining limb, to assist in toe clearance during the swing phase of gait. The consequence of this strategy, however, is a second biomechanical deficit—limb length discrepancy.[17]

Component Selection

The earliest hip disarticulation prosthesis designers insisted on locking all prosthetic joints. Later, proponents of free-axis joints for hip disarticulation prostheses advocated the use of only basic components, such as a single-axis knee and ankle. In recent years, a strong consensus has emerged that, to meet the patient's functional needs and goals fully, components for patients with hip disarticulation and transpelvic amputations should be selected for the same reasons and with the same criteria as for those with transfemoral and transtibial amputation.[18,19]

Choosing a Prosthetic Foot

All prosthetic feet have been successfully used for high-level amputations. Nonarticulating designs are often chosen because of their dependability, durability, and low maintenance; these designs rarely require servicing as a result of wear and tear. Single-axis feet (which allow the patient to quickly attain a stable foot-flat position) are used when enhanced knee stability is a concern. Multiaxial and dynamic response designs are usually reserved for higher-activity individuals who appreciate the added mobility of such components.[20]

Choosing a Prosthetic Knee Unit

The prosthetist selects a particular knee unit on the basis of the patient's functional needs. Because of the biomechanical stability of these prostheses, locked knee designs are rarely necessary. Locked knee designs have two additional drawbacks: they must be unlocked before sitting, and they may increase the risk of injury in the event of a fall. When stability is a primary concern, stance control or polycentric knees may be most appropriate. Single-axis knees, when properly aligned, also work well. The prosthetist might choose a pneumatic or hydraulic knee unit to provide fluid swing phase control for patients who are active and want the ability to change cadence.[19] Most recently, quite encouraging clinical results have been reported with a microprocessor-controlled, hydraulic stance and swing control knee, allowing active individuals to descend stairs foot-over-foot with a hip disarticulation prosthesis for the first time.[21]

Choosing a Prosthetic Hip Joint

The majority of patients with hip disarticulation benefit from a free-motion hip joint, although locking joints are still sometimes chosen for those with quite limited ambulation capabilities. Much effort has been made to provide some measure of active hip flexion motion in these prostheses because that would reduce or eliminate the key biomechanical deficits previously noted. In prior decades, modification of the hip joint by adding a coil spring mechanism that induced hip flexion when the prosthesis was unweighted was tried with some success, but maintenance and breakage of the spring precluded widespread acceptance. More recently, a flexible carbon fiber thigh "strut" that functions as a leaf spring has been used clinically in selected cases. Initial reports suggest that this approach increases cadence and that the improved swing clearance achieved by better prosthetic hip and knee flexion eliminates the need to shorten the prosthesis.[22] The use of vertical shock-absorbing shin elements and knees with stance flexion features is also being explored, with encouraging clinical acceptance.

Torque Absorbers

With the loss of three major biological joints of the lower limb, a corresponding loss of the body's ability to compensate for rotary motions inherent in gait occurs. For this reason, many prosthetists strongly recommend that a torque-absorbing device be included in these high-level prostheses. Torque absorbers typically improve both stride length and comfort by absorbing transverse forces that would otherwise be transmitted to the socket as skin shear.[23,24] Incorporation of a lockable turntable above the prosthetic knee is also suggested to facilitate common daily activities such as dressing and entering an automobile (Figure 25-3).

Energy Consumption

The major unresolved drawback to prosthetic fitting for those with high-level amputation is the tremendous increase in effort required to control a prosthetic limb with passive joints. Walking with a hip disarticulation or transpelvic prosthesis is much like controlling a flail biological leg. The concentration and energy required to ambulate makes short distance ambulation much more practical than distance walking for all but the most vigorous adult wearers.

Gait studies suggest that the use of a hip disarticulation prosthesis requires approximately 200% more effort than unimpaired walking.[25] This is approximately the same effort

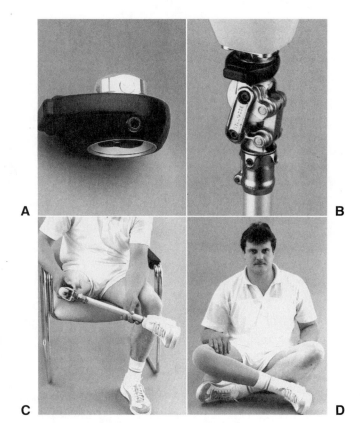

FIGURE 25-3 A lockable turntable **(A)** positioned in the prosthesis above the prosthetic knee **(B)** makes dressing, entering an automobile, and similar daily tasks much easier for individuals with high-level amputation **(C** and **D)**. A torsion adapter absorbs the torque forces generated during gait and decreases the stress on both the patient's skin and the prosthetic components. Such ancillary components should always be considered for patients with high-level amputations. (Courtesy Otto Bock Orthopedic Industry, Inc., Minneapolis, MN.)

required when using axillary crutches in single-limb gait. Because single-limb amputation with crutches tends to be faster than walking with a hip disarticulation prosthesis, the relatively high rejection rate of such prostheses is not surprising. Schnall and colleagues found that kinematic changes and energy expenditure increased 100% or more during ambulation in persons with hip disarticulation.[6]

Most rehabilitation professionals believe that any patient with an amputation who is physically and mentally capable of prosthetic use should, if interested, be fitted with an initial prosthesis. This recommendation is particularly true for those with high-level amputation who may feel "cheated" and become depressed if their clinical teams do not allow them to try prosthetic ambulation.

Socket Design

A variety of socket designs have been described in the clinical literature. The most critical factors for successful use are careful fitting and secure suspension, regardless of which socket design is selected. For patients with hip disarticulation, encapsulation of the ascending pubic ramus may add stability, although not every patient is able to tolerate a proximal trim

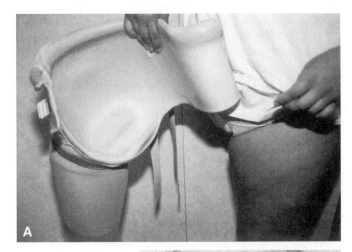

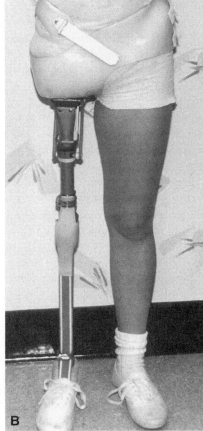

The transpelvic socket must fully enclose the gluteal fold and perineal tissues and completely contain the soft tissues on the amputated side. Full enclosure provides comfortable weight bearing on the residual limb tissues despite the absence of hemipelvis. Early transpelvic sockets extended upward to contain the lower ribs.[30] Clinical experience has shown that this may not always be necessary for relatively muscular or lean individuals. Failure to contain the transpelvic residuum adequately results in obvious protrusion where the trim lines are insufficient. Prosthetists modify the positive plaster model of the transpelvic residuum to incorporate a diagonally directed compressive force in the socket design to support and contain transpelvic tissues and eliminate the risk of perineal shear and tissue breakdown.[31]

For patients with translumbar amputation, weight bearing is achieved with a combination of soft tissue compression and thoracic rib support. Because of the loss of more than half of the body mass in this amputation, weight-bearing tolerance is better than might be expected. Designs that allow the patient to vary the compression by adjustable straps are often useful.[32]

Patients with translumbar amputation require a socket for effective seating and wheeled mobility (Figure 25-5). Many

FIGURE 25-4 A, The interior of a hip disarticulation socket fabricated from flexible silicone rubber. Note the contouring of the proximal brim to encase the crest of the ileum. **B,** Thermoplastic sockets are also used for hip disarticulation prostheses. (From Michael JW. Component selection criteria: lower limb disarticulations. *Clin Prosthet Orthot* 1988;12[3]:99-108.)

line in the perineum.[15,26] Flexible thermoplastic or silicone materials within a rigid laminated frame are more comfortable and increasingly popular than the more common hard plastic sockets (Figure 25-4).[27-29]

Suspension is achieved by carefully contouring the socket just proximal to the iliac crests whenever possible. When the patient is obese or has no ileum, shoulder straps may be necessary to minimize swing phase pistoning of the prosthesis.

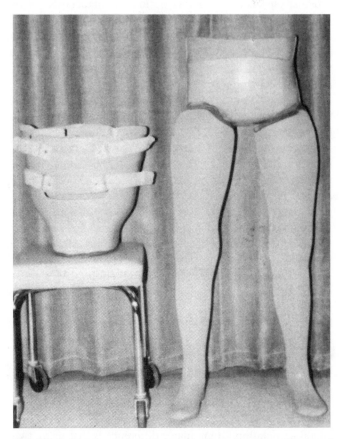

FIGURE 25-5 For patients with translumbar amputation, a laminated adjustable socket provides a stable base for sitting balance and wheeled stability (*left*). The socket can be positioned within an outer shell with bilateral prosthetic limbs (*right*) for cosmesis in sitting and for limited prosthetic ambulation. (From Gruman G, Michael JW: Translumbar amputation: prosthetic considerations. In Bowker JH, Michael JW [eds], *Atlas of Limb Prosthetics: Surgical, Prosthetic, and Rehabilitation Principles*, 2nd ed. St. Louis: Mosby-Year Book, 1992. pp. 563-568.)

patients with translumbar amputation successfully progress to ambulation for short distances with a prosthesis and choose to wear prosthetic limbs to enhance their cosmetic appearance and self-image. Long-term followup demonstrates positive prosthetic outcomes; return to work or school is usually a realistic goal.[33] For most patients, polycentric knees provide sufficient stability for the household ambulation typical of this population, making locking joints unnecessary.

Rehabilitation Outcomes After High-Level Amputation

Despite the obvious challenges that face patients with high-level amputation, a substantial percentage are able to manage a prosthetic device with appropriate training and long-term followup. Although the rate of prosthetic use varies, the trend is toward increasing functional use of a prosthesis.[6,7,34,35] Using a multidisciplinary team approach and fitting by an experienced prosthetist are believed to enhance the likelihood of success and to improve functional outcomes.

BILATERAL LOWER-LIMB LOSS

The loss of both lower limbs complicates the rehabilitation process, especially if the loss occurs simultaneously.[12,36] In North America, simultaneous bilateral loss is infrequent; such cases are typically the result of traumatic transportation or industrial accidents or electrocution. In the developing world, simultaneous limb loss is more frequent; in areas of armed conflict and postwar zones, roadside bombs and landmines are a major cause.[37,38] Fortunately, most patients with traumatic amputation are healthy and strong and generally have a good prognosis for the successful use of prostheses.

The major cause of bilateral lower-extremity limb loss is dysvascular disease. The Centers for Disease Control reports the number of hospital discharges for nontraumatic lower-extremity amputation with diabetes as a listed diagnosis increased from 45,000 in 1991 to 86,000 in 1996, when it peaked, and then decreased to 66,000 in 2006. From 1988 to 2006, the number of discharges increased by 20%.[39] When vascular disease affects both limbs, as is often the case, patients with a single dysvascular amputation face a significant risk of eventual bilateral limb loss. An incidence as high as 50% for contralateral limb loss over a 5-year period has been reported.[36,40] Clinical followup suggests that successful use of a unilateral prosthesis increases the likelihood of success with bilateral artificial limbs. For this reason, early fitting after initial amputation is strongly advocated, even when amputation of the opposite limb seems imminent.

The rehabilitation of persons with bilateral lower-extremity limb loss is similar to the rehabilitation of persons with unilateral amputation.[41] One major difference is that using two artificial limbs is physically more difficult; thus, the pace of advancement is slower and must be individualized according to the patient's strength, balance, and ability. Breaking down complex skills into small incremental tasks that can be more readily mastered is generally useful. Without the benefit of a sound limb, patients with bilateral loss can be expected to walk slowly and cautiously, often with a relatively wide-based

gait that maximizes their sense of stability. Su and colleagues investigated the gait characteristics of persons with bilateral transtibial amputations and found that persons with amputations walked at slower speeds and lower cadences, had shorter step lengths and wider step widths, and displayed hip hiking during swing phase.[42] Bilateral transfemoral amputees have even greater energy expenditure and lower rates of full time prosthetic use for functional ambulation.[12]

The use of balance aids such as canes are common, but not universal, in the gait training and mobility rehabilitation process for persons with bilateral amputation. Environmental barriers such as ramps, hills, irregular surfaces, and curbs or stairs present special challenges that must be identified and overcome. Specific training in sitting down, rising from a chair, falling in a controlled manner, and recovering from a fall are all important tasks to be mastered. Transfer with and without artificial limbs is also an important skill to foster independence. Persons with bilateral lower-limb amputation require a wheelchair for mobility for independent toileting in the night and for times when the prosthetic legs need repair.[12]

The rehabilitation of persons with bilateral lower-limb amputation occurs in various phases, including a preoperative phases, if time permits, an immediate postoperative phase, and acute rehabilitation phase. The rehabilitation process is patient centered and should be individualized for each patient, taking into account physical condition, biomechanical loss, and prosthetic needs. The reason for the amputations influences the pace and level of rehabilitation. Otherwise healthy individuals who sustain traumatic limb loss may be able to advance rapidly unless skin trauma is present on the residual limbs. Early prosthetic fitting is a critical factor in the long-term successful outcome for functional prosthetic use.[12]

Energy Cost

The effort required to use a unilateral prosthesis increases in direct proportion to the level of amputation: the longer the residual limb, the lower the energy cost of walking with a prosthesis.[43] Saving as much functional limb length as possible is therefore an axiom in amputation surgery. Although preservation of the anatomical knee joint is important for patients with unilateral amputation, it is a critical consideration when bilateral limb loss is present: When at least one biological knee joint remains, the chances for practical ambulation significantly increase.[12,44]

Energy cost of ambulation is also related to the reason for limb loss.[45,46] In general, patients with dysvascular amputation have lower energy reserves and expend more effort walking than those with traumatic amputation (Figure 25-6). Long-term use of bilateral transfemoral prostheses is uncommon, but not impossible, for elderly patients with dysvascular amputation.[47] In contrast, a significant number of those with traumatic bilateral transfemoral amputation successfully use prostheses long term.[48] Patients with bilateral transtibial ambulation tend to do well with prostheses regardless of reason for amputation. Interestingly, bilateral transtibial prostheses require less effort than a unilateral transfemoral

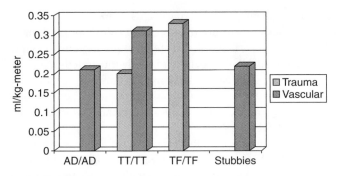

FIGURE 25-6 The energy (oxygen) cost of ambulation with bilateral prosthesis compared for patients with ankle disarticulation (*AD*), transtibial amputation (*TT*), and transfemoral amputation (*TF*) when using traditional transfemoral prostheses and *stubbies* (simplified prostheses consisting only of the transfemoral sockets attached to a stable base, without any prosthetic knee). Note that energy costs increase as the level of amputation moves proximally. Energy cost is also higher in dysvascular amputation compared with traumatic amputation. Ambulation requires less effort for patients with at least one anatomical knee joint than for those with bilateral transfemoral amputation. Preservation of an anatomical knee joint increases likelihood of independence in ambulation. (Modified from Waters RL. The energy expenditure of amputee gait. In Bowker JH, Michael JW [eds], *Atlas of Limb Prosthetics: Surgical, Prosthetic, and Rehabilitation Principles*, 2nd ed. St. Louis: Mosby-Year Book, 1992. pp. 381-387.)

prosthesis; this finding emphasizes the importance of retaining biological knee function whenever possible.

Component Selection

Selection of components for patients with bilateral lower limb amputation is made by the same guidelines as for unilateral limb absence. There are no unique or distinct components specifically designed or intended for use in bilateral prosthesis. The prosthetist should consider both prostheses together rather than simply generate a "right-side" and a "left-side" prescription recommendation. Prosthetists generally recommend that the same ankle-foot device be used on both sides so that gait mechanics are consistent, but this is not an absolute necessity. Some patients ambulate best with different prosthetic feet, depending on the level of amputations, the length and condition of the residual limbs, the nature of their preferred activities, and other individual characteristics.

The range of physical differences between two patients with bilateral lower-limb loss makes each patient and each prosthetic fitting a unique challenge. During the dynamic alignment procedure, a brief clinical trial with the recommended components is often helpful in confirming suitability for a specific individual before the prescription details are finalized. This trial is particularly helpful for experienced ambulators, who commonly develop strong preferences for a specific component after walking with it for many years.

Bilateral Transtibial Amputations

In North America, a solid-ankle, cushion-heel prosthetic foot is often chosen for patients with bilateral transtibial amputation because such feet offer predictable standing balance.

Most patients with bilateral amputation are concerned about falling backward. The prosthetist often chooses to use a slightly stiffer heel resistance to minimize the risk of backward falls. When concern about forward falls also exists, the prosthetist may also choose to use a slightly stiffer keel to offer additional resistance to falling forward. Patients classified as limited ambulators, those with poor postural responses, and those who walk with a very slow cadence often find this approach useful.

Active patients walk well with elastic keel and dynamic response feet or with multiaxial designs as long as they have sufficient strength and postural responses to manage these flexible components. Theoretically, single-axis feet are designed to generate an abrupt hyperextension moment at midstance, which loads the cruciate ligaments of the residual limb. In practice, little evidence exists that this loading is harmful; some patients with bilateral transtibial amputation prefer single-axis feet, choosing them over solid-ankle or dynamic-response designs. Patient preference is an important consideration in prosthetic prescription; preference is even more critical for patients with bilateral amputation who, literally, have no "good foot" to stand on other than prosthetic devices. If a patient expresses a definite dissatisfaction with a particular foot during the fitting process, an alternative component should be tried before proceeding further.

The consideration of ancillary components, such as torque absorbers or shock-absorbing pylons, is important for all patients with bilateral amputation. Because patients with bilateral amputation must bear all their body weight on prosthetic devices all the time, components that increase comfort or protect the skin are particularly appropriate. Lessening the weight of the prostheses, particularly at the ankle-foot area, is also important because lighter-weight prostheses are easier to control and increase acceptance of the device. Whenever possible, heavier components should be placed as close to the socket as possible.[49]

Bilateral Transfemoral Amputation

Postural responses are compromised in patients with bilateral transfemoral amputations because of the loss of both anatomical ankles and knees. For this reason, a primary goal of prosthetic prescription is stability in the stance phase of gait. One of the most effective prosthetic components for stance-phase stability during level walking is a polycentric knee unit. For those patients who have the potential to walk at varying speeds, the addition of fluid swing-phase control is recommended. Hydraulic stance and swing control units are also quite successful for this population. In recent years, microprocessor-controlled hydraulic knees offering both stance and swing-phase control have been well received clinically by this population, and many experts believe this technology offers more reliable stability and better mobility under real-world conditions than strictly mechanical knee mechanisms.[50] The risk of injury in a fall is greater if locking or stance control knees are used in both prostheses. For patients with significant stability issues, a locking or stance control knee may be used on one side. Because single-axis knees are stabilized by muscle control and postural responses at the hip, bilateral single-axis knees are often difficult to use safely in older adults with dysvascular amputation. Bilateral single-axis knees may be appropriate for small children because their short stature reduces the balance required to manage such components.

Ankle-foot components that emphasize stability and standing balances are typical for this group with bilateral loss. Solid-ankle designs predominate. Articulating designs are used less often; only those with very long transfemoral residual limbs and good muscle strength are typically able to control the added mobility provided by articulating ankle components. Many patients with bilateral transfemoral amputation use crutches or canes to assist with balance and postural control. Single-axis or multiaxial feet become easier to control if the patient leans forward slightly, shifting the center of gravity forward, so that the weight line falls anterior to the ankle axis at all times, eliminating the risk of falling backward.

Ancillary components, such as torque absorbers, often make walking easier and more comfortable for patients with bilateral transfemoral amputation. Some evidence exists that including components that permit controlled transverse rotation improves the gait kinematics of patients who wear two lower limb prostheses.[51] Locking rotation devices make many activities of daily living easier to accomplish.[52] Because the weight of such ancillary components must be considered, the perception of the artificial limb feeling heavy is minimized if the devices are positioned as far proximally within the prosthesis as possible.

Transfemoral–Transtibial Amputation

For patients with one transfemoral and one transtibial amputation, the preservation of one biological knee makes prosthetic use much easier and successful ambulation more likely.[53] For most patients, the transtibial side is the propulsive and balance limb and the transfemoral side supplements these functions. On the basis of these functional differences, the prosthetist may choose to use different prosthetic feet. When the transfemoral amputation is relatively short, for example, a single-axis foot and stance control knee might be recommended for the transfemoral prosthesis, whereas a dynamic response foot might be used in the transtibial prosthesis.

Socket Designs and Suspension

The person with bilateral lower-limb loss is constantly bearing full weight on artificial limbs while walking or standing. All options to increase skin protection and comfort should be actively considered, and suspension must be as secure as possible. A soft insert and flexible sockets may be used to enhance comfort during wear and reduce the likelihood that shear forces will be problematic for the skin. Suction suspension, with silicone sleeves or inserts as necessary, minimizes pistoning during swing and should be considered for the majority of patients with bilateral amputation.

Cotton or wool prosthetic socks are often used as an interface between the residual limbs and the sockets when suction suspension is not feasible. In that event, supracondylar wedge or cuff suspensions are typically used in transtibial prostheses; Silesian belts are often used in transfemoral designs. Because most patients with bilateral amputation use a pair of prostheses, suspension belts are usually integrated into a single assembly. Because thigh corsets with metal side joints, hip joints and pelvic bands, and waist belts can be cumbersome for donning and doffing, they are typically avoided unless absolutely necessary.

Ischial containment sockets are as effective for patients with bilateral amputation at the transfemoral level (of one or both limbs) as they are for patients with a single transfemoral amputation. Patients who have previously worn a quadrilateral transfemoral socket, and those who are limited ambulators, may be satisfied with a traditional quadrilateral design. Total contact of the residual limb in the socket is important for both ischial containment and quadrilateral socket skin integrity.

The loss of both feet and both knees makes the use of bilateral transfemoral prostheses quite challenging. For many adults with acquired limb losses, an initial fitting with sockets attached to special rocker platforms may be advocated to facilitate initial gait training (Figure 25-7). Such "stubbies" require less energy and balance than full-length prosthetic limbs and give the patient new to bilateral prostheses the best chance for successful ambulation.[54] Once the patient is able to balance effectively on the stubbies, the prostheses can be converted to use artificial feet with solid pylons, which are gradually lengthened to increase the height of the prostheses. If the patient is able to manage full-length prostheses, prosthetic knees can be incorporated and definitive prostheses with full components provided.

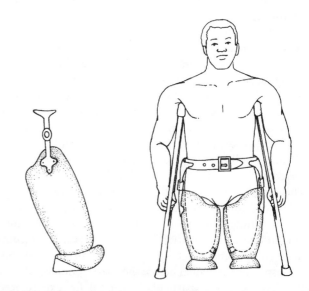

FIGURE 25-7 A pair of shortened prostheses, sometimes called *stubbies*, for early gait training for patients with bilateral traumatic transfemoral amputation. In these prostheses, patients can develop postural control without having to worry about the stability of prosthetic knee units. (From May BJ. Assessment and treatment of individuals following lower extremity amputation. In O'Sullivan SB, Schmitz TJ [eds], *Physical Rehabilitation: Assessment and Treatment*, 3rd ed. Philadelphia: Davis, 1994. p. 392.)

Not all patients with bilateral transfemoral amputation choose to pursue ambulation with prostheses. Some are unable to build the necessary muscular strength or postural control for a safe gait. Others find the energy cost of ambulation with prostheses excessive. In these cases, patients choose wheelchair mobility as a much less strenuous means of mobility and willingly adopt wheelchair use for the independence it provides.

Many patients with bilateral transfemoral amputation find a wheelchair most practical for long-distance mobility and use their limbs for walking short to moderate distances at home and work. Some patients accept the stubbies for long-term use, particularly if these devices allow them to remain independent in their home setting. Others choose to use their stubbies at home because they take less effort but wear full prostheses in public.

SUMMARY

Individuals with high-level or bilateral lower limb amputations are rare in the developed world. In North America, they are believed to represent fewer than 5% of all persons with amputation. Given these statistics, most prosthetists and therapists have limited opportunity to work with patients with such significant levels of limb loss. Although successful prosthetic training and rehabilitation for these patients are challenging, a large body of clinical information about managing such cases is available in the literature. This chapter highlights the key principles involved in rehabilitation of the person with high-level or bilateral lower-limb amputations.

Surgical technique during the amputation largely determines the potential for long-term ambulation. Gentle handling of soft tissues and careful preservation of all functional joints and bony length are essential. Anchoring functioning muscles to bone (myodesis) at their normal resting length is strongly encouraged whenever possible.

The socket design and suspension methods chosen for patients with high-level or bilateral amputation should incorporate strategies to protect the skin and maximize patient comfort, especially for individuals with bilateral amputation. Components reflect each individual's need for stability and responsiveness at the ankle-foot, knee, or hip joint level. Ancillary components to make the prosthesis more comfortable and easier to manage are advocated.

Although patients with bilateral transfemoral amputation caused by vascular disease often have difficulty mastering dual prosthetic devices, long-term use of functional prostheses is a realistic goal for patients with traumatic or tumor-related amputation who are otherwise healthy. With appropriate fitting and rehabilitation, many patients with hip disarticulation and transpelvic amputations continue to use their prostheses definitively. Even patients with translumbar amputation are able to return to productive education or work activities with an appropriate prosthesis for sitting or limited ambulation.

Despite the obvious physical and psychological challenges faced by patients with high-level or bilateral lower limb amputation, prosthetic rehabilitation must always be considered and is often successful, especially when offered by an experienced multidisciplinary team in a supportive setting. Although the sequelae from amputations of this magnitude present significant challenges, advances in surgical technique, prosthetic design and components, and rehabilitation contribute to successful outcomes for patients with high-level and bilateral amputation.

CASE EXAMPLE 1

A Patient with Traumatic Hip Disarticulation

J. S. is a 20-year-old man with a traumatic hip disarticulation amputation caused by a motorcycle accident 2 weeks ago. His residual limb is healed but complicated by multiple skin grafts and insensate areas in the abdominal region from the amount of trauma. He is eager to return to college as quickly as possible to avoid having to repeat this semester's courses but must walk several blocks to various buildings on the small, hilly campus. He has a lean, athletic build and demonstrates excellent balance and strength when ambulating on his remaining limb with bilateral forearm crutches.

Questions to Consider

- What additional information might be gathered to help determine J. S.'s potential to use a hip disarticulation prosthesis? How does his medical history and reason for amputation affect his rehabilitation prognosis?
- How should J. S.'s readiness to be fit with a prosthesis be determined? What tests and measures should be used?
- What major concerns or challenges will J. S., his prosthetist, and rehabilitation team face in fitting his hip disarticulation prosthesis?
- What options for socket and suspension will the team likely consider for J. S. given his functional needs and prognosis?
- What factors will influence the choice of knee units for J. S.'s prosthesis? What type of knee should be recommended? Why?
- What factors will influence the choice of a prosthetic foot for J. S.'s prosthesis? What type of foot should be recommended? Why?
- How should rehabilitation goals be prioritized as J. S. begins his prosthetic training? How should his rehabilitation progress? How should the efficacy of intervention be assessed to determine how well the goals have been met?

Recommendations

On the basis of findings during the evaluation and discussion with J. S. about his current functional needs and ultimate prosthetic goals, the team recommends an initial endoskeletal prosthesis with a foam-lined thermoplastic socket that includes additional gel padding in the region of the tender grafted skin, a microprocessor-controlled stance and swing-control hydraulic knee, dynamic-response foot,

Continued

and torque absorber. The clinical team considered first providing a less complex knee but decided against that option because it would require training to use a less-responsive prosthesis, then subsequent retraining with the microprocessor knee more appropriate for his projected functional abilities, thereby increasing the duration of his rehabilitation program.

Intensive inpatient therapy focuses on ambulation first within the parallel bars and then with his forearm crutches to facilitate J. S.'s return to campus. He will continue with outpatient therapy until his gait has matured and will likely learn to ambulate with no balance aids. When his socket no longer fits because of normal postoperative atrophy, he will receive a new custom socket and protective covering for the prosthesis but will continue to use the same functional components originally provided for as long as they are functionally appropriate for his needs.

CASE EXAMPLE 2

A Patient with Bilateral Lower-Extremity Amputations Caused by Chronic Dysvascular/Neuropathic Disease

R. W. is a 72-year-old woman who recently underwent an elective right transtibial amputation because of infection associated with diabetic neuropathy. Her residual limb is well healed and not unduly edematous, and she is eager to return to the condominium she shares with her daughter. Five years previously, R. W. underwent left transfemoral amputation after failed femoral-popliteal bypass surgery and has been a successful full-time prosthesis wearer until hospitalization for the recent amputation.

Questions to Consider

- What additional information might be gathered to help determine R. W.'s potential to use prostheses for her new right transtibial and existing left transfemoral residual limbs? How does her medical history and reason for amputation affect her rehabilitation prognosis?
- How should R. W.'s readiness to be fit with a transtibial prosthesis be determined? What tests and measures should be used to make this determination?
- What major concerns or challenges will R. W., her prosthetist, and rehabilitation team face in fitting the new transtibial prosthesis?
- What options for socket and suspension will the team likely consider for R. W.'s new transtibial and transfemoral prostheses, given her functional needs and prognosis?
- What factors influence the choice of knee units for R. W.'s transfemoral prosthesis? What type of knee should be recommended? Why?
- What factors influence the choice of a prosthetic foot for R. W.'s transtibial and transfemoral prostheses? What type of foot should be recommended for each prosthesis? Why?

- How should rehabilitation goals be prioritized as R. W. begins her prosthetic training? How should rehabilitation be assessed? Should the wearing schedules for her new transtibial limb be similar to or different from her transfemoral limb? Why or why not? How should the efficacy of intervention be assessed to determine how well the goals have been met?

Recommendations

Although her age and comorbidities make the use of two artificial limbs challenging, R. W. is a good candidate for bilateral fitting because of her motivation and proven success with a prior prosthesis. Her existing transfemoral prosthesis is well worn and no longer fitting optimally, so the prosthetic rehabilitation team recommends that two new prostheses be prescribed.

The transtibial prosthesis will provide primary balance and propulsion and enable her to rise from a seated position, applying significant forces to her residual limb. Her initial transtibial prosthesis will include a roll-on locking liner for suspension and a soft insert to protect the residual limb and provide added mediolateral stability at the knee through its supracondylar contours. She will use lightweight, solid-ankle dynamic response prosthetic feet on both artificial limbs because she prefers these components and has found them both stable and functional with her unilateral prosthesis.

Her new transfemoral prosthesis will be similar to what she has successfully worn, with a roll-on locking liner for suspension and a flexible ischial containment socket within a rigid frame for weight bearing and rotational stability. The roll-on suspension permits donning from a seated position, which is particularly advantageous for people with bilateral amputations. Initially, R. W. will wear an auxiliary elastic suspension belt for added security and rotational control.

Her unilateral prosthesis incorporated a single-axis knee with pneumatic swing control, but she will require a more mechanically stable design for bilateral stability. Because of cardiopulmonary restrictions and the loss of her second leg, the clinical team does not believe she will vary her walking pace as widely now, so the weight of a pneumatic swing-control unit is no longer necessary. R. W. will receive a stable polycentric knee in her new prosthesis and undergo gait training for several weeks.

Although she is eager to have her endoskeletal prostheses finished with protective covers that make them appear more lifelike, this fabrication step will be deferred until after she has completed gait training and mastered the use of bilateral artificial limbs. R. W.'s prosthetist will see her periodically to reevaluate the alignment of both prostheses as her gait pattern matures, making small alignment changes in response to her changing needs and balance. Once her gait pattern has stabilized, the final fabrication will be completed.

R. W. will also be prescribed a wheelchair with a posteriorly offset axle, which she will use for traversing long distances. Training in wheelchair transfers and mobility will also be an important part of her rehabilitation.

REFERENCES

1. Hermes LM. Military lower extremity amputee rehabilitation. *Phys Med Rehabil Clin N Am.* 2002;13(1):45–65.

2. Dillinger TR, Pezzin LE, Mackenzie EJ. Racial differences in the incidence of limb loss secondary to peripheral vascular disease: a population-based study. *Arch Phys Med Rehabil.* 2002;83:1252–1257.

3. Zeigler-Graham K, Mackenzie EJ, Ephraim PL, et al. Estimating the prevalence of limb loss in US 2005–2050. *Arch Phys Med Rehabil.* 2008;89(2):422–429.

4. Dillinger TR, Pezzin LE, Mackenzie EJ. Limb amputation and limb deficiency; epidemiology and recent trends in US. *South Med J.* 2002;95(8):875–883.

5. Group TG. Epidemiology of lower extremity amputation in centers in Europe, North America, and East Asia. The global lower extremity amputation group. *Br J Surg.* 2000;87(3):328–337.

6. Schnall BL, Baum BS, Andrews AM. Gait characteristics of a soldier with a traumatic hip disarticulation. *Phys Ther.* 2008;88(12):1568–1577.

7. Ferrapie AL, Brunel P, Besse W, et al. Lower limb proximal amputation for a tumor: retrospective study of 12 patients. *Prosthet Orthot Int.* 2003;27(3):179–185.

8. Katrak P, O'Connor B, Woodgate I. Rehabilitation after total femur replacement: a report of 2 cases. *Arch Phys Med Rehabil.* 2003;84(7):1080–1084.

9. Belthur MV, Grimer RJ, Suneja R, et al. Extensible endoprosthesis for bone tumors of the proximal femur in children. *J Pediatr Orthop.* 2003;32(2):230–235.

10. Burgess E, Romano RL. The management of lower extremity amputees using immediate postsurgical prostheses. *Clin Orthop.* 1968;57:137–146.

11. Cutson T, Bongiorni D, Michael JW. Early management of elderly dysvascular below-knee amputees. *J Prosthet Orthot.* 1994;6(3):62–66.

12. Davidson JH, Jones LE, Cornet J, et al. Management of the multiple limb amputee. *Disabil Rehabil.* 2002;24(13):688–699.

13. McLaurin CA. The evolution of the Canadian-type hip disarticulation prosthesis. *Artif Limbs.* 1957;4:22–28.

14. Radcliffe CW. Biomechanics of the Canadian-type hip disarticulation prosthesis. *Artif Limbs.* 1957;4:29–38.

15. Stark G. Overview of the hip disarticulation prosthesis. *JPO J Pract Orthot.* 2001;13(2):50–53.

16. Lehmann JR, Wareen CG, Hertling D. Craig-Scott orthosis: a biomechanical and functional evaluation. *Arch Phys Med Rehabil.* 1976;57(9):438–442.

17. Van der Waarde T, Michael JW. Hip disarticulation and transpelvic management: prosthetic considerations. In: Bowker JH, Michael JW, eds. *Atlas of Limb Prosthetics: Surgical, Prosthetic, and Rehabilitation Principles.* 2nd ed. St. Louis: Mosby-Year Book; 1992:539–552; reprinted 2002.

18. Michael JW. Component selection criteria: lower limb disarticulations. *Clin Prosthet Orthot.* 1988;12(3):99–108.

19. Michael JW. Prosthetic knee mechanisms. *Phys Med Rehabil State Art Rev.* 1994;8(1):147–164.

20. Michael JW. Prosthetic feet: options for the older client. *Top Geriatr Rehabil.* 1992;8(1):30–38.

21. Stinus H. Biomechanics and evaluation of the microprocessor controlled C-leg exoprosthesis knee joint. *Z Orthop Ihre Grenzgeb.* 2000;138(3):728–782.

22. Littig DN. Gait patterns in the unilateral hip disarticulation. *Z Orthop Ihre Grenzgeb.* 2000;42.

23. Knoche W. Welche vorteile bringt der einbau eines torsions adapters in beinprosthesn? *Orthop Tech.* 1979;30:12–14.

24. Jeffries GE, Angelico CP, Denison A, Kaiser J. Fitting for hip disarticulation and hemi-pelvectomy level amputations. *In Motion.* 1999;9(2). Available at: http://www.amputee-coalition.org/inmotion/mar_apr_99/pros_primer_hip_dis.html. Accessed 03.11.11.

25. Huang C-T. Energy cost of ambulation with Canadian hip disarticulation prosthesis. *J Med Assoc State Ala.* 1983;52(11):47–48.

26. Sabolich J, Guth T. The CAT-CAM HD: a new design for hip disarticulation patients. *Clin Prosthet Orthot.* 1988;12:119–122.

27. Madden M. The flexible socket system as applied to the hip disarticulation amputee. *Orthot Prosthet.* 1987;39(4):44–47.

28. Zaffer SM, Braddom RL, Conti A, et al. Total hip disarticulation prosthesis with suction socket: a report of two cases. *Am J Phys Med Rehabil.* 1999;78(2):160–162.

29. Carlson JM, Wood SL. A flexible air-permeable prosthesis for bilateral hip disarticulation and hemicorporectomy amputees. *JPO J Pract Orthod.* 1998;10(4):110–115.

30. Hampton F. A hemipelvectomy prosthesis. *Artif Limbs.* 1964;8(1):3–27.

31. Hampton F. Northwestern University suspension casting technique for hemipelvectomy and hip disarticulation. *Artif Limbs.* 1966;10(1):56–61.

32. Carlson MJ. A double socket prosthesis design for bilateral hip-to-hemi corporectomy amputation levels. *AAOP Proc.* 1997.

33. Gruman G, Michael JW. Translumbar amputation: prosthetic considerations. In: Bowker JH, Michael JW, eds. *Atlas of Limb Prosthetics: Surgical, Prosthetic, and Rehabilitation Principles.* 2nd ed. St. Louis: Mosby-Year Book; 1992:563–568.

34. Shurr DR. Hip disarticulation prostheses: a follow up. *Orthot Prosthet.* 1983;37(3):50–57.

35. McAnelly RD, Refaeian M, O'Connell DG, et al. Successful prosthetic fitting of a 73-year old hip disarticulation amputee patient with cardiopulmonary disease. *Arch Phys Med Rehabil.* 1998;79(5):585–588.

36. Rommers GM, Vos LDW, Groothoff JW, et al. Clinical rehabilitation of the amputee: a retrospective study. *Prosthet Orthot Int.* 1996;20:72–78.

37. Korver AJH. Amputees in a hospital of the International Committee of the Red Cross. *Injury.* 1993;24(9):607–609.

38. Shahriar SH, Masumi M, Edjtehadi F, et al. Cardiovascular risk factors among males with war-related bilateral lower limb amputation. *Mil Med.* 2009;174(10):1108–1112.

39. Centers for Disease control and Prevention. *Diabetes Complications.* Available at: http://www.cdc.gov/diabetes/statistics/complications_national.htm. Accessed April 10, 2012.

40. Anderson SP. Dysvascular amputee: what can we expect? *J Prosthet Orthot.* 1995;7(2):43–50.

41. Marzoug EA, Landham TL, Dance C, Bamj AN. Better practical evaluation for lower limb amputees. *Disabil Rehabil.* 2003;25(18):1071–1074.

42. Su PF, Gard SA, Lipschutz, Kuiken TA. Gait characteristics of persons with bilateral transtibial amputations. *J Rehabil Res Dev.* 2007;44(4):491–502.

43. Waters RL. The energy expenditure of amputee gait. In: Bowker JH, Michael JW, (eds.) *Atlas of Limb Prosthetics: Surgical, Prosthetic, and Rehabilitation Principles.* 2nd ed. St. Louis: Mosby-Year Book; 1992:381–387.

44. Schuling S, Greitemann B, Seichter C. Gehfahigkeit Beidseits beinamputierter nach prosthetischer versorgung. *Z Orthop Ihre Grenzgeb.* 1994;132(3):235–238.

45. Waters RL, Perry J, Antonelli D, et al. Energy cost of walking of amputees: the influence of level of amputation. *J Bone Joint Surg Am.* 1976;58:42–46.

46. Pinzur MS, Gold J, Schwartz D, et al. Energy demands in walking for dysvascular amputees as compared to level of amputation. *Orthopedics.* 1992;15(9):1033–1037.

47. Moore TJ, Barron J, Hutchinson F, et al. Prosthetic usage following major lower extremity amputation. *Clin Orthop Relat Res.* 1989;(238):219–224.

48. Dougherty PJ. Long term follow-up study of bilateral above-knee amputees from the Vietnam war. *J Bone Joint Surg Am.* 1999;81A:1384–1390.

49. Bach TM. Optimizing mass and mass distribution in lower limb prostheses. *Prosthet Orthot Aust.* 1995;10(2):29–35.

50. Gutfleisch O. Peg legs and bionic limbs: the development of lower extremity prosthetics. *Interdiscip Sci Rev.* 2003;28(2):139–149.

51. Schmidl H. Torsionadapter im kunstbein aus der sicht des technikers und des amputierten. *Orthop Tech.* 1979;30:35–38.

52. Torres MM, Esquanazi A. Bilateral lower limb rehabilitation: a retrospective review. *West J Med.* 1991;154(4):583–586.

53. Torres MM. Incidence and causes of limb amputations. *Phys Med Rehabil State Art Rev.* 1994;8:1–8.

54. Kruger LM. Stubby prostheses in the rehabilitation of infants and children with bilateral lower limb deficiencies. *Rehabilitation (Stuttg).* 1990;29(1):12–15.

26

Early Rehabilitation in Lower-Extremity Dysvascular Amputation

Julie D. Ries and Victor Vaughan

LEARNING OBJECTIVES

Upon completion of this chapter, the reader will be able to:

1. Organize and justify each component of a comprehensive physical therapy examination for the individual with transtibial and transfemoral amputation.
2. Utilize and synthesize data collected during the examination to establish diagnosis and prognosis for rehabilitation.
3. Create a well-defined and focused treatment plan that addresses the needs of the individual with transtibial and transfemoral amputation.
4. Identify, justify, and prioritize rehabilitation issues about which individuals with transtibial and transfemoral amputation must be educated.
5. Anticipate functional outcomes of an individual with transtibial or transfemoral amputation, based upon data collected and available evidence.
6. Identify and justify appropriate outcome measures for use with individuals with transtibial and transfemoral amputations.

Persons who have undergone transtibial or transfemoral amputation may approach rehabilitation with a sense of expectancy, excitement, and, often, apprehension. They may be relieved to have healed and curious about the prosthesis that they are about to receive. They may be anxious to commence their prosthetic rehabilitation and may have realistic or not so realistic expectations. To facilitate optimal rehabilitation outcome, the physical therapist must consider the patient's goals, physical abilities, and mobility needs, along with their previous functional level. This chapter explores the key components of successful rehabilitation for persons with transtibial and transfemoral amputation. It presents a model consistent with the *Guide to Physical Therapist Practice*,[1] with emphasis on the components of a thorough examination. It discusses the evaluation process, which is the synthesis of data to establish a diagnosis and prognosis. The chapter also provides a range of interventions for persons with a new transtibial or transfemoral amputation, from early physical therapy interventions that focus on preparing the limb for use of a prosthesis and building tolerance to prosthetic wear to more

functionally oriented activities aimed at ensuring safety and efficiency in gait and functional mobility skills. As prosthetic skills are mastered, interventions progress to more complex, higher-level bipedal activities. With many individuals, vocational, leisure, and sporting activities can be addressed to facilitate the return to a productive and enjoyable lifestyle. This chapter focuses primarily on strategies for initial and intermediate-level rehabilitation, with a short discussion on more advanced prosthetic training. Anticipated functional outcomes for the transtibial or transfemoral prosthetic user are also addressed.

Evidence-based practice requires the integration of best research evidence, clinical expertise, and patient values.[2] Although more research is needed to help to inform rehabilitation decisions for individuals with lower-extremity amputation,[3] limited research does support that individuals who participate in postamputation rehabilitation programs benefit from these programs.[4-6] The goal of this chapter is to provide a foundation for evidence-based practice in the management of individuals with either transtibial or transfemoral amputation.

COMPONENTS OF THE PHYSICAL THERAPY EXAMINATION

Effective physical therapy (PT) management for individuals with amputation begins with a thorough and comprehensive initial examination. In the PT examination, the physical therapist must obtain a patient history, conduct a systems review, and administer tests and measures to obtain baseline data. Ideally, data collected represents all levels of the World Health Organization's International Classification of Functioning, Disability, and Health (ICF)[7] including impairments, activity limitations, and participation restrictions, with attention toward contextual factors for the individual (environmental and personal modifiers).[8] This information allows the therapist to establish a diagnostic classification that provides the basis for accurately identifying the appropriate treatment interventions that will lead to optimum outcomes. The PT examination may occur preamputation, immediately following amputation, at the time of the prosthetic fitting, or after the individual has already obtained their prosthesis, depending upon the practice setting.

Patient History

The patient history is the collection of health-related data from the past and present. It helps to establish what brought the person to seek PT services and to highlight the individual's desires and expectations. The person's perspective of his or her illness, functional limitations, and possible disability has a powerful influence on the rehabilitation process. In fact, a positive outlook is associated with constructive coping and positive adjustment to amputation.[9,10]

A number of important areas must be explored while taking the patient history (Table 26-1). Although all the areas provide important information, several are very integral to the establishment of the diagnosis and the treatment plan. The person's general health status may impact the individual's overall health perception, physical functions, psychological functions, and role and social functions. Discussion of the current condition/chief complaint gives the therapist a sense of the individual's concerns, previous interventions, mechanism of injury or disease, and course of events. It also helps to understand what the goals and aspirations are for a person with a transtibial or transfemoral amputation. If the individual's initial goals appear to be over- or underambitious, the therapist can address these issues with education and interaction with peers as possible interventions.

The interview process provides valuable insights about the person's communication ability, emotional status, cognitive abilities, preferred coping strategies, insight into the rehabilitation process, and usual learning style, as well as the availability of emotional and instrumental support systems (assistance with activities of daily living). Information about the person's pre-amputation level of activity and mobility are helpful in establishing a realistic prognosis. Patients who are ambulatory prior to the amputation surgery are more likely to recover at least a modest degree of ambulation ability with their prosthesis.[11] Specific and probing interview questions are often helpful in obtaining clear and accurate information. Although many individuals are accurate historians, others may have an incomplete understanding or imprecise memory

TABLE 26-1   *Important Patient-Client History Component of Physical Therapy Examination*

Component	Issues to Consider
Social History	Cultural beliefs and behaviors Family and caregiver resources Social interactions, activities and support systems
Employment/work/leisure	Current and prior work Community and leisure activities Family/work roles
Living environment	Assistive devices and adaptive equipment Home environment (e.g., stairs? railings? shower vs. tub?) Projected discharge destination
General health status	General health perception Physical and psychological functions
Social health habits	Health risks (e.g. smoking, alcohol, or drug abuse) Level of physical fitness and exercise habits
Family history	Family medical history and health risks
Medical/surgical history	Prior hospitalizations, surgeries Preexisting medical and other health-related conditions
Chief complaint/current condition	Concerns that led patient or caregiver to seek PT services Any current medical or therapeutic interventions Mechanism of injury/disease including date of onset and course of events Patient/caregiver/family expectations and goals Patient/family/caregiver's perceptions of the person's emotional response to current situation Any previous occurrences of this problem and therapeutic interventions
Functional status and activity level	Current and prior functional status in self-care, home management activities and activities of daily living Current and previous functional status in work and community/leisure activities
Medications	Medications for chief complaint or other conditions
Other clinical tests	Laboratory and diagnostic tests Review of available records

Format and terminology consistent with *The Guide to Physical Therapist Practice.*[1]

of what has happened. It is always advisable to confirm information by interview with family members and review of the medical record.

The interview is a means to gather important information that is used to guide treatment interventions and to begin the process of education about amputation, treatment, and prosthetic training. Many individuals with transtibial or transfemoral amputation do not have a clear understanding of what to expect during rehabilitation or how their disease process might progress. Amputation is not selective to patients of a specific age group, cultural background, educational experience, or socioeconomic level. Every individual benefits by being well-educated about his or her condition and treatment. For many, the events that brought them to rehabilitation may be a blur of disjointed experiences and medical jargon, or a laundry list of conditions that seem unrelated or independent. The physical therapist can help individuals to place their history and experience in a meaningful context, which, in turn, assists them in forming realistic expectations, and may decrease the likelihood of a second amputation.

Systems Review

The systems review provides a gross and limited review of the anatomical and physiological status of the person's cardiopulmonary, musculoskeletal, integumentary, neuromuscular, endocrine, gastrointestinal, and urogenital systems. Cognitive screening is also an important part of the review of systems. This gross screening process aids in focusing and prioritizing the tests and measures portion of the examination. For instance, a gross screen of range of motion and strength of all uninvolved extremities may reveal findings to be within normal limits, eliminating the need for further assessment.

An integumentary screen may reveal an intact and healing surgical site, but a stage II sacral pressure ulcer, requiring further assessment and inclusion in the plan of care. The systems review helps to focus the rest of the examination in the most constructive and productive way.

Tests and Measures

The third component of the examination is the employment of appropriate tests and measures to gather objective data about the individual with amputation's various impairments and activity limitations. Combining this data with the history and systems review, the physical therapist is able to establish a working diagnostic hypothesis. The physical therapist chooses from among an array of possible tests and measures those that will best confirm or deny the developing diagnostic hypothesis. The information gathered in the interview, systems review, and examination allows the physical therapist to establish a suitable plan of care and develop the most appropriate interventions.[1] It is important to note that some assessments, such as strength testing or joint play motions, might require modification of technique because loss of limb length necessarily changes where the therapist is able to hold or resist the limb. Table 26-2 provides categories of tests and measures that might be appropriate for the patient with transtibial or transfemoral amputation and some detail of how the therapist might assess each area.

THE EVALUATION PROCESS

The process of evaluation requires the physical therapist to interpret and integrate the information obtained from the history, systems review and the tests and measures to identify

TABLE 26-2 *Tests and Measures Used in the Physical Therapy Examination*

Component	Issues to Examine
Aerobic capacity	During functional activities During standardized exercise testing Signs and symptoms of cardiovascular and/or pulmonary systems in response to increased oxygen demand during increased activity
Anthropometric characteristics	Body composition Body dimensions Edema
Arousal, attention, cognition	Motivation Ability to comprehend instructions Ability to problem solve Safety awareness and judgment
Assistive/adaptive devices	Equipment or devices used during functional activities Ability to care for devices or equipment Effectiveness of devices or equipment in correcting impairments, activity limitations or participation restrictions Safety during use of equipment or devices
Circulation	Cardiovascular signs Physiological responses to position changes

(Continued)

TABLE 26-2   *Tests and Measures Used in the Physical Therapy Examination—cont'd*

Component	Issues to Examine
Cranial/peripheral nerve integrity	Motor distribution and integrity Sensory distribution and integrity
Environmental barriers	Physical space and environment
Ergonomics/body mechanics	Functional and physical performance during work tasks Safety in work environment Specific work conditions/activities Tools, equipment, and workstation design used during job activities Body mechanics during home and work activities
Gait and balance	Static and dynamic balance with and without prosthesis Balance during functional activities with and without prosthesis Ambulation with and without prosthesis
Integumentary integrity	Activities and positioning that produce or relieve trauma to the skin Equipment, devices or prosthesis that may produce trauma to the skin Current skin characteristics and conditions Activities or positioning that may aggravate the wound or scar Presence of signs of infection Wound/scar characteristics (e.g., appearance, mobility, sensitivity)
Joint integrity and mobility	Joint play, including accessory movements
Motor function	Timing, coordination, and agility Hand function and dexterity
Muscle performance	Strength, power, and endurance Strength, power, and endurance during functional activities
Orthotic, protective, and supportive devices	Components, alignment, and fit of any orthotic or supportive devices Use during functional activities Effectiveness of devices in addressing activity limitations and participation restrictions Safety during use of devices
Pain	Location and description of pain with intensity ratings Current regime for management of pain and effectiveness
Posture	Postural alignment and positioning, static and dynamic Alignment of specific body parts
Prosthetic requirements	Components, alignment, fit and ability to care for prosthesis Use of prosthesis during functional activities Effectiveness of prosthesis at correcting activity limitations and participation restrictions Residual limb edema, strength, range of motion, and skin integrity Safety during use of prosthesis
Range of motion	Functional range of motion Active and passive joint movement Muscle length and flexibility, soft-tissue extensibility
Self-care and home management	Ability to access home Ability to perform self-care and home management activities Safety in home and self-care management
Sensory integrity	Superficial sensation Deep sensation Combined/cortical sensation
Work/community/leisure integration	Ability to return to work, community, and leisure activities Ability to access work site, community, and leisure activities Safety in work, community, and leisure activities

Format and terminology consistent with *The Guide to Physical Therapist Practice.*[1]

the primary areas of impairment, activity limitation, and participation restriction. The physical therapist uses professional judgment to predict or make a prognosis as to the likely functional outcome and time required for effective preprosthetic and prosthetic rehabilitation. The evaluation must include a summary of the individual's major problems and the presumed underlying cause(s). Problems are prioritized, with those that have the most significant functional implications receiving top priority. This is done within the personal and environmental context of the individual, as the same problem may affect different individuals in different ways. For instance, poor sensation of the residual limb in an individual who is cognitively intact may be easily resolved with education about compensating for the sensory deficit with visual inspection, effectively reducing the risk of compromise of skin integrity. Another individual with the same sensory deficit who also has cognitive impairment may require a more extensive educational intervention that is focused on residual limb care. This individual has a much higher risk of skin problems, and is likely to require the assistance of a caregiver to monitor skin integrity.

Physical therapists must also be skilled in determining the functional implications of specific problems. For instance, a slight knee flexion contracture can be accommodated for in transtibial socket alignment, whereas a significant knee flexion contracture prohibits prosthetic fitting with a conventional prosthesis. Prosthetic prescription and PT intervention may be quite different for two individuals who both present with knee flexion contractures.

ESTABLISHING A PHYSICAL THERAPY DIAGNOSIS

The establishment of the diagnosis for a person with lower extremity amputation is relatively straightforward. The diagnosis is determined by a collection of signs and symptoms that delineate the primary dysfunction of the individual. The physical therapist then directs interventions toward resolving that dysfunction. According to the *Guide to Physical Therapist Practice, Part 2*, the preferred practice pattern for a person with an amputation is "Impaired Motor Function, Muscle Performance, Range of Motion, Gait, Locomotion, and Balance Associated with Amputation."[1]

FORMULATING A PROGNOSIS

The physical therapist uses patient history information and specific test findings in the context of knowledge of previous outcomes for individuals with transtibial and transfemoral amputation, to predict each person's rehabilitation potential and probable functional outcome. Based on the individual's prognosis, measurable short-term and long-term goals are defined to guide planning for interventions. These goals are also used to inform assessment of outcomes as rehabilitation progresses. An important component of the prognosis is delineation of the likely time frame for achievement of

the optimal final outcome. A young, active, healthy person with traumatic transtibial amputation who has few postoperative complications is likely to progress through rehabilitation more quickly, achieving a high level of function in a short period of time. In contrast, a medically frail and deconditioned individual who has had a transfemoral amputation as a result of vascular compromise or nonhealing neuropathic ulcer will likely have a longer rehabilitation course, likely resulting in a less ambitious final functional outcome.

Research findings indicate several prognostic indicators of functional prosthetic use following rehabilitation. All of the following have been found to negatively affect functional prosthetic use, despite rehabilitation efforts: advanced age,[11-16] presence of comorbidities,[11-13] level of amputation (transfemoral vs. transtibial),[11-14,16] and cognitive and/or memory impairment.[11,12,17,18] This information is not intended to suggest the exclusion of individuals with any of these predictors from prosthetic rehabilitation efforts; in fact, there is evidence of successful prosthetic rehabilitation in even the oldest old,[19] but therapists need to be realistic in assessing the challenges facing each individual prosthetic user. It is generally accepted that the best predictor of postamputation mobility is the level of pre-amputation mobility. Patients who were ambulating prior to their amputation are much more likely to be able to use a prosthesis for ambulation postsurgery.[11,12] Consideration of all of these factors should be reflected in the plan of care, as well as the specific goals set and the anticipated rate at which goals will be met.

Plan of Care

The PT plan of care includes information about the frequency, duration, location, and specific PT interventions that are to be used. The plan of care is directly related to the goals delineated by the evaluation/prognostic process. The prioritized problem list provides a foundation for determination of functional short-term and long-term goals that, in turn, direct rehabilitation activities. If independent donning and doffing of a prosthesis are primary short-term goals, the associated treatment plan must include education strategies, opportunities to practice this skill, and remediation or adaptation of any movement components that, if missing, would compromise the individual's ability to perform this necessary task (e.g., the person may need to improve grip strength or intrinsic hand strength to manipulate prosthetic suspension). The plan includes information about equipment to be ordered, referrals to be made, and the ultimate PT discharge plan.

PREPROSTHETIC INTERVENTIONS

A variety of skills and physical/functional characteristics create the foundation for successful prosthetic use. These key areas include functional range of motion (ROM) of the hip and (if applicable) knee; functional strength of muscles at the hip and (if applicable) knee; adequacy of motor control and balance; aerobic capacity and endurance; effective edema control and maturation of the residual limb;

integrity of the skin and soft tissue; and sensory integrity of the residual limb. It is crucial to address these areas early in the rehabilitation process. Inability to achieve a certain status or level of performance in one area does not prohibit a good prosthetic outcome; however, difficulties in multiple areas have an impact on prosthetic candidacy and use. Each of these areas should be carefully evaluated and appropriate interventions undertaken to achieve at least minimal requirements for functional prosthetic use, if not optimal level of performance.

Range of Motion

Early and aggressive achievement of functional ROM of the involved lower extremity is of paramount importance. The flexor withdrawal pattern of hip flexion, abduction, and external rotation, and knee flexion, is a position associated with lower-extremity pain and is often a position of choice in individuals postsurgically. The elevation of the residual limb on pillows serves to reinforce this undesirable posture and puts these individuals at risk for contracture formation. The development of contractures or tightness of muscles consistent with this position of the residual limb, especially hip and knee flexors, can have a significant negative impact on ultimate prosthetic use.[11,20] Maintaining or increasing available ROM at the hip for persons with a transfemoral residual limb and at the hip and knee of the transtibial residual limb continues to be a primary treatment goal as the patient moves from preprosthetic into prosthetic rehabilitation. The prevention of loss of ROM is much easier than efforts to regain lost motion.[21] Prone positioning is an excellent strategy to combat contracture formation of the hip flexors and should be prescribed (60 minutes daily) as early as possible for all individuals who are able to tolerate this position. Low load, long duration stretch is safe and can yield significant elastic and plastic changes in soft tissues.[21] Active and passive stretching in the side-lying position may be used for those unable to lie prone. Full functional hip ROM into flexion, extension, and adduction is critical to achieving efficient ambulation and functional mobility with a prosthesis. Typical gait on level surfaces requires the hip to move from 30 degrees flexion to 10 degrees extension and requires adduction slightly beyond neutral.[22] More extreme ranges of hip flexion are required for transitioning sit to/from stand or reaching forward from a seated position.

To avoid knee flexion contracture in the individual with a transtibial amputation, a postoperative rigid dressing or knee extension splint or board (extending from under seating cushion) can be an effective technique early in the process to position the knee resting in an extended position while seated. Full knee extension ROM is required in typical ambulation on level surfaces[22] and for exploiting passive stability at the knee joint in static standing. Individuals with recent transtibial amputation should be encouraged to use the knee extension splint as long as tolerable throughout the day, supplemented with frequent active quadriceps exercises ("quad set"). The person must also be taught to regularly check the integrity of skin of the residual limb while using the splint or board,

to minimize risk of pressure-related skin damage that would delay use of the prosthesis.

For individuals with transtibial amputations, achieving knee flexion ROM is sometimes overlooked early in rehabilitation. Typical gait on level surfaces generally requires approximately 60 degrees of knee flexion,[22] and 90 degrees or more is required for efficient step-over-step stair ambulation, rising from a seated position, and high-level mobility activities such as kneeling or rising from the floor.

Assessment of ROM of the intact limb is also important, as loss of ROM of either limb has an impact on quality and energy efficiency of gait.[23] The importance of functional ROM is also emphasized in individual education and home exercise routines. Table 26-3 summarizes the potential prosthetic problems that are associated with loss of functional ROM. Utilization of a wide variety of active and passive ROM therapeutic exercise techniques is appropriate as early as possible. All exercises that are started during the preprosthetic phase are generally appropriate to continue as prescribed, or to be progressed as tolerated during the prosthetic training phase. Once full functional ROM is achieved, the person must be educated to maintain this level.

Strength

In a systematic review, van Velzen et al.[24] found several studies that demonstrated significant strength differences between muscles of the amputated limb as compared to the sound limb in subjects with transtibial and transfemoral amputations. Deficits in muscular endurance of the amputated limb as compared to the sound limb[25] and weakness of both the amputated and the sound limb in comparison to age-matched norms[26] have also been demonstrated. Although we cannot draw direct relationships between strength impairment and specific activity limitations, there has been some evidence to support the impact of weakness on activity level performance. For instance, hip extensor strength in persons with lower-extremity amputation has been identified as a useful predictor of performance on the 6-minute walk test,[27] and increased abductor strength in individuals with transtibial amputation is correlated with improved weight bearing on the prosthetic limb in quiet stance.[28]

Accurate strength assessment can help to elucidate the potential causes of gait deviations, as deviations are often related to strength deficits. Knowing which muscles are weak will serve to guide therapeutic exercise interventions. Gathering muscle strength measures in the initial stages of prosthetic training will also establish baseline strength levels against which progress can be demonstrated.

Early in the prosthetic training process, it is important to evaluate baseline strength in several ways. Assessing hip and, in persons with transtibial amputation, knee strength of the residual limb becomes somewhat more subjective, as the standard lever arm for providing resistance has been altered by the amputation. Isokinetic instrumentation or hand held dynamometers may be used to evaluate muscle strength, although the validity and reliability of these tests has not been well-established for this population.[26,29] Functional strength

TABLE 26-3 *Prosthetic Consequences of Limitations in Range of Motion*

Range of Motion Limitation	Potential Functional Limitation	Implication
↓ Hip extension	Inability to achieve upright posture in stance and inability to take advantage of extensor moment at hip; hip and low back extensors firing continually to maintain upright	Fatigue of hip and low back extensors
	Compensatory anterior pelvic tilt	Chronic low back pain
	Compensatory knee flexion in transtibial prosthetic	Instability during stance phase of gait
	Body cannot progress beyond prosthetic leg during gait	Decreased step and stride length of contralateral limb in gait
↓ Hip adduction	Abducted stance in gait (wide base of support)	Abductor lurch/lateral lean on ipsilateral side during stance decreasing gait efficiency
↓ Internal rotation	Toe-out stance and gait	Knee joint pain and/or pathology in transtibial prosthetic user because of lack of anterior/posterior orientation of knee joint
	Pelvic progression over stance limb in gait may be limited (contralateral pelvis rotates anteriorly from fulcrum of weight bearing hip; if limited internal rotation, this will impede pelvic rotation on fixed femur)	Decreased step and stride length of contralateral limb in gait
↓ Knee extension in transtibial prosthetic user	Limb functionally shorter	Gait deviations associated with leg length discrepancy
	Inability to take advantage of extensor moment at knee; knee extensors firing continually to maintain knee extension	Quadriceps fatigue, decreased midstance stability in gait
↓ Knee flexion in transtibial prosthetic user	Inability to place foot flat on the floor when sitting	Inability to weight bear through prosthesis during sit-to-stand transfers
	Inability to climb or descend stairs step over step	Limited to step-to-step method, which may be less efficient and slower

of the hip and knee during closed chain activities and eccentric control are equally important, as they reflect muscle activity during normal gait.

Although strengthening programs should address all muscles of the residual limb and sound limb, prioritizing exercises that address hip extensor strength in the amputated side is appropriate, as hip extension strength has been identified as a strong predictor of gait outcome in persons with amputation.[27,30] Hip abductor strength is a priority for frontal plane stability and knee extensor strength is key for knee stability in the sagittal plane in individuals with transtibial amputation, so these muscle groups must also be emphasized in a preprosthetic exercise program. Stability of the hip and pelvis, especially in stance on the prosthetic side, is one of the key ingredients in achieving effective forward progression over the prosthesis during gait. In persons with amputations appropriate hip extensor and abductor strength is critical to achieving stability of the pelvis over the prosthetic limb during single limb stance in gait.[27,30] Strengthening exercises targeting hip extensors and abductors should be initiated early and progressed appropriately.

Although pre-amputation weakness of proximal muscles is often subtle with little to no observable abnormalities in pre-amputation gait patterns, these impairments of strength and muscle endurance may be magnified in prosthetic gait. Periods of disuse prior to and following amputation typically produce further weakness in much of the involved limb's

musculature. Without adequate proximal muscle strength and with the loss of distal musculature because of the amputation, problems with gait are likely.

Attention to strengthening of the hip extensors, abductors, adductors, and, in the person with transtibial amputation, the quadriceps and hamstrings are paramount to achieving optimal ambulation abilities. This is best addressed in the early phases of rehabilitation but should continue throughout the rehab process. Core strengthening of the abdominal and paraspinal muscles is important to develop as a strong core is essential for trunk stabilization during mobility training for transfers and gait. The degree of strengthening for the extremities and the positioning of the individual's limb in gravity resistance or gravity neutral position will depend upon existing strength levels. Utilization of closed chain (e.g., residual limb on bolster or gymnastic ball, or individual in kneeling position if tolerated) and open-chain exercise techniques, with both concentric and eccentric muscle contractions, are appropriate and effective. Progressive resistance protocols are often used to improve strength and muscle endurance. Resistance may be applied manually or with equipment, such as cuff weights, elastic bands, or pulley weights. Using body weight is an effective way to introduce resistance training. Resistance is generally not applied at or near the suture line until the surgical wound is well healed. Basic physiological principles of strengthening (e.g., overload principle, specificity of training) are employed in the design of an appropriate resistance training program. Resistance exercises should specifically target muscles identified as weak in the examination and muscles that are functionally required in gait, transfer, and mobility activities. Strengthening within the context of functional activities is desirable. Correct exercise technique is critical to achieving the desired strength gains with the ultimate goal of minimizing an individual's activity limitations.

As an individual's strength improves, exercises become more functionally oriented as well as more intense. Closed-chain exercises can take on greater emphasis during the latter stages of rehabilitation as the intervention focus may be exclusively on upright functional activities. Table 26-4 highlights some exercises that may be helpful in strengthening an individual with transtibial or transfemoral amputation.

The strength requirements for ambulation with a prosthesis are similar but not identical to those of normal gait. Both the involved and intact lower extremities display increased muscle activity during their respective stance phases. Specifically, activity of the ipsilateral hip extensors and, in the case of transtibial amputation, knee extensors is increased

and prolonged during stance as compared to persons without amputation.[30,31] The intact limb is subject to increased ground reaction forces, presumably a result of the absence of the normal foot and ankle mechanism of the involved side.[32,33] Hip abductors and extensors and knee extensors of the intact limb must respond to these increased forces. They demonstrate an increase in power generation and muscle activity.[34]

It is clear that PT interventions must address the strength not only of the residual limb, but of the uninvolved limb and trunk as well. Persons with amputation often go through protracted periods of inactivity before and after amputation. Because of this "disuse," the patient often experiences generalized loss of strength. Adding exercises that address the trunk, upper extremities, and uninvolved limb will generally be beneficial to overall functional mobility as the demand on them will be increased during preprosthetic and prosthetic training.

Balance and Postural Control

Effective postural control during functional tasks has two fundamental components: (a) controlling the body's position in space for purposes of stability (maintaining center of mass over base of support) and (b) orientation of the trunk and limbs in space (appropriate relationship between body segments and between body and environment).[35] The normal balance mechanism relies on visual, vestibular, and somatosensory input. Visual and vestibular information add awareness of position in space with respect to objects in the environment and to gravity and somatosensation provides information about the positions of the joints of the lower extremity and the pressures through those joints. With loss of the distal limb to amputation, somatosensation and proprioception can no longer provide direct information about limb's interaction with support surfaces. Balance deficits are well documented in persons with amputation,[24,36] as are deficits in balance confidence.[37,38] Balance performance is associated with ambulation outcome following amputation[15,24,27,39] and reduced balance confidence has been linked to a loss of perceived ability with the prosthesis, a loss of performance with the prosthesis, and a reduction in a sense of social importance.[40] Additionally, the incidence of falls in persons with amputation is higher than in age-matched peers,[36,40] and many falls occur during the inpatient postoperative period,[41] especially during transitional movements such as transfers to/from wheelchairs.[42]

Before discussing standing balance, it is important to mention that some individuals will have difficulty adjusting to changes in sitting balance following transtibial or transfemoral amputation. Prior to receiving the prosthesis, lack of a second foot on the floor, or in the case of transfemoral amputation, loss of the surface area of the thigh on the seating surface, alters the base of support while sitting; and loss of the mass of the lower extremity impacts the location of the body's center of gravity in sitting. Most individuals adjust fairly quickly in achieving static sitting stability, but the inability to weight shift onto that foot can challenge dynamic sitting balance, especially with reaching tasks requiring movement anterior and ipsilateral to the amputated side. For this reason, seated reaching ability is evaluated during the initial

TABLE 26-4 *Examples of Therapeutic Exercises for Strengthening Used in Preprosthetic Training*

Muscle Group	Exercises
Hip extensors	Bridging with residual limb over ball, bolster, or padded stool Prone leg lifts with weights Manual resistance in prone or side lying, or even sitting (early in range) Supported standing (parallel bars) hip extension with pulley weights or elastic bands
Hip abductors	Side-lying bridges with small ball or padded stool under knee (TTA) or distal femur (TFA) of residual limb Hip abduction in side-lying with weights or manual resistance Supported standing hip abduction with pulleys or elastic bands
Hip flexors	Supine hip flexion (with knee extension for TTA) with manual resistance or weights Supported standing hip flexion with pulleys or elastic bands
Hip ER/IR	Seated or supine hip ER and IR with manual resistance or elastic bands
Knee extensors (TTA)	Seated knee extension, open chain with manual resistance or weights (long arc quad) Supine short arc quad over bolster
Knee flexors (TTA)	Seated knee flexion with manual resistance or elastic bands Prone knee flexion with manual resistance or weights

ER, external rotation; *IR*, internal rotation; *TFA*, transfemoral amputation; *TTA*, transtibial amputation.

examination and is addressed in treatment as necessary. Once an individual is training with a prosthesis, practicing dynamic sitting balance activities usually progresses quite quickly.

In the preprosthetic phase, standing balance assessment and training might include single-limb standing in the parallel bars or at a support surface with decreasing reliance on upper-extremity support. Ability to stand on the sound limb without upper-extremity support has been associated with better prosthetic gait outcomes in individuals with unilateral lower-extremity amputation,[15,24,27] making this an important skill to assess and train as early as possible.

In patients with transtibial amputation, if the individual can tolerate a kneeling position over the healed surgical site, or in individuals with either transtibial or transfemoral amputations, if they can tolerate gentle pressure to the healed distal end, the individual may stand with the intact limb on the floor and the residual limb resting on an elevated surface (low mat, gymnastic ball, or foam block) that allows minimal weight bearing and balance support. Preprosthetic gait training with an appropriate assistive device is another useful and functional approach to upright balance training.

Because sensory and proprioceptive input from the distal segment is absent after amputation, a new prosthetic user must learn to compensate for this lack of important postural information. In individuals with nonvascular amputations (sensory status of remaining limb presumed intact), quiet stance is characterized by asymmetrical weight bearing (sound limb greater than prosthesis) and an alteration of the location and trajectory of the center of pressure on both the prosthetic limb and the sound limb.[43] These sound limb variations are strategies to compensate for the prosthetic limb in maintaining upright balance. Because the vast majority of lower-extremity amputations are the result of vascular pathology, the underlying sensory mechanisms that help to inform the balance compensation cannot be presumed to be intact. Balance assessment and training is, therefore, a significant and justifiable component of the prosthetic rehabilitation process.

Prosthetic users may learn to deduce the position of the prosthetic foot and contact with the support surface by the angle of the hip or, in the case of the person with transtibial amputation, the knee, and/or pressures felt within the prosthetic socket. Early in gait training, the person with a transfemoral amputation may make an exaggerated effort to dig the prosthetic heel into the floor at initial contact, so as to use the resulting pressure at the posterior residual limb as an indicator of contact with the floor and to assure prosthetic knee extension. The individual may learn to interpret this sensory experience as the secure position for proceeding with loading response and progressing into midstance.

In addition to the loss of direct sensory knowledge of contact with the floor, the loss of muscles at the ankle often compromises postural responses. Nashner[44] describes three stereotypical motor responses that are used to ensure that the center of mass stays within the base of support in response to unexpected anteroposterior perturbations: ankle, hip, and stepping strategies. These postural strategies are also evident during functional activities, such as ambulation.[35] The ankle strategy movement pattern, evident in normal postural sway, requires intact ROM and strength of muscles at the ankle. After amputation, this strategy is no longer available to the involved limb, so that the person may not be able to resolve the balance perturbation using intact limb response only, and instead may need to rely on a hip strategy (movement of the trunk over the base of support) or a stepping strategy (moving the base of support under the center of mass) when a postural response is necessary.

Individuals with transtibial and transfemoral amputations must be able to respond to environmental demands during ambulation and other functional tasks in anticipatory (feed forward) and reactive (feedback) modes. Therapists can design activities to assess and encourage postural control in varying tasks and environments.[45] For example, successfully catching and throwing a ball requires the person to anticipate postural demands (in an effort to throw) and react to postural disruptions (in an effort to catch). Reaching activities in standing help individuals develop skill and confidence in their anticipatory postural responses and, should the reach distance be excessive, their reactive postural responses as well. Individuals with higher functional demands will require more advanced training. Therapists must consider the person's ultimate likely functional requirements and design a variety of balance tasks to help the individual achieve those levels.

Cardiovascular Endurance

A thorough assessment of a person's cardiovascular status followed by appropriate cardiovascular endurance training is an integral part of pre-prosthetic and prosthetic management. The energy requirements for an individual who is using a prosthesis for ambulation are higher than those of an individual who ambulates on two intact lower limbs. Aerobic capacity of persons with amputations has been demonstrated to be lower than age-matched peers, even in younger individuals with traumatic amputations.[46] An extensive literature review by Waters[47] identifies some of the key physiological considerations for gait in persons with prostheses:

- The energy cost of walking is greater in individuals with amputations than those without.
- Higher level amputations are associated with higher energy costs of walking than lower level amputations.
- Persons with amputations as a consequence of vascular pathology demonstrate greater energy cost of walking than those with traumatic amputations; this may likely be associated with overall fitness level.
- Customary walking speed decreases with higher level of amputation.
- Average rate of oxygen consumption during self-selected walking may not be significantly greater than normal, as users of prosthetics often adjust (decrease) their speed.
- It is generally more efficient for an individual with a prosthesis to ambulate with the prosthesis (with or without assistive device), than it is to ambulate with the

assistive device without the prosthesis. The one exception to this may be the person with a vascular transfemoral amputation, where the energy expenditure is similar with and without prosthesis, likely a result of the substantial dependency on the assistive device, even when using the prosthesis.

The energy expenditure for overground walking in people with unilateral transtibial amputation may be 10% to 36% higher than that of individuals without amputation,[48-52] with the lower end of the range representing those with non–vascular-related amputations, and subjects who were more physically active. Individuals with transfemoral amputations demonstrate even higher energy requirements, 27% to 65% higher than people without an amputation.[50,53-55] Physical conditioning is an essential component of rehabilitation for individuals with lower-extremity amputation, especially those with cardiopulmonary or vascular compromise. Individuals with vascular amputations are significantly less active than their peers.[56] Improving metabolic efficiency (aerobic capacity) has a direct impact on the potential for functional ambulation even for the frailest and most deconditioned individuals.[57] The ability to gain an exercise intensity of greater than or equal to 50% VO_2 has been associated with "successful" prosthetic outcome (i.e., ability to walk 100 m with or without cane) in older adults with high-level amputations (transfemoral and hip disarticulation).[58,59] Endurance activities during the preprosthetic rehabilitation phase (e.g., wheelchair propulsion, single-limb ambulation with an appropriate assistive device, bilateral upper or unilateral lower-extremity ergometry) can help improve cardiovascular status before prosthetic training. Individuals often continue these activities as they enter into the prosthetic phase of rehabilitation. As the condition of the person's residual limb and wearing tolerance permit, ambulation with the prosthesis can be used as an additional cardiovascular endurance activity. The 2-minute walk test with prosthesis may be a useful tool to document changes in functional exercise capacity for an individual with amputation.[60,61] For those whose endurance may be a limiting factor for prosthetic ambulation, the PT plan of care must include a cardiovascular exercise component as a priority. Individuals who are taught to monitor their own pulse, respiratory rate, and/or perceived rate of exertion are able to participate more fully in prosthetic rehabilitation and prosthetic training. To develop an effective cardiovascular conditioning program, the therapist uses knowledge of the person's past medical history and cardiovascular pathophysiology, adapting the program to provide an appropriate challenge without surpassing their physiologic capabilities. The therapist must recognize the influence of cardiopulmonary pathologies, such as unstable angina or advanced chronic obstructive pulmonary disease, on the individual's ability to improve his or her endurance and adjust goals and intervention strategies as appropriate. For individuals with few cardiovascular restrictions, more advanced cardiovascular exercises can be utilized as rehabilitation progresses. Brisk walking and/or use of exercise equipment (e.g., treadmill, stationary bicycle, stair climber, or elliptical machine) are excellent endurance training activities for the appropriate person. An amputation need not prevent individuals from participating in health and wellness exercise programs during and following their rehabilitation.

Edema Control of Residual Limb

Reduction of postsurgical edema is critical in the early postoperative rehabilitation phase. Use of rigid postoperative dressings (e.g., cast) after transtibial amputation appear to be superior to soft dressings (including ace wrapping) in controlling volume of the residual limb[62,63] and are associated with a shorter time frame from amputation to initial prosthetic fitting[64,65]; however, this type of postoperative care is not routinely used throughout the United States, perhaps because of physicians' hesitancy to be blinded to the surgical site for 5 to 7 days postsurgery. When the more common soft dressings are used, ace wrapping for compression is applied over the transtibial residual limb dressing. Ace wraps should be applied in oblique angles (not circumferentially, so as to avoid a tourniquet effect), with gradual increase in pressure from distal to proximal, and always extending above the knee (as the transtibial prosthetic socket engulfs the medial and lateral aspects of the knee). Patients and family members should be instructed in wrapping technique, as the Ace wrap typically needs to be reapplied several times per day.

The transfemoral residual limb does not lend itself to rigid postoperative dressings and is more challenging to Ace wrap, as it requires anchoring over the pelvis and it may be difficult for a patient to elevate the pelvis for wrapping. Nevertheless, efforts at compression wrapping postsurgically should be a part of the treatment plan.

After the staples or sutures are removed, use of a commercial pressure garment ("shrinker") is suggested for persons with either transtibial or transfemoral amputation. Residual limb edema plays a big role in determining when initial prosthetic fitting will take place—if the prosthesis is fitted too early and the residual limb is still substantially shrinking, this will affect the intimacy of prosthetic socket fit, making training more difficult and increasing the risk of complications caused by a poorly fitting socket.

Prerequisites for initial prosthetic fitting include sutures removed, surgical wound healed or healing, and edema controlled, with distal measurements less than or equal to proximal measurements. The importance of continued shrinking efforts, even after prosthetic training has begun, should be emphasized. Individuals usually must continue to wear a shrinker sock when they are not wearing their prosthesis, at least during early training efforts. If patients allow the edema to return to the limb the socket may no longer fit and aggressive efforts to reduce limb volume will need to precede any further prosthetic training.

Initiation of weight-bearing activities in the prosthetic socket significantly decreases limb edema and accelerates maturation of the residual limb as a result of total contact within the socket and the pumping of muscle contractions during weight-bearing activities and movement. Shrinking of the residual limb in early prosthetic training is accommodated for with the addition of layers of appropriate ply thickness of prosthetic socks to maintain a snug residual limb-prosthesis interface. Given fluctuations in residual limb size during early training and the need for an intimate socket fit, new prosthetic users must carry extra socks with them whenever they are going to be out for longer than 2 to 3 hours.

As mentioned, during early prosthetic rehabilitation, individuals continue to use a shrinker when not wearing the prosthesis to reduce the likelihood of insidious edema when the prosthesis is not being worn. Individuals prone to fluid volume fluctuations (e.g., those with kidney dysfunction or congestive heart failure) will likely need to use a shrinker indefinitely. For others, whose residual limb ultimately reaches a stable size and shape, a shrinker may not be necessary once the prosthesis is consistently being used. The decision to discontinue the use of a shrinker permanently is based on two factors: (a) consistency in the number of sock ply worn during the day and (b) the ability to don the prosthesis without decreasing the usual number of sock ply after a night's sleep without the shrinker.

Significant changes in body weight can also dramatically affect socket fit. Patients should be educated regarding the importance of limiting weight gain or loss so as not to compromise socket fit.

Soft-Tissue Mobility of Residual Limb

Soft-tissue and bony adhesions that limit tissue mobility around the incision scar and the surrounding area may have an impact on prosthetic tolerance, comfort, and use. Surgical amputation can include muscle-to-muscle (myoplasty), muscle-to-fascia (myofascial), and/or muscle-to-bone (myodesis) surgical fixations to stabilize the remaining muscle.[66,67] Scarring or adhesions can occur among any or all of these tissues. The normal stresses and shearing forces of cyclic loading and unloading during gait require that soft tissue throughout the residual limb be mobile. If the soft tissue is not able to move independently of the scar tissue or skeletal structures, the stress can lead to tissue breakdown and/or discomfort. Soft-tissue mobilization techniques early in the rehabilitation process can help establish appropriate tissue mobility in the residual limb. Once the surgical incision is securely closed, soft-tissue massage can be an effective tool in maintaining tissue mobility. Deep friction massage may be helpful in managing scar tissue that is restrictively adhered. Individuals can be instructed in the use of this modality with specific guidelines for proper technique. Appropriate deep friction massage targets movements between skin, subcutaneous soft tissue and fascia, and muscle layers. Improper deep friction massage technique is ineffective in managing scar tissue and potentially harmful for the person with fragile skin and soft tissue. Friction generated between the fingers and skin results in skin irritation, blistering, or breakdown and can delay prosthetic use until adequate healing occurs.

Sensory Status of Residual and Remaining Limb

Residual limb and sound limb sensibility is formally assessed during the initial PT examination. Standard sensation testing guidelines are used to assess all sensory modalities (pain, temperature, light touch, deep pressure, proprioception, vibration). Semmes-Weinstein monofilament testing may be used to assess for protective sensation of the sound limb. Several commonly occurring post-amputation sensory phenomena can have implications for functional outcome in patients with amputation. These include hyposensitivity, hypersensitivity, phantom sensations, and phantom limb pain.

Hyposensitivity

Hyposensitivity is most often encountered among those with a history of diabetes, neuropathy, traumatic nerve damage, or vascular disease. Limited research suggests that deep pressure remains intact, but superficial pain sensibility is impaired in transtibial residual limbs.[68] Individuals with amputation who have impaired sensation are at high risk for skin breakdown because they may not recognize discomfort associated with skin irritation resulting from repetitive stresses and pressures. Inclusion of education about the preventative need for visual inspection, and practice time to perform visual inspection of the residual limb for signs and symptoms of soft-tissue lesions can reduce the risk of skin breakdown. Adaptive equipment, such as mirrors, or the assistance of caregivers may be necessary for people with concurrent limitations in flexibility and/or visual impairment.

Hypersensitivity

Early in rehabilitation, it is not uncommon to encounter a generalized hypersensitivity of the residual limb. This hypersensitivity is thought to be a consequence of nerve damage from amputation surgery itself.[69] Hypersensitivity can be effectively managed by bombarding the residual limb with tactile stimuli using a variety of textures and pressures. Strategies for reducing hypersensitivity include gently tapping with the fingers, massaging with lotion, touching with a soft fabric (e.g., flannel or towel), rolling a small ball over the residual limb, and implementing a specific wearing schedule for shrinker socks and removable rigid dressings. Intensity of intervention is based on the individual's tolerance to the sensory stimulation. The techniques can be progressed in intensity, type of modality used, and duration of stimulus (e.g., touching the limb with a rougher fabric and increasing wearing time for the shrinker socks). Individuals with amputations are strongly encouraged to use these techniques independently as part of their home program. Over time these techniques should help reduce the hypersensitivity with the ultimate goal of tolerance to normal sensory input without discomfort. Physiologically, overloading the nervous system with sensory stimuli is thought to encourage habituation via downregulation of neural receptors.

Localized hypersensitivity may be an indication that a troublesome neuroma has developed at the distal end of a surgically severed peripheral nerve. A neuroma is suspected when localized tapping sends a shock sensation up the leg. If conservative clinical treatment is unsuccessful in reducing the hypersensitivity and pain caused by a neuroma, injection of a local anesthetic directly into the region or surgical removal may be necessary.

Phantom Limb Sensations

Phantom limb sensations are quite common after amputation.[70-72] Many individuals report experiencing feelings of itching, tingling, numbness, or sensations of heat and cold in the toes or foot of the limb that has been amputated. Although the sensation can include the entire missing extremity, proximal sensation often fades leaving only distal perceptions, a phenomenon known as "telescoping," presumably related to the large area of somatosensory cortex dedicated to the distal extremity.[72-74] Phantom limb sensation is a relatively harmless condition that tends to resolve in 2 to 3 years without treatment.[72] It has potential functional implications, as it may be useful in providing a semblance of proprioceptive feedback from the prosthesis. Be alerted, however, as to the importance of educating individuals of the potential danger of phantom limb sensations: nighttime falls are not uncommon when, half asleep, an individual attempts to stand and walk to the bathroom, expecting their phantom foot to make contact with the floor.

Phantom Limb Pain

Phantom limb pain occurs in 60% to 80% of all persons with amputation.[70,72,74,75] Incidence of phantom limb pain has been demonstrated to be higher with upper-extremity amputations as compared to lower-extremity amputations,[72,76,77] with proximal as compared to distal amputations,[72] and demonstrated to decrease over time.[70,72,74,76] When phantom pain occurs, it is most often described as a cramping, squeezing, aching, or burning sensation in the part of the limb that has been amputated. The spectrum of complaints may vary from occasional mild pain to continuous severe pain. The absence of observable abnormalities of the residual limb is common. Although the etiology of phantom pain is not definitively understood, changes in the peripheral nervous system, the spinal cord, and reorganization at the level of the cerebral cortex may all be involved in the perception of phantom limb pain.[70-72,74] The association between the etiology of amputation (vascular versus traumatic) and the incidence of phantom pain is unclear, but there does appear to be higher incidence of phantom pain in individuals who experienced pain in the limb prior to amputation.[70,74,78] Whatever the etiology and predisposing factors, phantom limb pain is challenging to manage and disabling if the pain is severe. Presently, there are no evidence based practice recommendations for the management of phantom limb pain. Clinically, strategies used to address phantom limb pain include medications (antidepressants, anticonvulsants, and analgesics), neural blockade, transcutaneous electrical nerve stimulators, heat and cold modalities, acupuncture, biofeedback, firm pressure applied to the residual limb (e.g., massage, compression or prosthetic socket), mirror box therapy, phantom exercises of the phantom limb, psychological treatment, and patient education.[70,72,73,79,80]

Residual Limb Pain

Residual limb pain is another potential limiting factor in persons after lower-extremity amputation. Common early after surgery, this pain usually subsides over time.[70,72,74] Ongoing complaints of residual limb pain should prompt careful inspection of the residual limb, as the therapist may pick up on signs of infection or small cutaneous or subcutaneous problems that could be manifesting as pain. This careful inspection and follow through is especially important in individuals with diabetes and vascular disease, as those who have an initial distal amputation at any level are at substantial risk of revision of amputation to a higher level. In a recent study of 277 subjects with diabetic amputation, 27% of patients required surgical revision by 1 year, and 61% by 5 years.[81]

Care of Sound Limb

Ongoing assessment of the intact lower extremity should be made the responsibility of the individual with the amputation, with support of the physical therapist. Individuals with diabetes, peripheral neuropathy, or peripheral vascular disease who have lost one leg as a result of the disease process have a significant chance of losing the other leg, given the symmetrical distribution of these disease processes and the increased functional demand on the remaining limb after the amputation. The added burden to the remaining limb extends beyond the preprosthetic period. Once ambulatory with a prosthesis, individuals will preferentially initiate level surface walking with the prosthetic limb, placing a larger burden on the sound limb for stability and propulsion.[82] And as an ambulatory individual makes adjustments to increase walking speed, this, too, will increased demands on the sound limb.[83]

Contralateral major limb amputation has long been known to be a very real threat in those with diabetes and vascular compromise,[84] and this is continually being reaffirmed. A 2006 study by Izumi demonstrated amputation of the contralateral limb of 12% of subjects with diabetes within 1 year of initial amputation, 44% within 3 years, and 53% within 5 years.[81] To minimize the risk of loss of the remaining limb, close monitoring of limb condition (especially for subtle or insidious trophic, sensory, or motor changes) and optimal foot care is essential. Ongoing, systematic, and frequent assessment of pulses, edema, temperature, and skin is suggested. Education about the importance of a daily routine of cleansing, drying, and closely inspecting the foot (including the plantar surface and between the toes) is crucial. Podiatric care of nails, corns, and plantar callus, appropriately fitting footwear or accommodative foot orthoses, and avoidance of barefoot walking are three additional imperatives for the longevity of the remaining foot. If unable to perform daily foot inspection independently because of disease or visual impairment or decreased agility, individuals must be able to direct a caregiver in inspecting the foot. Even if individuals are physically incapable of performing certain tasks for their own health and safety, they are ultimately responsible for their own care. Developing or improving on a person's skill at directing assistance is a useful and realistic PT treatment goal.

INITIAL PROSTHETIC TRAINING

Prosthetic fitting with an initial prosthesis (also called a temporary or training prosthesis) occurs when the surgical incision is healed (or healing without complications) and girth measurements at the distal residual limb are equal to or less than proximal girth measurements. The timeline from surgery to initial prosthetic fitting generally takes 6 to 12 weeks, although younger individuals with traumatic amputation and no other complications may be fitted as early as 2 to 3 weeks, and older dysvascular individuals may require substantially longer than 12 weeks, often because of delayed wound healing issues.

As a new residual limb matures and shrinks in size, the person will add additional ply (layers) of prosthetic sock to ensure adequate fit in the prosthesis. Typically, when the intimacy of fit within the socket is compromised by 15 or more ply of sock, a new prosthetic socket is indicated. How quickly the initial socket needs to be replaced varies depending on the pattern of shrinkage of the residual limb. For some, the first replacement socket may be necessary in 2 to 3 months, whereas others may use their initial socket for 6 months or more. The socket may be replaced several additional times as the residual limb continues to shrink in the first postoperative year. A definitive prosthetic socket is prescribed when the residual limb size is stable for an 8- to 12-week period, as indicated by girth measurements and by a consistent number of sock ply for prosthetic fit. Although some people are ready for their definitive prosthesis within 6 months after surgery, others do not achieve stable residual limb size for 12 to 18 months or longer. With each new socket, close monitoring of the residual limb throughout the adjustment period is necessary.

Several important components of rehabilitation involving prevention of skin breakdown and safe use of equipment can be effectively addressed in group classes or through printed materials. These components include care of the sound limb, donning and doffing the prosthesis, establishing a prosthetic wearing schedule, management and prevention of skin breakdown, positioning with the prosthesis, and care of equipment.

Prosthetic Prescription

The members of the interdisciplinary team involved in the care and rehabilitation of persons with amputation include the surgeon, a physiatrist, a prosthetist, a physical therapist, an occupational therapist, a social worker, a rehabilitation nurse, and a vocational rehabilitation counselor. Many hospitals and rehabilitation centers have established prosthetic clinics that bring together the appropriate professionals to address the needs and problems of prosthetic users. Determining prosthetic candidacy is the first major clinical decision to be made. Although the research literature has identified predictors of outcome of prosthetic use,[11,14,15,27] the team considers the individual's needs, motivation, and functional capacity in deciding about prosthetic candidacy. Factors that are most often considered in determining whether to fit an individual with a prosthesis include:

1. *Medical history:* Disabling medical conditions may prohibit successful prosthetic use. An earlier referenced systematic review by Sansam[11] suggests some studies relate increased number of comorbidities with poorer prosthetic outcome. Advanced cardiac or pulmonary disease that significantly impairs functional status before amputation has an impact on a person's prosthetic candidacy. A history of cerebrovascular accident with hemiplegia of the side opposite the amputation may limit functional prosthetic use, although some evidence suggests that degree of motor impairment is more predictive of outcome than the side of involvement.[11]

2. *Premorbid and present level of function:* An individual who required substantial assistance for functional mobility before amputation may have limited prosthetic training goals. Pre-amputation ambulation ability is predictive of prosthetic walking ability.[11,12] Additionally, individuals who are independent with functional activities, activities of daily living, and ambulation with an assistive device postamputation, will do well with a prosthesis.

3. *Body build:* Morbid obesity may pose significant challenges to prosthetic fitting. Individuals should not, however, be excluded from prosthetic fitting and training on the basis of their weight alone, as Kalbaugh and associates demonstrated that prosthetic outcome in overweight and obese individuals was comparable to that of a cohort of typical weight.[85] Interestingly, the study demonstrated that prosthetic outcome in the overweight and obese individuals was superior to individuals classified as underweight, although these findings were confounded by the increased numbers of comorbidities in the underweight group.

4. *ROM:* Significant hip and knee flexion contractures are best addressed prior to prosthetic fitting if an individual is to achieve efficiency and functional independence with a prosthesis, as contractures have been shown to have a negative impact on functional prosthetic outcome.[11,20]

5. *Support at home:* People who are likely to require assistance must depend on family members, significant others, or formal caregivers to help with one or more prosthetic tasks. The potential to be a limited household ambulator with a prosthesis may be important in reducing the burden of care for caregivers and may allow a person to remain at home with a caregiver as opposed to living in an institutional setting.

Because there is no definitive criteria for determining who is and is not a strong prosthetic candidate, careful consideration of the individuals' characteristics and situation are imperative. Some authors believe that even individuals who show limited/moderate potential for prosthetic success based upon our existing "criteria" should be fitted with a prosthesis and afforded the opportunity to try.[86,87] Should an individual be deemed a reasonable prosthetic candidate, these same considerations and others, are used in determining the specific prosthetic prescription for that individual.

The physical therapist must have a basic understanding of prosthetic components and design to be able to contribute to the prescription process. Because therapists spend a great deal of time working with people in one-on-one circumstances, they often have a better perspective about the individual's goals or needs than do other members of the team. The therapist may gain insight or information that is important in the decision-making process. If the therapist is familiar with prosthetic components, the therapist may be forming an opinion about the best prosthetic prescription for a person during the early rehabilitation phase. Physical therapists stay current with developments in prosthetic design and technology through professional interactions with prosthetists and by being critical consumers of the professional literature. For example, an understanding of the different characteristics of various prosthetic feet will help the therapist to work with the prosthetist in identifying the type of foot that is most suitable and economical to meet a specific patient's functional needs.

Therapists must also be familiar with the special needs of certain clinical populations so that they can assist in the optimal prosthetic prescription to meet any individual's needs. People with diabetes who are at great risk for additional skin breakdown and poor healing may benefit from a socket with a soft insert or from a silicone sleeve that is designed to reduce friction during prosthetic use. Frail or deconditioned individuals may reach higher levels of function if lightweight components are chosen and stability in prosthetic prescription is emphasized. Active children need durable components, but replacement costs must also be considered, as components will likely need to be replaced frequently to accommodate growth. Athletes with amputation desire durable, lightweight, high-technology components for a competitive edge in their sport performance.

Decisions to change socket design or suspension for long-term prosthetic users must be carefully considered. A person who has worn a particular type of prosthesis for a long period of time may have difficulty acclimating to a new type of device. If a person has no complaints about a prosthesis other than "it's worn out," it is advisable to use similar components for a replacement prosthesis. If a person is expressing interest in new goals or activities (e.g., a prosthetic user who has never run would like to try jogging), prosthetic prescription changes may be warranted. Hafner and Smith demonstrated that persons with transfemoral amputations originally classified as Medicare Functional Classification Levels (K Levels) 2 and 3 improved function and reduced the frequency of falls and transitioned to a higher Medicare Functional Classification Level when using an active microprocessor-controlled knee prosthesis,[88] and this advancement in Medicare Functional Classification Level with microprocessor-controlled knee joint has been identified as an incidental finding in another study as well.[89] This finding reminds therapists to suspend their biases that higher tech equipment should be reserved for younger individuals.

Medicare K levels are used to determine which prosthetic components are appropriate based on the persons with amputation's level of function. Components that are designed for higher activity levels would not be covered for payment under the Medicare policy. The physician determines the patient's functional ability level. If the patient's functional ability increases over time, the rating can be changed to a higher level.

Functional level 0: Patient does not have the ability or potential to ambulate or transfer safely with or without assistance and a prosthesis does not enhance his or her quality of life or mobility.

Functional level 1: Patient has the ability or potential to use a prosthesis for transfers or ambulation on level surfaces at fixed cadence—household ambulator.

Functional level 2: The patient has the ability or potential for ambulation with the ability to traverse low-level environmental barriers such as curbs, stairs, or uneven surfaces—limited community ambulator.

Functional level 3: The patient has the ability or potential for ambulation with variable cadence—advanced community ambulator who has the ability to traverse most environmental barriers and may have vocational, therapeutic, or exercise activity that demands prosthetic utilization beyond simple locomotion.

Functional level 4: The patient has the ability or potential for prosthetic ambulation that exceeds basic ambulation skills, exhibiting high-impact, stress, or energy levels—active children, young adults, and older adults engaged in recreational activities and sports.

The Preparatory Prosthesis

The initial socket is most often fabricated from high-temperature thermoplastic, but can be made of plaster of Paris, fiberglass, laminate, or other materials. The socket is connected to the prosthetic foot using an alignment system at either end of a metal or plastic pylon (pipe), and in the case of the transfemoral prosthetic, a knee joint. Endoskeletal modular prostheses are preferred to exoskeletal prostheses because alignment modification is likely early in the rehabilitation process. Some people are fitted with a permanent pylon and prosthetic foot at this early stage and progress through a series of sockets until their residual limb reaches its mature contours. Most often, a foam and stocking cosmetic prosthetic cover is not provided until the final socket fitting. Because of significant changes in residual limb size and shape, individuals may progress through two or three sockets before being fitted for the definitive socket or prosthesis.

Donning and Doffing the Prosthesis

Donning the prosthesis (Figure 26-1) should be taught through a series of steps including dressing the prosthesis; donning socks; donning a silicone liner, pull sock, or Dry-Lite lubricant; prepositioning the prosthesis while sitting; and then standing to weight bear through the prosthesis and adjust the suspension system. The steps for a given individual are dictated to a large extent by the prosthetic components. For instance, a roll-on liner with a pin-lock suspension system requires the individual to attend to the orientation of the distal pin when rolling the liner onto the residual limb, to adjust alignment and initiate the pin into the ring lock in a seated position, and stand for the final engagement of the suspension mechanism. A transfemoral prosthesis with a classic suction socket may require the individual to use a donning sleeve or pull sock to help ease the residual limb into the socket though a coordinated series of weighting and pulling maneuvers on the sleeve, which is threaded through the

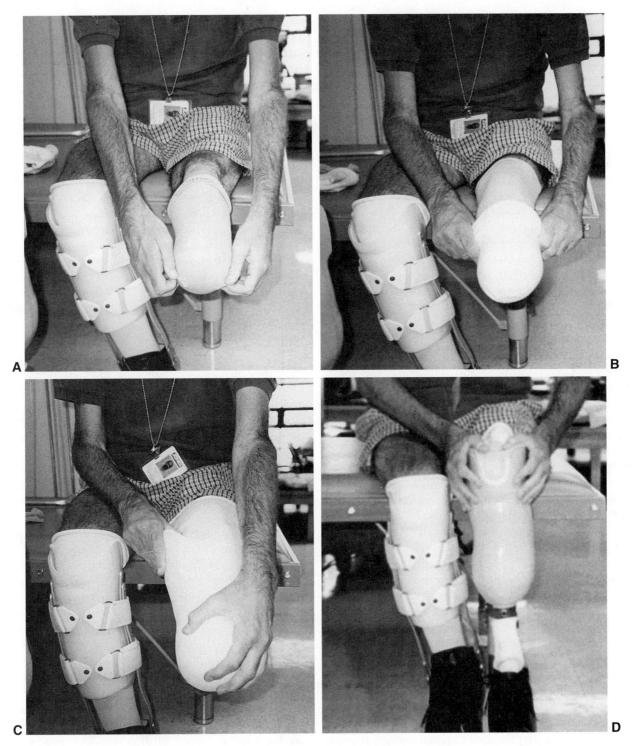

FIGURE 26-1 This patient with a recent transtibial amputation demonstrates the correct sequence for donning his prosthesis. **A,** First, he applies a nylon sheath, adjusting its fit to prevent formation of wrinkles or folds as additional layers of sock are added. Wrinkles result in uneven distribution of pressure and can increase the likelihood of residual limb discomfort and skin breakdown. **B,** Once the sheath is positioned, prosthetic socks are added, one at a time, and carefully adjusted for smooth fit until the desired number of ply is reached. The least possible number of socks is used to create a snug, comfortable prosthetic fit. **C,** This patient's prosthetic design includes a soft Pelite insert. The anterior trim line of the liner is cup shaped to accommodate the patella and is used to guide the position of the liner on the limb during donning. Patients are cautioned against using a twisting motion when applying the insert/liner, to avoid causing wrinkles in the underlying sheath or socks. **D,** The final step is to insert the residual limb with properly positioned socks and liner into the prosthesis. This patient dons the prosthesis in a sitting position, gradually increasing weight bearing to achieve the desired total contact fit. Note that a patellar tendon-bearing orthosis is used to support and protect his remaining limb, which is vulnerable as a result of Charcot arthropathy.

valve hole in the socket. Performed while standing, this donning procedure requires good balance and dexterity. Once the residual limb is deep into the socket and the air is expelled, the socket valve must be screwed into place. The chapters on prosthetic components elucidate further the donning requirements for specific types of prostheses.

One universal theme in donning of the prosthesis is to educate individuals to pay close attention to the orientation of socket in the horizontal plane. The contours of the socket are intimately designed to accommodate the patient's anatomical structures of the residual limb. In a person with a sensate residual limb, this may be constructive in assuring proper prosthetic alignment, as the socket will not "feel right" unless it is oriented appropriately; however, in the insensate limb, the patient must compensate with vision and palpation to assure proper alignment. Often, individuals use the prosthetic foot as a reference for horizontal plane alignment; static prosthetic alignment often places the foot in slight out-toeing in standing and the individual can use this visual cue as an affirmation of proper prosthetic alignment.

Teaching appropriate donning and fit of the transfemoral socket often requires the therapist to palpate the ischial tuberosity and potentially other structures (e.g., pubic rami, adductor tendons) for optimal positioning within the socket. This requires clear and professional patient and family education to clarify the purpose and process of a palpation that might be considered a serious invasion of personal space.

Prosthetic Sock Use

In early prosthetic rehabilitation, prosthetic socks are used to modify the fit between the socket and the shrinking residual limb. Proper use of prosthetic socks enhances residual limb weight bearing in pressure-tolerant areas, decreases the likelihood of skin breakdown in pressure-intolerant areas, and increases patient comfort during ambulation. Wool or cotton prosthetic socks are available in three different ply (thicknesses): 1 (thinnest), 3, and 5 (thickest). Many individuals with amputation who use a rigid or flexible socket will first apply a thin nylon sheath directly over the skin (under the socks) to minimize friction forces and wick moisture away from the skin. Cotton or wool socks of various ply (thickness) are then applied before the limb is placed in the socket. If a nylon sheath is not used, socks are applied smoothly directly onto the residual limb. When silicone suction suspension or a friction reducing liner that require skin contact is used, socks are applied after the sleeve or liner has been donned. For liners with a pin-lock mechanism, a small hole in the bottom of the socks will accommodate for engagement of the pin into its receptacle. Socks of various thicknesses are combined to create a snug and comfortable fit. Individuals are encouraged to don the fewest number of socks to achieve the same amount of thickness (e.g., one 3-ply sock is preferable to three 1-ply socks). Prosthetic socks can also be used creatively to solve problems with socket fit. If, for example, the person's distal residual limb girth has decreased more quickly than proximal girth, creating a pendulum effect within the socket during ambulation, one of the prosthetic socks can be cut to cover

just the lower half of the residual limb. When layered between two full-sized socks, the shorter sock helps to fill the extra space within the socket, ensuring total contact between the limb and socket.

Fluctuations in limb volume associated with edema in the first weeks and months after amputation often mean that the appropriate number of sock ply varies from day to day and perhaps within a given day. Because of this variability in limb size, choosing the correct number of prosthetic socks may be challenging for those new to prosthetic use. Limb size can change rapidly. Even a few minutes in a dependent position without a shrinker or Ace wrap in place can substantially increase residual limb size. For this reason, individuals must wear their compression device until the moment that they are ready to don the prosthesis. Therapists and prosthetists work with new prosthetic users to assist in the development of problem-solving skills and strategies to determine the appropriate number of socks to don.

Good prosthetic socket fit and satisfaction with the prosthesis is extremely important to individuals with amputations.[90,91] New prosthetic users must be educated on the principles of prosthetic fit and weight bearing. The optimal prosthetic fit is quite snug, like that of a custom-fit glove on the hand. Total contact between the residual limb and socket is very important and significant skin problems can occur when total contact is not achieved. Individuals must understand where weight-bearing pressures are best tolerated on the limb and where pressure sensitivity is likely to occur. Although they might initially expect to bear weight through the distal end of the limb, they must understand that sockets are designed to be total contact and to distribute weight-bearing forces across several areas. For the transtibial socket, these areas include the patellar tendon, anteromedial and anterolateral surfaces of the residual limb, medial tibial flare, and distal posterior aspect of the residual limb. For the ischial-ramal containment transfemoral socket, they include the posterior aspect of the residual limb with the pubic ramus (medially), ischial tuberosity (posteriorly), and greater trochanter (laterally) contained in the prosthetic socket. The ischial-ramal containment socket also distributes pressure through the lateral femur to increase the efficiency of the hip abductors in weight bearing. The quadrilateral socket utilizes pressure anteriorly on the Scarpa triangle, forcing the ischial tuberosity to rest on a posterior shelf of the socket.

A number of indicators are used to assess the adequacy of sock ply during prosthetic ambulation. If too few socks are used, the residual limb descends too far down within the socket. The individual may complain of pistoning during ambulation—that is, the prosthesis slips downward when unweighted during the swing phase and is pushed upward on the residual limb during weight bearing in stance. If pistoning is suspected, a pen or marker is used to mark the prosthetic sock at the anterior or posterior trim line of the socket. If the line becomes more visible when the individual lifts the limb (using a hip-hiking motion), it is likely that slippage is occurring, and additional sock layers are indicated. When the transtibial prosthesis and socks are taken off for inspection of the skin, reactive hyperemia (redness) is seen at the proximal patellar tendon and at the inferior border of the patella, as well as at the distal anterior residual limb. Redness may also be present on the fibular head, which contacted the socket below its intended relief area. These are all signs that thickness of the socks is inadequate and additional sock layers should be added. Too few ply socks in a transfemoral socket may result in increased weight bearing and hyperemia on the distal residual limb and complaints of pressure in the groin as the socket rides up higher than intended.

A different set of signs indicates that too many ply of sock have been donned. The person may feel that the prosthetic limb is difficult to don, fits too tightly, and is just slightly longer during forward progression at midstance and during foot clearance in swing. In the transtibial prosthetic user, when the skin is inspected after ambulation, reactive hyperemia is seen at the distal patellar tendon and the tibial tubercle. Redness may also be present at the head of the fibula, which contacted the socket above its intended relief within the socket. In the ischial containment transfemoral socket, too many socks will prohibit the residual limb from gaining good purchase within the socket and the patient will not feel "locked-in" to the socket; in the quadrilateral socket the ischial tuberosity will be elevated off of the posterior shelf. These are indications that one or more ply of socks should be removed to enhance socket fit. Although pistoning is usually an indication of too-few-ply socks, paradoxically, it might also be seen in a patient wearing too many ply, because the residual limb is never fully into the socket and therefore never gains good purchase and moves up and down with ambulation.

Most individuals become adept at judging the adequacy of sock ply when given the opportunity to practice and problem solve early in their rehabilitation. For the functional prosthetic user, donning and doffing the prosthesis becomes as second nature as donning and doffing one's pants or shoes. The initial instruction period in this skill, however, requires attention to detail. Individuals should be encouraged to establish a careful routine of donning the appropriate number of prosthetic socks, one layer at a time. The socks should be smoothed free of wrinkles, with any seams facing down and out so as to minimize pressure on the surgical scar.

Checking Adequacy of Suspension

Once the individual is comfortably in the socket, adjustment of the suspension device is necessary. Suspension options for transtibial prostheses include suspension sleeves, supracondylar straps with or without waist belt and auxiliary fork strap, supracondylar socket design, supracondylar/suprapatellar socket design, thigh corset with joint uprights, and suction liner with ridges or with pin in ring suspension. To complete the donning process, the person stands and weight bears through the socket to ensure proper positioning of the residual limb while adjusting the suspension system.

Roll-on silicone sleeves with pin-locking or shuttle-lock mechanisms are becoming one of the most commonly prescribed suspension systems. When rolling on the suspension sleeve, care must be taken that the pin is centered on the inferior surface of the distal residual limb. The appropriate number of socks is applied over the silicon sleeve by sliding the pin through the hole in each sock. The hard socket is donned as the individual aligns the pin with the socket receptacle and pushes into the socket; the pin should click into place. Once the residual limb is seated in the hard socket, the individual stands and weight bears through the prosthesis; the pin should further depress into the ring mechanism, confirmed with three to five audible clicks. If more clicks are audible upon initial weight bearing than anticipated, this is an indication that more ply of sock may be required.

Prevention and Management of Residual Limb Skin Problems

Because prolonged wound healing and development of new skin irritation can delay prosthetic training, the prevention and management of skin breakdown on the residual limb represent important goals. The prevalence of skin problems on the residual limb in prosthetic users has been reported to be between 36% and 64%.[92-94] Especially vulnerable to skin issues are very active prosthetic users[92] and individuals with impaired hand function.[95] Residual limb skin issues have been demonstrated to have an impact on functioning in daily life for the prosthetic user.[96]

In the new prosthetic user, skin issues can preclude weight-bearing and gait-training activities. Pressure, friction, or shearing forces are the primary etiologies of skin breakdown related to prosthetic wear. If, during weight bearing, external pressure exceeds capillary refill pressure (25 to 32 mm Hg) for an extended period of time, the delivery of oxygen and nutrients and the removal of waste products from active tissues are interrupted. If relief of pressure is provided, this local ischemia is followed by a reactive vasodilation or hyperemia. This is the mechanism that produces the redness over weight-bearing areas, such as the patellar tendon and medial tibial flare and shaft, that is observed in new transtibial prosthetic users. A blanchable area of redness over weight-bearing areas, which returns to normal skin coloration within 10 minutes, is to be expected in early prosthetic training and indicates normal reactive hyperemia.[97] If redness persists or does not blanch on firm palpation, tissue damage has likely occurred, and the risk of skin breakdown increases significantly.

It is important that therapists and individuals with amputation recognize the different implications of redness over pressure-tolerant versus pressure-sensitive areas of the residual limb. If a pressure-tolerant area shows evidence of excessive pressure, socket fit and alignment may be appropriate, but the amount of weight bearing or duration of wearing time may need to be decreased. If pressure-sensitive areas are showing signs of too much pressure, it is more likely that socket fit or alignment needs to be adjusted. When excessive redness is observed, successful problem solving dictates changing a single variable at a time and assessing the impact of this one change on the prosthetic problem. If multiple changes are made at the same time (e.g., wearing time, alignment, and socket fit are all altered), it is not clear which change actually solved the problem, if indeed the problem is solved.

If the problem is not solved, there is no way of knowing if the interventions may have been more successful independent of one another.

An individual's risk for skin breakdown on the residual limb is determined by physiologic and mechanical factors. The vascular, sensory, and musculoskeletal conditions of the residual limb are the physiologic determinants, whereas socket fit, socket alignment, amount of weight bearing, and duration of weight bearing are the mechanical determinants. Each of these risk factors may have clinical implications. A conservative prosthetic wearing schedule and frequent residual limb inspection may be indicated for those with skin breakdown caused by any of the physiological risk factors. If poor scar and soft tissue mobility of the residual limb leads to tissue breakdown, deep friction massage over the involved area (after healing) and/or application of a nylon sheath under prosthetic socks may be appropriate interventions.

Improper socket fit or alignment can result in increased weight bearing to pressure-sensitive areas of the residual limb and may result in skin breakdown. If poor fit or alignment is suspected, the first step in problem solving is a thorough reevaluation of donning technique and the number of socks used. Prosthetic fit is then reassessed to determine if total contact between the residual limb and socket has been achieved. If all of these areas are sufficient, potential problems with prosthetic alignment are investigated. It is important to note that increasing duration of prosthetic wearing too quickly in a well-aligned and appropriately fitting prosthesis can also result in skin breakdown to pressure-tolerant areas of the residual limb. An individual who has been ambulating with partial weight bearing using axillary crutches without any problems with skin integrity may, when progressed to full-time unilateral crutch use, present with skin breakdown over a pressure-tolerant area as a result of increased weight bearing.

The presence of skin breakdown is not a direct contraindication to further use of the prosthetic device. The first priority should be to identify the cause of breakdown and eliminate it by making the appropriate changes. Close observation and ongoing assessment and treatment of any lesions using appropriate nonadherent dressings inside the socket should allow prosthetic training to continue. Certainly, if a lesion becomes progressively worse despite clinical management during prosthetic training, a hiatus from prosthetic use may be indicated. In the example presented previously, a return to bilateral crutch use and diminished prosthetic wearing time may be indicated until the lesion is healed. After healing, ambulation time might be divided between bilateral and unilateral crutch use, to build tolerance for increased weight bearing before full-time unilateral crutch use is attempted once more. If the area does not show signs of healing or becomes worse with increasing lesion size or signs of inflammation or infection, prosthetic use may need to be discontinued altogether for healing to occur.

As a person begins to ambulate over different terrains, the magnitude and direction of weight-bearing pressures within the socket may change as well, presenting additional mechanical risk factors for skin breakdown. Descending stairs using a step-to-step pattern protects the residual limb by leading with the prosthetic leg; when advancing to a step-over-step technique, the residual limb experiences a different pattern of pressure distribution. Depth of stairs also has an impact on pressure distribution within the socket: As step height increases, so does the total excursion through ROM necessary to descend the stairs. Ambulation on uneven terrain, such as grass or gravel, produces different pressures within the prosthetic socket than walking on a predictable, level surface. When evaluating potential causes of skin breakdown, it is important to consider the characteristics of the environments and the task demands of the activities in which the individual has been engaging. Changing task technique by adapting the movement strategy or the environment, or adding an assistive device can provide just enough protection for the residual limb to prevent skin irritation and breakdown.

If localized increased pressure is determined to be the cause of tissue breakdown, pressure relief is the goal, and socket modification by the prosthetist may be necessary. Certain methods of pressure relief are inappropriate and should be avoided. The use of "donut" padding around an area of breakdown or potential breakdown is counterproductive for three reasons. A donut pad (a) increases pressure to the area surrounding the lesion when the limb is placed in the socket, (b) increases the ischemic effect of weight bearing, and (c) potentially leads to edema or extrusion of the vulnerable tissue through the "hole" of the donut. Any adhesive materials that are in contact with skin should be used with extreme caution. A nylon sheath can be used to hold a dressing in place under the prosthetic socks. Finally, the abrasive quality of certain dressings, including standard gauze, must be avoided inside the socket. Nonadherent dressings or nonstick pads tend to be less textured and less abrasive to an area of skin breakdown. Many new products are available that are thin and self-adherent, but not noxious to the skin, effectively providing another "tissue" layer to an area that is threatening breakdown or in the process of healing.

Dressings should be used sparingly inside a prosthetic socket, as the socket fit is designed to be snug, and any padded dressing increases pressure over the affected area, which is counterproductive to the goal of wound healing. The therapist must reevaluate the prosthetic fit if a dressing is used within the socket, recognizing that the application of even a thin dressing may require the removal of one ply layer of socks.

Prosthetic Wearing Schedule

After the evaluation of socket fit and alignment has been completed and any adjustments have been made, it is time to begin prosthetic training. Constant reassessment of socket fit and alignment is necessary during the entire training phase because of changes in residual limb shape and size. The duration of time for initial prosthetic wearing is usually conservative, especially for individuals with a history of skin integrity problems. Often, the first prosthetic weight-bearing activities are closely supervised, lasting no longer than 5 to 10 minutes in between skin inspections. Once individuals are tolerating 30 to 60 minutes in the prosthesis without problems, total time in the prosthesis is gradually increased, often in increments of 15 to 30 minutes, as skin condition permits. People with no history of skin integrity problems (e.g., after traumatic amputation or revision of congenital limb anomaly) often progress quickly with wearing activities, whereas those with sensory impairment or peripheral vascular disease may need to be progressed much more cautiously.

Inspection of the residual limb after the first few minutes of weight bearing should reveal redness of the skin in predictable pressure-bearing regions. Because both the transtibial and transfemoral sockets are intended to have total contact with the residual limb, the entire limb may develop a mild reactive hyperemia that is apparent when the socket is first removed. Increasing wearing time requires continued, frequent skin inspection. It is vital that the individual understand the importance of gradual progression of wearing time. If a person is allowed to initiate prosthetic wearing unsupervised or does not take the wearing schedule seriously, the potential for skin breakdown is greatly increased.

It is optimal, but not always possible, for the prosthetist and physical therapist to both be present for the delivery of the prosthesis to the patient with amputation, so that both may be involved in the final fitting and alignment checkout. After delivery of the prosthesis, the physical therapist and person with amputation may determine that it is safest to use the prosthesis only when supervised by the therapist during the first week or more of therapy. Once the patient is cleared to use the prosthesis at home, an individualized written wearing schedule (Figure 26-2) is used to guide

prosthetic wear and prevent misunderstandings about the time permitted for prosthetic use.

Positioning

People will often need instruction about positioning of the lower extremity in the prosthesis when seated. The trim lines of the transtibial socket are designed for optimal pressure distribution during upright weight-bearing activities. The high posterior wall of the socket is necessary to provide counterpressure to the anterior weight-bearing surface in stance, but can provide undue pressure to the hamstring tendons in sitting. The patellar tendon indentation in the prosthesis is designed to take weight in standing but can provide pressure to the anterior aspect of the tibial tuberosity if the prosthesis slips down when the patient is seated. Similarly, the transfemoral socket can shift or lose suction in sitting which can result in undue pressure if maintained over an extended period. It is optimal that when seated, the individual's prosthetic foot should rest flat on the floor or foot plate of the wheelchair so that the residual limb remains in total contact with the socket. This helps avoid the risk of undue pressure and decreases the chance of gapping between the prosthesis and the residual limb that may allow edema to collect. This becomes especially difficult when sitting on low surfaces and for individuals with transfemoral prosthesis since the socket is often moved because of the posterior pressure in sitting.

Additionally, although some individuals may be anxious to carry out exercise programs with the prosthesis in place, they must understand that using the prosthesis for activities other than walking (e.g., weighted long-arc quad exercise) changes the magnitude and direction of forces on the residual limb and may increase the possibility of skin breakdown.

PROSTHESIS WEARING SCHEDULE

Patient Name: _____

Your wearing schedule for your prosthesis is _____ on and _____ off.

Check your skin every time you take your prosthesis off. You are looking for areas of redness that

do not go away within 10 minutes, areas of blistering or abrasions, or pain in your residual limb.

If you have any of these problems, or any questions, call your therapist at the number below and

do not wear your prosthesis again until the problem is addressed with your therapist.

If you do not have any of the problems above, in two (2) days you can increase the "on time"

to _____ and maintain the off time as above.

Next scheduled appointment: _____

Therapist name & phone number: _____

FIGURE 26-2 Example of a wearing schedule used to guide the patient's use of the new prosthesis at home, early in rehabilitation.

Care of Prosthetic Equipment

People with amputations also require explicit instructions about the proper care and maintenance of their prosthetic equipment. The prosthetic socket and liner should be wiped daily with a damp cloth. Prosthetic socks should be washed daily and laid flat to dry (wool socks shrink when dried in an electric clothes dryer). When not being worn, most prosthetic devices (with the exception of those with hydraulic mechanisms) should be stored in a flat position to minimize the risk of damage should they fall over (hard sockets are particularly vulnerable to traumatic cracks).

PROSTHETIC FIT AND ALIGNMENT

As new prosthetic users become comfortable and confident with their prosthetic limb, changes in socket fit and alignment may be necessary to achieve the most energy-efficient and cosmetic gait. Ideally, the prosthetist, the person with amputation, and therapist work as an interdisciplinary team to solve problems with socket fit and alignment as they arise. The physical therapist ought to have a thorough foundational knowledge of optimal socket fit and alignment in order to recognize and troubleshoot problems and be ready to refer the patient to the prosthetist should alignment need adjustment.

The Prosthetic Socket

An intimate fit between the residual limb and the socket is necessary for successful prosthetic training. The total contact socket is designed to distribute the load of weight bearing over the residual limb to assist in venous blood return from the limb, provide some sensory feedback to the prosthetic user through the residual limb, and provide an efficient transfer of muscle function to the prosthetic device. Although the socket is prepared over a positive model of the patient's limb, either through casting or computerized technology, as a result of

early changes in the residual limb it is not uncommon for the socket to be modified in the early days of prosthetic training. Frequent and careful inspection of the residual limb and verbal feedback from the user both help to assess socket fit and patient tolerance to prosthetic wear.

Alignment

Prosthetic alignment is evaluated in quiet standing (statically) and during gait activities (dynamically). Static alignment refers to assessment of the relationships between the socket, prosthetic knee joint (if applicable), pylon, prosthetic foot, and floor; the length of the prosthesis; and the overall fit of the socket on the residual limb. Dynamic alignment includes those concepts as well as prosthetic considerations as they relate to suspension, symmetry of gait, and energy requirements of gait.[98] Because static alignment assessment is the first standing activity in which a patient engages, it is prudent to carry this out in the parallel bars or with substantial support if parallel bars are not readily available. Information gleaned from alignment assessment can reveal clues about pressure distribution on the tissues of the residual limb inside the socket. Problems with alignment affect not only pressures within the socket but also the biomechanics of gait and the translation of forces from the prosthetic foot up the kinematic chain. Both static and dynamic alignment must be evaluated from an anterior, posterior, and lateral (prosthetic side) view. For a thorough review of prosthetic alignment, see componentry chapters; Table 26-5 provides a basic rationale for standard transtibial and transfemoral static prosthetic alignment.

PROSTHETIC GAIT TRAINING

The ability to move within and over one's base of support with efficient timing and sequencing of muscle activity and appropriate postural control is the key determinant of functional

TABLE 26-5   *Static Prosthetic Alignment and Rationale*

Alignment	Rationale for Alignment
POSTERIOR VIEW	
Prosthetic height (symmetrical leg length)	• Prevents gait deviations associated with leg length discrepancy • Provides optimal weight bearing through the socket to prevent pain or skin issues • Prevents sound limb orthopedic deformity associated with leg-length discrepancy
Plumb line: midsocket to slightly lateral to midheel	• In the transtibial prosthesis, creates slight varus moment during stance, as in normal gait • In the transtibial socket, directs compressive forces to pressure-tolerant areas at medial proximal (medial tibial flare, medial femoral condyle) and lateral distal (fibular shaft) residual limb and minimizes compressive forces on nontolerant areas at lateral proximal (fibular head) and medial distal residual limb • In the transfemoral socket, directs forces onto the residual lateral femoral shaft
Slight adduction of transfemoral socket	• Adduction of the transfemoral socket serves to improve length tension relationship and efficiency of the hip abductors in maintaining a level pelvis during unilateral stance
LATERAL VIEW	
Transtibial socket in 5 to 10 degrees of flexion (anterior tilt of socket, encouraging slight knee flexion) when in a midstance position	• Distributes weight bearing forces to anterior, pressure tolerant aspect of transtibial residual limb • Limits vertical displacement of center of gravity at midstance to decrease energy cost of gait • Allows for controlled knee flexion in loading response and late stance, as in normal gait • Prevents abnormal hyperextension of the knee in midstance

TABLE 26-5 *Static Prosthetic Alignment and Rationale—cont'd*

Alignment	Rationale for Alignment
Transfemoral socket in 5 degrees of flexion (posterior tilt of socket, encouraging hip flexion) with the knee in full extension at the midstance position	• Serves to improve length tension relationship and efficiency of the hip extensors during stance phase of gait • Distributes weight bearing forces to posterior, pressure tolerant aspect of transfemoral residual limb
Plumb line: midsocket to anterior edge of heel	• In transtibial alignment, allows for knee flexion from mid to terminal stance • In transtibial alignment, prevents hyperextension of the knee in stance
Assessment of trochanter-knee-ankle line	• In transfemoral alignment, provides assessment of the location of the center of rotation of the knee joint in the transfemoral prosthesis relative to hip and ankle, which dictates the stability of prosthetic knee extension during stance and the ease of prosthetic knee flexion in preparation for swing

ambulation across the wide variety of environments that are encountered in daily life. Many prosthetic users have the potential to ambulate with a near-normal symmetrical gait pattern that is free of significant gait deviations and independent of assistive devices.[23] To do this, however, the person must meet a variety of challenges, including (a) building tolerance to prosthetic wear and weight bearing through the residual limb; (b) controlling dynamic weight shifting through the prosthesis in all planes of movement; and (c) reintegrating postural control and balance with respect to the lack of ankle, and in the case of transfemoral amputation, knee joint sensory and proprioceptive input, muscle control, and ROM.

An individual's fears and concerns influence determination and motivation. Fear and concern are powerful determinants of the ability to ambulate and perform other important functional activities.[38,40] An individual with an amputation who is otherwise functionally capable of safe ambulation in the community may choose not to venture outside of their home because they lack confidence in their physical ability or are fearful of being identified as disabled or different. In contrast, a person whose clinical picture is less promising for functional prosthetic use but who is determined to return to a busy and productive life "on two feet" may very well do so.

Initial Training

For the new prosthetic user, initiation of gait training typically starts with ambulation on level surfaces with few environmental demands. Gait training often begins in the parallel bars, as a protected environment, because it provides a stable and secure setting with minimal environmental challenges. Countertop or table support, raised mats, plinths or chairs, even assistive devices can all be appropriate alternatives if parallel bars are unavailable. When training does begin in the parallel bars, individuals are encouraged to use a relaxed and open handed grip on the bars, as the tendency to pull and rely heavily on the secure bars is a difficult habit to "untrain" when transitioning out of the bars. When an individual receives the prosthesis and is excited to take the first steps, it is useful to limit cues and simply allow the individual to walk in the parallel bars. It is valuable to educate the person regarding what to expect with their first attempts at ambulation with a

prosthesis: The socket may feel tight, almost as if it is squeezing the residual limb because of the nature of the total contact of the socket, and weight bearing through the prosthesis may feel strange initially.

Ambulation in the parallel bars helps the therapist to identify gait deviations early in training before maladaptive habits become problematic. Based on this preliminary gait assessment, individual problem areas can be addressed with exercise activities and gait training. Early therapeutic activities will progress from initially supporting and later challenging the individual's postural stability. Progressing from weight bearing and gait activities with significant bilateral upper extremity support to minimal or no support is a common early goal in the rehabilitation process of both transtibial and transfemoral prosthetic users. A typical progression of early prosthetic training activities might include:

1. Static weight bearing with decreasing dependency on upper extremity (UE) support (e.g., progressing from bilateral open-handed UE support, to contralateral open-handed UE support, to ipsilateral open-handed UE support, to static standing activities without support).

2. Simple dynamic weight-shifting activities, consisting of loading and unloading body weight through the prosthesis in multiple directions (anterior/posterior, medial/lateral, and diagonal patterns) as is required in gait and functional activities. These tasks are progressed by decreasing UE support and varying foot positions (parallel stance, step-stance, tandem stance). It may be helpful to cue the individual to think about the weight going through the "ball" or "heel," or the medial or lateral surface of the prosthetic foot as they shift weight in different directions. This may help to correlate sensations within the prosthetic socket with former somatosensory experiences of the foot. Another important cue during these activities may be to have the individual focus on the pelvic position versus the prosthesis during weight shifting activities. The focus on the pelvis is important for several reasons: (a) the pelvis has been found to be less stable in upright standing in persons with transfemoral amputations than

in individuals without amputations[99]; (b) the pelvis is key to stability in the upright position, so the patient is cued in to this important locus of control; (c) by focusing on the pelvis, the patient is being directed to control a part of the body that is intact and "whole," and although some individuals have not focused on pelvic awareness prior to prosthetic rehabilitation, this takes the focus off of the prosthesis and the "new" challenges that the patient is facing; and (d) awareness of pelvic position in early weight-shifting activities may make later gait demands, such as emphasizing pelvic rotation, easier for the patient to grasp. In controlling the pelvis during weight-shifting activities, the patient might envision the pelvis as a table top and a very tall vase centrally located on the table, so if the pelvis tips in any direction, the vase will fall and break; or they may imagine a ball on that table and regardless of the direction of the weight shift, they must not let the ball roll off of the table. These cues are intended to encourage anterior, posterior, and lateral translational movements of the pelvis, but without substantial anterior, posterior, or lateral tilting of the pelvis.

3. Standing reaching activities that require the person to reach to a variety of heights and directions within a functional context. These activities are progressed by increasingly challenging reaching limits in all directions, varying foot position and decreasing UE support. These early reaching activities are prerequisites to very functional goals such as reaching to high shelves and lifting something of substantial weight or picking up a heavy object from the floor.

4. Repeated stepping activities (e.g., breaking down gait cycle into its component parts) in all directions with decreasing UE support. The focus here may be in loading and offloading the prosthetic limb with good proximal/pelvic control.

5. Stepping with the uninvolved limb onto an elevated surface (begin with a low surface and progress height and/or begin with stable surface, such as stepstool, and progress to less stable surface, such as small ball) forcing increased weight bearing through the prosthetic limb with progressively decreasing UE support.

6. Gait training to minimize gait deviations inside, or progressing out of the parallel bars. Early in training, individuals often benefit from cues to make firm contact with the prosthetic heel during initial contact to enhance awareness of the location of the prosthetic foot on the floor and assure stability of the prosthetic knee of the transfemoral prosthesis with active hip extension.

7. Sit-to-stand and stand-to-sit activities, to enhance the ease and independence of transitional movements. Persons with transtibial amputations are encouraging to integrate partial weight bearing through the prosthesis; whereas a transfemoral prosthesis is much more difficult to weight during transitional movements. Beginning training to/from high surfaces with arm rests and progressing to lower surfaces without arm

rests, and varying training to include different types of support surfaces will enhance the individual's ability to generalize the skill to a variety of settings. Figure 26-3 depicts some of these early prosthetic training activities.

Although use of specific weight-bearing activities outside of functional tasks may be contrary to fundamental motor learning principles of encouraging action-directed performance versus motor performance, activities that encourage weight bearing can be successfully practiced and then integrated into functional gait and mobility skills. Repetitive loading of the prosthesis is an appropriate task, even without translation of weight over the foot as in the intact gait cycle. Once the individual becomes accustomed to accepting the weight (as in initial contact through loading response of the stance phase of gait), the individual may then progress to practicing more full-weight-bearing activities in preparation for the single-limb support phase of gait and finally integrate the activity into the full gait cycle. Regardless of the focus of the intervention (weight bearing, balance, postural control, or coordination and sequencing), the activity can and should be integrated into the gait cycle or the functional task within the same treatment session. Interventions are most effective if they are ultimately done within the context of functional tasks.[35] A typical and detrimental mistake often made in rehabilitation is implementing a treatment plan that is beneath the capabilities of the patient. Therapists are reminded that physically and functionally challenging the person training with a prosthesis is vital to reaching the person's full potential.

Progressing prosthetic training requires increasing challenges to postural control and balance. Dynamic activities without UE support and activities that require both anticipatory and reactive balance strategies (e.g., playing catch) can be used to prepare the prosthetic user for more open, unpredictable environments.[45] Again, challenging the individual is important to their long-term balance success. New prosthetic users must be allowed to find their limits of stability in the upright position. If the individual is not challenged to really test the limits of the individual's stability, because they are always permitted the use of UE support and/or the therapist is guarding very closely and intervening with even the slightest loss of balance, the person will likely not learn their own zone of stability and may never have the opportunity to develop their own confidence in their ability to monitor and maintain their own balance. Figure 26-4 depicts some balance activities. Coordination and sequencing of an appropriate assistive device and activities to promote timing and fluidity of gait (e.g., use of cues, for instance a metronome, to facilitate symmetrical timing of steps) as well as to encourage appropriate weight bearing (e.g., use of audio biofeedback for weight bearing) are other areas that can be included in this phase of prosthetic training. During all activities with the new prosthetic user, the therapist must remain cognizant of the need for frequent skin checks for signs of pressure intolerance and skin irritation.

Some individuals will have difficulty accepting weight through the prosthetic limb even during static standing activities. They may rely heavily on weight bearing through

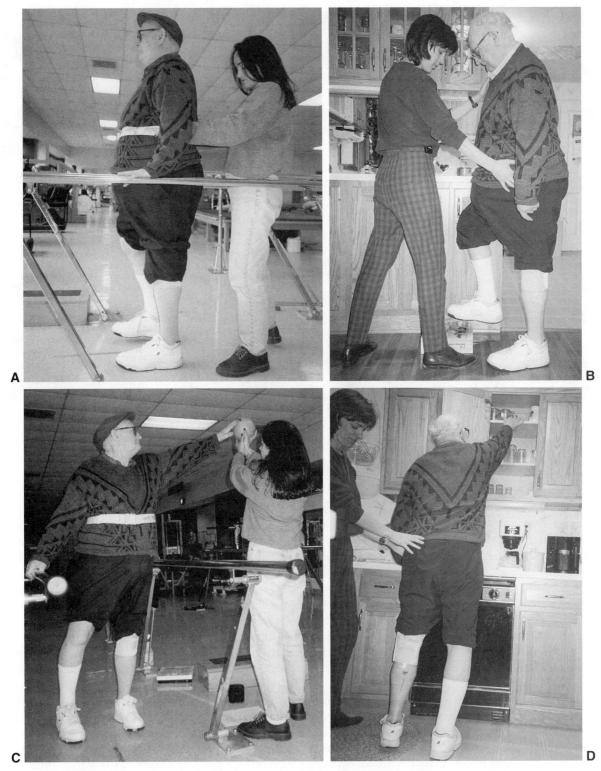

FIGURE 26-3 Weight-bearing, weight-shifting, and balance activities in early prosthetic training. **A,** A new prosthetic user practices loading weight onto the prosthesis by repeatedly practicing single steps (forward and backward) with the intact limb. Note full weight bearing through the prosthesis, demonstrating good prosthetic alignment and erect trunk and head posture, with a gentle open-handed grip on the parallel bars. **B,** Stepping up onto a phone book or low stool can increase weight bearing through the prosthesis. **C,** Reaching activities, using all planes of movement, encourage weight shifting onto and off of the prosthesis and can challenge balance and postural control. Early on, the opposite hand grip on the parallel bar compensates for decreased balance and postural control. This activity can be progressed by decreasing, and ultimately eliminating, upper extremity support. **D,** Reaching activities in a functional context should be integrated early in the rehabilitation process.

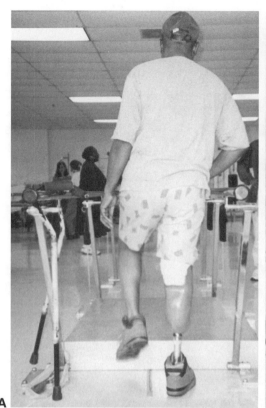
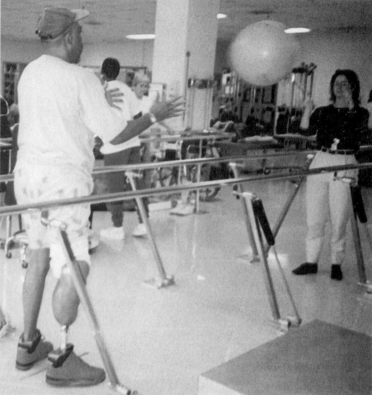

A   B

FIGURE 26-4 Progression of weight-shifting and balance activities in prosthetic training. **A,** Stepping activities become more challenging without the use of the upper extremities for balance or support. **B,** Throwing and catching activities encompass balance (feed-forward and feedback), coordination, postural control, and weight bearing through the prosthesis.

the upper extremities in the parallel bars, and express hesitancy or simply be unable to put all of their weight through the prosthesis. Ironically, individuals who have been especially active and functional during the preprosthetic phase, ambulating with crutches or a walker may find weight bearing through a prosthesis difficult. During the preprosthetic phase, the sound limb often gravitates to a more central location under the individual so that their center of gravity is directly over their base of support. This puts the remaining limb in an adducted position and the amputated limb in an abducted position. These individuals must reorient their lower-extremity positioning when training with a prosthesis.

Individuals with hip and/or knee strength deficits may also struggle with weight bearing through the prosthesis and/ or decreasing reliance on upper extremities during standing activities. A long history of vascular disease that has progressively limited physical activity may likely impact strength of the lower extremities, which can affect stance stability of the prosthetic limb. Ambulation without an assistive device will not be possible unless functional levels of strength are recovered. Individuals who are hesitant to weight bear through the prosthesis, whether because of weakness or fear or habitual patterns, may be tempted to use the prosthesis as an "assistive device" for ambulation rather than a true replacement limb. Having the individual step onto a bathroom scale to provide objective feedback regarding weight bearing through

the prosthesis may be useful with these individuals who are having difficulty loading the limb. The use of mental imagery of successful mastery of all weight-bearing and ambulation activities may be an appropriate adjunct to PT.[100] It is important for both therapist and new prosthetic wearer to recognize that improved prosthetic weight bearing allows for decreased mechanical stresses on the sound limb,[34] which often has vascular compromise.

Other intervention strategies that might be useful in early gait training include verbal cueing to progress the pelvis toward the parallel bars (laterally) and anteriorly during stance on the prosthetic side over a stable foot, and tactile cueing of the therapist's hand placed on the anterolateral aspect of the involved hip to facilitate anterior progression.

In persons with transfemoral amputations, early gait training presents some additional challenges since prosthetic knee stability and mobility are directly related to prosthetic alignment and strength and motor control of the hip musculature. Although this focus on pelvic control is presented in the context of helping to control the prosthetic knee in persons with transfemoral amputations, those with transtibial amputations will also benefit from improved pelvic control as facilitated by verbal and tactile cues during gait training.

The transfemoral prosthesis is aligned to provide stance stability through the knee joint during weight bearing. In unilateral stance on the prosthetic limb, the person must be able to stabilize and control their trunk and pelvis over the prosthesis, which requires adequate strength in the hip abductors (to counteract the gravitational adduction torque at the hip) and hip extensors (to maintain the hip and trunk in an upright and extended position). Forward progression while weight bearing on the prosthetic limb is a challenge that requires a focus on pelvic position and movement. Active hip abduction and extension and forward pelvic progression are vital to stance stability. There is often a tendency for the prosthetic stance limb to display posterior pelvic rotation or to let the pelvis "drift" posteriorly during stance—the swing-side pelvis should be rotating forward at this time, but the stance-side pelvis should not be rotating posteriorly. This posterior pelvic position makes smooth transition over the prosthetic limb impossible as it disrupts the normal forward progression.

The therapist can facilitate forward pelvic progression during stance using principles of proprioceptive neuromuscular facilitation (PNF) with deliberate application of hand position and input to muscles (e.g. resistance, quick stretch). Pelvic movement can be successfully encouraged from in front of or behind the patient (Figure 26-5). Swing phase likewise requires training to facilitate the correct motion. An effective swing will allow for correct step length and facilitates a smooth transition into stance phase. Symmetrical step lengths are conducive to a smooth and energy efficient gait pattern. There are two specific cues that may help individuals with transfemoral prostheses to achieve a good swing of the prosthetic limb. Initially the person needs to be encouraged to step forward with a normal step on the uninvolved side. Prosthetic users are often hesitant to do this—when they have an asymmetrical gait pattern, it is often because the prosthetic step is very large (because they are comfortable taking weight through the sound limb) and the sound limb step is very small (because they are not comfortable taking weight through the prosthesis). A full-size sound limb step creates more hip extension and posterior pelvic transverse rotation on the involved side. Because of the design of many prostheses, anterior pelvic rotation in the transverse plane at preswing will facilitate "knee break." This effectively shortens the limb to allow clearance during swing phase. Persons with transfemoral amputations should be cued to rotate the pelvis forward, which will swing the prosthetic limb forward and extend the knee, allowing for full knee extension at initial contact. Early gait training with a transfemoral prosthesis might involve practice and perhaps facilitation of this forward pelvic translation to help the person get the feeling of the knee break and initial swing. The same types of PNF techniques that are used to facilitate stability of the pelvis during weight bearing can be used to facilitate active movement of the pelvis for swing. Forceful hip flexion in the absence of pelvic rotation to advance the prosthesis forward prohibits normal step length. Likewise vaulting, hip hiking, and circumduction are not efficient methods of forwarding the prosthesis during swing phase. These are common gait deviations that should be eliminated as quickly as possible.

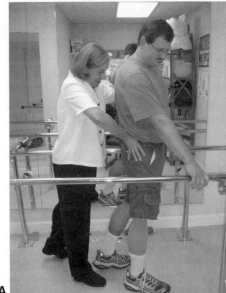

A

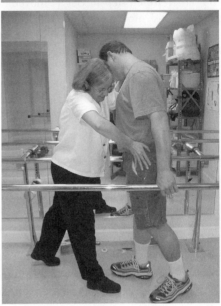

B

FIGURE 26-5 Facilitation of forward pelvic motion for efficient prosthetic gait. **A,** The therapist can use manual techniques to cue pelvic position from behind. **B,** The therapist can also use proprioceptive neuromuscular facilitation manual contacts and appropriate resistance, asking the patient to move the pelvis upward and forward as he or she steps with either limb.

Assistive Devices

Assistive devices can provide help with balance only (i.e., single-point cane or quad cane) or with weight bearing and balance (i.e., standard walker, rolling walker, axillary crutches, or Lofstrand crutches). The goals of assistive device use are to provide only the amount of support that is necessary to protect the healing residual limb and to reduce the risk of falling without hampering the individual's willingness or ability to load the prosthesis. It may be prudent to spend time on prosthetic weight-bearing and weight-shifting activities in the parallel bars or at a stable surface to allow the person to progress directly to an assistive device that aids in balance only.

Optimally, the prosthetic limb can tolerate 100% weight bearing, so that UE weight bearing through an assistive device is unnecessary. Individuals who demonstrate good weight bearing, strength, and balance may progress directly from the parallel bars to the use of a single-point cane or no assistive device. Quad canes should be prescribed with caution, as they are frequently misused as weight-bearing devices and the wide base can create a fall hazard. For those who are unable to achieve early full weight bearing through the prosthesis and require a weight-bearing assistive device, the devices of choice are a rolling walker or axillary or Lofstrand crutches. Crutches allow individuals to progress to a two-point gait using a step-through gait pattern, which closely approximates a normal sequence and pattern of gait. Individuals may begin with bilateral support and progress to unilateral support with crutches as prosthetic weight bearing improves.

Standard walkers impede progression of an efficient reciprocal gait pattern because they limit forward progression to a "step-to" rather than "step-through" movement strategy. This interrupts fluid movement, hampers smooth forward progression of the center of gravity over the base of support, and precludes an effective terminal stance and preswing. Standard walkers are used only when individuals are long-term users and/or are resistant to transitioning to a new device. A wheeled walker can minimize interruptions to the gait cycle if it is advanced between each step or if the person is weight bearing only slightly through the walker (i.e., pushing the walker like a grocery cart).

Although persons with amputation who also have physical or medical frailty may require assistive devices for household ambulation, many individuals with transtibial amputation reach functional independence without any assistive device, or choose to use just a straight cane for "balance assist" when walking on unpredictable surfaces or in crowded environmental conditions. Depending on age, balance abilities and strength, and fear of falling, persons with transfemoral amputation may walk with or without an assistive device.

Prosthetic Gait

An understanding of the biomechanics of normal gait is crucial for physical therapists, as it provides the standard by which prosthetic gait is measured. The main objective of static and dynamic prosthetic alignment and PT intervention is to optimize the energy efficiency, biomechanics, and cosmesis of gait. The ultimate goal is a gait that is safe, energy efficient, and symmetrical. When deviations from the norm are observed, the therapist and prosthetist seek to discover and resolve the underlying cause(s) of the problem.

It is well documented that gait speed of persons with amputations is slower than in persons without amputation[24,30,101,102] and that symmetry of gait is affected by amputation.[24,83] Biomechanically speaking, there are several well-documented changes in comparing prosthetic gait to gait of able-bodied individuals. In persons with transtibial amputation, the lack of plantar flexors is thought to be the most influential component driving gait changes,[31,103,104] and this is compensated for by increased activity and power of the muscles around the hip

of the prosthetic limb, most notably the hip extensors. In persons with transfemoral amputation, the strength, endurance and power demands on musculature of the hip are higher still, as the hip also must compensate for the missing knee.

There is conflicting information about whether specific prosthetic devices have a significant impact on efficiency and quality of prosthetic gait. Some studies support the benefit of microprocessor-controlled knees[105-107] and dynamic response feet[33,108] in enhancing gait mechanics and/or efficiency, whereas others have had more equivocal findings.[52,107] A full discussion comparing and contrasting different prosthetic componentry is beyond the scope of this chapter, but the therapist should work closely with the prosthetist in identifying the best prosthetic prescription for patients based upon their ambulation and functional goals.

Commonly observed prosthetic gait deviations have many different potential contributors. Gait deviations may be a product of intrinsic factors (pertaining to the individual using the prosthesis), or extrinsic factors (pertaining to the prosthesis and/or environmental factors). The observed deviation may be a primary gait problem, caused directly by an intrinsic or extrinsic factor, or a compensatory strategy, a result of the individual's attempt to avoid a primary deviation. If a new prosthetic user is observed to ambulate with a forward-leaning trunk throughout the stance phase of gait, the therapist must determine if this is a primary or a compensatory problem. It may be a primary gait deviation resulting from a hip flexion contracture that limits the individual's ability to achieve upright posture. Or it may be a compensatory strategy of the person who is fearful of knee instability during prosthetic stance; by using a forward-leaning trunk, the individual's line of gravity is dropped anterior to the knee joint, improving stability at the knee by creating an extensor moment at that joint.

During initial gait training, prosthetic alignment issues may not be immediately evident. Hesitancy to fully load the prosthesis and UE weight bearing through the parallel bars or assistive device will affect the resulting gait pattern. As the individual becomes more willing to bear weight through the residual limb, a "truer" gait pattern will emerge and the function of the prosthesis becomes more critical. The therapist, along with the prosthetist, must be attentive to the potential emerging need to correct prosthetic alignment as the individual improves in prosthetic weight bearing and as impairments improve (i.e., changes in strength, ROM, or balance might warrant prosthetic alignment changes).

When problem solving, the clinician must think about why certain gait deviations might occur and whether they are primary or compensatory. Answering these questions allows the therapist to focus treatment on the most salient issues. Table 26-6 describes some of the more common prosthetic gait deviations and their most likely potential causes.

Consider an individual who shows knee instability during loading response and throughout midstance, as evidenced by lack of knee extension or excessive knee flexion. The therapist must use deductive reasoning to identify what the true sources of the problem might be. If the instability is occurring

TABLE 26-6 *Prosthetic Gait Deviations*

Gait Deviation	Phase of Gait	Category*	Possible Causes
GAIT DEVIATIONS COMMON TO TRANSTIBIAL AND TRANSFEMORAL PROSTHETIC USERS			
Lateral trunk lean toward prosthetic side	Loading response through terminal stance	Intrinsic	Lacking hip abductor strength and/or timing on prosthetic side (compensate with lateral lean to avoid Trendelenburg)
			Abductor contracture on prosthetic side
			Hip joint pain on prosthetic side
			Very short transfemoral residual limb (poor purchase in socket, poor leverage)
		Prosthetic (extrinsic)	Prosthesis too short
			Foot too outset
			Transfemoral socket medial wall trim line too high
			Transfemoral socket places femur in abduction
			Transfemoral socket lateral wall fails to provide adequate femoral support/stabilization
		Environmental (extrinsic)	Uneven terrain
Anterior trunk lean	Loading response through terminal stance	Intrinsic	Hip flexion contracture
			Lacking knee extensor strength and/or timing in individual with transtibial amputation (compensate with forward lean to provide knee stability)
			Fear of instability of physiological or prosthetic knee
			Insufficient hip extensor strength or lumbar extensor strength making maintenance of an upright trunk difficult
		Prosthetic (extrinsic)	Transtibial socket set too posterior (forcing knee hyperextension)
			Transtibial socket lacks anterior tilt
			Transfemoral prosthetic knee positioned too anterior (trochanter-knee-ankle line not providing stability)
		Environmental (extrinsic)	Walking up incline
Insufficient weight bearing through prosthesis	Loading response through terminal stance	Intrinsic	Residual limb pain or hypersensitivity
			Excessive upper-extremity weight bearing on assistive device
			Instability of the physiological or prosthetic knee joint
			Decreased muscle strength of residual limb
			Fear of falling/lack of confidence in prosthesis
		Prosthetic (extrinsic)	Prosthesis is too long
			Poor socket fit
		Environmental (extrinsic)	Walking uphill
			Walking on rugged terrain

(Continued)

TABLE 26-6 *Prosthetic Gait Deviations—cont'd*

Gait Deviation	Phase of Gait	Category*	Possible Causes
Inadequate prosthetic foot clearance†	Throughout swing phases	Intrinsic	Poor hip stabilization on sound limb (pelvic drop on prosthetic side during swing)
			Lacking active anterior pelvic rotation strength and/or timing required to initiate prosthetic swing
			Lacking hip flexor strength and/or timing required to initiate prosthetic swing
			Lacking knee flexor strength and/or timing to contribute to prosthetic swing in transtibial amputation
		Prosthetic (extrinsic)	Prosthesis too long
			Transfemoral prosthetic knee with excessive friction
			Prosthetic foot/ankle too plantar flexed
		Environmental (extrinsic)	Uneven terrain with unexpected elevations
Pistoning (downward translation of prosthesis on residual limb when unloaded)	Throughout swing phases	Intrinsic	Error in sock application (too few or too many plies)
		Prosthetic (extrinsic)	Inadequate suspension
			Poor socket fit
		Environmental (extrinsic)	Muddy or wet environment can create pull on prosthesis

GAIT DEVIATIONS COMMON TO TRANSTIBIAL PROSTHETIC USERS

Gait Deviation	Phase of Gait	Category*	Possible Causes
Excessive knee flexion/knee instability	Initial contact or loading response to midstance	Intrinsic	Knee or hip flexion contracture
			Lacking knee or hip extensor strength and/or timing
			Anterior distal residual limb pain
		Prosthetic (extrinsic)	Excessive dorsiflexion of the prosthetic foot
			Excessive transtibial socket flexion (anterior tilt)
			Transtibial socket positioned anterior to prosthetic foot
			Excessive heel cushion stiffness (SACH foot)
		Environmental (extrinsic)	Prosthesis too long
			Walking down inclines
Excessive knee extension (no shock absorption)/hyperextension	Initial contact or loading response to midstance	Intrinsic	Lacking knee extensor strength and/or timing (hyperextend knee as compensation)
			Cruciate ligament insufficiency
			Lacking hip extensor strength and/or timing
			Posterior distal residual limb pain
		Prosthetic (extrinsic)	Excessive plantar flexion of prosthetic foot
			Lacking appropriate socket flexion (posterior tilt)
			Excessively soft heel cushion (SACH foot)
			Socket positioned posterior to prosthetic foot
			Prosthesis too short
		Environmental (extrinsic)	Ascending inclines/walking uphill

Gait Deviation	Phase	Category	Possible Causes
Genu valgus moment at knee	Midstance	Intrinsic	Medial collateral ligament insufficiency Coxa vara at hip Medial distal residual limb pain
		Prosthetic (extrinsic)	Excessive outset of prosthetic foot Tilt of transtibial socket in frontal plane
		Environmental (extrinsic)	Walking on uneven surfaces
Excessive genu varus moment at knee	Midstance	Intrinsic	Lateral collateral ligament insufficiency Coxa valga at hip Lateral distal residual limb pain
		Prosthetic (extrinsic)	Excessive inset of prosthetic foot Tilt of transtibial socket in the frontal plane
		Environmental (extrinsic)	Walking on uneven surfaces
Early heel rise/early knee flexion or "drop off"	Midstance to preswing	Intrinsic	Hip and/or knee flexion contracture Weakness of hip extensor muscles Anterior/distal residual limb pain
		Prosthetic (extrinsic)	Excessive dorsiflexion of prosthetic foot Socket positioned anterior to prosthetic foot Too much socket flexion (anterior tilt) The opposite prosthetic problems (plantar flexed foot, socket positioned posteriorly, not enough socket flexion) can all cause this same gait deviation if the person is working to "overcome" being forced into hyperextended knee position by the prosthesis.
		Environmental (extrinsic)	Walking down inclines or hills
Delayed heel rise/delayed knee flexion	Terminal stance to preswing	Intrinsic	Knee hyperextension as compensation for instability or weakness earlier in stance makes transition to knee flexion difficult Decreased anterior weight shift (weight through heel of prosthesis) Posterior/distal residual limb pain
		Prosthetic (extrinsic)	Excessive plantar flexion of prosthetic foot Socket positioned posterior to prosthetic foot Insufficient socket flexion Excessively long keel of prosthetic foot
		Environmental (extrinsic)	Walking up inclines/uphill

GAIT DEVIATIONS COMMON TO TRANSFEMORAL PROSTHETIC USERS

Gait Deviation	Phase	Category	Possible Causes
Excessive anterior pelvic tilt/lumbar lordosis	Initial contact through preswing	Intrinsic	Hip flexion contracture Weak hip extensors and/or abdominals Effort to shift center of gravity anteriorly for stability at prosthetic knee
		Prosthetic (extrinsic)	Insufficient flexion (posterior tilt) of socket Trochanter-knee-ankle line does not provide adequate knee stability
		Environmental (extrinsic)	Walking up inclines/uphill

(Continued)

TABLE 26-6 *Prosthetic Gait Deviations—cont'd*

Gait Deviation	Phase of Gait	Category*	Possible Causes
Abducted gait	Initial contact through preswing	Intrinsic	Hip abduction contracture Adductor tissue roll/redundant tissue Impaired balance (compensatory widened base of support)
		Prosthetic (extrinsic)	Distal femur pain Prosthesis too long Socket alignment places femur in abduction Medial socket wall too high
		Environmental (extrinsic)	Uneven terrain
Delayed prosthetic knee flexion	Terminal stance to preswing	Intrinsic	Lacking active anterior pelvic rotation strength and/or timing required to unload prosthesis Lacking hip flexor strength and/or timing required to initiate forwarding of prosthesis
		Prosthetic (extrinsic)	Trochanter-knee-ankle line providing excessive knee stability Excessive plantar flexion of prosthetic foot or excessively soft heel cushion (SACH foot)
		Environmental (extrinsic)	Walking up inclines
Medial heel whip	Preswing to early swing	Intrinsic	Loose residual limb tissue that rotates freely around femur Patient improperly dons socket in internally rotated position
		Prosthetic (extrinsic)	Prosthetic knee oriented in external/lateral direction Prosthetic foot oriented laterally Prosthetic foot toe break oriented laterally
		Environmental (extrinsic)	Rugged terrain
Lateral heel whip	Preswing to early swing	Intrinsic	Loose residual limb tissue that rotates freely around femur Patient improperly dons socket in externally rotated position
		Prosthetic (extrinsic)	Prosthetic knee oriented in internal/medial direction Prosthetic foot oriented medially Prosthetic foot toe break oriented medially
		Environmental (extrinsic)	Rugged terrain
Terminal swing impact		Intrinsic	Excessive anterior pelvic rotation and/or hip flexion to assure knee extension in swing
		Prosthetic (extrinsic)	Insufficient knee friction Extension aid too strong
		Environmental (extrinsic)	Environment demands rapid movement

*Intrinsic problems are a result of patient-related factors. Extrinsic problems are associated with prosthetic issues (alignment or fit) or environmental issues (best understood by analyzing the specific conditions or activity in which they are observed).

†Possible compensations for inadequate prosthetic swing-phase clearance include a lateral lean of the trunk toward the sound limb, vaulting on the sound limb, hip hiking or circumduction of the prosthetic limb, and, in the case of transtibial amputation, a high steppage gait.

on level surfaces, environmental causes of the problem can be ruled out. If evaluation of the static alignment of the prosthesis reveals appropriate alignment of the foot and pylon but the socket is set in excessive knee flexion, this could contribute to the problem. Thorough evaluation of the problem requires assessment of potential intrinsic causes as well. If examination reveals full, strong, active ROM at the knee and no complaints of pain, the therapist must look to the joints proximal to the problem. Assessment of the hip may reveal a hip flexion contracture that leads the person to maintain knee flexion as a compensatory strategy to maintain upright posture. When these two (excessive socket flexion and hip flexion contracture) distinct potential causes of the problem are identified, the therapist can then prioritize and address each cause. Initiation of a stretching intervention to address the ROM limitation can be started immediately, but likely will not have an immediate effect, but perhaps an effect over time. Prosthetic extrinsic causes can be modified immediately: if quality of gait improves and deviations are eliminated after realignment (typically the responsibility of the prosthetist), this suggests that alignment was the factor underlying the gait deviation. If a socket alignment adjustment does not have a significant impact, magnifies the observed gait problem, or leads to a new gait deviation, the underlying cause is likely to be an intrinsic issue needing PT intervention.

Gait Training on Alternate Surfaces

To adapt to and meet environmental demands, the individual with a prosthesis must be able to adjust his or her step length and cadence while ambulating in response to environmental conditions or circumstances. The PT program might begin with practice opportunities until the person is able to achieve a normal cadence. It might then progress to activities that demand an increased or decreased cadence, and transitional gait movements, such as sidestepping, turning, and walking backward. These skills can initially be practiced in the clinic with minimal environmental demands. They can be progressed to situations in which the environment presents a challenge, such as crossing a street in a timely manner, getting on and off an elevator or escalator, walking through a crowded corridor in a busy store, or walking to a seat in the middle of an aisle in an auditorium or theater. Successful community ambulation also requires management of many different ground surfaces, including steps, curbs, ramps, and varied terrain. In providing therapeutic practice opportunities for a person who is new to prosthetic use, the therapist considers the following important extrinsic variables:

1. Level of assistance required for safe performance;
2. The specific demands of the environment, such as depth or height of steps and curbs, or degree of slope of a ramp;
3. The need for an assistive device or railing;
4. The optimal technique for performing the task safely; and
5. The ability to superimpose an additional activity while walking or moving in the environment.

An initial goal might be to decrease the level of assistance on these alternative surfaces. This can be accomplished by simplifying one or more of the other variables of the task, such as decreasing the depth of the step/curb, allowing the use of sturdy rail versus crutch or cane, and/or allowing the sound limb to "lead" or dominate the task. As skill improves, the task demands are increased. Early skills in stair climbing are generally developed in a step-to gait pattern with the sound limb leading in ascent and the prosthetic limb leading in descent. Advanced gait training activities may instead require the patient to use the prosthetic limb first while ascending and the sound limb first while descending; these skills are necessary if the patient is to master a step-over-step pattern for stair ascent/descent. Placement of the prosthetic forefoot off of the step for step-over-step stair descent allows the forward progression of the prosthetic shank, mimicking ankle dorsiflexion required to lower the body onto the next step. In persons with transfemoral amputation using a microprocessor-controlled knee or some pneumatic/hydraulic knees step-over-step descent of stairs or curbs may be possible as the servomechanism in the knee mimics eccentrically controlled knee flexion.

Managing slopes, inclines, and ramps are challenging for persons with both transtibial and transfemoral amputation. In both situations, the relative stiffness of the ankle that will not allow for fully functional dorsiflexion or plantar flexion creates a lack of adaptability to the incline or decline surface. In the person with a transfemoral prosthesis the loss of the knee joint and accompanying quadriceps control compounds the challenge. Most people with transfemoral prosthesis navigate inclines, declines, ramps, and slopes using one of two methods (or some combination of the two). They will either shorten the step length of the involved limb to help compensate for the lack of quadriceps contraction and ankle mobility and continue with an asymmetrical step-to-step pattern or they will turn partially sideways and employ a sidestepping pattern leading with the uninvolved limb going up and prosthetic limb going down. By reorienting the axis of rotation for knee motion in this manner, there is less of a risk of the slope directly impacting knee position or stability. The method used is generally determined by patient preference and the grade of the slope. As in stair descent, if the person has a microprocessor-controlled knee, then angled surfaces are more easily managed by the computer control of the knee, especially descending.

Treadmill training has become a popular mechanism for gait training in many PT clinics, both with and without partial body-weight support. Although partial body-weight support treadmill training has not been studied with this population, treadmill training has been compared to overground gait training. Self-selected comfortable gait speed on the treadmill has been demonstrated to be significantly slower than overground walking at the same energy cost, which suggests a higher energy cost of walking on the treadmill than overground.[109] A small case series suggests that movement strategies may be altered in walking on a treadmill as compared to overground.[110] If a treadmill is to be used in training, these considerations may be important, as is special consideration to safety and guarding technique.

The ultimate goal is to provide a repertoire of strategies for the individual to choose from to respond to environmental demands. For example, when crossing the street, it is ideal if one can ascend the curb without disrupting gait cadence, even if this means leading with the prosthetic foot. The unpredictable surface of uneven terrain encountered in walking across a lawn can challenge postural responses significantly if no assistive device is used. Sidestepping is a skill needed in environments such as theaters and can be practiced when the theater is empty or when people are seated. A supervised community outing is an excellent strategy for addressing and achieving high-level ambulation goals.

Curtze demonstrated that when transtibial prosthetic users were faced with the challenge of rough terrain versus smooth surfaces, arm swing speed increased (presumably to assist with balance) and gait speed decreased slightly, but other gait parameters were not significantly altered.[111] Vrieling and colleagues concluded that specific training for prosthetic gait initiation, termination, obstacle crossing, and incline and decline management should be a purposeful component of the rehabilitation regime, as movement strategies of these functional tasks are different than those of able-bodied individuals,[82,112-115] and addressing these tasks in rehabilitation has the potential to impact safety and confidence.

Superimposing functional activities on gait during therapeutic treatment prepares patients for the daily "real-world" challenges that they are sure to encounter. The variety of functional tasks practiced by the patient may be driven by specific patient goals. Safe ambulation while carrying objects of varying weights and sizes is an important functional skill and an appropriate PT activity. The individual's specific goal may be to carry a full laundry basket down the hall or a cup of hot coffee from the kitchen to the living room. As individuals become functional prosthetic users, household tasks and leisure or work activities may guide their therapeutic needs. Safe ambulation while doing more dexterous skills, such as using a mobile phone or texting is another very likely patient goal.

High-level activities, such as running and athletic endeavors, are appropriate and attainable goals for many prosthetic users. Some individuals with amputation may wish to resume certain sports or leisure activities that they participated in prior to their amputation. With current advances in prosthetic components a person can enjoy a multitude of athletic and recreational activities. Individuals with amputation are returning to basketball, running, rock climbing, and cycling; and some are taking up these sports for the first time as prosthetic users! With the technological advances in prosthetics and the growth and exposure of the Paralympics, high-level athletics are no longer limited to a small elite group of prosthetic users. Table 26-7 describes some more advanced rehabilitation activities that can help individuals prepare to take part in their chosen activity.

Functional Activities

Prosthetic training is not just a matter of teaching an individual to ambulate but includes a variety of other functional activities, such as transfer training from a variety of surfaces, picking up objects from different levels and surfaces, kneeling, management of falls, and rising from the floor. Motor learning theory supports that prescriptive instruction on different functional tasks such as these may not be the most effective way to assist individuals in developing these skills; rather, encouraging individuals to solve their own motor problems and figure out how to best perform a given functional task allows them to "own" the task and to better generalize to other related tasks.[35] The skilled therapist will design an environment for success when introducing new skills and

---

TABLE 26-7   *Advanced Exercises and Activities for Individuals with Lower-Extremity Amputation*

Range of motion	Independent stretching of hip flexors, abductors, external rotators are top priority for all levels of amputation; for transtibial amputation, add stretching of hamstrings and quadriceps Stretching of hip extensors, adductors and internal rotators will also be part of a comprehensive stretching program; however, these muscles pose a lower risk of developing contractures
Strengthening	Resistance training of hip musculature, and in the case of transtibial amputation, quads and hamstrings Closed-chain exercises with prosthesis: step-ups, leg press, wall or ball squats, involved limb stance with opposite limb resistance exercises, multiple plane stepping exercises with Thera-Band resistance, involved limb lunges, advance to using handheld weights to increase resistance
Balance and coordination	Standing activities with balance challenges including compliant surface (foam) or mobile surface (Biomechanical Ankle Platform System [BAPS] board, rocker board); catching and throwing balls of different shapes and weights and throwing variable distances Involved single-limb stance, with stool stepping with uninvolved limb, progress to stepping on less stable surface (foam, ball); catching and throwing with staggered stance (involved limb on step/stool/ball) Dynamic challenges to upright balance: functional multidirectional walking, avoiding obstacles, picking up objects from floor, narrow base or support or beam walking, starts and stops and turns in rapid progression
Speed and agility	Figure-eight walking, progressing to running, shuttle walk to run, sprinting, obstacle course
Cardiovascular activities	Swimming, running, cycling, treadmill walking, stair climbing or stepper

*Some activities and exercises adapted from Gailey RS, Gailey AM. *Prosthetic Gait Training Program for Lower Extremity Amputees.* Miami FL: Advanced Rehabilitation Therapy, 1989.[122]

should have suggestions and ideas to offer, if needed, to the patient who is attempting new tasks. Additionally, the therapist should creatively progress the demands of the task as appropriate, always working to challenge the individual in working toward realistic and functional goals. Specific functional tasks should also be designed to address unique goals as they relate to activities of daily living, job-related activities, or recreational activities. Occupational therapists have excellent knowledge of adaptive devices and skill in environmental adaptation, thus working with these team members may prove to be very helpful.

For many people with amputation there is a strong desire or need to return to work and leisure activities. The successful return to employment of persons with amputation has been studied[18,116] and a review article by Burger and Marincek puts the return to work rate at approximately 66% for persons with lower-extremity amputation.[117] Factors found to be associated with success in returning people to work after lower-extremity amputation include younger age at the time of amputation, lower level of amputation, higher education level, good prosthetic comfort, and higher gross annual income.[18,116,117] Certainly, no individual who is motivated to return to work should be discouraged based upon not meeting these criteria. Functional tasks that simulate job or leisure activities would be very appropriate to incorporate into the PT plan of care. Couture and associates found that, while individuals with lower-extremity amputations may demonstrate a decrease in participation of leisure activities, their satisfaction with activities remains high.[118] In progressing functional, vocational, and leisure activities, the art of designing interventions that are task oriented and that help to develop the person's problem-solving skills is the goal. Challenging individual's problem solving skills and assisting them in the development of creative solutions when they are faced with new challenges is a rewarding and important component of prosthetic rehabilitation.

Outcome Assessment

Recognizing and measuring the effectiveness of PT interventions is an important component of the patient/client management model in PT.[1] The overriding goal of the rehabilitation plan of care is to return the person with amputation to the highest functional level attainable with the best possible outcome. The ICF framework reminds us that it is important to assess performance at different levels of the ICF paradigm: the body function level (impairments), the activities level (activity limitations), and the participation level (participation restrictions). Recent publications reviewing outcome measures in amputation rehabilitation at both the body function and activity levels of the ICF[119,120] concluded that there are few outcome measures in amputation rehabilitation that demonstrate strong validity within the body function domain, and while there may be more methodological studies supporting use of outcome measures in the activities domain, the responsiveness of these tools requires further study. There are no definitive guidelines as to what outcome measures should be used with persons with amputation who

are undergoing rehabilitation[119-121]; however, careful documentation of performance in each domain of the ICF can be useful. Impairment level changes that may be measured in the individual with transtibial or transfemoral amputation might include increases in ROM, strength or balance. Activity limitation level changes might include improvements in transfer ability (less assistance or improvement in varied surfaces) or ambulation (less assistance, change in assistive device or increased distance and/or speed) or activities of daily living (less assistance or improved endurance). Participation restriction level changes might include improved satisfaction with ability to carry out specific life's roles in the family or with respect to social/work/leisure activities.

Some of the outcome measures that have been used in amputation rehabilitation are amputation specific (e.g., Amputation Mobility Predictor or the Prosthetic Evaluation Questionnaire [PEQ]) and others are broader rehabilitation outcome measures that have been used with this population (e.g., Activity-Specific Balance Confidence Scale, Functional Independence Measure [FIM]). Standardized walking tests that have been used in the amputation rehabilitation research include 2-Minute Walk Test, 6-Minute Walk Test, Timed Up and Go, 10-Meter Walk, and instrumented walkways. Although normative values for individuals with amputations have not been well established for these outcome measures, there are norms available for the older adult that can be useful in monitoring change over time and assessing performance relative to age-matched peers. Gait speed has been routinely linked to function in the rehabilitation of the older adult, and gait speed has been studied repeatedly in persons with amputations. Table 26-8 demonstrates the consistent findings that self-selected gait speed is slower in persons with vascular versus traumatic amputation, and slower in persons with transfemoral versus transtibial amputation.

Minimal detectable change (MDC) scores are becoming an increasingly popular way to demonstrate change in performance in physical therapy. MDC provides the amount of change required to represent "true" change in performance, more than what would be expected in measurement error and patient variability of performance. Table 26-9 displays test-retest reliability and MDC scores of outcome measures that might be useful in monitoring progress of persons with lower limb amputation.

SUMMARY

Prosthetic rehabilitation of individuals with lower-extremity amputation is both challenging and rewarding. Early in the rehabilitation process, concerns for the integrity of the suture line and skin are a major determinant of progression of time in the prosthesis and the types of activities that are appropriate. As the residual limb matures, emphasis is placed on the quality of ambulation and on developing adaptive motor skills that enable the patient to function safely during a variety of activities under many different environmental conditions. The diversity of people with amputation requires that the therapist carefully consider individual circumstances to

TABLE 26-8   *Published Gait Speed Findings in Persons with Amputation*

Author (year), Brief Description of Participants	Vascular Amputation Etiology Mean ± Standard Deviation (if reported) (m/sec)	Nonvascular Amputation Etiology Mean ± Standard Deviation (if reported) (m/sec)	Normals/controls (if included in study) Mean ± Standard Deviation (if reported) (m/sec)
Waters (1976)[123] 13 participants with vascular TTA (mean age 63 with mean 1.4 years prosthetic use) and 13 with vascular TFA (mean age 60 with mean 1.2 years prosthetic use); 14 participants with traumatic TTA (mean age 29 with mean 9.5 years prosthetic use) and 15 with traumatic TFA (mean age 31 with mean 10 years prosthetic use); gait speed calculated from final 2 minutes of 5 minute walk	TFA 0.60 ± 0.25* TTA 0.75 ± 0.15*	TFA 0.87 ± 0.23* TTA 1.18 ± 0.17*	1.37*
Lemaire (1993)[124] 8 male participants with traumatic TTA; mean age 65; long term prosthetic use (>40 years); "walkway" length for data collection not specified	N/A	TTA 1.20 ± 0.18	N/A
Boonstra (1993)[125] 16 participants with TFA (etiology of amputation not specified; but mean age 40 suggests non-vascular etiology) and 15 controls (mean age 30); gait speed data collected in 7m of 10m walkway	N/A	TFA 1.04 ± 0.214	1.45 ± 0.175
Hermodsson (1994)[126] 24 male participants with TTA (12 with vascular amputation and 12 with traumatic amputation; mean age 67) and 12 age matched persons without amputation; gait speed data collected on 8 m walkway	TTA 0.85 ± 0.2	TTA 0.99 ± 0.2	1.42 ± 0.2
Isakov (2000)[127] 14 male participants with traumatic TTA (mean age 45, with mean prosthetic use 16.5 years); gait speed data collected on 3.6 m walkway	N/A	TTA 1.25*	N/A
Hagberg (2007)[128] 41 participants with non-vascular TFA (mean age 49) and 22 age-matched controls; gait speed calculated from 5 minute walk	N/A	TFA 1.03 ± 0.21*	1.50 ± 0.21*
Su (2008)[129] 10 participants with bilateral traumatic TTA (mean age 43) and 9 participants with bilateral vascular TTA (mean age 64); lab database of 14 control subjects (mean age 26); "walkway" length for data collection not specified	Bilateral TTA 0.69	Bilateral TTA 1.11	1.20
Hoffman (1997)[130] 5 participants with bilateral TFA for trauma or congenital malformation (mean age 22) and 5 matched controls; gait speed calculated from 6 minute walk (unclear if calculated from full 6 minutes or final 2-3 minutes)	N/A	Bilateral TF 0.82 ± 0.28 (mean speed 0.70 when single outlier eliminated)	1.04 ± 0.07

TF, Transfemoral amputation; *TT*, transtibial amputation.
*Values published in m/min and converted to m/sec for this chart.

TABLE 26-9 *Outcome Measures for Persons with Lower-Extremity Amputations*

Outcome Measure	Test-Retest Reliability Intraclass Correlation Coefficient (95% confidence interval)	Standard Error of Measurement (SEM)	Minimal Detectable Change (calculated at 90% confidence interval)$_{90}$
Two Minute Walk Test[121]	.83 (.71-.90)	14.8 m	34.3 m
Six Minute Walk Test[121]	.97 (.95-.99)	19.4 m	45.0 m
Timed Up and Go[121]	.88 (.80-.94)	1.6 sec	3.6 sec
L test[131]	.96 (.94-.97)[§]	3.0 sec	7.0 sec*
Amputee Mobility Predictor[121]	.88 (.79-.93)	1.5 U	3.4 U
Activities specific Balance Confidence (ABC) Scale[132]	.91 (.84-.95)	6.0 U	14.0 U*

*Calculated from SEM data using: $MDC_{90} = SEM \times 1.65 \times \sqrt{2}$.

§Authors focused on intra- and inter-rater reliability; inter-rater reliability listed here as it was used by authors to determine SEM.

guide prosthetic prescription and progression of the rehabilitation program. Effective education strategies and opportunities for practice of a variety of skills in a variety of settings are essential for mastery of mobility skills and optimal outcomes for rehabilitation.

REFERENCES

1. American Physical Therapy Association. Guide to physical therapist practice. 2nd ed. *Phys Ther.* 2001;81(1):9–746.
2. Sackett D, Strauss S, Richardson W, et al. *Evidence-Based Medicine: How to Practice and Teach EBM.* 2nd ed. New York, NY: Churchill Livingstone; 2000.
3. Cumming JCO, Barr S, Howe TE. Prosthetic rehabilitation for older dysvascular people following a unilateral transfemoral amputation. *Cochrane Database Syst Rev.* 2006;(4): CD005260.
4. Johannesson A, Larsson G-U, Ramstrand N, et al. Outcomes of a standardized surgical and rehabilitation program in transtibial amputation for peripheral vascular disease: a prospective cohort study. *Am J Phys Med Rehabil.* 2010;89(4):293–303.
5. Stineman M, Kwong P, Kurichi J, et al. The effectiveness of inpatient rehabilitation in the acute postoperative phase of care after transtibial or transfemoral amputation: study of an integrated health care delivery system. *Arch Phys Med Rehabil.* 2008;89(10):1863–1872.
6. Stineman M, Kwong P, Xie D, et al. Prognostic differences for functional recovery after major lower limb amputation: effects of the timing and type of inpatient rehabilitation services in the Veterans Health Administration. *PM R.* 2010;2(4):232–243.
7. WHO. *International Classification of Functioning, Disability and Health.* Geneva, Switzerland: World Health Organization; 2001.
8. Jette AM. Toward a common language for function, disability, and health. *Phys Ther.* 2006;86(5):726–734.
9. Unwin J, Kacperek L, Clarke C. A prospective study of positive adjustment to lower limb amputation. *Clin Rehabil.* 2009;23(11):1044–1050.
10. Folkman S. The case for positive emotions in the stress process. *Anxiety Stress Coping.* 2008;21(1):3–14.
11. Sansam K, Neumann V, O'Connor R, et al. Predicting walking ability following lower limb amputation: a systematic review of the literature. *J Rehabil Med.* 2009;41(8):593–603.
12. Taylor SM, Kalbaugh CA, Blackhurst DW, et al. Preoperative clinical factors predict postoperative functional outcomes after major lower limb amputation: an analysis of 553 consecutive patients. *J Vasc Surg.* 2005;42(2):227–235.
13. Geertzen JH, Martina JD, Rietman HS. Lower limb amputation. Part 2: rehabilitation—a 10 year literature review. *Prosthet Orthot Int.* 2001;25(1):14–20.
14. Raichle KA, Hanley MA, Molton I, et al. Prosthesis use in persons with lower- and upper-limb amputation. *J Rehabil Res Dev.* 2008;45(7):961–972.
15. Schoppen T, Boonstra A, Groothoff JW, et al. Physical, mental, and social predictors of functional outcome in unilateral lower-limb amputees. *Arch Phys Med Rehabil.* 2003;84(6):803–811.
16. Davies B, Datta D. Mobility outcome following unilateral lower limb amputation. *Prosthet Orthot Int.* 2003;27(3):186–190.
17. O'Neill B, Evans J. Memory and executive function predict mobility rehabilitation outcome after lower-limb amputation. *Disabil Rehabil.* 2009;31(13):1083–1091.
18. Schoppen T, Boonstra A, Groothoff JW, et al. Factors related to successful job reintegration of people with a lower limb amputation. *Arch Phys Med Rehabil.* 2001;82(10):1425–1431.
19. Graham LA, Fyfe NCM. Prosthetic rehabilitation of amputees aged over 90 is usually successful. *Disabil Rehabil.* 2002;24(13):700–701.
20. Munin MC, Espejo-De Guzman MC, Boninger ML, et al. Predictive factors for successful early prosthetic ambulation among lower-limb amputees. *J Rehabil Res Dev.* 2001;38(4):379–384.
21. Kisner C, Colby L. *Therapeutic Exercise: Foundations and Techniques (Therapeutic Exercise: Foundations & Techniques).* 5th ed. Philadelphia, PA: F.A. Davis; 2007.
22. Perry J, Burnfield J. *Gait Analysis: Normal and Pathological Function.* 2nd ed. Thorofare, NJ: Slack; 2010.
23. Rose J, Gamble JG. *Human Walking.* 3rd ed. Baltimore, MD: Lippincott Williams & Wilkins; 2005.
24. van Velzen JM, van Bennekom CAM, Polomski W, et al. Physical capacity and walking ability after lower limb amputation: a systematic review. *Clin Rehabil.* 2006;20(11):999–1016.
25. Moirenfeld I, Ayalon M, Ben-Sira D, et al. Isokinetic strength and endurance of the knee extensors and flexors in trans-tibial amputees. *Prosthet Orthot Int.* 2000;24(3):221–225.
26. Pedrinelli A, Saito M, Coelho RF, et al. Comparative study of the strength of the flexor and extensor muscles of the knee

through isokinetic evaluation in normal subjects and patients subjected to trans-tibial amputation. *Prosthet Orthot Int.* 2002;26(3):195–205.

27. Raya MA, Gailey RS, Fiebert IM, et al. Impairment variables predicting activity limitation in individuals with lower limb amputation. *Prosthet Orthot Int.* 2010;34(1):73–84.

28. Nadollek H, Brauer S, Isles R. Outcomes after trans-tibial amputation: the relationship between quiet stance ability, strength of hip abductor muscles and gait. *Physiother Res Int.* 2002;7(4):203–214.

29. Moirenfeld I, Ayalon M, Ben-Sira D, et al. Isokinetic strength and endurance of the knee extensors and flexors in trans-tibial amputees. *Prosthet Orthot Int.* 2000;24(3):221–225.

30. Powers CM, Boyd LA, Fontaine CA, et al. The influence of lower-extremity muscle force on gait characteristics in individuals with below-knee amputations secondary to vascular disease. *Phys Ther.* 1996;76(4):369–377 discussion 378–385.

31. Winter DA, Sienko SE. Biomechanics of below-knee amputee gait. *J Biomech.* 1988;21(5):361–367.

32. Snyder RD, Powers CM, Fontaine C, et al. The effect of five prosthetic feet on the gait and loading of the sound limb in dysvascular below-knee amputees. *J Rehabil Res Dev.* 1995;32(4):309–315.

33. Powers CM, Torburn L, Perry J, et al. Influence of prosthetic foot design on sound limb loading in adults with unilateral below-knee amputations. *Arch Phys Med Rehabil.* 1994;75(7):825–829.

34. Nolan L, Lees A. The functional demands on the intact limb during walking for active trans-femoral and trans-tibial amputees. *Prosthet Orthot Int.* 2000;24(2):117–125.

35. Shumway-Cook A, Woollacott MH. *Motor Control: Translating Research into Clinical Practice.* 4th ed. Philadelphia, PA: Lippincott Williams & Wilkins; 2011.

36. Miller WC, Speechley M, Deathe B. The prevalence and risk factors of falling and fear of falling among lower extremity amputees. *Arch Phys Med Rehabil.* 2001;82(8):1031–1037.

37. Miller WC, Deathe AB. A prospective study examining balance confidence among individuals with lower limb amputation. *Disabil Rehabil.* 2004;26(14–15):875–881.

38. Miller WC, Speechley M, Deathe AB. Balance confidence among people with lower-limb amputations. *Phys Ther.* 2002; 82(9):856–865.

39. Matjačić Z, Burger H. Dynamic balance training during standing in people with trans-tibial amputation: a pilot study. *Prosthet Orthot Int.* 2003;27(3):214–220.

40. Miller W, Deathe A, Speechley M, et al. The influence of falling, fear of falling, and balance confidence on prosthetic mobility and social activity among individuals with a lower extremity amputation. *Arch Phys Med Rehabil.* 2001;82(9):1238–1244.

41. Yu JC, Lam K, Nettel-Aguirre A, et al. Incidence and risk factors of falling in the postoperative lower limb amputee while on the surgical ward. *PM R.* 2010;2(10):926–934.

42. Dyer D, Bouman B, Davey M, et al. An intervention program to reduce falls for adult in-patients following major lower limb amputation. *Healthc Q.* 2008;11(3 Spec No.):117–121.

43. Rougier PR, Bergeau J. Biomechanical analysis of postural control of persons with transtibial or transfemoral amputation. *Am J Phys Med Rehabil.* 2009;88(11):896–903.

44. Nashner L. Sensory, neuromuscular, and biomechanical contributions to human balance. In: Balance: Proceedings of the APTA Forum. Alexandria VA: American Physical Therapy Association; 1989:5–12.

45. Gentile A. Skill acquisition: action, movement, and neuromotor processes. In: Carr JH, Shepherd RB, eds. *Movement Science: Foundations for Physical Therapy in Rehabilitation.* 2nd ed. Gaithersburg, MD: Aspen Publishers; 2000:111–187.

46. Chin T, Sawamura S, Fujita H, et al. Physical fitness of lower limb amputees. *Am J Phys Med Rehabil.* 2002;81(5):321–325.

47. Waters RL, Mulroy S. The energy expenditure of normal and pathologic gait. *Gait Posture.* 1999;9(3):207–231.

48. Gailey RS, Wenger MA, Raya M, et al. Energy expenditure of trans-tibial amputees during ambulation at self-selected pace. *Prosthet Orthot Int.* 1994;18(2):84–91.

49. Gonzalez EG, Corcoran PJ, Reyes RL. Energy expenditure in below-knee amputees: correlation with stump length. *Arch Phys Med Rehabil.* 1974;55(3):111–119.

50. Waters RL, Perry J, Antonelli D, et al. Energy cost of walking of amputees: the influence of level of amputation. *J Bone Joint Surg Am.* 1976;58(1):42–46.

51. Torburn L, Powers CM, Guiterrez R, et al. Energy expenditure during ambulation in dysvascular and traumatic below-knee amputees: a comparison of five prosthetic feet. *J Rehabil Res Dev.* 1995;32(2):111–119.

52. Hsu M-J, Nielsen DH, Lin-Chan S-J, et al. The effects of prosthetic foot design on physiologic measurements, self-selected walking velocity, and physical activity in people with transtibial amputation. *Arch Phys Med Rehabil.* 2006;87(1):123–129.

53. Traugh GH, Corcoran PJ, Reyes RL. Energy expenditure of ambulation in patients with above-knee amputations. *Arch Phys Med Rehabil.* 1975;56(2):67–71.

54. Gitter A, Czerniecki J, Weaver K. A reassessment of center-of-mass dynamics as a determinate of the metabolic inefficiency of above-knee amputee ambulation. *Am J Phys Med Rehabil.* 1995;74(5):332–338.

55. Gailey RS, Lawrence D, Burditt C, et al. The CAT-CAM socket and quadrilateral socket: a comparison of energy cost during ambulation. *Prosthet Orthot Int.* 1993;17(2):95–100.

56. Bussmann JB, Grootscholten EA, Stam HJ. Daily physical activity and heart rate response in people with a unilateral trans-tibial amputation for vascular disease. *Arch Phys Med Rehabil.* 2004;85(2):240–244.

57. Ward KH, Meyers MC. Exercise performance of lower-extremity amputees. *Sports Med.* 1995;20(4):207–214.

58. Chin T, Sawamura S, Fujita H, et al. %VO2max as an indicator of prosthetic rehabilitation outcome after dysvascular amputation. *Prosthet Orthot Int.* 2002;26(1):44–49.

59. Hamamura S, Chin T, Kuroda R, et al. Factors affecting prosthetic rehabilitation outcomes in amputees of age 60 years and over. *J Int Med Res.* 2009;37(6):1921–1927.

60. Brooks D, Hunter JP, Parsons J, et al. Reliability of the two-minute walk test in individuals with transtibial amputation. *Arch Phys Med Rehabil.* 2002;83(11):1562–1565.

61. Brooks D, Parsons J, Hunter JP, et al. The 2-minute walk test as a measure of functional improvement in persons with lower limb amputation. *Arch Phys Med Rehabil.* 2001;82(10):1478–1483.

62. Smith DG, McFarland LV, Sangeorzan BJ, et al. Postoperative dressing and management strategies for transtibial amputations: a critical review. *J Rehabil Res Dev.* 2003;40(3):213–224.

63. Nawijn SE, van der Linde H, Emmelot CH, et al. Stump management after trans-tibial amputation: a systematic review. *Prosthet Orthot Int.* 2005;29(1):13–26.

64. van Velzen AD, Nederhand MJ, Emmelot CH, et al. Early treatment of trans-tibial amputees: retrospective analysis of early fitting and elastic bandaging. *Prosthet Orthot Int.* 2005;29(1):3–12.

65. Taylor L, Cavenett S, Stepien JM, et al. Removable rigid dressings: a retrospective case-note audit to determine the validity of post-amputation application. *Prosthet Orthot Int.* 2008;32(2):223–230.

66. Friedmann LW. *The Surgical Rehabilitation of the Amputee.* Springfield, IL: Charles C. Thomas Publisher; 1978.

67. Smith D, Michael J, Bowker J. *Atlas of Amputations and Limb Deficiencies: Surgical, Prosthetic, and Rehabilitation Principles.* 3rd ed. Rosemont, IL: American Academy of Orthopaedic Surgeons; 2004.

68. Kosasih JB, Silver-Thorn MB. Sensory changes in adults with unilateral transtibial amputation. *J Rehabil Res Dev.* 1998;35(1):85–90.

69. Kempczinski RF. *The Ischemic Leg.* Chicago, IL: Year Book Medical Publishers; 1985.

70. Casale R, Alaa L, Mallick M, et al. Phantom limb related phenomena and their rehabilitation after lower limb amputation. *Eur J Phys Rehabil Med.* 2009;45(4):559–566.

71. Melzack R. Phantom limbs. *Sci Am.* 1992;266(4):120–126.

72. Manchikanti L, Singh V. Managing phantom pain. *Pain Physician.* 2004;7(3):365–375.

73. Chapman S. Pain management in patients following limb amputation. *Nurs Stand.* 2011;25(19):35–40.

74. Nikolajsen L, Jensen TS. Phantom limb pain. *Br J Anaesth.* 2001;87(1):107–116.

75. Ephraim PL, Wegener ST, MacKenzie EJ, et al. Phantom pain, residual limb pain, and back pain in amputees: results of a national survey. *Arch Phys Med Rehabil.* 2005;86(10):1910–1919.

76. Bosmans JC, Geertzen JHB, Post WJ, et al. Factors associated with phantom limb pain: a 3 1/2 -year prospective study. *Clin Rehabil.* 2010;24(5):444–453.

77. Davidson JH, Khor KE, Jones LE. A cross-sectional study of post-amputation pain in upper and lower limb amputees, experience of a tertiary referral amputee clinic. *Disabil Rehabil.* 2010;32(22):1855–1862.

78. Hanley MA, Jensen MP, Smith DG, et al. Preamputation pain and acute pain predict chronic pain after lower extremity amputation. *J Pain.* 2007;8(2):102–109.

79. Mulvey MR, Bagnall A-M, Johnson MI, et al. Transcutaneous electrical nerve stimulation (TENS) for phantom pain and stump pain following amputation in adults. *Cochrane Database Syst Rev.* 2010;(5): CD007264.

80. Ulger O, Topuz S, Bayramlar K, et al. Effectiveness of phantom exercises for phantom limb pain: a pilot study. *J Rehabil Med.* 2009;41(7):582–584.

81. Izumi Y, Satterfield K, Lee S, et al. Risk of reamputation in diabetic patients stratified by limb and level of amputation: a 10-year observation. *Diabetes Care.* 2006;29(3):566–570.

82. Vrieling AH, van Keeken HG, Schoppen T, et al. Gait initiation in lower limb amputees. *Gait Posture.* 2008;27(3):423–430.

83. Nolan L, Wit A, Dudziñski K, et al. Adjustments in gait symmetry with walking speed in trans-femoral and trans-tibial amputees. *Gait Posture.* 2003;17(2):142–151.

84. Reiber G, Boyko E, Smith D. Lower extremity foot ulcers and amputations in diabetes. In: Harris MI, Cowie CC, Stern MP, et al.*Diabetes in America.* 2nd ed.Bethesda, MD: National Institutes of Health; 1995.

85. Kalbaugh CA, Taylor SM, Kalbaugh BA, et al. Does obesity predict functional outcome in the dysvascular amputee? *Am Surg.* 2006;72(8):707–712; discussion 712–713.

86. Fortington LV, Rommers GM, Geertzen JH, et al. Mobility in elderly people with a lower limb amputation: a systematic review. *J Am Med Dir Assoc..* 2011. Mar 15. [Epub ahead of print] http://www.ncbi.nlm.nih.gov/pubmed/21450239. Accessed 05.04.11.

87. Green GV, Short K, Easley M. Transtibial amputation. Prosthetic use and functional outcome. *Foot Ankle Clin.* 2001;6(2):315–327.

88. Hafner BJ, Smith DG. Differences in function and safety between Medicare Functional Classification Level-2 and -3 transfemoral amputees and influence of prosthetic knee joint control. *J Rehabil Res Dev.* 2009;46(3):417–433.

89. Kahle JT, Highsmith MJ, Hubbard SL. Comparison of non-microprocessor knee mechanism versus C-Leg on Prosthesis Evaluation Questionnaire, stumbles, falls, walking tests, stair descent, and knee preference. *J Rehabil Res Dev.* 2008;45(1):1–14.

90. Asano M, Rushton P, Miller W, et al. Predictors of quality of life among individuals who have a lower limb amputation. *Prosthet Orthot Int.* 2008;32(2):231–243.

91. Legro MW, Reiber G, del Aguila M, et al. Issues of importance reported by persons with lower limb amputations and prostheses. *J Rehabil Res Dev.* 1999;36(3):155–163.

92. Dudek NL, Marks MB, Marshall SC, et al. Dermatologic conditions associated with use of a lower-extremity prosthesis. *Arch Phys Med Rehabil.* 2005;86(4):659–663.

93. Meulenbelt HE, Geertzen JH, Jonkman MF, et al. Skin problems of the stump in lower limb amputees: 1. A clinical study. *Acta Derm Venereol.* 2011;91(2):173–177. http://www.ncbi. nlm.nih.gov/pubmed/21290085 Accessed 04.0311.

94. Meulenbelt HE, Geertzen JH, Jonkman MF, et al. Determinants of skin problems of the stump in lower-limb amputees. *Arch Phys Med Rehabil.* 2009;90(1):74–81.

95. Baars ECT, Dijkstra PU, Geertzen JHB. Skin problems of the stump and hand function in lower limb amputees: A historic cohort study. *Prosthet Orthot Int.* 2008;32(2):179–185.

96. Meulenbelt HE, Geertzen JH, Jonkman MF, et al. Skin problems of the stump in lower-limb amputees: 2. Influence on functioning in daily life. *Acta Derm Venereol.* 2011;91(2):178–182.

97. Bullock BL. *Pathophysiology: Adaptations and Alterations in Function.* Philadelphia, PA: JB Lippincott; 1996.

98. New York University Medical Center. *Lower-Limb Prosthetics.* New York, NY: New York University Medical Center; 1983.

99. Goujon-Pillet H, Sapin E, Fodé P, et al. Three-dimensional motions of trunk and pelvis during transfemoral amputee gait. *Arch Phys Med Rehabil.* 2008;89(1):87–94.

100. Malouin F, Richards CL. Mental practice for relearning locomotor skills. *Phys Ther.* 2010;90(2):240–251.

101. Isakov E, Keren O, Benjuya N. Trans-tibial amputee gait: time-distance parameters and EMG activity. *Prosthet Orthot Int.* 2000;24(3):216–220.

102. Su P-F, Gard SA, Lipschutz RD, et al. Differences in gait characteristics between persons with bilateral transtibial amputations, due to peripheral vascular disease and trauma, and able-bodied ambulators. *Arch Phys Med Rehabil.* 2008;89(7):1386–1394.

103. Soares ASO de C, Yamaguti EY, Mochizuki L, et al. Biomechanical parameters of gait among transtibial amputees: a review. *Sao Paulo Med J.* 2009;127(5):302–309.

104. Sadeghi H, Allard P, Duhaime PM. Muscle power compensatory mechanisms in below-knee amputee gait. *Am J Phys Med Rehabil.* 2001;80(1):25–32.

105. Highsmith MJ, Kahle JT, Bongiorni DR, et al. Safety, energy efficiency, and cost efficacy of the C-Leg for transfemoral amputees: A review of the literature. *Prosthet Orthot Int.* 2010;34(4):362–377.

106. Kaufman KR, Levine JA, Brey RH, et al. Gait and balance of transfemoral amputees using passive mechanical and microprocessor-controlled prosthetic knees. *Gait Posture.* 2007;26(4):489–493.

107. Schmalz T, Blumentritt S, Jarasch R. Energy expenditure and biomechanical characteristics of lower limb amputee gait: the influence of prosthetic alignment and different prosthetic components. *Gait Posture.* 2002;16(3):255–263.

108. Graham LE, Datta D, Heller B, et al. A comparative study of oxygen consumption for conventional and energy-storing prosthetic feet in transfemoral amputees. *Clin Rehabil.* 2008;22(10–11):896–901.

109. Traballesi M, Porcacchia P, Averna T, et al. Energy cost of walking measurements in subjects with lower limb amputations: a comparison study between floor and treadmill test. *Gait Posture.* 2008;27(1):70–75.

110. Button C, Moyle S, Davids K. Comparison of below-knee amputee gait performed overground and on a motorized treadmill. *Adapt Phys Activ Q.* 2010;27(2):96–112.

111. Curtze C, Hof AL, Postema K, et al. Over rough and smooth: amputee gait on an irregular surface. *Gait Posture.* 2011;33(2):292–296.

112. Vrieling AH, van Keeken HG, Schoppen T, et al. Gait adjustments in obstacle crossing, gait initiation and gait termination after a recent lower limb amputation. *Clin Rehabil.* 2009;23(7):659–671.

113. Vrieling AH, van Keeken HG, Schoppen T, et al. Uphill and downhill walking in unilateral lower limb amputees. *Gait Posture.* 2008;28(2):235–242.

114. Vrieling AH, van Keeken HG, Schoppen T, et al. Obstacle crossing in lower limb amputees. *Gait Posture.* 2007;26(4):587–594.

115. Vrieling AH, van Keeken HG, Schoppen T, et al. Gait termination in lower limb amputees. *Gait Posture.* 2008;27(1):82–90.

116. Hebert J, Ashworth N. Predictors of return to work following traumatic work-related lower extremity amputation. *Disabil Rehabil.* 2006;28(10):613–618.

117. Burger H, Marincek C. Return to work after lower limb amputation. *Disabil Rehabil.* 2007;29(17):1323–1329.

118. Couture M, Caron C, Desrosiers J. Leisure activities following a lower limb amputation. *Disabil Rehabil.* 2010;32(1):57–64.

119. Hebert J, Wolfe D, Miller W, et al. Outcome measures in amputation rehabilitation: ICF body functions. *Disabil Rehabil.* 2009;31(19):1541–1554.

120. Deathe A, Wolfe D, Devlin M, et al. Selection of outcome measures in lower extremity amputation rehabilitation: ICF activities. *Disabil Rehabil.* 2009;31(18):1455–1473.

121. Resnik L, Borgia M. Reliability of outcome measures for people with lower-limb amputations: distinguishing true change from statistical error. *Phys Ther.* 2011;91(4):555–565. http://www.ncbi.nlm.nih.gov/pubmed/21310896. Accessed 09.03.11.

122. Gailey RS, Gailey AM. *Prosthetic Gait Training Program for Lower Extremity Amputees.* Miami FL: Advanced Rehabilitation Therapy Incorporated; 1989.

123. Waters RL, Perry J, Antonelli D, et al. Energy cost of walking of amputees: the influence of level of amputation. *J Bone Joint Surg Am.* 1976;58(1):42–46.

124. Lemaire ED, Fisher FR, Robertson DG. Gait patterns of elderly men with trans-tibial amputations. *Prosthet Orthot Int.* 1993;17(1):27–37.

125. Boonstra AM, Schrama J, Fidler V, et al. The gait of unilateral transfemoral amputees. *Scand J Rehabil Med.* 1994;26(4):217–223.

126. Hermodsson Y, Ekdahl C, Persson BM, et al. Gait in male trans-tibial amputees: a comparative study with healthy subjects in relation to walking speed. *Prosthet Orthot Int.* 1994;18(2):68–77.

127. Isakov E, Keren O, Benjuya N. Trans-tibial amputee gait: time-distance parameters and EMG activity. *Prosthet Orthot Int.* 2000;24(3):216–220.

128. Hagberg K, Häggström E, Brånemark R. Physiological cost index (PCI) and walking performance in individuals with transfemoral prostheses compared to healthy controls. *Disabil Rehabil.* 2007;29(8):643–649.

129. Su P-F, Gard SA, Lipschutz RD, et al. Differences in gait characteristics between persons with bilateral transtibial amputations, due to peripheral vascular disease and trauma, and able-bodied ambulators. *Arch Phys Med Rehabil.* 2008;89(7):1386–1394.

130. Hoffman MD, Sheldahl LM, Buley KJ, et al. Physiological comparison of walking among bilateral above-knee amputee and able-bodied subjects, and a model to account for the differences in metabolic cost. *Arch Phys Med Rehabil.* 1997;78(4):385–392.

131. Deathe AB, Miller WC. The L test of functional mobility: measurement properties of a modified version of the timed "up & go" test designed for people with lower-limb amputations. *Phys Ther.* 2005;85(7):626–635.

132. Miller WC, Deathe AB, Speechley M. Psychometric properties of the Activities-specific Balance Confidence Scale among individuals with a lower-limb amputation. *Arch Phys Med Rehabil.* 2003;84(5):656–661.

27

Advanced Rehabilitation for People with Microprocessor Knee Prostheses

Christopher Kevin Wong and Joan E. Edelstein

LEARNING OBJECTIVES

On completion of this chapter, the reader will be able to do the following:

1. Provide a chronology for the development of prosthetics research leading to the microprocessor knee prostheses.
2. Compare knee control function for a variety of microprocessor knee prostheses.
3. Explain functional ambulation skills and activities of daily living that are challenging for users of transfemoral prosthesis or higher that do not have microprocessor knee.
4. Apply Medicare K-level requirements when considering microprocessor knee prostheses for patients.
5. Explain the similarities and differences of microprocessor knee prostheses.
6. Describe how a microprocessor knee unit can benefit the user during gait, stair climbing and ramp negotiation, transfers, and stumbling.
7. Discuss prosthetic and training solutions for common gait deviations which microprocessor knee prostheses can significantly benefit.
8. Evaluate a variety of physical therapy interventions that can be applied when rehabilitating individuals with transfemoral amputation who use microprocessor knee prosthesis.
9. Describe the evidence to support use of microprocessor knee prostheses.

HISTORICAL DEVELOPMENT

Since Ambroise Parè's sixteenth century articulated transfemoral prosthesis,[1] surgeons, patients, and engineers have attempted to imitate the function of the human leg. In the United States, scientific prosthetics development began in 1945 with the establishment of the Prosthetic Appliance Service of the Veterans Administration and the research and development program of the National Academy of Sciences.[2] Early versions of sophisticated knee units include the 1942 Filippi hydraulic stance control unit[3] and the hydraulic swing and stance control knee unit patented by engineer Hans Mauch and radiologist Ulrich Henschke in 1949.[4] The Veterans Administration approved the first hydraulic swing-phase control mechanism in 1962; the component linked a hydraulic knee unit to a single-axis ankle.[5] This chapter discusses the unique features of microprocessor knee (MPK) prostheses that are increasingly used, and provides prosthetic and training solutions for persons with common gait deviations that can be reduced by using a MPK.

Research beginning in the 1970s led to the 1993 introduction by Blatchford (Basingstoke, England) of the first commercially available microprocessor-controlled prosthetic knee: the Endolite Intelligent Prosthesis. The Endolite Intelligent Prosthesis required a wired connection to program the variable swing-phase control. The Adaptive Prosthesis followed in 1998, allowing wireless programming and featuring an onboard processor that controlled adjustment of the hybrid pneumatic/hydraulic MPK; Endolite Intelligent Prosthesis (sixth generation) MPK is the Orion (Figure 27-1).[6] Since introduction of the Endolite Intelligent Prosthesis, at least six other companies have joined the marketplace in offering MPK prostheses. Otto Bock (Duderstadt, Germany) initiated the hydraulic C-Leg MPK in 1997.[2,7-10] Other manufacturers presented comparable units. Össur (Reykjavik, Iceland) launched the Rheo Knee in 2006 and the Power Knee in 2009.[11] Freedom Innovations (Irvine, CA) recently introduced the Plié MPK unit.[12] The Nabtesco Corporation of Japan also offers MPK units through the Swedish distributor, Centri AB.[13]

OVERVIEW OF NONMICROPROCESSOR KNEE PROSTHESES

After amputation that includes the knee joint, people face significantly more difficulty in mobility tasks than those whose knees remain intact. Without the knee and the muscles that control it, the prosthesis user must control knee flexion in new ways to avoid falling. The simplest way to remain stable is to use a mechanically locked knee unit. Some older first-time prosthesis users prefer the security of a locked knee to one that is unlocked.[14] If the knee is not locked, knee stability can be maintained simply through alignment of the joint

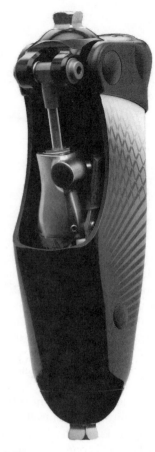

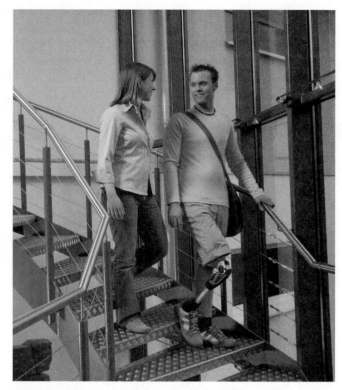

FIGURE 27-2 Prosthetic and sound foot placement for stair descent. (Courtesy Otto Bock Health Care, www.ottobockus.com.)

FIGURE 27-1 Orion: a pneumatic microprocessor knee unit with stance and swing-phase control. (Courtesy Endolite, www.endolite.com.)

axes combined with significant residual limb gluteal muscle power. However, many prosthesis users who wish to walk in the community with additional stability benefit from more sophisticated non-MPK units.

Weight-activated friction brake knees are non-MPK units that control knee flexion upon initial loading and through most of stance phase. Weight bearing on the prosthesis activates strong braking resistance to knee flexion even when the knee is slightly bent. If the knee is flexed more than 20 degrees, no flexion resistance is provided making stair descent or stumble recovery difficult. Hydraulic non-MPK units provide sufficient resistance to weight bearing knee flexion beyond 20 degrees to allow step-over-step descent of stairs or curbs (Figure 27-2).[15] Hydraulic or pneumatic knees also provide variable levels of resistance to knee flexion during swing phase to minimize asymmetry between sound and prosthetic knee flexion at different gait speeds.

The two different resistance modes in hydraulic knees make these units ideal for those who are able to move at different speeds and traverse a variety of surfaces such as encountered in the community. However, these knees require specific motions during gait to provide the mechanical cue, such as a firm knee hyperextension force of at least 0.1 second in terminal stance phase,[11] to switch between the two different

levels of resistance required for weight-bearing stance phase and non–weight-bearing swing phase. If a sufficient cue is not achieved at the end of the swing phase, the appropriate resistance to support the weight-bearing limb will not be applied and a fall may occur. Alternatively, if the cue is not achieved at the end of stance phase, the leg may remain stiff in the swing phase, leading to an awkward gait pattern. As a result, the user must be careful to move with adequate hip action to prevent stumbles.

Users of non-MPK prostheses must use compensatory techniques for other activities. For instance, to go from sit-to-stand, the wearer generally places more weight on the sound limb and depends on that leg, and arms as needed, to raise themselves to standing. When sitting, unweighting the prosthetic leg is required in order for the knee to bend easily. Such basic activities place extra stress on the sound limb, which can contribute to the frequent reporting of low back and sound limb pain among prosthesis users.[16] Another example is descending slopes, a notoriously difficult activity for users of transfemoral prostheses. A step length matching that of the sound limb often results in a prosthetic knee angle that exceeds the approximately 20-degree safety range of a hydraulic stance phase control or a weight-activated knee unit. Thus, most prosthesis users learn to take very short steps. Finally, ascending stairs step-over-step is very difficult for any transfemoral prosthesis user, generally requiring use of a banister if the step is of standard height.

INTRODUCTION TO MICROPROCESSOR KNEE PROSTHESES

Unlike non-MPK prostheses that use alignment, locked knees, or weight-activated friction brakes, and hydraulic or pneumatic mechanisms, MPK prostheses incorporate an onboard microprocessor to compute data from various electronic sensors and provide real-time adjustments during the user's activities. The computer's processor enables rapid adjustments in knee resistance during both swing and stance phases control, usually with pneumatic or hydraulic components. The speed of current microprocessors allows data sampling from sensors in the MPKs at speeds of up to 50 times per second[17] to provide more responsiveness to individual movements than can be offered by non-MPK pneumatic and hydraulic knee prostheses. Based on input from various combinations of joint position and motion sensors, pressure sensors, and gyroscopes, proprietary software algorithms determine the phase of gait or function of the leg to provide real-time adjustment of resistance within the MPK unit to facilitate the optimal walking pattern.

The prosthetist performs the initial MPK calibration for the wearer's typical use patterns with software specific to the MPK manufacturer. Calibration requires that the wearer walk at slow, normal, and fast speeds for approximately 12 m (40 ft). Then the wearer negotiates stairs and ramps so that the appropriate knee resistance levels can be set. Additional adjustments may be necessary as the user bears more weight on the prosthesis and participates in more activities.

MPKs offer a variety of swing and stance phase control functions, including resisted swing-phase knee extension and knee flexion, resisted stance-phase knee flexion, powered stance-phase knee extension, locked or unlocked (free) knee motions, and various combinations for specific functional applications. MPKs offer stance-phase knee resistance within a 0- to 35-degree range (Table 27-1).[6]

As with the non-MPK units that have both swing- and stance-phase control functions, the MPK must switch between different functions. MPK units receive data from various sensors, such as plantar pressure on different foot regions, that indicate the portion of stance phase, especially initial loading. Some MPKs, like the C-Leg and the Rheo Knee, allow controlled knee flexion upon initial loading to reduce vertical shock impact. Angle and velocity of the knee indicate the oncoming of terminal swing. A MPK like the Genium has

a gyroscope, which senses the direction of movement and determines when the user lifts the leg to ascend stairs or to step over an obstacle (Figure 27-3).

In general, manufacturers suggest that MPKs with stance-phase control be prescribed for Medicare K2- and K3-level users (Table 27-2) whereas MPKs with both stance- and swing phase-control be prescribed for K3- and K4-level users who will utilize different walking speeds.[11,17] However, all currently available MPKs are designed for low to moderate impact activities (Table 27-3).[11,17] Processor and actuator

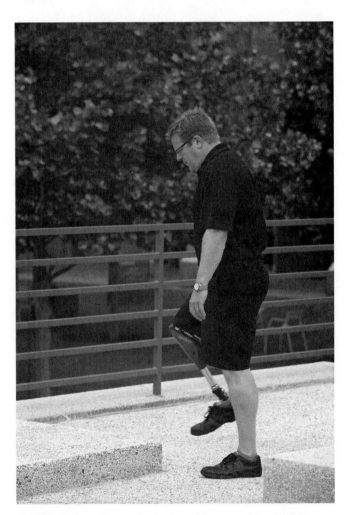

FIGURE 27-3 Genium microprocessor knee with gyroscope, accelerometer, and angle sensors responds to movement in all directions. (Courtesy Otto Bock Health Care, www.ottobockus.com.)

TABLE 27-1 *Microprocessor Knee Prostheses Offer a Variety of Knee Control Functions*

| Gait-Phase Controlled | Manufacturer | | | | |
	Endolite	Freedom Innovations	Nabtesco	Otto Bock	Össur
Swing only	Smart IP		Intelligent Hybrid		
Stance only				Compact	
Swing and stance	Smart Adapt, Orion	Plie 2.0		C-Leg, Genium	Rheo Knee, Power Knee
Stair ascent (powered assist)					Power Knee

TABLE 27-2   *Medicare Functional Levels for People with Unilateral Transtibial and Transfemoral Amputation*

Level	Typical User Profile	Functional Abilities with Prosthesis
K1	Household ambulator	Has ability or potential to transfer and ambulate on level surfaces at slow speeds with fixed cadence. Time and distance severely limited.
K2	Limited community ambulator	Has ability or potential to ambulate and traverse common environmental barriers such as curbs, stairs, or uneven surfaces. Time and distance often limited.
K3	Community ambulator	Has ability or potential to ambulate at faster speeds with variable cadence and traverse most environmental barriers. Can undertake vocational, therapeutic, or exercise activity that demands use beyond ambulation. Time and distance still somewhat limited.
K4	Active user (child, active adult, athlete)	Has the ability or potential for prosthetic use that exceeds ambulation, including high impact, torsion, or energy levels common to sport. Time and distance essentially unlimited.

speeds are insufficient for high-speed activities and, as with all electronic devices, MPKs are vulnerable to overheating. Prosthesis users at the K4 level who engage in high impact activities, such as running or jumping, are more suited to hydraulic non-MPK designs like the Mauch Knee.

In addition to different combinations of swing- and stance-phase control, the commercially available MPKs have other options. For instance, the Plie 2.0 knee utilizes a pneumatic mechanism that the user pumps regularly to adjust resistance levels (Figure 27-4).[12] The pneumatic hybrid is available with both single and multiaxis knee joints that allow up to 160 degrees of flexion.[13] MPKs, however, generally provide a knee flexion range from 120 to 140 degrees, which exceeds that of most non-MPKs like the Mauch Knee. MPKs generally dampen knee extension to minimize terminal knee extension impact as well as to adjust the arc of shank swing to the speed of walking, but not early swing phase knee flexion. The C-Leg and Genium have dampened swing phase knee flexion to approximate the 60 degrees normal in level walking.[17,18] The Power Knee offers powered robotic assistance in sit-to-stand and stair ascent functions (Figure 27-5).[11]

All MPKs have some common characteristics. Although technical specifications of individual MPKs vary, all are powered by batteries that must be charged 4 to 14 hours for use limited in general to 1 to 5 days. The Power Knee, the only MPK to provide robotic assistance to movement, maintains its charge for only 12 hours.[11] Depending on use intensity, the Smart Adaptive MPK can maintain charge for up to 14 days.[6] The battery and hydraulic mechanisms do not function in all environments and are limited to operating temperatures ranging from -10° C (14° F) to 60° C (140° F) for the C-Leg,[17] sufficient for most people's requirements. As with other electronic devices, such as laptop computers, MPKs are also vulnerable to sand, debris, and water—especially salt water. The most water-resistant MPK, the Plie knee, is purported to be able to withstand occasional submersion in water up to 0.5 m (1.64 ft) in depth (see Figure 27-4).

Electronic signals, such as repeated beeps or vibrations, warn the user of impending shutdown because of computer or hydraulic overload or other malfunction, as well as changes in mode of function. The wearer must learn the meaning of the different signals to assure proper use. Upon shutdown, MPK will default to various states. Most default to swing phase control, which allows knee bending in swing phase but can also permit collapse in stance phase. The C-Leg and Power Knee default to stance-phase resistance, which causes the knee to lock and protects against falls if the microprocessor receives abnormal input such as can occur during a stumble or step onto an obstacle or uneven surface. A stance-phase resistance default setting, however, requires circumduction, hip hiking, or vaulting in swing phase until normal MPK function is restored.

The battery and other electronic components add weight, causing MPKs to be heavier than hydraulic non-MPK units. Weights for MPK units range from 1145 g (2.5 lb) for the C-Leg to 3200 g (7.1 lb) for the more complicated Power Knee; compared to the hydraulic non-MPK units such as the SR95[17] at 360 g (12.6 oz) or the Mauch knee which weighs 1140 g (2.5 lb).[11] While the Mauch Knee Plus can accommodate high impact use by users weighing to 166 kg (366 lb),[11] MPKs are generally designed for low to moderate impact use by individuals who weigh less than 125 kg (275.6 lb). The newly available Genium can support people up to 150 kg (330.7 lb).[17] Typical MPK units cost $16,000 to $18,000, with total cost of the prosthesis as much as $50,000 in 2004,[19] with 3-year warranties standard; Otto Bock offers an extended 6-year warranty for the Genium.[17] Cost can be two to three times the cost of a non-MPK unit. However, in a cost analysis of Dutch transfemoral prosthetic users, total intervention costs were only 23% more because associated rehabilitation expense was less. When patient and family expenses, such as housekeeping and decreased work productivity, were included, the cost to MPK users was roughly half of non-MPK users although the two groups both averaged 47 years of age and had similar work profiles and amputation etiologies.[20]

Any MPK can be integrated with many other prosthetic components. Endoskeletal construction is typically employed to save weight and provide space for componentry. Each company recommends integrating its MPK with an energy-storing foot selected from its catalog. The difference between feet may not make a substantial difference[21] and can be individually determined based on the judgment of the prosthetist, patient, physician, and therapist.

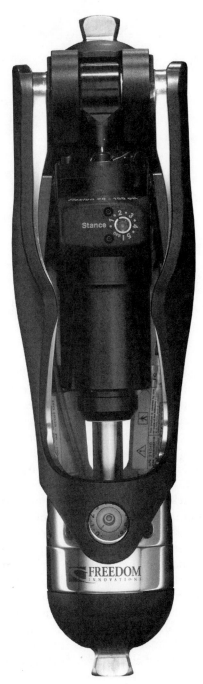

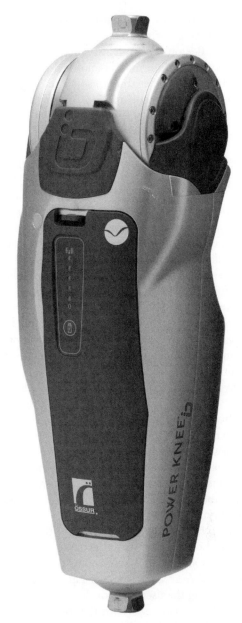

FIGURE 27-5 Power Knee provides assisted knee extension. (Courtesy Össur Americas, www.ossur.com.)

FIGURE 27-4 Plie 2.0, a water-resistant pneumatic microprocessor knee unit. (Courtesy Freedom Innovations LLC, www.freedom-innovations.com.)

When integrating a MPK into a hip disarticulation prosthesis, some shank, feet, or hip joint units may provide functional benefits. Particularly useful are shank devices that provide transverse plane rotation, such as the Delta Twist, which can dampen over 20 degrees of rotation and can be combined with the C-Leg. The Ceterus foot,[11] for instance, also may help provide transverse plane rotation accentuated by the longer step lengths that sometimes result when using a MPK.[22] The Helix3D hip joint provides transverse plane rotation unlike other prosthetic hip joints.

MICROPROCESSOR KNEE PROSTHESES CONTROL MECHANISMS

The MPK works by sensors transmitting input to the microprocessor, which converts the data so that the appropriate output can be provided. In some cases, artificial intelligence allows the MPK to adapt to the user's movements in different activities. Two types of mechanisms provide input to the MPK namely, computational and interactive.[23]

Computational control mechanisms use sensors to detect movement and forces and send this information to a computer that processes the information and adjusts the resistance provided by the knee mechanism to accommodate for variations determined by the data. For instance, 70% body weight borne through the weight-bearing foot will be interpreted as occurring during stance phase leading to full resistance to knee flexion. This intrinsic mechanism is so-called because the sensory information and decision-making process is intrinsic to the knee unit sensors and microprocessor, which prompts an automatic reaction. It is the most common form of input mechanism.

Interactive control mechanisms, more common to upper-limb myoelectric prostheses, integrate the user's conscious initiation. Pattern recognition or electromyographic signal sensors detect the movement initiation. Upper-limb prosthetic function is distinctly different from lower-limb function. Arm movement is modulated primarily by the cognitively variable central nervous system to perform complex acts like grasping a variety of foods. In the lower-limb, most everyday function involves walking, which is modulated by the spinal cord and central pattern generators without many fine motor variations.

While the prosthesis user would not want to think about each of the average 6000 steps taken each day,[24] the future may bring interactive control of the prosthesis through myoelectric input. Preliminary experiments with people with lower-limb amputations using myoelectric technology in a virtual environment demonstrate that electrodes imbedded in muscles of the residual lower limb can be used to facilitate specific movements, as is typically done in myoelectric upper-limb prostheses. However, the time to complete simple tasks in the experiments, like extending and relaxing the knee in sitting, exceeded 1.5 seconds.[25] Perhaps myoelectrically driven intrinsic control mechanisms may eventually assist slow and deliberate non–weight-bearing tasks for people with leg amputation.

Currently, the Proprio foot, outfitted with an accelerometer, joint sensor, and motorized actuator, can plantar and dorsiflex the foot in non–weight-bearing positions upon receiving the correct cues (by heel tap or wireless remote control), enabling the user to sit or don trousers more easily (Figure 27-6). Other functions for the transfemoral prosthesis user, such as rotating the leg to place it on the knee to don shoes and socks, would be the kind of action such an interactive control system may perform in the future.[11]

Once the sensor data has been input and the microprocessor has determined what function is occurring, the MPK can provide two types of knee movement output: resistance or powered assistance. Most commonly, MPKs resist movement, which can be thought of as an eccentric force. Most knee function in gait is eccentric, whether resisting knee flexion in early stance or resisting knee extension in terminal swing phase. By providing the appropriate amount of resistance through the required range of motion, the MPK can assist the wearer to walk at varied speeds and descend stairs and ramps with less difficulty.

Powered MPKs can also assist movement, comparable to a concentric force. Such a force can be helpful in ascending stairs and rising from a chair, especially for those with bilateral limb loss or a weak intact limb. Although powered assistance provides the potential for the most complete replication

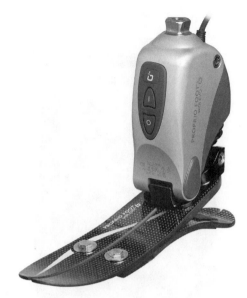

FIGURE 27-6 Proprio foot. (Courtesy Össur Americas, www.ossur.com.)

of normal leg function, this potential is limited by actuator technology and electromechanical speed. For instance, the human knee moves more than 300 degrees per second in walking[26] and can increase to over 600 degrees per second in running.[27] It would be difficult for actuators that have activation times only as fast as 10 milliseconds[12] to create such high velocities, without overheating when maximum speeds are maintained.

Artificial intelligence is used in MPKs to varying degrees. Standard setup includes initial programmed learning while the wearer walks with the MPK at various speeds and negotiates ramps and stairs. Setup programming prepares the prosthesis for normal function but may not provide sufficient information for the knee to respond appropriately during unexpected events, such as stepping into a divot. Although technically possible, most MPKs do not use real-time accommodation, as it is unnecessary for ordinary use. For instance, even unexpected situations such as stumbles cause predictable inputs that are anticipated by default settings.

COMMON MOBILITY PROBLEMS AND POTENTIAL SOLUTIONS

Despite sophisticated technology, prosthesis users face a variety of problems in moving around the community. Some problems can be significantly improved by MPK use, although users who are transitioning from non-MPK prostheses may have developed habits that must be unlearned. To illustrate how a MPK unit can benefit the user, common problems in gait, stair and ramp negotiation, transfers, and stumbling are presented.

Despite rigorous training and dedicated practice, some gait deviations persist.[15,28] The most common deviations that MPKs can significantly benefit are discussed here with prosthetic and training solutions.

Stance Phase

Loading Response

A common stance-phase deviation is decreased prosthetic knee flexion during loading response. Decreased knee flexion develops because amputation of the knee robs the lower limb of the eccentric function of the quadriceps, which typically absorbs impact shock as the knee flexes approximately 15 degrees during initial loading.[29] Knee buckling in loading response is a primary concern in early prosthetic training. The experienced non-MPK user prevents collapse and potential falls by keeping the knee extended in loading response. Decreased prosthetic knee flexion, however, diminishes shock attenuation and transmits stress up the kinetic chain to the hip, pelvis, and spine.[30] Weight-activated friction brakes stabilize the knee when in the safe 0 to 20-degree knee flexion range. Hydraulic units provide graded resistance to knee flexion within the 0 to 20-degree range for descent of stairs, but will buckle readily beyond this range. Although this range of support is usually adequate for level walking, more range is required when descending a steep ramp, stepping on uneven surfaces, or when missteps occur. Lacking graded eccentric knee flexion control upon initial loading, the user learns to walk with a habitually extended knee.

Prosthetic Solutions

Some MPKs, like the C-Leg and Rheo Knee, allow knee flexion upon loading to provide the normal shock-absorbing function of the anatomic knee upon heel strike. For experienced prosthesis users who have learned to walk with the prosthetic knee extended upon initial contact, this function may seem strange. Indeed, the transfemoral amputation limb generates substantial hip extension power in the initial loading phase of gait particularly on the amputated side to push the thigh posterior and maintain the knee extended as well as to power the body forward over the stance limb.[31] The new MPK user transitioning from a non-MPK unit must unlearn old habits and let the knee bend upon initial contact to benefit from the MPK's capacity for greater shock absorption. The prosthetist can adjust the level of resistance as the user adapts.

Training Solutions

Whether learning to walk with a prosthesis for the first time or transitioning to an MPK that allows dampened knee flexion upon initial contact, prosthetic training should develop both movement ability and trust in the leg. Although strengthening gluteus maximus is always beneficial to increase eccentric motor control that can support knee flexion control, the major factor is developing the trust in the MPK to allow knee flexion. Initially standing in parallel bars to provide security, the MPK user can step forward onto the prosthesis, perceiving the resistance to knee flexion as weight progresses from the heel to the toe. Repeatedly leaning on the prosthetic foot to rock from heel to toe as the knee bends gives the MPK user awareness of the strength of knee resistance and helps foster trust in the leg (Figure 27-7). Training can progress to practice stepping performed with knee flexion upon heel contact as the

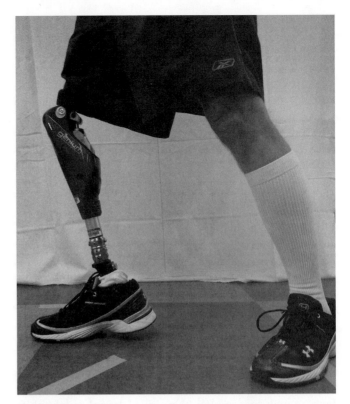

FIGURE 27-7 Rocking onto toes to feel the microprocessor knee flexion resistance.

body advances over the prosthetic foot causing knee extension, similar to able-bodied gait. This can be practiced in the parallel bars and later advanced to walking with initial knee flexion upon heel contact, guarded by the physical therapist who can insure that the knee unit will progress into extension as in normal gait. Training proceeds to ramp descent—best begun using a railing with therapist assistance. Developing the confidence to descend ramps while the MPK flexes through initial loading can seem like a leap of faith at first. Making the transition from walking with a hyperextended prosthetic knee to allowing the knee unit to flex during loading response can be difficult. Nevertheless, as few as 10 weeks has been needed to acclimate to the MPK.[32]

Asymmetric Step Length

Various physical impairments make asymmetric step length a common deviation for prosthesis users. The sound limb step is typically shorter than that of the prosthesis. Amputated side hip extensor weakness, uncertain balance, and limited hip extension range of motion, further restricted by the 10-degree hip flexion built into the transfemoral socket bench alignment, all cause a briefer sound limb swing time and shorter step length. Decreased hip rotation and concomitant lessened contralateral pelvic rotation also contribute to shorter prosthetic steps. Increasing hip extension range of motion and hip strength improves balance and facilitates longer prosthesis stance time. Practice walking with shorter sound limb step lengths can also reduce asymmetry.[22]

Gluteus maximus strength is critical during initial loading to generate the hip extension force in early stance that lifts the center of gravity from lowest to highest point and converts stance limb torque from internal to external rotation. Extensor strength is the strongest predictor of prosthetic walking speed.[33] In the absence of quadriceps and with the inevitable atrophy of the hamstrings,[34] hip extension and abduction display the greatest strength loss after amputation.[35] Atrophy of gluteal fast twitch fibers explains the slower gluteal contraction latency periods observed in amputated limbs.[36] Greater demand and slower contractions on the weakened amputated side hip extensors decrease the user's ability to quickly raise the center of gravity from the lowest point in dual limb stance to the highest point by midstance,[33] particularly if long prosthetic steps are emphasized early in the rehabilitation process when gluteal strength is weakest. As a result, prosthetic stance time is significantly briefer than on the sound side, leading to shorter sound limb swing phase duration and step lengths.[37,38]

Hip abductor weakness reduces the ability to maintain the body in prosthetic limb stance. This leads to a similar scenario in the frontal plane that also contributes to shorter sound limb steps.[39] Insufficient gluteus medius strength also diminishes the confidence to maintain single limb stance long enough to complete the normal lateral weight shift. The prosthesis user compensates by placing the sound foot farther from the midline, widening the base of support. The wide base shortens the gluteus medius length–tension relationship, further impairing hip abduction strength while simultaneously requiring a larger lateral weight shift. Hip abductor weakness also plays a role in step-length asymmetry, with weakness correlating with slower gait, shorter steps on both sides, and decreased weight bearing on the prosthesis.[39] Those with shorter amputation limbs have more abductor weakness, demonstrated in midstance by faster and/or greater pelvic drop.[40,41] In both situations, longer and/or wider steps disadvantage the gluteal muscles and can undermine balance confidence.

In terminal stance, decreased prosthetic side hip extension restricts the body's advance over the prosthetic foot causing the sound limb to take a shorter step forward. Lack of sufficient hip extension because of hip flexor contracture occurs in able-bodied people but is more prevalent among people with lower-limb amputation. Prolonged sitting during the rehabilitation process that can continue at home because of decreased activity is common after amputation.[24] The standard flexed bench alignment of the transfemoral socket can accommodate mild hip flexion contractures but reduces hip extension excursion.[38]

In the presence of limited hip extension range of motion, users attempt to advance the body over the prosthesis by exaggerating anterior pelvic tilt[40,41] with accentuated lumbar paraspinal muscle use, leading to greater lumbar extension compared to able-bodied people.[42] Such compensation may lead to lower back strains; people with both amputation and low back pain had weaker back extensors.[43] Increased demand for hip and lumbar extension strength and range of motion might be met with extra training to guard against low back pain. Abdominal

and hip strength is also critical to protect end-range lumbar extension as well as to assist atrophied hip flexors.[44]

In normal gait, stance phase hip extension occurs with rotation around the stance hip.[29] Although often observed as contralateral forward pelvic rotation, the rotation occurs primarily at the hip. After amputation, hip extension and contralateral forward rotation around the prosthesis are greatly reduced compared to the sound limb,[40] because transection through the femur minimizes transverse plane bony leverage. As a result, translation of rotary forces from the limb to the socket is greatly reduced because the femur rotates within the soft tissues of the thigh. Any looseness in socket fit reduces the translated forces even more. In fact, unlike sound side or able-bodied individuals, prosthetic stance phase is marked by internal, rather than external, torque,[41] which decreases trunk counterrotation and arm swing (Figure 27-8). Less trunk rotation is needed to counterbalance pelvic rotation when the individual wears a prosthesis. Nevertheless, when pelvic rotation is decreased, trunk rotation for prosthesis users is also diminished by limited joint mobility, weaker abdominal strength, incoordination between pelvis and trunk, and habit.

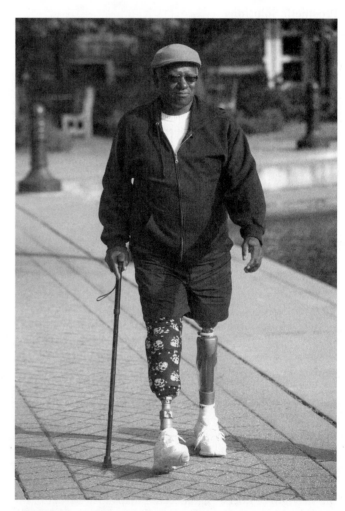

FIGURE 27-8 Excessive internal rotation and lack of hip extension in gait. (Courtesy Otto Bock Health Care, www.ottobockus.com.)

Lessened trunk rotation decreases the alternating forward momentum that normally drives arm swing, leading to decreased shoulder movement. The ipsilateral upper limb may be unconsciously held posterior to the hip axis to maintain a hip extension moment for enhanced stability (Figure 27-9).

For more experienced and usually healthier users who have more confidence in the prosthesis and have striven to walk faster, prosthetic steps may be shorter than those of the sound limb.[18,45] Multiple years of hip flexor stretching increases hip extension range.[43] However, the iliopsoas often atrophies and weakens,[44] providing insufficient power to protect the hip and lumbar spine and to enable uniform step lengths. Increased lumbar rotation that compensates for limited hip rotation after amputation may exacerbate low back pain.[42] Regardless of which step is shorter, coordination of trunk and pelvis is important to stabilize the lumbar spine dynamically and produce sufficient trunk and pelvic rotation to achieve symmetrical step length.

Prosthetic Solutions

The enhanced stance-phase stability of an MPK obviates the need to use the arm to maintain a hip extension moment throughout stance and allows the user to spend more time on prosthetic single-limb stance, thus equalizing step lengths and restoring the normal external rotation torque in stance phase. A torque adaptor in the shank can augment the limited contralateral forward pelvic rotation around the prosthesis to position the foot in normal toe out at initial loading. Regardless of the type of knee unit, significant hip abductor strength is required for single-limb stance on the prosthesis without contralateral pelvic drop or ipsilateral trunk lean.

Training Solutions

Developing symmetry in prosthetic gait requires a comprehensive approach that reduces underlying joint and muscular impairments to optimize functional outcomes.[46] For the experienced wearer, the habit of keeping the arm behind the hip is likely to be ingrained. Focused training is required to restore normal trunk counterrotation and arm swing. To enable the user to walk with as much symmetry as possible, the person should have normal range of motion throughout the lower limb, particularly the hip. Anterior hip capsular tightness limiting hip extension range is common, being a result of prolonged sitting. Anteriorly directed hip mobilization can help restore hip extension and rotation range (Figure 27-10).[47] Additional mobilization of the sacroiliac and lumbar joints may also be beneficial. Soft-tissue mobilization or trigger-point therapy for the iliopsoas followed by stretching[48] can help maintain hip flexor flexibility[49] and can be performed in the prone position or with the patient lying prone with the sound foot on the floor to help maintain or increase hip range (Figure 27-11). Hip mobilization may also result in gluteal strengthening.[50,51]

Once joint motion is optimized, gluteal strengthen must be increased. These muscles minimize lumbar extension and frontal plane gait compensations that typically result from hip weakness. In addition to residual limb hip abduction exercise performed side lying against a bolster,[52] the person can wear the prosthesis to perform closed chain exercises. Forward step-ups are a challenge; however, lateral step-ups on a low platform activate the gluteus medius.[53] To progress

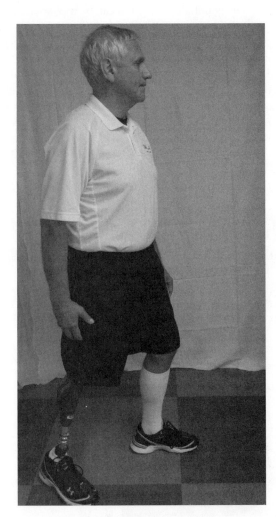

FIGURE 27-9 Reduced prosthetic side arm swing provides a hip extension moment but causes gait asymmetry.

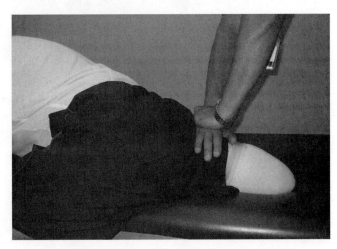

FIGURE 27-10 Anterior hip joint capsule mobilization.

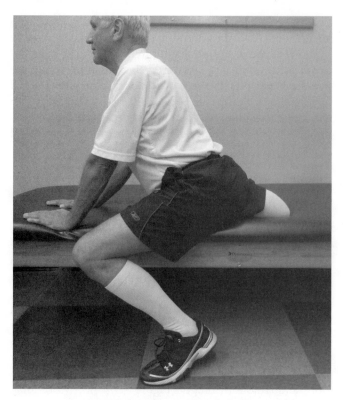

FIGURE 27-11 Hip flexor stretch.

a user's efforts, increase the step height gradually. Activities involving prolonged stance on the prosthesis also develop prosthetic side hip strength, especially hip abductors, for example, standing on the prosthesis while pushing in the opposite direction against a wall (Figure 27-12). More dynamic activities include standing on the prosthesis while using the sound limb to roll a ball on the floor, kicking against Theraband,[54] reaching in different directions around a circle like the star excursion balance test,[55] or maintaining the sound limb on a stool or unstable surface while throwing a ball (Figure 27-13). Using one hand to lightly maintain balance is important for safety; however, if both hands are required, the activity is probably too difficult and should be modified.

In addition to unilateral trunk bridging that focuses on gluteus maximus strengthening and control, hip extensor strength can be developed wearing the prosthesis while standing or simulating gait positions. One method to activate the gluteus maximus is to stand with hands in front pushing forward against a wall or kitchen counter, while leaning forward far enough to lift the prosthetic heel off the floor. As the trunk shifts forward over the forefoot, a hip flexion moment is created that must be maintained with hip extensors to keep the heel high (Figure 27-14). Promoting forefoot loading facilitates gluteus maximus activation and trains the user to activate MPK functions. Developing sufficient prosthetic side hip power to take long sound limb steps can be performed by standing with the prosthetic foot ahead of the intact foot facing a low stool. The wearer steps forward with the sound limb progressing to higher steps. This activity exaggerates the demands on the gluteus maximus during initial loading and can be used to develop the power needed for more challenging activities (Figure 27-15).

Strengthening the gluteus maximus, the primary external rotator of the hip, is also vital in transforming the leg torque from internal to external rotation after initial loading. Activities described above such as the sound limb star balance excursion test or exaggerated step lengths to ever higher steps increase gluteal strength and develop pelvic rotation around the prosthetic stance limb. Exercises that empha-

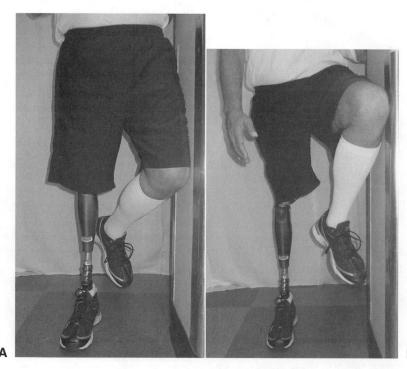

FIGURE 27-12 Isometric hip abduction (**A**) and isometric hip external rotation (**B**) against a wall.

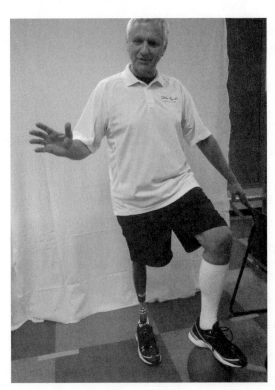

FIGURE 27-13 Step standing with sound limb on an unstable surface.

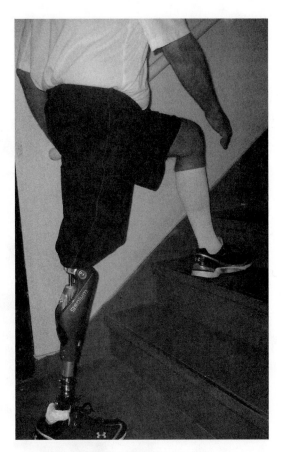

FIGURE 27-15 Sound limb to high step.

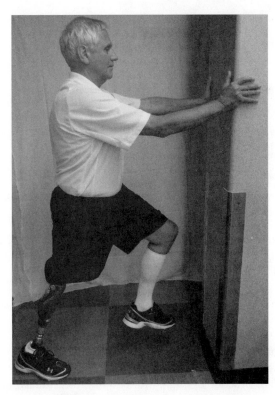

FIGURE 27-14 Pushing forward against wall while rising onto the forefoot for hip extension and external rotation.

size hip rotator strength include pressing the contralateral arm or leg back against a wall to promote isometric contralateral trunk rotation (see Figure 27-12, *B*). Active rotation around the prosthesis can be performed by turning the pelvis to point the sound foot as far around as possible in each direction and then maintaining the position, using the hands of a clock as a visual cue (Figure 27-16). Rotational activities can be progressed by pivoting on both heels to turn the toes in and out. Even more challenging is weight bearing through the forefeet while turning first one then both heels medially and laterally (Figure 27-17). Pivoting with weight on the toes develops hip strength and assists functional use of the MPK during turns and sidesteps. For effective neuromuscular reeducation and activation of the hip rotators, the therapist may use cueing or apply resistance through the sound limb (Figure 27-18). Pelvic rotation contributes to the overall goal of uniform step length with faster gait speeds although specific pelvic motions may become less symmetrical.[40]

More advanced gluteal strengthening activities can integrate trunk and upper-extremity function through exaggerated elements of gait. One method is to face a wall, then press only the ipsilateral hand against the wall while simultaneously lifting the prosthetic heel off the floor and flexing the sound hip as high as possible (see Figure 27-14). Avoid lumbar hyperextension to protect the back. Maintaining this position with spinal stability activates the abdominal muscles and helps promote contralateral pelvic rotation around the prosthesis with upper trunk counterrotation and arm swing often impaired in gait.

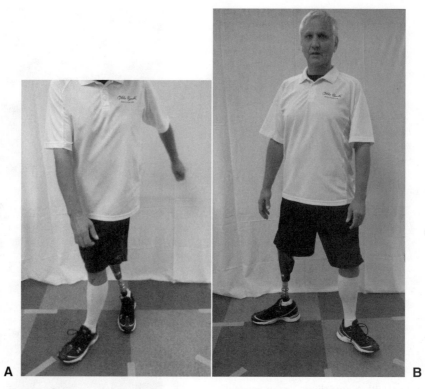

FIGURE 27-16 Stepping and holding in hip rotation: internal (**A**) and external (**B**).

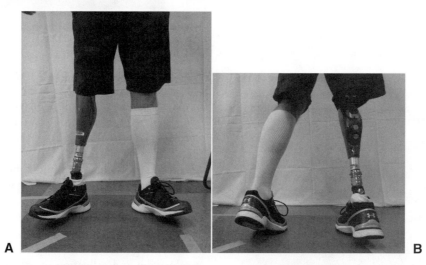

FIGURE 27-17 Pivoting in and out on both heels (**A**) and toes (**B**).

Spinal stabilization exercises increase prosthetic step length and gait speed.[45] Strengthening the hip flexors of both limbs also helps protect the hip and spine as they extend in terminal stance phase. Hip flexion generates power through swing phase. Hip strengthening and functional proficiency are important for both legs because sound limb hip rotation adds impetus to prosthetic swing phase, trunk counterrotation, and arm swing.

In addition to pelvic and trunk rotation training, additional practice may be necessary to make arm swing natural. For example, facilitating arm swing through the shoulders or with canes held in each hand by both user and therapist while

walking in synchronicity can help. Pelvic and trunk rotation in gait can be progressed using resisted gait techniques. With user and therapist facing each other, the therapist provides manual resistance to the user's pelvis or hands so that while the user walks forwards they must push the therapist back to integrate trunk counterrotation and arm swing (Figure 27-19).

Functional activities to develop transverse plane rotation and gait symmetry that can eventually be used for independent practice by highly functioning individuals include tandem balancing (Figure 27-20) and walking or grapevine walking to encourage rotation around each hip as well as

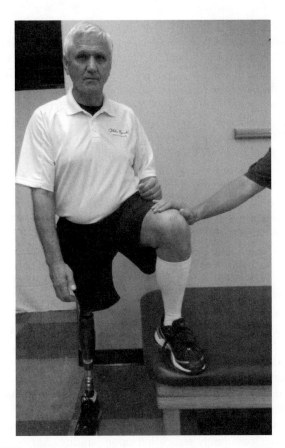

FIGURE 27-18 Resisted hip external rotation by therapist through the sound knee.

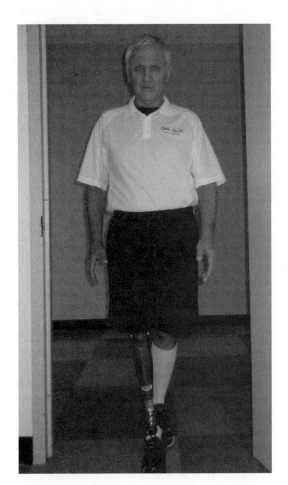

FIGURE 27-20 Tandem stance in a doorway.

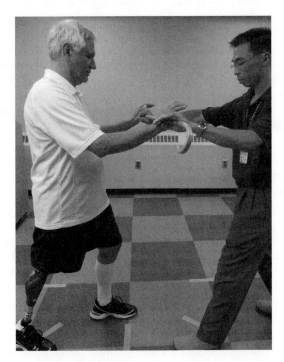

FIGURE 27-19 Resisted gait with cane.

decrease the base of support. Floor markers placed evenly apart can serve as visual cues for uniform step lengths while a full-length mirror at the end of a walkway allows the prosthesis user to check the symmetry of arm movements and general symmetry. A metronome provides an audible cue to rectify asymmetric stance times. A treadmill can be used to train progressive and consistent gait speed on level and inclined surfaces. As the patient builds strength, confidence, and awareness of muscle function and the limit of stability, the ability to take normal length steps during functional activities improves.

Other stance phase deviations discussed elsewhere in this text, such as wide base of support and lateral trunk lean or Trendelenburg, are unlikely to be affected specifically by MPK use, but may benefit from the proposed training solutions. Regardless of prosthetic components, training is required to minimize gait deviations and maximize function.

Swing Phase

Gait asymmetry can be affected by the difficulty transitioning from stance to swing phase. For able-bodied individuals, ankle plantarflexion prior to swing phase raises the body, providing much of the propulsive power.[29] Hip flexors contract to decelerate end range hip extension, then initiate swing phase with the adductors. The flexing hip and the forward propulsion of the body create momentum that first passively flexes the knee from heel off to early swing then extends the knee through terminal swing when hip flexion is reversed by the hip extensors. When momentum is reduced, as in slow gait, the hamstring muscles flex the knee to assure toe clearance augmenting foot dorsiflexion.

Amputation eliminates active ankle plantarflexion. Work shifts to the iliopsoas muscle increasing power derived from the hip flexor group by more than 50%.[31] Without active knee flexion, the hip flexors must contract even stronger to supply sufficient momentum to advance the limb through swing phase. Unfortunately, the ipsilateral iliopsoas atrophies.[44] Developing hip flexor strength can be difficult, especially with shorter amputation limbs. The new user can have difficulty advancing the limb, leading some to exaggerate hip flexion by kicking the leg laterally to initiate swing. Exaggerated kicking can lead to swing phase deviations like steppage (exaggerated hip and knee flexion) that can linger long after sufficient strength is restored.

Non-MPK hydraulic knee users must also switch their knees from stance phase control knee flexion resistance to swing phase resistance. This is generally accomplished in knees such as the Mauch at the end of stance phase when the wearer applies a knee hyperextension force with strong hip extension contraction or at the end of swing phase by achieving full knee extension for at least 0.1 second.[11] Although unnatural at first, prosthesis users learn to perform the knee extension motion without much thought.[56] However, swing phase is delayed and stance times asymmetric.[37] When momentum is not directed forward, such as when turning or sidestepping, transition between stance and swing phase knee resistance can be ineffective resulting in occasional circumduction, hip hiking, or vaulting if adequate swing resistance is not activated. Knee collapse and falling may occur if stance resistance is not activated.

Prosthetic Solutions

For the MPK user, transition between resistance phases is initiated intrinsically in response to electronic sensors. In the C-Leg, the user must achieve knee extension for 0.1 second with 70% body weight forefoot loading to disengage stance control and allow swing-phase knee flexion. The amount of body weight required can be adjusted depending on the user's needs. Default settings of the specific MPK determine what happens if the criteria are not met. For instance, the C-Leg defaults to stance-phase control to protect the wearer from knee collapse, a significantly improved safety feature compared to non-MPK prostheses. Other MPK units, like the Rheo Knee, default to swing-phase control to avoid toe drag in swing phase.

Training Solutions

To insure that the user is comfortable bearing weight through the prosthetic forefoot, activities involving forefoot loading are critical. Pivoting can be practiced with weight on both forefeet to allow rapid swing phase action during turns (see Figure 27-17, *B*). Lateral weight shifts onto the toes with one or two quick bounces can help prepare for side-stepping. Forefoot bouncing can also be useful, as some MPKs, like the Power Knee, use forefoot bounces as mechanical cues to change knee resistance modes. Pushing off the forefoot to kick into swing phase can assist forward walking or the quick transition into swing phase necessary for a brief jog.

For those with decreased pelvic and trunk motion, abdominal muscles may be recruited to assist swing phase, particularly for people with amputation limbs shorter than 57% of the sound length where hip flexors are weaker. Shorter limb length correlates with increased pelvic tilting during gait even after traumatic amputation.[57] Core abdominal mobility exercises are even more important after hip disarticulation or higher amputations that deprive the user of all active hip motion.

Stairs and Ramps

Descents

Stairs and ramps remain difficult even for experienced users. Descents and ascents pose different problems. As in walking, limited prosthetic knee flexion is a particular problem when descending stairs and declines. Limited shock attenuation is particularly evident upon landing on the prosthetic limb when descending stairs, curbs, or declines. Because the wearer descends stairs onto the heel, not the forefoot as able-bodied individuals do, more shock is transmitted to the extremity; the user commonly feels a jolt upon landing. Although the prosthetic limb is subjected to less vertical force than a normal limb upon landing, this force is more poorly attenuated without the normal knee flexion and ankle dorsiflexion upon loading. The hip on the prosthetic side must exert double the extension force to control the knee. On the sound limb, the relative lack of prosthetic knee flexion results in approximately 50% greater vertical impact forces as the body lowers from a greater height.[58,59] In fact, all sound limb joints experience increased stress in gait, exposing the sound side to more risk of injury.[30] As a result, most people with transfemoral or higher amputations instinctively take smaller steps of shorter duration to decrease ground reaction forces and muscle demand on ramps whether descending or ascending.[60] The new wearer usually takes short prosthetic steps to prevent accidental collapse and compensates with longer sound limb steps to maintain speed, making gait asymmetrical.

Non-MPK hydraulic stance-control knees provide graded resistance to knee motion beyond 20 degrees flexion, giving time for the sound limb to alight onto the next lower step in a step-after-step pattern, but most users still have noticeably decreased prosthetic stance time when descending stairs.[59] Descending ramps is more difficult than stairs because to place the prosthetic foot flat on the ground without the normal ankle plantarflexion range, the prosthetic shank must be thrust forward downhill creating a rapid, sizeable knee flexion moment (Figure 27-21). Knee flexion resistance in a non-MPK hydraulic stance control unit can be adequate on shallow ramps, but knee flexion resistance is not always sufficient on steeper ramps. Prosthetic users often hesitate when descending ramps.

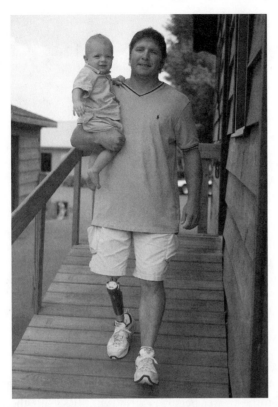

FIGURE 27-21 Descending slopes creates large knee flexion moments that can be controlled with the C-Leg. (Courtesy Otto Bock Health Care, www.ottobockus.com.)

Prosthetic Solutions

As in level walking, MPK sensors provide data used to adjust the real-time resistance needed for descent. For the typical MPK, full knee extension at terminal swing combined with prosthetic heel weight bearing triggers knee flexion resistance to match the individual's body weight, angle of descent, and gait speed through a greater range of motion (30 to 35 degrees) than provided by non-MPK units.[22] Slow, interrupted, or unsteady stair descent may cause insufficient momentum to create full knee extension, thereby leaving MPKs with swing-phase resistance default settings unready to provide stance-phase stability; this deficiency can lead to knee collapse. Collapse is less of a problem for the C-Leg, which defaults to stance-phase knee resistance, even in knee flexion ranges of 36 to 55 degrees.[58] Prosthesis users functioning at the Medicare K2 or K3 levels (see Table 27-2) performed better on stairs and declines with MPK compared to non-MPK hydraulic knees.[61] After the MPK software is adjusted and the user develops confidence and balance through training, the wearer can descend steep declines with significantly longer prosthetic steps that promote less asymmetry and faster speeds.[22]

Training Solutions

To descend stairs, the MPK user must learn to place only the rearfoot on the lower step and load substantial body weight through the heel (see Figure 27-2). This foot placement triggers the graded knee flexion resistance needed while leaving the toes

to angle down and progress to the next step as the knee bends. To step down stairs onto the heel in this manner can be anxiety producing for the new MPK user and should be practiced initially on the bottom step using a banister with guarding.

The prosthesis user can mitigate some of the impact shock to the residual limb by reaching the entire leg down toward the next step so the foot meets the lower stair with less impact. Pelvic anterior depression[62] enables positioning the foot forward and down. This motion, derived from proprioceptive neuromuscular facilitation, can be practiced on level ground or by standing on a low platform to reach the heel forward and down with a pelvic motion before returning to the starting position.

Taking long prosthetic steps when descending a ramp is unnatural to the person who has habitually used a non-MPK prosthesis. This habit may be overcome. Training the MPK user to (a) utilize pelvic anterior depression in terminal swing, (b) activate the hip extensors to advance the body forward during initial loading, (c) rotate the contralateral pelvis around the stance hip in midstance, and (d) maintain weight bearing through the prosthetic forefoot in terminal stance facilitate a longer step on descent. A banister provides safety during the training process until the new wearer develops confidence to progress to resisted training and finally unassisted declines.

Ascents

Most people with transfemoral amputation ascend stairs in step-to fashion. A similar gait pattern is used for steep inclines. When ascending, the wearer typically flexes the sound limb more to make up for the lack of prosthetic side elevation normally provided by ankle plantar flexion.[60] In the community, some people ascend stairs two steps at a time with the sound limb to maintain the same speed as companions. Greater knee flexion, however, increases forces on all sound limb joints when climbing stairs.[59] In the stance phase of ramp ascent, the prosthetic shank is thrust backward making it difficult to advance the body forward and causing a short step on the intact side.

Prosthetic Solutions

When ascending ramps, forefoot weight-bearing causes the shank to be thrust backward exerting a strong knee extension moment. On stairs an MPK can sense increased knee extension force and trigger the stair ascent mode that gives less swing-phase resistance to knee flexion to help the foot clear the edge of the next step. Software can be adjusted to the user's needs. Once the foot is on the next step, however, the user must exert considerable hip extensor power to lift the body onto the next step, which is typically accomplished with the assistance of a hand on a banister. In the absence of a banister, step-over-step stair ascent is very difficult for most users.

The Power Knee provides powered assistance to ascent. The user must stop at the bottom stair for 3 seconds to default to the standing state before ascending. Initiating knee extension activates the assisted knee extension function.

Data sent wirelessly from sensors strapped to the sound leg help match prosthetic movement to the sound limb. At the top of the stairs, the user must pause again for 3 seconds to reset the MPK before walking. The powered mechanism makes sounds noticeable to passersby; the noise bothers some users.

The Genium uses a gyroscope and accelerometers to recognize that the user is ascending a step. A quick hip extension movement to drag the foot off the ground followed by quick hip flexion lifts the foot to the next step with prosthetic hip and knee flexion. Once the foot is on the next higher step, the Genium provides maximal resistance to further knee flexion upon bent-knee weight bearing. Placement of the heel slightly off the step augments the knee extension moment powered by hip extensors contraction and the body's forward momentum.

Training Solutions

Because of hip flexor weakness, the prosthesis user may have to elevate or tilt the pelvis posteriorly using the abdominals to gain sufficient elevation and to compensate for limited prosthetic ankle dorsiflexion on stairs and inclines. If the user stops on a step, restarting swing phase up the stairs is difficult. Turning 45 degrees allows space for foot to clear after a stop on the stairs without excessive hip hiking. Ascending step-over-step requires great hip extensor strength and usually the assistance of a banister. New MPK designs, including the Power Knee and Genium, meet this challenge. With these units, placing only the forefoot on the next step with the heel off the step can help extend the knee. The Power Knee only requires the user to initiate knee extension with the hip extensors. Step-over-step ascent with the Genium requires significant hip extensor strength and is recommended only for active users at the K3 and K4 levels (see Table 27-2).

Sitting and Squatting

Although navigating stairs can be difficult for people using prosthetic knees, any knee bending and straightening activities like rising from a chair or squatting demands compensatory movements, which imposes added stress to the sound limb. Many prosthetic knees require unloading the prosthesis to allow the knee unit to bend so that the user can sit at a speed similar to able-bodied individuals. As a result, many prosthesis wearers stand with 10% to 30% more body weight on the sound limb than on the prosthesis.[39,63] Squatting with both legs can be useful. For instance, the prosthesis user may want to squat to reach down to a child (Figure 27-22) or pick up something from the floor without bending from the waist to avoid low back pain, which occurs in more than 80% of people using transfemoral prostheses.[44] After 30 degrees knee unit flexion, most MPKs provide insufficient flexion resistance to prevent collapse.[58] Thus, for many users, sit–stand transitions, especially squatting, become single-limb activities that place substantial stress on the sound limb. Potential solutions for sit-to-stand transitions and squatting follow.

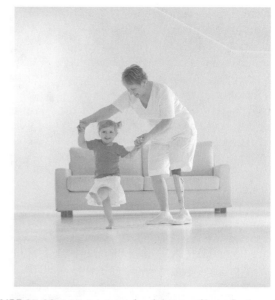

FIGURE 27-22 Maintaining a fixed degree of knee flexion with the stand feature of the Compact C-Leg. (Courtesy Otto Bock Health Care, www.ottobockus.com.)

Prosthetic Solutions

When the wearer begins to sit down, MPKs like the C-Leg and Rheo Knee provide controlled resistance to knee flexion activated by prosthetic weight bearing. MPKs allow symmetrical distribution of weight between the feet to reduce stress on the sound limb; resistance settings can be adjusted to the needs of the user. Whether using non-MPK or MPK prostheses, wearers continue to bear weight asymmetrically and sit slower than able-bodied individuals.[63] To sit rapidly without adjusting the resistance, MPKs that have swing-phase default settings can be offloaded; this shifts stress to the sound limb as with non-MPKs.[30] Although MPKs allow symmetrical weight bearing during stand-to-sit transitions, the user must be trained to bear more weight on the prosthesis by sitting down against the inner posterior socket wall with a hip extension force to offload the sound limb.

Most MPKs do not assist sit-to-stand activity; the user depends greatly on sound limb strength to rise. The Power Knee, however, assists user-initiated knee extension. A push up from the chair armrests activates the assisted sit-to-stand function. As compared with those wearing unpowered knee units, prosthesis users rising with the Power Knee move with greater symmetry with hip force closer to that exhibited by able-bodied individuals.[63] To sit using a Power Knee, the user must pause to activate the default standing mode, then slowly lower the body to the chair. If the sitting motion is stopped midway, the Power Knee will support the user in a squat until the prosthesis is unweighted. Transferring the weight to the sound limb allows further knee unit bending.

Some MPKs provide special function modes that allow squatting or prolonged standing. The C-Leg, for instance, permits prosthetic weight bearing with the knee unit flexed to any angle between 7 and 70 degrees, allowing maximal support for squatting or bent-knee standing.

The Compact knee, designed for K2-level users, offers the same function in a 0- to 30-degree range. This mode is activated by handheld wireless remote control unit, with predetermined physical cues such as bouncing quickly on the forefoot, but also more intuitively by lowering the body to the desired degree of knee flexion and then slightly straightening the prosthetic knee to turn on the maximal knee flexion resistance needed to squat.[17] The Power Knee facilitates squatting by locking when the user stops the stand-to-sit motion at the desired degree of knee flexion.[11]

Training Solutions

When sitting, placing the MPK user's hands on the arm rests enhances safety and decreases the chance that the user will fall backward. Using arm rests, however, shifts the body weight backward onto the heels rather than forward onto the forefeet, as in able-bodied sit-to-stand transitions. For those who demonstrate the potential to stand unassisted, transferring weight forward over the forefeet can be practiced from surfaces of decreasing height as the person improves. The user's hands can be positioned anteriorly or on the thighs while arising. Placing both feet behind the knees helps advance weight over the forefeet, but can be difficult because of limited prosthetic ankle dorsiflexion. The Proprio Foot user can dorsiflex the prosthetic ankle by tapping the heel or signaling with the wireless remote to position the foot for sit-to-stand transitions. Keeping the spine straight minimizes patellar compressive forces and back pain. Practicing at different speeds on different seat heights and while holding objects of different weights can prepare the user for a range of functional activities.

To develop the strength and control to master the squatting feature of the C-Leg or Power Knee, the user should practice single-limb squats with the sound limb. If unable, the wearer can start by performing a wall squat with a chair at hand for support. Methods to stimulate greater contribution of hip extensors on the amputated side will help in controlling the descent to the desired knee flexion angle. Squats on an unstable surface, such as a cushion or tilt board, performed between parallel bars and with appropriate guarding for safety, can be effective. Step-ups with the prosthesis leading also help enable knee unit extension through forceful hip extensor contractions. Gluteal strengthening exercises are essential.

Fall Protection

People with leg amputation have a greater risk of falling than do able-bodied individuals, with reported incidences of 20% to 32% during rehabilitation[64,65] and 52% within the community.[66] Falls occur when the wearer unexpectedly bears weight on the flexed prosthetic knee, as can happen when a user slips, stubs a toe, or steps on a rock unbalancing the prosthetic foot and causing the knee unit to bend. Stepping onto a flexed knee can also occur when the user turns, takes small sidesteps, or stops suddenly preventing the knee unit from fully extending and activating

stance-phase control. When using a hydraulic non-MPK, tripping or stepping on an object leads to swing-phase knee-flexion resistance and increases the risk of falls.[67] Slips may occur upon heel strike onto slick surfaces such as ice. A slip causes very high demand for gluteal muscle strength that must respond rapidly to the anteromedial shear upon landing.[68] The muscles of prosthetic users, including postural muscles like the erector spinae and oblique abdominal muscles, do not consistently contract when walking and respond to slips and trips slower than the muscles of sound limbs or able-bodied people.[68] The wearer may adapt to the risk of unexpected knee instability by taking shorter prosthetic steps, which results in slow, asymmetrical gait.

Prosthetic Solutions

Whether a stumble or fall will result from an unexpected step onto a flexed knee depends greatly on the MPK default setting. MPKs with swing phase knee resistance default settings require great compensatory movements; otherwise, falls occur even in younger people whose amputation etiologies were nondysvascular.[58] Knee collapse can also occur when knee unit flexion exceeds the 30- to 35-degree range programmed for stance-phase resistance capacity.[58] The Power Knee and C-Leg default to stance-phase knee resistance and will prevent collapse even after swing phase is interrupted.[67] In everyday situations, stance-phase default C-Leg users report significantly fewer stumbles and falls[69] and a safer experience compared to non-MPK.[70]

Training Solutions

Because stumbling is unexpected, it is difficult to prepare the new user. However, most slips result from the foot sliding upon initial contact rather than in terminal stance. Thus, the gluteal muscles are the most important group to strengthen and the hip flexors are a secondary concern. Consistent contraction of the core muscles throughout gait, not typically present in prosthesis users, should be developed and strengthened to allow stronger and faster response to postural disturbances.[68] Methods for strengthening gluteal muscles and integrating abdominal contractions in gait have been presented in training solutions for asymmetric steps.

Practice in functional activities encountered in real life also prepares users to respond to stumbles and falls. Obstacle courses should include different walking surfaces and stepping up, over, and onto obstacles. Carrying items and performing dual tasks can develop overall functional ability. With training, MPK users can negotiate obstacle courses quickly with fewer steps compared to those wearing non-MPK prostheses.[71] Practice on outdoor terrain can enable the wearer to participate fully in daily activities.

Other Activities

The user may wish to participate in activities that require free-swinging knee function like biking, or locked knee function like prolonged standing.

Prosthetic Solutions

Non-MPK hydraulic or pneumatic knees sometimes have a manual switch at the back of the knee that will switch the knee to different modes of function.[11] MPKs offer various modes of function, but eliminate the need to operate a switch manually. A physical cue like pushing down on the toes three times followed by unweighting the leg for 1 second switches the mode of operation from walking to free swinging for biking or maximal knee resistance for prolonged standing.[17] Regardless of whether wireless remote or leg movements are used to switch functional modes, an electronic signal, either a series of beeps or vibrations, confirms the change in setting to the user. The Proprio Foot uses heel tapping to trigger the ankle to drop into plantarflexion when the wearer sits and return to dorsiflexion before the person stands. The user can also activate these functions by a handheld wireless remote.[11]

Training Solutions

Remembering how to switch modes, performing the physical cue, and hearing or feeling the confirming electronic signals varies among users. As with gait training, forefoot weight-bearing practice is a fundamental skill to develop. Heel tapping to signal the Proprio Foot requires hip flexor strength and coordination to move the prosthesis up and down. Having the user practice initiating the cues and perceiving the signals is important to the smooth, effective use of these MPK features.

Although clinicians may focus on gait deviations that persist despite dedicated training for even the most experienced and high-level users, wearers themselves tend to focus more on their functional abilities. Even active prosthesis users typically take part in bouts of activity lasting less than 2 minutes and averaging only 17 steps per minute. Most wearers only engage in activity lasting more than 15 continuous minutes only once per day.[72] Functional ability and attitude towards the prosthesis are the strongest predictors of patient satisfaction.[73] Prosthetic outcomes can be maximized through a clinical approach that addresses range of motion and strength impairments while integrating functional abilities to optimize participation in the pleasures and challenges of real life.

OUTCOMES

Success of prosthetic fitting can be measured by objective factors, principally energy consumption, walking velocity, and step symmetry, as well as subjective responses such as falls history and quality-of-life questionnaires. Overall, prosthesis users perform somewhat better and report greater satisfaction when wearing MPK prostheses, than with less-sophisticated components. A few investigators compared function of people wearing prostheses with various units. Even in the presence of laboratory evidence regarding the biomechanical characteristics of MPK units, clinicians' and wearers' subjective reactions remain the mainstay of formulating prosthetic prescription and thus determining prosthetic rehabilitation outcomes.[73,74]

Physical characteristics appear to outweigh the importance of a particular prosthetic component in determining the individual's performance. Review of combat-associated amputations reveals that function and amputation limb length are directly correlated, while energy consumption and length are inversely related.[75] Preserving the knee joint is critical because energy consumption of men with unilateral transfemoral amputation exceeded that of subjects with transtibial amputation during slow and fast level walking and traversing slopes of two different inclines.[76] People with mid length or longer thighs, however, showed that no significant kinematic or kinetic gait differences.[57]

Gait Studies

Laboratory comparisons of performance with prostheses equipped with the C-Leg and the Mauch Swing and Stance hydraulic knee units generally indicate that subjects walked faster with the C-Leg by as much as 21%, depending on terrain.[18,69] Faster self-selected walking speed with a C-Leg did not necessarily come at higher energy costs.[77] One research team, however, reported no significant differences in free walking speed.[56] Faster gait speeds obtained with people after transfemoral amputation using the C-Leg compared to non-MPK prostheses have also been documented in a case report of one person with bilateral knee disarticulations.[78] Laboratory comparison of subjects wearing the Endolite Intelligent Prosthesis and non-MPK units reveal similar results as those involving C-Leg.[79]

A goal of prosthetic fitting is to enable the patient to walk as inconspicuously as possible. People wearing the C-Leg exhibited less step-length asymmetry than when using a hydraulic non-MPK unit.[18,40,45] Kinematic analysis of subjects walking with MPK units showed less delay between late swing-phase knee extension and heel contact than with other units.[37]

Optimum rehabilitation restores the individual's ability to walk greater distances without appreciable fatigue. In one study, subjects who wore prostheses with step counters and distance monitors took similar numbers of steps and walked for equivalent durations in the home and community environments whether using the C-Leg or Mauch knee units,[72] while another group reported that wearing a MPK prosthesis was associated with greater physical activity in the community.[80] Much research involves measuring oxygen consumption. Some investigators detected no significant difference in oxygen cost of walking when comparing performance of subjects wearing the C-Leg and hydraulic non-MPK units,[77] whereas others suggest that walking with C-leg is more energy efficient.[71,81,82] Although metabolic demand when wearing the microprocessor Adaptive Knee was comparable to that of a hydraulic non-MPK unit,[83] use of the Intelligent Prosthesis was associated with slightly reduced oxygen consumption.[84-87] Four young adults with traumatic amputation alternated wearing the C-Leg and the Intelligent Prosthesis; their oxygen consumption was similar, although much higher than required by the able-bodied control subjects.[79] Metabolic demand with the Rheo Knee unit was slightly less than with the C-Leg.[88] In general, any MPK reduces energy consumption modestly compared to a non-MPK, confirmed by laboratory comparison of adults walking with several types of MPKs.[58]

Performance in other ambulatory activities: Sit-to-stand transitions required less hip force for subjects wearing the Power Knee as compared with performance with the C-Leg or the Mauch Swing and Stance Control unit, although all participants relied primarily on the intact limb.[63] The C-Leg offers more protection against tripping as compared with non-MPK units. Three subjects participated in a randomized study in which the examiner tugged on a cord in an attempt to cause prosthetic knee flexion. Unlike other knee units, the C-Leg either produced rapid knee extension or supported the wearer on the flexed knee.[67] Performance on stair and ramp descent was safest with the C-Leg, as compared with the Rheo Knee, Adaptive 2 Knee, and Hybrid Knee.[58] On hill and stair descent, MPK users exhibited smoother maneuvering over obstacles, fewer stumbles, and superior multitasking ability allowing many to advance to a higher Medicare functional level.[61] The Rheo Knee and the C-Leg were associated with smoother gait and decreased hip power generation as compared with performance with the Mauch Swing and Stance Control unit.[88] Subjects who walked on a treadmill while solving mental problems swayed less when tested with the Intelligent Prosthesis, suggesting that it was not as cognitively demanding as less-sophisticated knee units.[89]

Several research teams administered questionnaires to people who wore prostheses equipped with C-Legs. Respondents praised confidence, gait, and maneuverability,[70] as well as overall satisfaction.[22] Scores on the Prosthesis Evaluation Questionnaire were higher.[69,71] Subjective response to the Intelligent Prosthesis was also favorable, with users preferring it to nonmicroprocessor units when walking at different speeds and greater distances with less fatigue.[90] Survey respondents commended increased quality of life when wearing MPKs.[80]

Although many studies of adults wearing MPKs have been published, none has addressed such issues as mechanical durability, effect of unit weight on performance, and whether the cost of the units equates to substantially greater benefit. Ideally, future research would involve larger sample sizes. Nevertheless, at the present time, one can conclude that MPK units can improve the quality of life of many people with transfemoral amputation.

PRESCRIPTIVE CASES

Selecting the prosthesis that matches an individual's needs requires taking into account the person's general health, level and status of the residual limb, history of prosthetic use, features and limitations of the available prosthetic components, impact level of the intended use, and the individual's functional level. Manufacturers recommend MPKs for low to moderate impact activities (Table 27-3) by users at the Medicare K2 to K4 functional levels (see Table 27-2), regardless of insurance company policies. After transfemoral amputation many people may not attain the functional ability to become K2 community ambulators, walking at 3 km/h (1.9 mph) and negotiating steps and curbs. Because gait speeds are low for K2-level walkers, MPK units like the C-Leg Compact with stance-phase control only are appropriate. Prosthesis users who walk 5 km/h (3.1 mph), traverse daily distances of 5 km (3.1 miles) including stairs, and engage in moderate impact activities are at the K3 to K4 functional level, thus both stance- and swing-phase features are recommended. In addition to matching prosthetic components to the individual's physical and functional needs, another inescapable consideration is the cost of incorporating a MPK. Insurance will often reimburse the price of a MPK only for users at the K3 to K4 levels. The cases that follow highlight important considerations relevant to MPK prescription.

Those with hip disarticulation or higher amputations can be considered at the K2 level if walking independently, regardless of speed, although Medicare K levels are not published for people other than unilateral transtibial and transfemoral amputation.

TABLE 27-3 *Impact Levels*

Levels	Target Activity	Typical Use
Low	Walking with small cadence variations	Daily walking with low foot forces. Examples: household tasks, gardening, shopping, and occasional nonimpact sports such as golf and leisure walking.
Moderate	Walking with variable cadence	Daily walking of long durations with moderate forces. Examples: aerobics, jogging, sports like tennis, and vocational activities like lifting/carrying.
High	High cadence walking	Daily activities involving vigorous and repetitive actions with fast speeds and high loading forces. Examples: distance jogging, running, jumping, sports like basketball, and vocational activities like construction work.
Sport-Extreme	High impact sports and activities	Daily activities with high or extreme forces common in repetitive, fast, and/or sustained activities. Examples: sprinting, long-distance running, active military service.

CASE EXAMPLE 1:

The Active Athlete

A 29-year-old 110 kg (245 lb) former college athlete has a transfemoral amputation resulting from a motorcycle accident 5 years ago. He has been using a non-MPK hydraulic knee prosthesis for his everyday life, which includes work as a sales representative during the week and recreational basketball and tennis on the weekends. He jogs proficiently using the skip-hop style but has gotten interested in more sports activities and wants to run step-over-step and potentially compete in athletic contests. He is ready for a new prosthesis that can facilitate reaching his goals.

Questions to Consider
- What type of knee unit best matches his needs?
- What is his K level?
- How does his weight factor into the decision making about which prosthesis to recommend?
- How does his recreational and exercise activity factor into the recommended prosthesis?

Recommendation

His activities show K4 level functioning and would qualify him for reimbursement of a MPK prosthesis by many insurance companies. Although a MPK would be an excellent choice for his everyday activities, MPKs are designed for low-to-moderate-impact activities and could be overloaded by the sustained and high-impact nature of his intended sports. If he is going to proceed with only one prosthesis, one with a non-MPK hydraulic knee unit such as the Mauch Knee Plus may serve him best to meet his athletic goals. Such a knee could be paired with a heavy-duty energy-storing foot designed to absorb shock like the Re-Flex VSP.

CASE EXAMPLE 2:

At Risk to Fall?

A 65-year-old woman underwent transfemoral amputation 4 years ago resulting from a thrombosis associated with peripheral vascular and cardiovascular disease. She was active prior to amputation. Her activity has increased since the amputation and she has returned to work as a school administrator using a weight-activated friction brake knee unit. She gardens and enjoys leisure walking in the community, although her strength and endurance limit her from walking as fast or as far as she would like and she has fallen twice in the past year. She has recently qualified for Medicare and wants a prosthesis that can help her reach her goals.

Questions to Consider
- What type of knee unit best matches her needs?
- What is her K level?
- What is her fall risk?
- How does her leisure and exercise activity factor into the recommended prosthesis?

Recommendations

Her activities demonstrate K2-level prosthetic functioning with K3-level potential. Medicare and her employer-based insurance may not approve a MPK because her functional activities do not demand a varied cadence or fast walking speed. Her age and general health status may also mitigate against her efforts to get reimbursed for the cost of a MPK. However, community ambulating prosthesis users are at heightened fall risk.[66] Falls within her age group have annual incidence rates from 19% to 60%, with as many as 32% reporting injury.[91] Although current reimbursement practice often does not include a MPK for a K2-level patient/client, she would benefit from using a MPK, particularly its stumble and fall protective features.

CASE EXAMPLE 3:

After Higher Amputation

A 44-year-old man had a hemipelvectomy 3 months ago as a consequence of chondrosarcoma. His incision has healed and he is ready for fitting. He has never used a prosthesis but was very active until 1 year ago when he underwent tumor resection and internal hemipelvectomy and suffered a bout of depression. After the resection, he limited activity to working in an office and curtailed most sporting activities other than occasional walks in the park. Since his amputation, he has returned to work as an accountant and is adept with crutches, which he uses for light sports activities such as soccer with his children. He uses a wheelchair for traversing long distances. He complains that it is difficult to rise from a chair or hold something in his hands while using crutches. He lives with his wife and teenage sons in a suburban two-story house. He is insured through his employer and his prosthetist is confident that a MPK prosthesis will be covered by insurance. His goals are to continue work and family life with greater ease.

Questions to Consider
- What type of knee unit best matches his needs?
- What is his K level?
- What is his fall risk?
- How does his difficulty with rising from the seated position factor into the recommended prosthesis?

Recommendations

As a previously active adult who is able to walk after hemipelvectomy, he is comparable to the K2 functional level. His status has been changing and his medical and prosthetic prognoses remain unclear. He may achieve K3-level functioning. A MPK would allow him to descend stairs and slopes with safety on two legs and walk without crutches at work and social functions. However, most MPKs will not provide assistance for rising from a chair or ascending stairs at the same pace as his peers. Difficulty rising from a chair, walking, and negotiating stairs are complicated by fit problems common to people with hemipelvectomies who fluctuate in body weight. He may benefit from a temporary prosthesis with a non-MPK to determine his level of prosthetic use before expending the cost of a MPK prosthesis.[92]

REFERENCES

1. Murphy EF. Lower extremity components. In: *American Academy of Orthopaedic Surgeons. Orthopaedic Appliances Atlas.* vol. 2. Ann Arbor, MI: Edwards; 1960.
2. McAleer J. Mobility redux: post World War II prosthetics and functional aids for veterans, 1945 to 2010. *J Rehabil Res Dev.* 2011;48:vii–xvi.
3. Filippi P. U.S. Patent 2,305,291. December 15 1942.
4. Henschke U, Mauch H. U.S. Patent 2,490,806, December 13 1949.
5. Erback JR. Hydraulic prostheses for above-knee amputees. *J Am Phys Ther Assoc.* 1963;43:105–110.
6. Endolite. *User manuals and technical information, and history.* Available at: http://www.endolite.com/products/knees/. Accessed 07.07.11.
7. Aeyels B, Peeraer L, Vander Sloten J, Van der Perre G. Development of an above-knee prosthesis equipped with a microcomputer-controlled knee joint: first test results. *J Biomed Eng.* 1992;14:199–202.
8. Bar A, Ishai G, Meretsky P, Koren Y. Adaptive microcomputer control of an artificial knee in level walking. *J Biomed Eng.* 1983;5:145–150.
9. Berry D. Microprocessor prosthetic knees. *Phys Med Rehabil Clin N Am.* 2006;17:91–113.
10. Dietl H, Kaitan R, Pawlik R, Ferrara P. The C-Leg®: a new system for fitting of transfemoral amputees. *Orthopädie-Technik (English).* 1998;49:197–211.
11. Össur. *User manuals, technical information, and impact level descriptions.* Available at: http://www.ossur.com/?PageID=12643; Accessed 07.07.11.
12. Freedom Innovations, LLC. *User manuals and technical information.* Available at: http://www.freedom-innovations.com/knees/index.html. Accessed 15.07.11.
13. Centri AB. *User manuals and technical information located at: Prosthetic knee systems—Nabtesco.* Available at: http://www.centri.se; Accessed 07.07.11.
14. Devlin M, Sinclair LB, Colman D, et al. Patient preference and gait efficiency in a geriatric population with transfemoral amputation using a free-swinging versus a locked prosthetic knee joint. *Arch Phys Med Rehabil.* 2002;83:246–249.
15. Seymour R. *Prosthetics and Orthotics: Lower Limb and Spinal.* In: Baltimore, MD: Lippincott Williams & Wilkins; 2002:144–159 213, 230–234.
16. Taghipour H, Moharamzad Y, Mafi AR, et al. Quality of life among veterans with war-related unilateral lower extremity amputation: a long-term survey in a prosthesis center in Iran. *J Orthop Trauma.* 2009;23:525–530.
17. Otto Bock Health Care. *User manuals, technical information, and mobility grading system.* Available at: http://www.ottobockus.com/cps/rde/xchg/ob_us_en/hs.xsl/589.html. Accessed 07.07.11.
18. Segal AD, Orendurff MS, Klute GK, et al. Kinematic and kinetic comparisons of transfemoral amputee gait using C-Leg® and Mauch SNS prosthetic knees. *J Rehabil Res Dev.* 2006;43:857–870.
19. Zamiska N. Bionic knee "learns" how to walk. *Wall St J [Midwest Ed]* July 6, 2004;. Available at http://online.wsj.com/ad/article/philips/SB108907039283655627.html. Accessed 07.07.11.
20. Seelen HAM, Hemmen B, Schmeets AJ, et al. Costs and consequences of a prosthesis with an electronically stance and swing phase controlled knee. *Technol Disabil.* 2009;21:25–34.
21. Graham LE, Datta D, Heller B, Howitt J. A comparative study of conventional and energy-storing prosthetic feet in high-functioning transfemoral amputees. *Arch Phys Med Rehabil.* 2007;88:801–806.
22. Hafner BJ, Willingham LL, Buell NC, et al. Evaluation of function, performance, and preference as transfemoral amputees transition from mechanical to microprocessor control of the prosthetic knee. *Arch Phys Med Rehabil.* 2007;88:207–217.
23. Martin J, Pollock A, Hettinger J. Microprocessor lower limb prosthetics: review of current state of the art. *J Prosthet Orthot.* 2010;22:183–193.
24. Stepien JM, Cavenett S, Taylor L, et al. Activity levels among lower-limb amputees: self-report versus step activity monitor. *Arch Phys Med Rehabil.* 2007;88:896–900.
25. Hargrove LJSA, Lipschutz RD, Finuncane SB, Kuiken TA. Real-time myoelectric control of knee and ankle motions for transfemoral amputees. *JAMA.* 2011;305:1542–1544.
26. Richards JD, Pramanik A, Sykes L, et al. A comparison of knee kinematic characteristics of stroke patients and age-matched healthy volunteers. *Clin Rehabil.* 2003;17:565.
27. Kellis E, Liassau C. The effect of selective muscle fatigue on sagittal lower limb kinematics and muscle activity during level running. *J Orthop Sports Phys Ther.* 2009;39:210–220.
28. Psonak R. *Transfemoral Prosthetics.* Boston: Butterworth Heinemann; 2000 491–520.
29. Olney SJ. Gait. In: Levangie PK, Norkin CC, eds. *Joint Structure and Function.* 4th ed. Philadelphia: Davis; 2005:517–563.
30. Nolan L, Lees A. Functional demands on the intact limb during walking for active trans-femoral and trans-tibial amputees. *Prosthet Orthot Int.* 2000;24:117–125.
31. Sadeghi H, Allard P, Duhaime M. Muscle power compensatory mechanisms in below-knee amputee gait. *Am J Phys Med Rehabil.* 2001;80:25–32.
32. Kaufman KR, Levine JA, Brey RH, et al. Gait and balance of transfemoral amputees using passive mechanical and microprocessor-controlled prosthetic knees. *Gait Posture.* 2007;26:489–493.
33. Raya MA, Gailey RS, Fiebert IM, et al. Impairment variables predicting activity limitation in individuals with lower limb amputation. *Prosthet Orthot Int.* 2010;34:73–84.
34. Jaegers SM, Arendzen JH, de Jongh HJ. Changes in hip muscles after above-knee amputation. *Clin Orthop Relat Res.* 1995;319:276–284.
35. Jandrić S. Isometric hip muscle strength in posttraumatic below-knee amputees [in Serbian]. *Vojnosanit Pregl.* 2007;64:807–811.
36. Burger H, Valencic V, Marincek C, et al. Properties of musculus gluteus maximus in above-knee amputees. *Clin Biomech (Bristol, Avon).* 1996;11:35–38.
37. Mâaref K, Martinet N, Grumillier C, et al. Kinematics in the terminal swing phase of unilateral transfemoral amputees:

microprocessor-controlled versus swing-phase control prosthetic knees. *Arch Phys Med Rehabil.* 2010;91:919–925.

38. Peterson AO, Comins J, Alkjaer T. Assessment of gait symmetry in transfemoral amputees using C-Leg® compared with 3R60 prosthetic knees. *J Prosthet Orthot.* 2010;22:106–112.

39. Nadollek H, Brauer S, Isles R. Outcomes after trans-tibial amputation: the relationship between quiet stance ability, strength of hip abductor muscles and gait. *Physiother Res Int.* 2002;7:203–214.

40. Sjodahl C, Jarnlo G-B, Soderberg B, Persson BM. Pelvic motion in trans-femoral amputees in the frontal and transverse plane before and after special gait re-education. *Prosthet Orthot Int.* 2003;27:227–237.

41. Goujon-Pillet H, Sapin E, Fodé P, et al. Three-dimensional motions of trunk and pelvis during transfemoral amputee gait. *Arch Phys Med Rehabil.* 2008;89:87–94.

42. Morgenroth DC, Orendurff MS, Shakir A, et al. The relationship between lumbar spine kinematics during gait and low-back pain in transfemoral amputees. *Am J Phys Med Rehabil.* 2010;89:635–643.

43. Friel K, Domholdt E, Smith DG. Physical and functional measures related to low back pain in individuals with lower-limb amputation: an exploratory pilot study. *J Rehabil Res Dev.* 2005;42:155–166.

44. Kulkarni J, Gaine WJ, Buckley JG, et al. Chronic low back pain in traumatic lower limb amputees. *Clin Rehabil.* 2005;19:81–86.

45. Corio F, Troiano R, Magel JR. The effects of spinal stabilization exercises on the spatial and temporal parameters of gait in individuals with lower limb loss. *J Prosthet Orthot.* 2010;22:230–236.

46. World Health Organization. *Classifications: International Classification of Functioning, Disability and Health (ICF).* Available at: http://www.who.int/classifications/icf/en/. Accessed 12.07.11.

47. Hoeksma HL, Dekker J, Ronday HK, et al. Comparison of manual therapy and exercise therapy in osteoarthritis of the hip: a randomized clinical trial. *Arthritis Rheum.* 2004;51:722–729.

48. Ingber RS. Iliopsoas myofascial dysfunction: a treatable cause of "failed" low back syndrome. *Arch Phys Med Rehabil.* 1989;70:382–386.

49. Selkow NM, Grindstaff TL, Cross KM, et al. Short-term effect of muscle energy technique on pain in individuals with nonspecific lumbopelvic pain: a pilot study. *J Man Manip Ther.* 2009;17:E14–E18.

50. Yerys S, Makofsky H, Byrd C, et al. Effect of mobilization of the anterior hip capsule on gluteus maximus strength. *J Man Manip Ther.* 2002;10:218–224.

51. Makofsky H, Panicker S, Abbruzzese J, et al. Immediate effect of grade IV inferior hip joint mobilization on hip abductor torque: a pilot study. *J Man Manip Ther.* 2007;15:103–111.

52. Thompson DM. Rehabilitation for persons with transfemoral amputation. In: Lusardi MM, Nielsen CC, eds. *Orthotics and Prosthetics in Rehabilitation.* Boston: Butterworth Heinemann; 2000:521–542.

53. Mercer VS, Gross MT, Sharma S, et al. Comparison of gluteus medius muscle electromyographic activity during forward and lateral step-up exercises in older adults. *Phys Ther.* 2009;89:1205–1214.

54. Gailey RS. Ten exercises to maximize the performance of your prosthetic feet. *In Motion.* 2001;11:1–3.

55. Leavey VJ, Sandrey MA, Dahmer G. Comparative effects of 6-week balance, gluteus medius strength, and combined programs on dynamic postural control. *J Sport Rehabil.* 2010;19:268–287.

56. Williams RM, Turner AP, Orendurff MS, et al. Does having a computerized prosthetic knee influence cognitive performance during amputee walking? *Arch Phys Med Rehabil.* 2006;87:989–994.

57. Baum BS, Schnall BL, Tis JE, et al. Correlation of residual limb length and gait parameters in amputees. *Injury.* 2008;39:728–733.

58. Bellmann M, Schmalz T, Blumentritt S. Comparative biomechanical analysis of current microprocessor controlled prosthetic knee joints. *Arch Phys Med Rehabil.* 2010;91:644–652.

59. Schmalz T, Blumentritt S, Jarasch R. A comparison of different prosthetic knee joints during step over step stair descent. *Orthopädie-Technik (English).* 2002;7:586–592.

60. Vrieling AH, van Keeken HG, Schoppen T, et al. Uphill and downhill walking in unilateral lower limb amputees. *Gait Posture.* 2008;28:235–242.

61. Hafner BJ, Smith DG. Differences in function and safety between Medicare Functional classification level-2 and -3 transfemoral amputees and influence of prosthetic knee joint control. *J Rehabil Res Dev.* 2009;46:417–434.

62. Adler SS, Beckers D, Buck M. *PNF in Practice: An Illustrative Guide.* 2nd ed. Berlin, Germany: Springer; 2000 82.

63. Highsmith MJ, Kahle J, Carey SL, et al. Kinetic asymmetry in transfemoral amputees while performing sit to stand and stand to sit movements. *Gait Posture.* 2011;34:86–91.

64. Pauley T, Devlin M, Heslin K. Fall sustained during inpatient rehabilitation after lower limb amputation: prevalence and predictors. *Am J Phys Med Rehabil.* 2006;85:521–532.

65. Gooday HMK, Hunter J. Preventing falls and stump injuries in lower limb amputees during inpatient rehabilitation: completion of the audit cycle. *Clin Rehabil.* 2004;18:379–390.

66. Miller WC, Speechley M. The prevalence and risk factors of falling and fear of falling among lower extremity amputees. *Arch Phys Med Rehabil.* 2001;82:1031–1037.

67. Blumentritt S, Schmalz T, Jarasch R. The safety of C-Leg®: biomechanical tests. *J Prosthet Orthot.* 2009;21:2–15.

68. Yang J, Jin D, Ji L, et al. The reaction strategy of lower extremity muscles when slips occur to individuals with trans-femoral amputation. *J Electromyogr Kinesiol.* 2007;17:228–240.

69. Kahle JT, Highsmith MJ, Hubbard SL. Comparison of nonmicroprocessor knee mechanism versus C-Leg® on prosthesis evaluation questionnaire, stumbles, falls, walking tests, stair descent, and knee preference. *J Rehabil Res Dev.* 2008;45:1–14.

70. Berry D, Olsen M, Larntz K. Perceived stability, function, and satisfaction among transfemoral amputees using microprocessor and nonmicroprocessor controlled prosthetic knees: a multicenter survey. *J Prosthet Orthot.* 2009;21:32–42.

71. Seymour R, Engbretson B, Kott K, et al. Comparison between the C-Leg® microprocessor-controlled prosthetic knee and nonmicroprocessor control prosthetic knees: a preliminary study of energy expenditure, obstacle course performance, and quality of life survey. *Prosthet Orthot Int.* 2007;31:51–61.

72. Klute GK, Berge JS, Orendurff MS, et al. Prosthetic intervention effects on activity of lower-extremity amputees. *Arch Phys Med Rehabil.* 2006;87:717–722.

73. Kark L, Simmons A. Patient satisfaction following lower-limb amputation: the role of gait deviation. *Prosthet Orthot Int.* 2011;35:225–233.

74. Van der Linde H, Hofstad CJ, Geurts AC, et al. A systematic literature review of the effect of different prosthetic components on human functioning with a lower-limb prosthesis. *J Rehabil Res Dev.* 2004;41:555–570.

75. Fergason J, Keeling JJ, Bluman EM. Recent advances in lower extremity amputations and prosthetics for the combat injured patient. *Foot Ankle Clin.* 2010;15:151–174.

76. Goktepe AS, Cair B, Yilmaz B, et al. Energy expenditure of walking with prostheses: comparison of three amputation levels. *Prosthet Orthot Int.* 2010;34:31–36.

77. Orendurff MS, Segal AD, Klute GK, et al. Gait efficiency using the C-Leg®. *J Rehabil Res Dev.* 2006;43:239–246.

78. Perry J, Burnfield JM, Newsam CJ, et al. Energy expenditure and gait characteristics of a bilateral amputee walking with C-Leg® prostheses compared with stubby and conventional articulating prostheses. *Arch Phys Med Rehabil.* 2004;85:1711–1717.

79. Chin T, Machida K, Sawamura S, et al. Comparison of different microprocessor controlled knee joints on the energy consumption during walking in trans-femoral amputees: intelligent knee prosthesis (IP) versus C-Leg®. *Prosthet Orthot Int.* 2006;30:73–80.

80. Kaufman KR, Levine JA, Brey RH, et al. Energy expenditure and activity of transfemoral amputees using mechanical and microprocessor controlled prosthetic knees. *Arch Phys Med Rehabil.* 2008;89:1380–1385.

81. Highsmith MJ, Kahle JT, Bongiorni DR, et al. Safety, energy efficiency, and cost efficacy of the C-Leg for transfemoral amputees: a review of the literature. *Prosthet Orthot Int.* 2010;34: 362–377.

82. Schmalz T, Blumentritt S, Jarasch R. Energy expenditure and biomechanical characteristics of lower limb amputee gait: the influence of prosthetic alignment and different prosthetic components. *Gait Posture.* 2002;16:255–263.

83. Jepson F, Datta D, Harris I, et al. A comparative evaluation of the Adaptive knee and Catech knee joints: a preliminary study. *Prosthet Orthot Int.* 2008;32:84–92.

84. Buckley JG, Spence WD, Solomonidis SE. Energy cost of walking: comparison of "Intelligent prosthesis" with conventional mechanism. *Arch Phys Med Rehabil.* 1997;78:330–333.

85. Chin T, Sawamura S, Shiba R, et al. Effect of an Intelligent Prosthesis (IP) on the walking ability of young transfemoral amputees: comparison of IP users with able-bodied people. *Am J Phys Med Rehabil.* 2003;82:447–451.

86. Taylor MB, Clark E, Offord EA, et al. A comparison of energy expenditure by a high level trans-femoral amputee using the Intelligent Prosthesis and conventionally damped prosthetic limbs. *Prosthet Orthot Int.* 1996;20:116–121.

87. Datta D, Heller B, Howitt J. A comparative evaluation of oxygen consumption and gait pattern in amputees using Intelligent Prostheses and conventionally damped knee swing-phase control. *Clin Rehabil.* 2005;19:398–403.

88. Johansson JL, Sherrill DM, Riley PO, et al. A clinical comparison of variable-damping and mechanically passive prosthetic knee devices. *Am J Phys Med Rehabil.* 2005;84:563–575.

89. Heller BW, Datta D, Howitt J. A pilot study comparing the cognitive demand of walking for transfemoral amputees using the Intelligent Prosthesis with that using conventionally damped knees. *Clin Rehabil.* 2000;14:518–522.

90. Datta D, Howitt J. Conventional versus microchip controlled pneumatic swing phase control for trans-femoral amputees: user's verdict. *Prosthet Orthot Int.* 1998;22:129–135.

91. Muir SW, Berg K, Chesworth B, et al. Use of the Berg Balance Scale for predicting multiple falls in community-dwelling elderly people: a prospective study. *Phys Ther.* 2008;88:449–459.

92. Yari P, Dijkstra PU, Geertzen JHB. Functional outcome of hip disarticulation and hemipelvectomy: a cross-sectional national descriptive study in the Netherlands. *Clin Rehabil.* 2008;22:1127–1133.

28

Athletic Options for Persons with Amputation

Mark Anderson and Carol Dionne

LEARNING OBJECTIVES

Upon completing the chapter, the reader will:

1. Discuss the relationship of physical exercise and sports to health and prevention of "hypokinetic" disease.
2. Describe barriers that contribute to lack of participation in athletics for persons with disabilities.
3. Identify organizations that support athletic participation for persons with disabilities.
4. Compare the different sports and recreation activities available for persons with limb loss.
5. Describe prosthetic components available to active participation in sports of varying types.

"Games, sport, that is what we must have."
Sir Ludwig Guttman,[1] Founder, Paralympic Games

The importance of participation in sports, recreation, and/or physical activity for all is well understood. Numerous authors have extolled the virtues of being physically active for both physical and mental health, as well as the prevention of "hypokinetic diseases," such as obesity, diabetes, hypertension, and cardiovascular disease. Benefits for individuals who participate in sports or recreational activities include maintenance of normal muscle strength, flexibility, and joint structure and function.[2,3] These benefits are essential with the slowing of the functional decline often associated with normal aging or the presence of a disabling condition. Therefore, the goals for increased physical activity for individuals with a disability are to reverse deconditioning secondary to impaired mobility, to optimize physical functioning, and to promote overall well-being.[4]

In addition to the physical benefits, participation in sports or recreational activities has a significant psychological benefit for both able-bodied and disabled individuals. Both body image and quality-of-life scores have improved in individuals with disability who participate in physical activity and sports.[5-7] Participation in regular sport or vigorous recreational activity has favorable effects on the emotional state of adolescents.[8] Many psychological constructs, such as improved social acceptance, improved physical self-concept and self-esteem, increased self-efficacy and self-confidence,

and a greater locus of control build upon the physical performance accomplishments of the athlete with a disability.[9] Even though the benefits of participation in sports and physical activity are well recognized, there is still a disconnect between knowledge and action. This chapter discusses the importance of athletics for persons with disabilities and describes athletic activities and opportunities for active engagement in sports and recreation available to persons with amputation and disabilities associated with loss of limb.

More than half of the adults with disabilities in the United States do not participate in any leisure-time physical activity compared to one-third of adults without disability.[10] This reinforces the notion that on average, people with a disability are more inactive than the general population, which leads to the questions, "What are the barriers for those with a disability to their participation in sports or physical activities?" and, "What motivates those with disabilities to participate in sports and recreational activities?" The most common barriers[11] to sports participation for individuals with a disability are lack of money, unsuitable local facilities, and health concerns. Additional barriers are lack of local sports facilities, transportation issues, lack of sports offerings for those with a disability, and lack of peer with which to participate. Only 10% of those with a disability report lack of motivation as a barrier to participate. Reasons for participation include health benefits, a feeling of accomplishment after participation, social contacts, and recommendation from a physician or health care professional. In those with limb deficiencies, age, level of amputation, and etiology of amputation do not appear to be related to sports participation following lower-extremity amputation. However, a history of sports participation prior to the amputation increases the likelihood of sports participation following amputation.

OPPORTUNITIES FOR SPORTS OR RECREATION PARTICIPATION

Sports for athletes with physical disabilities are governed by various disabled sports organizations and national governing bodies which are disability-specific. In the United States, the disabled sports organizations for athletes with amputation is Disabled Sports, USA (www.dsusa.org/). The motto of Disabled Sports, USA is, "If I can do this, I can do anything!" and its mission is "to provide national leadership and opportunities for individuals with disabilities to develop independence, confidence, and fitness through participation in community sports, recreation, and educational programs."[12] Disabled Sports, USA is comprised of a nationwide network of community-based chapters that offer a variety of sports/recreational programs. In many instances, sports and recreation participation are the final step in the rehabilitation process of individuals following amputation. Sports participation not only improves sports skills, but it allows individuals to experience the emotional highs and lows of winning and losing, which prepares them to face daily challenges and changes following rehabilitation. Disabled Sports, USA, along with other disabled sports organizations, is a member of the United States Paralympic Committee, which sanctions and conducts competitions and training camps to prepare athletes to represent the United States at the Summer and Winter Paralympic Games. The Paralympic Games are the major international multisports event for athletes with physical disabilities, and are second to only the Olympic Games in number of athletes participating. These Games are organized and conducted under the supervision of the International Paralympic Committee and other international sports federations. For athletes with amputation, there are opportunities to compete in 16 different Summer Paralympic sports and five different Winter Paralympic sports.

The U.S. Paralympics Committee also offers an Emerging Sport Program, which is designed to identify, recruit, track, support, and retain Paralympic-eligible athletes with physical disabilities seeking to become internationally competitive. The success of this program depends on the collaboration between community and military programs, partner organizations, military and veteran facilities, and national governing bodies.

Athlete recruitment and identification begins at the local level. Potential athletes are identified in a variety of ways, including military sport camps, site coordinators for specific sports or events, community programs, coaches, technical officials, or current athletes. Once an athlete is identified as having high performance potential, the Emerging Sports manager facilitates appropriate communication between athlete(s) and local program(s), as well as with the appropriate Paralympic sport coaches and high performance directors. Assistance is provided to these athletes by way of connections to local training resources, participation in select emerging and/or national U.S. Paralympics Team camps and competitions, as well as information regarding able-bodied competitions, events and other general sport program opportunities for developing and emerging athletes.

Summer Paralympic Sports

Summer Paralympic sports[12] include archery, athletics (track and field), cycling, equestrian, fencing, powerlifting, rowing, sailing, shooting, swimming, table tennis, tennis, sitting volleyball, and wheelchair basketball. In 2016, triathlon and canoe will make their Paralympic debut. Each sport has its own unique set of requirements, which may necessitate a modification of the traditional rules of the sport to allow the disabled athlete to compete.

Archery

Archery has been a medal sport since the first Paralympic Games in Rome in 1960. Athletes with physical disabilities demonstrate their shooting precision and accuracy from either a standing or seated (wheelchair) position, in men's and women's categories. Paralympic competition format is identical to that of the Olympic Games. Paralympic archers shoot 72 arrows from a distance of 70 m at a target of 122 cm (approximately 48 inches), using a recurve bow (Figure 28-1, *A*). For competitions other than the Paralympics, athletes shoot at each of four distances. Thirty-six arrows are shot at each distance. The two longest distances use a 122 cm target; the two shorter distances

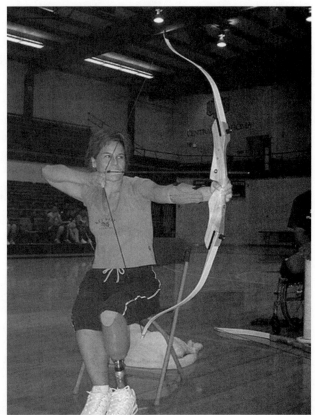

A

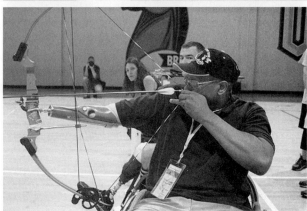

B

FIGURE 28-1 Archery using **(A)** a recurve bow and **(B)** a compound bow. (Courtesy Disabled Sports, USA.)

use an 80 cm target (approximately 36 inches). Distances are 90, 70, 50, and 30 m for men; 70, 60, 50, and 30 m for women. Depending upon their classification based upon level and number of amputations and the athletes' functional ability, athletes competing in other than the Paralympic Games may use either a recurve bow or a compound bow (Figure 28-1, *B*). Archery competition is open to male and female athletes with upper or lower-extremity amputation/limb loss. Specialized devices are also available to assist athletes with upper-extremity prostheses in drawing back the bow and releasing the string.

Athletics (Track and Field)

Athletics events are open to athletes in all disability classes and have been a part of the Paralympic program since the first Paralympic Games in Rome, Italy, in 1960. Events include track (Figure 28-2, *A*) (running distances from 100 m to 10,000 m, plus 4 × 100 m and 4 × 400 m relays), throwing (Figure 28-2, *B*) (shot put, discus, and javelin), jumping (high jump, long jump, and triple jump), pentathlon (long jump, shot put, 100 m, discus and 400 m) and the marathon. The rules of Paralympic track and field are almost identical to those of its nondisabled counterpart. Paralympic track and field competition is open to male and female athletes with upper- and or lower-extremity single or multiple amputation/limb loss. Prosthetic devices may be used. These have been specifically developed to withstand the demands of sports competition. International Paralympic Committee rules require the use of leg prostheses in track events; however, the use of prostheses in field events is optional.

Cycling

Cycling was first introduced as a Paralympic sport in 1984 in Mandeville, England, and involved only those athletes with cerebral palsy. However, it wasn't until 1992 that athletes with amputation competed at the Paralympic Games in cycling. At the 2004 Paralympic Games in Athens, handcycling (for wheelchair users) made its debut as a medal event.

Athletes compete in both track (velodrome) and road events. Track events generally consist of sprints as short as 200 m to time trials and pursuits up to 4 km. Relay races consisting of three-person teams are also contested on the track. Competition on the roads consists of time trials and road races. In time trials, athletes start individually in staggered intervals, racing mostly against themselves and the clock. Road races consist of mass starts. Distances vary based on the host country's discretion. Distances range from 5 km to 65 km in length. Paralympic cycling competition is open to male and female athletes with upper- and/or lower-extremity single or multiple amputation/limb loss (Figure 28-3).

Equestrian

Equestrian made its debut appearance at the Paralympic Games in 1996 with riders from 16 countries competing. By the Paralympic Games in 2008, in Beijing, that number had grown to 73 riders from 28 countries. Riders compete in two dressage events; a championship test of set movements and

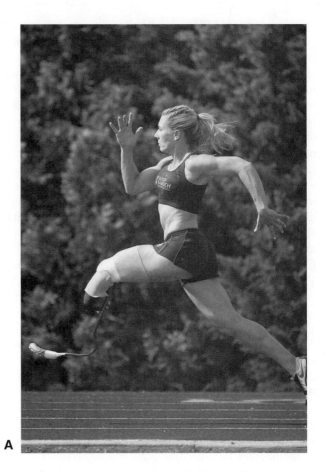

A

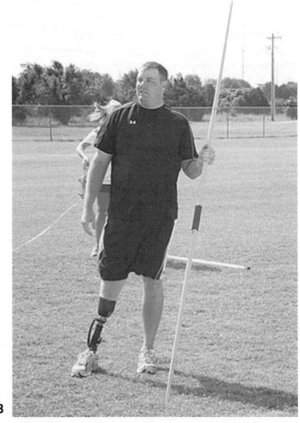

B

FIGURE 28-2 Paralympic athletic events include **(A)** running track and **(B)** javelin.

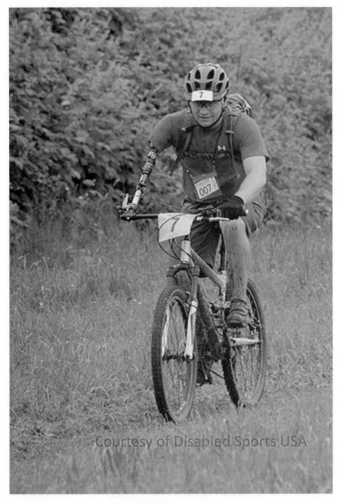

FIGURE 28-3 Cycling.

a freestyle test to music. There is also a team test for three or four riders. Competitors are judged on their display of horsemanship skills demonstrated through their use of commands for walk, trot, and canter. Paralympic equestrian competition is open to male and female athletes with upper- and/or lower-extremity single or multiple amputation/limb loss.

Fencing

Fencing has been part of the Paralympic Games since 1960. Athletes compete in wheelchairs that are fixed to the floor. They rely on ducking, half-turns and leaning to dodge their competitors' touches. However, fencers can never rise up from the seat of the wheelchair. The first fencer to score five touches is declared the winner. Athletes play the best out of three rounds and compete in single and team formats. Weapon categories for men include foil, epee and sabre. Women compete in foil and epee. Paralympic fencing competition is open to male and female athletes with upper- and/or lower-extremity single or multiple amputation/limb loss.

Powerlifting

Powerlifting is one of the fastest growing Paralympic sports. Paralympic athletes have been competing in powerlifting since 1964; however, it was initially offered only to lifters with

spinal cord injuries. Currently, athletes from many different disabled sports groups participate in the sport, assimilating rules similar to those of nondisabled lifters. Athletes compete only in the bench press, and they draw lots to determine order of weigh-in and lifts. After the athletes are categorized within the 10 different weight classes (male and female), they each lift three times (competing in their respective weight class). The heaviest "good lift" (within the weight class) is the lift used for final placing in the competition. Paralympic powerlifting competition is open to male and female athletes with upper- and/or lower-extremity single or multiple amputation/limb loss. There is currently a move to include the single-arm press in powerlifting competitions for those individuals with upper-extremity amputation, with the hope of making this a Paralympic sport.

Rowing

Rowing is a relatively new Paralympic sport, making its first appearance in Beijing in 2008. The sport was selected for Paralympic inclusion in 2005, just 3 years after adaptive rowing made its debut on the world championship level in 2002. The rowing events include the men's and women's single sculls, the trunk-arms double sculls and the legs-trunk-arms mixed four with coxswain (Figure 28-4). Paralympic rowing competition is open to male and female athletes with upper- and/or lower-extremity single or multiple amputation/limb loss.

Sailing

Sailing first became a medal sport for the 2000 Paralympic Games in Sydney, Australia. Three boat types raced at the 2008 Paralympic Games in Beijing: the 2.4mR, a single-person keelboat; the SKUD-18, a two-person keelboat; and the Sonar, a three-person keelboat, along with the high performance SKUD-18 m, which must include one female and one person deemed a Functional Classification System "1," or severely disabled, such as an athlete with quadriplegia. Sailors are seated on the centerline for Paralympic events, but the boat can be sailed with or without either of the seats and configured to suit different sailors' needs. Because of its design and control, the

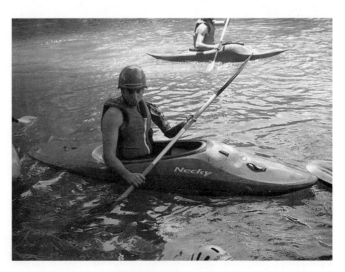

FIGURE 28-4 Kayaking.

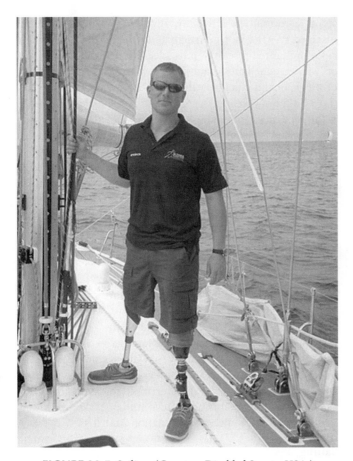

FIGURE 28-5 Sailing. (Courtesy Disabled Sports, USA.)

2.4mR was selected for single-person races. The boat's ease of use allows for a level playing field, making tactical knowledge the dominant factor in competition. The Sonar uses a versatile crew-friendly design that is accommodating to athletes with physical disabilities. It is used by sailors of all experience and ability levels, from the novice to international competitors (Figure 28-5). Paralympic sailing competition is open to male and female athletes with upper- and/or lower-extremity single or multiple amputation/limb loss.

Shooting

Shooting, divided into rifle and pistol events, air and .22 caliber, has been a Paralympic sport since 1976. The rules governing Paralympic competition are those used by the International Shooting Committee for the Disabled. These rules take into account the differences that exist between disabilities allowing ambulatory and wheelchair athletes to compete shoulder to shoulder. Shooting matches athletes of the same gender, with similar disabilities, against each other, both individually and in teams. Paralympic shooting competition is open to male and female athletes with upper- and/or lower-extremity single or multiple amputation/limb loss.

Swimming

Swimming for men and women has been a part of the Paralympic program since the first Games in 1960 in Rome, Italy. Races are highly competitive and among the largest and most popular events in the Paralympic Games. Paralympic swimming competitions occur in 50-m pools and, while competing, no prostheses or assistive devices may be worn. Athletes compete in the following events: 50 m, 100 m and 400 m Freestyle; 100 m Backstroke; 100 m Breaststroke; 100 m Butterfly; 200 m Individual Medley; 4 × 100 m Freestyle Relay and 4 × 100 m Medley Relay. Paralympic swimming competition is open to male and female athletes with upper- and/or lower-extremity single or multiple amputation/limb loss.

Table Tennis

Table tennis has been a part of the Paralympic program since the inaugural Games in 1960. Rules governing Paralympic table tennis are the same as those used by the International Table Tennis Federation, although slightly modified for players using wheelchairs. Athletes must use the same quick technique and finesse in the games of competitors from various disability groups, including men's and women's competitions, as well as singles, doubles, and team contests. All matches are played best-of-five games to 11 points. Paralympic table tennis competition is open to male and female athletes with upper- and/or lower-extremity single or multiple amputation/limb loss.

Tennis

Wheelchair tennis first appeared at the Paralympic Games in Barcelona in 1992 and is played on a standard tennis court and follows many of the same rules as tennis. However, in wheelchair tennis, a player is allowed to let the ball bounce twice if necessary before hitting a return shot and the doubles court lines are used for both singles and doubles. Also, the athlete's wheelchair is considered to be a part of the body, so rules applying to the player's body apply to the chair as well. Paralympic wheelchair tennis competition is open to male and female athletes with upper- and/or lower-extremity single or multiple amputation/limb loss.

Sitting Volleyball

Instituted in 1976 as a standing Paralympic sport, Paralympic volleyball has now become exclusively a sitting sport. Paralympic volleyball follows the same rules as its able-bodied counterpart with a few modifications to accommodate the various disabilities (Figure 28-6). In sitting volleyball, the net is approximately 3.5 feet high, and the court is 10 × 6 m with a 2-m attack line. Players are allowed to block serves, but one "cheek" must be in contact with the floor whenever they make contact with the ball. Paralympic volleyball competition is open to male and female athletes with upper- and/or lower-extremity single or multiple amputation/limb loss.

Wheelchair Basketball

Basketball has been a part of the Paralympic Games since 1960 and originally played only by men with spinal cord injuries. Now both men's and women's teams throughout the world, with a variety of disabilities, compete in the sport. Many of the same rules from its counterpart apply in the wheelchair game. Although plays and tactics are similar, special rules,

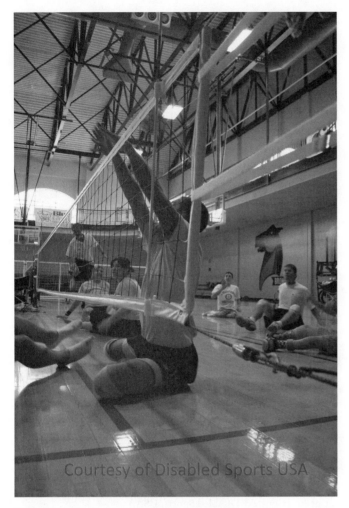

FIGURE 28-6 Sitting volleyball. (Courtesy Disabled Sports, USA.)

such as those to accommodate dribbling from a wheelchair, are also in place. The sport is governed by the International Wheelchair Basketball Federation. The International Wheelchair Basketball Federation governs all aspects of the game, including court size and basket height, which remain the same as able-bodied basketball. Athletes in this event are grouped by demonstrated playing ability, rather than strictly by medical classification. Paralympic basketball competition is open to male and female athletes with upper- and/or lower-extremity single or multiple amputation/limb loss.

Winter Paralympic Sports

Just like the Summer Paralympic Games, the Winter Paralympic games[12] are held every 4 years following the conclusion of the Winter Olympic Games in the host city of the Olympics. Paralympic athletes with amputations compete in five winter sports: alpine skiing; biathlon; cross-country skiing; curling; and sled (sledge) hockey.

Alpine Skiing

Paralympic alpine skiing competition is open to male and female athletes with amputation. There are four individual events in alpine skiing: downhill, which started as a demonstration event at the 1980 Paralympic Games in Norway;

slalom; giant slalom, which was introduced as a demonstration event in 1984; and super-G. Mono-skiing (Figure 28-7, *A*) was introduced in both alpine and Nordic events in 1988 at the Games in Innsbruck, Austria. Skiing equipment varies, depending on the athlete's level and number of amputations. Athletes with double-leg amputation above the knee (transfemoral) typically use two skis with two outriggers but may also choose to sit ski in a mono-ski. Athletes with single transfemoral amputation often use one ski with two outriggers (Figure 28-7, *B*). Athletes with double-leg below-knee (transtibial) amputation and those with single-leg transtibial amputation may use two skis with two ski poles. Athletes with double-upper-extremity amputations, regardless of level, ski with two skis but no ski poles while single-upper-extremity amputee athletes use two skis and one ski pole. If athletes have one upper-extremity and one lower-extremity amputation, they may use ski equipment that facilitates the athletes' best function.

Nordic Skiing

Paralympic Nordic skiing is a Winter Paralympic sport consisting of two events: biathlon and cross country skiing. Biathlon (Figure 28-8) combines elements of cross-country skiing and target shooting. Athletes ski three 2.5-km loops (7.5 km total), stopping after the first two loops to shoot at five targets (10 targets total). One minute is added to the athlete's finishing time for each miss. Biathlon has been a part of the Paralympic Winter Games since 1992. Cross-country skiing started with the Paralympic Games in Sweden in 1976. Cross-country races range from 2.5 km to 20 km depending on disability and gender. Paralympic Nordic skiing competition is open to male and female athletes with amputation/limb loss.

Curling

Paralympic curling is a wheelchair sport that was introduced at the 2006 Paralympic Winter Games. As in able-bodied curling, teams are composed of two competitors who throw "stones" by hand or by the use of a stick towards a target at the opposite end of the ice. However, there is no sweeping and only competitors in wheelchairs are allowed to compete. The object of the game is to get a team's stones as close to the center of the target (the "house") as possible. Six ends are played with a possible extra end if the teams are tied after six. Paralympic wheelchair curling competition is open to male and female athletes with amputation/limb loss.

Sled (Sledge) Hockey

Sled hockey is a variation of ice hockey in which the athletes compete on the ice by means of a sled. Just as in ice hockey, sled hockey is played with six players (including a goalie) at a time. Players propel themselves on their sled by use of spikes on the ends of two three-foot-long sticks, enabling players to push themselves as well as shoot and pass the puck. Rinks and goals are regulation Olympic-size, and games consist of three 15-minute stop-time periods. Sledge hockey became a medal sport in the 1994 Paralympic. Paralympic sled hockey competition is open to male athletes with amputation/limb loss.

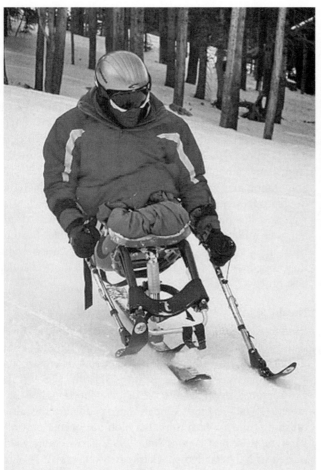
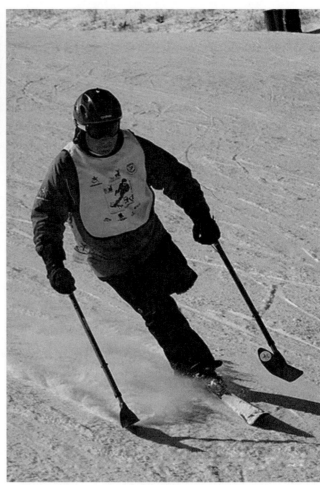

A   **B**

FIGURE 28-7 Alpine skiing. **A,** Mono-ski. **B,** Outriggers. (Courtesy Disabled Sports, USA.)

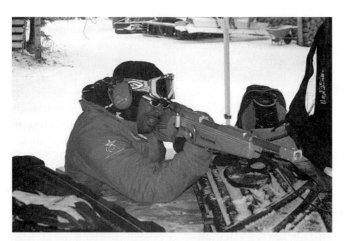

FIGURE 28-8 Target shooting component of a Nordic skiing-shooting biathlon. (Courtesy Disabled Sports, USA.)

Nonparalympic Sports and Recreational Activities for Individuals with Amputation

Although Paralympic sports are popular among individuals with amputation, there are many other sports and recreational activities available to this population. Many of these sports require little or no adaptation for participation by those with amputation, allowing competition between able-bodied and disabled individuals.

Badminton

Disabled badminton [13] is played by people with many different disabilities, including those with both upper- and lower-extremity amputation. Participants may compete either standing or in a wheelchair. Disability badminton provides players of different disabilities and backgrounds an opportunity to participate in a common sport. Although more common in Europe, most people in the United States become involved in badminton through word of mouth and people introducing others to the sport. It is a growing sport with an increasing number of participants taking up the game either socially or competitively, or both. Both men and women in all age groups participate in badminton, and the sport is in the process of being evaluated for possible inclusion in the Paralympic Games.

Fishing

Fishing [14] is a sport that can be enjoyed by anyone. There are many different types of specialized equipment available to the disabled angler, including rods, reels, line, rod holders, and tackle, including easy cast and electric fishing reels for individuals who may have difficulties casting and reeling in a fish. There are also harness rod holders which can mount on a wheelchair or the side of a boat and allow an individual with limited use of their arm(s) to participate in recreational fishing. Pontoon boats can provide easy accessibility for those in wheelchairs. The Paralyzed Veterans of America sponsors a variety of fishing tournaments for people with disabilities, and there are disability fishing groups and clubs that cater for children with disabilities who enjoy fishing. They offer several bass fishing tournaments where those interested in fishing can learn new skills or improve old ones. The Paralyzed Veterans of America Bass Tour offers Team/Open Competition, pairing disabled anglers with able-bodied boat partners. Those who prefer not to fish from a boat can participate in the Bank Competition. Both novice and experienced anglers can compete for significant cash and other prizes. Fishing Has No Boundaries, Inc. is another nonprofit organization for all persons with disabilities that has grown into a national organization with 23 chapters in 11 states. Fishing Has No Boundaries enables thousands of people with disabilities to participate fully in the recreational activity of fishing.

Hunting

As with fishing, hunting [13] is a recreational activity that can be enjoyed by all, and any disability can be offset by adaptive hunting equipment and adaptive hunting techniques. There are many different types of adaptive equipment that can be used by either gun or bow hunters with either upper- or lower-extremity amputation. This includes hunting blinds that are more wheelchair friendly, protective clothing to make cold weather hunting more enjoyable, adaptive tree stands, tripod-mounted crossbow or gun rests, and wheelchair-based gun rests. Federal, state, and local governments are providing easier access to thousands of acres of trails, parks, and wilderness areas. There are organizations and clubs with programs for persons with disabilities who want to participate in hunting activities.

Golf

Just about anyone, regardless of ability level, can participate in golf [15]. This makes it one of the best sports for people with disabilities, especially those with amputation (Figure 28-9). All amputees can successfully play golf, including those with lower-extremity prostheses, where a torsion absorber and rotator allow them to pivot to finish their swing. For those with upper-extremity amputation, they may play with just one arm, or if they play with one arm and a prosthesis, there are a number of pieces of adaptive hardware that allow them to attach their prosthetic arm to their club, allowing them to swing with both hands. If they are unable to walk a full 18-hole course, they may play golf from a seated position on a single-rider golf cart. Numerous other devices exist to help golfers with amputation tee-up and retrieve their ball, better grip the club, and aid their game.

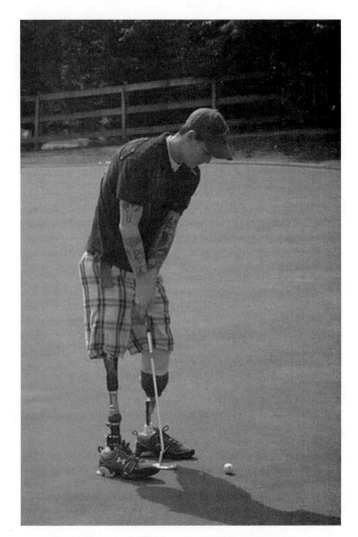

FIGURE 28-9 Golf. (Courtesy Disabled Sports, USA.)

Trail Orienteering

Conventional orienteering combines fast running with precise navigation, typically through forests or over moorland. Trail orienteering [16] is a discipline of the sport designed so that people with disabilities could have meaningful orienteering competitions (Figure 28-10). It completely eliminates the element of speed over the ground, but makes the map-interpretation element much harder. Able-bodied people can compete on equal terms with the disabled. Depending on the level of difficulty, up to five control markers are hung at each site and only one will correspond exactly with the control description and control circle position. Sites are chosen so that they can be seen from a wheelchair-navigable path or area, but they may be quite a distance into the forest or over nonnavigable terrain. The only special equipment needed is a compass. An escort can give the competitor physical help—pushing a chair, holding and orienting map and compass, even marking the control card with the decision according to the competitor's instructions. However, it is an important rule that escorts must not help in the decision-making process; they can give as much physical help as may be necessary,

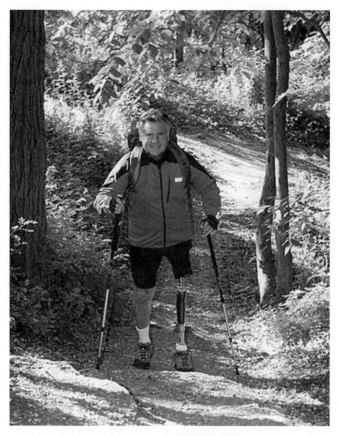

FIGURE 28-10 Trail orienteering. (Courtesy Disabled Sports, USA.)

but must not offer advice or opinions to the competitor. For serious competitions, escorts are "swapped" so they do not know the competitor they are helping.

Along with trail orienteering, other ambulatory sports/ activities may be appropriate for individuals with amputation. For those who enjoy the outdoors, hiking (Figure 28-11, *A*), mountain climbing (Figure 28-11, *B*), rock climbing (Figure 28-11, *C*), and ropes courses (Figure 28-11, *D*) are popular, as is snowboarding (Figure 28-11, *E*) during the winter months. These activities are easily done with able-bodied friends and can be done safely as long as normal outdoor precautions are observed. For those activities that require additional training or practice, there are many qualified instructors available at most recreational areas for lessons or instructions to increase enjoyment and reduce the likelihood of injury while participating in these sports.

Sky Diving

Skydiving[17] is a sport that can involve skydivers who have one or more amputated limbs. Because of their prosthetic devices, amputee skydivers often have to compensate for the change in weight with the positioning of their body for both themselves and other divers in a formation. Many of these individuals begin skydiving in tandem, making jumps while attached to a certified jump instructor. However, as individuals become more experienced, many progress to solo (accelerated free fall) jumps. Modifications to prosthetic devices, particularly lower-extremity prostheses, may need to be made because of the forces incurred during landing after the jump.

Additional Water Sports and Activities

Besides swimming, there are numerous other water sports in which individuals with amputation may participate. These include surfing, windsurfing, water skiing, kayaking, and scuba diving. Surfing[18] for individuals with amputation can be a fun and exciting sport (Figure 28-12, *A*). Individuals may begin surfing while lying on the board, progressing to seated, quadruped, kneeling, and finally standing. Once standing, individuals may choose to surf with our without their prosthetic device.

Until recently, windsurfing[19] has been an inaccessible sport to people with amputations. However, equipment modifications have made windsurfing accessible to people with all types of disabilities. One may begin to windsurf in a fixed or swivel seat attached to the windsurfing board. Outriggers or flat-bottom pontoons can be attached to the sides of the windsurfing board to provide additional stability. A standing rail can be used on the board for someone to stand with an instructor for support. One or two sails can be used so that instructors can be on the windsurfing board to help assist. Such adaptations open the sport up to men and women with all types of disabilities, including amputation.

Water skiing[20] has been adapted so that physically disabled individuals can participate and compete (Figure 28-12, *B*). Competition is held in three events, slalom, tricks and jumping for lower-extremity amputees (above and below knee), upper-extremity amputees, and individuals with both arm and leg amputations. The skiers compete with the same water ski equipment used by able-bodied skiers; however, the use of a prosthetic device is optional.

Kayaking may be done solo or in tandem. To avoid entrapment, individuals with lower-extremity amputations should not wear a regular prosthesis in the kayak. A water-sports prosthesis that can be strapped to the outside of the boat for easy access is recommended. For those with upper-extremity amputations, one-handed paddles may be used, or individuals may practice paddling using heavy tape or rubber rings to secure their grip on the paddle, as conventional terminal devices are not designed to hold paddles. Rowing prosthetics also are available for amputees using other types of water crafts. For safety, wetsuits, helmets, and flotation devices are recommended for all participants.

Scuba diving can be an excellent recreational activity for individuals with amputation (see Figure 28-12, *C*). Because of the buoyancy provided by the water, mobility issues are significantly reduced, and scuba diving can be taught to swimmers with both upper- and lower-extremity amputation with virtually no modifications. For some, scuba diving represents total freedom because it affords one the opportunity to move about without an assistive device in a barrier-free, gravity-free environment. Many individuals choose to scuba dive without their prostheses, but water-sport prostheses are available in desired. As with able-bodied divers, the same basic safety and equipment concerns apply to everyone.

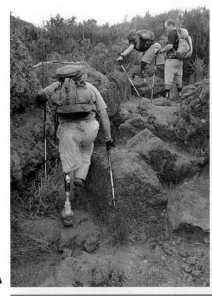

A

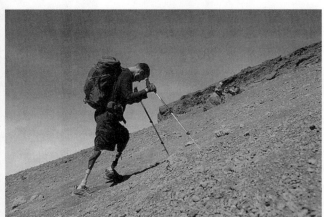

B

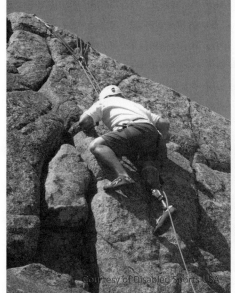

C

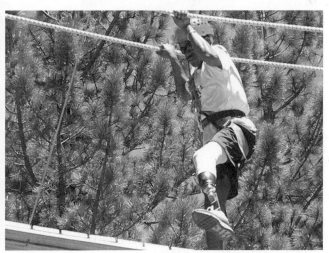

D

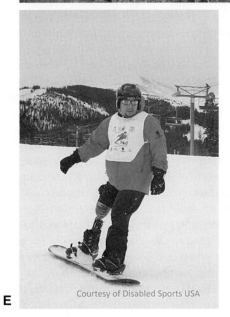

E

FIGURE 28-11 Outdoor activities. **A,** Hiking. **B,** Mountain climbing. **C,** Rock climbing. **D,** Ropes course. **E,** Snowboarding. (Courtesy Disabled Sports, USA.)

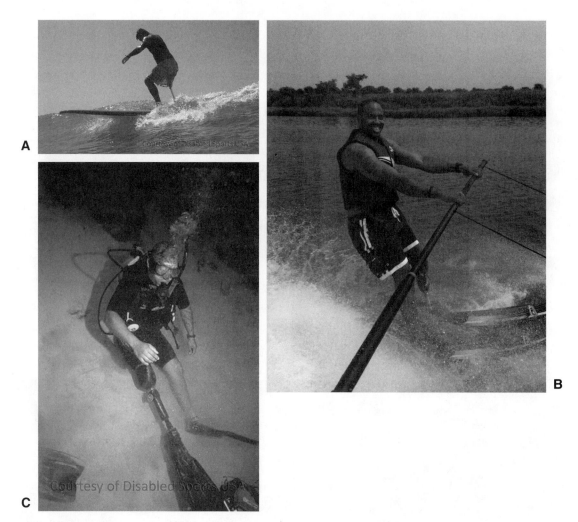

FIGURE 28-12 Water sports. **A,** Surfing. **B,** Water skiing. **C,** Scuba diving. (Courtesy Disabled Sports, USA)

PROSTHETIC COMPONENTS FOR ATHLETES WITH AMPUTATION

Historically, people with amputation were considered disabled. Without exception, they were marginalized in activities of everyday life, most notably so in participation in recreational and competitive sports. Exoskeletal prosthetics, essentially the only choice of artificial limb design available at the time, were heavy and difficult to manage while attempting to throw a ball or move at a varied pace required in any skilled sport.[21] Now, with the advent of inclusion of people with all levels of ability, people with amputation are part of the societal mainstream. Most people with amputation receive rehabilitation to improve overall function in order to return to the family, to a workplace, and, more recently, to sport-related activity. Moreover, motivated people with amputation have formed sport-enthusiast groups that have created the market demand for improvement and acceleration of modifications to everyday use prosthetic limbs and creation of more sport-specific designs.

Prosthetic Components for Athletes with Lower-Limb Amputation

Lower-limb prosthetics are commonly composed of a means of suspension, a prosthetic socket, joint articulation (as needed), shaft (or pylon), and foot. Prosthetics have now become modular in construction such that the athlete can still use the prosthetic socket of choice and interchange certain components to meet the demands of a specific sport. Even recreational athletes with amputation can enjoy sports using their usual prosthetics with additional or interchangeable modification. However, committed athletes with amputation must consider the biomechanical demands of their sport and apply the components that allow safe and competitive participation, and choose prosthetic components accordingly.[13] For example triathletes may choose to use a swimming prosthetic leg or opt not to use a prosthetic limb during the swimming portion of the competition. Additionally, prosthetic design has advanced to the creation of sport-specific prosthetics, such as for bicycling, swimming and track and field competition. However, affordability of these devices poses as a barrier to common accessibility.

Once the residuum has sufficiently matured to be able to accept the shear, torsion, and load demands playing in a desired sport, athletes with amputation can be fitted with prosthetics to help meet the rigors of training. Considerations must be made for sports that demand high levels of shear, such as those that involve running or cutting.[22] These excessive forces increase the risk of soft-tissue breakdown, pain, time out of the prosthesis, and away from the sport. High levels of activity also increase added perspiration within the prosthetic socket, increasing the risk of infections and related skin problems.[23] Regardless of choice of prosthetic components, proper prosthetic management and skin care are essential in sport.

Suspension and Sockets

If people recovering from limb amputation surgery set a goal for participation in sport, they should closely consult with the rehabilitation team, composed of the surgeon, physical therapist, and specifically, the prosthetist, to create a prosthesis to meet that goal. Added prosthetic suspension (cuff, straps, sleeve) may be required for the prosthesis to remain intimate to the residual limb, in light of expected changeable limb volume during play.[24] And, as previously stated, the residuum skin must be protected during participation in recreational sports as well as every-day activities. Gel liners or sleeves provide a protective socket-residuum interface to minimize shear and other loading factors, particularly during the early phases of recovery or during repetitive movements in play.[25] Thus, gel liners are also recommended for the higher-level athletes. Special accommodation for boney areas at the socket-residuum interface should be considered and is usually warranted. Total-surface-bearing prosthetic sockets are recommended because they are designed to disperse forces evenly over the entire surface area of the residuum-socket interface to minimize risk for soft-tissue breakdown.[16,26]

Knee Joints

There are a variety of computerized knee joints on the market that are designed for user-matched walking speeds. However, there has yet been a computerized knee joint designed to withstand the rigors of "stop-start" running, cutting, jumping, or swimming. The athlete with transfemoral amputation can choose to use a mechanical running limb because it is a simpler, more reliable knee joint design that can be controlled in "real time." Usually, however, the athletes depend on the energy-storing running foot and the power of the hip extensors to substitute for natural knee function. Alternatively, athletes can choose to use no articulation at all, like when competing in track and field events (Figure 28-13).

Lower Leg/Foot/Ankle Components

Prosthetics have now become modular in construction such that the athlete can still use the socket of best fit and change out the prosthetic components to minimize risk of injury and maximize performance. Application of the appropriate prosthetic foot to maximize efficiency towards symmetrical step lengths during varied walking speeds enables the

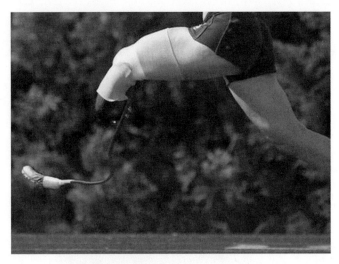

FIGURE 28-13 Prosthetic suspension.

recreational amputee to participate in higher levels of activity. In some cases, prosthetic foot/ankle/knee components can be interchanged using a "quick-release" coupler for use in specific sport-like activities. Forces that may negatively impact the residual limb must be minimized with proper selection of prosthetic components. Pylons, special-design prosthetic ankles and heels that absorb and dissipate energy during loading, are important considerations. Athletes with either transtibial or transfemoral amputation who wish to run or sprint typically use an energy-storing foot. This specialized foot is constructed of materials that essentially "store" the energy during locomotion and transfer energy with significant efficiency to propel the athlete forward in walking or running gait. This particular prosthetic foot is attached posterior to the prosthetic socket. For the athletes involved in running or sprinting, these high-performance carbon fiber foot components are essential. This design enables the athlete with bilateral or unilateral, transtibial or transfemoral, amputation to participate and successfully compete in sports never before considered. However, there are limitations to these designs. For those who play sports on uneven ground and need ankle designs that simulate foot pronation and supination, athletes must depend on the older, mechanical designs to compete with less risk for injury and falls.[14]

Athletes with Upper-Limb Amputation

Although there are fewer people with upper-limb amputation than with lower-extremity amputation, there is a growing number of those who are competing in sports who require skilled use of the arms and hands. As with computerized lower-extremity prosthetics, computerized upper-extremity prosthetics pose an even more daunting obstacle for pragmatic use in sport. So, prosthetic designers have created, with use of the human-powered prosthesis, terminal devices that are used to throw and catch a ball or hold a bow and arrow. The devices do not simulate human anatomy, but are designed for performance in sport, not cosmesis (Figure 28-14).[16]

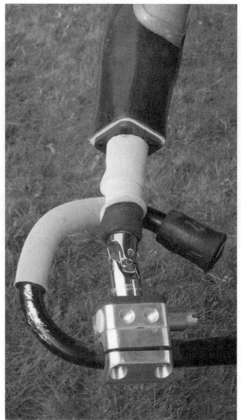

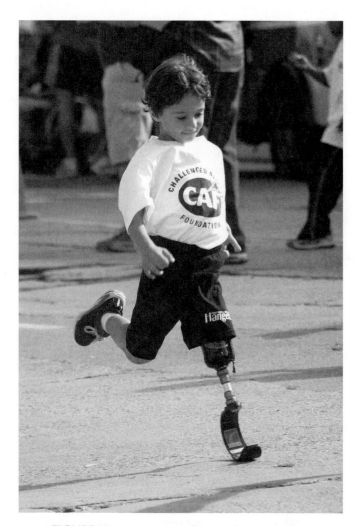

FIGURE 28-15 Sports prosthesis without knee joint.

CHILDREN WITH AMPUTATION IN SPORT

It is very important for children with amputation to be physically active and fit to meet the added energy expenditure of playing and competition using artificial limbs. This poses a daunting challenge to those who create prosthetics for these children. Typically, the prosthetic design is essentially of simpler construction for use when the children are very young. But, as children develop and grow, more complicated, adult-level components are added to the prostheses. For example, current pediatric knee components usually provide control, shock absorption, and freedom to move like a growing child. Use of carbon-fiber energy-storing prosthetic feet is considered the norm. However, these components must be light, yet strong and sufficiently durable to enable the young athlete to compete (Figure 28-15).[27]

PROSTHETICS IN SPORTS: WHAT IS BEST?

Despite many advances in the design and composition of either upper- or lower-extremity prosthetic limbs, there is no tangible evidence as to which component designs are best

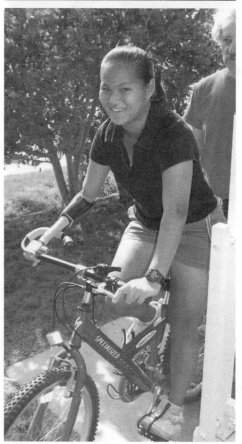

FIGURE 28-14 Upper-limb sports prosthesis.

suited for any particular sport or amputee consumer group. According to systematic review, there have been several studies whose aims were to determine the effectiveness of a group of prosthetic foot-ankle or knee joint designs, but, because of the poor quality and incomparability of research designs, no conclusions could be drawn. Thus, choice of sports prosthetic is currently made on an individualized, case-by-case, expert opinion basis for those in competitive sport.[18]

SUMMARY

The value of active engagement in physical activity that includes participation in sports and recreation for all individuals has been determined as an essential component of healthy living. Persons with disabilities should have the opportunity to participate in athletics of varying types and engage in competitive sports. This chapter provides information on the many competitive and noncompetitive athletic options available to persons with disabilities associated with limb loss. Health care providers working with persons with amputation are encouraged to facilitate active involvement in physical exercise by means that involve participation in sports and recreational activities. Physical therapists, occupational therapists, prosthetists, and orthotists should work together with the individual with special needs to assure that the most favorable equipment and materials and instructions for use are provided for maximum participation.

REFERENCES

1. Whitteridge D, Guttmann L. 3 July 1899–18 March 1980. In: *Biographical Memoirs of Fellows of the Royal Society*. Vol 29. London: The Royal Society; 1983:226–244.
2. Pringle D. Winter sports for the amputee athlete. *Clin Prosthet Orthot*. 1987;11(3):114–117.
3. Nolan L. Lower limb strength in sports-active transtibial amputees. *Prosthet Orthot Int*. 2009;23(3):230–241.
4. Murphy NA, Carbone PS. Promoting the participation of children with disabilities in sports, recreation, and physical activities. *Pediatrics*. 2008;121:1057–1061.
5. Tatar Y. Body image and its relationship with exercise and sports in Turkish lower-limb amputees who use prosthetics. *Science Sports*. 2010;25:312–317.
6. Deans SA, McFadyen AK, Rowe PJ. Physical activity and quality of life: a study of a lower-limb amputee population. *Prosthet Orthot Int*. 2008;32(2):186–200.
7. Groff DG, Lundberg NR, Zabriskie RB. Influence of adapted sport on quality of life: perceptions of athletes with cerebral palsy. *Disabil Rehabil*. 2009;31(4):318–326.
8. Steptoe A, Butler N. Sports participation and emotional wellbeing in adolescents. *Lancet*. 1996;347:1789–1792.
9. Hutzler Y, Bar-Eli M. Psychological benefits of sports for disabled people: a review. *Scand J Med Sci Sports*. 1993;3:217–228.
10. Rimmer JH, Wolf LA, Sinclair LB. Physical activity among adults with a disability—United States, 2005. *MMWR Morb Mortal Wkly Rep*. 2007;56(39):1021–1024.
11. Finch N, Lawton D, Williams J, et al. *Young disabled people and sports. Disability Survey 2000: Survey of young people with a disability and sport*. www.sportengland.org. Accessed 15.04.11.
12. *Disabled Sports USA*. http://www.dsusa.org/.
13. *Badminton*. http://www.activeamp.org/badminton.
14. Take it Outside—Hunting, Fishing Adapt to Meet Physical Abilities and Enhance Experience. *Challenge Magazine*. 2005; 10(2):29–31.
15. Golf is for Everyone. *Challenge Magazine*. 2005;10(1):23–26.
16. *Trail Orienteering*. http://www.trailo.org.
17. *Amputee Skydiving*. http://atwiki.assistivetech.net/index.php/Amputee_skydiving.
18. *AmpSurf*. http://ampsurf.org.
19. *Windsurfing*. http://www.activeamp.org/sport_dir.htm.
20. *Disabled Water Skiing*. http://waterski.teamusa.org/sport-disciplines/disabled-water-skiing.
21. Prince F, Allard P, Therrien RG, et al. Running gait impulse asymmetries in below-knee amputees. *Prosthet Orthot Int*. 1992;16:19–24.
22. Klute GK, Berge JS, Orendurff MS, et al. Prosthetic intervention effects on activity of lower extremity amputees. *Arch Phys Med Rehabil*. 2006;87:717–722.
23. Lyon CC, Kulkarni J, Zimerson E, et al. Skin disorders in amputees. *J Am Acad Dermatol*. 2000;42:501–507.
24. May BJ, Lockard MA. *Prosthetics & Orthotics in Clinical Practice: A Case Study Approach*. Philadelphia: Davis; 2011.
25. Tazawa E. Analysis of torso movement of transfemoral amputees during level walking. *Prosthet Orthot Int*. 1997;21:129–140.
26. Van der Linde H, Hofstad CJ, Geurts AC, et al. A systematic literature review of the effect of different prosthetic components on human functioning with a lower-limb prosthesis. *J Rehabil Res Dev*. 2004;41(4):555–570.
27. Wind WM, Schwend RM, Larson J. Sports for the physically challenged child. *J Am Acad Orthop Surg*. 2004;12:126–137.

29

Rehabilitation for Children with Limb Deficiencies

JOAN E. EDELSTEIN

LEARNING OBJECTIVES

On completion of this chapter, the reader will be able to do the following:

1. Relate developmental milestones to the habilitation of children with congenital limb deficiency and rehabilitation of those with amputation.
2. Describe how prostheses can be designed to accommodate longitudinal and circumferential growth so that fit remains comfortable and the child can attain maximum function.
3. Outline the ways a clinician can address psychosocial concerns for infants, toddlers, school-age children, and adolescents.
4. Compare prosthetic options for children of various ages who have upper- or lower-limb deficiencies.
5. Specify the training goals for children of various ages fitted with upper- and lower-limb prostheses.
6. Design a habilitation program for an infant born with multiple limb deficiencies.

Maria, who was born without a left forearm and hand, Bobby, who caught his foot in a powered lawn mower, and George who is recovering from femoral sarcoma have different skeletal, neuromuscular, learning, and psychosocial challenges from those of adults with amputation. Children share some rehabilitation issues with adults, particularly the basic components of the prosthesis and the essential elements of postoperative care. Other considerations, however, are unique. Because children are smaller than adults, the choice of prosthetic components is not as broad. Youngsters grow and develop through the rehabilitation process. In addition, young people legally, financially, and emotionally depend on adults for their medical, surgical, and rehabilitation care.

Clinicians concerned with comprehensive management of children with limb deficiencies need to consider the causes of limb deficiency, the relationship of developmental milestones to prosthetic selection and use, and the psychosocial factors that affect children in order to design optimal programs.[1-3] Care of the infant born with a limb anomaly is habilitation, whereas management of someone who undergoes amputation because of trauma or disease is rehabilitation.

Unless the distinction is relevant, however, habilitation and rehabilitation are used interchangeably in this chapter. Similarly, limb deficiency is used to designate both congenital and acquired limb absence. The overall goal of physical therapy is to facilitate the normal developmental sequence and prevent the onset of secondary impairments and functional limitations such as contractures, weakness, and dependence in self-care.

COMPREHENSIVE CONSIDERATIONS IN CHILDHOOD

The philosophy of this chapter is that the child with a limb deficiency is first and foremost a person, with the beauty, delight, and promise inherent in all young people.

Classification and Causes of Limb Deficiencies

The International Organization for Standardization approved a system of limb deficiency classification in 1989 (Figure 29-1).[4] Congenital limb anomalies are described anatomically and radiologically as transverse, in which no skeletal elements exist below the level of normal development, or longitudinal, in which a reduction or absence of elements is present within the long axis of the limb, with normal skeletal elements usually present distal to the affected bone (Figure 29-1). This system replaces older terms, such as phocomelia (distal segments attached to the torso), amelia (complete absence of a limb), and hemimelia (partial absence of a limb).

Limb deficiency is caused by congenital deficiency, trauma, cancer, and disease. In the total U.S. population, peripheral vascular disease among adults accounts for more than 80% of amputations, with a greater than 25% rate of increase in the latter half of the twentieth century. Rates of trauma- and cancer-related amputations are declining, whereas the incidence of congenital deficiencies remains stable.[5] A recent survey of all children with lower-leg deficiencies in The Netherlands indicated 73% with congenital deficiencies and 27% with amputations as a result of malignancies (9%), trauma (8%), infection (4%), and other pathologies (6%).[6]

Among those with congenital limb anomalies, transverse deficiency of the upper limb, especially the left extremity, is the most common.[7] McGuirk and associates found the overall prevalence of limb deficiency among 161,252 newborns to be 0.7 per 1000 births. Thirty percent of the defects were

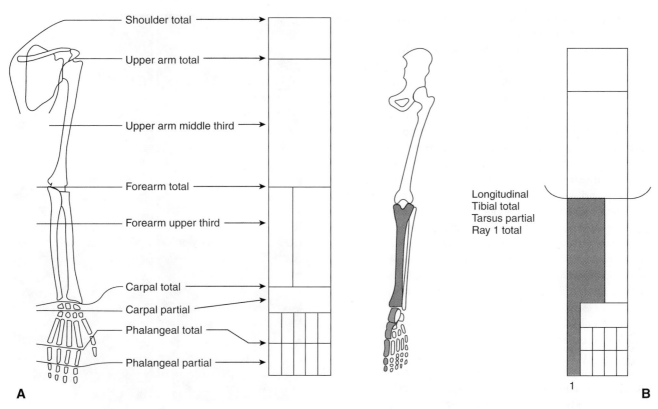

FIGURE 29-1 A, International Organization for Standardization/International Society for Prosthetics and Orthotics system for classifying upper-limb congenital limb deficiencies. Lower-limb transverse deficiencies are named in a similar fashion. Levels can also be described by naming the absent bone(s). **B,** Lower-limb longitudinal limb deficiency. The *shaded area* represents missing segments. (Reprinted with permission from Murdoch G, Wilson AB (eds). *Amputation: Surgical Practice and Patient Management.* Oxford, UK: Butterworth Heinemann, 1996. p. 352.)

caused by genetic factors, 4% by teratogens, 35% by vascular disruption, and 32% by an unknown cause.[8]

Powered lawn mowers[9-11] and all-terrain vehicles[12] are responsible for many traumatic amputations among children and adolescents.

Long-term followup of the Childhood Cancer Survivor Study, which is composed of 14,054 individuals who have survived for 5 or more years after cancer treatment, indicates that osteosarcoma or Ewing sarcoma of the lower limb or pelvis is the most common tumor; the median age at diagnosis is 14 years.[13] Some patients with tumor are treated by various limb-sparing procedures, and others undergo amputation. Long-term outcome is similar, although more patients with amputation used walking aids and were less satisfied with their status as children.[14-19]

Developmental Milestones

Motor skills develop in a predictable sequence, with well-established milestones that mark achievement of important functional abilities.[20-22] In the absence of cerebral maldevelopment or malformation, the infant born with a limb anomaly or a young child who undergoes amputation demonstrates physical control at approximately the same time as an unaffected child does. Limb deficiency, however, often alters how the developmental tasks and activities are

performed. For example, the 5-month-old infant who has only one intact leg will develop a distinctive style of crawling. Therapists who conduct initial evaluations of these children focus on muscle strength, range of motion, gross motor patterns, coordination, attention span, and interests.

All children, not just those with limb deficiency, display varying rates of neuromuscular development. Chronological age cannot provide a complete picture of a child's developmental level. In this chapter, milestones pertaining to upper and lower limb development are related to habilitation of children with limb disorders.

Physical conditioning programs, especially active sports, are important to enhance general health and endurance, particularly for those who wear a prosthesis. Play and games increase coordination and improve strength. Swimming is particularly beneficial because it does not traumatize the limbs and does not require a prosthesis; nevertheless, some children may be reluctant to display an anomalous limb.

Accommodating Growth

All children grow, regardless of congenital anomalies or amputations. Prosthetic planning should incorporate measures to maintain comfortable socket fit and symmetrical limb length. The preschool-age child may need a new prosthesis almost yearly. Those in grade school often require a new prosthesis every 12 to 18 months, and teenagers outgrow prostheses every 18 to 24 months.[1]

Longitudinal growth is typically more rapid than circumferential growth, a troublesome fact for children with lower-limb deficiency. Reconstructive surgery, especially circular (Ilizarov) fixation, suits children with minimal length discrepancy, whereas amputation remains preferable for those with severe limb loss.[23] Too short a lower-limb prosthesis disturbs the quality and efficiency of gait and substantially increases energy cost. In contrast, an upper limb prosthesis that is slightly short will probably not present a noticeable asymmetry and will have little effect on bimanual activities. Endoskeletal prosthetic components facilitate lengthening and substitution of more sophisticated components.

Vigorous play causes considerable wear of the mechanical parts of prostheses. These parts are also vulnerable because of their small size and the sand, grass, and mud which children find inviting. Youngsters are likely to wear out prostheses from everyday use before circumferential growth necessitates a change. Signs of an outgrown socket include a tendency of the residual limb to slip out of the socket, pain or skin reddening caused by socket tightness, and a flesh roll around the margin of the socket. Socket liners are a convenient way to accommodate circumferential growth; as the child grows, liners can be removed. Alternatively, the prosthesis can be fitted with several layers of socks; the child eventually wears fewer socks to accommodate the added residual limb girth. Flexible sockets fitted to extra-thick frames are another way to accommodate growth. To fit the larger residual limb, a new flexible socket is made and material is ground from the frame.[23]

Prosthetic alignment should complement the immature skeleton and joint capsules. Children with surgical amputations through the bony diaphysis or metaphysis may have terminal bony overgrowth (Figure 29-2). As these children grow, terminal periosteal new bone may protrude beneath the terminal subcutaneous tissue and skin. Without treatment, a bursal sac forms and the skin becomes ecchymotic and hemorrhagic. The underlying bone then ruptures the bursal sac, and infection can occur.[1] Overgrowth is a particular problem when the adolescent growth spurt begins. Customary treatment is excision of the periosteal sac, transection of the distal 2 to 3 cm of bone, and primary closure of the incision. Children may require this procedure several times during the growth period.[24] Another approach is continuous skin traction, which can be used to maintain skin and soft-tissue coverage over the distal end of the residual limb until skeletal growth is complete. The difficulties of keeping distal force on the limb day and night usually preclude this method. Disarticulation preserves the distal epiphyseal plate and thus is not associated with overgrowth.

Near-normal range of joint motion is an important determinant of effective prosthetic use in children with limb deficiencies, as well as in adults with amputation. Active therapeutic exercise designed to increase joint excursion is preferable to passive stretching, especially in the presence of congenital contracture.[2]

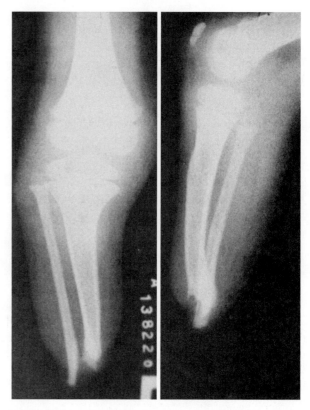

FIGURE 29-2 Bony overgrowth of the fibula in the transtibial amputation limb of a 7-year-old child. In the original amputation surgery, the fibula was slightly shorter than the tibia. (Courtesy J. E. Edelstein.)

Postoperative Care

Postoperative care is simpler for young children who undergo amputation than for adolescents and adults. Ordinarily the residual limb presents little or no edema and the wound heals rapidly. Phantom pain can occur and is associated with the extent of preoperative pain. Approximately one-fourth of those with congenital limb deficiency or amputation before the age of 6 years have phantom sensation, with far fewer reporting phantom pain.[25] A pain diary may help older children and adolescents cope with phantom pain from traumatic amputation.

Psychosocial Factors in Habilitation and Rehabilitation

Habilitation amounts to more than selecting a suitable prosthesis and devising appropriate training. All children have personalities that develop along with their physical growth. Optimal emotional development occurs when parents and clinicians promote wholesome interactions. The essential message is that the child has a unique personality and that independence commensurate with age can be fostered.

Infants

Infants learn trust when their basic needs are met. The baby with limb anomaly has as much need for trusting, responsive care as does the infant with normal limbs. Infants respond to the anxieties of parents and others who interact with them. Successful habilitation depends on the parents' replacing the expectation of a "perfect" infant with the reality of a baby who happens to have a limb deficiency. Birth of a baby with a limb deficiency can elicit intense emotion. Because such an event is rare in any hospital, medical staff may display shock and feelings of helplessness or revulsion. Some parents characterize the first few weeks after birth as a nightmare. They believe they are alone with a unique and hopeless problem when questions go unanswered or evaded. Reactions of the infant's grandparents, siblings, and other family members influence habilitation. Mourning for the loss of the ideal child is part of the coping process.[1]

Newborns are too young for prosthetic fitting; nevertheless, early referral to a specialized clinic is highly desirable. The core team is composed of a pediatrician, physical therapist, occupational therapist, and prosthetist. The team should be able to draw on the expertise of psychologists, social workers, orthopedists, and engineers, depending on the needs of the child and family.[2] Effective clinical team management involves the family in rehabilitation decisions and weighs management recommendations in light of the immediate impact on the child's welfare and the long-term consequences on his or her appearance and function as an adult. An important resource is the Association of Children's Prosthetic-Orthotic Clinics (6300 North River Road, Suite 727, Rosemont, IL 60018-4226; www.acpoc.org). The association, founded in 1958, has held an annual interdisciplinary conference since 1972.

The clinical team creates an atmosphere in which parents and their baby are welcome, encouraging conversation about feelings and obtaining answers to questions. The team's approach aims to maximize the child's function, while learning the parents' style of dealing with unexpected events. Team members should empathize with parents' grief, which can bear little relation to the extent of the infant's disability.[1] Some parents resist holding the baby, hide the deformity, avoid direct contact, or withdraw into silence. When clinicians hold the baby, parents usually realize that the infant really is lovable. Rather than denying any difference, the team fosters the attitude that, yes, they know the child is different, but they recognize and accept the baby for what the baby is and what the baby can do.

CASE EXAMPLE 1

A Newborn with Congenital Transradial Limb Deficiency

Mr. and Mrs. M. anticipated the birth of their second child with great eagerness. Mrs. M. had excellent prenatal care and an easy pregnancy. The couple prepared their 2-year-old daughter for her new role as "big sister," encouraging her to feed her dolls bottles and push them in a stroller. Their daughter also moved to a junior bed with a coverlet that she chose. Mr. and Mrs. M. repainted the crib and hung new curtains in the nursery. The grandparents flew to town to await the birth and to help care for the older child and the new baby.

S. M. was born a few days later in the local hospital. She was a healthy, term infant with lusty lungs. The obstetrical nurse wrapped her in a receiving blanket and presented her to her proud parents. Mrs. M. was wheeled to her room for an overnight stay. Once settled in her room, Mr. and Mrs. M. unwrapped the baby, only to discover a left transradial limb deficiency. Mrs. M. shouted to the nurse on duty that someone had made a mistake. The nurse checked identification bracelets and confirmed that S. M. was indeed her daughter. Both Mr. and Mrs. M. were distraught that the baby's left hand was missing. In his grief and anger, Mr. M. threatened the nurse, medical staff, and hospital administration with legal action. Mrs. M., meanwhile, was silent, turning her head to the wall, refusing food and medication. Discharge to home with the baby is planned for the next morning.

Questions to Consider

- Given Mrs. M.'s depression and Mr. M.'s anger, how should the attending physician and nursing staff proceed?
- What should the social worker or psychologist do to provide appropriate guidance for the parents?
- How might the grandparents and older sister help Mr. and Mrs. M. when they return home with their new daughter?
- What is the most constructive response the physical therapist can give when first meeting S. M. and her parents?
- How can the physical therapist and occupational therapist facilitate positive immediate and long-term family interaction?

Families may be interested in seeing pictures or examples of the type of prosthesis that the child will probably use. Expectations regarding the extent of prosthetic restoration, however, may be unrealistic. Parents should understand what prosthetic and surgical possibilities exist so they can make rational decisions for their child. Infants usually receive the first prosthesis at approximately 6 to 9 months of age.[2,25] Comparing the performance of children fitted with an upper-limb prosthesis before 1 year of age with those fitted later indicates no difference in satisfaction with the prosthesis nor functional use.[26] Some parents find it difficult to accept the prosthesis, believing that it draws attention to the limb deficiency.

The team can also help parents of children who undergo amputation because of trauma or disease cope with feelings of guilt and shock. Team members assist the family in realizing that they were not negligent in protecting the child against injury or not recognizing symptoms of a disease process early enough to prevent amputation.

In addition to clinical team management, families benefit from participating in peer support groups in which they can share concerns, exchange information, and observe children of various ages playing with and without prostheses. Some groups publish newsletters that share information with those who live too far from the meeting site. The Amputee Coalition of America (900 East Hill Avenue, Suite 205, Knoxville, TN 37915; www.amputee-coalition.org) is a peer advocacy organization that produces a magazine, monographs, and videos; has annual conferences; operates the National Limb Loss Information Center; sponsors a youth camping program, national peer network, and limb-loss education and awareness program, among many other activities.

Parental acceptance of and active cooperation in the training program are the most important factors in its success and largely determine whether the child regards the prosthesis as a tool in daily activities.[1] Families need to learn skin care, prosthetic operation, maintenance, and the capabilities and limitations of the prosthesis. Outpatient training is preferable to avoid homesickness, which can interfere with the child's learning. In addition, the constant presence of one or both parents during therapy sessions enables the entire family to learn about prosthetic use and maintenance. Putting a prosthesis on an active child is a skill that takes time for parents to master. Scheduling appointments after naps and meals is generally more productive than attempting to coerce a tired and hungry child to participate in therapy. Clinicians should incorporate many brief activities in the treatment session, recognizing that infants have short attention spans. Therapists who treat infants need to interpret nonverbal indications of comfort or discomfort and satisfaction or dissatisfaction with the prosthesis. For example, the infant who coos, smiles, and engages in play is probably content with the prosthesis and the function it offers, whereas a cranky, crying child may be contending with an ill-fitting socket. As with all patients, the clinician must frequently examine the child's skin, with particular attention to persistent redness, indicating high pressure, and irritation, which may signal dermatitis.

CASE EXAMPLE 2

A Child with Congenital Transradial Limb Deficiency

S. M. eats heartily, allows her older sister to sprinkle talcum powder on her, and is developing normally. She smiles and gurgles when someone approaches her. By 6 months she is sitting independently and can use both arms to clutch stuffed toys. She grabs the railings of her crib, attempting to pull herself to standing. The physical therapist recommended that the family take S. M. to a rehabilitation center that specializes in caring for children with amputations. At the center, Mr. and Mrs. M. overcame their initial hesitation and now participate enthusiastically in a peer support group, in which a dozen parents of children with limb deficiency trade advice and provide emotional support.

Mr. and Mrs. M. are concerned about unwelcome comments regarding their daughter's appearance, both with an empty sleeve and with the possibility of a hook terminal device. They tried to persuade the clinical team to provide

S. M. with an infant passive mitt, which would disguise the anomaly. The therapist showed Mr. and Mrs. M. that the mitt has no prehensile capability. One of the members of the support group extolled the virtues of a myoelectric hand, so Mr. and Mrs. M. then argued that S. M. should be provided with "only the best," regardless of cost. Support group members pointed out that S. M. was too small for myoelectric fitting but might be a candidate in another year or two. S. M. is fitted with a simple transradial prosthesis consisting of infant voluntary-opening hook, wrist unit, socket, and infant harness. The prosthesis does not have a cable.

Questions to Consider
- What activities in the clinic would help S. M. acclimate to her new prosthesis?
- What activities would be appropriate for a home program for the first week after prosthetic fitting?
- What types of bimanual activities can be accomplished with a transradial prosthesis with a passive hand rather than a cable-controlled terminal device?
- What toys can be recommended to the grandparents that will help S. M. incorporate the prosthesis in her play time?
- How can the prosthesis facilitate S. M.'s physical and psychological development?

Toddlers

Toddlers must develop self-control to acquire the autonomy necessary to cope with their environment. The interval between 1 and 3 years of age is characterized by the development of language and functional communication, assertion of independence, and interpersonal control. Children as young as 3 years should be informed of any impending surgery, whether to revise a congenital anomaly or treat disease or injury. Doll play can help the child understand surgery and rehabilitation. Special dolls that depict amputations at various levels, with and without prostheses, are available.

Children must resolve feelings of deprivation and resentment that accompany the visible alteration of their bodies.[1] Mobility, control, exploration, initiative, and creativity are prime emotional developmental milestones for older toddlers and young school-age children. Parents and professional staff should encourage the child's independence. Facile use of a prosthesis can help children maximize their psychological potential. Children compare themselves with others and ask, "Where is my other hand (or leg)?" Children form two body images, one with and the other without the prosthesis. Parents should be able to give a simple and truthful answer, clearly stating that the child will not grow another hand, saying something like "you were born this way."[1] Similarly, children who undergo amputation need a realistic answer to the question, "What happened to you?" The child may engage parents in a power struggle regarding prosthetic wearing. A firm yet gentle approach with a range of acceptable choices usually enables the child to incorporate autonomy needs while gaining prosthetic proficiency.

The clinical team should value the parents' comments about their child and involve the family in all aspects of care. The waiting room should have a variety of safe toys to make visits more pleasant. Parents should be present during the child's examination and prosthetic fitting to increase communication and thereby reduce anxiety and maximize effectiveness of the prosthetic prescription and fitting process.

School-Age Children

School-age children need to become industrious and engaged in planning and executing tasks. The upper- or lower-limb prosthesis can be instrumental in fostering this important psychological task. The clinical team can help prepare the child and family for encounters with teachers, scout masters, clergy, and other adults.

In group experiences, the child may have to deal with feelings of social devaluation. The teacher or other group leader is in a position to bolster the child's sense of self-worth. The first day at school or camp can be the occasion when the child displays the prosthesis and demonstrates its function. The presentation usually dispels the mystery of the appliance and shows that the prosthesis is simply a tool that makes it easier for its wearer to engage in certain activities. The teacher should be aware of the appearance of the residual limb, the child's function with and without the prosthesis, any environmental or programmatic adaptations that the child may need, and how to cope with prosthetic malfunction. Anticipating awkward situations helps develop coping strategies. For example, in a circle game, classmates may be reluctant to hold hands with someone who wears an upper-limb prosthesis. If the teacher holds the child's prosthetic hook, the other students are likely to realize that it is not scary or unacceptable to do so. School officials may be concerned about the ability of a child with a prosthetic leg to maneuver in the classroom and playground. Classmates' natural curiosity should be dealt with through honest, simple answers. Although teasing is inevitable, the young child who feels secure understands that taunts are merely crude expressions of interest.

Among school-age children with limb deficiencies, demographic variables (such as age, sex, socioeconomic status, and degree of limb loss) are not significant predictors of self-esteem. In contrast, social support, family functioning, self-perception, and microstressors affect the child's adaptation. Many school-age and older children respond favorably to scouting, camping, and other group recreational activities. Sports programs, such as skiing, horseback riding, and track events, are fun and give children with disabilities pride in athletic achievement.

Older Children and Adolescents

Adolescents face the critical step of developing a satisfying identity within themselves and with their peer groups. The teenager may select times when prosthetic wear is not desirable, for example, eschewing an upper limb prosthesis during a football game or discarding the leg prosthesis when swim-

ming or playing beach volleyball. Adults should nurture young adults so they develop sufficient self-esteem to make satisfying decisions about when to use or remove the prosthesis. Teenagers with limb loss must cope with being visibly different. Young adults have to adapt to a culture designed for those who do not have a disability and must evaluate whether people relate to them as individuals or as people with handicaps. During adolescence, feelings such as "Why did this happen to me?" are often intensified. Adolescents constantly reexamine their body image; group showering after physical education class may be especially stressful for those with limb loss. Other developmental concerns in which limb loss plays a role are choosing a vocation, obtaining a driver's license, and engaging in sexual activity. The clinical team needs to be sensitive to concerns about privacy, confidentiality, and independence.

Adolescents with bone cancer who undergo an amputation typically pass through a stage of initial impact when they learn that the treatment plan includes amputation. This news may be met with despair, discouragement, passive acceptance, or violent denial. Informing the adolescent of the rehabilitation process and the achievements of others can be helpful. The next stage is retreat, during which the adolescent experiences acute grief. Anger may be part of the coping process. The goal of grieving is relinquishing hope of retrieving the lost object. The staff can reinforce the patient's strengths and encourage maximal independence. The third stage is acknowledgment, when the adolescent is willing to participate in rehabilitation and has incorporated the changed appearance into his or her body image. Reconstruction, the final stage, involves the return to developmentally appropriate activities, such as school, sports, and dating.

CASE EXAMPLE 3

An Adolescent with Osteogenic Sarcoma

E. K., who is 15 years old, is scheduled tomorrow to have surgical ablation of his right arm at the level of the humeral epicondyles to remove an osteogenic sarcoma. Six months ago he fractured his right radial head. Although the fracture healed well, he noticed persistent tenderness at the elbow with a firm mass that was increasing in size. His physician referred him to an orthopedist. After a series of bone scans and biopsies, the orthopedist confirmed the diagnosis of osteogenic sarcoma and recommended immediate amputation. E. K. and his parents refused the surgery and traveled to four clinics in the surrounding states seeking advice regarding treatment of the tumor. They explored alternate methods of treatment, including herbal preparations to shrink the sarcoma, en bloc resection with implantation of an endoprosthetic elbow joint, and amputation of the arm distal to the epicondyles. After meeting with the clinical team at the children's medical center and speaking with several patients who had had surgery and rehabilitation, they reluctantly agreed to amputation during his summer vacation.

An excellent student, E. K. is also the shortstop on his high school varsity baseball team and plays the tuba in the marching band. For the past two summers he has been a counselor at a sports- and computer-oriented camp. The family is committed to devoting all its financial and emotional resources to enable E. K. to resume a full agenda of academic and recreational activities. E. K. has compiled considerable information regarding prostheses from the Internet.

Questions to Consider
- What postoperative management would foster wound healing and enable E. K. to become accustomed to a prosthesis?
- How can the occupational therapist and physical therapist help E. K. cope with loss of his dominant hand?
- Compare the advantages of a cable-controlled prosthesis with a prosthesis having a myoelectrically controlled terminal device and cable-controlled elbow unit.
- What terminal device would be most suitable for E. K.?
- How can the clinical team guide E. K. when he returns to school in September?
- In what recreational activities can E. K. engage after his amputation?

REHABILITATION AND PROSTHETIC DECISION MAKING

Not all children with limb deficiency benefit from prostheses. With certain upper-limb anomalies, the remaining portion of the limb is more functional when bare than it would be if it were covered by a prosthesis.[1,25] Some children who are born with bilateral arm absence generally use their feet to play and can do almost everything they need to without using complicated and heavy prostheses.[25,27,28] In one large study, approximately half of the children with unilateral congenital deficiencies and two-thirds of those with amputation received prostheses. By the age of 12 years, two-thirds of those who had prostheses were still using them.[29]

Rehabilitation of Children with Upper-Limb Amputation

Because functional use of an upper-limb prosthesis often involves control of a terminal device (substitute for the missing hand), the prosthetic design and the rehabilitation program should be appropriate for the child's level of motor, cognitive, and perceptual development.

Infants

Prosthetic fitting and training should complement an infant's development. Although a prosthesis usually is not fitted until babies are at least 6 months of age, earlier developmental accomplishment paves the way for successful prosthetic use.

The average 2-month-old infant can hold objects with both hands. The baby who lacks one or both hands typically attempts to hug a stuffed animal with the forearms or upper arms, capitalizing on the tactile sensitivity of the skin. The normal 3-month-old can bring grasped objects to the mouth. Three months is also the age when babies attempt two-handed prehension, although this skill is not perfected until the child attains sitting balance at age 6 to 9 months.[3]

The 4-month-old infant props on the forearms, shifts weight to reach, and usually enjoys shaking noisy rattles by using rapid elbow flexion and extension. An important developmental step is reached at approximately the same age when the child can manipulate objects with one hand while the other hand stabilizes the toy. Simultaneous sitting and manipulating are still challenging at this age. Increased trunk strength enables the baby to reach unilaterally and bilaterally. Bilateral coordination at 4 months allows the infant to reach objects at the midline. Two-handed holding of a bottle typically occurs at approximately 4.5 months.[22]

By the fifth month, the infant can transfer toys from one hand to the other and is thus aware of the usefulness of holding objects. The infant's dominant interest is in getting food; exploring surroundings; and making social contact with those who feed, hold, and provide care. Holding a large ball encourages the infant to clasp objects between the arms. Manipulating blocks or beads promotes stabilization of proximal body parts to allow fine movements with distal parts. Although a baby with intact limbs can get to the quadruped position and shift weight from side to side,[22] the infant who is missing one or both arms will probably find that crawling is impossible and will have difficulty coming to a sitting position and pulling to a standing position.

Six months is generally considered the optimal age for upper-limb prosthetic fitting (Figure 29-3).[1] The baby with unilateral amputation has achieved good sitting balance, can free the sound hand for manual activities while sitting, and is actively engaged in exploring the environment. The prosthesis restores symmetrical limb length and enables the infant to hold stuffed animals and similar toys at the midline. The prosthesis also accustoms parents to the concept that a prosthesis will likely be a permanent part of their child's wardrobe. Fitting can assuage parental guilt or shame regarding their infant's abnormal appearance by replacing negative reactions with a constructive device that enhances the baby's development. Many parents seek a prosthetic hand to disguise the limb anomaly. Early fitting provides experience that will be the basis for the young person's later decision regarding whether to continue with prosthetic use. Fitting earlier to a rapidly growing infant makes the maintenance of socket fit difficult. In addition, a younger baby may find the prosthesis a hindrance during rolling maneuvers. Infants who are much older than 6 months may resist a prosthesis that deprives them of using the tactile sensation at the end of the residual limb. Initial fitting after 2 years tends to result in greater rejection of the prosthesis because by then the child has developed compensatory techniques.

At 8 months, most babies sit while manipulating objects with both hands by using gross palmar grasp and controlled release. A prosthesis aids in clasping large objects and stabilizing smaller ones while the sound hand explores them.

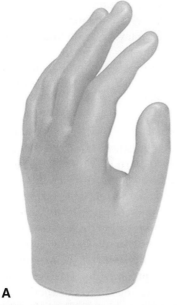

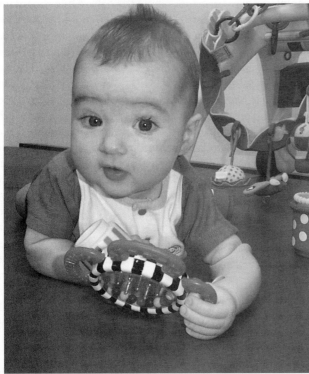

FIGURE 29-3 Infant prosthetic hands. **A,** Centri passive hand. **B,** Infant playing with Alpha hand. (A, Courtesy Fillauer Companies, Inc., Chattanooga, TN.; B Courtesy TRS, Inc., Boulder, CO.)

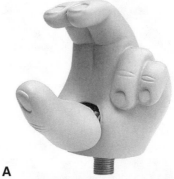

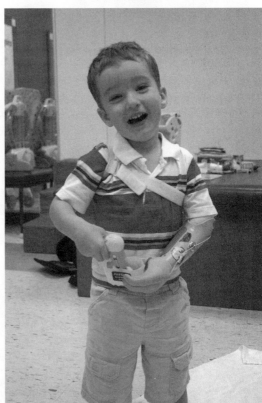

FIGURE 29-4 Children's terminal devices. **A,** Voluntary-closing hand. **B,** Boy wearing CAPP (Child Amputee Prosthetics Project) Voluntary-opening terminal device on a transradial prosthesis (A, Courtesy TRS, Inc., Boulder, Colo.; B, Courtesy Fillauer Companies, Inc., Chattanooga, TN)

By 15 months, most children can place a pellet in a small container and use crayons for scribbling and a spoon for feeding. These skills can also be performed with a prosthesis.

The first prosthesis is usually passive, that is, it does not have a cable or other operating mechanism. The terminal device may be a hook or a passive mitt. The hook is covered with pink or brown resilient plastic to disguise its mechanical appearance. The plastic also blunts the impact of the hook as infants explore with it, swiping themselves and others in the

vicinity. The hook may be a voluntary-opening design, without a cable. Parents can place a rattle or other object in the hook to acquaint the baby with prehension on the deficient side. A few children start with the Child Amputee Prosthetics Project (Los Angeles, CA) terminal device (Figure 29-4), which functions in the voluntary-opening mode. Some infants have a voluntary-closing hook on the first prosthesis (Figure 29-5); in the absence of a cable, the hook holds the toy secured with tape or a rubber band. The three options offer little difference in function. A fourth terminal device option is the infant passive mitt. The mitt has a less-mechanical appearance than other terminal devices but has no prehensile function; objects can be taped to it for the amusement of the baby. The absence

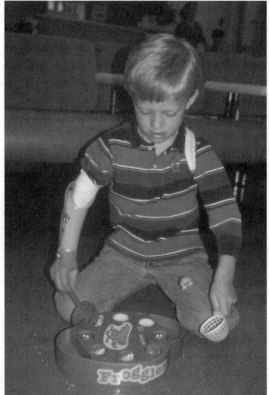

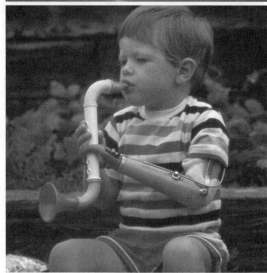

FIGURE 29-5 Voluntary-closing terminal devices on prostheses. **A,** Lite-Touch hand. **B,** Adept hook. (Courtesy TRS, Inc., Boulder, CO.)

does not have an elbow unit even if the anomaly is comparable to transhumeral amputation.

Regardless of the level of limb loss, the prosthetic socket is suspended on the infant's torso by a harness, which typically has more straps than an adult harness. The toddler harness inhibits the infant's attempts to remove the prosthesis, whether deliberately or inadvertently during rolling and crawling.

Clothing problems arise when a prosthesis is worn. The rigid parts of the prosthesis eventually wear holes in fabric. Shirts and blouses worn over the prosthesis should be loose fitting; sleeves set at the natural shoulder line can interfere with cable operation, thus raglan sleeves are preferable.

Training the infant fitted with a passive prosthesis usually begins with two sessions in a 1-week period and then at periodic followup appointments. The first meeting should be held when the baby is well rested and content. The therapist or parent puts the prosthesis on the baby, who is then placed on the floor with various toys. The therapist encourages the parents to play with and handle the baby while the infant is wearing the prosthesis. The baby may ignore the prosthesis because its socket eliminates the sense of touch and because the length of the prosthesis feels awkward. Parents should present large toys that require the use of both arms. The basic prosthesis allows the infant to cuddle a teddy bear, swat at a dangling toys, and use both upper limbs for rolling and crawling. Training involves instructing the parents and other caregivers to gain familiarity with the prosthesis, care for the infant's skin by making certain that the socket and harness do not exert undue pressure, and provide toys that require bimanual prehension (Box 29-1). Placing a rattle in the terminal device is another way of acquainting the infant with grasp on the side of limb deficiency. At the end of the session, the therapist and parent remove the prosthesis to inspect the child's skin for signs of irritation from the socket or harness. Parents learn how to apply the prosthesis and how to encourage full-time wear except during baths, naps, and bedtime. The baby may be rather awkward when sitting and moving while adjusting to the weight of the prosthesis. Toys suitable for the infant's developmental level, such as large balls, dolls,

of a hooked configuration hampers use of the mitt when the baby attempts to pull to standing at the side of the crib or playpen. Whatever the design, the terminal device is generally fitted into a wrist unit at the distal end of the socket.

The thermoplastic socket is custom molded to a plaster model of the child's residual limb. A fabric sock protects the skin from pressure concentration imposed by the socket. A snug fit is needed around the humeral epicondyles to stabilize the prosthesis on the child's residual limb. Depending on the rate of growth, changes may be needed every 2 to 4 months. If the anomaly is higher, the first prosthesis usually

---

BOX 29-1   *Prosthetic Training Goals for Infants*

Therapy sessions are designed to increase the infant's
- Comfort with the prosthesis
- Wearing tolerance
- Ability to clasp large objects
- Ability to use the prosthesis to aid in sitting and crawling

Parents of an infant with a prosthesis should do the following:
- Apply and remove the prosthesis correctly
- Care for the child's skin
- Care for the prosthesis
- Recognize and report to the clinical team any problems with the prosthesis or child

stuffed animals, balloons, xylophones, and other noisy and colorful objects, provide incentives for enjoying the prosthesis. Parents can put a mallet or other toy in the hook so that the infant can obtain pleasure from using the prosthesis. Push and pull toys are appropriate when the child is able to stand and cruise.[25]

Printed instructions, augmented by audiotapes or videotapes, are useful guides for the family. Instructions can address parental concerns regarding the possibility that the child may catch the prosthesis on table legs or use it to strike themselves or others; children recover balance readily, and peers are usually able to defend themselves.

At the second training session a few days later, the therapist can assess the parents' experiences. Donning and doffing the prosthesis should be reviewed. Initially, the infant may tolerate the prosthesis only for a few minutes. It should be frequently applied during the day. Eventually, the child should be able to wear it most of the day, except when sleeping and bathing.

Subsequent followup sessions focus on the adequacy of prosthetic fit and the child's readiness for the addition of a cable to the prosthesis, substitution of a myoelectrically controlled prosthesis for a passive one, or, in the case of the child with transhumeral amputation, the addition of an elbow unit.

Toddlers

When the child is between the ages of 15 and 18 months, control cables may be added to traditional, body-operated prostheses (Figure 29-6). Active control may not become reliable until the toddler is approximately 2.5 years of age, when the understanding of cause and effect is established. Readiness for the cable is indicated when the child wears the prosthesis full time, can follow simple instructions, has an attention span of at least 5 minutes, and will allow the therapist and prosthetist to handle him or her. A toddler who resists instruction from someone other than the parent may be too immature to learn to control the prosthesis.

If the prosthesis has a voluntary-opening hook, it should be fitted with a half- or a quarter-width rubber band to facilitate opening. The tension in the terminal

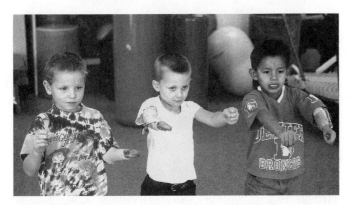

FIGURE 29-6 Children learning that shoulder flexion produces terminal device operation because flexion tenses the control cable. (Courtesy of TRS, Inc., Boulder, CO.)

Therapy sessions are designed to increase the toddler's
- Control of the terminal device
- Control of the elbow unit
- Use of the prosthesis in bimanual prehension
- Use of the prosthesis in functional activities

Parents of toddlers with prostheses should do the following:
- Provide toys that require bimanual prehension
- Encourage use of the prosthesis as an assistive device
- Inspect the skin to determine whether the prosthesis causes undue irritation

device should be sufficient to let the child hold objects but not so great that opening the hook is difficult. Young children appear to use the voluntary-closing hook with as much ease as the more traditional voluntary-opening terminal devices. Box 29-2 summarizes the goals of prosthetic training for toddlers.

The training environment should be quiet, with a low table holding a few toys that require bimanual grasp, such as large beads and a string with a rigid tip. For the child with unilateral amputation, the terminal device serves to hold an object, such as a bead, while the child threads the string through the bead. The therapist is on the child's prosthetic side, holding the child's forearm at 90 degrees of elbow flexion, the optimal position of cable operation. This position also keeps the terminal device and the grasped object within the child's view. The adult moves the child's forearm forward, flexing the shoulder, tensing the cable, and causing the hook to operate. When the arm is moved back (shoulder extension), the terminal device changes position. A voluntary-opening hook opens with shoulder flexion, whereas a voluntary-closing hook closes with shoulder flexion. The therapist encourages the child to help with the control motion. With either design, the initial training involves placing a toy in the hook and encouraging the child to discover how to keep it in place. With a voluntary-opening hook, the child simply relaxes to allow the rubber bands or springs to keep the hook fingers closed. The voluntary-closing hook requires that the wearer exert tension on the control cable by the harness to keep the hook closed. Children use the same control motions as do adults, namely shoulder flexion or shoulder girdle protraction for terminal device operation. The toddler may revert to the earlier practice of opening the terminal device with the sound hand; eventually he or she will find that cable operation is more efficient, allowing more complex bimanual play maneuvers.

Reaching for objects with the sound hand is the child's initial preference. To provide the child the necessary practice with the prosthesis, the therapist or parent should offer large objects or toys that require bimanual grasp to operate. Another technique to encourage prosthetic use is to have the child hold one object in the sound hand and another in the prosthesis. For example, two hand bells make twice as much sound as one. With some young patients, prosthetic training merely involves using the terminal device as a stabilizer rather than as a prehensile tool; for example, the child may lean the prosthesis onto a replica of a mailbox while placing objects in the slot with the sound hand. The prosthesis also serves to stabilize paper while the child draws and colors pictures.

Although children as young as 18 months have been fitted with myoelectrically controlled transradial prostheses,[30] those who are at least 3 years of age have an easier time learning to contract the appropriate flexors and extensors to close and open the hand (Figure 29-7). The prosthesis is relatively heavy, susceptible to breakdown, and needs more maintenance than does a cable-operated device. To prepare the child for a somewhat heavier myoelectric prosthesis, weight should be gradually added to the passive prosthesis. Rudimentary training begins with practice with the prosthesis off the arm. At first, the therapist may place an electrode on the sound forearm and ask the child to flex and extend the wrist to close and open the fingers of the prosthetic hand. The therapist then places an electrode on the forearm on the amputated side and encourages the child to discover that contraction of the forearm musculature on that side achieves the same results. Motorized toys can be used to help the child practice deliberate contraction of flexors and extensors to cause an electric train, for example, to go backward and forward, depending on which electrode is stimulated. When the child gains reasonable proficiency, the prosthetic socket can be made with the electrodes embedded in it. Care must be taken to achieve and maintain snug fit so that the electrodes are in constant contact with the skin.

Whether the prosthesis is cable or myoelectrically controlled, practice to gain prosthetic proficiency is the same. The beginner experiences many instances of dropping objects while learning the amount of muscle contraction or cable tension needed to maintain suitable terminal device closure. The ability to close the terminal device around an object develops before active release. Grasping an object from the tabletop is difficult. Children attempting to put objects into their mouths discover that the change in shoulder position alters the tension on the control cable. Similarly, children who drop toys and try to retrieve them from the floor discover how to hold the shoulder to maintain adequate cable tension. Those who are wearing myoelectrically controlled prostheses also notice that the prosthesis is easier to operate in some forearm positions than in others.

Moving pegs on a board affords the child practice in opening and closing the terminal device. Tossing a beanbag is useful for teaching terminal device opening, as is playing cards. Cutting paper is another satisfying activity. The child holds the paper in the terminal device and uses the scissors in the sound hand. Prosthetic training should acquaint the child with objects of various textures, sizes, and shapes. Resilient foam toys are easier to grasp than are those made of rigid plastic, wood, or metal. Playing with sewing cards, nested barrels, and snap-apart beads; removing a toy from a drawstring bag; opening a zipper; removing loose clothing; opening small boxes of raisins; opening and closing felt-tipped pens; and playing the xylophone entice the child to attempt grasping,

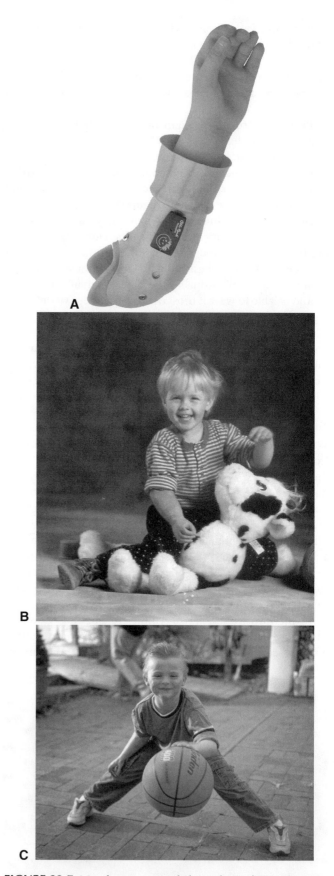

FIGURE 29-7 Myoelectric transradial prosthesis. **A,** Prosthesis. **B,** Boy wearing right prosthesis playing with stuffed toy. **C,** Boy wearing right prosthesis playing basketball. (Courtesy Otto Bock Orthopedic Industry, Inc., Minneapolis, MN.)

holding, and releasing motions with the terminal device.[31] Moving checkers or other markers from one location to another on a game board is a good drill. The prosthesis is helpful when swinging and climbing on the playground, rolling a wheelbarrow or doll carriage, jumping rope, and riding a tricycle. Children with unilateral amputation usually regard the intact limb as the dominant one. Many children with unilateral amputation refer to the prosthesis as the helper, which correctly identifies its role as a device that assists the intact hand.

Functional training depends on the child's ability to reach the mouth, waist, hips, feet, and perineum. Feeding, dressing, writing, and personal hygiene are incorporated at the appropriate times. Thirty-month-old children can throw and catch a ball, start uncomplicated dressing, and eat with a spoon with little spillage. Children play in sand, earth, and water and engage in rough-and-tumble activities, which can damage the prosthesis and the skin. Daily inspection and attention to minor problems help avoid major prosthetic repairs and skin disorders.

A 2-year-old with transhumeral amputation may have a prosthesis with an elbow unit, although mastery of the elbow-locking cable is unlikely to occur before the third birthday. Strategies to self-manage donning and doffing the prosthesis can be introduced to children as young as 3 years. They find removing the prosthesis easier than applying it.

At 3 years of age, the child may begin to be curious about the rotational possibilities of the wrist unit. Objects of various shapes within reach oblige the child to turn the terminal device in the wrist unit to the suitable position. Most objects can be manipulated with the terminal device in the pronated position; however, thin disks are more easily managed with the terminal device in midposition, and small balls are best cradled in the terminal device when it is rotated to the supinated position. Holding the handlebars of a tricycle or manipulating hand controls in other wheeled toys helps the child learn how to use terminal device rotation in the wrist unit. Prosthetic activities for the toddler should include eating, drinking, dressing, and managing crayons and other writing implements. Three-year-olds blow soap bubbles, pull up pants, pull a belt through loops in pants, and fill a cup with water from a spigot.[31]

Throughout the toddler phase, work periods should alternate with free play that may or may not involve the prosthesis. Weekly training sessions are effective. Parents should inspect the axilla; persistent redness indicates that the harness is applying undue pressure. The home program should include written suggestions regarding activities to promote bimanual prehension, instructions concerning the care of the prosthesis and the care of the child's skin, terminology pertaining to parts of the prosthesis, and ideas regarding clothing that will not impede prosthetic function.

School-Age Children

An important consideration for the growing child is a socket large enough for comfortable fit and adequate prosthetic control.

The 4-year-old child is usually coordinated enough to grasp fragile objects without breaking or crushing them.

With a voluntary-opening hook, the child must maintain tension on the control cable to prevent the hook fingers from snapping shut. A voluntary-closing terminal device necessitates application of gentle tension on the cable rather than forceful shoulder motion. With a myoelectrically controlled hand, the child must minimally contract flexors so that the fingers close on the object without undue pressure (Figure 29-8). Four-year-olds can pour from containers, peel a banana, sharpen a pencil with a hand-held sharpener, sew, hammer nails, and apply adhesive bandages (Figure 29-9). The average 5-year-old can open a milk container and sweep with a brush and dust pan.[31] Box 29-3 summarizes the goals of prosthetic training for school-age children.

The pediatric prehension assessment provides a standard clinical assessment of children with transradial amputation by objectively scoring activities of daily living that require repetitive use of a terminal device. Three test batteries correspond to age groups of 2 to 3 years, 4 to 5 years, and 6 to 7 years. In test 1, the child is asked to string four large beads, open four 35-mm film cans, separate three nested screw-top barrels, assemble 10 interlocking beads, and separate a five-piece notched plastic block. In test 2, the child uses a sewing card, strings 10 small beads, sticks an adhesive bandage to the table, cuts a paper circle and glues it to another paper, and opens a small package of tissues. In test 3, the child is asked to cut modeling plastic with a knife and fork, cut paper, discard five playing cards from a hand of 10 cards, lace a shoe and tie a bow, and wrap a book.[31]

Card games often fascinate children in elementary school. Maintaining several cards in the terminal device and then releasing the desired card involves a gradation of tension on the control cable for prostheses equipped with a voluntary-opening or -closing terminal device. Card playing is more difficult with a myoelectrically controlled prosthesis because the child must contract the forearm flexors and extensors with the correct amount of force at the appropriate time.[32] The 5-year-old should be independent in dressing, except for buttons, shoelaces, and pullover shirts and sweaters. The child

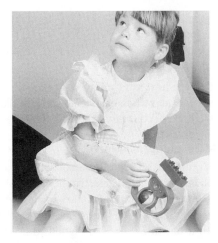

FIGURE 29-8 Girl contracting forearm muscles to operate a myoelectrically controlled terminal device. (Courtesy Otto Bock Orthopedic Industry, Inc., Minneapolis, MN.)

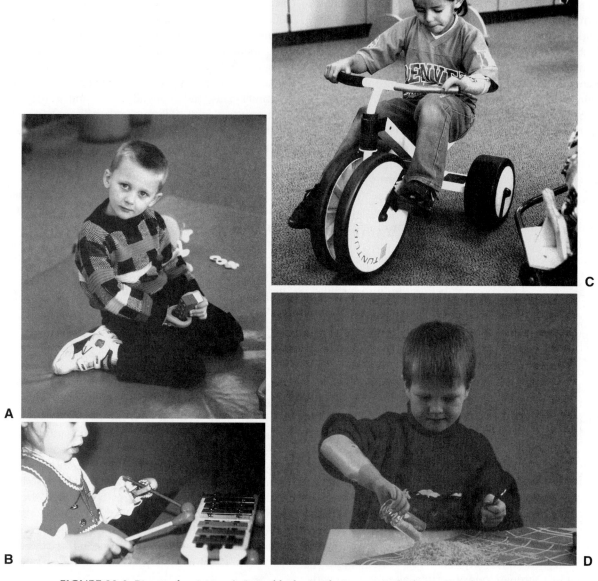

FIGURE 29-9 Bimanual activities. **A,** Large blocks. **B,** Playing a toy xylophone. **C,** Riding a tricycle. **D,** Boy wearing right prosthesis pouring rice from a glass. (A and C, Courtesy TRS, Inc., Boulder, CO; B, Courtesy J. E. Edelstein; D, Courtesy Otto Bock Orthopedic Industry, Inc., Minneapolis, MN.)

also needs to learn how to take care of the prosthesis, keep it clean, and ask for help when parts malfunction. Skin inspection is an essential part of training.

Older Children and Adolescents

Many older children are able to incorporate the prosthesis in school activities. A myoelectric hook terminal device (Figure 29-10) may be practical for the teenager who is interested in repairing bicycles and cars. Sports prostheses, such as those with a terminal device designed to hold a basketball, give wearers more opportunities to participate in group activities (Figure 29-11).[33] Teenagers may find that playing a musical instrument is pleasurable. Simple adaptations, such as fingering a trumpet with the sound hand and supporting it with the prosthesis, can open a world of enjoyment to the musician.[34] Older adolescents should have vocational exploration, vocational assessment, and, when indicated, job training. Obtaining a driver's license is a meaningful event for most teenagers. The use of a prosthesis does not influence the capacity to drive, although those with upper-limb deficiency are more likely to use adaptive devices when driving than those with lower-limb deficiency.[35]

Some adolescents with unilateral limb deficiency seek escape from parental control by abandoning their prostheses, preferring to manage with the intact limb. A few young people ultimately resume prosthetic wear on a full-time or

BOX 29-3 *Prosthetic Training Goals for School-Age Children*

Therapy sessions assist the school-age child to do the following:

- Maintain proper prosthetic fit
- Grasp firm and fragile objects without dropping or crushing them
- Open and close the terminal device reliably
- Don and doff the prosthesis independently
- Dress independently
- Recognize when the prosthesis needs repair or alteration

Parents of school-aged children with prostheses should do the following:

- Be independent in daily activities and play

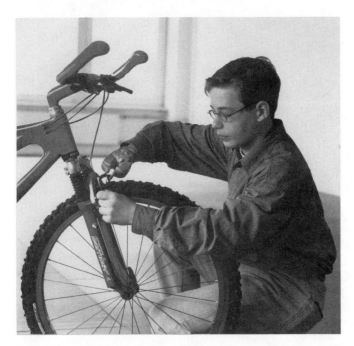

FIGURE 29-10 Myoelectric Greifer terminal device on right transradial prosthesis. (Courtesy Otto Bock Orthopedic Industry, Inc., Minneapolis, MN.)

occasional basis. Certain activities are more easily accomplished without the prosthesis or cannot be done with a prosthesis. For example, prostheses are not worn when showering. Individuals with transradial amputation may prefer to stabilize objects in the antecubital fossa, using elbow flexion, rather than use a prosthetic terminal device. Sometimes simple equipment adaptation facilitates one-handed performance, such as the use of a book holder, guitar pick band, or camera grip. Some people become quite facile with the remaining upper limb, learning to hit a baseball, and fold laundry with one hand.

Functional outcome evaluation of children fitted with unilateral upper prostheses is aided by the Prosthetic Upper Extremity Functional Index administered to parents and older children.[36] Long-term followup of children with unilateral

transradial deficiency indicates that approximately 40% use a passive prosthesis, 40% use a voluntary-closing terminal device, and 15% use a myoelectrically controlled prosthesis.[37] Of those trained to use a myoelectrically controlled prosthesis, most report satisfaction with it even though many do not wear it.[38] Rejection of a prosthesis is somewhat less among children who had been fitted at younger than 2 years of age[39,40] or prior to the age of 3 years.[41] Prior to kindergarten, children wear the prosthesis for an average of nearly 6 hours a day.[42] Studies of older children suggest that quality of life is about the same for those who do and do not wear prostheses,[43] with prostheses used for specific activities.[44] Overall, children with upper-limb deficiency are as socially competent as able-bodied peers.[45]

Rehabilitation of Children with Lower-Limb Loss

Children with lower-limb deficiencies deserve clinic team management similar to that described for those with upper-limb deficiencies. Early referral to a clinical team is equally important for the family with a child who has a lower-limb amputation or limb deficiency. Peer support is also invaluable for parents who need to share concerns, suggestions, and camaraderie with others who coping with a similar situation. Treatment should suit the patient's developmental stage so that prosthetic use fosters achievement of key milestones. Parents serve as the primary instructors of their children, with the guidance of the physical therapist and other members of the clinical team.

Infants

Sitting balance is a major guide to lower-limb prosthetic fitting.[1] The average age when babies accomplish independent sitting is 6 months. Sitting depends on postural control and antigravity muscle strength. Sitting balance and trunk stabilization are also important for freeing the hands to explore the environment.[22] Box 29-4 summarizes the goals of rehabilitation of infants with lower-limb malformation or amputation.

Infants who are 5 to 7 months of age discover the mobility possibilities of crawling and creeping, moving from supine to four-point and sitting positions, and moving to the hands and knees from the sitting position.[29] Crawling involves the alternate action of the opposite arms and legs in a manner similar to walking. Hip extensors strengthen during crawling and kneeling. Rocking on four points before launching into crawling is another important precursor to walking.

Most babies are able to overcome gravity to pull up to a standing position and rise from kneeling to standing at approximately 8 months. When pulling to a standing position, the baby expends great energy bouncing and actively disturbing balance. Bouncing gradually gives way to shifting weight from side to side. The initial standing posture is wide based, with the hips abducted, flexed, and externally rotated. The base accommodates the child's new center of gravity position, which is higher than when crawling. Maintaining upright posture depends on sufficient maturity of the visual, proprioceptive, and vestibular systems.

Stepping movements are common among 7-month-olds who are supported. Cruising along furniture is a preferred mode

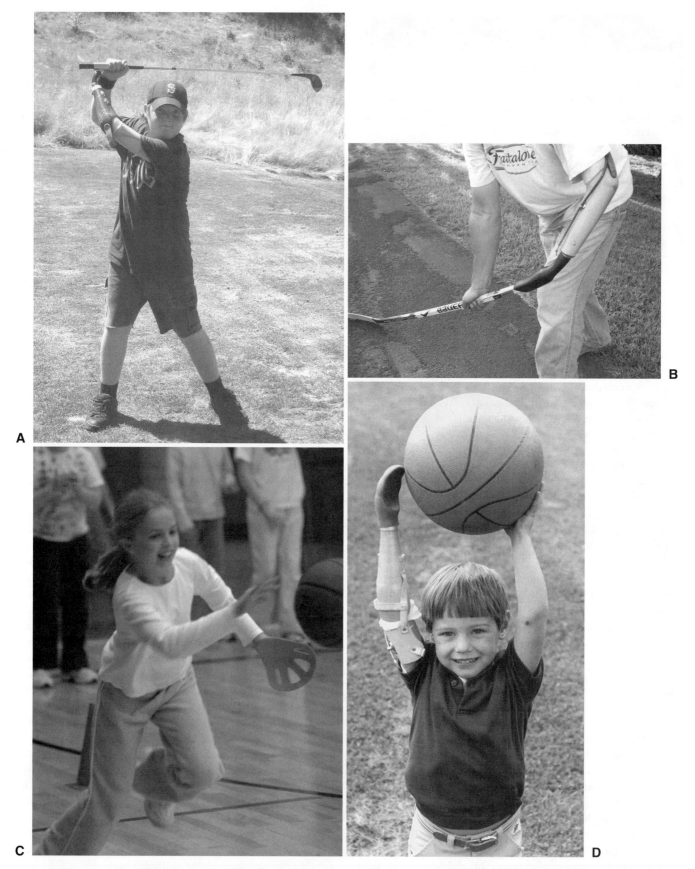

FIGURE 29-11 Activity-specific terminal devices. **A,** Boy swinging golf club with GolfPro terminal device. **B,** Adolescent playing hockey with PowerPlay Hockey terminal device. **C,** Girl playing basketball wearing left transradial prosthesis with Mill's ReBound-Pro terminal device. **D,** SuperSport terminal device. (Courtesy TRS, Inc., Boulder, CO.)

of locomotion when the child is approximately 10 months old. Cruising strengthens the hip abductors. The typical nondisabled child stands alone at approximately 11 months and walks alone at 12 months.[20,46] The urge to walk is the culmination of the endless pulling and standing activity that has occupied the baby for several preceding months.

Some infants undergo surgery either to transform a congenitally anomalous limb into one that is more suitable for a prosthesis, or as part of the treatment of a limb that has been involved in trauma or in the presence of tumor. Skin grafting in these instances does not result in adverse functional outcome.[47] Another intervention applicable to a few children is limb lengthening using an Ilizarov apparatus. Long-term outcomes are favorable, with average to above-average quality of life.[48–50] A very few children with myelodysplasia undergo amputation of lower limbs that are severely contracted or have intractable ulcers. Those with transtibial or more distal amputation readily become prosthesis wearers.[51]

Regardless of the etiology of limb deficiency, the goal of prosthetic fitting is to facilitate the child's attainment of motor milestones.[52] The infant who is missing a lower limb should have prosthetic restoration at approximately 6 months, when the baby has enough trunk control for sitting and is ready to pull to a standing position. A simple prosthesis fosters symmetrical sitting balance and aids the baby's attempts to pull to standing. In addition, the prosthesis equalizes leg length, adds weight to the anomalous side, and obviates the tendency to compensate with a one-legged standing pattern. Reducing the weight asymmetry inherent in limb deficiency facilitates rotational control of the trunk. The prosthesis enables standing and walking. Otherwise, the world is circumscribed by the confines of the stroller or playpen, and the deficiency becomes a source of shame. Fitting before 6 months might hinder the baby's efforts to turn from prone to supine position and back again.

The first prosthesis includes a solid-ankle, cushion-heel (SACH) foot, the smallest foot manufactured (Figure 29-12). Rubber-soled shoes give the infant more traction and are therefore preferable to leather-soled shoes. The initial transtibial prosthesis usually has a thigh corset (Figure 29-13),

primarily to help the child retain the prosthesis on the amputation limb. The prosthesis must be comfortable when the baby stands, sits, squats, crawls, and climbs. A silicone socket liner (Figure 29-14) may be desirable to protect sensitive skin from chafing in the socket. The toddler with transfemoral amputation starts with a prosthesis having a locked knee. By 3 years, most can manage an unlocked knee (Figure 29-15). Polycentric knee units, with or without stance control, are appropriate for school-age youngsters (Figure 29-16).[53,54]

During the first training session, the therapist and parent confirm that the prosthesis fits comfortably, without redness of the residual limb. Most of the handling of the child should be done by the parent, rather than the therapist, so that the family gains confidence in managing the child at home. Useful equipment includes a play table, an elevated sandbox, a floor mat, a rolling stool, a full-length mirror, steps, and a ramp. The parent should encourage the child's standing on both feet by first supporting the trunk and then gradually reducing the support. The young child gains prosthetic tolerance and standing balance by being near the table. Initially, the child may lean the torso against the table while manipulating toys that require use of both hands. Toys should be moved to places on the table where the child has to reach in different directions, shifting weight. Eventually, the child will move along the periphery of the table to place objects in the desired location. When first learning to walk with a prosthesis, the child moves cautiously. Initially, the child takes small steps and has a wide base, keeping the trunk upright and arms abducted. The new prosthesis wearer resembles normal peers who begin walking with increased hip and knee flexion, full-foot initial contact, short stride, increased cadence, and relative foot drop on the sound side in swing phase.[20–22]

At home, a sturdy table that is chest high to the child encourages standing balance and cruising during play with toys placed on the table. Raised sandboxes, blocks, finger paints, and pans of water with floating toys all promote standing balance. A playpen is a good environment to enable the baby to pull to standing, cruise the perimeter, and sit when the baby wishes. Balls are useful in prosthetic training. Kicking a ball requires balance on one leg and flexion of the other leg. The baby starts by holding on to a stable object with both hands, then with one, and eventually letting go. Throwing a ball requires good balance and usually sustains the infant's interest. Wheeled toys, such as a doll carriage, enable the child to walk with a modicum of support. Placing toys where the child must take a few steps to reach them fosters independent walking.

Young children frequently revert to crawling and sitting on the floor as they grow accustomed to the prosthesis. Falling is seldom a problem, inasmuch as the child generally lands on the buttocks as an able-bodied child would. When the child falls or tries to retrieve a toy on the floor, the parents and therapist should let the young person explore the movement and not be overly protective. Just as other children learn to walk by supporting themselves on furniture, the child who wears a prosthesis should have the same experience to develop confidence. Parallel bars, walkers, and harnesses are seldom advisable for children with unilateral amputation or bilateral transtibial amputation.

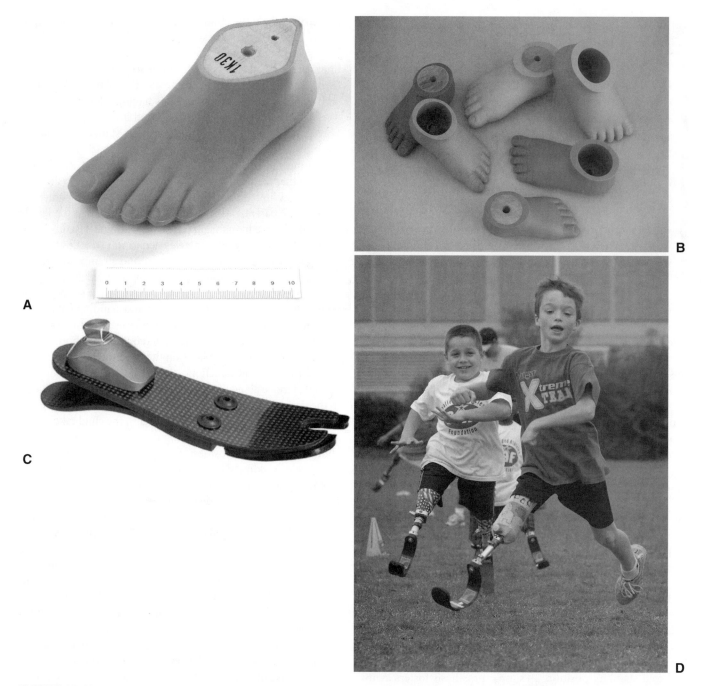

FIGURE 29-12 Children's prosthetic feet. **A,** Solid-ankle, cushion-heel (SACH) foot. **B,** SACH feet adaptable for crawling and walking. **C,** Flex Foot Junior. **D,** Boys running while wearing transfemoral prostheses with Flex-Run feet. (A, Courtesy Otto Bock Orthopedic Industry, Inc., Minneapolis, MN; B, Courtesy TRS, Inc., Boulder, CO; C and D, Courtesy Össur Americas, www.ossur.com.)

A prosthesis imposes weight-bearing loads on portions of the leg not ordinarily used for this purpose. Consequently, building tolerance to prosthetic wear is important so that skin over weight-bearing areas can adjust to the pressure. During the first week most infants tolerate 1 hour of wear, after which the prosthesis should be removed and the skin examined. After a 10- to 15-minute rest period, the prosthesis can be reapplied for another hour. Signs of fatigue, limping, and the avoidance of standing on the prosthesis indicate that the prosthesis is irritating and should be removed. The infant with a transfemoral prosthesis should be checked to determine whether skin near the proximal part of the prosthesis is irritated by urine or feces, which may leak from the diaper.

Toddlers

By 15 months, toddlers are upright and mobile. The heel-toe sequence replaces flat-foot contact during the second year. Neurological maturation, changes in physique, and improved strength are evident as the child's base of support narrows. Muscular activity has matured into the adult pattern. Goals for rehabilitation (Box 29-5) reflect the developmental activities of a preschool-age child.

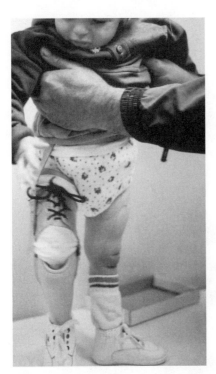

FIGURE 29-13 Transtibial prosthesis with thigh corset and a solid-ankle, cushion-heel (SACH) foot. (Courtesy J. E. Edelstein.)

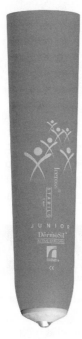

FIGURE 29-14 Silicone socket liner. (Courtesy Össur Americas, www.ossur.com.)

Another milestone expected of all children, including the child with a prosthesis, is running, which begins between 2 and 4 years of age. The flight phase (double float), the period when both feet are off the ground, occurs by strong application of propulsive force during late stance. The prosthetic foot offers much less energy storage and release compared with the gastrocnemius. Consequently, the child with a prosthesis adopts

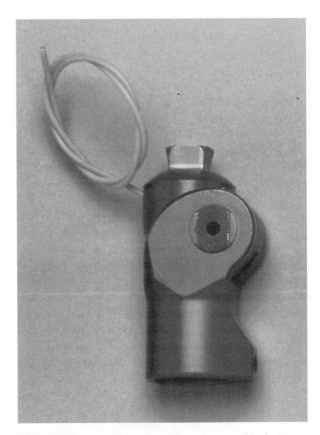

FIGURE 29-15 Single-axis knee units with manual lock. (Courtesy Otto Bock Orthopedic Industry, Inc., Minneapolis, MN.)

an asymmetric running gait that emphasizes propulsion on the sound side. Two-year-olds can kick a ball accurately, steer a push toy, and jump. As with running, jumping with a prosthesis is primarily an action of the sound side. Games of throwing and catching a ball or beanbag and tossing darts help the toddler refine balance with the prosthesis.

The 3-year-old will probably leap, jump, gallop, climb stairs step over step, and ride a tricycle. The tricycle pedal should have a strap to secure the prosthetic foot. Jumping from a step and hopping are other toddler stunts. Playground equipment, such as a jungle gym, slide, swing, seesaw, sandbox, and tunnels, is enticing. Children with unilateral transtibial amputation achieve an almost normal gait and have no difficulty in climbing inclines and stairs. Opportunities for kneeling, managing various types of chairs, and getting to and from the floor are additional elements in rehabilitation. The child will need help in removing and donning the prosthesis.

School-Age Children and Adolescents

By 4 years of age, most children can descend stairs step over step, ride a bicycle, and roller skate. Skates that clip on the shoe are preferable to shoe skates; the latter require that the prosthetic foot accommodate the height of the heel in the shoe skate. Five-year-olds skip rope and play dodge ball. Accurate kicking demonstrates balance on one foot while transferring force to the ball. By age 6 years, most children can don and doff the prosthesis independently. They can start, stop, and change direction with ease as well

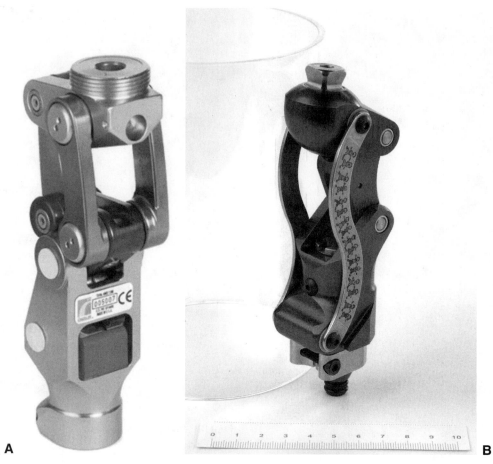

FIGURE 29-16 Polycentric knee units. (A, Courtesy Össur Americas, www.ossur.com. B, Courtesy Otto Bock Orthopedic Industry, Inc., Minneapolis, MN.)

as skip and hop for long distances. The child moves toward independence in prosthetic management as well, taking more responsibility for donning and doffing, skin inspection, and maintenance of the prosthesis (Box 29-6).

Children who undergo lower-limb amputation after 5 years may respond favorably to balance and gait training similar to that appropriate for adults. Physical therapy emphasizes dynamic stability, weight shifting, control of the

prosthetic foot, and, in the case of the child with transfemoral amputation, the knee unit (Figures 29-17 and 29-18).

Sports are particularly useful for developing self-esteem as well as strength and coordination. Most children with amputations take part in physical education classes at school, sometimes with modified activity. Carbon acrylic or graphite

---

BOX 29-5   *Prosthetic Training Goals for Toddlers with Lower-Limb Deficiency*

Goals of rehabilitation for toddlers with lower-limb deficiency include the following:
- Full-time wear of the prosthesis, except for bathing and sleeping
- Use of the prosthesis in age-appropriate ambulatory activities

Parents of toddlers with lower-limb prostheses should do the following:
- Encourage use of the prosthesis
- Provide toys and equipment that require age-appropriate activities
- Inspect the skin to determine whether the prosthesis causes undue irritation

---

BOX 29-6   *Goals for School-Age Children and Adolescents with Lower-Limb Deficiency*

In later childhood and adolescence, rehabilitation includes the following:
- Monitoring and maintaining proper prosthetic fit
- Inspecting the skin
- Donning and doffing the prosthesis independently
- Dressing independently
- Engaging in the full range of ambulatory activities with the prosthesis
- Recognizing when the prosthesis needs repair or alteration

Parents of school-age children and adolescents with lower-limb prostheses should do the following:
- Encourage the young person's independence
- Provide opportunities for sports participation

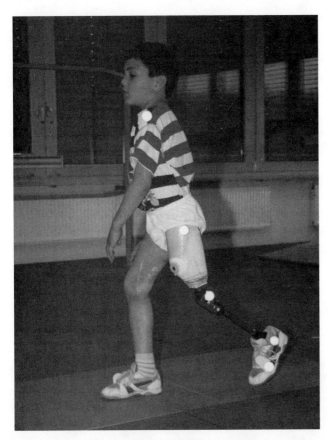

FIGURE 29-17 Boy wearing transfemoral prosthesis walking in a gait laboratory; prosthesis has reflective markers to aid gait analysis. (Courtesy Otto Bock Orthopedic Industry, Inc., Minneapolis, MN.)

CASE EXAMPLE 4

A Child with Traumatic Transfemoral Amputation

P. J., who is 4.5 years old, was riding his bicycle on the street in front of his home at twilight when an automobile turned the corner and struck him. In the police statement, the driver said he did not notice the child. P. J.'s father rushed him to the local hospital, where the boy was admitted to have his leg and thigh wounds debrided and dressed. Despite meticulous care at the hospital, the thigh wound became necrotic. The attending pediatrician arranged a consultation with the surgeon, who advised amputation at the transfemoral level immediately proximal to the femoral condyles. The family consented to the surgery, which proceeded uneventfully.

P. J.'s amputation wound was covered with an Unna dressing and healed rapidly. He is scheduled to come to the prosthetic clinic this morning.

Questions to Consider

- Describe the postoperative program that will enable P. J. to achieve the most rapid rehabilitation.
- What components (foot, shank, knee unit, socket, and suspension) would suit P. J. in his first prosthesis?
- Outline the steps in training P. J. to use his prosthesis.
- In addition to walking on level surfaces, what other activities should the physical therapist include in the initial rehabilitation program?
- How will P. J. resume riding his bicycle?
- What knee unit would suit P. J. when he enters junior high school?

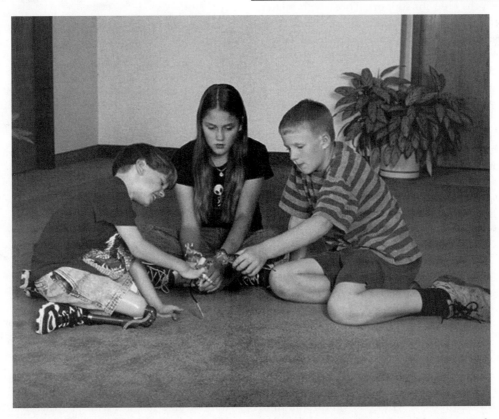

FIGURE 29-18 Boy sitting on floor, wearing transfemoral prosthesis with single-axis knee unit with extension aid. (Courtesy Otto Bock Orthopedic Industry, Inc., Minneapolis, MN.)

reinforcements enable the prosthesis to withstand extremely high stresses. The child should understand that shoes must always be worn; the plantar surface of most prosthetic feet is not durable enough to withstand abrasion by a sidewalk, and the alignment of the foot is intended for a shoe.

Some activities are more easily performed without a prosthesis or do not require a prosthesis. Children should learn how to use crutches as an alternate mode of locomotion when the prosthesis is being repaired. Bathing is facilitated either by sitting on the shower floor or by using a sturdy bath seat. Most people prefer to swim and scuba dive without a prosthesis. They hop or use crutches to get from the dressing room to the water's edge. Sports prostheses, such as a swimming prosthesis with a fin in place of the foot, can be constructed. Bicycling, skiing, and mountain climbing are other sports that can be enjoyed with or without a prosthesis.

Rehabilitation of Children with Multiple Limb Amputation

Babies who have lower-limb deficiency, together with anomalies of one or both upper limbs, generally do best by being fitted first with simple lower-limb prostheses to foster sitting balance. The introduction of upper- and lower-limb prostheses simultaneously is apt to overwhelm the infant.

When both upper limbs are anomalous, a simple bilateral fitting counteracts the tendency toward development of positional scoliosis. The baby with bilateral upper-limb deficiency should receive prostheses after independent walking is established; otherwise, prostheses make it more difficult to crawl, move about on the floor, and pull to standing with the chin for support. Those with bilateral upper-limb deficiency become quite skillful with foot prehension. The extent to which foot use should be encouraged is controversial. Foot prehension is so rarely observed in public that the child who does use the feet may experience unwanted stares. Nevertheless, feet have the tactile sensation and considerable dexterity that prostheses lack. Children with bilateral longitudinal deficiencies have partial or complete hands; they would be encumbered by wearing prostheses. Functional activities with and without prostheses should be introduced according to the physical and emotional maturity of the child. Adaptive aids may be required for some functions, such as personal hygiene.

Infants with trimembral or quadrimembral limb deficiency, possibly as a result of meningococcal septicemia,[55] move about by rolling along the floor. They need opportunities to look at objects and manipulate toys with their mouths and their residual limbs. Most infants develop good sitting balance and can scoot along on their buttocks. Because of the drastic reduction in body surface, these children can easily become overheated. They should be dressed very lightly to enable heat dissipation. Young children with bilateral transfemoral deficiency usually begin with a pair of prostheses that do not have knee units (Figure 29-19). They may walk indoors without any assistive devices; however, few are willing to venture outdoors and across streets without at least one cane. In adolescence,

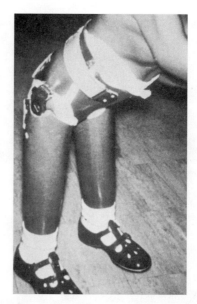

FIGURE 29-19 Bilateral transfemoral prostheses without knee units for a toddler who is beginning to walk. (Courtesy J. E. Edelstein.)

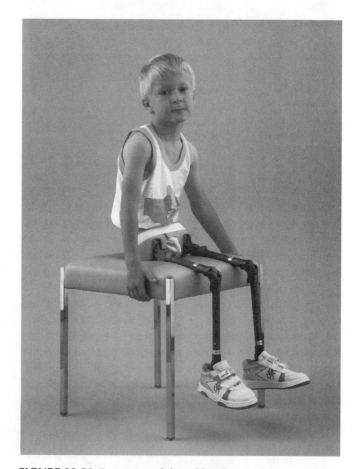

FIGURE 29-20 Boy wearing bilateral hip disarticulation prostheses. (Courtesy Otto Bock Orthopedic Industry, Inc., Minneapolis, MN.)

many find that a wheelchair provides more efficient mobility. Those with bilateral hip disarticulations (Figure 29-20) may be able to walk with prostheses at home, but usually rely on a wheelchair for community travel.

SUMMARY

Rehabilitation of children with limb deficiencies can be most gratifying. The physical therapist, together with all members of the clinical team, should design the rehabilitation program to assist the child in achieving developmental milestones associated with maturing upper and lower limb function. Psychosocial factors govern the behavior of all children, although it appears that those with limb deficiency behave in a comparable manner to able-bodied peers.[56,57] Peer support is very helpful for children and parents. Clinic team members need to recognize the basis for parental distress while fostering realistic expectations for the child's function by demonstrating that the child is lovable regardless of the condition of the limbs.

REFERENCES

1. Blakeslee B, ed. *The Limb-Deficient Child.* Berkeley, CA: University of California; 1963.
2. Setoguchi Y, Rosenfelder R. *The Limb-Deficient Child.* Springfield, IL: Thomas; 1982.
3. Stanger M. Limb deficiencies and amputations. In: Campbell SK, Vander Linden DW, Palisano RJ, eds. *Physical Therapy for Children.* 2nd ed. Philadelphia: Saunders; 2000:370–397.
4. Fisk JR. Terminology in pediatric limb deficiency. In: Smith DG, Michael JW, Bowker JH, eds. *Atlas of Amputations and Limb Deficiencies: Surgical, Prosthetic, and Rehabilitation Principles.* 3rd ed. Rosemont, IL: American Academy of Orthopaedic Surgeons; 2004:779–781.
5. Dillingham TR, Pezzin LE, MacKenzie EJ. Limb amputation and limb deficiency: epidemiology and recent trends in the United States. *South Med J.* 2002;95:875–883.
6. Rijnders LJ, Boonstra AM, Groothoff JW, et al. Lower limb deficient children in The Netherlands: epidemiological aspects. *Prosthet Orthot Int.* 2000;24:13–18.
7. Jain S, Lakhtakia PK. Profile of congenital transverse deficiencies among cases of congenital orthopaedic anomalies. *J Orthop Surg (Hong Kong).* 2002;10:45–52.
8. McGuirk CK, Westgate MN, Holmes LB. Limb deficiencies in newborn infants. *Pediatrics.* 2001;108:E64.
9. Conner KA, et al. Pediatric traumatic amputations and hospital resource utilization in the United States, 2003. *J Trauma.* 2010;68:131–137.
10. Nguyen A, et al. Lawn mower injuries in children: a 30-year experience. *ANZ J Surg.* 2008;78:759–763.
11. Vollman D, Smith GA. Epidemiology of lawn-mower-related injuries in children in the United States, 1990–2004. *Pediatrics.* 2006;11:273–278.
12. Bhatta ST, et al. All-terrain vehicle injuries in children: injury patterns and prognostic implications. *Pediatr Radiol.* 2004;34:130–133.
13. Nagarajan R, Neglia JP, Clohisy DR, et al. Education, employment, insurance, and marital status among 694 survivors of pediatric lower extremity bone tumors: a report from the Childhood Cancer Survivor Study. *Cancer.* 2003;97:2554–2564.
14. Ginsberg JP, et al. A comparative analysis of functional outcomes in adolescents and young adults with lower-extremity bone sarcoma. *Pediatr Blood Cancer.* 2007;40:964–969.
15. Refaat Y, Gunnoe J, Hornicek FJ, et al. Comparison of quality of life after amputation or limb salvage. *Clin Orthop.* 2002;397:298–305.

16. Nagarajan R, Neglia JP, Clohisy DR, et al. Limb salvage and amputation in survivors of pediatric lower extremity bone tumors: what are the long-term implications? *J Clin Oncol.* 2002;20:4493–4501.
17. Robert RS, Ottaviani G, Huh WW, et al. Psychosocial and functional outcomes in long-term survivors of osteosarcoma: a comparison of limb-salvage surgery and amputation. *Pediatr Blood Cancer.* 2010;54:990–999.
18. Ottaviani G, Robert RS, Huh WW, et al. Functional, psychosocial and professional outcomes in long-term survivors of lower-extremity osteosarcomas: amputation versus limb salvage. *Cancer Treat Res.* 2009;152:421–436.
19. Hopyan S, Tan JW, Graham HK, et al. Functional and upright time following limb salvage, amputation, and rotationplasty for pediatric sarcoma of bone. *J Pediatr Orthop.* 2006;26:405–408.
20. Edelstein JE. Developmental kinesiology. In: Smith DG, Michael JW, Bowker JH, eds. *Atlas of Amputations and Limb Deficiencies.* 3rd ed. Rosemont, Ill: American Academy of Orthopaedic Surgeons; 2004:783–788.
21. Campbell SK. Understanding motor performance in children. In: Campbell SK, Vander Linden DW, Palisano RJ, eds. *Physical Therapy for Children.* 2nd ed. Philadelphia: Saunders; 2000:3–45.
22. Cech D, Martin S. *Functional Movement Development across the Life Span.* 2nd ed. Philadelphia: Saunders; 2001.
23. Fishman S, Edelstein J, Krebs D. ISNY above-knee prosthetic sockets: pediatric experience. *J Pediatr Orthop.* 1987;5:557–562.
24. Fixsen JA. Major lower limb congenital shortening: a mini review. *J Pediatr Orthop.* 2003;12:1–12.
25. Patton JG. Training the child with a unilateral upper-extremity prosthesis. In: Atkins DJ, Meier RH, eds. *Functional Restoration of Adults and Children with Upper Extremity Amputation.* New York: Demos; 2004:297–316.
26. Huizing K, Reinders-Messelink H, Maathuis C, et al. Age at first prosthetic fitting and later functional outcome in children and young adults with unilateral congenital below-elbow deficiency: a cross-sectional study. *Prosthet Orthot Int.* 2010;34:166–174.
27. Edelstein JE. Rehabilitation without prostheses. In: Smith DG, Michael JW, Bowker JH, eds. *Atlas of Amputations and Limb Deficiencies.* 3rd ed. Rosemont, Ill: American Academy of Orthopaedic Surgeons; 2004:745–756.
28. Stoeker W. Foot skills and other alternatives to hand use. In: Meier RH, Atkins DJ, eds. *Functional Restoration of Adults and Children with Upper Extremity Amputation.* New York: Demos; 2004:133–134.
29. Kuyper MA, Breedijk M, Mulders AH, et al. Prosthetic management of children in The Netherlands with upper limb deficiencies. *Prosthet Orthot Int.* 2001;25:228–234.
30. Sorbye R. Myoelectric prosthetic fitting in young children. *Clin Orthop.* 1980;148:34–40.
31. Krebs D, ed. *Prehension Assessment: Prosthetic Therapy for the Upper-Limb Child Amputee.* Thorofare, NJ: Slack; 1987.
32. Edelstein JE, Berger N. Performance comparison among children fitted with myoelectric and body-powered hands. *Arch Phys Med Rehabil.* 1993;74(4):376–380.
33. Fernandez A, Lopez MJ, Navarro R. Performance of persons with juvenile-onset amputation in driving motor vehicles. *Arch Phys Med Rehabil.* 2000;81:288–291.
34. Walker JL, Coburn TR, Cottle W, et al. Recreational terminal devices for children with upper extremity amputations. *J Pediatr Orthop.* 2008;28:271–273.
35. Edelstein J. Musical options for upper-limb amputees. In: Lee M, ed. *Rehabilitation Music and Human Well-Being.* St. Louis: MMB Music; 1989.

36. Wright FV, Hubbard S, Naumann S, et al. Evaluation of the validity of the prosthetic upper extremity functional index for children. *Arch Phys Med Rehabil.* 2003;84:518–527.

37. Crandall RC, Tomhave W. Pediatric unilateral below-elbow amputees: retrospective analysis of 34 patients given multiple prosthetic options. *J Pediatr Orthop.* 2002;22:380–383.

38. Routhier F, Vincent C, Morissette MJ, et al. Clinical results of an investigation of paediatric upper limb myoelectric prosthesis fitting at the Quebec Rehabilitation Institute. *Prosthet Orthot Int.* 2001;25:119–131.

39. Meurs M, Maathuis CG, Lucas C, et al. Prescription of the first prosthesis and later use in children with congenital unilateral upper limb deficiency: a systematic review. *Prosthet Orthot Int.* 2006;303:165–173.

40. Postema K, van der Donk V, van Limbeek J, et al. Prosthesis rejection in children with a unilateral congenital arm defect. *Clin Rehabil.* 1999;13:243–249.

41. Davids JR, Wagner LV, Meyer LC, et al. Prosthetic management of children with unilateral congenital below-elbow deficiency. *J Bone Joint Surg Am.* 2006;88:1294–1300.

42. Egermann M, Kasten P, Thomsen J. Myoelectric hand prostheses in very young children. *Int Orthop.* 2009;33:1101–1106.

43. James MA, Bagley AM, Brasington K, et al. Impact of prostheses on function and quality of life for children with unilateral congenital below-the-elbow deficiency. *J Bone Joint Surg Am.* 2006;88:2356–2365.

44. Buffart LM, Roebroeck ME, van Heijningen VG, et al. Evaluation of arm and prosthetic functioning in children with a congenital transverse reduction deficiency of the upper limb. *J Rehabil Med.* 2007;39:379–386.

45. Hermansson L, Eliasson AC, Engstrom I. Psychosocial adjustment in Swedish children with upper-limb reduction deficiency and a myoelectric prosthetic hand. *Acta Paediatr.* 2005;94:479–488.

46. Chambers HG. Pediatric gait analysis. In: Perry J, Burnfield JM, eds. *Gait Analysis: Normal and Pathological Function.* 2nd ed. Thorofare, NJ: Slack; 2010:341–363.

47. Parry IS, Mooney KN, Chau C, et al. Effects of skin grafting on successful prosthetic use in children with lower extremity amputation. *J Burn Care Res.* 2008;29:949–954.

48. El-Sayed MM, Correll J, Pohlig K. Limb sparing reconstructive surgery and Ilizarov lengthening in fibular hemimelia of Achterman-Kalamchi type II patients. *J Pediatr Orthop B.* 2010;19:55–60.

49. Walker JL, Knapp D, Minter C, et al. Adult outcomes following amputation or lengthening for fibular deficiency. *J Bone Joint Surg Am.* 2009;91:797–804.

50. Busse JW, Jacobs CL, Swiontkowski MF, et al. Complex limb salvage of early amputation for severe lower-limb injury: a meta-analysis of observational studies. *J Orthop Trauma.* 2007; 21:70–76.

51. Alan RK, Brown JP, Pugh LI, Stasikelis PJ. Function of children with myelodysplasia and lower extremity amputations. *J Pediatr Orthop.* 2007;27:51–53.

52. Nelson VS, Flood KM, Bryant PR, et al. Limb deficiency and prosthetic management. 1. Decision making in prosthetic prescription and management. *Arch Phys Med Rehabil.* 2006;87:S3–S9.

53. Andrysek J, Naumann S, Cleghorn WL. Design characteristics of pediatric prosthetic knees. *IEEE Trans Neural Syst Rehabil Eng.* 2004;12:369–378.

54. Andrysek J, Naumann S, Cleghorn WL. Design and quantitative evaluation of a stand-phase controlled prosthetic knee joint for children. *IEEE Trans Neural Syst Rehabil Eng.* 2005;13:437–443.

55. Lowe KG, Boyce JM. Rehabilitation of a child with meningococcal septicemia and quadrilateral limb loss: a case report. *Arch Phys Med Rehabil.* 2004;85:1354–1357.

56. Boonstra AM, Rijnders LJ, Groothoff JW, et al. Children with congenital deficiencies or acquired amputations of the lower limbs: functional aspects. *Prosthet Orthot Int.* 2000; 24:19–27.

57. Michielsen A, Van Wijk I, Ketelaar M. Participation and quality of life in children and adolescents with congenital limb deficiencies: a narrative review. *Prosthet Orthot Int.* 2010;34:351–361.

30

Prosthetic Options for Persons with Upper-Extremity Amputation

JOHN R. ZENIE

LEARNING OBJECTIVES

On completion of this chapter, the reader will be able to do the following:

1. Compare and contrast prosthetic needs and expected functional outcomes for individuals with upper-extremity amputations at various levels.
2. Compare and contrast the fitting and control issues for individuals with various etiologies of amputations and residual limb lengths.
3. Describe the factors that determine recommendations for prosthetic options (no prosthesis, passive prosthesis, body-powered prosthesis, externally powered systems, or hybrid prosthetic systems).
4. Compare and contrast options for donning and suspension of a prosthesis for individuals with upper-extremity amputations of various levels.
5. Describe the biomechanical principles of transradial and transhumeral body-powered prosthetic control systems and the movement strategies necessary for control of electric terminal devices (TDs), elbow units, and other prosthetic components.
6. Explain the basic principles of myoelectric control, including determining electrode placement and the types of muscle contractions used to operate or switch among TDs, electric elbow units, and other electric prosthetic components.

IMPACT OF TECHNOLOGY

Prosthetic management of individuals with upper-extremity amputations presents all allied health professionals, including prosthetists, with a set of unique challenges. For those wearing an upper–extremity limb, the TD of the prosthesis is not covered or obscured by clothing in the same way that a lower-extremity prosthesis is "hidden" by pants, socks, and shoes. By the virtue of its level, the person with upper-extremity amputation must cope with not only physical appearance changes, but the loss of some of the most complex movement patterns and functional activities of the human body.

In addition, limb deficiency in the upper extremity deprives the patient of an extensive and valuable system of tactile and proprioceptive inputs that previously provided "feedback" to guide and refine functional movement.[1,2] Even the simplest tasks related to grasp and release become challenging. The ability to position prosthetic limb segments in space, as well as the ability to maintain advantageous postures needed to manipulate objects, challenge the medical community to continuously improve the functional and aesthetic outcomes of prosthetic replacement for patients in this population.[3-5]

Many of these challenges have been addressed with new and emerging technologies. These new technologies have made it possible, in some circumstances, to successfully "fit" a patient with high-level amputation who previously would have little or no reasonable expectation to succeed with traditional technology and fitting techniques.[2,6,7] Advanced socket interface designs and material science have afforded prosthetists the ability to offer stronger, more stable platforms for all levels of amputation, while in most cases saving substantial amounts of weight. Similarly, more innovative suspension strategies and interface mediums have increased the functional ranges of motion a patient can comfortably achieve.[8]

These advancements have had a profound and positive effect on the comfort, function, and compliance of both conventional body-powered and externally powered prostheses at all levels of amputation. Furthermore, the huge strides made in the externally powered arena have in large part been driven by these advancements and technological breakthroughs.

LENGTH OF THE RESIDUAL LIMB

Amputations to the upper extremity can be classified or named by the limb segments affected (Figure 30-1). The most distal are at the finger, partial hand or transcarpal levels. Amputations that separate the carpal bones from the radius and ulna are referred to as wrist disarticulations. Amputations that occur within the substance of the radius and ulna are classified as transradial amputations. When the humerus is preserved but the radius and ulna are removed, the amputation is referred to as an elbow disarticulation. Those that leave more than 30% of humeral length are designated as transhumeral amputations. Shoulder disarticulations are those in which less than 30% of the proximal

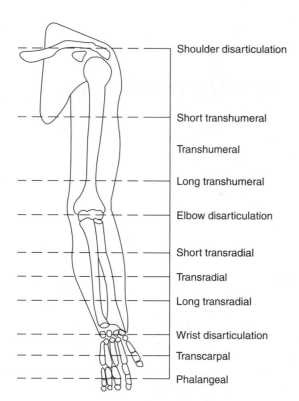

FIGURE 30-1 Classification of upper-extremity amputation and residual limbs. (From Murdoch G, Wilson AB, *Amputation: Surgical Practice and Patient Management.* Oxford, UK: Butterworth, 1996. p. 308.)

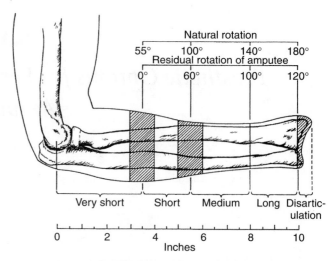

FIGURE 30-2 Potential for pronation and supination of transradial residual limbs of differing lengths. (From Taylor CI. The biomechanics of control in upper extremity prosthetics. *Orthot Prosthet* 1981;35:20.)

humerus remains. More proximal amputations that invade the central body cavity, resecting the clavicle and leading to derangement of the scapula, are described as forequarter amputations or scapulothoracic amputations. In clinical prosthetic and rehabilitation practices, transradial and transhumeral amputations account for nearly 80% of all upper-extremity amputations.[6]

All patients who have amputations of the upper extremity require a complete and thorough examination at the levels of involvement and of associated functional and physiological deficits associated with that specific amputation. For patients with partial hand amputations, the range of motion (ROM) of any remaining digits and the condition of the structural bones of the hand have a profound effect on the selection of possible prosthetic options. The inclusion or absence of an intact thumb also dictates the parameters of fitting.

For those with transverse amputations of the forearm, the length of the residual limb affects the amount of functional elbow flexion and forearm pronation and supination that will be retained independent of prosthetic intervention.[1] Articulations between the radius and the ulna along the entire forearm are necessary to provide for natural anatomical movements in supination and pronation; as the level of amputation moves proximally from the styloid process of the radius toward the elbow, the ability to perform and to use pronation and supination during functional activities is progressively lost (Figure 30-2). When the residual forearm is extremely short, all transverse motion is essentially lost, and it is difficult to gain any active functional forearm rotation for prosthetic use.

Amputations at the level of the elbow (elbow disarticulation) derive little functional benefit from the added length because the length of the limb limits options for cosmetic and functional placement of elbow units within the prosthesis, without substantially improving functional leverage.

Although the primary concern of surgeons who perform an upper-extremity amputation is adequate closure of the wound, they must also consider the potential advantages of a fairly long lever arm, balanced by an understanding of the space requirements for prosthetic components. Provided that adequate skin and tissue viability are not compromised, consideration should be given to adequate room for a full array of prosthetic componentry.

UPPER-EXTREMITY PROSTHETIC COMPONENT

Prosthetic components can be thought of as a means to replace lost functional capacity associated with the anatomical loss of limb segments. A TD is employed to replace grasp and release. An elbow mechanism is used to replace the humeral-ulnar articulation; a shoulder mechanism is placed proximally to provide humeral orientation in space at the shoulder disarticulation and scapulothoracic amputation levels. Rotators can be placed in the forearm of the prosthesis to substitute for pronation and supination or above the elbow unit to substitute for internal and external rotation of the shoulder as well.[9,10]

Partial Hand, Transcarpal, and Wrist Disarticulation

Until recently, patients with digit, partial hand, or transcarpal amputations were often offered passive (nonfunctioning) cosmetic prostheses (restorations).[11] Depending on the characteristics of the residual limb, a functional prehensile post might have been fabricated to regain some grasp and release capability of the affected limb. Recent advances in technology and microprocessors have made externally powered options

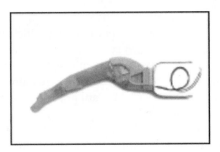

FIGURE 30-3 Example of an externally powered prosthetic hand used for individuals with a partial hand amputation or wrist disarticulation.

more readily available (Figure 30-3).[12] These advances permit electric control despite the extremely distal amputation site. Consideration must be given preoperatively to any remaining functional digits. The status of sensation and mobility of these digits should not be understated. If functional range and sensation are inadequate, the surgeon considers a more proximal level of amputation.

The wrist disarticulation residual limb provides a long and functional lever for prosthetic use.[13] If the radial and ulnar styloid processes are preserved, then the prosthetist can use a positive suspension strategy over these prominences to keep the prosthesis and stable suspended on the residual limb, making harnesses unnecessary. The disadvantage of wrist disarticulation, however, is limitation in room to fit a wrist and hand unit into a cosmetically acceptable prosthesis. If the styloid processes have been modified or removed during surgery, more aggressive proximal suspension strategies are necessary. In addition, the extra residual limb length leads to a difference in arm length once the wrist and prosthetic hand unit is in place, which might be cosmetically unacceptable to the patient. In such cases, a more proximal amputation would allow for a full complement of prosthetic options.

Transradial and Transhumeral Considerations

For most adult transradial prostheses, nearly 8 inches of space is necessary beyond the distal residual limb for the prosthetic wrist rotator and TD or hand.[13] Similarly, at the transhumeral level, approximately 6 inches of space must be present beyond the distal residual limb to accommodate a mechanical elbow mechanism within the prosthesis.[14] For patients with a short residual humerus, a conventional (body-powered) prosthetic system may not be realistic, and even an externally powered prosthesis may be difficult or problematic to fit, suspend, and control. When the residual humerus is short, it may be necessary to treat a transhumeral amputation functionally as a shoulder disarticulation (Figure 30-4).

Positive models to fabricate any contemporary prosthesis can be secured with conventional plaster direct molding techniques similar to those used for lower-extremity amputations. Model acquisition and data collection are also possible using computer-aided design. Both direct contact and optical methods are finding ever-increasing utility in modern practice. This technology is particularly valuable as a means to quantify and document volume and shape changes, enhancing fit and function for optimal clinical outcomes (Figure 30-5).

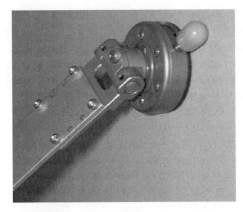

FIGURE 30-4 Example of a prosthetic shoulder joint used in individuals with a shoulder disarticulation or extremely short transhumeral residual limb.

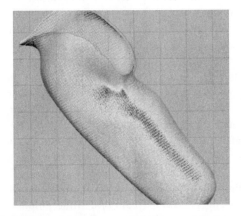

FIGURE 30-5 A computer-assisted design model of a transradial prosthetic socket. Note the aggressive anatomical contouring of the socket and the anteroposterior force system (between the anterior cubital fossa and olecranon) that will be used to suspend the socket on the residual limb. (Courtesy CPS, Branford, CT.)

ETIOLOGY OF UPPER-EXTREMITY AMPUTATION

The etiology of upper-extremity amputations varies widely. The earliest recorded use of limb prosthesis was that of a soldier who reportedly amputated his own limb around 484 BC.[15] One of the earliest known prostheses was fabricated of copper around 300 BC.[16] These early attempts at prosthetic management predate early surgical considerations for lifesaving reasons by many decades. Ambrose Pare, whom many consider the father of modern orthopedic surgery, introduced early surgical techniques around 1529.[17] Public belief is that Pare performed the earliest upper-extremity amputation, an elbow disarticulation, late in 1536. The incidence and prevalence of upper-extremity amputation over the past several centuries is attributed to advances in the pharmacological and surgical management of disease, as well as trauma.[18] Upper-extremity trauma related to industry, mechanized farming, and armed conflict has been the catalyst for medical and prosthetic advancements in the twentieth century.[6]

The National Center for Health Statistics reports approximately 50,000 new amputations every year in the United States. With a ratio of 1:4 upper-extremity to lower-extremity amputations the number of existing and new upper-extremity amputees is both significant and most likely a population that is underserved. As the number of upper limb cases is relatively small in comparison to lower-limb cases, many prosthetic practitioners who are highly skilled and qualified in the arena of lower-limb prosthetics, have far lesser experience and confidence when dealing with complex upper-limb management. Furthermore, in the realm of externally powered prosthetics, fewer practitioners still have the additional education and certifications to work with these complex systems.

Of the approximately 54 million persons in the United States with disabilities, at least 10% have had amputations.[19] Although the exact number of patients with amputations is unknown, the number of patients with acquired and congenital amputations is significant. Of all persons with amputations, the number of patients with amputations to the upper extremity is small in comparison to all total amputations.[19] Compelling evidence suggests an estimated 10,000 new amputations to the upper extremity each year.[20] These numbers represent a large number of individuals who require prosthetic intervention.

The primary cause of acquired amputations is trauma.[6] Other causes of upper-extremity amputation are the various sarcomas, as well as congenital limb deformities, including amelias and phocomelias.[21-23] Amputations to address congenital limb deficiencies are most often performed on individuals younger than 15 years old, while amputation after traumatic injury is most often performed on those between 15 and 45 years old.[24] Seventy percent of all upper-extremity amputations occur in persons younger than 64 years of age.[6,24] Because trauma is more likely to occur in the operation of machinery or in combat, many more amputations occur among males than females.[24]

PREPROSTHETIC CARE

All patients with upper-extremity amputation, regardless of cause, require some degree of preprosthetic management. This is particularly essential with a recent amputation but includes even those persons who have worn prosthetic devices previously. Comprehensive preprosthetic and prosthetic management is a strong predictor of optimal rehabilitation outcomes.[25,26] After amputation surgery, facilitation of wound healing and effective pain management are the foundations for all other types of preprosthetic care. Care is most effective if coordinated through a multidisciplinary team— the prosthetist, surgeon, nurses, physical and occupational therapists, counselors, and others as necessary.[7]

Edema and Volume Control

Edema and volume control are additional key elements of preprosthetic care. If the wound site is adequately protected and bandaged, compressive wraps or shrinkers should be used as soon as possible. In most cases, multidirectional shrinker garments are more effective than other methods, including elastic bandages.[27] Shrinkers appear to more efficiently control volume and shape the residual limb. When donned properly, shrinkers have far less tendency to migrate or shift position on the residual limb. In addition, shrinkers are more effective at creating the consistent distal toward proximal pressure gradient that is most effective. The compressive garment should terminate proximal to the joint above the amputation site when possible. With the transhumeral amputation, this requires the shrinker to include a modified shoulder cap. Such a device is rarely commercially available and usually requires custom fabrication on site. This additional effort has been shown to produce favorable results in comparison with shrinkers that terminate more distally.[26] Due diligence must be exercised to ensure that appropriate tension and compression gradients are achieved and maintained. Effective and timely volume management influences more than the residual limb volume and shape; many patients report that this compression is a surprisingly efficient tool in the management of phantom sensation.[27]

Skin Care, Desensitization, and Range of Motion

The services of a skilled therapist have proven invaluable in the areas of skin care, desensitization, and scar mobilization. Preprosthetic ROM and strengthening should be undertaken concurrently as tolerated.

Skin care can present some significant challenges, particularly when an individual has sustained a traumatic amputation. Chemical and electrical injuries with associated skin grafts can become problematic, particularly when irregular and uneven surface topography is present.[28] Maintaining skin integrity throughout both the fitting and postdelivery phase of rehabilitation is extremely important. The appropriate medical professional should carefully assess any postoperative open lesions. Blast and percussion injuries also present a complex array of socket interface and electrical conductivity issues.[29] This type of injury frequently displays an unusual soft tissue consistency. The tissue is unlike that of crushing, degloving injuries. Tissues exposed to the enormous energy associated with blast injuries frequently respond to the outside compressive forces of shrinkers and preparatory sockets much more dramatically than do tissues injured by other sources. This phenomenon must be considered carefully, as its effects profoundly affect any rehabilitation plan.

The nature of any volume management protocol in and of itself begins the limb maturation and desensitization process simultaneously. Further and more focused efforts must be undertaken to assure that limb volume is both stabilizing and fostering a limb shape or contour that is favorable to donning, wearing, and operating a prosthetic device.[28] Limbs with large longitudinal contours or bulbous distal contours are least desirable. Residuum with insignificant tissue or skin coverage should also be avoided whenever possible. Ideally the residual limb is long enough to provide a functional lever arm but not so long as to preclude the use of a wide array of prosthetic components. Residual limbs with effective myodesis frequently display smaller myoelectric artifact without any apparent or material loss of volitional potential.

Preprosthetic ROM should be maximized regardless of the planned prosthetic intervention. Strengthening of the muscles about and proximal to the amputation is paramount. However, a more global approach to strengthening affords the patient a more expeditious and complete rehabilitation. These efforts to maximize ROM and increase volitional power should not overlook the secondary movers or accessory stabilizers. For patients with transradial amputations, for example, maximizing ROM and strength of pronation and supination is an important determinant of positive functional outcomes.

Adaptation Process

Patients and families facing amputation, whether congenital or acquired, adjust and cope with absence or loss of the limb differently.[30] The extent or level of involvement often has little to do with the complexity of the adaptation process. All persons must find ways to deal with the functional and aesthetic issues related to limb loss. Adaptation is an ongoing process rather than a specific event. In many cases the services of a qualified psychotherapist are valuable, providing the patient and caregivers are amenable to such intervention.

Most professionals agree that there is a fairly short window of opportunity within which the prospects for successful rehabilitation are greatest, although there is disagreement about the duration of this "optimal rehabilitation" period. In most circumstances the earlier a patient can be evaluated, fitted, and trained, the more likely a positive rehabilitation outcome occurs.[6] Malone and colleagues[25] suggest high levels of success with patients fit within the first 30 days following amputation. In addition, individuals fit with a prosthesis as early as possible return to work quickly, many within 4 months of injury.[6,25]

PROSTHETIC EXAMINATION AND EVALUATION

Examination of persons with upper-extremity amputations should include complete documentation of the involved limb's ROM. Care should be exercised to identify both the active and passive ranges. Volitional muscle control should be evaluated and documented. Limb shape and contour, as well as tissue consistency, are important elements in the evaluation. Particular attention must be paid to any grafts, scars, or painful areas of the residuum. Pertinent medical history must be duly noted, as it may affect not only prosthetic development but all phases of the rehabilitation protocol.

The past medical history must adequately address any injuries or pathologies on both sides of the body. For patients with high-level amputations, the prosthesis, regardless of configuration or power source, ultimately has some integrated components across one or both of the axilla, as well as the thoracic wall.

The objective of all prosthetic interventions should be to restore as much functional potential as possible.[31] This is best accomplished by using components, materials, and interface designs to most closely approximate the lost body segments and functions. The appropriateness of any design should address the patient's vocational, recreational, and aesthetic needs. The needs of most patients can be met with one or more prosthetic options.

PROSTHETIC OPTIONS

Depending on the patient's situation, the prosthetist and rehabilitation team can make a number of recommendations. These include not providing a prosthesis, providing a passive prosthesis or cosmetic restoration, designing a conventional body-powered system, or providing a sophisticated myoelectrically controlled prosthetic limb with multiple components.

No Prosthesis

A significant percentage of patients with upper-extremity amputations elect not to use a prosthesis on a regular basis.[6] In many cases this decision can be traced to a poorly conceived or executed prosthetic device that was provided early in the patient rehabilitation process.[25] Some potential wearers report that the devices they have been exposed to are uncomfortable, heavy, and too slow during use or difficult to don and suspend.[6] The advent of advanced materials has enabled prosthetists to build lighter, stronger, and more comfortable systems, as well as extremely cosmetic restorations. Despite these advancements, not all individuals with amputations integrate a prosthesis into their body image. The prosthetist or rehabilitation team should follow patients who choose not to use a prosthesis initially at regular intervals (often yearly) to ensure that their functional needs are being met. Given the rate of technological development, new components or devices are likely to become available to address problems the patient might have had at an earlier time.

Passive Prostheses and Restorations

This category of prosthesis consists of systems that do not possess the ability to actively position a mechanical elbow in space or actively provide grasp and release function, or both. The absence of these properties does not, however, render the prosthesis as passive as the name would suggest. These devices are extremely functional in terms of supporting objects or stabilizing items during bimanual tasks and activities, especially for young children with congenital deficiencies.[32,33] These systems most frequently have a self-suspending design and use a realistic hand as a TD. Suspension is achieved either with specific socket interface geometry or suction negative pressure. The absence of operational mechanical components generally results in an extremely lightweight prosthesis.

The finish of these devices varies widely. Production latex cosmetic gloves provide an cost-effective medium for many patients. Many individuals, however, seek out more realistic restorations (Figure 30-6). These restorations require substantially greater investments in time and financial resources. This investment is most often rewarded with an extremely aesthetic, very natural appearing device. Silicone is the media of choice for these cosmetic limbs, primarily because it is practically impervious to outside contaminants. Where latex readily stains and deteriorates in ultraviolet light, silicone does not mark and, for all practical purposes, is inert. Generally, the

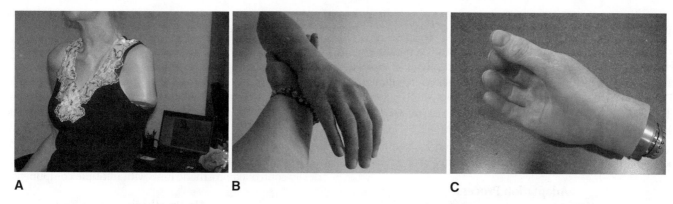

A   **B**   **C**

FIGURE 30-6 Passive prostheses and restorations (A, Courtesy CPS, Branford, CT; B, Courtesy Alternative Prosthetics).

additional cost of silicone is mitigated by its superior cosmesis, durability, and increased coefficient of friction (Figure 30-6).

Laser scanning and computer modeling to create near perfect "mirror" images of high level amputations, such as shoulder disarticulations, and scapulothoracic amputations (see Figure 30-6, *A*).

Conventional Body-Powered Systems

Conventional (body-powered) systems include any prosthesis that uses a control cable system to translate volitional muscle force and shoulder or arm movement to operate a TD or prosthetic elbow.[34] The patient must use specific strategies in order to effectively create enough excursion in the cable to control the TD or preposition the forearm in space. In most instances the glenohumeral joint contributes the largest amount of excursion in conventional prosthetic control. Glenohumeral flexion typically has more than ample excursion and satisfactory power to provide useful motors for this type of control. Additional excursion can be achieved through scapular and biscapular abduction (scapular protraction). These secondary movements allow a well-trained and skilled prosthetic wearer to increase the functional work envelope, the space in which the wearer can effectively control the TD.

For most conventional upper-extremity prostheses, the functional envelope is limited to a relatively small area below the shoulders, above the waist, and not far outward past shoulder width.[34] Many prosthetic wearers have significant difficulty with tasks that involve grasp-and-release tasks above the head or down near the feet. Because the control strategy involves generating cable excursion through flexion or protraction, or both, tasks and activities occurring behind the back are impossible. Despite these functional limitations, conventional prostheses have provided many patients with reliable and durable prosthetic systems.

Figure-of-Eight Suspension and Control Cable

The foundation of all conventional body-powered prostheses is a harnessing system that provides both a firm anchor for the control cables and, in many cases, a stable means of suspension. Most conventional systems use a figure-of-eight–style harness (Figure 30-7). The terminal ends of the figure-of-eight are formed by means of an axillary loop that is fit over the opposite shoulder, a control attachment cable, and an

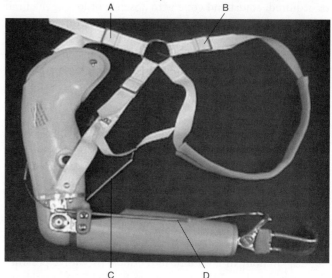

A   **B**

C   **D**

FIGURE 30-7 The figure-of-eight harness with posterior ring and cable control systems used in a conventional (body-powered) transhumeral prosthesis includes an anterior suspension loop **(A)**, the contralateral axillary loop **(B)**, a cable to control locking and unlocking of the elbow mechanism **(C)**, and a cable that will lift the forearm if the elbow unit is unlocked or operate the terminal device if the elbow unit is locked **(D)**.

anterior suspension component on the amputated side. Most prosthetists recommend that the center of the figure-of-eight be positioned just below the seventh cervical vertebra and slightly toward the sound side.[34] The straps of the two axillary loops can be mobile by means of attachment to a circular ring or fixed with a sewn cross point. The use of a center ring often makes the donning process less difficult and appears to provide the most satisfactory ROM. Harnessing materials are most frequently constructed of medium weight Dacron webbing with both leather and plastic integrated components.

Cable Control for Self-Suspending Sockets

If the prosthetist recommends a self-suspending socket, the anterior suspension of a figure-of-eight harness is not necessary. In these instances a figure-of-nine harness, consisting mainly of the contralateral axillary loop, is used to minimize cumbersome harnessing while still maximizing a firm anchor for the control cable. Self-suspending sockets may be of an anatomically contoured design or that of a flexible silicone interface, with either a locking or suction valve mechanism.

Control and Suspension for Bilateral Prostheses

For patients with amputation of both upper extremities, careful clinical consideration must be given to achieving an easily donable and highly functional prosthetic system. Instead of using a traditional figure-of-eight harness with a contralateral axillary loop for each prosthesis, the two anterior suspension components are linked.[35] In this arrangement, the bilateral prosthetic system is effectively stabilized by the equal counteracting forces from each prosthesis. On the basis of the patient's functional needs, the prosthetist may use either a single- or dual-ring system to maximize the efficiency of the conventional prostheses (Figure 30-8). The second ring in the system, mounted below the primary ring, is used exclusively

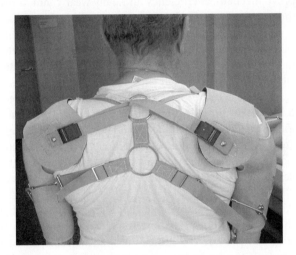

FIGURE 30-8 The harness system used for conventional (body-powered) bilateral transhumeral prostheses includes an upper ring that stabilizes the prostheses on the trunk and a lower ring that anchors the cable control systems (Courtesy CPS, Branford, CT).

for the control attachment straps. The more proximal ring is used for the anterior suspensor straps and, for patients with bilateral transhumeral residual limbs, the connection of elbow locking straps.

Some patients with bilateral amputations opt to use separate and completely independent harness systems for their prostheses, especially if they sometimes wear only one prosthesis or if their prostheses are dissimilar. An individual with bilateral transradial amputations, for example, might elect to use a conventional cable-driven system on the nondominant side and a self-suspending externally powered prosthesis on the dominant residual limb.

Triceps Cuff in Conventional Transradial Prosthesis

Individuals with transradial amputations using a conventional harness suspension control the TD by means of a single cable.[34] In most instances a triceps cuff is used to secure the cable housing in an optimal position, as well as provide an integral link to the forearm section (Figure 30-9). Several mechanisms of connection are available between the triceps cuff and the forearm. Flexible Dacron hinges provide satisfactory suspension and ROM for most midlength transradial amputations. Steel cable hinges can be substituted in circumstances where extremely heavy axial loads can be expected (i.e., if a wearer must carry or move heavy objects at work). For those with short and extremely short transradial amputations, metal hinges provide better medial lateral stability at the elbow, as well as functional stop at full extension to protect the residual limb.

Cable Systems to Control a Prosthetic Elbow

Patients with transhumeral amputations need a dual-cable system; an anterior cable controls the locking and unlocking of the elbow mechanism, while the other cable controls the TD (if the elbow is locked) or moves the prosthetic forearm (if the elbow is unlocked).[36] The second (longer) cable that

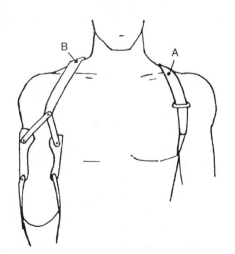
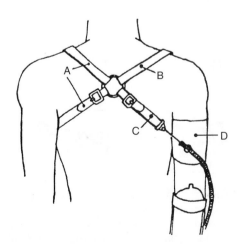

FIGURE 30-9 Anterior and posterior view of a figure-of-eight harness system for a transradial prosthesis, with the axillary loop **(A)**, the anterior support strap that provides stability during a downward pull **(B)**, the attachment strap for cable control of the terminal device **(C)**, and the triceps pad that anchors the control cable in the most effective position **(D)**. (Modified from the Northwestern University Printing and Duplicating Department, Evanston, IL, 1987.)

attaches to the TD requires a split-cable housing system. The proximal portion of the housing is attached to the humeral section, while the distal portion is attached at a location and height anterior to the elbow center.

Most elbow mechanisms have multiple locking positions at equally spaced intervals moving from full extension to flexion. The locking mechanism is most frequently activated using a rapid and forceful shoulder extension and abduction (Figure 30-10). When the elbow mechanism is "locked" in any given position, this quick down and back movement elongates an anterior cable that releases the lock; subsequent shoulder flexion or scapular abduction (protraction) affecting the posterior cable repositions the prosthetic forearm in space. This happens because the cable running to the TD is aligned anterior to the axis of rotation of the elbow mechanism; when the elbow is unlocked, tension through this cable causes the forearm to rise in flexion. When the forearm reaches the desired inclination for the task at hand, another quick down and back motion will reengage the lock. Once the elbow mechanism is locked, cable control is transferred to the TD, and subsequent shoulder flexion or protraction operates the prosthetic hook or hand. Because this control strategy is always sequential in nature, careful consideration and assessment must be given to the force excursion ratio. Failure to maximize these criteria results in incomplete elbow flexion or incomplete TD control.

Cables and Cable Housings

For both transradial and transhumeral prostheses, the cable and housings should traverse as straight a path as practical. An abrupt or sharp radius creates excessive and unnecessary drag as the cable passes through the housing. The mechanical

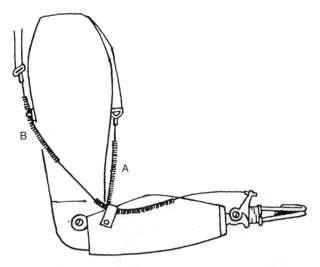

FIGURE 30-10 Dual control cable and lift loop of a conventional (body-powered) transhumeral prosthesis. Quick and forceful downward and backward shoulder motion operates the elbow locking and unlocking mechanism via the anterior cable (**A**). The second cable system (**B**) operates the terminal device if the elbow is locked or lifts the forearm if the elbow is locked. This occurs because the TD control cable is positioned anterior to the axis of the mechanical elbow joint. (Modified from Northwestern University Printing and Duplicating Department, Evanston, IL, 1987.)

efficiency of the system is critical to successful operation, particularly for those patients with limited strength or ROM.[37] Steel cable has been used successfully for many years in prosthetic practice. Steel cable is available in several thicknesses so as to meet the needs of all types of users. Clearly the heaviest cables are well suited to heavy-work applications and are often used for individuals wearing prostheses for both upper extremities.

Low-friction linings are often added to the interior surfaces of the cable housing to improve the mechanical efficiency.[38] This technique effectively decreases the coefficient of friction of the stainless cable as it passes through the metal cable housing. Typically, the low-friction linings wear and require replacement before cable failure.

Recently, nonmetallic cable media with both high strength and low coefficients of friction became available; these improve mechanical efficiency and daily wear characteristics of the prosthetic system.[39] When nonmetallic cables are used with low coefficient linings, the result is often an extremely smooth and highly efficient cable system. These nonmetallic cable alternatives are not mechanically swedged to the attachment hardware used at each end of a prosthetic cable system. Instead, cable connections are made by using highly specialized knots that provide a reliable connection with a smooth profile. Should a nonmetallic cable fail, it is possible for the wearer (with some assistance) to complete emergency repairs without returning the facility. Furthermore, nonmetallic cables do not leave dark residue and stains typically associated with steel cables.

Although these nonmetallic cables are every bit as strong as their steel counterparts, one important drawback is that they do not provide any indication that the cable is nearing the end of its service life. Conversely, steel cables typically become rough and begin to drag as the individual strands of the cable part. Despite this single drawback, nonmetallic cables are strongly recommended in most clinical applications. Further consideration should be given to provide all patients with additional backup cables for times when immediate access to prosthetic repair services is not available.

TERMINAL DEVICES FOR CONVENTIONAL PROSTHESES

The TDs most often used for conventional body-powered prostheses are either a hook (Figure 30-11) or hand (Figure 30-12).[34,40] Both are available as a voluntary opening system (the TD is closed at rest, and the wearer opens the hand by means of the cable) or as a voluntary closing system (the TD is open at rest, and the wearer closes the hand by means of the cable). Each configuration has its own inherent strengths and weaknesses.

Voluntary opening devices enable the wearer to apply volitional force and excursion of the cable (using shoulder flexion or abduction) to open the TD. Once tension is released from the cable system, the object being grasped is "trapped" in the device, allowing the wearer to position the object in space as the task demands. The prehensile

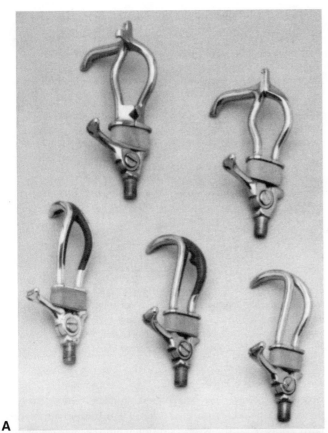

A

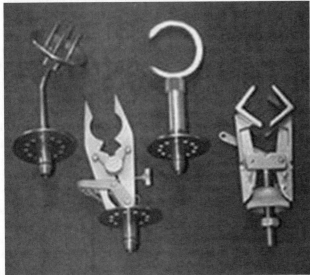

B

FIGURE 30-11 A, Various conventional "hooks" are available to meet the functional needs of individuals using conventional (body-powered) prostheses. The top row of these voluntary opening terminal devices, designed for children, has a "thumb post," as well as coated grip surfaces that are held closed by rubber bands at the base of the hook. Adult hooks are available in a number of configurations to meet the functional and vocational needs of the wearer. **B,** Terminal devices have also been designed for occupations that require stabilizing objects, carrying objects, or holding cylindrical or spherical objects. (A, Courtesy Hosmer Dorrance, Campbell, CA; B, Courtesy Otto Bock Healthcare, Minneapolis, MN.)

force (grip strength) is dictated by some external closing mechanism, most frequently springs or elastic bands (see Figure 30-11). Significant prehensile forces can be generated by using multiple layers of elastic bands or multiple springs but must be matched to the wearer's ability to create and sustain cable excursion. Because grip strength is determined by the number of elastics or springs used, it is constant and cannot be voluntarily modified when handling heavy or fragile objects. The mechanical inefficiency and friction inherent in a cable control system increase the force necessary to open the TD above the closing force achieved by the rubber bands or spring systems. Finding the right combination of external closing mechanism strength and user's motor control and excursion for the many different daily functional tasks can be challenging. Several manufacturers market voluntary opening prehensors with settings the wearer can adjust to light or forceful grip strength.[41]

In voluntary closing TDs, the volitional force and excursion supplied by the wearer closes the TD from its normally open position.[42] The key advantage of a voluntary closing TD is the ability to volitionally grade prehensile force, adapting it to the characteristics of the object to be held.[43] When a voluntary closing TD is used, significantly higher forces can be applied through the cabling system. In fact, with most voluntarily closing TD and cable systems, voluntary prehensile force is limited only by the motor powers available from the wearer or by discomfort of the residual limb. In this control strategy the patient must maintain both excursion and power so as to retain the object in the TD.

Voluntary closing devices are not often chosen for individuals with transhumeral amputations because the limited cable excursion available to them is also being used to preposition the forearm in space. Functionally, much of the cable excursions would be used to close the TD so that less would be available to move the forearm. Although those with transhumeral amputation frequently have adequate motor control to position the forearm in space, many are quite challenged to produce enough excursion to effectively operate the elbow throughout full ranges of motion while maintaining a graded prehension of the TD. These actions become even more challenging if the residual transhumeral limb is relatively short. The external passive closure of a voluntary opening TD tends to be more functional for these individuals. Because cable excursion is typically limited for those with bilateral amputations, voluntary opening devices are also the TDs of choice if bilateral conventional prostheses are recommended.

Socket Configurations

The transhumeral and transradial prosthetic sockets used in contemporary prosthetic practice have evolved from non-anatomically and functionally based designs to highly contoured, skeletally correct and intimately fitting designs. A significant portion of these anatomically contoured socket advancements have come as a direct result of changes in material technology. Until recently, upper-extremity prosthetic sockets were fabricated using thermal setting resins

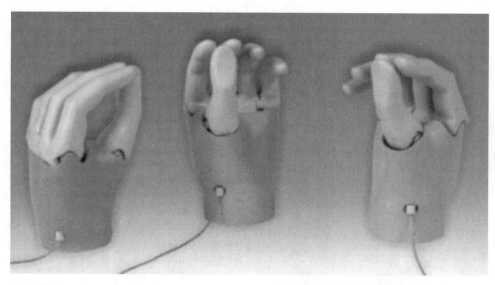

FIGURE 30-12 Examples of mechanical hands for a conventional (body-powered) prosthesis. Tension of the cable opens the hand to grasp an object using a mechanical "three jaw chuck" grasping pattern. Release of tension on the cable passively holds an object between the thumb and first two digits. To release a held object, the wearer applies tension to the cable once again, to open the mechanical hand. The fourth and fifth fingers are passive and prepositioned in slight flexion but are not part of the grasp and release function of the mechanical hand.

for structural integrity and finish. By nature these materials were hard and did not yield effectively to changes in muscle contour as the wearer used the limb in functional activities. With the advent of moldable thermoplastics and advanced anatomically contoured socket designs, improvements in intimacy of fit and functional ROM have been achieved.

Most contemporary upper-extremity prosthetic sockets use some type of flexible interface with a rigid frame exterior. The interface material is often composed of a high silicone content elastomer. These elastomers have dramatically improved patients' perceptions of fit and function with regard to comfort.

Socket Transradial Self-Suspending Sockets

Many patients with transradial amputations are now fit with self-suspending sockets that both increase functional ROM during activity and, more importantly, improve wearer acceptance and compliance.[6] Highly specialized bone and muscle contour promote effective control in both conventional body-powered and myoelectrically controlled prostheses. Historically, self-suspending transradial sockets encase the medial and lateral humeral condyles to provide suspension.[34] The nature of this medial-lateral compression inherently decreased ROM, particularly in terminal flexion. New designs are becoming less dependent on the condyles and are using higher anteroposterior forces between the anterior fossa and olecranon of the elbow to achieve suspension. This strategy increases the wearer's ability to fully extend the elbow.

Advances in Donning Techniques

As the intimacy of socket designs has increased, so has the need for more effective donning techniques. Historically, cotton stockinettes or elastic bandages were adequate for drawing tissue into prosthetic sockets and allowed for satisfactory donning.

Because these materials have high coefficient friction, they can be difficult to pull from the socket. High friction also can be fairly abrasive on the wearer's residual limb. A new generation of pull socks made of low-friction cloth have been developed (). Many have coatings impregnated into the cloth during manufacture to allow for effective, nonabrasive donning of intimately contoured prosthetic sockets. With the initial tension as it is first pulled through the opening in the socket, the pull sock encases the soft tissue of the residual limb as if it were a cylindrical cone. As the pull sock is drawn through the opening, it positions the soft tissue of the residual limb as intended by the contour of the socket. These donning tools have also enabled some individuals with bilateral amputations to independently don aggressive self-suspending sockets.

Advances in Transhumeral Socket Design

Whereas the traditional transhumeral prosthesis had an over-the-shoulder cap socket design, recent advances in socket design have resulted in sockets with lateral trim lines below the acromion process. The additions of anterior and posterior stabilizer extensions that cross toward the midline on the amputated side provide superior rotational stability.

CASE EXAMPLE 1

An Individual with Traumatic Transradial Amputation

P. C., 34, sustained a severe crush injury to his left hand, wrist, and lower forearm when a rock wall he was building in his backyard collapsed as he was working on it. The team at the trauma center determined that he was not a candidate for limb salvage and recommended transradial amputation. Now it is 8 weeks after the surgery. P. C. has been consistent with compression of his residual limb and his upper-extremity home-exercise program. He is referred for prescription of a transradial prosthesis. Clinical examination reveals a well-healed incision, with a skin graft over the anterior surface of the cubital fossa and residual limb. Tissue density is relatively firm. Touch and pressure sensation is slightly diminished in the area of the skin graft. P. C. can fully extend his elbow but lacks the final 25 degrees of elbow flexion. He has minimal pronation and supination ability in his residual limb. Shoulder ROM and strength are within normal limits. The residual limb measures 16 cm from the lateral epicondyle to the distal end and 12.5 cm from the cubital fold to the distal end.

P. C. is right-hand dominant. He works as a self-employed building contractor, with a small business focused on home remodeling. He lives with his wife and three elementary school–age children in a three-story Victorian home that he is in the process of rehabilitating. He is an avid water skier in the summer and downhill skier in the winter. P. C. is apprehensive about his ability to return to work and support his family.

Questions to Consider

- Given the condition and function of his residual limb, what type of socket and interface might the team might recommend for P. C. from among available options? Why would these be the optimal choices? What factors are likely to influence clinical decision making in this case?
- Given his employment and vocational interests, what type of suspension and control system might the team recommend for P. C. from among available options? Why would these be the optimal choices? Will a conventional cable control system allow P. C. the "work envelope" required for his job as a builder? Given his skin condition, would a myoelectrically controlled prosthesis be possible? How would the team determine this?
- Given his employment and vocational interests, what type of terminal device (or hand) and wrist unit might the team recommend for P. C.? Why would these be the optimal choices? What are the benefits and drawbacks of a "quick disconnect" wrist unit and having activity-specific TDs?

Recommendations

After much discussion P. C. and the team decide that a self-suspending transradial prosthesis with a flexible socket in a rigid frame is most appropriate. Given his role as a builder and the need to work overhead and have sufficient grip force to hold and manipulate lumber and other building materials, the team recommends a myoelectrically powered prosthesis with a power wrist control unit and a Griefer as a terminal device to be used in his work setting. P. C. inquires whether TDs might be interchangeable so that he can have a prosthetic hand with a silicone glove to wear when he is not at work.

EXTERNALLY POWERED SYSTEMS

All externally powered systems share a single common denominator: an electric power cell that provides electrical current to prosthetic components (Figure 30-13).[44] Cell technology has dramatically improved in the past decade. Traditional technology involved rechargeable nickel cadmium batteries that, in addition to environmental concerns on disposal, are vulnerable to a memory effect. Cell memory effect occurs when batteries are charged before reaching a fully discharged state. As batteries incur greater and greater amounts of memory, the maximal charge the battery accepts decreases. As maximal charge decreases, so does the maximal time a patient can expect service from the battery. As a practical matter, a patient cannot reasonably be expected to use the battery until full discharge is achieved, and therefore a rechargeable battery in this state is impractical.

As the medium that promotes electrical charge in prosthetic batteries has changed, memory effect has been virtually eradicated. Batteries made with lithium, lithium ion, have no memory effect and supply significantly higher amounts of current, while simultaneously decreasing the weight of the battery. An active prosthetic user can now use an externally powered prosthesis more than a full day on a single charge. Because lithium-based cells are smaller and lighter, they are also less challenging to "fit" cosmetically into the prosthesis.

Other than having an electric cell, externally powered prostheses may have little in common with each other by classification. Electric TD componentry is available in many forms, including hooks, hands, and specially developed work tools. These tools can be oriented in space using electric rotators that can substitute effectively for lost pronation and supination.[9]

Electric and electronic elbow mechanisms are also readily available. These mechanisms provide powered flexion and extension at the elbow joint (Figure 30-14). Substitution for internal and external rotation of the shoulder is more difficult. Most systems integrate a passive friction humeral rotator; this allows the patient to reposition the distal extremity in the desired amount of internal or external rotation.[10] Although actively powered humeral rotation has been problematic in terms of design and function, much research and development is under way.

For patients with exceptionally short transhumeral limbs and shoulder disarticulation, most prostheses use a mechanical device to replace the shoulder joint that can be passively prepositioned.[45] Electrically actuated locks are available for clinical use and provide an effective means of locking the position of the humerus relative to the midline of the body for individuals with high-level amputations.

DECISION MAKING

The decision process on what input devices will provide control to externally powered components is a complex one. Full assessment and evaluation of the available motors, ROMs, electromyographical signal, signal separation, and limb length and skin integrity must be considered.[46] The choice of input devices for externally powered devices represents a broad and

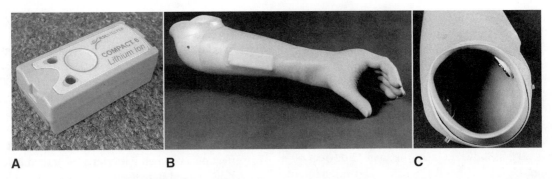

A   **B**   **C**

FIGURE 30-13 A, An example of a lithium power cell used in a myoelectric prosthesis. This cell must be fit somewhere within the prosthesis (**B**) to power terminal devices and other prosthetic components, on the basis of signals received by the myoelectrodes (**C**) embedded in the walls of the socket. (Courtesy Liberating Technologies, Boston, MA.)

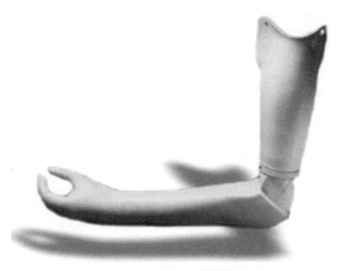

FIGURE 30-14 An example of a myoelectrically controlled transhumeral prosthesis with electric elbow and hand. The socket brim has anterior and posterior "wings" to stabilize the prosthesis on the residual humerus. Myoelectrodes over the residual biceps are used to flex the elbow or close the hand, while those over the residual triceps extend the elbow or open the hand. Quick cocontraction of biceps and triceps will switch control from elbow to hand mode. (Courtesy Motion Control, Salt Lake City, UT.)

wide-reaching array of control strategies that allow nearly all patients the opportunity to successfully control a prosthesis. The most common and preferred means to control a prosthesis is with the electromyographic (EMG) signal. This technology uses the small electrical potentials generated by contraction of the residual muscles to operate one or more devices. Modern circuitry and sophisticated filters allow most patients, even those with small signals, the potential for reasonable control.

MYOELECTRIC CONTROL SYSTEMS

Ideally, the prosthetist tries to identify two independent signals in a set of physiologically paired (agonist and antagonist) muscles. The wearer can activate these signals over a wide spectrum of contraction intensity to use them as electrode sites. For those with transradial limbs, electrodes are typically positioned over flexor muscle residuum in the forearm to control grasp (closing of the TD) and the extensor

muscle residuum to control release (opening of the TD).[47] Many patients who, with sufficient training, master independent contraction of these muscle groups are candidates for even more sophisticated control.

The prosthetist selects the most appropriate myoelectrodes from the many sizes and numerous configurations that are manufactured. The prosthetist also chooses electrodes on the basis of whether they require a remote or nonremote placement of the preamplification electronics. In selecting the myoelectrode and preamplification system, the prosthetist must carefully consider the location, function, and components (TD, elbow, locking mechanism, and rotators) to be used. Because nonremote sensing electrodes house the preamplifier in the bundle of the electrode, less space is necessary to house electronics in the prosthesis. Placing the preamplifier close to the electrode, however, increases the risk that perspiration will disrupt electronic function. Electrode selection should consider the amount of soft tissue present on the residual limb, the presence or absence of scar tissue, and the material medium with which the interface will be constructed.

Many components can interpret large or small, fast or slow muscular contractions and respond prosthetically in a proportional fashion, linking speed and force of device operation to speed and amplitude of muscle contraction under the myoelectrode site.[47] This graded control enables a patient to develop extremely precise speed and grip strength strategies. The well-developed independent control of antagonistic muscles also is a prerequisite for mode selection, which uses different types of contraction of the same muscle groups for dissimilar tasks. Many patients wearing a transradial myoelectrical prosthesis use a quick cocontraction of forearm muscle residuum to switch between control of the hand and the wrist unit. For those with transhumeral prostheses, quick cocontraction of shoulder flexors and extensors is used to switch between control of the electronic elbow and hand. Effective mode selection with cocontraction requires a patient to fire antagonistic muscles above a predetermined threshold at nearly the same instant.[47] Many patients find this technique challenging as control training begins. Mode selection is based on nearly simultaneous timing of contraction of agonistic and antagonistic muscles. Early in training, however, many new myoelectric prosthetic users focus on forcefulness of contraction in an effort to increase amplitude of the signal, rather than on producing the desired quick cocontraction.

If a patient struggles or is unable to master cocontraction mode selection, alternative strategies are always available. The prosthetist can use programmable controllers to allow complex muscle activity not generally associated with everyday tasks as the mode selection trigger. Additionally, many systems allow the user a default mode (usually to the TD) to which the mode selector reverts after a predetermined time interval.

Programmable microprocessors have had an additional impact on prosthetic fitting; they allow the prosthetist to experiment with multiple strategies without having to replace hardware. Before programmable microprocessors were available, myoelectric components were secured for individual patients without the benefit of real-time clinical assessment. Microprocessor control has allowed the prosthetist to maximize the patient's rehabilitation potential within a single hardware construct. Enormous benefit is also derived from the ability to save, recover, and manipulate software configurations easily and quickly with immediate patient feedback. This allows prosthetic users to experiment with a strategy for control and then progress to alternative strategies with the luxury of returning to the precise original strategy and settings quickly. Programmable controllers allow individuals with recent amputations to maximize their current physiological control and then progress to significantly more complex and involved strategies without having to replace components or relinquishing a prosthesis for modification.

Three basic approaches are used to program the microprocessor. In the first approach, adjustments to electronics are made through a direct connection to a laptop or similar computer using a graphical interface. Wireless interface communication or the implementation of coding plugs enables efficient assessment and modification of control strategies. For some individuals with new amputations who are candidates for early postoperative fitting, a myoelectrically controlled TD may be integrated in a rigid dressing immediately after surgery. The psychological and physiological benefits of early fitting have been well demonstrated.[25]

ALTERNATIVE CONTROL STRATEGIES

If effective myoelectric control is too difficult to master for a patient immediately after amputation surgery (or is inappropriate because of cocontraction problems), the prosthetist may opt to use switch control as an alternative means of operating electric prosthetic components.[48] Switch control does not require myoelectric sensors against the skin. In addition, switch control of functional grasp and release can be mastered fairly readily by most new prosthetic users, without the appreciable training time required for myoelectric systems. Switch control systems require extremely small movement to trigger—typically an excursion in millimeters and a force in fractions of pounds.[49] This makes it much more functional than early postoperative devices with body-powered components that required larger cable excursions to operate TD or lock or unlock the prosthetic elbow. The small excursion and light force required to engage switch control makes prosthetic use feasible for individuals with limited ROM or strength. This

technique allows for early intervention with limited exposure to the stresses on the recently amputated residual limb . It also allows new users to develop functional grip strength within a short time. When switches are used to trigger externally powered prosthetic components, however, proportional control (graded action where the action of the device is proportional to the effort made to trigger its operation) is not possible.

Several other control systems are available as well. Force sensitive resistors (FSRs, also called touch pads) have found great utility as a primary control driver in instances when other signals are not readily available. FSRs are designed to interpret surface pressure on the pad and supply a resultant proportional output. Because these devices are extremely flat and small in diameter, they are well suited for applications such as residual limb buds in children with congenital limb deficiencies. Special consideration must be given, however, to the location and preparation of sites in which an FSR is to be used. These devices can become problematic if the base on which they are placed is not perfectly flat. Even a small radius can cause the conductive gel inside the sensor to fail. The location must be placed strategically to allow any perspiration to settle away from the sensor. Failure to adequately address this strategic locating of the device may cause the FSR to fail.

In addition to being used in early postoperative fittings, switches can also be used in definitive prostheses. Although most switches are activated by pulling a cable or strap, other applications are activated by depressing a lever or button. Some switches are complex in nature because they have numerous functions that are dictated by the position of the switch. Most switches do not have the capacity to provide proportional output to control electric components. The absence of proportionality can be viewed as a limiting factor in many switch control applications.

To achieve true proportionality, a servo-resistor or other sensing resistor would be necessary. These devices interpret the travel (excursion) applied to the system and translate this input quantitatively with predetermined electrical outputs. These devices can also translate force simultaneously or independently with excursion to create a proportional output.

Proportional control of all electrically powered devices (especially of elbows and the TDs) has enabled patients to achieve unprecedented levels of fine motor control and speed variability for skilled activity.[50,51] Technology has enabled this proportional control to further expand the functional envelope of the prosthesis, with higher-speed drive motors and clutches that allow extremely responsive and rapid control (Figure 30-15). When proportional control is coupled with circuitry designed to create and maintain stable prehensile patterns within the TD, wearers can achieve increasingly complex and sophisticated tasking patterns.

ELECTRIC TERMINAL DEVICES

Electric TDs are available in many configurations; the most commonly used is an electric hand (Figure 30-16).[52] Most hands are available in an array of sizes, from those designed to fit young children (Figure 30-16) with congenital limb

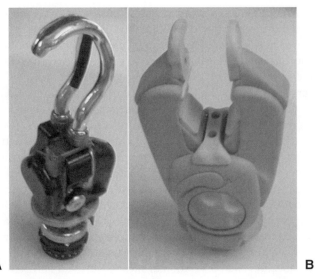

FIGURE 30-15 A and **B,** Examples of terminal devices that allow proportional control of grasp on the basis of muscle contraction speed at the myoelectrode site or the use of programmable microprocessor controllers. (A, Courtesy Motion Control, Salt Lake City, UT; B, Courtesy Otto Bock Healthcare, Minneapolis, MN.)

deficiencies to those that fit adults with traumatic amputations. Most hands use a "three jaw chuck" grasping pattern of the thumb and first two digits. The remaining fingers (digits four and five) follow passively but in a similar pattern to the active first two digits opposing the thumb. Significant grasp pressures can be achieved with most electromechanical hands; in fact, pressures can be so significant that patients must be cautioned during early training about the amount of force possible. In myoelectric prostheses with proportional control, maximum grip strength is achieved with corresponding maximum input signal generated by forceful muscle contraction. Proportionality of input signal translates to both the speed of finger movement and the terminal force applied to the object being grasped. In a nonproportionally based system (such as simple switch control), maximum grip strength is achieved on a time-dependent basis. Recently, circuits have been added to provide slip control. This allows objects to be retained in the grasp without conscious control from patient input. Objects of a soft nature can also be manipulated more effectively without being crushed with such slip-sensing technology. Excellent cosmesis can be achieved in these systems with the implementation of a custom sculpted and painted silicon outer shell (see Figure 30-6, *A*).

Although hands make up the majority of externally powered prostheses with TDs, other highly functional TDs are readily available.[52] These devices range from tools that closely resemble portable vices to terminal hardware that closely mimics the functional characteristics of an electric hook. As most prostheses include a quick-disconnect option for the TD, prosthetic wearers can easily change TDs to suit their functional demands. Many of the non–hand-type TDs can generate even greater forces than the corresponding hands. The geometries of the opening mechanism allow these alternative tools to easily grasp larger, cylindrical, and more irregularly shaped objects. The smaller tips of some of these tools allow patients to grasp smaller and flatter objects as well. When these alternative TDs are used, there is less obstruction of the visual field. As a result, many have better functional efficiency than possible with a prosthetic hand. To date no system is commercially available that satisfactorily replicates the lost proprioception and sensation of the fingers and anatomical hand. The size and location of the visual field blocked by the palmar surface of the hand and outstretched mechanical fingers has a significant impact on function.

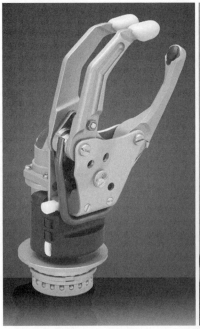
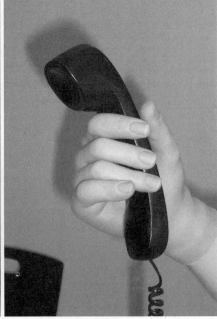
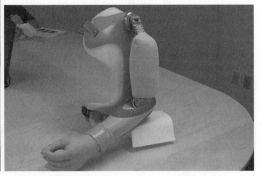

FIGURE 30-16 Examples of electric terminal devices.

Until recently most externally powered hands utilized a three jaw chuck prehension pattern. In this highly functional grasp pattern, the active grasp is generated between the thumb and first two fingers. Patients now can utilize more compliant hands that have active motion in all five fingers. This advancement permits many prosthetic hand tasks that were previously impossible to be executed with ease. Generally speaking, the maximum grip force of a multidexterous or compliant hand is somewhat lower than the noncompliant hand. The reduced grip force is offset by the additional surface area and contour of multiple fingers around an object (see Figure 30-16).

TDs (hands and design tools) with wrist flexion potential can provide the patient with advantageous approaches for improved grasp. Wrist flexion also assists, in a small way, in restoring the visual field when using electromechanical hands.

Electric Elbow Components

A number of externally powered elbow components are commercially available, but many require that the prosthetist be specially trained in their implementation and usage.[53,54] Each of the commercially available electromechanical elbows uses proprietary signal processing and drive mechanisms to achieve design-specific functional attributes. In selecting an externally powered elbow unit, the prosthetist considers the specific functional needs of individual patients. The type of inputs necessary to control the elbow mechanism, the location of myoelectrodes, and the number of inputs necessary to control both the elbow and TD must be weighed in the decision on what elbow mechanism is most appropriate. Most commercially available elbow systems incorporate microprocessors that are compatible with a large array of input devices and can be programmed to use wrists and TDs from a large selection of manufacturers. Most prosthetists are no longer constrained to develop prosthetic recommendations from a single manufacturer product line; in fact, doing so often limits possibilities and therefore functional outcome.

Dual-Control Strategies

Microprocessor control has assisted control strategies that can be better customized to individual patient needs.[47] The traditional control strategy for an individual using an externally powered transhumeral prosthesis might include one myoelectrode to capture EMG signals of the residual biceps and a second myoelectrode over the residual triceps. Assuming both signals are of satisfactory amplitude and differentiation, successful myoelectric control of two devices—an electrically powered elbow and an electrically powered TD—can be successfully achieved. To grasp an object, the patient purposefully contracts the biceps; an EMG signal from the biceps is programmed to promote elbow flexion. This physiologically correct application uses the biceps in a fashion similar to preamputation status. A signal is provided continuously until the forearm and elbow reach the desired position in space. The mechanism can be locked in this position by holding the elbow steady (no longer flexing or extending) through a predetermined (see Figure 30-16) and programmed time interval. The system then cycles to TD (hand) control, using the same to EMG inputs. The most commonly employed combination is contraction of the triceps to open the hand or extend the elbow and contraction of the biceps to close the hand or flex the elbow.

Sequential and Simultaneous Control Strategies

Myoelectric control of prosthetic pronation and supination can be added using an electric wrist rotator.[9] Under the constraints of a two-electrode system, the rotator is frequently controlled using a momentary contact switch mounted on the medial side of the humeral section, where it can be easily bumped against the body. In this configuration, three inputs, two EMG and one switch, control forearm position in space, pronation, and grasp and release. This type of control strategy is often referred to as sequential because one task must be completed before the next is executed (see Figure 30-16).

Recent developments in microcircuitry and microprocessors have made simultaneous control of more than one device possible. For simultaneous control, the same two myoelectrode EMG signals at the biceps and triceps are used. A wrist rotator and TD are also installed, but the momentary contact switch that previously controlled wrist position is removed. Instead, control of pronation and supination is triggered to the EMG inputs. Patients use their biceps to close the TD and pronate the prosthetic forearm and use the triceps to open the TD and supinate the prosthetic forearm. Mode selection, via cocontraction of the biceps and triceps, determines whether opening and closing of the TD or pronation and supination of the forearm will be triggered by subsequent EMG signal. Many individuals with upper-extremity amputations can master mode selection using this control strategy.

Simultaneous control of the elbow and TD can now be accomplished by adding a proportional input to the system. Great success can be achieved by inserting a linear potentiometer or strain gauge into the harnessing of the transhumeral prosthesis. As the wearer generates excursion in either humeral flexion or scapular protraction, the input device translates this movement or force into a usable signal to control position in space of the elbow mechanism. This makes both nonsequential and simultaneous control of the TD and elbow possible. This is advantageous as a patient can approach an object by bringing the forearm into the appropriate position while concurrently opening the hand in preparation for grasp.

The combination of greater TD speeds and long battery life enables myoelectrically controlled upper-extremity prosthetic wearers to control multiple devices through ever-increasing functional planes. They can do so over time durations compatible with most everyday needs. The number of combinations of myoelectrodes and control strategies becomes limitless as more manufacturers develop modular componentry that is compatible with most commercially available systems.

HYBRID PROSTHESES

For some individuals, the integration of technology from both the conventional and externally powered systems provides the greatest potential for functional outcome. Prosthetic systems

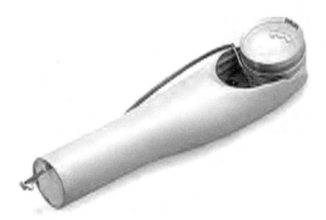

FIGURE 30-17 This externally powered elbow and terminal device configuration includes a myoelectrically controlled elbow and a cable for body-powered operation of the terminal device.

can be configured to use an electrically powered elbow with a body-powered mechanical TD (Figure 30-17) or an electrically powered TD with a nonpowered elbow. Compelling arguments can be made for both control strategies; the ultimate decision for componentry and control systems must be based on a patient's ability to use proprioceptive feedback from the cable system, as well as available inputs for the electromechanical system. Consideration should also be given to the motivating factors to use a hybrid. Frequently, hybridized systems are sought because insufficient range or strength is available to provide complete functional control at the elbow joint and TD with conventional systems. This may be the result of a frozen shoulder, an unstable joint that is vulnerable to frequent subluxation, or shoulder disarticulation (Figure 30-18). If the musculature in the residual limb can generate satisfactory EMG signals despite the more proximal shoulder involvement, then myoelectric control of the TD can be achieved despite impairments limiting the strong volitional movements at the shoulder necessary to control a conventional system. Placement of the forearm in space can then be assisted using a large variety of spring-assisted or forearm-balancing mechanical devices. These technologies allow patients with varying degrees of functional capacity to be fitted successfully with components from two different arenas.

Activity-Specific Prostheses

Most of this chapter's discussions have revolved around functions that relate to activities of daily living and vocational pursuits. Most individuals with upper-extremity amputations want to be involved in various pursuits beyond activities of daily living and vocational activities, just as they were before their amputations. A number of unique prosthetic applications, as well as adaptations and assistive tools for an existing prosthesis, can effectively address the recreational and avocational desires of individual patients.[55] Although conventional wisdom suggests that these pursuits not proceed until complete maximal rehabilitation has occurred with the primary prosthetic device, this is not always the case; being

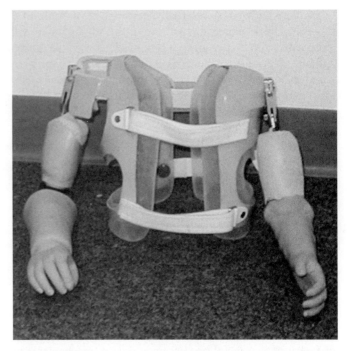

FIGURE 30-18 Example of a hybrid prosthesis designed for an individual with bilateral shoulder disarticulation as a result of congenital deficiency. Suspension is provided by a thermoplastic "jacket." A conventional shoulder joint is used on the right, while a myoelectric system incorporated on the left controls elbow motion, forearm rotation, and operation of the terminal device operation on the left.

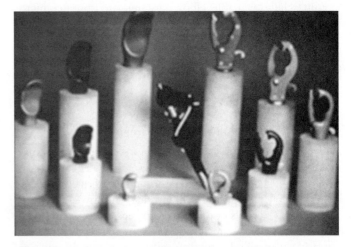

FIGURE 30-19 Examples of terminal devices that might be used for vocational and leisure activities. Passive terminal devices *(left)* are often chosen for young children or for individuals involved in sports that require ball handling. Voluntary closing terminal devices *(right)* allow graded prehension for various skilled activities. (Courtesy TRS.)

able to return to an important avocational activity might be a major motivating factor in rehabilitation. However, few patients have the financial resources for specialized prostheses for vocational and avocational activities. Most prosthetists make every attempt to implement activity-specific devices within the primary prosthetic design. Because the array of activities in which persons participate is limitless, so too is the creation of specific tools and adaptations to accommodate these needs. Quick-disconnect wrists allow for a myriad of options in place of the existing TD. Commercial application of TDs can include nearly any imaginable adaptation for sport and recreational pursuits (Figures 30-19 and 30-20). Specific challenges such as exposure to the elements, vibration, and impact may require more significant modification to ensure acceptable durability to the device.

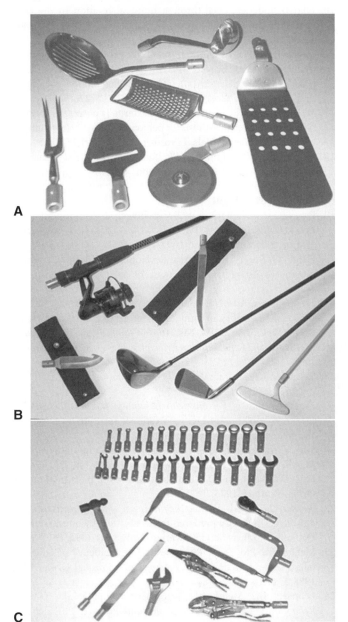

FIGURE 30-20 Examples of activity- or function-specific terminal devices that can be used in a prosthesis with "quick disconnect" attachment for the terminal device. **A,** A variety of kitchen utensils and cooking tools. **B,** Devices for leisure and sport activities such as fishing and golf. **C,** Carpentry and mechanical tools such as hammers, files, pliers, wrenches, ratchets, and saws. The prosthetic wearer disconnects the conventional terminal device or prosthetic hand and attaches the tool temporarily while involved in a given activity. (Courtesy of Texas Assistive Devices, Brazoria, TX.)

An Individual with Traumatic Transhumeral Amputation

E. S., 29, has been employed since high school in maintenance and mechanics and is responsible for cleaning and repairing the presses during the night shift at a paper manufacturing plant. Six months ago, while cleaning a press that had been improperly shut down, the sleeve of his sweatshirt became entangled in a press. His right arm was drawn into the press almost to the level of the axilla before his coworker could activate the safety stop mechanism. The crush and degloving injuries were so severe that the only option was amputation at a short transfemoral level. In addition, steady traction on his arm while being drawn into the press damaged his brachial plexus, and E. S. has significant weakness in residual muscles controlling his shoulder. His residual arm measures 14 cm from acromion to distal end. ROM is limited by 50% in shoulder flexion, extension, and abduction. For 4 months, he has been wearing a body-powered dual-cable control prosthesis suspended with a figure-of-eight harness, including a locking elbow and voluntary opening hook, but is not satisfied with the functional level this prosthesis allows him. He has developed signs of axillary compression (sensory impairment) in his intact left upper extremity. He is referred for evaluation for a myoelectrically controlled prosthesis.

Since the accident, E. S. has been living with his sister and her family, but he is eager to return to his own home, a cabin on a lake several hours from the rehabilitation and prosthetic center where he has been receiving care. He is seriously considering returning to college to study electrical engineering or material sciences, with the goal of becoming a prosthetist.

Questions to Consider

- Given the condition and function of his residual limb, what type of socket and interface might the team recommend for E. S. from among available options? Why would these be the optimal choices? What factors are likely to influence clinical decision making in this case?
- Given his brachial plexus injury and contralateral axillary compression, what type of suspension and control system might the team recommend for the patient E. S. from among available options? Why would these be the optimal choices? How would the team determine if a myoelectrically controlled prosthesis would be possible? Should other options for external power also be considered?
- What type of prosthetic elbow, wrist unit, and terminal device (or hand) and wrist unit might the team recommend for E. S.? Why would these be the optimal choices? What are the benefits and drawbacks of each unit?
- How would you apply the ICF framework to E.S.?

Continued

Recommendations

E. S. has not been able to fully use his initial prosthesis effectively because of inadequate cable excursion as a consequence of limitations in ROM and strength. His effort to maximize cable excursion has resulted in compression injury of his remaining arm, compromising function of his left hand. The team determines that there is sufficient myoelectric signal to operate a power elbow, forearm rotator, and TD or hand. They recommend his harness suspension system be replaced with a custom-fit shoulder saddle to avoid further compression in the left axilla. The prosthesis will have a flexible socket with rigid frame; electrodes will be incorporated into the walls of the socket. A linear potentiometer will be used to provide full ROM of the prosthetic elbow, with simultaneous myoelectric control of the TD.

SUMMARY

Prosthetic rehabilitation of persons with upper-extremity amputations is both challenging and rewarding. Success is often difficult to measure purely in clinical terms; however, maximizing individual functional potential and providing the appropriate amount of technology to assure acceptable outcomes are highly predictive of success. In addition to understanding the patient's needs, consideration of the needs and expectations of spouses, children, and extended family is also important. Once the patient's requirements are completely understood, careful and thoughtful rehabilitation plans can be developed. An effective prosthetic prescription will detail (a) the power source and control system (conventional or externally powered) that will operate prosthetic components, (b) the elbow design (for transhumeral or higher amputations), (c) the socket type and interface medium, (d) the appropriate TD (hook, hand, or specialized tools), and (e) the alignment of components. Each of these five categories can be subdivided into additional criteria-based items, the number of divisions based upon the complexity of the case and the clinical resources that are available. Following these guidelines will eliminate unnecessary difficulties and challenges during the design process.

REFERENCES

1. Baumgartner RF. Upper extremity amputation and prosthetics. *J Rehabil Res Dev.* 2001;38(4):vii–x.
2. Childress DS. Historical aspects of powered-limb prostheses. *Clin Prosthet Orthot.* 1985;9(1):2–13.
3. Millstein SG, Heger H, Hunter GA. Prosthetic use in adult upper limb amputees. *Prosthet Orthot Int.* 1986;10(1):27–34.
4. Durance J, O'Shea P. Upper limb amputees: a clinical profile. *Int Disabil Stud.* 1988;10(2):68–72.
5. Sherman RA. Utilization of prostheses among US veterans with traumatic amputation: a pilot survey. *J Rehabil Res Dev.* 1999;36(2):100–108.
6. Atkins DJ, Heard DC, Donovan WH. Epidemiologic overview of individuals with upper limb loss and their reported research priorities. *J Prosthet Orthot.* 1996;8(2):2–11.
7. Vacek KM. Transition to a switch activated 3-S transhumeral prosthesis: a team approach. *J Prosthet Orthot.* 1998;10(3):56–60.
8. Daly W. Clinical application of roll-on sleeves for myoelectrically controlled transradial and transhumeral prostheses. *J Prosthet Orthot.* 2000;12(3):88–91.
9. Sears HH, Shaperman J. Electric wrist rotation in proportional control systems. *J Prosthet Orthot.* 1998;10(4):92–98.
10. Ivko JJ. Independence through humeral rotation in the conventional transhumeral prosthetic design. *J Prosthet Orthot.* 1999;11(1):20–22.
11. Michael JW. Partial hand amputations: prosthetic and orthotic management. In: Bowker JH, Michael JW, eds. *Atlas of Limb Prosthetics: Surgical, Prosthetic, and Rehabilitation Principles.* 2nd ed. St. Louis: Mosby-Year Book; 1992:217–226.
12. Weir RF, Grahn EC, Duff SJ. A new externally powered myoelectrically controlled prosthesis for persons with partial hand amputations at the metacarpals. *J Prosthet Orthot.* 2001;13(2):26–33.
13. Burkhalter WE, Hampton FL, Smeitzer JA. Wrist disarticulation and below elbow amputation. In: American Academy of Orthopedic Surgeons. *Atlas of Limb Prosthetics.* St. Louis: Mosby; 1981:183–191.
14. Fryer CM, Michael JW. Body powered components. In: Bowker JH, Michael JW, eds. *Atlas of Limb Prosthetics.* 2nd ed. St. Louis: Mosby; 1992.
15. Fliegel O, Feuer SF. Historical development of lower extremity prostheses. *Arch Phys Med Rehabil.* 1966;47(5):275–285.
16. Magee R. Amputation through the ages: the oldest major surgical operation. *Aust N Z J Surg.* 1998;69(9):675–678.
17. Wilson AB. History of amputation surgery and prosthetics. In: Bowker JH, Michael JW, eds. *Atlas of Limb Prosthetics: Surgical, Prosthetic, and Rehabilitation Principles.* 2nd ed. St. Louis: Mosby; 1992:3–13.
18. Robinson KP. Historical aspects of amputation. *Ann R Coll Surg Engl.* 1991;73(3):134–136.
19. *Digest of Data of Persons with Disability; Mathematical Policy Research.* Washington DC: US National Institute on Disability and Rehabilitation Research; January 1992.
20. Torres MM. Incidence and causes of limb amputations. *Phys Med Rehabil: State Art Rev.* 1994;8:1–8.
21. Kay HW, Newman JD. Relative incidences of new amputation. *Orthot Prosthet.* 1975;29(2):3–16.
22. Nielsen CC. *Issues affecting the future demands for orthotists and prosthetists.* A study prepared for the National Commission on Orthotic and Prosthetic Education, November 1996.
23. McDonnell PM, Scott RN, McKay LA. Incidence of congenital upper limb deficiencies. *J Assoc Child Prosthet Orthot Clin.* 1988;23:8–14.
24. Leonard JA, Meier RH. Prosthetics. In: DeLisa JA, ed. *Rehabilitation Medicine: Principles and Practice.* Philadelphia: Lippincott; 1993:330–345.
25. Malone JM, Flemming LL, Robertson J, et al. Immediate, early, and late postsurgical management of upper-limb amputation. *J Rehabil Res Dev.* 1984;21(1):33–41.
26. Manella KJ. Comparing effectiveness of elastic bandages and shrinker socks for lower extremity amputees. *Phys Ther.* 1981;61(3):334–337.
27. Halburt J, Crotty M, Cameron ID. Evidence for the optimal management of acute and chronic phantom pain: a systematic review. *Clin J Pain.* 2002;18(2):84–92.

28. Hunter GA. Amputation surgery of the arm in adults. In: Murdock G, Wilson AB, eds. *Amputation: Surgical Practice and Patient Management*. Oxford, UK: Butterworth-Heinemann; 1996:305–312.

29. Robinson KP. The problem amputation stump. In: Murdock G, Wilson AB, eds. *Amputation: Surgical Practice and Patient Management*. Oxford, UK: Butterworth-Heinemann; 1996:285–299.

30. Pucher I, Kickinger W, Frischenschlager O. Coping with amputation and phantom limb pain. *J Psychosom Res*. 1999;46(4):379–383.

31. Dykes WG. Biomechanics and prosthetics. In: Murdock G, Wilson AB, eds. *Amputation: Surgical Practice and Patient Management*. Oxford, UK: Butterworth-Heinemann; 1996: 334–341.

32. Michael JW. Prosthetic considerations during the growth period. In: Murdock G, Wilson AB, eds. *Amputation: Surgical Practice and Patient Management*. Oxford, UK: Butterworth-Heinemann; 1996:232–240.

33. Thornby MA, Krebs DE. Bimanual skill development in pediatric below-elbow amputation, a multicenter cross sectional study. *Arch Phys Med Rehabil*. 1992;73(8):697–702.

34. Brenner CD. Prosthetic principles: wrist disarticulation and transradial amputation. In: Bowker JH, Michael JW, eds. *Atlas of Limb Prosthetics: Surgical, Prosthetic, and Rehabilitation Principles*. 2nd ed. St. Louis: Mosby-Year Book; 1992:241–251.

35. Miguelez JM. *Management of the bilateral upper limb deficient individual*. Retrieved 2001. http://www.oandp.org.

36. Smith DJ, Michael JW, Bowker JH, eds. *Atlas of Amputation and Limb Deficiencies*. Rosemont, IL: American Academy of Orthopaedic Surgeons; 2004.

37. Carlson LB, Veatch BD, Frey DD. Technical forum: efficiency of prosthetic cable and housing. *J Prosthet Orthot*. 1995;7(3):96–99.

38. Sammons F. The use of low-friction housing liner in upper extremity prostheses. *Bull Prosthet Res*. 1983;10(4):77–81.

39. Exparza W, Ivko JJ. Technical note: friction free cable system; alternative cable system for transhumeral level conventional prosthesis. *J Prosthet Orthot*. 1997;9(3):135–136.

40. Billock JN. Upper limb terminal devices: hand versus hooks. *Clin Prosthet Orthot*. 19(2):57–65.

41. Frey DD, Carlson LE, Ramaswamy V. Voluntary opening prehensors with adjustable grip force. *J Prosthet Orthot*. 1995;7(4):124–130.

42. Radocy B. Voluntary closing control: a successful new design approach to an old concept. *Clin Prosthet Orthot*. 1986;10(2): 82–86.

43. DeVisser H, Herder JL. Force-directed design of a voluntary closing hand prosthesis. *J Rehabil Res Dev*. 2000;37(3):261–271.

44. Heger H, Millstein S, Hunter GA. Electrically powered prostheses for the adult with an acquired upper limb amputation. *J Bone Joint Surg*. 1985;67B:278–281.

45. Miguelez JM. Critical factors in electrically powered upper extremity prosthetics. *J Prosthet Orthot*. 2002;14(1):36–38.

46. Sears HH. Approaches to prescription of body powered and myoelectric prostheses. *Phys Med Rehabil Clin N Am*. 1991;2(2): 1047–1051.

47. Speigel SR. Adult myoelectric upper limb prosthetic training. In: Atkins DJ, Meier RH, eds. *Comprehensive Management of the Upper Limb Amputee*. New York: Springer-Verlag; 1989.

48. Berbrayer D, Farraday WT. Switch-activated electrically controlled prosthesis following a closed head injury: a case study. *J Prosthet Orthot*. 1994;6(2):48–51.

49. Upper limb electronic technology moves forward. *O&P Bus News*, December 20-23, 1999.

50. Eledstein JE, Berger N. Performance comparison among children fitted with myoelectric and body powered hands. *Arch Phys Med Rehabil*. 1993;74(4):376–380.

51. Stein RB, Walley M. Functional comparison of upper extremity amputees using myoelectric and conventional prostheses. *Arch Phys Med Rehabil*. 1983;64(6):243–248.

52. Heckathorne C. Components for adult externally powered systems. In: Bowker JH, Michael JW, eds. *Atlas of Limb Prosthetics*. 2nd ed. St. Louis: Mosby-Year Book; 1992:151–174.

53. Sears HH, Andrews JT, Jacobsen SC. Experience with the Utah arm, hand and terminal device. In: Atkins DK, ed. *Comprehensive Management of the Upper Limb Amputee*. New York: Springer Verlag; 1989:194–210.

54. Williams TW. Use of Boston elbow for high level amputees. In: Atkins DK, ed. *Comprehensive Management of the Upper Limb Amputee*. New York: Springer Verlag; 1989:211–226.

55. Rubin G. Devices enable persons with amputation to participate in sports. *Arch Phys Med Rehabil*. 1983;64(1):37–40.

31

Rehabilitation for Persons with Upper-Extremity Amputation

MARGARET WISE

LEARNING OBJECTIVES

On completion of this chapter, the reader will be able to do the following:

1. Compare the roles and goals of rehabilitation in adult patients with new upper-extremity amputation in the acute, preprosthetic, initial prosthetic training, and advanced skill phases of rehabilitation.
2. Identify the key components of examination and evaluation for patients with new upper-extremity amputation in each of the phases of rehabilitation.
3. Discuss factors, including those in the psychosocial and affective domains, that influence the prognosis for successful prosthetic training for patients with upper-extremity amputation.
4. Suggest an appropriate plan of care for patients with new amputation in each of the phases of rehabilitation, including wound and skin care, pain and edema management, and strategies to enhance range of motion and strength.
5. Discuss the pros and cons of the six prosthetic options the team and family consider in prosthetic planning.
6. Identify therapeutic activities and interventions to facilitate functional independence in activities of daily living.
7. Explain the process of selection of electrode placement and functional training for patients with electrically controlled upper extremity prostheses.

"Hands can do all kinds of things…change a tire, bake a pie, fly a kite or catch a fly, plant a seed and help it grow, point the way for feet to go….Rough hands, smooth hands, plump hands, thin hands like wrinkled apple skin. Hands can do most anything…wear a ring, wear a glove, most important… hands can love!"[1]

EDITH BAER

REHABILITATION AFTER UPPER-EXTREMITY AMPUTATION

Human hands are wonderfully complex sensory and motor organs, capable of interpreting and interacting with the environment. The fine manipulative skills and intricate grasp patterns of the hand cannot be duplicated. When a hand is lost, the ability to perform normal daily tasks is greatly changed.

Although a prosthesis cannot duplicate hand function, it can help substitute for basic grasp in the performance of normal daily activities and help maintain bilateral hand function.

This chapter discusses the treatment of adults with amputations, including aspects of acute care, preprosthetic care, basic prosthetic training, and advanced functional skills training. Working with patients with upper limb amputation can be quite rewarding for therapists, who must draw on manual and orthopedic skills, functional skills for training in activities of daily living, and counseling skills to respond to psychosocial needs.

INCIDENCE AND CAUSES OF UPPER-EXTREMITY AMPUTATION

The primary cause of upper-limb amputations is trauma; most commonly crush injuries, electrical burns that occur at work, or, in times of war, traumatic injuries sustained in combat. Congenital anomalies, infections, and tumors are other causes of amputation. Because upper-extremity amputations are typically occupation related, they primarily occur in young adults between the ages of 20 and 40 years; the ratio of men to women is 4:1. Dillingham[2] reports approximately 18,500 new upper-extremity amputations per year. Just fewer than 2000 of these are at wrist level or higher. The ratio of upper-extremity amputations to lower-extremity amputations is 1:9.[2,3]

CLASSIFICATION AND FUNCTIONAL IMPLICATIONS

The remaining part of the amputated limb is referred to as the residual limb. The broad categories used to describe levels of upper-extremity amputation include transphalangeal, metacarpal–phalangeal, transcarpal, wrist disarticulation (styloid), transradial, elbow disarticulation, transhumeral, humeral neck, shoulder disarticulation, and intrascapulothoracic (Figure 31-1).[2-5]

Functionally speaking, the more proximal the level of amputation, the greater the loss of range of motion (ROM) and strength that results. Of particular importance are the loss of supination and pronation in amputations approaching the mid-forearm and the loss of shoulder rotation as the amputation approaches the axillary fold. Although a longer

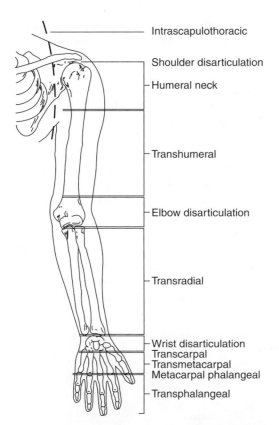

Intrascapulothoracic
Shoulder disarticulation
Humeral neck

Transhumeral

Elbow disarticulation

Transradial

Wrist disarticulation
Transcarpal
Transmetacarpal
Metacarpal phalangeal
Transphalangeal

FIGURE 31-1 The upper-extremity residual limb is described by the bony limb segment at which amputation occurred. (Modified, with permission, from Kottke F, Lehman JF [eds], *Krusen's Handbook of Physical Medicine and Rehabilitation*, 4th ed. Philadelphia: Saunders, 1990. p. 1011.)

residual limb provides better mechanical advantage for prosthetic use, limb length does not always correspond to better prosthetic function. The length of the residual limb in an elbow disarticulation or long transhumeral length amputation, for example, limits the space available for an electric elbow unit and affects both cosmesis and function of the prosthesis.

STAGES OF REHABILITATION

The rehabilitation of individuals with upper-extremity amputation can be divided into four phases: acute care, preprosthetic rehabilitation, basic prosthetic training, and advanced functional skills training. Although certain goals and activities are unique to each phase, the ultimate goal is to enhance function so that patients with upper-extremity amputation can return to the activities most important to them.

Acute Care

Often the most pressing issue in the first days to weeks after traumatic upper-extremity amputation is saving the patient's life. The patient may return to the operating room several times for surgeons to clean the wound or perform revision surgery. The patient usually has intravenous lines for antibiotics and pain medications; special infection control

procedures may also be in place. The patient may not be fully alert or even have full recollection of what took place the first weeks after injury.

The initial goals of therapy may be quite basic and must be modified to be appropriate to the patient's medical status. Goals of the acute phase of rehabilitation include the following:

- To perform a screening evaluation to identify immediate priorities and help predict eventual outcome.
- To develop rapport with the family and patient.
- To control pain effectively.
- To promote wound healing.
- To establish a strategy for effective edema control.
- To preserve as much passive ROM of the residual limb as possible.

Screening Evaluation

Even though the patient may not be able to participate fully during an evaluation, the therapist can begin to gather information to guide the early rehabilitation process. Important facts to discern are the patient's medical status, presence of associated injuries, wound status, ROM, and whether a myodesis (when remnants of major muscles are surgically attached to the bone) or myoplasty (when muscle remnants of the antagonist muscles are sutured to each other) was performed on major antagonist muscle groups during surgery. This basic information helps the therapist develop an intervention plan for early care to facilitate further rehabilitation as the patient's medical status improves.

Rapport

During the acute care stage, when the patient's condition is likely to be quite serious, the family suddenly faces many difficult issues and often experiences emotional crisis. Establishing rapport with and providing necessary support to the family are key elements of the acute care stage. Family members may be struggling with questions such as, "How did this happen?" "Why did it happen?" and "What can the future hold?" The family may be overwhelmed by all the medical procedures being performed on their loved one. The therapist should take time to talk with the family, hear their concerns, and explain the goals for the current stage of rehabilitation as well as the long-range prognosis. During this period of crisis, neither the family nor the patient is ready to hear details about all types of prostheses available, but rather may be comforted to know that general prosthetic plans are being made and that the clinical team is working to help achieve a positive outcome that includes a bright future. Rapport with patients can be developed as they become more alert.

Pain Control

During this early phase, pain is primarily controlled by intravenous medication. Strong pain medication may influence the patient's affect and attitude; the apparent anger and unwillingness to cooperate shown by patients with traumatic amputation may be associated with the pain medication being used. Effective edema control also contributes to pain management. During these first few days, when many professionals are treating the patient day and night, sleep is often interrupted. Coordination of schedules with nursing helps maintain rest periods, which in turn may have a positive effect on pain management.

Wound Healing

Early wound healing and edema control go hand in hand. Wound care protocols may vary depending on physician preference but generally include keeping the wound clean and dry. If a skin graft has been used to close the wound, the limb must be positioned to prevent tension over the suture lines (Figure 31-2). Initial bandage changes may be quite painful for the patient. During the acute period, some physicians prescribe pain medications before bandage changes. Unless contraindicated, a nonadherent dressing such as Xeroform (Kendall, Mansfield, MA) or Adaptic (Johnson & Johnson, New Brunswick, NJ) can be used directly over the wound and then covered with sterile bandages. Soaking adherent areas with saline can ease removal of the dressing.

Edema Control

Effective edema control helps reduce the chance of adhesion formation along the healing suture line, aids in wound healing, and management of pain. Edema may initially be controlled by bulky bandages and elevation. When the patient is able to tolerate pressure, elastic bandages may be applied in a figure-of-eight style, with gentle compressive pressure over the distal end that gradually tapers proximally. Ideally, the bandage should continue up and over one joint proximal to the amputation (e.g., above the elbow in transradial amputation) (Figures 31-3 and 31-4). Elastic wraps must be frequently checked for proper placement and compression; close communication with nurses involved in the patient's care can facilitate this. As wounds heal and are able to tolerate greater compression, elastic wraps are replaced with a "shrinker" or a roll-on liner.

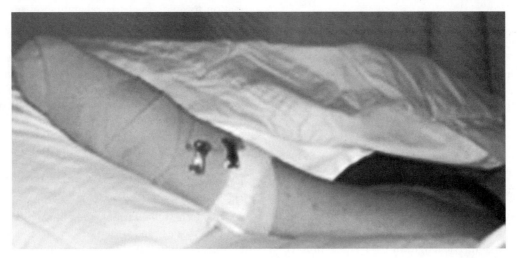

FIGURE 31-2 In the days after amputation surgery, the transradial residual limb is wrapped in a compressive dressing and a slightly elevated position is maintained to manage edema and control pain. Note the fully extended elbow.

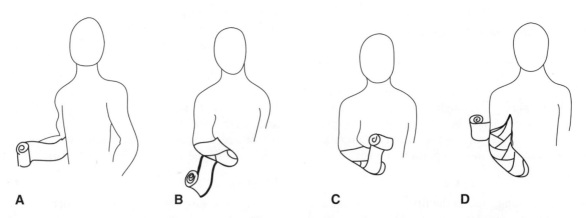

FIGURE 31-3 A, To apply a compressive wrap to a transradial residual limb, the patient anchors the elastic bandage between the elbow and trunk and wraps it around the distal end of the limb. Next, a series of overlapping figure-of-eight layers of the wrap (**B** and **C**) are applied, creating a distal-toward-proximal pressure gradient. The wrap should continue proximally for several inches above the elbow joint (**D**).

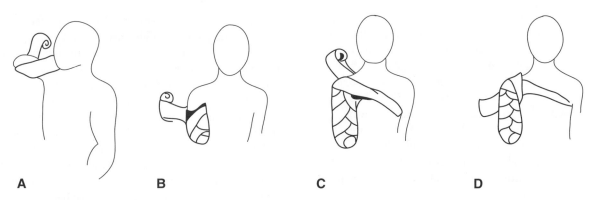

FIGURE 31-4 A, To apply a compressive wrap to a transhumeral residual limb, the patient anchors the elastic bandage between the chin and clavicle and wraps it over and behind the distal end of the residual limb. **B,** Once the initial figure-of-eight layer is applied to anchor the end of the bandage, the patient continues to apply overlapping layers, creating a distal-toward-proximal pressure gradient. The wrap continues up and over the shoulder (**C**), over the anterior chest wall under the contralateral axilla, and then around the back, over the residual shoulder and under the axilla, before being secured in place (**D**).

Range of Motion

After injury, patients tend to hold their residual limb in a position of comfort; the arm typically adducted toward the body, the forearm supinated and elbow flexed. Soft-tissue contractures begin to develop if the limb is consistently held in this position. In patients with transhumeral amputation, limitations of shoulder flexion, abduction, and external rotation are likely to occur. For those with transradial amputation, limitations in elbow extension and pronation are also likely to develop.

Early passive ROM exercise to gently elongate tissues of joints most at risk of contracture formation is essential and can be carefully performed even when intravenous lines are in place. Passive stretching should be performed slowly and gently, just to the point where the therapist begins to feel tension on the muscle or the patient begins to feel pain. Generally, with acute injuries, performing passive ROM twice daily is sufficient to increase motion. If, however, progress is not being made within 2 weeks, the therapist should consider static splinting as an adjunct to passive ROM.

CASE EXAMPLE 1

A Patient with Bilateral Traumatic Amputation of the Forearm

T. M. is a 17-year-old high school soccer player who underwent traumatic amputation of his right and left forearms when the sleeves of his winter jacket became caught in the blades of a running snow blower that had jammed, then suddenly released, as he was trying to clear the mechanism. T. M. was home alone when the accident occurred and had significant blood loss before he was able to reach a neighbor's home for assistance. At the local hospital, tourniquets were placed to control blood loss, wounds were flushed and cleaned, intravenous fluids with antibiotics and packed red blood cells were begun, and morphine was administered. T. M. was prepared for emergency transfer to the nearest trauma center.

On arrival at the trauma center, he was immediately taken to surgery for debridement and closure of his wounds. His parents arrived at the trauma center while he was in surgery. The right transradial residual limb has 3 inches of radius and ulna preserved and required a split-thickness skin graft to close (the donor site was the anterior right thigh). The left transradial residual limb had 7 inches of radius and ulna preserved and was closed without skin graft.

Two days have passed since T. M.'s surgery, and he is recovering in the surgical intensive care unit. His white blood cell count and temperature are moderately elevated. His residual limbs are in bulky dressings with elastic compressive wraps, with significant serosanguineous drainage noted at dressing changes. A morphine pump is being used for pain management. T. M. is currently receiving supplemental oxygen by nasal cannula and is sleeping fitfully. On questioning, he is semialert, oriented to family members and place, but not to others or time.

Questions to Consider

- What tests and measures are most appropriate to include in the screening evaluation at this point in the acute phase of T. M.'s care? What is the evidence of reliability and validity of these screening instruments? How will the information collected guide the development of a plan of care for this young man?
- What immediate concerns will T. M.'s parents likely express? In what ways can the team help establish an effective relationship with T. M. and his parents in these early days of care? What information is most important to help the family cope with this crisis situation and prepare for the days ahead? How will the rehabilitation team assess the family's understanding of the situation and need for emotional support?

Continued

- What specific intervention strategies should the rehabilitation team use to address issues of pain control, limb volume and edema, and wound healing in the next 2 to 5 days? How should patient and family education be best integrated with these strategies? How should the team assess whether these strategies are effective?
- What specific ROM is most important to target for this young man with a short transradial residual limb on the right and a long transradial residual limb on the left, anticipating the need for bilateral prostheses in his future? Which upper-extremity joints are most at risk of contracture formation and why? What specific intervention strategies should the therapists initiate to preserve as much functional ROM as possible? How might pain, medications, and level of consciousness influence the potential development of soft tissue contractures?
- What postsurgical complications is the team most likely to be concerned about? What are the warning signs of these complications? What members of the team are responsible for monitoring the development of these complications?
- What influence will immobility and pain have on T. M.'s ability to learn, endurance and physiological function, and emotional status during this early phase of rehabilitation?

Preprosthetic Rehabilitation

In many facilities, only when wound closure has occurred are patients with new upper-extremity amputation referred for rehabilitation care. During the preprosthetic therapy phase, the patient's medical condition is often stable enough to begin an active role in care. Education of referral sources about goals of the preprosthetic phase can result in early referrals.

Goals for preprosthetic rehabilitation include the following:

- Establish good rapport and trust with the patient and family.
- Complete a comprehensive evaluation to guide the team in determining an appropriate prosthetic plan.
- Shape and control volume of the residual limb effectively.
- Minimize adhesive scar tissue.
- Desensitize the limb in preparation for prosthetic wear.
- Achieve full ROM in remaining joints of the residual limb.
- Strengthen the muscles of the residual limb to maximize potential for effective prosthetic use.
- Provide appropriate intervention for rehabilitation of associated injuries.
- Help the patient develop some independence in performing basic activities of daily living.

Rapport

In the acute phase of care, when the patient is quite ill, rapport is primarily established with family members. These relationships can help facilitate trust between the therapist and the patient during the early preprosthetic period. Upper-extremity amputation is a major traumatic event that affects the family as well as the patient. As all those involved grapple with the changes and challenges they are facing, the rehabilitation team encourages them to express their hopes, concerns, and fears.

Psychological counseling is considered an integral part of the early rehabilitation program and should be made available for the family and the patient.[6] Some patients may benefit from talking to individuals with amputations of a similar level. Speaking with peer counselors can be helpful; however, rehabilitation professions should screen potential peer counselors carefully. Some individuals who sustained amputations in previous years might not have had a good rehabilitation experience or have not had the benefit of more recent prosthetic design and components. A professional should be sure that peer counselors are offering objective and current information.

Comprehensive Evaluation

Before prosthetic options are discussed, a comprehensive examination and evaluation is required. In specialized centers a multidisciplinary team that includes the physical and occupational therapists, a prosthetist, the surgeon or physician, and a psychologist or counselor completes the examination and evaluation. In other facilities the therapists and prosthetists are responsible for completing a comprehensive assessment.

The preprosthetic comprehensive examination begins with a good history and the gathering of preliminary or background data, including the following:

- The cause and date of amputation
- Any associated injuries that might influence the rehabilitation process
- Hand dominance
- All medications the patient is currently taking

The examination continues with an assessment of the psychosocial environment as a resource for rehabilitation and eventual discharge. The therapist assesses the following patient characteristics:

- The availability of family and other support systems
- Living situation
- Level of education
- Prior occupation and leisure interests

The therapist then considers the condition of the residual limb, documenting the following:

- The presence and description of any phantom limb sensation
- The presence and description of any pain the patient is experiencing
- The length of the residual limb
- The presence of edema, measured by limb circumference
- Skin condition and the presence of scar tissue or soft tissue adhesion
- Detailed ROM of the residual limb to identify any contractures that may have developed during the acute care phase
- Evaluation of upper extremity strength
- Evaluation of possible sites for placement of electrodes for myoelectric control

The comprehensive examination concludes with a consideration of mobility and functional status, including the following assessments:

- Posture and skeletal alignment as a result of the missing limb
- Pertinent limitations of the lower extremity
- Postural control (static, anticipatory, and reactionary balance)
- Current and potential abilities to perform activities of special interest to the individual, e.g., self-care, work, leisure activities

If the patient previously used a prosthesis, a prosthetic history also includes the type of prosthesis used, how long the prosthesis was worn each day, and how the prosthesis was used in instrumental and other activities of daily living. The team should determine the patient's opinions regarding the positive and negative aspects of a previous prosthesis as well as any different or additional functions that the patient wants to achieve.

Edema Control and Limb Shaping

As the patient's medical status improves, bulky bandages are removed and the patient becomes more mobile. The patient must continue to use some type of compression on the limb nearly 24 hours a day, removing it only for wound care and bathing. At this point, elasticized shrinker socks or a roll-on liner may replace the elastic figure-of-eight bandages because they are more convenient and provide more consistent compression (Figure 31-5). For those with transradial residual limbs, the shrinker should extend at least 2 inches above the

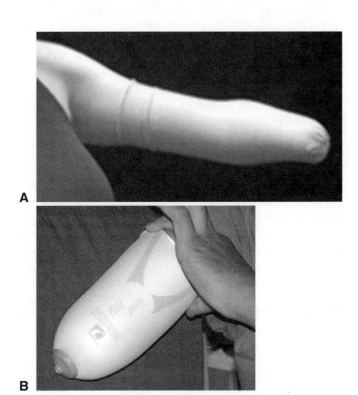

FIGURE 31-5 An appropriately applied commercially available transradial (**A**) and transhumeral (**B**) elasticized shrinker garment.

elbow. For those with transhumeral residual limbs, the sock extends as high as possible on the humerus with a strap going across the chest to anchor it in place.

As limb volume decreases, the shrinker sock should be made smaller (leaving the seam on the outside of the sock) or replaced with a smaller size garment so that it still compresses the residual limb. If shrinker socks are not available or the patient is not yet able to tolerate the compressive force provided by a shrinker, tubular elastic bandaging, such as Compressogrip (Knit-Rite, Kansas City, KS) or Tubigrip (Seton Healthcare Group, Oldham, England), is an alternative. Typically a double layer of bandage is worn, with the layer underneath longer and extending 2 inches further proximally than the second layer.

Edema can further be reduced through soft-tissue mobilization and retrograde massage. Soft-tissue mobilization around areas of adherent tissue through gentle friction massage helps enhance circulation and increase flexibility. Ending treatment with retrograde massage with gentle stroking techniques in the direction of lymphatic flow also helps control edema.[7] Heat modalities may be useful as a preparation for subsequent massage and active exercises.

Elevation, while still important, becomes more difficult to enforce with a mobile patient. Raising the residual limb over the head and performing contractions of remaining musculature at least once an hour during the day also helps control edema (Figure 31-6). Active participation in self-care and use of the arm as an assist during functional activities is also helpful.

Management of the Incision and Scar

When the incision lines are adequately closed and sutures have been removed, scar management becomes a primary concern. When adherent scar tissue forms, the tissue of the residual limb does not move freely. Adherent scar tissue near the end of the bone is a particular problem that may lead to skin breakdown because of friction across the scar when the prosthesis is worn. Scar tissue adherence can be minimized by active ROM and gentle friction massage. Circular massage directly over the incision line, with pressure increasing as tolerated, is also a way of minimizing adherent scar formation. A slightly sticky cream or oil, such as pure lanolin or vitamin E oil, is preferred so the scar can be more easily mobilized over underlying tissue. Silicone gel sheeting can be used under bandages to apply pressure directly over the scar to deter adherent scar formation. Kinesio Tex Tape (Bailey Manufacturing, Atlanta, GA) has also been helpful in softening scar tissue.

Desensitization

Persons with recent amputation often have altered sensation or dysesthesias, including incisional pain, phantom sensation, phantom pain, and hypersensitivity. Incisional pain is treated with pain medications and effective edema control. Incisional pain typically subsides as the wound heals and begins to mature and stabilize.

Phantom sensation is a normal phenomenon experienced by most patients with recent amputation. Patients typically report that they "feel" all or part of their amputated limbs.

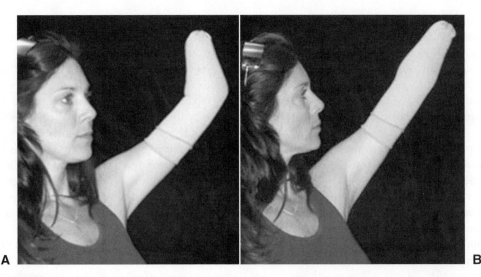

FIGURE 31-6 In the preprosthetic stage of rehabilitation, patients with transradial amputation are able to take a more active role in their program, such as active ROM **(A)** and isometric exercise **(B)**, emphasizing elbow extension as a strategy to minimize risk of elbow flexion contracture.

Some describe a pulling, tingling, or burning sensation in the missing limb. Most describe the feeling of a tight fist or a tight band around the arm. Phantom sensation is usually more annoying than painful. Many patients are hesitant to discuss these sensations for fear of sounding "crazy." For this reason, the likelihood of experiencing phantom sensation should be discussed with the patient as early in the rehabilitation process as possible. As rehabilitation progresses to more motion and prosthetic use, phantom sensation typically decreases to a point at which it is not significantly annoying, but it does not usually disappear entirely.

Phantom pain does not occur in all patients, but when it does it is extremely problematic. Unlike phantom sensation, phantom pain is a pathological condition that may persist long after amputation, hindering functional prosthetic use and lifestyle. A number of treatments have been suggested, including heat, desensitization techniques, imagery, mirror therapy, limb revision, and neurosurgery. Effectiveness of these techniques vary with each patient. Other issues that may be confused with phantom pain include proximal nerve damage and neuromas, which may require limb revision or neurosurgical intervention.[8–10]

Hypersensitivity is increased sensitivity to stimuli. Light touch is often particularly uncomfortable for the patient with a hypersensitive residual limb. Hypersensitivity can be effectively treated with a systematic and structured program that includes firm massage, various textures stroked on the limb, submersion of the residual limb in various graded media (e.g., dried beans, rice, and popcorn), fluidotherapy, vibration, transcutaneous electrical nerve stimulation, and increased functional use of the residual limb during daily activities.[11]

Enhancing Range of Motion

Having as close to full upper-extremity ROM as possible allows the patient to use the prosthesis to its full capability. Elbow flexion contracture and loss of supination and pronation are common occurrences in patients with transradial amputation. Patients with transhumeral amputation may lose scapula mobility and all shoulder motions, especially external rotation and horizontal adduction. Interventions such as heat modalities, soft-tissue mobilization, gentle stretching, and active ROM exercise can often quickly improve motion in patients with recently developed tissue tightness and ROM restriction. Long-term contractures may require static or static progressive splinting or casting and may take longer to resolve.

The possible loss of lower-extremity ROM caused by immobility and reduced activity during the acute and early rehabilitative phases of care should also be addressed. Limitations in lower-extremity range may affect balance and impede good body mechanics. For those with bilateral upper-extremity amputation, good balance and lower-extremity ROM are essential for the performance of most basic and instrumental activities of daily living.

Strengthening

When the wound has healed and pain is decreasing, strengthening is initiated for all muscles of the residual limb and for major muscle groups of the other extremities. For intact musculature, initial strengthening may be achieved through isometric contraction or active motion. The patient usually quickly progresses to active resistive exercises by using manual resistance, weight cuffs, elastic bands, weight machines, and functional activities.

Management of Concurrent Injuries and Limitations

Traumatic upper-extremity amputations seldom occur in isolation. When an upper extremity is caught in a press or other apparatus, the injured person struggles to get out of the machine by pulling and twisting and even using other extremities to extricate the arm from the machine. The patient can have obvious injuries such as fractures and soft tissue and muscle damage. Other injuries are often present but are not obvious on initial investigation. Painful and limiting rotator cuff injuries of the injured limb or the contralateral shoulder are not uncommon.

Myofascial trigger points are almost always present. Travell and Simons[12] describe a myofascial trigger point as a "hyperirritable locus within a taut band of skeletal muscle, located in the muscular tissue and/or its associated fascia. The spot is painful on compression and can evoke characteristic referred pain and autonomic phenomena." For patients with upper-extremity amputation, trigger points are often found bilaterally in the upper trapezius, rhomboid, and teres minor muscles. Those with transhumeral amputations may have additional trigger point pain in all three portions of the deltoid as well as the biceps, and triceps muscles. Individuals with transradial amputations may have additional trigger point pain in the wrist and finger flexors or extensors. All associated injuries must be treated so the patient can more fully participate in prosthetic training.

Basic Training in Activities of Daily Living

When the dominant hand is amputated, most persons with unilateral amputation choose to change hand dominance for activities requiring fine coordination and manipulative skills, such as writing and eating. Drawing, craft activities, and computer games can all contribute to developing hand coordination and change of hand dominance.

Patients with an upper-extremity amputation are anxious to quickly gain as much independence as possible in basic or survival functional skills such as eating, dressing, and hygiene. Initially adaptive equipment such as modified utensils, button hooks, and writing adaptations may be needed. Assuring the patient that most adaptive equipment will not be needed when they are proficient in prosthetic use helps establish an expectation that the patient will soon be using two "hands." Remaining bimanual is important for ease of performance and for minimizing risk of overuse syndrome of the remaining extremity.

CASE EXAMPLE 2

A Patient with Transhumeral Amputation

R. O. is a 37-year-old automobile mechanic who underwent a transhumeral amputation of the right upper extremity 3 weeks ago after he sustained a crush injury when a car slipped off the jack while he was changing its tire in a neighbor's driveway, pinning him at the elbow. While struggling to get out from under the vehicle, he seriously strained his right rotator cuff. At this point, all surgical drains and sutures have been removed, and the wound has closed except for a ¼-inch area on the medial, distal humerus that continues to leave slight signs of clear drainage on the nonadherent dressing. R. O. is currently using a double layer of elasticized Tubigrip (Seton Healthcare Group, Oldham, England) for volume control. He reports a sensation of a tight constrictive cuff around his "missing" right elbow and a somewhat unpredictable shooting

"electric" sensation into his missing forearm and hand. He tends to hold his residual limb diagonally across his lower chest. R. O. experiences pain in his right shoulder with movement in all planes.

Active and passive ROM is evaluated with R. O. in the supine position. Active ROM at the shoulder is currently 0 to 90 degrees of flexion, 0 to 70 degrees of abduction, 0 degrees of internal rotation, and 0 to 25 degrees of external rotation. His shoulder and residual limb can be passively moved into 115 degrees of flexion, 90 degrees of abduction, 10 degrees of internal rotation, and 40 degrees of external rotation.

R. O. is having a difficult time imagining how he will be able to return to work to support his young family (a wife and two preschool-age children). He is discouraged and impatient with his postoperative pain and phantom sensation. He is reluctant to allow his residual limb to be moved, passively or with active assistance, toward any end ROM at the shoulder because of impingement pain. He is discouraged with the skill level he has reached in self-care with his nondominant left upper extremity.

Questions to Consider

- What are R. O.'s most immediate educational and support needs now that he has begun the early rehabilitative, preprosthetic period of care? What strategies would help strengthen rapport with R. O., help him understand the next steps in the process, and enhance his outlook and motivation?

- What tests and measures are most important to use in the comprehensive examination and evaluation of R. O.'s residual limb and potential for prosthetic rehabilitation? What is the evidence of reliability and validity of these measures? How will the results of the assessment influence immediate and long-term therapeutic goals?

- Given the length of his residual limb and the status of his incision line, what specific strategies for volume control, edema, and limb shaping should be recommend at this time? How should effectiveness of the recommended volume control and limb shaping interventions be assessed? What are the indicators of readiness for prosthetic fitting?

- Given the status of his incision line, what strategies are now appropriate to reduce likelihood of scar formation along the incision line? Why is expecting R. O. to be responsible for this aspect of his care important?

- Given the dysesthesia that R. O. is currently experiencing, what interventions might be used to help his residual limb become less hypersensitive to sensory stimulation? What is the evidence of efficacy of the interventions available? Why is addressing dysesthesia important, on both a functional and psychological level, for patients such as R. O. with recent amputation?

- Given his current level of discomfort and the concurrent rotator cuff dysfunction, what contractures are most likely to develop at R. O.'s shoulder? Considering

Continued

his hopes to return to work as an auto mechanic, what shoulder motions would be most important to preserve and enhance in preparation for prosthetic training? What specific strategies should be used to accomplish this?

- What impact might a rotator cuff injury have on R. O.'s potential to use a prosthesis successfully? How should the severity of his rotator cuff impairment be assessed? What strategies could be used to improve the function of his shoulder, given the acuity of his rotator cuff injury?
- What types of muscle performance are most important to address at this point? What strategies should be used to address strength, power, and control of the various types of muscle contraction that R. O. will need to use his prosthesis effectively?
- What basic activities of daily living skills should be priorities for functional training at this point? What strategies should be used to enhance motor learning of skilled activity with his left (nondominant) hand? How might his residual limb be incorporated during these functional activities?

Determining a Prosthetic Plan

Comprehensive examination and evaluation by the members of the multidisciplinary team, which includes physician and surgeon, therapists, prosthetists, and other team members, determine prosthetic options that can be discussed with the patient and family. Factors such as the patient's strength, ROM, handedness, and other physical and psychological findings, as well as vocational pursuits and long-term goals, are important determinants of an individual prosthetic plan. The patient, family, and team members decide from the following options:

1. No prosthesis
2. A passive prosthesis to meet the patient's need for cosmesis and function
3. A body-powered prosthesis
4. An externally powered prosthesis
5. A hybrid prosthesis (combination body-powered and externally powered)
6. One or more activity-specific prostheses

The prosthetist and therapist discuss the pros and cons of the various control schemes available to operate the prosthesis with the patient and family, with the goals of selecting the control schemes that will allow the patient to become the most functional. The prosthetist may begin fabrication of the prosthesis as the therapist and patient work to achieve important preprosthetic goals. At this point the patient and family see more fully the patient-centered team in action. Involvement of the patient and family from the beginning of the rehabilitation process helps the patient accept and participate in the needed training and eventually accept the prosthesis.

Motions Required to Operate a Body-Powered Prosthesis

If plans are to use a body-powered prosthesis, strengthening shoulder joint and shoulder girdle musculature in both upper extremities is important. For maximal use of the prosthesis with minimum effort, the patient must be able to isolate muscle function with subtle, fluid motion. The patient needs to be able to perform the following motions, through as large a ROM as possible:

- Shoulder protraction or biscapular abduction
- Shoulder flexion
- Shoulder depression, extension, and abduction

The additional motions of elbow flexion and extension, forearm supination and pronation, and shoulder internal and external rotation should also be strengthened. Patients with very high levels of amputation or those with brachial plexus injuries may need to use chest expansion to operate the prosthesis. Chest expansion involves having the patient inhale deeply to expand the chest and then slowly exhale.

Muscle Requirements for a Hybrid Prosthesis

The hybrid is a common and reliably used prosthesis. It is operated by a combination of control systems. For example, a hybrid transhumeral prosthesis may use a body-powered elbow and forearm lock while using myoelectric control for the hand or other terminal device. Motions required to operate a hybrid prosthesis are a combination of those needed for the body-powered and myoelectric prostheses and require similar strength and control. The patient, prosthetist, and therapists work together to determine the most efficient control scheme for the prosthetic user.

Muscle Requirements for a Myoelectric Prosthesis

When a muscle contracts, it generates an electromyographic signal. The electromyographic signals produced by contracting muscles can be detected by surface electrodes placed in the socket of the prosthesis and are used to control mechanical functions of the prosthesis. Whenever possible, with adults, two separate muscles are used to operate the prosthesis.[13] The therapist is often called on to work with the prosthetist in selecting the most appropriate electrode sites. For those with transradial amputation, the sites most often selected are over the muscle bellies of the wrist flexors and extensors. For those with transhumeral residual limbs, the most frequently used sites for electrode placement are over the biceps and triceps.

Selecting Electrode Sites

An optimal electrode site for a myoelectrically controlled prosthetic component has seven characteristics.[13,14]

1. The site must be located over superficial muscles, preferably not over heavy adipose tissue or graft sites.
2. The patient must have sufficient muscle strength to activate the prosthesis without undue fatigue.
3. The sites must use motions reasonable to learn and relate to normal movement (e.g., wrist extensors for opening the terminal device [TD] and wrist flexors for closing the TD).
4. The site must use muscles that the patient can control independently of other motions.
5. The site must use muscles that, when activated, will not interfere with, or inhibit, normal activity.

6. If dual control is desired, the sites must use two sets of muscles that the patient can physiologically contract together as well as independently of each other.

7. The electrode sites must be able to be contained within the critical constraints of the socket.

Precise electrode placement makes it easier for a patient to use a myoelectric prosthesis. The therapist palpates the most likely spot while the patient contracts the desired muscle to test for strength and consistency of the contraction. Once a potential site is located, the skin is cleaned and moistened with water and a surface electrode is positioned over the muscle, parallel to the muscle fibers. The electrode is connected to biofeedback equipment, such as a Myolab (Motion Control, Salt Lake City, UT) or the Myoboy (Otto Bock HealthCare, Vienna, Austria) (Figure 31-7). The strength of the signal can be read from the meter, and precise electrode placement is adjusted as necessary. Once the electrode site is determined for one muscle, the second electrode site is found over the antagonist in a similar manner.

Control Site Training

Once the best electrode sites have been located, the patient must learn to control consistency of muscle contraction. For effective use of a myoelectrically controlled prosthesis, good muscle control is more important than overall strength of contractions. During control site training, the patient should learn three patterns of muscle activation:

1. To contract one muscle (muscle A, agonist) to a specific level, while leaving the other (muscle B, antagonist) at rest or in a quiet state.

2. To contract muscle B to a specific level while leaving muscle A at rest or in a quiet state.

3. To perform quick and equal cocontractions of muscles A and B.

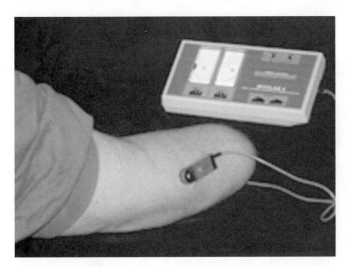

FIGURE 31-7 Surface electrodes are used to locate potential myoelectric control sites and provide biofeedback to help patients master the types of contractions necessary to control actions of the terminal device, wrist unit, and forearm motion and elbow lock (for those with transhumeral limbs).

Biofeedback equipment, or muscle trainers, greatly facilitate this training to master effective, efficient muscle control. Once patients can consistently produce isolated muscle signals on command without undue fatigue, they are ready to proceed with myoelectric prosthetic training.

Basic Prosthetic Training

When the patient receives the prosthesis, the basic prosthetic training phase of care begins. Goals in basic prosthetic training include the following:

- To become independent in skin care of the residual limb.
- To increase wearing tolerance of the prosthesis sufficiently for daily functional use.
- To become independent in donning and doffing the prosthesis.
- To understand the function and operating schemes of various prosthetic components.
- To develop necessary skills to use and control the prosthesis effectively.

Learning to operate the basic controls of a body-powered prosthesis is, of course, different from learning to operate a myoelectrically controlled prosthesis. Once basic operations are mastered, however, training methods of using the prosthesis are fairly similar. People with bilateral amputations may even have a different control scheme on each side. Gaining basic control of one prosthesis at a time is most often less frustrating for the person than trying to master both at once.

Skin Care

Most therapists prefer that the patient wear a T-shirt under the harness of a body-powered prosthesis, in early prosthetic training, to prevent skin irritation when learning to operate the cable system. As skin tolerance develops, the T-shirt becomes optional. For the externally or myoelectrically powered prosthesis, direct contact must be made between the skin and electrode sites. Regardless of the control system being used, the residual arm and axilla must be washed daily with mild soap and water, and the socket of the prosthesis must be wiped clean with a damp cloth. The harness should be removed and cleaned as needed. Patients using a body-powered prosthesis often wear prosthetic socks as an interface between the skin and socket surface. A fresh, clean sock should be used each day; in hot weather, the sock may need to be changed several times per day. For those using a myoelectric prosthesis, the electrodes may need to be cleaned several times each day to ensure effective contact between control site and the electrode. Although skin pliability is important, the application of moisturizers or lotions before donning the prosthesis is generally not recommended and is contraindicated with a myoelectric prosthesis.

New prosthetic users must understand that skin irritation, if not quickly addressed, may lead to a prolonged period out of the prosthesis. New users are counseled to notify the physician, prosthetist, or therapist as soon as any rash, pressure points, or sign of infection is noted.

Wearing Tolerance

In early prosthetic training, the prosthetic wearing period is typically limited to 30 to 45 minutes at a time. After each wearing period, the prosthesis is removed and skin condition carefully examined. Areas of redness (reactive hyperemia) that persist for more than 20 minutes after the residual limb is out of the socket may indicate areas of high pressure; the prosthetist should be consulted for possible modification of the socket. For those wearing a body-powered prosthesis, the skin of the sound axilla must also be examined. Until skin tolerance is developed, padding placed in the axillary region under the harness may increase comfort and allow longer wearing time. Wearing time is gradually increased, according to the patient's tolerance, skin condition, and need for prosthesis use.

Donning and Doffing

Full prosthetic use includes independence in donning and doffing. Both body-powered and myoelectric prostheses can be donned by either the push-in or pull-in method. Unless a roll-on liner with pin lock is used, the pull-in method is the preferred method for several reasons (Figure 31-8). It offers the advantage of distributing tissue equally in the socket; equal and consistent tissue placement is especially important for those using an electrically powered prosthesis. Pulling-in to the socket is accomplished in the following manner:

1. The patient applies a low-friction sleeve (often made of parachute-type material) over the residual limb.
2. The distal end of the sleeve is positioned through a "pull hole" in the wall of the prosthesis.
3. The patient then gently pulls each side of the sleeve, equally and repeatedly, until the sleeve completely comes out of the pull hole and the arm is pulled into the socket.

Alternative methods of donning may be required for patients with high levels of amputation. Those with very high bilateral transhumeral amputation may need special equipment for independence in donning and doffing. Some individuals with very high bilateral amputation may decide that the effort required to don the prostheses independently is not worth the energy expenditure.

Control of the Body-Powered Prosthesis

In the body-powered prosthesis, forces generated by gross body motions are translated through the harness and cable system to activate the forearm and TD (Figure 31-9). The individual with transradial amputation only needs to learn to operate the TD. Any motion that puts tension on the cable operates the TD (either hook or hand). A body-powered hand is usually considered passive in nature rather than functional as it requires a considerable amount of tension on the cable to operate. In voluntary-opening TDs, tension on the cable opens the TD and either rubber bands or springs close the TD. The addition of rubber bands or springs increases pinch power. In voluntary-closing TDs, the TD remains open until tension is applied on the cable; then the device closes in proportion to the amount of tension on the cable.

Control movements to operate the TD for the transradial prosthesis include shoulder flexion on the sound side, shoulder flexion of the amputated side, or biscapular abduction (shoulder protraction).

Individuals with long transradial limbs typically retain active forearm supination and pronation; this active movement can be used to position the TD for function. If active movement is lost or severely limited, the TD must be passively rotated in the wrist unit. Wrist flexion units are typically operated manually; the patient changes the angle of the TD with the opposite hand.

The patient with transhumeral amputation must be able to control the TD, forearm motion (flexion and extension to lift and reach), and the elbow locking and unlocking mechanism. When the elbow component in a transhumeral prosthesis is *locked*, the TD operates exactly as the TD in the transradial prosthesis—by using shoulder flexion or biscapular abduction. When the elbow component is *unlocked*, however, tension on the cable created by these movements causes the

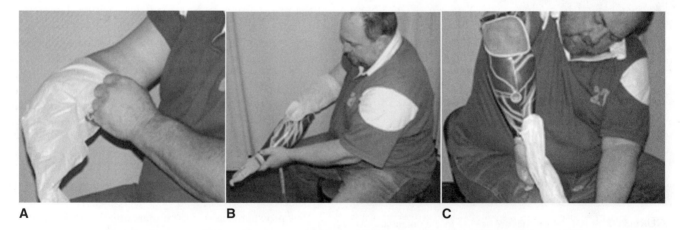

FIGURE 31-8 This patient is donning his myoelectric transradial prosthesis. First, he positions his pull-in sleeve on the residual limb (**A**), leaving a distal "tail" that he will thread through the distal opening in the socket (**B**). Once his limb is positioned in the socket, he gently tugs the sleeve out through the opening so that total contact between skin and socket surface is achieved (**C**).

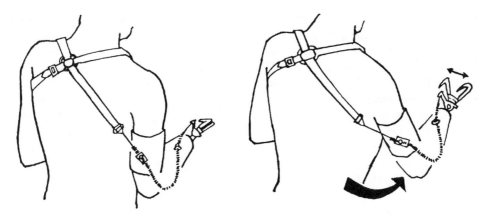

FIGURE 31-9 The harness and cable system of a body-powered transradial prosthesis. Glenohumeral flexion and scapular abduction (protraction) increase tension on the control cable to operate this voluntary-opening terminal device during activities performed away from the center of the body. Bilateral scapular (biscapular) abduction increases cable tension for fine motor activities performed near the midline or closer to the trunk. The same motion would allow graded prehension in a voluntary-closing terminal device. (Modified with permission, from Northwestern University Printing and Duplicating Department, Evanston, IL, 1987.)

forearm of the prosthesis to flex. When tension on the cable gradually releases (by using eccentric contraction of these muscles) the elbow returns to extension.

The elbow component of a transhumeral prosthesis is locked or unlocked with a combination of motions, unlike the motion used to operate the TD. This motion is simultaneous humeral abduction, extension, and depression—a quick, "move down, and back" motion of the arm. The use of a very different movement strategy helps ensure that the elbow component will not unintentionally unlock during functional activities with the TD.

To position the TD optimally for the functional task, passive motion (either with the intact limb or pressure against a stable surface) is used to rotate the TD in the wrist unit. Similarly, internal and external rotation of the prosthesis is passively controlled by rotation at the elbow turntable. Consider a carpenter wearing a transhumeral prosthesis who wants to hold a nail steady on a piece of lumber while working at his bench. First, he might catch his hook on the edge of the bench and rotate it to a proper position to hold the nail. Then, with the elbow of his prosthesis unlocked, he uses biscapular abduction to flex the forearm of his prosthesis into the desired position to accomplish his task. Finally, he locks the elbow to hold the forearm in proper position so that he is able to control opening of the terminal device to grasp the nail. A new prosthetic user may have to think carefully and perform each of these motions deliberately, but an experienced prosthetic user can perform all these motions fluidly in a matter of seconds.

Control of the Electric Prosthesis

Electric prostheses can be controlled in a variety of ways. Depending upon the patient's physical and cognitive presentation, the prosthetist may choose from surface electrodes, touch pads, switches, rockers, and other input devices. Myoelectric control is often used to operate the prosthesis. Control of

the myoelectric prosthesis involves deriving myoelectric signals from the voluntary contraction of muscles. Surface electrodes implanted in the walls of the prosthetic socket record electrical signals generated by muscle contraction. These signals are processed and used to control mechanical functions of the prosthesis.[13] A wide variety of components is available to prosthetists, providing many types of control schemes. The therapist must consult with the prosthetists on every patient regarding the exact controls used so that the best functional outcome can be achieved. The patient with a long transradial amputation usually retains control of some supination and pronation of the forearm. The patient with a shorter forearm amputation requires a wrist rotation unit to achieve forearm supination or pronation. Several options exist for control of wrist and forearm rotation. The wrist unit can be passively positioned by using the intact hand to position the TD for task-specific function. Alternately, the wrist rotator can be myoelectrically controlled.

Although multisite control systems are available, currently two sites are most commonly used. When using a two-site control system the individual with a transradial amputation must switch from hand (or other TD) mode to wrist mode. One way to accomplish this is for the individual to quickly and simultaneously contract forearm flexors and extensors. Once the unit is in wrist mode, contraction of the extensors rotates the hand in one direction and contraction of the flexors rotates the wrist in the other direction, effectively causing supination and pronation. When strength of a contraction signal is weak, control schemes can be altered; muscles with the most consistently reliable control should operate the function deemed most important.

Patients with transhumeral myoelectric prostheses have to manage the additional complexity of controlling the forearm (for flexion and extension) and the elbow (for lock and unlock function) as well as the TD and wrist rotator. Commonly used transhumeral control schemes use contraction of the biceps and triceps to operate the prosthetic TD and forearm. When the elbow unit is locked, contraction of one muscle opens the terminal device. Contraction of the opposite muscle signals closure of the TD. When the elbow is unlocked, contraction of the control muscle flexes the forearm. The speed of operation is matched to the rapidity and strength of the myoelectric signal generated by muscle contraction. Graded prehension and elbow motion is possible with practice.

Functional Changes

Engineers have realized the complexity of motions the prosthesis must perform for fluid, functional, upper-extremity motion. They are working with prosthetists, therapists, and patients to develop new components, terminal devices, and control schemes for more functional prostheses. In the past, most prostheses required the elbow unit to be locked to operate the TD. In the past 7 to 10 years several manufacturers developed transhumeral prosthesis with simultaneous control of the elbow and hand. These include the Dynamic Arm by Otto Boch and the Utah Arm-3 by Motion Control. Both of these prostheses have contributed to a more normal pattern of use.

New or improved terminal devices have also come on the market. The Electronic Terminal Device introduced by Motion Control is water resistant. This has allowed people greater use of their TD near water at work or at home. The Electronic Terminal Device, for example, may be used to wash dishes.

Wrist flexion adds greatly to a person's ability to position the terminal device for functional activities. It allows better ergonomic positioning of the upper extremity, affords better vision, and increases function for many activities. Both locking and multiflex (by Motion Control) wrists are available.

An exciting development in prosthetic control is targeted muscle reinnervation. "Targeted muscle reinnervation (TMR) is a new elective surgery that increases the number of [electromyographic] control signals, thus improving the potential for enhanced prosthetic function."[15] The surgery involves transferring nerves that previously innervated muscles distal to the amputation to denervated areas of unused muscles such as portions of the pectoralis major. These re-innervated muscles can then provide additional available electromyographic control sites. Although not commonly seen in practice, "TMR is now being performed as a clinical device, not just as research protocol. To date, TMR programs have been developed in six different centers around the world."[16] A greater number of electromyographic signals available may translate into simultaneous control of the elbow and hand and also power a wrist.

Skills Training

After mastering operation of all individual components, the next step in training is learning to integrate individual movements into smooth prosthetic operation. Similar training principles are used whether the control system is body powered, hybrid, or myoelectric.

Actual skills training for bilateral amputees is similar to that for unilateral users. The bilateral user, however, requires more time, effort, and patience. Bilateral training is further complicated by lack of sensation and proprioception in either hand; it takes some time for visual clues and "the feel of the prosthesis" to begin to compensate for sensation. The new prosthetic user must learn how to control the terminal device selectively so that it is opened just enough to grasp the intended object while maintaining just enough tension on the muscle or cable to hold the object without squeezing it. Practice using different sponges or soft toys give visual feedback as to grasp pressure. Another fundamental skill to master is the ability to operate the terminal device at various heights and in various positions. These positions may include tasks requiring the elbow to be flexed to 90 degrees while the arm is held at the side of the body; tasks requiring a forward or upward (above waist height) motion for grasping, lifting or carrying; and tasks requiring picking objects up from a lower surface, such as the floor. Most people find control of the TD in a stooped position, such as needed for tying shoes, very difficult.

Practicing how to grasp with the TD pre-positioned prevents unnecessary or awkward movements. Pre-positioning involves actively or passively turning the TD prior to reaching for an object. As progress is made in developing simultaneous controls of the elbow, wrist, and hand, prepositioning of the TD may become unnecessary.

After learning basic control moves, the patient is ready to begin incorporating prosthetic use in activities of daily living which may include:

- Using utensils to eat, cutting food
- Making a sandwich or basic meal
- Opening and closing various types of packages, boxes, jars, and other containers
- Brushing teeth
- Cleaning and clipping fingernails
- Holding a hairdryer while styling hair
- Bathing with or without assistive devices
- Dressing with or without adaptive equipment
- Fastening a jacket zipper
- Tying shoes
- Toileting

The amount of training and types of adaptive equipment needed depends largely on the level of amputation, whether the person has unilateral or bilateral amputations, and if there are concomitant injuries.

Persons with unilateral amputation, either transradial or transhumeral, and without other injuries can usually achieve independence in activities of daily living with the need for minimal adaptive equipment. Some helpful products include:

- Bath mitts or brushes
- Suction nail brush and clippers
- Suction cutting board with aluminum nails
- Rocker knives
- Tripin or spinner knob

A person with bilateral amputations faces a much greater challenge to gain independence in activities of daily living. The patient requires a greater amount of training and often more adaptive equipment than a person with a unilateral amputation. Good balance and core muscle strength, along with full lower-extremity ROM is helpful in gaining independence in activities of daily living.

Self-feeding, dressing, and toileting are especially important to individuals with bilateral amputations and deserve special attention. Difficulty in accomplishing these tasks increases with the level of amputation. It is important that the prosthetist understand motions required to accomplish specific tasks, as prosthetic design can make the difference between independence and dependence in certain tasks. For example, slight radial deviation of the prosthetic forearm and wrist make self-feeding easier.

Self-Feeding

Activity analysis will show self-feeding to be a complicated task. For a person with transhumeral amputation this activity requires shoulder flexion (and or abduction), locking/unlocking of the elbow, wrist rotation (supination/pronation), wrist positioning, and grasp release of a utensil. Initial training may require the use of a swivel spork, and be further facilitated by turning the hand off while eating to prevent dropping the utensil. With progress, all but the highest level amputee should be able to grasp and release utensils and finger food independently. Persons with high transhumeral or shoulder disarticulation amputations may choose to have help with eating. Helpful equipment may include:

- Swivel spork
- Rocker knife
- Long straw
- T-handle cup

Self-Dressing

The person with bilateral transradial amputations may initially require 30 minutes to just don their pants. This is a very frustrating and seemingly impossible activity. Guidance, assurance, and talking with persons of similar level of amputations helps to encourage the patient to work until independence is achieved. Most often persons with bilateral transradial amputations can learn to dress and perform grooming activities within 30 minutes. This skilled independence may not be achieved during the initial therapy sessions, but rather on a return visit 3 to 6 months after initial discharge.

Equipment that may be helpful for dressing include:

- Velcro fastenings
- Various types of button hooks
- Loops sewn inside pants
- Zipper pulls
- Custom-fabricated dressing racks

Although persons with all levels of amputation may become independent in dressing, no value judgment should be placed on the individual who chooses to save time and energy by accepting help from others.

Self-Toileting

Independence in toileting is always one of the first activities in which patients are interested, but not always easy to achieve. This activity requires good balance, good ROM, independence in managing clothing at the toilet, and a willingness to consider alternate ways of task accomplishment. Although it is not really healthy to do so, many people limit fluid intake when away from home to limit the need to go to a public bathroom. Amputees often plan a bowel program to coincide with showering so that they may clean themselves in the shower. When possible, a person with bilateral amputations will choose to use a bidet at home. Alternatively, if a person has enough ROM, toilet paper can be wrapped around the terminal device and moved back and forth until clean. A flushable wet wipe can also be placed on the edge of the toilet bowl for the person to move back and forth for cleaning. Finally, toilet paper or a wet wipe (or if at home, a damp washcloth) can be carefully placed over the heel of the foot with the foot propped on the toilet seat for similar cleaning.

CASE EXAMPLE 3

A Patient with Bilateral Upper-Extremity Amputation After Electrocution

E. H. is a 19-year-old college freshman studying to become a marine biologist. Six months ago, he participated in a school project on a boat with an instructor and other students to measure lake depth and take samples of underwater plants. The day before, the local power company had begun stringing power lines that extended over the edge of the lake and inadvertently left these wires lower than intended. E. H. was using an aluminum pole to measure water depth and accidentally touched these live wires with the pole. He was immediately electrocuted, rendered unconscious, and fell into the water. The other students pulled him from the lake and resuscitated him in approximately 4 minutes. He was medically evacuated to the trauma center, where he was found to have burns on both hands and forearms. The entrance wound, where the electrical current entered his body, was in his right (dominant) hand. The exit wounds were in his left forearm and thigh. As result of the burns and subsequent tissue damage, amputation was necessary on the right side at the midtransradial level and on the left at midhumeral level; he received a skin graft on his left thigh and left arm.

E. H. was hospitalized for 2 months near his home and then discharged to live with his family (parents and brother) and receive outpatient therapy. At the time of discharge, in addition to bilateral upper extremity ROM limitations, E. H. had severe balance deficits and limited lower-extremity strength and flexibility bilaterally. He was completely dependent in activities of daily living.

Three months later he is referred to an outpatient prosthetic center for prosthetic fitting and therapy. The goal is to train him to use his prostheses to become as independent as possible, including returning to school to pursue his career in marine biology. E. H.'s wounds are well healed. His arms are well contoured, show minimal edema, and have few adhesions and full ROM. Hip flexion is limited to 85 degrees, extension to neutral. He is able to stand on the right

Continued

foot for 20 seconds and the left for 5 seconds. Because of inactivity, E. H. is 40 lb overweight. E. H. receives his prostheses 3 weeks after beginning prosthetic rehabilitation.

Questions to Consider

- What is the stage of E. H.'s rehabilitation? What tests and measures are appropriate at this time? What is his prognosis for prosthetic use and return to functional independence at home and school? What are the most important goals that he needs to accomplish in his early prosthetic rehabilitation? How will his goals change as prosthetic rehabilitation progresses? How many weeks will likely be required?
- What effect will his impairments and limitations in balance and lower extremity ROM have on upper extremity prosthetic training and future activities of daily living skills? How might interventions to address these impairments and functional limitations be incorporated in the plan of care?
- What factors should be considered when planning prosthetic options? What are the pros and cons of body-powered or electrically controlled prostheses for E. H.? Will one type of prosthesis meet his needs? Why or why not?
- Should his initial prosthetic training be unilateral or bilateral? Why? If beginning training with a single prosthesis, which side should be targeted? Why? What basic components should be recommended for each of his prostheses?
- How can the team assist E. H. in learning to use his electrical hands or hooks? What control motions are needed for the right (transradial) side? What motions are needed for the left (transhumeral) side? How might E. H. progress from simple activity to more complex and realistic activities with his terminal devices to facilitate learning while minimizing frustration?
- What effect does elbow function have on hand positioning? How will elbow function affect the use of his transradial prosthesis? What is the sequence that E. H. needs to master to control elbow function of his transhumeral prosthesis? What kinds of activities would help him master elbow control in both single-limb and bimanual tasks? How would training tasks be graded to ensure success?
- Are E. H.'s goals of returning to college to study marine biology realistic? What problems might he face?

ADVANCED FUNCTIONAL SKILLS TRAINING

The full understanding of all components and the ability to operate them to the fullest extent are necessary before discharge from therapy. For example, using the forearm and hand for fluid reach and grasp and walking with a near-normal arm swing are important, as is using the prosthesis for independence in self-care and basic activities of daily living. For most people, this is not enough. The person with an amputation

wants to participate in activities having special meaning to them. These activities may include child care, homemaking, home maintenance, work, sports, and other recreational activities. To help achieve full independence in instrumental activities of daily living the prosthetist, therapist, and other team members must listen to the patient's desires and help achieve their goals.

SUMMARY

New advances in prosthetics are achieved every year, resulting in better socket design, increased comfort, reduced weight, advanced componentry, and better cosmesis. These changes have resulted in better patient satisfaction and increased use. Therapists must help assure that patients are aware of available prostheses, that the prostheses fit and operate well, and that the patients receive comprehensive training by knowledgeable therapists. This chapter presents management aspects for the treatment of adults with upper-extremity amputation, including acute care, preprosthetic care, basic prosthetic training, and advanced functional skills training. The technology available in body powered and myoelectric prosthetics provides individuals with upper-extremity amputation the opportunity to become skillful users of prosthetic devices that enhance function and facilitate participation in activities of daily living. Rehabilitation professionals working together can advocate for persons with upper-extremity amputation to assure that the best rehabilitation outcomes are achieved.

REFERENCES

1. Baer E. *The Wonder of Hands*. New York: MacMillan; 1992.
2. Dillingham TR. Rehabilitation of the upper limb amputee. In: Dillingham TR, Belandres RV, eds. *Rehabilitation of the Injured Combatant*. Washington, DC: Office of the Surgeon General, Department of the Army; 1998:33–73.
3. Dillingham TR, Pezzin LE, MacKenzie EJ. Limb deficiency and amputation: epidemiology and recent trends in the United States. *South Med J*. 2002;95(8).
4. Atkins DJ, Meier RH. *Comprehensive Management of the Upper-Limb Amputee*. New York: Springer-Verlag; 1989.
5. Olivett BL. Conventional fitting of the adult amputee. In: Hunter J, Mackin E, Callahan A, eds. *Rehabilitation of the Hand and Upper Extremity*. 4th ed. St. Louis: Mosby; 1995:1223–1240.
6. Desmond D, MacLachlan M. Psychosocial issues in the field of prosthetics and orthotics. *J Prosthet Orthot*. 2002;14(1):19–21.
7. Colditz JC. Therapist's management of the stiff hand. In: Hunter J, Mackin E, Callahan A, eds. *Rehabilitation of the Hand and Upper Extremity*. 5th ed. St. Louis: Mosby; 2002:1021–1049.
8. Brown PW. Psychologically based hand disorders. In: Hunter J, Mackin E, Callahan A, eds. *Rehabilitation of the Hand and Upper Extremity*. 5th ed. St. Louis: Mosby; 2002:9–19.
9. Shenaq S, Meier R, Brotzman B, et al. The painful residual limb: treatment strategies. In: Atkins DJ, Meier RH, eds. *Comprehensive Management of the Upper-Limb Amputee*. New York: Springer-Verlag; 1989:72–78.
10. Chan BL, Witt R, Charrow AP, et al. Mirror therapy for phantom limb pain. *N Engl J Med*. 2007;357:2206–2207.

11. Waylett-Rendall J. Desensitization of the traumatized hand. In: Hunter J, Mackin E, Callahan A, eds. *Rehabilitation of the Hand and Upper Extremity*. 4th ed. St. Louis: Mosby; 1995:693–700.

12. Travell JG, Simons DG. *Myofascial Pain and Dysfunction: The Trigger Point Manual*. Baltimore: Williams & Wilkins; 1983.

13. Hubbard S. Myoprosthetic management of the upper limb amputee. In: Hunter J, Mackin E, Callahan A, eds. *Rehabilitation of the Hand and Upper Extremity*. 4th ed. St. Louis: Mosby; 1995:1241–1252.

14. Proceedings from the University of New Brunswick's Myoelectric Controls/Powered Prosthetics Symposium, Fredricton, New Brunswick, Canada, August 25-27, 2002.

15. Stubblefield KA, Miller LA, Lipschutz RD, et al. Occupational therapy protocol for amputees with targeted muscle reinnervation. *J Rehabil Res Dev*. 2009;46(4):481–488.

16. Englehart K, Hudgins B, Chan ADC. Continuous multifunction myoelectric control using pattern recognition. *Technol Disabil*. 2003;15(2):95–103.

ADDITIONAL RESOURCES

Bhella S, Berbrayer D. Pain in a traumatic upper extremity amputee. *Univ West Ont Med J*. 2006;75(1):S17–S19.

Biddiss E, Chau T. Upper-limb prosthetics: critical factors in device abandonment. *Am J Phys Med Rehabil*. 2007;86:977–987.

Daly W. Clinical application of roll-on sleeves for myoelectrically controlled transradial and transhumeral prostheses. *J Prosthet Orthot*. 2000;12(3):88–91.

Jones LE, Davidson JH. Save that arm: a study of problems in the remaining arm of unilateral upper limb amputees. *Prosthet Orthot Int*. 1999;23(1):55–58.

Kisner C, Colby LA. *Therapeutic Exercise Foundations and Techniques*. 3rd ed. Philadelphia: Davis; 1996.

Lake C, Miguelez JM. Comparative analysis of microprocessors in upper limb prosthetics. *J Prosthet Orthot*. 2003;15(2):48–63.

Miguelez JM, Miguelez MD. The Micro Frame: the next generation of interface design for glenohumeral disarticulation and associated levels of limb deficiency. *J Prosthet Orthot*. 2003;15(2):66–71.

Muzumdar A, ed. *Powered Upper Limb Prostheses, Control, Implementation and Clinical Application*. Berlin, Germany: Springer-Verlag; 2004.

Proceedings from the University of New Brunswick's Myoelectric Controls/Powered Prosthetics Symposium, Fredricton, New Brunswick, Canada, August 25-27, 2002.

Smith D, Michael J, Bowker J, et al., eds. *Atlas of Amputations and Limb Deficiencies: Surgical, Prosthetic, and Rehabilitation Principles*. 3rd ed. Alexandria, VA: American Academy of Orthopaedic Surgeons; 2004.

Smurr LM, Gulick K, Yancosek K, et al. Managing the upper extremity amputee: a protocol for success. *J Hand Ther*. 2008;21:160–176.

Soltanian H, de Bese G, Beasley R, et al. Passive hand prostheses. In: Brown RE, Neumeister MW, eds. *Hand Clinics: Mutilating Hand Injuries*. Vol. 19. Philadelphia: Saunders; 2003:177–183.

Supan T. Active functional prostheses. In: Brown RE, Neumeister MW, eds. *Hand Clinics: Mutilating Hand Injuries*. Vol. 19. Philadelphia: Saunders; 2003:185–191.

Zeigler-Graham K, MacKenzie EJ, Ephraim PL, et al. Estimating the prevalence of limb loss in the United States: 2005 to 2050. *Arch Phys Med Rehabil*. 2008;89:422–429.

Index

Note: Page numbers followed by *f* indicate figures, *t* indicate tables and *b* indicate boxes.